AF677109

Kistner's Gynecology

PRINCIPLES AND PRACTICE

SIXTH EDITION

Kistner's Gynecology

PRINCIPLES AND PRACTICE

KENNETH J. RYAN, M.D.
Kate Macy Ladd Distinguished Professor
of Obstetrics, Gynecology, and Reproductive Biology
Brigham and Women's Hospital
Harvard Medical School
Boston, Massachusetts

ROSS S. BERKOWITZ, M.D.
William H. Baker Professor of Gynecology
Director of Gynecology and Gynecologic Oncology
Department of Obstetrics, Gynecology
and Reproductive Biology
Brigham and Women's Hospital
Harvard Medical School
Boston, Massachusetts

ROBERT L. BARBIERI, M.D.
Kate Macy Ladd Professor
Department of Obstetrics, Gynecology
and Reproductive Biology
Chairman
Department of Obstetrics, Gynecology
and Reproductive Biology
Brigham and Women's Hospital
Harvard Medical School
Boston, Massachusetts

Mosby

St. Louis Baltimore Boston Carlsbad Chicago Naples New York Philadelphia Portland
London Madrid Mexico City Singapore Sydney Tokyo Toronto Wiesbaden

Mosby
Dedicated to Publishing Excellence

A Times Mirror
Company

Editor: Susie Baxter
Developmental Editor: Anne Gunter
Project Manager: Linda McKinley
Designer: Page Two Associates, Inc.
Production: Page Two Associates, Inc.

SIXTH EDITION

Copyright © 1995 by Mosby-Year Book, Inc.

Previous editions copyrighted 1986, 1990

All rights reserved. No part of this publication may be reproduced, stored in a retrieval system, or transmitted, in any form or by any means, electronic, mechanical, photocopying, recording, or otherwise, without prior written permission from the publisher.

Permission to photocopy or reproduce solely for internal or personal use is permitted for libraries or other users registered with the Copyright Clearance Center, provided that the base fee of $4.00 per chapter plus $.10 per page is paid directly to the Copyright Clearance Centre, 27 Congress Street, Salem, MA 01970. This consent does not extend to other kinds of copying, such as copying for general distribution, for advertising or promotional purposes, for creating new collected works, or for resale.

Printed in the United States of America

Mosby-Year Book, Inc.
11830 Westline Industrial Drive
St. Louis, Missouri 63146

Library of Congress Cataloging in Publication Data

Kistner's gynecology: principles and practice—6th ed.
[edited by] Kenneth J. Ryan, Ross S. Berkowitz, Robert L. Barbieri
p. cm.
Includes bibliographical references.
ISBN 1-8151-7479-9
I. Ryan, Kenneth J. II. Berkowitz, Ross S.
III. Barbieri, Robert L.

DNLM/DLC
for Library of Congress

96 97 98 99 / 9 8 7 6 5 4 5 3 2

CONTRIBUTORS

ROBERT L. BARBIERI, M.D.
Kate Macy Ladd Professor
Department of Obstetrics, Gynecology
and Reproductive Biology
Chairman
Department of Obstetrics, Gynecology
and Reproductive Biology
Brigham and Women's Hospital
Harvard Medical School
Boston, Massachusetts

BERYL R. BENACERRAF, M.D.
Co-Director, High-Risk Obstetrical Ultrasound
Department of Obstetrics, Gynecology
and Reproductive Biology
Brigham and Women's Hospital
Clinical Professor
Department of Obstetrics, Gynecology
Brigham and Women's Hospital
Harvard Medical School
Boston, Massachusetts

JOAN M. BENGTSON, M.D.
Gynecology Specialist
Department of Obstetrics and Gynecology
Harvard Community Health Plan
Division of Obstetrics and Gynecology
Brigham and Women's Hospital
Assistant Professor
Department of Obstetrics, Gynecology
Harvard Medical School
Boston, Massachusetts

ROSS S. BERKOWITZ, M.D.
Director of Gynecology and Gynecologic Oncology
Co-Director of New England
Trophoblastic Disease Center
Department of Obstetrics, Gynecology
and Reproductive Biology
William H. Baker Professor of Gynecology
Brigham and Women's Hospital
Harvard Medical School
Boston, Massachusetts

DANIEL W. CRAMER, M.D., Sc.D.
Director, Epidemiology
Associate Professor
Department of Obstetrics, Gynecology
and Reproductive Biology
Brigham and Women's Hospital
Harvard Medical School
Boston, Massachusetts

JANIS H. FOX, M.D.
Instructor
Department of Obstetrics, Gynecology
and Reproductive Biology
Brigham and Women's Hospital
Harvard Medical School
Boston, Massachusetts

ANDREW J. FRIEDMAN, M.D.
Chief, Division of Reproductive Endocrinology and Infertility
Associate Professor
Department of Obstetrics, Gynecology
and Reproductive Biology
Brigham and Women's Hospital
Harvard Medical School
Boston, Massachusetts

DONALD P. GOLDSTEIN, M.D.
Director of New England Trophoblastic Disease Center
Assistant Clinical Professor
Department of Obstetrics, Gynecology,
and Reproductive Biology
Harvard Medical School
Boston, Massachusetts

HOWARD M. GOODMAN, M.D.
Division of Gynecologic Oncology
Assistant Clinical Professor
Department of Obstetrics, Gynecology
and Reproductive Biology
Brigham and Women's Hospital
Harvard Medical School
Boston, Massachusetts

CONTRIBUTORS

R. IAN HARDY, M.D., Ph.D.
Clinical Fellow
Department of Obstetrics, Gynecology,
and Reproductive Biology
Brigham and Women's Hospital
Harvard Medical School
Boston, Massachusetts

JOSEPH A. HILL, M.D.
Associate Professor
Department of Obstetrics, Gynecology
and Reproductive Biology
Brigham and Women's Hospital
Harvard Medical School
Boston, Massachusetts

MARK D. HORNSTEIN, M.D.
Assistant Professor
Department of Obstetrics, Gynecology,
and Reproductive Biology
Brigham and Women's Hospital
Harvard Medical School
Boston, Massachusetts

SUSAN CARUSA KLOCK, Ph.D.
Associate Psychologist in Medicine
Division of Psychiatry
Brigham and Women's Hospital;
Instructor
Department of Psychiatry
Harvard Medical School
Boston, Massachusetts

MARC R. LAUFER, M.D.
Director, Pediatric Adolescent Gynecology
Instructor
Department of Obstetrics, Gynecology,
and Reproductive Biology
Brigham and Women's Hospital
Harvard Medical School
Boston, Massachusetts

MICHAEL G. MUTO, M.D.
Assistant Professor
Division of Gynecologic Oncology
Department of Obstetrics, Gynecology
and Reproductive Biology
Brigham and Women's Hospital
Harvard Medical School
Boston, Massachusetts

RAPIN OSATHANONDH, M.D.
Medical Director, Family Planning
Associate Professor
Department of Obstetrics, Gynecology
and Reproductive Biology
Brigham and Women's Hospital
Harvard Medical School
Boston, Massachusetts

MITCHELL S. REIN, M.D.
Assistant Professor
Department of Obstetrics, Gynecology,
and Reproductive Biology
Brigham and Women's Hospital
Harvard Medical School
Boston, Massachusetts

LAUREL W. RICE, M.D.
Associate Professor
Department of Obstetrics and Gynecology
Division of Gynecologic Oncology
University of Virginia Health Science Center
Charlottesville, Virginia

KENNETH J. RYAN, M.D.
Kate Macy Ladd Distinguished Professor
of Obstetrics, Gynecology, and Reproductive Biology
Brigham and Women's Hospital
Harvard Medical School
Boston, Massachusetts

CONTRIBUTORS

ISAAC SCHIFF, M.D.
Chief, Vincent Memorial Obstetrics and Gynecology Service
Massachusetts General Hospital
Joe Vincent Meigs Professor of Gynecology
Harvard Medical School
Boston, Massachusetts

ELLEN E. SHEETS, M.D.
Assistant Professor
Division of Gynecology Oncology
Director of Pap Smear Evaluation Center
Department of Obstetrics, Gynecology and Reproductive Biology
Brigham and Women's Hospital
Harvard Medical School
Boston, Massachusetts

FREDERICK H. SILLMAN, M.D.
Associate Professor
Department of Obstetrics, Gynecology and Reproductive Biology
Brigham and Women's Hospital
Harvard Medical School
Boston, Massachusetts

BARBARA L. SMITH, M.D., Ph.D.
Director, Comprehensive Breast Health Center
Assistant Professor of Surgery
Massachusetts General Hospital
Harvard Medical School
Boston, Massachusetts

ELIZABETH A. STEWART, M.D.
Instructor
Department of Obstetrics, Gynecology and Reproductive Biology
Brigham and Women's Hospital
Harvard Medical School
Boston, Massachusetts

RUTH TUOMALA, M.D.
Director, Infectious Disease
Assistant Professor
Department of Obstetrics, Gynecology and Reproductive Biology
Brigham and Women's Hospital
Harvard Medical School
Boston, Massachusetts

EBOO VERSI, M.A., D.Phil, M.B. B.Chir, MRCOG
Director, Urogynecology
Associate Professor
Department of Obstetrics, Gynecology and Reproductive Biology
Brigham and Women's Hospital
Harvard Medical School
Boston, Massachusetts

BRIAN W. WALSH, M.D.
Director of Menopause Unit
Assistant Professor
Department of Obstetrics, Gynecology and Reproductive Biology
Brigham and Women's Hospital
Harvard Medical School
Boston, Massachusetts

LOUISE WILKINS-HAUG, M.D.
Director, Antenatal Diagnostic Center
Assistant Professor
Department of Obstetrics, Gynecology and Reproductive Biology
Brigham and Women's Hospital
Harvard Medical School
Boston, Massachusetts

JOHN YEH, M.D.
Assistant Professor
Department of Obstetrics, Gynecology, and Reproductive Biology
Brigham and Women's Hospital
Harvard Medical School
Boston, Massachusetts

PREFACE TO SIXTH EDITION

Kistner's Gynecology: Principles and Practice has been a standard text and reference for over 30 years, designed to serve the needs of medical students, interns, residents, and especially practicing physicians in the field of gynecology and its subspecialties. As originally conceived, the book was an outgrowth of the teaching and practice of physicians at the Free Hospital for Women in Brookline, Massachusetts, and followed in the tradition of the textbook of gynecology of Dr. William Graves, the first professor and chief of gynecology at Harvard Medical School and the Free Hospital. Dr. Robert Kistner was a very skilled and popular gynecologic surgeon, endocrinologist, and teacher at Harvard and the Free Hospital for Women who first distilled his command of the field into his writing of this text in 1964. As the field expanded, he engaged his colleagues to help him in preparing the text of subsequent editions. This Sixth Edition is a continuation of the tradition by editors and authors with roots in the original Free Hospital and the successor institutions, The Boston Hospital for Women, and now the Department of Obstetrics and Gynecology of the Brigham and Women's Hospital. Many of the authors have worked with or were students of Dr. Robert Kistner and are proud to be able to carry on the tradition.

For this new updated and revised edition, we have added completely new chapters on science-based practice (Chapter 1), ethics (Chapter 2), epidemiology (Chapter 15), psychosomatic disease (Chapter 17), and urogynecology (Chapter 18). These and several other chapters are the equivalent of specialized monographs in such fields as ultrasonography, pediatric and adolescent gynecology, and gynecologic infections. An attempt has been made to adequately cover the field of gynecology and especially the subspecialties of reproductive endocrinology and gynecologic oncology.

The editors wish to express their appreciation to the authors of this sixth edition for their hard work and scholarship and to acknowledge our debt to contributors to previous editions that helped provide the standards we are trying to maintain. We also wish to recognize the central role and organizing skills of Mary Ann Murphy in coordinating the preparation of the book and for help in editing, communicating with the publisher and authors, and handling manuscripts.

Kenneth J. Ryan
Ross S. Berkowitz
Robert L. Barbieri

PREFACE TO FIRST EDITION

This work is designed both as a textbook and as a general reference book of gynecology to meet the needs of undergraduate medical students, young practitioners of gynecology, and specialists in this field. The format of each chapter is similar, the purpose being to provide a uniform and organized approach to the understanding of multiple disease processes of each organ of the female genital tract. Thus, in each chapter the embryology, anatomy, and histology are correlated with specific malformations. Morphologic variations are correlated with physiologic alterations. Recent advances in the diagnosis and therapy of infectious processes are described in detail. Particular emphasis has been given to the relationship of premalignant to malignant neoplasms, and methods for the prophylaxis of certain tumors are suggested. Because of the importance and increasing incidence of endometriosis a separate chapter on this disease is included. Particular emphasis has been placed on hormonal therapy, and details of management outlined.

Because of my interest in the practical endocrinologic aspects of gynecology, a chapter is devoted to steroid therapy. In this chapter an attempt is made to obviate many of the difficulties of administration associated with the new synthetic preparations. I have included (1) a brief résumé of basic steroid chemistry, (2) a summation of the pharmacology and physiology of androgens, estrogens, and progesterone, together with a similar discussion of the synthetic progestins, and (3) a discussion of proved and proposed indications for the use of these steroids, with specific contraindications and optimum dosage.

The observations and opinions expressed in this text summarize the sum and substance of the teaching and practice at the Free Hospital for Women during the past 15 years. This hospital was opened on November 2, 1875, and has been in continuous operation since that time. It is the only remaining specialty hospital in the United States whose primary objective is the diagnosis and treatment of medical and surgical diseases of the female.

The Free Hospital for Women became internationally known because of the *Textbook of Gynecology* written by Dr. William P. Graves, formerly Professor of Gynecology at Harvard Medical School. Although the fourth and last edition of Graves' textbook appeared in 1928, since that time a multiplicity of original and important contributions has been published by the members of the staff. Outstanding among these have been the innumerable works of Drs. George and Olive Smith concerning the measurement and metabolism of ovarian steroids and gonadotropic hormones during the menstrual cycle, the period of conception, and subsequent pregnancy. During the years 1938 through 1957 Drs. John Rock and Arthur T. Hertig accomplished their monumental studies on the earliest stages of human growth following fertilization. From 1928 through 1958 Dr. Rock directed intensive study and research projects relating to the etiologic factors in infertility. The pathogenesis of carcinoma in situ of the cervix and its relationship to invasive carcinoma have undergone thorough investigation and evaluation by Drs. Paul Younge, Arthur T. Hertig, and Donald G. MacKay. During the past seven years the synthetic progestational agents have been subjected to extensive clinical investigation in specific gynecologic disorders such as endometriosis and endometrial carcinoma.

In preparing a work of this type, material must be gathered not only from the author's personal experience but to a still greater extent from the work of others. I have, therefore, attempted to include the important observations of numerous authors who have published data concerning the clinical material at the Free Hospital for Women. From the great number of publications consulted there have been several to which I have had frequent recourse, both for new material and for corroboration of personal observations. I must, therefore, express a general acknowledgement of indebtedness to Drs. George and Olive Smith, Arthur T. Hertig, Christopher J. Duncan, Paul A. Younge, Donald G. MacKay, and John Rock. I have also drawn on the writings of the late Joe V. Meigs and Langdon Parsons, both former residents at the Free Hospital for Women. In writing the sections on the relationship of endocrinology to gynecology I have received the greatest assistance from the excellent works, *Endocrine and Metabolic Aspects of Gynecology* by Joseph Rogerts, *Human Endocrinology* by Herbert S. Kupperman, and *The Endocrinology of Reproduction*, edited by Joseph T. Velardo. The reader is referred to these publications for additional and specific details.

I am indebted to Mrs. Edith Tagrin for the excellent illustrations and to Mr. Leo Goodman and Dr. Robert Ehrmann for the photomicrographs. Dr. Arthur T. Hertig and Dr. Hazel M. Gore have also kindly given their excellent photomicrographs previously published in *Tumors of the Female Sex Organs*, published by the Armed Forces Institute of Pathology. The student is advised to refer to these fascicles for a complete survey of the pathology of tumors of the female genital tract.

I also wish to acknowledge a deep indebtedness to the tireless fingers and indefatigable efforts of my secretaries, Mrs. Ann Gregory Metzger, Mrs. Constance M. Rakoske, Mrs. Linda Angelico, and Mrs. Rachel Markiewicz. Valuable assistance has been given to me by the Administrator of the Free Hospital for Women, Miss Lillian Grahn. Finally, the courtesies of the staff of Year Book Medical Publishers have made the final preparation of this manuscript a pleasant task.

Robert W. Kistner

ACKNOWLEDGMENT

The Sixth Edition of *Kistner's Gynecology: Principles and Practice* has developed and grown from the legacy and scholarly contributions of the earlier editions. The first few editions were primarily the work of Robert Kistner, M.D., who was later joined by other invited participants who contributed to the book. Some of the authors of the previous editions have not written for the Sixth Edition and we wish to acknowledge that material from prior editions and authors may have been carried forward to this work in terms of content, figures, organizational structure, and concepts. We wish to express appreciation and indebtedness to the following:

Richard W. Erbe, M.D. – Genetics
Stephen Evans, M.D. – Infertility
Neil J. Finkler, M.D. – Uterine Corpus
C. Thomas Griffiths, M.D. – Cervix and Ovary
Robert C. Knapp, M.D. – Cervix
Thomas Leavitt, Jr., M.D. – Vulva
Patricia M. McShane, M.D. – Oviduct and Ectopic Pregnancy
Wayne A. Miller, M.D. – Genetics
Veronica A. Ravnikar, M.D. – Habitual Abortion, Endocrine Disorders, and Infertility Treatment
Isaac Schiff, M.D. – Menopause
Robert L. Shirley, M.D. – Breast
Phillip G. Stubblefield, M.D. – Conception Control
Robert M. Wah, M.D. – Infertility Treatment

CONTENTS

DETAILED CONTENTS

4 The vulva 50

5 The vagina 79

6 The cervix 103

7 The uterine corpus 137

8 The fallopian tube and ectopic pregnancy 166

9 The ovary 187

20 Medical genetics 461

21 Gynecologic infections 496

22 Conception control 532

23 Pediatric and adolescent gynecology 571

Chapter 1

THE CHANGING NATURE OF GYNECOLOGIC PRACTICE

Putting Science in Gynecologic Practice

Kenneth J. Ryan

Medicine has always portrayed the image that it is based on science. Over the centuries medicine has tried to supplant faith healing, witchcraft, religious fatalism, and homeopathy in combating disease. However, it is only in the past half century with the advent of antibiotics and advances in molecular biology and genetics that a true understanding and an effective means of dealing with disease have unfolded. In fact it is only in the past decade and a half that rigorous criteria for evaluating the value and effectiveness of diagnosis and treatment have appeared. The new techniques for determining the quality of medicine have included the following: (1) use of scientific evidence to justify medical interventions as exemplified by the U.S. Preventive Services Task Force Reports[12]; (2) the use of meta-analyses to evaluate common therapies as demonstrated in the two volume work, *Effective care in pregnancy and childbirth*, from Oxford University[2]; and (3) *Users' guides to the medical literature* as described by the evidence-based medicine working group from McMaster University.[4-7,10] The last group portrayed this move to evidence-based medicine as a paradigm shift in the Kuhnian sense of a scientific revolution.[3] As our mathematical tools and knowledge of human biology has expanded, along with the ability to custom design drugs and therapies, a standard of what constitutes "good" medicine has emerged.

Scientific basis for clinical recommendations

The method used by the U.S. Preventive Services Task Force to evaluate the scientific basis for recommending a clinical test or procedure should be useful in evaluating any type of clinical strategy.[12] The strength of a recommendation is graded from A to E based on whether evidence is good, fair, or poor for justifying or not justifying a screening procedure, test, or therapy (Table 1-1). Although evidence might be poor, since much in medicine is not yet validated, there may be enough justification for a risky procedure if the potential benefits outweigh all possible harm. On the other hand an A-strength recommendation would place a burden on the physician to explain why that procedure should not be performed. Meanwhile an E-strength

Table 1-1. Strength of recommendations for diagnostic, preventive, and therapeutic medical procedures

Grade	Recommendations
A	There is GOOD evidence for performing a procedure
B	There is FAIR evidence for performing a procedure
C	There is POOR evidence for performing a procedure
D	There is FAIR evidence against performing a procedure
E	There is GOOD evidence against performing a procedure

From: U.S. Preventive Services Task Force: *Guide to clinical preventive services*, Baltimore, 1989, Williams & Wilkins.

Box 1-1. Quality of evidence that backs up strength of recommendations

I	Randomized controlled studies
II-1	Controlled trial without randomization
II-2	Cohort or case-control analytic studies
II-3	Uncontrolled experiments
III	Expert opinions, descriptive epidemiology

From U.S. Preventive Services Task Force: *Guide to clinical preventive services,* Baltimore, 1989, Williams & Wilkins.

recommendation would force the physician to explain why that procedure should not be avoided. The data that back up the A to E recommendations are characterized by the number and quality of studies available, from well-conducted randomized clinical trials to more subjectively based expert opinions or clinical intuition (Table 1-2). In the end the studies still have to be evaluated and even randomized. Controlled trials may have design problems that can limit their usefulness, as will be noted later.[13] The process of evaluating a medical intervention by the U.S. Preventive Services Task Force is quite involved. This evaluation includes a thorough literature search, an evaluation of the accumulated material by a consensus development panel that writes the recommendations, followed by a critical appraisal after the report is completed. Using this system of grading, the strength of recommendations and the quality of the studies in the literature provide a means of expressing the degree of confidence in any medical action contemplated or taken. A primer on evaluating papers is included in the section below on evidence-based medicine. In the future such evaluation will extend beyond just preventive medicine and become routine for diagnosis and therapy as well.

Meta-analysis

Effective Care in Pregnancy and Childbirth is a two volume collection of meta-analyses of controlled trials of clinical interventions during pregnancy and the peripartum period. This sets a standard for evaluating the quality of obstetrical practice.[2,8] A comparable collection for gynecological practice does not exist yet but will undoubtedly be developed. Meta-analysis of clinical trials does not replace clinical judgment in deciding how to practice medicine but rather becomes one important factor that must be considered. One still has to evaluate the quality of the meta-analysis and the individual studies that come under scrutiny. Meta-analysis involves review of several clinical trials in which odds ratios and confidence limits for or against the effectiveness of a medical intervention exist. The process sums these statistics and increases the power of the individual studies. Sometimes the combined data allow a definitive judgment about whether a procedure is effective.

Some examples of the meta-analyses already performed should be instructive.[2] In studies analogous to randomized controlled trials of prophylactic use of antibiotics in hysterectomy, there have been a total of 43 adequately controlled trials of the use of antibiotics in cesarean section after the cord is clamped. It is clear from meta-analysis that serious infection and endometritis in the postpartum mother are significantly reduced in all of these studies. The odds that the patient will benefit are so great that it should indicate to the prudent clinician that *not* using prophylactic antibiotics would now have to be justified. It should not be necessary to do 43 studies before a therapy becomes a standard of practice and a technique of cumulative meta-analysis has been introduced.[9]

The therapeutic maneuver of using progesterone-like drugs to prevent miscarriage has been a subject of considerable controversy in the past. When subjected to a meta-analysis of some 17 studies, the odds ratio is 1.01. This ratio suggests that there is no evidence progesterone affects the outcome of the pregnancy. It would be difficult to recommend the use of progesterone to prevent miscarriage without some special justification. Even proposing a new study suggests that something was missing from the prior 17 trials.

In the widely accepted therapy of postpartum prophylaxis for Rh disease, only 9 controlled clinical trials were evaluated. Aside from one of the studies, which had only 26 subjects in each arm and was marginal in outcome, the remaining studies had 95 to 1000 subjects in the treatment and control arms. As a result the meta-analysis revealed extreme effectiveness that now justifies this intervention as routine treatment.

Scanning the other meta-analyses, 31 studies indicate that x-ray pelvimetry is of little help and 2 studies show that shaving the perineum prior to delivery makes little difference in infection. There are no good data to justify the use of routine iron in pregnancy, whereas the data (not from meta-analysis) on the value of folic acid supplementation are increasing. Physicians must still be prepared to defend their actions in the care of individual patients. Meta-analyses provide us with valuable help if properly conducted and use strict guidelines for the selection of studies included in the analysis.[8]

The advent of evidence-based medicine

In the past much of the practice of medicine has been based on cumulative clinical experience and the text book writings and opinions of experts.[3] Randomized, controlled clinical trials are of relatively recent origin, and they have not always provided definitive answers. It is still often said that every patient is an "experiment" in that one can never predict outcomes with certainty. This mind set has typified the approach to medicine in the past. Outcomes can now be predicted, but they are statistical predictions and not absolute ones. For example, a practitioner in the 1960s protested that oral contraceptives could not cause emboli because he had not seen one in his practice. The individual clinician must learn how to deal with the disparity between personal experience and the collective experience in which rare events and most clinical effects must be evaluated. Many gynecologists denied the relationship of estrogens to endometrial cancer until sufficient studies were completed. The use of estrogen treatment in menopause has been validated for hot flushes by randomized, blinded, and controlled cross-over studies in spite of a considerable placebo effect. The value of estrogen in preventing osteoporosis was proved only by carefully controlled studies. The area of gynecological practice that has been most difficult to validate has involved indications for surgery and the type of operative procedure used. Operative techniques such as pelviscopy have been introduced into practice before sufficient study, but even here progress is made by critically evaluating the experience. Evidence-based medicine has come to gynecology and is important in all other branches of medicine as well. Searching and evaluating the literature are becoming important components of practicing medicine.

EVALUATING THE LITERATURE FOR GYNECOLOGIC THERAPIES

To adequately practice gynecology today, the clinician must be aware of what is available in the literature and be able to critically evaluate the validity of studies that are the basis of contemporary practice. Reports from the U.S. Preventive Task Force[12,13] and the meta-analyses noted above[2] include examples of evaluation of the literature on specific topics. Practice guidelines issued by the government and technical bulletins issued by the American College of Obstetricians and Gynecologists provide annotated references.[1] A series of articles in the *Journal of the American Medical Association* from the evidence-based medicine working group provides a guide to the use of the medical literature that should prove helpful.[4-7,10] Their thesis is that throw-away journals, drug detailing, and advertising should not constitute the first line of information used by the clinician.

Most physicians have access to a medical library and with the computer, on-line literature searches are increasingly available. One can also start with standard up-to-date texts (such as this one) and review articles to obtain references on a specific topic. The best bet is to look for randomized-controlled trials and then make a decision about their validity. The questions to ask include the following:

1. Were the patients truly randomized? There are examples of surgical operations that were widely accepted as effective, such as extracranial-intracranial bypass to prevent stroke, shown to be ineffective after a multicenter randomized trial was completed. The only effect of surgery was to make the patient worse immediately after the procedure. Another surprise after a randomized clinical trial overthrew conventional wisdom was that steroids may increase rather than reduce mortality in patients with infection.[4] Randomization limits bias in subject selection and evenly distributes other factors that might influence the outcome of the study. An absence of randomization limits the validity of any study. Nonrandomized studies are more apt to show false-positive treatment effects that are inevitably misleading.
2. Were the inclusion and exclusion criteria for randomization reasonable and were the treatment and control arms comparable? Factors such as age, gender, socioeconomic factors, and the degree of disease involvement may all influence the outcome.
3. Were all randomized subjects accounted for at the end of the study? It is necessary to account for drop-outs or individuals who do not complete a study because of irregularities or complications that might skew the results.
4. Were the research personnel and the patients blinded? Blinding limits bias that can creep into studies because of the enthusiasm of the subjects or the scientists and controls for placebo effects. When possible, blinded cross-over studies, where patients are their own controls, provides some additional assurance of the validity of effects. This was used to good effect with the role of estrogens in controlling hot flushes.
5. Were the two arms of the study treated equally except for the treatment? It is not enough to have randomization to be assured of a valid outcome. The U.S. Preventive Task Force evaluation of home uterine activity, which monitors for preterm labor,[13] found in a randomized study (grade I evidence) that the monitored group showed benefit over the controls and reached an increased age of gestation. When they critiqued the study, they found that there were small numbers in each arm, the investigators were not blinded, the treatment-arm subjects were contacted daily, and the control group was contacted twice a week. So in spite of poor grade I evidence, they assigned a "C" grade for strength of recommendation.
6. What is the magnitude of the treatment effect? What is the power of the study? These questions can be answered when relative risk or odds ratios and confidence limits are known. The size of the study is an important component of this, and when results are intriguing but not clear cut, the above-mentioned meta-analyses should be of help.

LABORATORY TESTING AND DIAGNOSES IN GYNECOLOGY

Evaluation of the literature for effectiveness of diagnostic procedures involves a different set of criteria from that used for therapy.[6,7] Very often there is a reference standard against which the diagnostic procedure is judged. Does the patient have the disease if the result is positive and not have the disease if the test is negative? Very often diagnostic laparoscopy or operative specimens have to be referred to for the answers. Important questions include the following: can the beta-subunit predict an ectopic pregnancy? can ultrasonography or OC-125 diagnose ovarian cancer? For these questions, sensitivity, specificity, predictive values, and probabilities, as discussed by Dr. Cramer in his chapter on principles of biostatistics for gynecologists are important. Note also that Dr. Benacerraf in her chapter on pelvic sonography gives such statistics for some of her studies. The evidence-based medical group recommends use of likelihood ratios in judging whether the test can identify the disease in question.[7]

In gynecology it has been traditional to use a fair number of endocrine tests looking for the etiologies in patients with amenorrhea, hirsutism, or infertility. The justification of many such tests would be suspect if measured against the critical standards to which they refer.

GYNECOLOGY IN PRIMARY CARE AND HEALTH CARE REFORM

"Health care reform" has raised the issues of quality in medicine and the need to address the important issues of primary health care. The motivation for health care reform in the United States in the 1990s has been to provide universal coverage of all citizens regardless of socioeconomic status. High quality medical services are combined with ease of access and reduced costs. Central to this effort is an increased emphasis on managed care, with the central role played by the primary care first-contact physician. This physician provides continuity in medical services, preventive services, education on health promotion and disease prevention, counseling, and appropriate referral to a limited panel of specialists. It is necessary for the primary care physician to be enough of a generalist to provide direct care for most of the medical problems confronting patients. Thus an essential component of managed care is that once the patient selects a primary care physician, all other access to health care services is via that physician. Exceptions have occasionally been made for an annual or biennial eye exam and for an annual visit to the obstetrician-gynecologist, if the patient desires this. Patients can also opt out of managed plan restrictions by paying extra for selecting their own referrals. However, managed care plans try to discourage doctor shopping and excessive use of costly hospital emergency services as "walk-in" clinics and try to provide incentives to such patients and physicians to use cost-effective diagnostic and treatment strategies. The virtues of the "managed" system are based on both economics and enhanced quality of care, with emphasis on continuity of care, on prevention, and on limited use of higher cost specialists, diagnostic tests, and facilities. The limitations of the system are the restricted options for the patient and the necessity for individual or group practice physicians or specialists to restructure how they refer or receive patients. The full impact of the managed way of practicing medicine will not be felt until it becomes the predominant or only way of providing health care services in any given area.

While family practice physicians, internists, and pediatricians have all laid claim to functioning as primary care physicians, many obstetrician-gynecologists either function or would like to work in the expanded primary care role for women.[1] Obstetricians caring for a pregnant patient often fulfill without question the primary care role during the pregnancy. Many women in the reproductive years already use their obstetrician-gynecologist as their sole primary care provider. Aside from obstetrical care, a majority of women in the reproductive years see the gynecologist for a general check-up, for family planning services, and for the Papanicolaou smear. Attention to perimenopausal and postmenopausal years, with concerns about hormone replacement therapy, carries the concerns of the gynecologist into the care of aging women as well.

Gynecology refers to the medical discipline concerned with the prevention, diagnosis, and treatment of diseases of the female reproductive system. While the field is recognized for this specialty function and for subspecialty roles in urogynecology, infertility, and oncology, special attention is now being directed to the primary health care role of the gynecologist. The interest in primary care is not shared by all gynecologists. Some want to keep the discipline limited to a referral and consultative practice, but the national societies in obstetrics and gynecology have been encouraging a primary care option within the specialty.[1] Whether in specialty or primary care, there has also been new emphasis on the scientific or evidence-based practice noted above and measures of cost-effectiveness and outcome. This has led to the creation of clinical practice guidelines, especially in preventive services, many of which have a direct relevance to gynecology practiced either as a specialty or as primary care.

The review of clinical practice with respect to disease prevention started with the Canadian Task Force on the Periodic Health Examination.[11] This was extended by a U.S. Preventive Services Task Force in the 1970s and 1980s.[12] Their reports concluded that the patient's personal health behaviors were more important in terms of morbidity and mortality than most interventions performed in the periodic health examination. They observed that most screening was not useful and that physicians might have more impact on health if they provided patient education and counseling on personal health behaviors instead of tests. Routine blood counts, screening for diabetes in nonpregnant women, chest x-rays, and electrocardiograms have not been shown to be effective. The Papanicolaou smear performed every 1 to 3 years, breast palpation, and mammograms annually over age 50 are essentially all that remain of helpful tests directed to the female reproductive system. Cervical cancer mortality has declined over 70% in the last 40 years. A major contribution to the decline has been early detection of a precancerous lesion. However, screening has not been effective for ovarian cancer, a major cause of death in women. Counseling on sexual practices and contraception to avoid unintended pregnancies and sexually transmitted diseases remain important contributions of the gynecologist either as a specialist or as a primary care physician.

The rank order of age-adjusted death rates in the United States are heart disease, lung cancer, and cerebrovascular disease for both African-American and Caucasian women. Hence, screening for high blood pressure and serum cholesterol and counseling on nutrition, smoking, and physical activity could be effective. Smoking is a factor in one of every six deaths resulting from cancer, coronary and cerebrovascular disease, and chronic obstructive pulmonary disease. Deaths from chronic lung disease, pneumonia, and influenza are sufficiently high to justify annual immunizations for influenza and the administration of pneumococcal vaccine, depending on age and other risk factors. In the reproductive years, motor vehicle accidents, homicide, and acquired immunodeficiency syndrome are major causes of death for women. Thus showing sensitivity to and intervention in domestic physical abuse and violence, counselling on drug use, encouraging the use of seat belts, warning about drinking and driving, and advising about safe sexual practices are important. Whether the gynecologist functions as a specialist or a primary care provider must be made explicit to the patient. The expanded responsibilities of the primary care role must not be left to chance encounters. It should be clear from the foregoing that much of what the gynecologist normally does falls within the description of primary care.[1] To this must be added further training and an emphasis on ambulatory medicine, especially on diseases common to women, such as hypertension, coronary disease, lung disease, thyroid disorders, diabetes, arthritis, and depression.

THE RELATIONSHIP BETWEEN GYNECOLOGY AND OBSTETRICS

Even though the American Board of Obstetrics and Gynecology was founded in 1930 to provide examination and certification in a combined discipline, separate departments of obstetrics and gynecology in both hospitals and medical schools had preceded and followed the establishment of the Board. Although German universities had established combined departments by the end of the nineteenth century, programs in England, France, and the United States stubbornly remained divided until the mid-twentieth century. The division seems to have been more over tradition and self-image than of substance. Because of the need for emphasis on specialist training and practice, some of the arguments for separation have been answered at the subspecialty level. Since the 1970s, there have been the subspecialties of maternal-fetal medicine, reproductive endocrinology, and gynecological oncology. On the other hand, there is a natural affinity between obstetrics and gynecology at the generalist level because of the shared anatomy, endocrinology, and physiology; the interrelatedness of health and disease processes in women cannot be neatly divided between the pregnant and the nonpregnant state. What must not be lost sight of is the way obstetrics and gynecology and their subspecialties overlap in terms of patient needs and in the requirement of knowledge and clinical skills by any practitioner who cares for women. The gynecologist must consider the reproductive consequences of all gynecologic care including surgery, chemotherapy, radiation, and the expanded options for assisted reproduction. The obstetrician must be concerned with the impact of pregnancy and its management on the woman's subsequent health and function. The obstetrician must also recognize that not only prenatal care but also interconceptional care can be important for pregnancy outcomes. In the reproductive years, amenorrhea or bleeding should always raise questions about a normally implanted or ectopic pregnancy in the differential diagnosis. An unsuspected pregnancy must always be considered prior to the use of medication or tests. Finally, as a combined practitioner, the obstetrician-gynecologist can bring more to the primary care of women than by restricting practice to one or the other specialty.

REFERENCES

1. ACOG Task Force on Primary and Preventive Health Care: *The obstetrician-gynecologist and primary-preventive health care*, Washington, DC, 1993, American College of Obstetricians and Gynecologists.
2. Chalmers I, Enkin M, Keirse MJ: *Effective care in pregnancy and childbirth*, 2 vols, New York, 1989, Oxford University Press.
3. Evidence-Based Medicine Working Group: Evidence-based medicine: a new approach to teaching the practice of medicine, *JAMA* 268:2425, 1992.
4. Guyatt GH, Sackett DL, Cook DJ: Users' guides to the medical literature. II. How to use an article about therapy or prevention. A. Are the results of the study valid? *JAMA* 270:2598-2601, 1993.
5. Guyatt GH, Sackett DL, Cook DJ: Users' guides to the medical literature. II. How to use an article about therapy or prevention. B. What were the results and will they help me in caring for my patients? *JAMA* 271:59-63, 1994.
6. Jaeschke J, Guyatt GH, Sackett DL: Users' guides to the medical literature. III. How to use an article about a diagnostic test. A. Are the results of the study valid? *JAMA* 271:389-391, 1994.
7. Jaeschke J, Guyatt G, Sackett DL: Users' guides to the medical literature. III. B. What are the results and will they help me in caring for my patients? *JAMA*: 271:703-707, 1994.
8. Kassirer JP: Clinical trials and meta-analysis. What do they do for us? *N Eng J Med* 327:273-274, 1992.
9. Lau J et al: *N Eng J Med* 327:248-254, 1992.
10. Oxman AD, Sackett DL, Guyatt GH: Users' guides to the medical literature. I. How to get started, *JAMA* 270:2093-2095, 1993.
11. Task Force Report: The periodic health exam, *CMA* 121:1193-1254, 1979.

12. U.S. Preventive Services Task Force: *Guide to clinical preventive services,* Baltimore, 1989, Williams & Wilkins.

13. U.S. Preventive Services Task Force: Home uterine activity monitoring for preterm labor, *JAMA* 270:371-376, 1993.

Chapter 2

MEDICAL ETHICS AND THE PRACTICE OF GYNECOLOGY

Kenneth J. Ryan

Medical ethics has been shaken to its Hippocratic roots in the last half of the twentieth century.[8,9] Advances in medical technology, such as in vitro fertilization, organ transplantation, and life support practices, have raised new ethical problems for doctors and patients on how much one should intrude into nature at the beginning and at the end of life. Even while technology was advancing, the public in the 1960s and 1970s rebelled against the controls that government and medicine had over their lives. People began to insist on newly formulated patient's rights, women's rights, and reproductive freedoms that required a fresh look at our moral rules and presumptions. As conflicts between medical institutions and patients or their families arose over these issues, the courts were used to resolve disputes and set precedents. For example, in the Karen Ann Quinlan case, the New Jersey Supreme Court allowed the parents to order withdrawal of a respirator from their daughter who had been in a prolonged coma. In deciding this case, the court suggested the use of an ethics committee to determine the patient's prognosis. This has since triggered the creation of ethics committees in essentially all hospitals throughout the United States concerned with moral questions about medical practice and research and technology assessment. Bioethics thus came into being in the 1960s.[4,6] While the explicit teaching of medical ethics had long been neglected in medical schools prior to 1970, the extensive publicity about moral dilemmas in medical practice and research resulted in formal courses in medical ethics in essentially all institutions. The supreme court decision on *Roe v. Wade* in 1973 set the stage for the ensuing public debate over abortion and increased public interest in medical ethics in general.

The practice of gynecology has had more than its fair share of ethical concerns and problems. These ethical issues have included the following: justification for abortion; whether or not to provide contraceptives to minors without parental consent; the issue of assisted reproduction not only for married couples but also for single and gay couples; and the failure of physicians in the past to recognize the wide extent of abuse and sexual assault of women. Then there is the long-standing discrimination against women by the pharmaceutical industry in medical research because of the problems associated with hormonal effects during the menstrual cycle or with birth control pills. Investigators are afraid of harming the fetus or of being sued in case of an inadvertent pregnancy during a drug trial. As a consequence, women to a large extent are therapeutic orphans and often have to be treated for medical problems on the basis of drug studies using only the male. Finally, dealing with terminal care for patients with end-stage malignancy has always been a tough problem for gynecologists; now they have to deal with advanced directives, proxies, and the controversies over euthanasia and assisted suicide as well.

MORAL THEORIES AND PRINCIPLES

The writings of Hippocrates and the Hippocratic Oath have been an integral part of medical ethics for at least 2500 years. These medical ethics still apply and include requirements of confidentiality, of not "abusing (sexually) the bodies of man or woman, bond or free," trying to help the sick and avoiding injury and wrong-doing, and not administering a poison.[6] The admonitions against abortion and surgery have much less force today, but it is not known how widely any of these recommendations were followed in ancient Greece. While the Hippocratic tradition championed the concepts of helping and not harming the patient as the ultimate obligation, it also supported the elitist and paternalistic aspects of medicine that were challenged in the 1960s. In addition, the ethical guidance of these writings seemed inadequate to deal with the advances of technology that raised questions not even thought of by the Greeks.

When bioethicists entered the medical scene, they looked toward ethics and moral philosophy to provide guidance about what to do in any given situation. Unfortunately, most bioethicists looked backward to the two major competing theories about morality: utilitarianism as advanced by John Stuart Mills in the nineteenth century and deontology as advanced by Immanuel Kant in the eighteenth century.[6] Utilitarianism is the most prominent method of deciding whether something is good or bad, right or wrong, based on the *outcome* or end result (also known as teleological or consequentional). In this theory one tries to create the most good for the most people as a guide to ethical behavior. On the other hand, deontology is generally a rule or obligation-based ethic that does not rely on the outcome so much, as the means used in achieving it. In Kant's formulation, an ethical guide would be the categorical imperative: act only on maxims that are universal, (e.g., never tell a falsehood, and to use people as ends and never as means, thereby exalting the value of being a rational human being). Other deontological ethical theories have been proposed, such as Ross' *prima facie* duties.[6] The problem with trying to follow only one or another of any of these theories as the bioethicists first advised is that they do not conform to the way most individuals deal with ethical problems. We are more apt to follow the admonition of the American pragmatist philosopher, John Dewey, i.e., (to consider *both* means and ends and to use judgment in trying to decide when the ends or the outcome do not justify the means and when following rules would create an unacceptably bad outcome). These theories are also sufficiently abstract in that they provide only general guidance.[6]

When Congress asked the National Commission for the Protection of Human Subjects of Biomedical and Behavioral Research, chaired by the author, which ethical principles should underlie the conduct of research or the provision of medical care, the response was the following three principles as published in the Belmont Report[7]: (1) respect for persons (sometimes expressed as respect for autonomy), (2) beneficence, and (3) justice. The Commission went on to interpret the application of these in the following ways: respect for a person or their autonomy is shown by obtaining informed consent from them; beneficence is shown by doing the risk-benefit calculus and trying to provide benefit while keeping harm to a minimum—sometimes expressed by a separate principle of nonmaleficence; concern for justice is shown by treating the patient fairly in all respects—an outgrowth of the influence of *Justice*, the major work of the Harvard philosopher, John Rawls. The three principles are quite general and should be used as just one of several inputs against which ethical actions are judged. It should be noted that when principles conflict, there is not necessarily a prearranged priority. In general the desire to help a patient (to be beneficent) cannot in morality or law ordinarily override the need to respect the patient's right to autonomy. In other words the patient should never be forced to undergo a procedure or treatment she refuses, even if she would benefit. This statement is a reflection of the widely accepted move away from paternalism, aided and abetted by the outcome of many court cases in which the requirement for informed consent is taken as overriding.

Making moral judgments and resolving conflict

From the foregoing discussion of moral theories and principles, it should be apparent that there are no "cook book" procedures for deciding which course of action to take. The objective of moral education, as President Bok of Harvard once commented, is not to make an ethical person out of a blackguard but more modestly to teach students how to recognize moral issues when they arise, to teach proper reasoning about moral issues (simply the same as proper reasoning about any subject in a relevant and logical manner), and to at least exhort students to make consideration of ethics important in their lives. When asked by physicians how in general to approach an ethical dilemma, the following is recommended: accumulate all of the facts of the case and be sure of the facts; try to define the specific ethical issues in question; use analogy to other comparable, ethically troubling, situations read about or experienced; explore the differences between various options; and test the choices against commonly accepted moral principles, guides, or rules. Discuss difficult cases with other members of the health care team or colleagues, and ask for a hospital ethics committee consultation when wider discussion would be helpful. Reading ethical case studies and reviewing the arguments that others have made in support of or against a given course of action also provide a good background for dealing with ethical issues in medicine.

ETHICAL ISSUES IN GYNECOLOGIC PRACTICE

The doctor-patient relationship

The primary focus of ethics in medical practice has been the doctor-patient relationship. In its 1980 book, *Principles of Medical Ethics*, the American Medical Association asks that physicians provide competence, honesty, compassion, and respect for human dignity in caring for their patients.[6] Developed in 1973 by the American Hospital Association, a Patient's Bill of Rights for hospitalized patients stresses considerate and respectful care, complete disclosure of information by the physician to the patient on medical status, and also disclosure of sufficient information on which to base truly *informed* consent for any anticipated procedure, treatment, or alternatives. As indicated earlier the trend is away from paternalism and toward empowering the patient to assume responsibility for her care. It is not permissible to involve patients in teaching exercises or research without their knowledge and consent, and patients still expect privacy and confidentiality.

Ethical issues in assisted reproduction

Away from the traditional doctor-patient relationship, the major ethical issues involve societal values and priorities about the uses of medicine. In gynecology a major concern has been over assisted reproduction.[10,11] When in vitro fertilization was first being developed in the 1970s, the major arguments against it were that it was unnatural and its safety had not been established in the human. The concerns about safety have since been dispelled as thousands of infants have been born by this technique without an increase in congenital defects. The argument over what is natural and acceptable continues to this day. The Vatican position still maintains that only coitus by a married couple is licit in the creation of children. There were also concerns about freezing embryos and discarding those that could not be used. The status of the early embryo was disputed. Some wanted it to have the absolute value afforded to persons, while others felt that the objective of providing children for childless couples justified manipulating embryos for this purpose. In spite of these issues, in vitro fertilization has become widely used and generally accepted. The arguments about what is natural have abated somewhat. Much of what civilization and modern medicine achieves is the protection of people against the misfortunes inflicted by nature.

Although first used only for married couples, infertility services are now sought by single and homosexual individuals. The technology allows individuals to bypass customary social taboos and depersonalize the reproductive process, which would not occur if normal sexual relations were required. There is much controversy over whether this should be allowed; a counterargument has been made about the sad state of society, the high divorce rate, and the general breakdown of family values even with customary reproduction. In vitro fertilization has permitted requests to be made for donation of eggs and spare embryos as well as the traditional use of sperm for artificial insemination. These expansions of infertility services raise questions about the importance of two heterosexual parents and the concepts of family and personal identity. Recently, women in their 50s, beyond their normal reproductive years, have received transfer of embryos and had normal pregnancy and delivery. Since sources of ova donation are limited, an argument is raging about using ova from aborted fetuses or cadavers. The arguments about how assisted reproduction should be used depend to a large extent on an individual's religious and social views. It is likely controversy will continue over whether infertility services should be offered in such cases. The issue of recruiting women for surrogate gestation has not been mentioned, but this has also caused much argument and distress, since it often involves class differences and suggestions of economic coercion. The author uses a straight forward test whenever any form of infertility services are requested. If a child is truly wanted, if it will be given a good home and loving care, and if there is no exploitation of anyone in the process, including the expected child, the infertility service should be morally acceptable. In other words, most of these cases have to be judged on their own merits.

Abuse of women

The extent of domestic violence and physical abuse of women in our society has until recently been largely overlooked. In a recent article on ethics, Ruth Macklin reviewed the situation.[5] Apparently, attacks by husbands, ex-husbands, and lovers cause more injury to women than auto accidents, muggings, and sexual assault combined. There are 4 million batterings and 4000 deaths of women by close acquaintances each year. One fifth to one third of all women will be physically abused in domestic violence in their lifetimes. While there is a limit to what a gynecologist can do to alleviate this problem, it has been suggested that gynecologists should screen for this and play essentially the same role for abused women that pediatricians play in calling attention to child abuse. Women caught in such situations are often socially isolated, severely intimidated, and undergo both physical and psychological abuse. These women often have a low self-esteem and difficulty in breaking out of this environment. Gynecologists should be aware of the community resources available to help such women.

Pain, euthanasia, suicide, and terminal care

Dr. Jack Kevorkian, the "suicide" doctor from Michigan, has been in the news a good deal since 1990. He has assisted in 20 suicides of men and women who wanted to end their lives because of incurable illnesses. Dr. Kevorkian is a retired pathologist who publicized his activities to force a change in laws prohibiting physician-assisted suicide and euthanasia. He hardly knew any of the individuals he assisted to their deaths, and because of this and his lack of direct patient care experience, this serious issue became a media event.[12] Recent initiatives to legalize euthanasia have been narrowly defeated on several state ballots. In the Netherlands, however, a permissive environment for active euthanasia by physicians has existed for quite some time.

In this country opinion has evolved to the point where "passive euthanasia," or letting the patient die, has become generally acceptable for patients in the terminal days of their illnesses and for patients in persistent and irreversible coma. It started with the Karen Ann Quinlan case referred to earlier and progressed to the Cruzan case where the U.S. Supreme Court acknowledged that individuals can control their own destinies and forgo medical therapy, including food and fluid.[1,13] The tendency to use "do not resuscitate" orders more frequently in terminal illness is consistent with a trend to avoid futile treatment and to avoid the delay of death.

The range of feelings about these options involves general acceptance of the patient's or the family's choice about forgoing therapy in terminal illness, to some discord in withdrawing support from the nonterminal comatose patient in the persistent vegetative state, to bitter disagreement on active euthanasia and assisted suicide. There is the argument that passive and active euthanasia do not differ that much from an ethical perspective, since the objective of both is to avoid unnecessary suffering. This is obviously a utilitarian idea. There is the counterargument that it should always be possible to relieve pain and suffering by good hospice care and thereby avoid the need for active euthanasia or for doctors' involvement in direct killing. This has a brutalizing effect, and there is always the possibility of abuse. The public and physicians are divided on the issue.

One initiative that has gained popular support is to discuss terminal care with patients before it becomes an issue and to ask patients in advance for directives on how they wish to be treated. The Cruzan case makes it clear that the courts will abide by what the patient desires. In addition, patients should be encouraged to provide a health care proxy in case they cannot represent their own interests.

Another side to this issue is the question of pain relief for cancer patients. Physicians, in general, do a poor job in providing pain relief. As a result, new guidelines have been released by the Agency for Health Care Policy and Research of the U.S. Department of Health and Human Services to deal specifically with the problem. Undertreatment of pain is largely due to inadequate information from physicians and a need for better assessment of pain and its management. It is also necessary to overcome the negative feelings about the use of drugs for pain relief by patients and doctors alike. Pain can in fact be relieved in up to 90% of patients with cancer by simple means.[3] This being the case, a good argument can be made for worrying less about euthanasia and more about providing effective pain relief.

Abortion as an aberration for an ethical dispute

There is not much one can add that is new on the abortion controversy. Those who champion fetal rights and interests are pitted against those who support the rights and interests of the pregnant woman. Since the 1973 U.S. Supreme Court decision in *Roe v. Wade*, which made abortion legal, the country has been divided. Physicians are also in disagreement on this issue. It is one of the few morality instances where both sides can be "right." Each side legitimately defends its point of view based on differing starting premises. The pro-life position is that life from conception is sacred and absolute. However, if the pregnant woman's rights are considered superior to the life developing within her, the pro-choice position is defensible. A goal of convincing one side or another of their error is no longer realistic. The most that can be hoped for is civilized respect for the opposing positions. A book, *Life's Dominion*, by Ronald Dworkin, has tried to address the issues of both abortion and euthanasia and to offer some arguments that will bring the two sides closer together.[2] Undoubtedly, it will not be the last book on the subject.

REFERENCES

1. Bopp J Jr: Choosing death for Nancy Cruzan, *Hastings Center Report* 20:42-44, 1990.
2. Dworkin R: *Life's dominion*, New York, 1993, Alfred A Knopf.
3. Jacox A, Carr DB, Payne R: New clinical-practice guidelines for the management of pain in patients with cancer, *N Engl J Med* 330:651-655, 1994.
4. Jonsen AR: The birth of bioethics: special supplement, *Hastings Center Report* 23, No 6, 1993.
5. Macklin R: Women's health: an ethical perspective, *The Journal of Law, Medicine & Ethics* 21:23-29, 1993.
6. Mappes TA, Zembaty JS: *Biomedical ethics*, ed 3, New York, 1991, McGraw-Hill.
7. Pellegrino ED: The metamorphosis of medical ethics, *JAMA* 269:1158-1162, 1993.
8. Ryan KJ: Ethics in obstetrics & gynecology, *Am J Ob Gyn* 151:840-843, 1985.
9. Ryan KJ: Ethical issues in reproductive endocrinology and infertility, *Am J Ob Gyn* 160:415-417, 1989.
10. Ryan KJ: Ethics of the current reproductive technologies. In Soules MR, editor: *Controversies in reproductive endocrinology and infertility*, New York, 1989, Elsevier.
11. National commission for the protection of human subjects of biomedical and behavioral research, The Belmont Report: *DHEW Publication No (OS)* 78-0012, Washington, DC, 1978, US Govt Printing Office.
12. Trial is ordered for suicide doctor, *New York Times National*, p 9, Feb 19, 1994.
13. Wolf SM: Nancy Beth Cruzan: in no voice at all, *Hastings Center Report*, 20:38-41, 1990.

Chapter 3

THE MENSTRUAL CYCLE

Robert L. Barbieri
Kenneth J. Ryan

There are two views of the menstrual cycle: (1) the clinical view of cyclic bleeding and (2) the more theoretical, basic neuroendocrine view of the cycle. There is a science to both the clinical and basic views of the cycle, and an attempt will be made in this chapter to integrate the two perspectives.

CLINICAL MENSTRUAL CYCLE

Menstruation is the cyclic uterine bleeding experienced by most women of reproductive age. Normal menstruation represents the cyclic shedding of the uterine secretory endometrium because of a decline in estradiol and progesterone production caused by a regressing corpus luteum.

Duration of the cycle

The association of menstruation with the lunar cycle is a romantic notion. Contrary to popular belief, the menstrual cycle of most women does not repeat like "clockwork." To establish some sense of normalcy, the gynecologist routinely asks each patient about the menstrual interval, regularity of menstrual intervals, duration of menses, and volume of menstrual flow.

Treloar et al reported on the menstrual interval and regularity of menstrual intervals in Caucasian women who attended the University of Minnesota.[53] Data were collected prospectively over 30 years, and 275,947 menstrual cycles were available for analysis. Table 3-1 summarizes the results of this study. The cycle length usually varies by 1 to 2 days each month, and only 50% of women have a cycle within the 26- to 30-day range that encompasses the so-called typical 28-day interval. For most women, menses starts for the first time at age 13 years (normal range 8 to 16 years) and stops by age 52 years (normal range 45 to 55 years). Over the age range of 20 to 40 years, women have the tightest regularity to their cycles, with more variability in the immediate postmenarche and premenopause years. However, the median "normal" cycle length actually declines from 28.87 (± 2.75) days at age 20 years to a median of 26.8 (± 2) days by age 40 years. In this population of normal women, cycle lengths ranged from 25.4 to 34.7 days at age 20 years and from 24.4 to 30.3 days by age 40 years. By observing a large number of healthy women over 30 years, the investigators observed that cycle lengths cluster around a normal biologic distribution curve; individual women tend to vary around a cycle length that is usual for them. During the first few years after menarche and just before menopause, women experience wider deviation from the mean. The concept of "normalcy" encompasses variations that include 50% of women at age 25 years who have cycle lengths either less than 27 days or more than 31 days.

Table 3-1. Median and 5% upper and lower bounds on menstrual interval in days from 275,947 menstrual cycles

	Menstrual interval (Days)		
Chronologic age (yr)	**5% Lower bound**	**Median**	**5% Upper bound**
17	22	28	40
25	23	28	37
33	22	27	34
41	22	26	32
49	15	27	>80

Adapted from Treloar AE et al: Variation of human menstrual cycle through reproductive life, *Int J Fert* (12):77-126, 1962.

By reference to such studies of a large number of women over a considerable period of time, the limits of normalcy have been defined. In general, cycle lengths less than 24 days are considered polymenorrhea, and those more than 35 days are considered oligomenorrhea (Table 3-1). It has subsequently been established that most ovulatory cycles (as determined by a luteinizing hormone [LH] surge and normal luteal-phase progesterone) vary from 24 to 35 days. The variability of the menstrual cycle within this range is both a common and a normal event from a biologic perspective.[27] The average duration of menstruation is between 3 and 7 days, and shorter (hypomenorrhea) or longer (hypermenorrhea) than this is considered abnormal.

Amount of menstrual flow

The normal duration of menstrual flow ranges from 3 to 7 days, and the amount of total blood loss is generally 80 mL or less. It has been established that women vary widely from one another in the amount of blood lost at menstruation, but each woman is fairly consistent from month to month in her individual loss. This pattern has been established for women in several parts of the world in which the average loss and variation are strikingly similar. The method used to measure blood loss involves extracting blood from tampons and pads with a solution of sodium hydroxide and converting heme chromogens to a form that can be measured on a spectrophotometer. When menstrual blood loss exceeds 80 mL in an individual, there is a good correlation with anemia (hemoglobin value less than 12 gm) and with low plasma iron values.[18] Since trying to determine the extent of menstrual blood loss by patient estimates is difficult, checking for anemia is one practical way to monitor the extent of menstrual flow.

BIOLOGIC BASIS OF THE MENSTRUAL CYCLE

To explain why menstrual bleeding occurs at all and why it is cyclical, one must understand the role of hormones and peptide growth factors in controlling cell division and differentiation of the endometrial lining of the uterus and its vasculature. Menstrual bleeding occurs only in higher apes and humans, whereas most mammals do not slough the lining of their uterus at the end of each nonfertile cycle. This striking difference in the reproductive process is probably related to the evolution of viviparity and the unique placentation of primates. In early human pregnancy, there is an extensive invasion by the placenta deep into the endometrial layer so that the cotyledons can be bathed in maternal blood. Each month that pregnancy does not occur, the thick endometrial layer and its spiral blood vessels lose their hormonal support and the endometrium is sloughed, resulting in menstrual flow. In other mammals, the endometrium is not similarly developed or there is no luteal hormone released unless pregnancy occurs. Although there are no menstrual periods in other mammals, some do have cyclic bleeding at the time of ovulation and sexual receptivity (heat). This is typically seen in the domestic dog.

Prior to the early twentieth century, it was taught that human ovulation occurred at the time of menses. This resulted in the development of a rhythm method for family planning that could not have been further off the mark. It was only after the correct temporal relationships of endometrial changes to menstruation were described by Hitschmann and Adler[20] that others determined the relationship between ovulation and the secretion of ovarian estradiol and progesterone and their subsequent hormonal effects on the endometrium. This was followed in 1932 by an understanding of the reciprocal relationships between the pituitary gland and the gonads, and isolation of the pituitary and ovarian hormones. Subsequently the classic concept of the menstrual cycle evolved. This first model included only the interaction of the pituitary, ovary, and endometrium with the release of pituitary follicle-stimulating hormone (FSH) and luteinizing hormone (LH). This release of hormones caused follicular estrogen secretion and endometrial proliferation in the first half of the cycle followed by a surge of LH. As a result, ovulation with secretion of progesterone and estrogen occurred and resulted in a secretory endometrium in the second half of the cycle (Fig. 3-1). The relationship of the pituitary and ovary was characterized as a closed-loop negative feedback system, like the relationship of a thermostat to a heating system. The FSH and LH stimulated the secretion of ovarian hormones that in turn kept the FSH and LH levels in the right range. When the corpus luteum regressed, the cycle started over.[17,44] This was an oversimplified explanation and was ultimately corrected by the discovery of the role of the hypothalamus in reproduction, the discovery of the positive feedback of estrogen to cause the LH surge and ovulation, and finally the isolation of gonadotropin-releasing hormone (GnRH) in the early 1970s.[30,49] Our current understanding of the complex neuroendocrine interactions that regulate the menstrual cycle is now sufficiently detailed to be clinically applicable to the gynecologist taking care of patients with menstrual problems.

INTEGRATION OF THE MENSTRUAL CYCLE

The menstrual cycle depends on a complex interaction between the brain (of which the hypothalamus is a part), the pituitary, the ovaries, and the endometrium. Generally, input to the system comes from environmental cues (nutrition, stress, emotion, light, smell, and sound) via the central nervous system (CNS) to the hypothalamus, which transforms neural signals into a neuropeptide (GnRH) output. This in turn causes the pituitary to secrete gonadotropins, which stimulate the ovaries. The ovaries respond by undergoing gametogenesis (developing an oocyte for ovulation) and secreting steroids. The ovarian steroid hormones, estradiol and progesterone, stimulate the endometrial lining for pregnancy and give feedback to both the hypothalamus and pituitary to keep gonadotropins at the right level. If pregnancy does not occur, the endometrium is sloughed and the cycle repeats itself.[43]

The complexity of the relationships between the higher brain centers, hypothalamus, pituitary, ovaries, and endometrium can best be illustrated by comparison to the multiple components of a modern hi-fi stereo system. Tuners, tape decks, preamplifiers, amplifiers, and speakers depend on the radio station transmitter for input signals. Meanwhile, the receiving "end-organ" listener sits with a remote control for feedback to switch stations, adjust the volume, and turn the system on and off. With the hi-fi set, all the components have to be in place and connected for music to be heard. Many things can go wrong when any one of the components malfunctions. This is also true for the neuroendocrine system in its control of the normal ovulatory menstrual cycle. The gynecologist repairs menstrual dysfunction similar to the radio repair expert who fixes stereo systems. Both must know all of the components in the system: how each component works; how each is "connected" to the others; how to diagnose malfunctions; and how to correct them. For this reason, we will review the anatomy and function of the neuroendocrine system organ by organ and hormone by hormone.

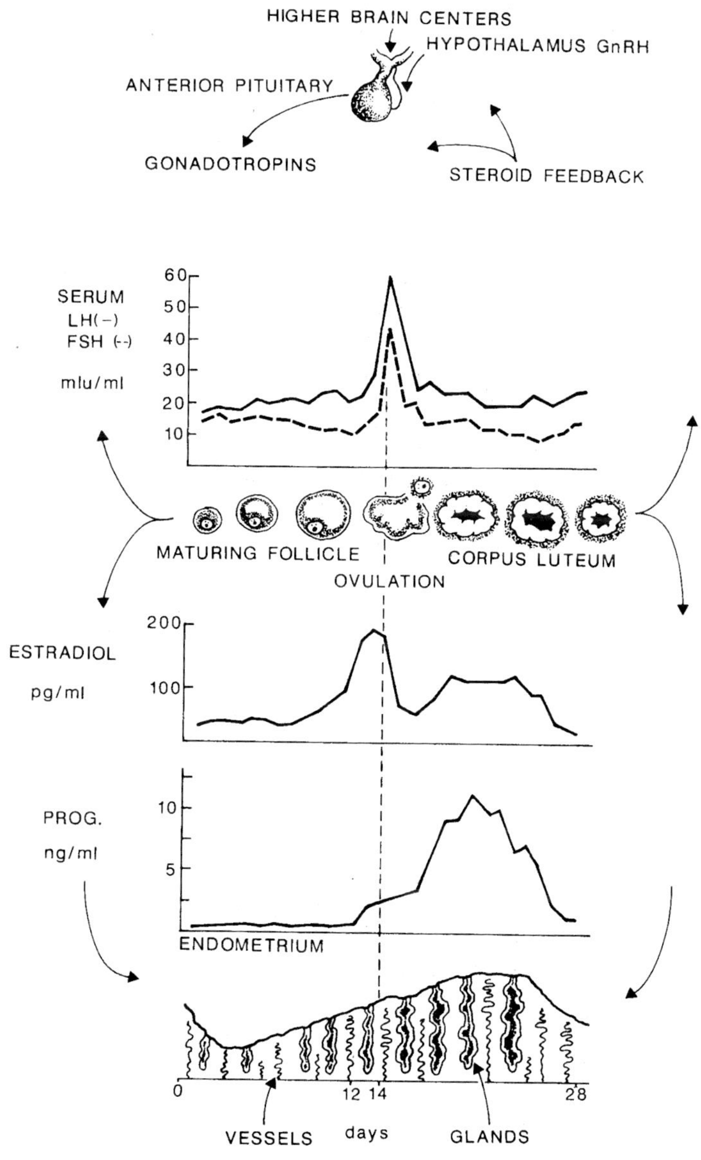

Fig. 3-1. Diagrammatic representation of the menstrual cycle showing the temporal relationships of the pituitary gonadotropins FSH and LH with the ovarian follicular estradiol, and luteal progesterone and estradiol, and the progressive response of the endometrium to the sequential change in steroids.

Hypothalamus and gonadotropin-releasing hormone

The hypothalamus and its pulsatile release of gonadotropin-releasing hormone (GnRH) regulates pituitary gonadotropin secretion and thereby controls ovarian cyclicity and the menstrual cycle. The hypothalamus is an evolutionally ancient part of the brain concerned with regulating the primitive functions needed for survival such as appetite, temperature control, salt and water regulation, growth, and metabolism as well as reproduction. There are two-way neural connections between the hypothalamus and other parts of the nervous system. With all of these activities concentrated in one small area of the brain, it is not surprising that there is an interaction between control of the menstrual cycle, behavior, and other metabolic functions. The hypothalamic nerve cells are derived from the embryonic ventral diencephalon and migrate during early development to form clusters of neurons that constitute the named "nuclei" of the adult hypothalamus. Each nucleus is composed of neurons devoted to regulation of one or more of the specific functions previously noted. The hypothalamus sits at the base of the brain bounded anteriorly just rostral to the optic chiasm and extending caudad to the mammillary bodies. The dorsal portion of the hypothalamus constitutes the floor of the third ventricle and its lateral walls. The base of the hypothalamus or infundibulum contains the infundibular stalk and hypothalamic-hypophyseal portal vascular system leading into the pituitary gland.[43] Although it was initially thought that the pituitary was the master gland that controlled the reproductive system, it was finally demonstrated by Harris that the pituitary required a specific anatomic relationship to the hypothalamus to function and to secrete gonadotropins as well as other hypophyseal hormones.[19] The hypothalamus was then demonstrated to produce several releasing and inhibiting hormones that reached the pituitary via the privileged access of the portal vessels and could thereby control pituitary function.[30] One of these releasing substances, GnRH, was isolated by both Guillemin's group[3] and by Schally et al[50] for which they each subsequently received the Nobel prize.[50,3]

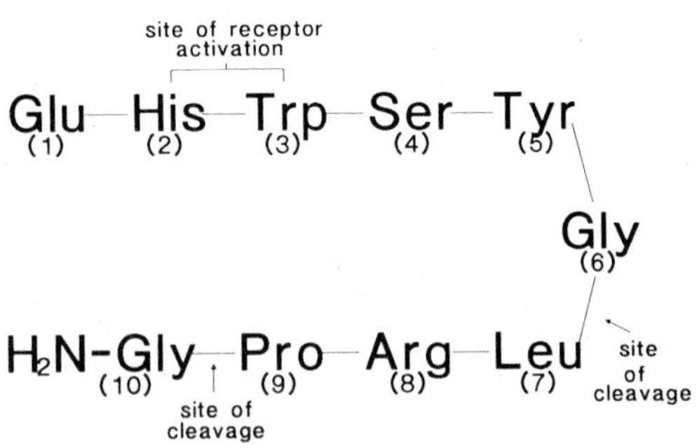

Fig. 3-2. Chemical structure of GnRH with arrows at points critical for receptor binding and cleavage inactivation (From Friedman AJ, Barbieri RL: Leuprolide acetate: applications in gynecology, *Curr Probl Obstet Gynecol Fertil* 6:209, 1988.

GnRH is a decapeptide (Fig. 3-2) that has now been synthesized.[13,31] The neurons producing GnRH are localized to the hypothalamic preoptic and arcuate nuclei. The arcuate nucleus is located in the ventral hypothalamus just above the median eminence.

In classic experiments on the Rhesus monkey, Knobil demonstrated that if the arcuate nucleus is destroyed, the pituitary can no longer secrete gonadotropic hormones.[24] The cycling of ovarian function stops, and in the absence of ovarian hormones, endometrial stimulation and regression cease. However, administration of hourly pulses of GnRH could restart the system. It had been observed previously that FSH and LH are normally secreted in pulses with intervals of approximately 90 minutes. If GnRH was given continuously, gonadotropin secretion would stop, or if the interval of administration of GnRH was too short or too long, the response of the pituitary was impaired. Knobil has since identified a pulse-generating signal that normally stimulates the release of pulsatile GnRH from the arcuate nucleus of the hypothalamus. It is presumed that each pulse reaches the pituitary resulting in the intermittent pulses of LH and FSH.[6] Since it has not been possible to easily measure GnRH levels in peripheral blood, confirmation for pulsatile secretion of GnRH has come from animal studies in which sampling directly from the hypophyseal portal system provides evidence for the pulse.

The hypothalamus acts like a transducer to convert neuronal impulses into pulses of neuropeptides such as GnRH to which the pituitary can respond. The neurons of the hypothalamus are highly specialized. Not only do they synthesize and package these neuropeptides, but also transport them down their axons to be released into the portal vessels that carry the hormones to the pituitary cells where they will act. The signal to these GnRH-secreting neurons comes from other hypothalamic neurons or afferent neural connections via neurotransmitters (Fig. 3-3). In addition to the releasing factors, neurotransmitters are produced and released by hypothalamic neurons to influence other neurons, and sometimes the pituitary as well. One neurotransmitter that acts this way is dopamine. It can act in the hypothalamus and also be released into the hypophyseal portal vessels to inhibit the secretion of prolactin in the pituitary. Dopamine, norepinephrine, and serotonin are three neurotransmitters produced or released in the hypothalamus that can directly or indirectly affect GnRH production and secretion.[33] There are also receptors for the ovarian steroids estradiol and progesterone on hypothalamic neurons. It is believed that the steroids modulate the menstrual cycle not only by effects on the pituitary but also by effects on the hypothalamic nerve cells, which in turn regulate the pulse frequency of GnRH release. These effects of the steroids are in addition to their generally accepted feedback actions at the level of the pituitary and are probably achieved via the intermediacy of the

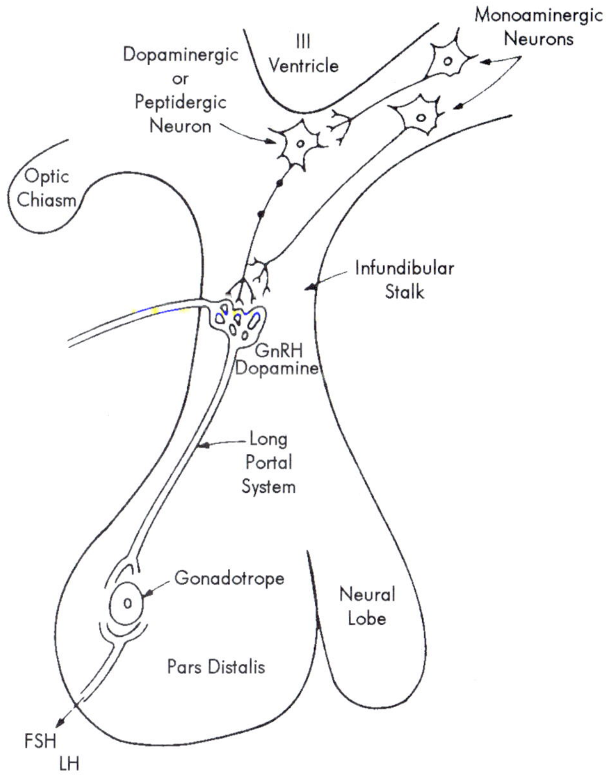

Fig. 3-3. Diagrammatic representation of the relationship of hypothalamic neurons to hypophyseal portal blood vessels that have privileged access to pituitary gonadotropes (From Ryan KJ: The endocrine pattern and control of the ovulatory cycle. In Insler V, Lunenfeld B, editors: *Infertility: male and female,* New York, 1986, Churchill Livingstone.)

neurotransmitters previously described. Finally, endogenously released opioid peptides such as β-endorphin also influence GnRH pulses by action in the hypothalamus, which normally results in a decline in LH pulse frequency during the luteal phase of the cycle.[58] This also provides a clue to the yet unexplained relationship of emotional problems with menstrual irregularity.

Abnormalities in GnRH pulse frequency are associated with menstrual dysfunction. In the monkey, abnormalities in menstrual function can be induced by experimental manipulations that decrease or increase GnRH pulse frequency. In the human, decreased GnRH pulse frequency is associated with oligomenorrhea or amenorrhea, and increased GnRH pulse frequency is associated with the polycystic ovary syndrome. Since GnRH is not present in high concentration in the peripheral circulation, LH pulses are measured as a proxy for GnRH pulses. Khoury et al measured LH pulses in 14 women with amenorrhea and in 25 women with normal ovulation.[23] The ovulating women had an LH pulse every 90 minutes. The anovulatory women had an LH pulse every 480 minutes. Administration of the opioid antagonist, naloxone, increased LH pulse frequency to one pulse every 140 minutes. This study suggests that low GnRH pulse frequency contributes to the development of some cases of amenorrhea. This study also suggests that high hypothalamic opioid activity may contribute to the low GnRH pulse frequency observed in amenorrheic women.

The polycystic ovary syndrome (PCOS) is characterized by irregular menses, oligoovulation or anovulation, and hyperandrogism. In many women with PCOS, GnRH pulse frequency is significantly increased. Waldstreicher et al measured LH pulse frequency in 12 women with PCOS and 21 ovulatory women during the follicular phase.[55] In women with normal ovulatory women the mean LH interpulse interval was 90 minutes in the early follicular phase. In the women with PCOS the mean LH interpulse interval was 60 minutes. The LH pulse frequency correlated positively with circulating estradiol. This study suggests that the elevated GnRH pulse frequency may contribute to the development of PCOS.

Pituitary: major link of the brain to ovarian function

The pituitary with its pulsatile secretion of gonadotropins is the major link of the brain to ovarian function. During embryonic development, the anterior lobe of the pituitary is derived from a pinching off of a portion of the oral cavity, whereas the posterior lobe is an extension of the neural tissue linked to the hypothalamus. The two lobes come into apposition to form the definitive adenohypophysis attached to the median eminence by the infundibular stalk, which is surrounded by some anterior pituitary cells and designated the pars tuberalis. The adult pituitary is 10 by 13 by 6 mm and weighs 0.5 gm. The anterior pituitary composes three fourths of the total gland. The gland sits in the sphenoid bone in a cavity known as the *sella turcica* and is separated from the cranial cavity by the dura mater, which the pituitary stalk and blood vessels penetrate. The anterior pituitary is comprised of a range of cell types, each type specific for one or more of the pituitary hormones. It is believed that one cell type is specific for both LH and FSH (gonadotropes), and another is specific for prolactin (lactotrope).[43]

The pituitary cells receive signals from the hypothalamus in the form of pulsatile GnRH secretion and in response synthesize and secrete FSH and LH in pulses to match the GnRH signal. The secretion of gonadotropins by the pituitary is also modulated by the negative feedback of steroid hormones, especially ovarian estradiol, which keeps FSH and LH levels in the 10 to 20 mIU/mL range during most of the cycle. When estradiol is no longer secreted at the menopause or after oophorectomy, gonadotropins are released from negative feedback control and rise to more than 50 mIU/mL.

The gonadotropins are glycoproteins, each composed of two subunits bound together noncovalently. The subunits are designated as alpha and beta. FSH and LH each contain the same alpha subunit containing 89 amino acids (in common with thyroid-stimulating hormone [TSH] and human chorionic gonadotropin [hCG]). It is the beta subunit that is different for each of these four hormones and confers to them their biological and immunological specificity.[4]

Ovarian development

During embryonic development, primitive germ cells migrate from the yolk sac to the mesonephric ridge where the definitive ovary develops. The primitive germ cells, or oogonia, divide by mitosis and increase their numbers to several million until about 6 months of intrauterine development, when mitotic division stops. Starting at 8 to 13 weeks, oogonia also continually enter meiosis until all are converted to oocytes, which are arrested in the dictyate stage. The process is completed by 6 months postpartum. Oocytes remain arrested in meiotic prophase until stimulated to resume meiosis during the preovulatory period of each ovulatory cycle in response to the LH surge. The number of oocytes continually declines during life, by puberty only 300,000 remain, of which only a few hundred will be ovulated over the life of the woman.

The earliest stage of follicular development is designated the primordial follicle, which consists of the oocyte surrounded by a basal lamina and some spindle-shaped cells. When the oocyte becomes surrounded by cuboidal granulosa cells, the structure is designated a *primary follicle*. In going from a primordial to a developed follicle, the oocyte grows, becomes invested with a clear band called the *zona pellucida*, and is surrounded by a dividing layer of granulosa cells, all without benefit of gonadotropin stimulation. It is at this point that follicles are recruited for each ovarian cycle during active reproductive life.[41]

Follicular development

Resting follicles are recruited into a cohort of follicles, only one of which will be destined to ovulate, with the remainder undergoing atresia. The follicles each start out with an oocyte surrounded by a band of granulosa cells, which is surrounded by a band of modified fibroblast-like cells called *theca interna*. Both FSH and LH are necessary for the follicle to develop. LH stimulates the thecal cells to divide and produce androgens, which can be converted to estrogens by the granulosa cells. FSH stimulates the granulosa cells to divide and to increase the enzymes necessary to convert thecal androgens to estradiol (aromatization). The granulosa cell numbers increase dramatically to 50 million in the dominant follicle. The follicle increases in volume by forming a fluid-filled cavity or antrum of about 5 mL, and its diameter increases some 400-fold to 2.5 cm. The follicle destined to ovulate can be identified by the following characteristics: it has FSH in its antral fluid; it has the optimal number of granulosa cells for its size; and it produces estradiol in preference to androgens.

The follicles destined for atresia have not captured enough FSH to accomplish maturation. They have fewer granulosa cells and more androgen than estrogen in their follicular fluid, which is associated with atresia.[32] Oocytes derived from the mature healthy follicle will resume meiosis more often than oocytes derived from follicles destined for atresia.

The follicular development of the dominant follicle thus creates an environment in which the oocyte matures and is ready to resume meiosis. Enough estradiol is secreted from its granulosa cells to trigger the LH surge of the pituitary by positive feedback, which will cause the follicle to ovulate at a time when it is "ripe." The estradiol produced by the same follicle induces endometrial proliferation, which prepares the uterus for further development if conception occurs. It has been demonstrated that if the ripe follicle is destroyed, the estradiol level drops quickly; the FSH level rises in response to a transient release from negative feedback, and it takes 2 weeks for another follicle to develop to the same stage. In other words the 2-week timing of the follicular phase of the cycle depends on the ability of the ovary to respond. The "clock" is in the ovary, even though it depends on the pituitary to make it run.[8]

Follicular microenvironment

An important feature of the ovarian follicle is that the granulosa cells and oocyte are separated from the systemic circulation by a basement membrane. All proteins entering the follicle must pass through the basement membrane and granulosa cells. This feature allows each follicle to develop a unique microenvironment. Two adjacent follicles may have markedly different microenvironments. Many studies suggest that follicles which create a microenvironment rich in FSH and estradiol are the follicles most likely to grow rapidly, gain dominance, and ovulate. This is not surprising since FSH and estradiol are potent stimulators of granulosa cell mitosis. Follicles that contain low concentrations of FSH and estradiol grow poorly and undergo atresia (follicular demise). The factors that regulate the development of the microenvironment have not been fully delineated. However, follicles that capture a large percentage of total ovarian blood flow appear to be at an advantage in the race to produce a microenvironment rich in FSH. Although each follicle is exposed to the same circulating concentration of FSH, the follicle with the greatest total blood flow receives the largest flux of FSH.

Selection and dominance

At the beginning of the follicular phase of the cycle (day 1 of menses), there are about four antral follicles 4 mm in diameter in the ovaries. By day 12 of the cycle there is only *one* large antral follicle 20 mm in diameter remaining. The process by which the four small antral follicles are "winnowed" to one large, preovulatory antral follicle is called the process of "selection." The mechanisms underlying the process of selection have not been fully characterized. However, the status of the follicular miroenvironment is probably crucial to the process of selection. The small antral follicle that is able to create a microenvironment optimally conducive to growth will achieve dominance and go on to ovulate. At day 4 of the follicular phase, no one follicle has achieved dominance. Once a dominant follicle is established, no new large antral follicles can appear until that dominant structure undergoes atresia at the end of the luteal phase. The dominant follicle prevents the growth of other new structures by steroids (estrogen, progesterone) and protein (inhibin, follicle-regulatory protein) secretions. Surgical removal of the dominant follicle is followed by the growth of a new cohort of small antral follicles that compete to become dominant. The processes of selection and dominance help ensure that, on the average, only one egg is ovulated each cycle.

Ovulation

The timing of ovulation is determined by the dominant ovarian follicle. When the dominant ovarian follicle produces enough estrogen to sustain a circulating estradiol concentration in the range of 300 pg/mL for 48 hours, the hypothalamic-pituitary unit responds by secreting a surge of gonadotropins. The gonadotropin surge is characterized by an increase in LH pulse frequency (implying an increase in GnRH pulse frequency) and amplitude, resulting in a marked increase in serum LH. The gonadotropin surge is characterized by modest increases in serum FSH. The LH surge stimulates four events in the ovary that result in ovulation. The events initiated by the LH surge include the following: (1) an increase in intrafollicular proteolytic enzymes (plasmin), that destroy the basement membrane and allow follicular rupture; (2) luteinizating of the granulosa cells and theca, resulting in increased progesterone production; (3) resumption of meiosis in the oocyte, thus preparing it for fertilization; and (4) an influx of blood vessels into the follicle, preparing it to become a corpus luteum. Both the granulosa cells and the theca contribute to the total mass of the corpus luteum. The beginning of the LH surge *precedes* ovulation by about 36 hours. The temporal relationship between the LH surge and ovulation is used to great advantage in programs of in vitro fertilization (IVF). In most IVF programs, oocyte harvesting is scheduled for 34 to 36 hours after the administration of exogenous hCG gonadotropin. This allows the eggs to fully mature prior to harvesting but prevents the eggs from being ovulated into the peritoneal cavity.

Luteal phase of the cycle

Following ovulation, the follicle collapses and undergoes reorganization. There is an ingrowth of the thecal cells and blood vessels, and the granulosa cells luteinize. They increase in size and develop characteristic morphological changes. The lutein cells develop receptors on their cell surface to bind and internalize serum cholesterol bound to low-density lipoprotein (LDL-cholesterol). This cholesterol becomes the major precursor for the production of the increased amounts of progesterone now synthesized by the corpus luteum. This progesterone induces a secretory change in the estrogen-primed endometrium to prepare it for pregnancy. Estradiol is also produced by the corpus luteum, and the production of both steroid hormones is dependent on continued stimulation by pituitary LH. If pregnancy occurs, the corpus luteum will be stimulated by fetal hCG; this will extend the life span of the corpus luteum until the placenta can assume its endocrine function at about 7 to 8 weeks of pregnancy. In the absence of pregnancy, the corpus luteum regresses. The lowered level of steroid hormones induces the pituitary to increase gonadotropin secretion, and a new cycle of follicular recruitment begins. The lowered steroid hormone levels also cause collapse of the endometrial vasculature, and menstruation is the result. Why the corpus luteum regresses in the primate at the end of each nonfertile cycle is not completely understood. In many animals, prostaglandin produced in the uterus in response to progesterone reaches the corpus luteum and causes luteolysis in a form of negative feedback. In these animals simple hysterectomy will prolong the life of the corpus luteum. It is believed that in the primate, prostaglandin produced locally in the corpus luteum causes its own destruction.

Ovarian compartments

It should be apparent from the foregoing description of ovarian function during the menstrual cycle that the ovary is a dynamic organ with cyclic changes in morphology and hormone secretion. The ovary can be thought of in terms of three major compartments: (1) the follicles, (2) the corpora lutea, and (3) the stroma. The follicular compartment contains all the primordial and primary follicles that are hormonally and structurally quiescent until they are recruited into the cohort of growing follicles for a given cycle by pituitary FSH and LH. The follicular compartment also includes the growing follicles that are actively secreting hormones. From the pool of growing follicles, the dominant follicle will be selected for ovulation and the others will regress in atresia. The estradiol secreted from the ovary during the follicular phase of the cycle is derived predominantly from the cohort of developing follicles. The ovulatory follicle, however, provides the bulk of the estradiol. After the LH surge is released just prior to ovulation, estradiol production declines rapidly, leading to ovulation itself. Ovarian steroid production is next dominated by the corpus luteum, in turn derived from the ruptured follicle. This compartment makes progesterone and estradiol until it regresses in response to prostaglandin signal. Follicles and corpora lutea in various stages of development are distributed in the stromal compartment of the ovary, which consists of largely dense fibroblast-like cells. The stroma itself produces androgens, that become the dominant secretory product of the ovary whenever follicles or corpora lutea are not functional. This can occur in anovulatory states and after menopause when follicles and oocytes are depleted.[47,48]

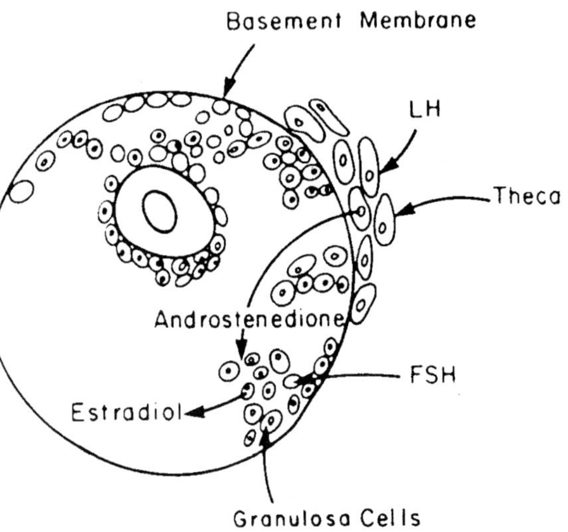

Fig. 3-4. Diagram of relationship of granulosa and thecal cells of the follicle. Note LH-stimulated thecal androstenedione being transported to FSH-stimulated granulosa cell for aromatization to estradiol (From Ryan KJ: The endocrine pattern and control of the ovulatory cycle. In Insler V, Lunenfeld B, editors: *Infertility: male and female*, New York, 1986, Churchill Livingstone.)

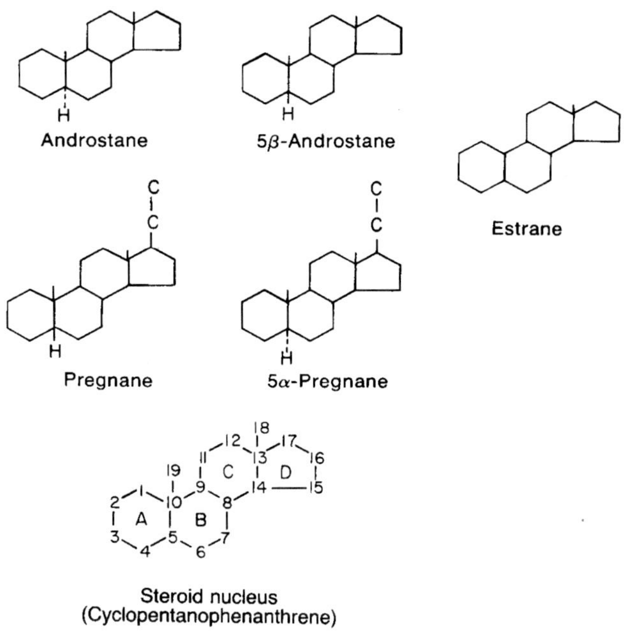

Fig. 3-5. Structural formula showing the basic steroid nucleus with appropriate numbering of the carbon atoms. The basic C-18 steroid estrane, the C-19 steroids, androstane and 5β- androstane, and the basic C-21 steroids, pregnane, and 5α- pregnane, are illustrated.

Two-cell theory

The concept of ovarian compartments evolved from studies on isolated follicles, corpora lutea, and stroma studied in vitro. From such studies it was discovered that thecal cells had LH receptors and could make androstenedione and testosterone. Granulosa cells, on the other hand, had FSH receptors, and when stimulated with FSH, responded by increasing their ability to metabolize androgens to estrogens. This explained the need for both LH and FSH for follicular development.[9] A theory evolved that the theca makes androgens in response to LH, which is transported to the granulosa cells. Under the effect of FSH, the androgen is converted to estrogen (Fig. 3-4). The dominant preovulatory follicle does this better than follicles destined for atresia, which can produce androgen but failing adequate conversion of androgen to estrogen, undergo degeneration under the influence of their own accumulating androgens.[41]

Steroid structure

The cyclopentenophenanthrene-ring structure is the basic carbon skeleton for all steroid hormones. The carbon skeleton consists of a five-carbon cyclopentane ring conjoined to a phenanthrene molecule, which is itself made up of three six-carbon rings configured as shown in Fig. 3-5. The carbons are shared where each of the rings meet one another so that carbons 5, 10, 8, 9, 13, and 14 are common to adjoining rings. The rings are designated A, B, C, and D. The numbering of the carbons of the skeleton is important for indicating where hydroxyl groups, side chains, and other additions are added to the ring to define a specific hormone. The numbering allows precise designation of the steroid structure and hence should be kept in mind to distinguish between the hormones, which are all closely related. Since the ring systems are relatively planar and rigid, stereoisomers that need to be distinguished also occur. In general, molecules or atoms that extend in space above the plane of the ring are designated β, and those below the plane are designated α. Axial and equatorial designations are also used to specify a more exact configuration and relationship of one insertion on the carbon to the other.

There are three physiologically important steroid nuclei: estrane (18 carbon atoms), androstane (19 carbon atoms), and pregnane (21 carbon atoms) (Fig. 3-5). All the important gonadal steroids are derivatives of these three steroid nuclei. Specific suffixes and symbols are used to indicate changes in these basic structures. For example, when the C-4 and C-5 carbon bond is unsaturated and a double bond is present, the suffix "ene" replaces the "ane" ending. If a keto (= O) group is substituted for two hydrogens, the suffix "one" is used together with the number of the carbon to which it is attached. The 4-ene-3-one grouping is present in many biologically active steroids (testosterone, progesterone, cortisol). If a hydroxy (OH) group is substituted for a hydrogen, the suffix "ol" is used.

In Fig. 3-6 the structural formula for progesterone is shown. Progesterone is a derivative of the C-21 compound pregnane. Since there is a double bond in ring A, the term pregnane is changed to pregnene. The position of the double bond (between carbon atoms 4 and 5) is designated as Δ^4. Two ketone groups are present: one on the carbon 3 and another on the carbon 20 atom, thus 3, 20-dione (meaning two ketone groups). Therefore the systematic name for progesterone is Δ^4- pregnene-3, 20-dione. Fig. 3-6 also shows the structure and systematic name for 17-hydroxyprogesterone. Note that the OH group at the C-17 position is below the plane of the carbon ring and is therefore designated 17-α-ol.

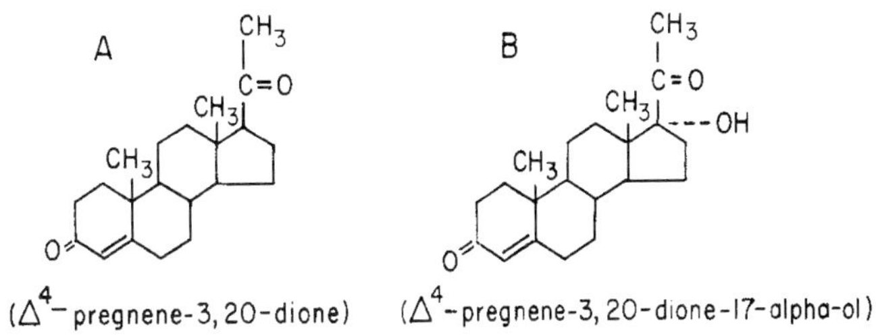

Fig. 3-6. Structural formulas for **A**, Progesterone, and **B**, 17α-hydroxyprogesterone.

Biochemistry of steroid biosynthesis

The quantitatively important sources of steroid production are the ovaries, the testes, and the adrenals. Each of these glands makes hormones that are unique to that gland. For example, the ovary secretes large amounts of estradiol. The testis secretes large amounts of testosterone. The adrenal gland is responsible for the production of cortisol and aldosterone. In addition to these unique steroid products, each gland can produce some common "core" steroids: progesterone, 17-hydroxyprogesterone, and androstenedione (Fig. 3-7). These core steroids are the important precursors for the production of all gonadal steroids, glucocorticoids, and mineralocorticoids. Discussion of the biosynthesis of these core steroids follows.

Cholesterol is the parent steroid from which all the gonadal steroids, glucocorticoids, and mineralocorticoids are derived. Classical concepts of steroidogenesis state that the steroid-producing glands, such as the ovaries synthesize cholesterol from acetate and then utilize the cholesterol to produce progestins, estrogens, and androgens. However, recent evidence suggests that plasma cholesterol is the precursor for some adrenal and ovarian steroid hormones. In the circulation, cholesterol is carried in lipoprotein packages that consist of a core of apolar cholesterol and cholesterol esters surrounded by a shell of amphoteric phospholipids and apoproteins. The LDLs and the high-density lipoproteins (HDLs) contain most of the cholesterol present in the circulation. The adrenal and ovarian cells responsible for steroidogenesis have membrane receptors for the LDL lipoprotein package. The circulating LDL binds to these receptors and becomes incorporated into the cell by a process of endocytosis. The cholesterol from the LDL is released for utilization by the cell by the action of lysosomal enzymes.

Once cholesterol is released from the lipoprotein package, it must be transported to the mitochondria where it binds to the cholesterol cleavage enzyme and is metabolized to pregnenolone (Fig. 3-8). Pregnenolone is then metabolized to the other core steroids (progesterone, 17α-hydroxyprogesterone, and androstenedione) by three enzyme systems (see Fig. 3-7). In turn, progesterone can be secreted or metabolized to the important mineralocorticoid aldosterone. 17α-hydroxyprogesterone can be secreted or metabolized to the important glucocorticoid cortisol. Androstenedione can be secreted or metabolized to the gonadal steroids testosterone and estradiol (Fig. 3-9).

There are only three types of reactions that all steroids can undergo: (1) removal or addition of hydrogen, as in the conversion of pregnenolone to progesterone (3β-hydroxysteroid dehydrogenase); (2) hydroxylations (addition of OH), as occurs in the conversion of progesterone to 17α-hydroxyprogesterone [17α-hydroxylase]; and (3) conjugation reactions, such as sulfoconjugates and glucuroconjugates.

The conversion of cholesterol (C-26) to progesterone (C-21), to androstenedione (C-19), and finally to estradiol (C-18), requires the sequential removal of different carbon side chains. These cleavage reactions are accomplished by multiple hydroxylations of neighboring carbon bonds. This produces a highly unstable intermediate compound that reaches a lower energy state by separation of the carbon side chain from the parent steroid nucleus. For example, in the conversion of cholesterol to pregnenolone, multiple hydroxylations occur at the C-20 and C-22 carbon bonds that lead to a breakdown of the parent compound to pregnenolone and the isocaproic aldehyde side chain (Fig. 3-8). The following enzymes involve cleavage of carbon side chains from the parent molecule: cholesterol cleavage enzyme, 17, 20-lyase, and aromatase (Figs. 3-7 to 3-9).

Steroid hormones are produced in the gonads and adrenals and secreted in the circulation. In the circulation, steroids are transported to peripheral tissues where further chemical transformations can occur. In the liver, multiple hydroxylation, hydration, and conjugation reactions occur that lead to loss of steroid activity. However, in some peripheral tissues potent steroid agonists can be locally produced from weak precursors. For example, the weak androgen androstenedione can be converted in fat tissue to the important estrogen, estrone, by the enzyme aromatase. In the pilosebaceous unit, the weak androgen, androstenedione, can be converted to the potent androgen dihydrotestosterone. This *peripheral conversion* is of utmost importance in such disease states as polycystic ovarian disease and endometrial hyperplasia.

Another important peripheral conversion is that of androstenedione into the potent androgen testosterone. In

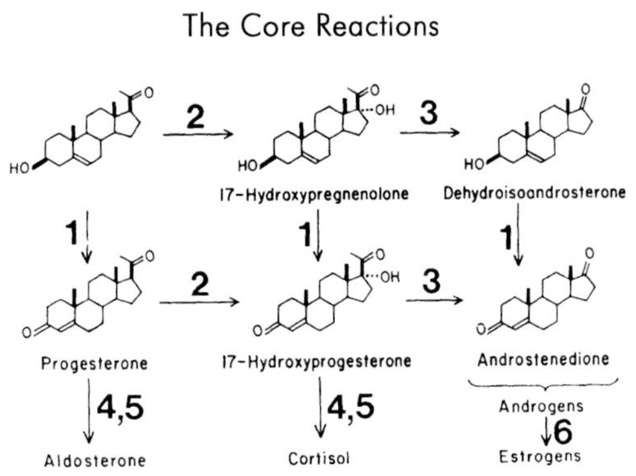

Fig. 3-7. The ovary, the testis, and the adrenal produce six common core steroids. The core Δ^5 steroids are pregnenolone, 17α-hydroxypregnenolone, and dehydroepiandrosterone. The core Δ^4 steroids are progesterone, 17α-hydroxyprogesterone, and androstenedione. The core steroids are the important precursors for the production of all gonadal steroids, glucocorticoids, and mineralocorticoids. Progesterone is an important gonadal steroid and is the precursor for all mineralocorticoids. 17α-hydroxyprogesterone is the precursor for all glucocorticoids. Androstenedione is the precursor for the androgens and estrogens. Enzyme no. 1 is 3β-hydroxysteroid-dehydrogenase-isomerase; enzyme no. 2, 17α-hydroxylase; enzyme no. 3; 17, 20-lyase; enzyme no. 4, 21-hydroxylase; enzyme no. 5, 11β-hydroxylase; and enzyme no. 6, aromatase.

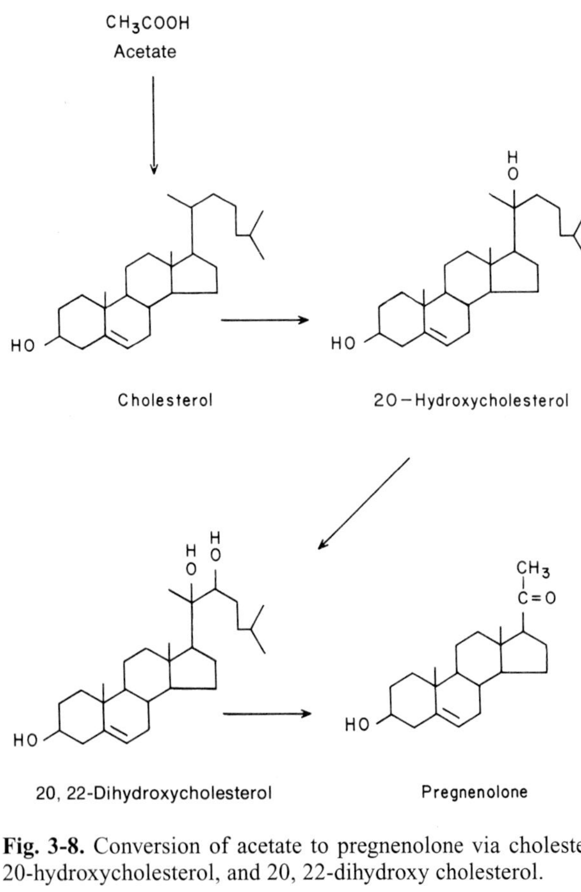

Fig. 3-8. Conversion of acetate to pregnenolone via cholesterol, 20-hydroxycholesterol, and 20, 22-dihydroxy cholesterol.

normal women, 50% of circulating testosterone arises from the peripheral conversion of androstenedione derived from the ovary and the adrenal.

Steroid pathways in the ovarian follicle and corpus luteum

Steroid biosynthetic pathways were defined for the human ovarian follicle based on enzymatic studies of tissue in vitro and by studies on isolated and recombined granulosa and thecal cells.[46,47] The pathway involves the steps just described. The 2-carbon acetate molecule can be converted to the 27-carbon cholesterol molecule by a series of complex reactions. There is then a loss of part of the cholesterol side chain to form the 21-carbon pregnenolone. Pregnenolone is converted to progesterone. In a side chain cleavage the pregnenolone and progesterone are converted to form 19-carbon androgens which are then transformed to 18-carbon estrogens. Although both theca and granulosa can carry out all of these steps, the theca is most facile in taking acetate to androgens, and the granulosa cells are most facile in the last aromatization step to form estrogens from androgens.[47] In the corpus luteum, a new form of steroid production takes place. The acetate to cholesterol steps are bypassed, and the cell uses preformed cholesterol obtained from the blood stream to make progesterone. This probably accounts for the jump in progesterone production in the transition from the follicle to the corpus luteum. To sequester cholesterol, the luteal cells develop receptors that can bind LDL-cholesterol for internalization and processing.[54] Estrogens can then be formed in the corpus luteum as a further metabolic step from progesterone.

Ovarian regulatory proteins

Many functions that occur in the follicle and corpus luteum cannot be readily explained by the direct action of gonadotropins or steroids. This includes such phenomena as the life-long meiotic arrest of oocytes until they are ready to be ovulated, and then meiosis resumes. This includes development of the rich blood supply of the dominant follicle, further vascularization of the corpus luteum, and then vascular regression each month. It has long been known that isolated granulosa cells cannot be made to divide in vitro by either steroids or gonadotropins. There was a growth factor in pituitary gonadotropin extracts that made granulosa cells divide in vitro, but it disappeared on purification of the gonadotropins. This led to the discovery of the fibroblast growth factor (FGF), isolated first from the pituitary and since known to be made in the ovary. The fibroblast growth factor is not only a potent mitogen for the granulosa cells, but also the angiogenic factor that is probably responsible for marked vascular proliferation of folliculogenesis and corpus luteum formation.

Inhibins and activins have also been isolated from the ovary. These proteins may have both local effects on the ovary and distant effects on the pituitary. Inhibin is the long-sought nonsteroidal feedback substance that controls the level of

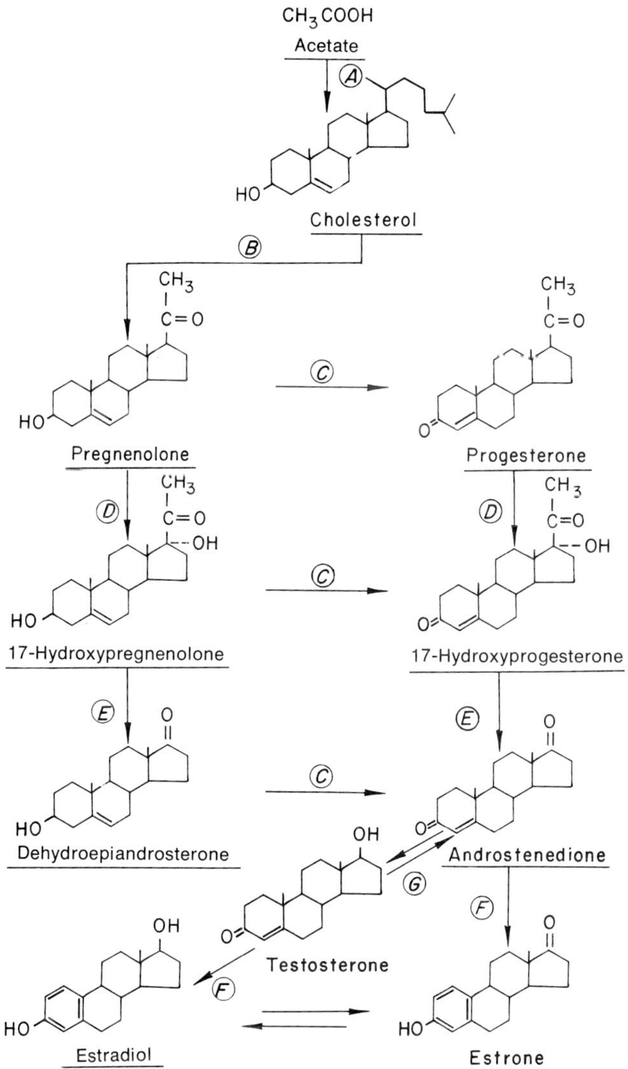

Fig. 3-9. Possible metabolic pathways for the ovarian biogenesis of estrogens. Letters above arrows denote the following metabolic pathways and the enzyme systems involved: **A**, Formation of the sterol nucleus; **B**, Cleavage of cholesterol side chain with formation of C-21 steroid; **C**, Isomerase reaction with changing of double bond from C-5 to C-4, and dehydrogenation at C-3: 3β-ol dehydrogenases; **D**, 17α-hydroxylation (i.e., introduction of hydroxy radical in a position on C-17); **E**, Cleavage of side chain, converting C-21 to C-19 steroids; **F**, Aromatization (i.e., introduction of double bonds into *ring A* with conversion of C-19 to C-18 steroids); **G**, 17β-ol dehydrogenase reactions (reversible) (i.e., conversion of hydroxy radical in β position on C-17 to ketone group, or vice versa). (From Smith OW, Ryan KJ: *Am J Obstet Gynecol* 84:141, 1962.)

FSH by a direct negative feedback on the pituitary. Although long predicted as important in the male reproductive system, inhibin was isolated first from follicular fluid. Inhibin seems to be secreted by the dominant follicle along with estradiol. Its production is stimulated by FSH action on the granulosa cell.

A host of other regulatory proteins identified in other cells and biologic systems have since been shown to be made in the ovary also. These include the epidermal growth factor first isolated from the salivary glands of mice, which is also a potent mitogen for granulosa cells and is believed to be made in the ovarian follicle. Transforming growth factors first found in viral-transformed cells are now also known to be made in the ovary. Transforming growth factor beta is believed to have an effect on augmenting resumption of meiosis. Müllerian-inhibiting substance, so important for embryonic male development, is also synthesized in the ovarian follicle and is considered as a possible oocyte meiosis inhibitor. The insulin-like growth factors (IGFs) are also synthesized in the follicle and appear to have an effect on granulosa cell function. It is still too early to define the role, if any, that each of these regulatory proteins plays in normal ovarian development and hormonal activity. There are receptors for essentially all of these factors on granulosa cells, and they are synthesized by either granulosa or thecal cells. They therefore function as autocrine (effect on cell of origin) or paracrine (effect on adjoining cells) regulators that have to be considered along with the endocrine steroids and gonadotropins as major players in the complex control of the reproductive cycle. Another fascinating aspect of these regulatory proteins is that many are related to one another by interesting homologies in their amino acid sequences. Transforming growth factor beta, inhibins, and müllerian-inhibiting substance all share common amino acid sequences. This will make study more difficult and identification of the natural ligand problematic if they bind to one another's receptors and act as agonist or antagonist.[45]

Relaxin, a protein hormone with a long history but no well-defined role in primate reproduction is now known to be made in the ovary, predominantly in the corpus luteum, with greater production in early pregnancy.[56] Relaxin shares interesting homologies with insulin, but its role in the ovary or in the menstrual cycle has not been established. Both renin and angiotensin have also been found in follicular fluid and are believed to be made locally in the ovary.[28]

Insulin-like growth factors. The development of the dominant follicle is critically dependent on the pituitary hormones FSH and LH. Growth factors such as the IGF can modulate the action of FSH and LH by amplifying (or attenuating) their stimulatory signals. IGF-I is produced in granulosa cells from healthy follicles and can stimulate expression of IGF-I receptors on granulosa cells. IGF-I acts synergistically with FSH to stimulate cAMP, estradiol, and progesterone. In turn, FSH and estradiol increase the amount of granulosa cell IGF-I receptor, and estradiol increases the amount of IGF-I synthesized by the granulosa cell.[15,60]

Insulin-like growth factor binding proteins (IGFBPs). The ovary is capable of producing most of the IGFBPs. IGFBPs bind IGFs and most often act as IGF antagonists. For example, in the porcine ovary IGFBP-3 is capable of blocking the ability of FSH to stimulate estradiol and progesterone secretion in granulosa cells, probably by binding and inactivating IGF-I.[51] These observations suggest that some of the IGFBPs may be FSH antagonists. The release of the IGFBPs in the rat ovary are highly regulated. IGFBP-2 and IGFBP-6 are released in the theca. IGFBP-3 is released in the corpora lutea during luteolysis. IGFBP-4 and IGFBP-5 are released from some atretic granulosa cells. IGFBP-1 is not detectable.[10,11]

Inhibins, activin, and follistatin. The inhibins are dimer proteins composed of alpha and beta subunits that are each encoded by unique genes. There are two forms of the beta subunit (ßa and ßb) that are closely related in structure. The alpha-beta (α-ß) heterodimer, "inhibin," suppresses basal and GnRH stimulated FSH secretion.

Inhibin is produced by granulosa cells and the corpus luteum. Blood levels of inhibin rise during the follicular phase and peak near ovulation. In the luteal phase, serum inhibin levels parallel the changes observed in progesterone, including a midluteal peak. Inhibin and estradiol are the two ovarian hormones involved in suppressing pituitary secretion of FSH.[52]

The beta-beta dimers are referred to as activins. Activins can stimulate pituitary secretion of FSH. Activins do not circulate at significant levels.[7] Activins are present in ovarian follicular fluid and probably play an important role in oocyte growth.

Follistatin is a protein unrelated to inhibin or activin that is present in follicular fluid and can suppress pituitary FSH secretion by binding and inactivating activin.[35]

Estrogen and progesterone effects on the endometrium

The bottom line for endocrine function in the menstrual cycle is the mechanism by which hormones cyclically stimulate the endometrial lining in preparation for pregnancy and cause its regression if pregnancy does not occur. Estradiol stimulates proliferation and gland formation as well as vascular growth in the endometrial cells. It increases its own intracellular receptor, which augments its response. In addition, progesterone receptors are developed in the cells in response to estrogen. It is highly likely that estrogen does not directly cause mitosis in the cells but achieves this secondarily via regulatory proteins like those described for the ovary. In humans, estrogen development of the endometrium clearly anticipates being augmented by progesterone after ovulation. If ovulation does not occur and no progesterone is secreted, the endometrium may continue to proliferate under a constant estrogen level into a form of hyperplasia frequently seen in anovulatory states. At a constant estrogen level, or if the estrogen level declines or is withdrawn completely, the endometrium cannot be maintained and starts to bleed. This estrogen withdrawal, or breakthrough bleeding is typified by being variable in duration and amount depending on the prior level of hyperplasia. It is not menstrual bleeding from a secretory endometrium, and it is the most common basis of dysfunctional bleeding.

The proliferative phase of the endometrium under the effect of estrogen is followed sequentially by postovulatory progesterone stimulation of the estradiol-primed endometrium. Spotting at the time of ovulation may represent an endometrial response to the sharp drop in the estrogen level just before the corpus luteum is formed and before progesterone can further develop the cells. After ovulation the endometrium is ready to respond to progesterone since progesterone receptors were developed by estradiol in the early phase of the cycle. Progesterone causes gland development and deciduation of the stromal cells with a further spiraling and tortuosity of the underlying vasculature. This clearly is a suitable lining for implantation and placentation if pregnancy occurs. In the sterile cycle, both progesterone and estrogen production by the corpus luteum declines as a result of luteolysis and menstrual bleeding with the collapsing of blood vessels and sloughing occurs. This is true menstrual bleeding of a well-developed secretory endometrium after progesterone withdrawal, which is generally more orderly in duration and amount than withdrawal bleeding from estrogen alone. This is the basis for treating anovulatory bleeding with progesterone.

Much of our knowledge of the effects of the steroid hormones on endometrium has come from the pioneering animal studies of Hisaw and Greep.[17] In addition, Markee studied the changes in the endometrium of the monkey as transplanted to the anterior chamber of the eye where it could be observed throughout the cycle in response to specific hormones.[44] Noyes et al made the correlation between the histologic appearance of human endometrial specimens obtained at surgery with the day of the menstrual cycle (i.e., day 1, day 2, and so on).[36] They defined the range of effects that can be observed when the estrogen of the follicular phase of the cycle is followed by progesterone during the luteal phase.

Dating the endometrium

Specific changes occurring in the stromal and glandular elements of the endometrium during the menstrual cycle have been of interest to both the pathologist and the clinician. By close scrutiny of these changes, it has been possible to date the endometrium (within a range of about 48 hours), particularly in the postovulatory phase of the cycle. This correlation between the date of the cycle and the histologic appearance of the endometrium has particular importance in the study of the infertile patient. For simplicity, a 28-day cycle with ovulation occurring on the 14th day will be described. The first day of the menstrual period will be considered the first day of the cycle with menstrual flow lasting 4 days. The *proliferative phase* of the cycle then begins at the termination of the *menstrual phase*. The postovulatory phase, or

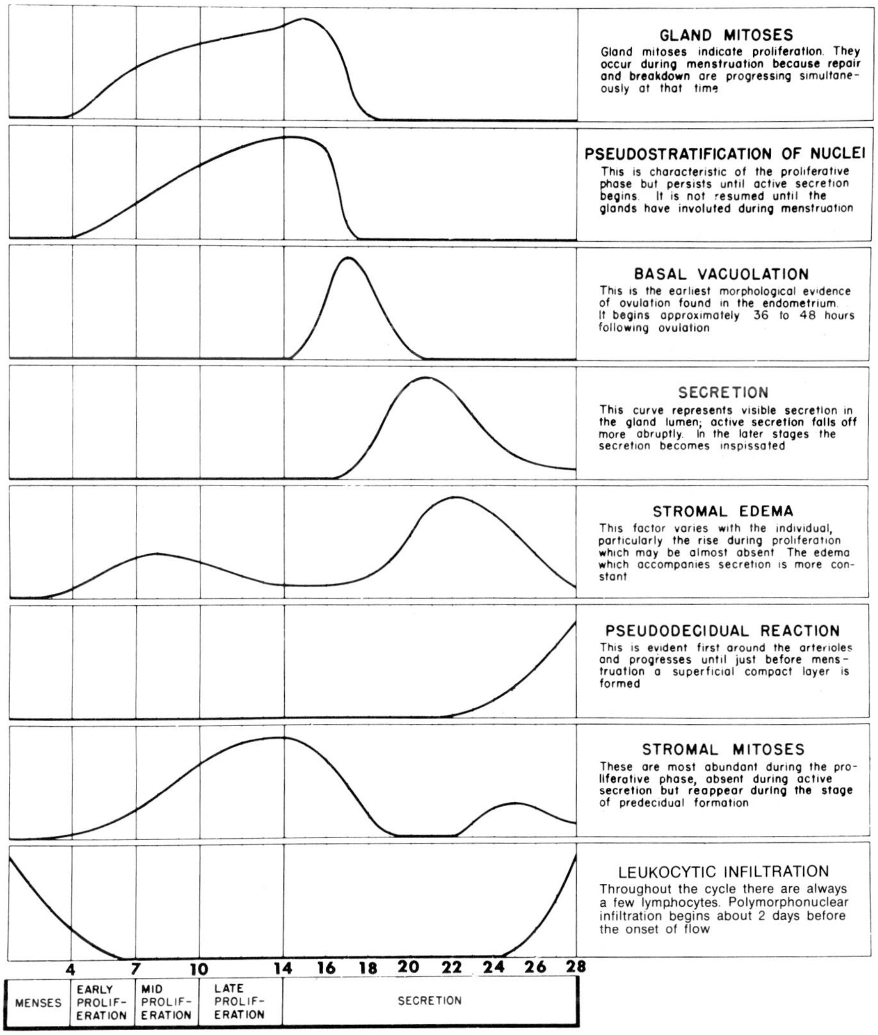

Fig. 3-10. Changes in various morphologic features utilized in dating the endometrium; graphs correlate with their appearance and disappearance during the menstrual cycle. (From Noyes RW, Hertig AT, Rock J: Dating the endometrial biopsy, *Fertil Steril* 1:3, 1950.)

secretory phase, of this cycle extends from day 14 to day 28. It should be remembered that the changes to be described occur only in the functional layers of the endometrium and not in the basal layer or in the lower uterine segment. Biopsies of the endometrium therefore have significance only if an adequate amount of functional endometrium is obtained. It is recognized that all parts of the endometrium do not undergo simultaneous change. Tissue responsiveness will vary, depending on blood supply, adjacent leiomyomas, and so forth. In the normal cycle, however, an approximation of dating within 48 hours is frequently of considerable help.

Proliferative phase. Under the stimulation of estrogen, the endometrium gradually rebuilds its substance. The early proliferative phase extends from day 4 through day 7, the middle proliferative phase extends from day 8 through day 10, and the late proliferative phase lasts from day 11 until the time of ovulation on day 14 (Fig. 3-10). Discussion of the histologic characteristics of each preparation phase follows.[36]

Early proliferative phase (Fig. 3-11). The glands of the endometrium are short and narrow. With mitotic activity, some glands remaining from the menstrual phase may show secretory exhaustion. The surface epithelium is regenerating between the openings of the glands. The stroma is compact with few mitoses. Stellate or spindle-shaped cells contain very little cytoplasm and large nuclei.

Middle proliferative phase (Fig. 3-12). The glands are longer with a slightly curved effect. There is early pseudostratification of the nuclei that appear superimposed in layers,

Text continued on p. 30.

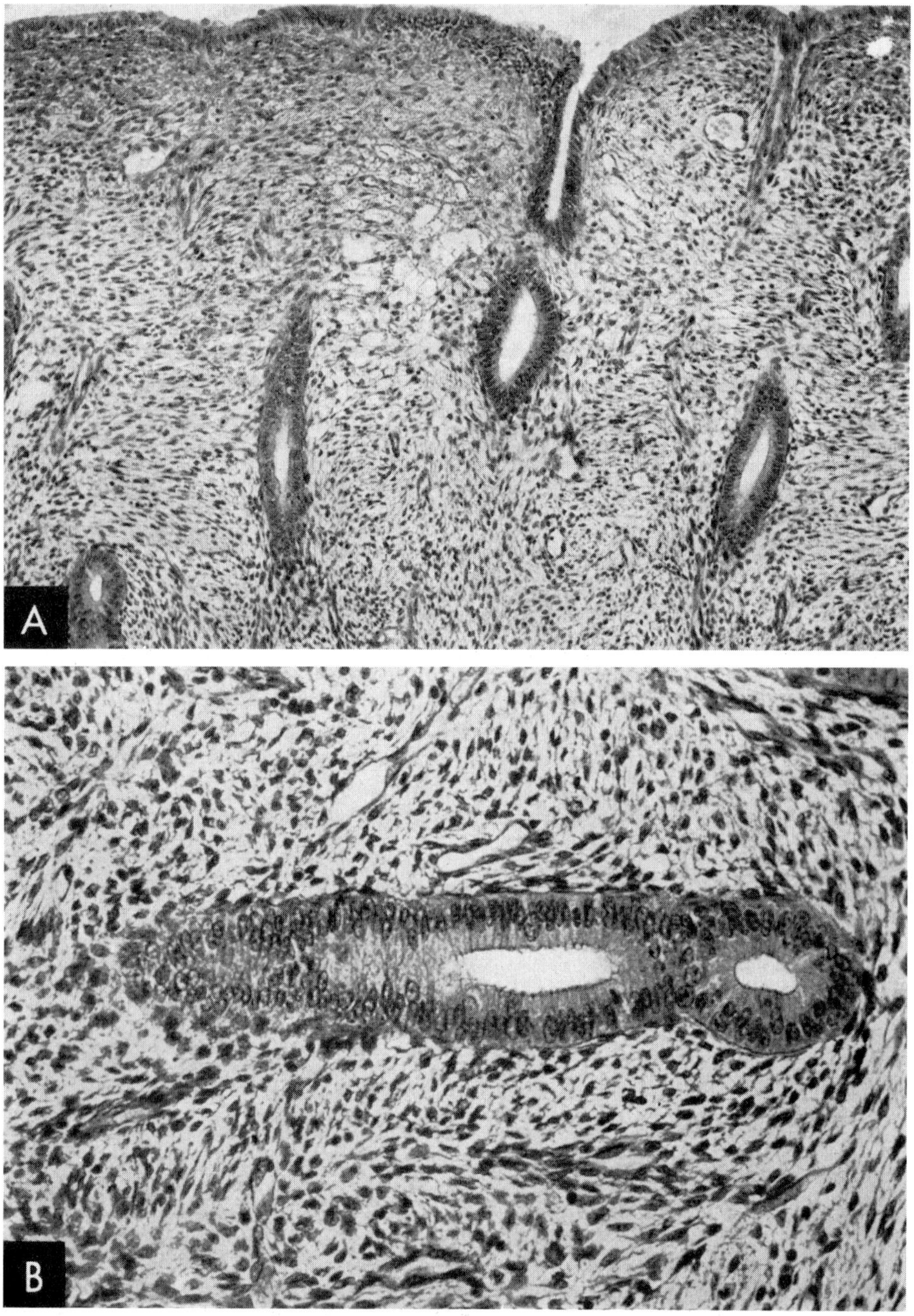

Fig. 3-11. Early proliferative endometrium. **A**, Surface epithelium thin; glands sparse, narrow, and straight. (× 150.) **B**, Few mitoses in glands and stroma; little pseudostratification of gland nuclei. (× 400.) (From Noyes RW, Hertig AT, Rock J: Dating the endometrial biopsy, *Fertil Steril* 1:3, 1950.)

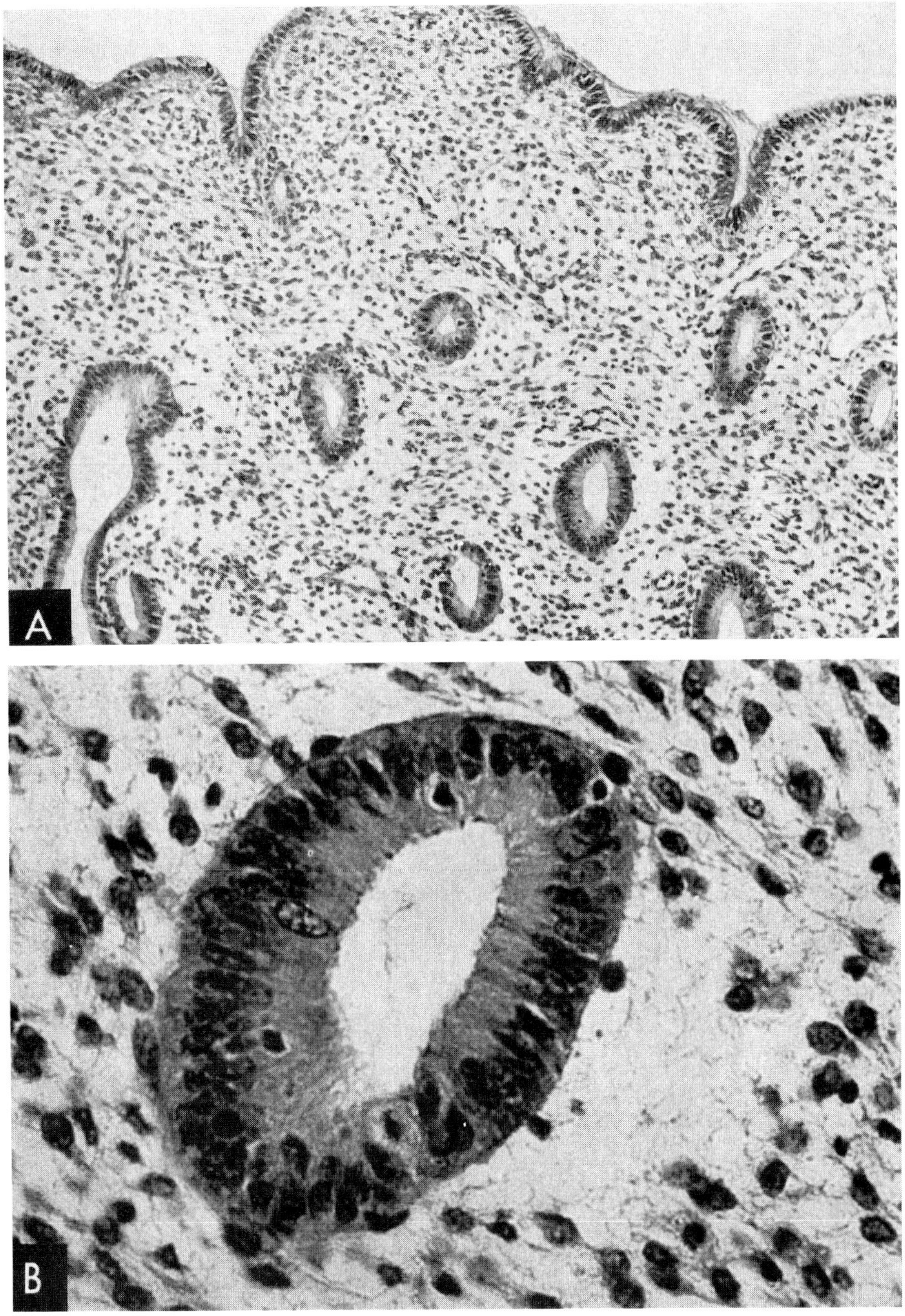

Fig. 3-12. Endometrium showing intermediate degree of proliferation. **A**, Glands slightly tortuous; tall columnar surface epithelium. Extracellular fluid is not always as marked as in this section. (× 150.) **B**, Glands show numerous mitoses with pseudostratification becoming marked. Note the "naked nucleus" type of stromal cell with fine anastomosing processes. (× 400.)

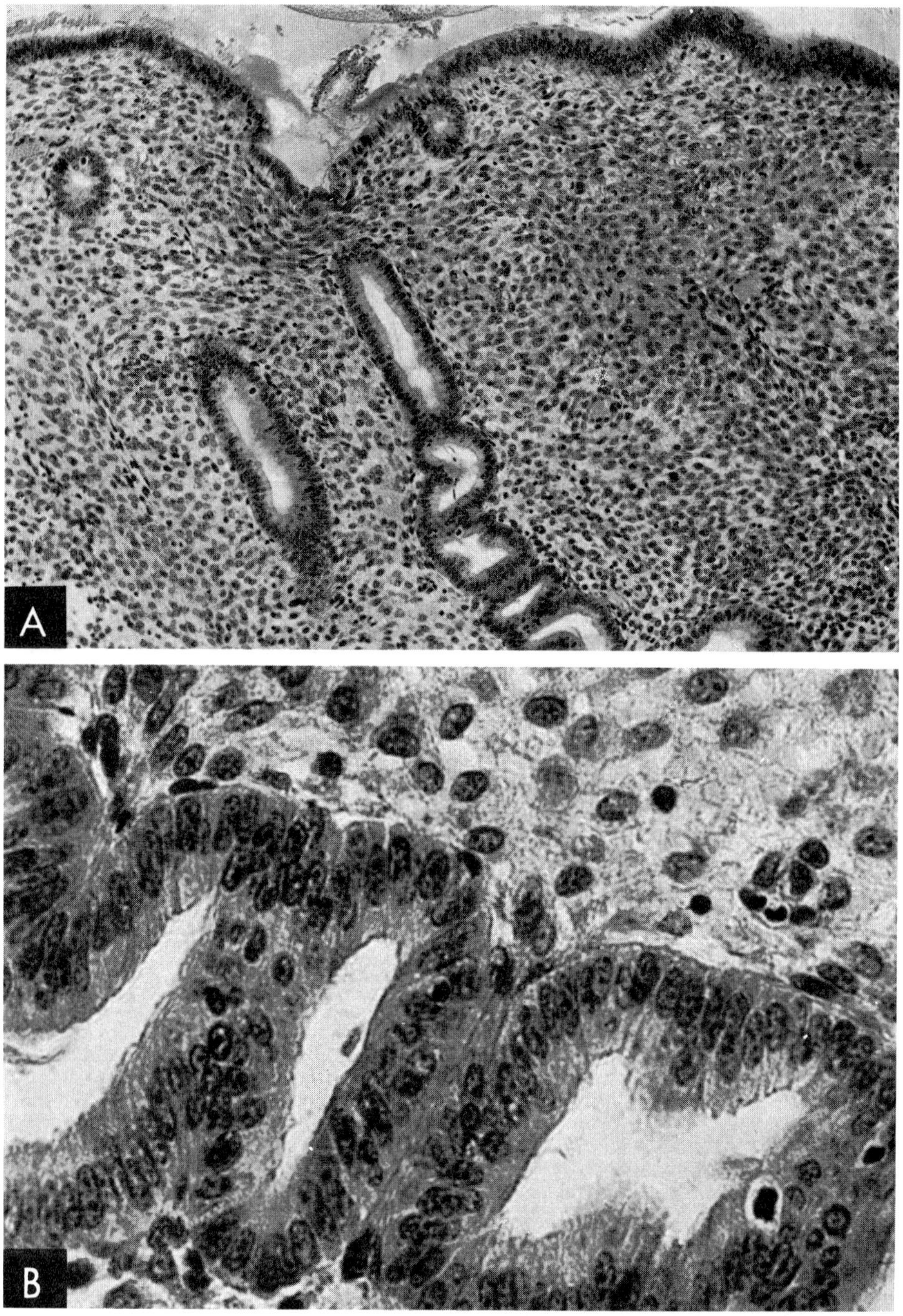

Fig. 3-13. Late proliferative endometrium. **A**, Glands tortuous; stroma usually quite dense. (× 150.) **B**, Epithelial nuclei are pseudostratified and oval in shape. (× 400.) (From Noyes RW, Hertig AT, Rock J: Dating the endometrial biopsy, *Fertil Steril* 1:3, 1950.)

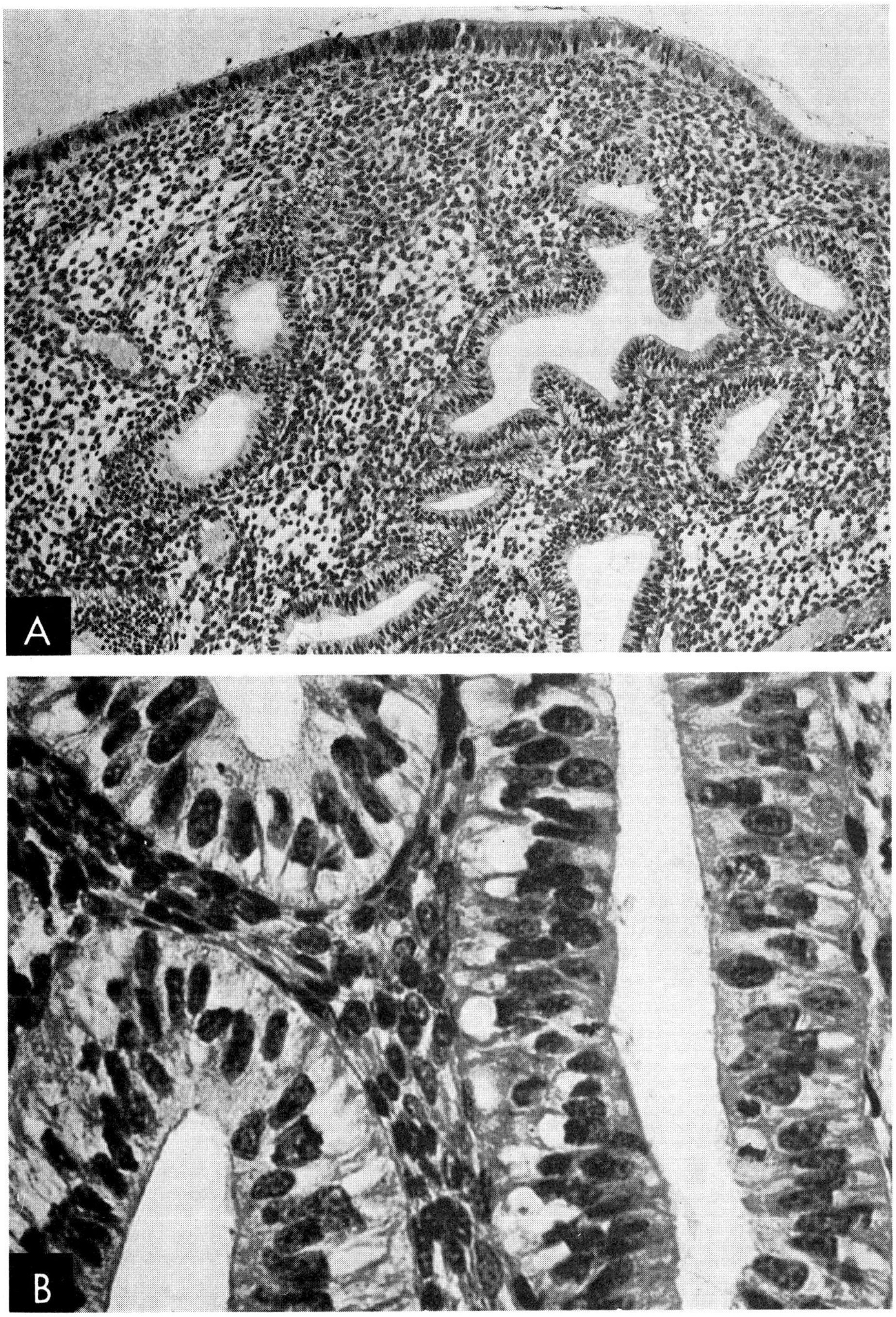

Fig. 3-14. Second postovulatory day. **A**, Glands tortuous; stroma dense; cells consist of nearly naked nuclei. (× 150.) **B**, Gland mitoses very numerous; pseudostratification of nuclei exaggerated by subnuclear vacuoles. (× 400.) (From Noyes RW, Hertig AT, Rock J: Dating the endometrial biopsy, *Fertil Steril* 1:3, 1950.)

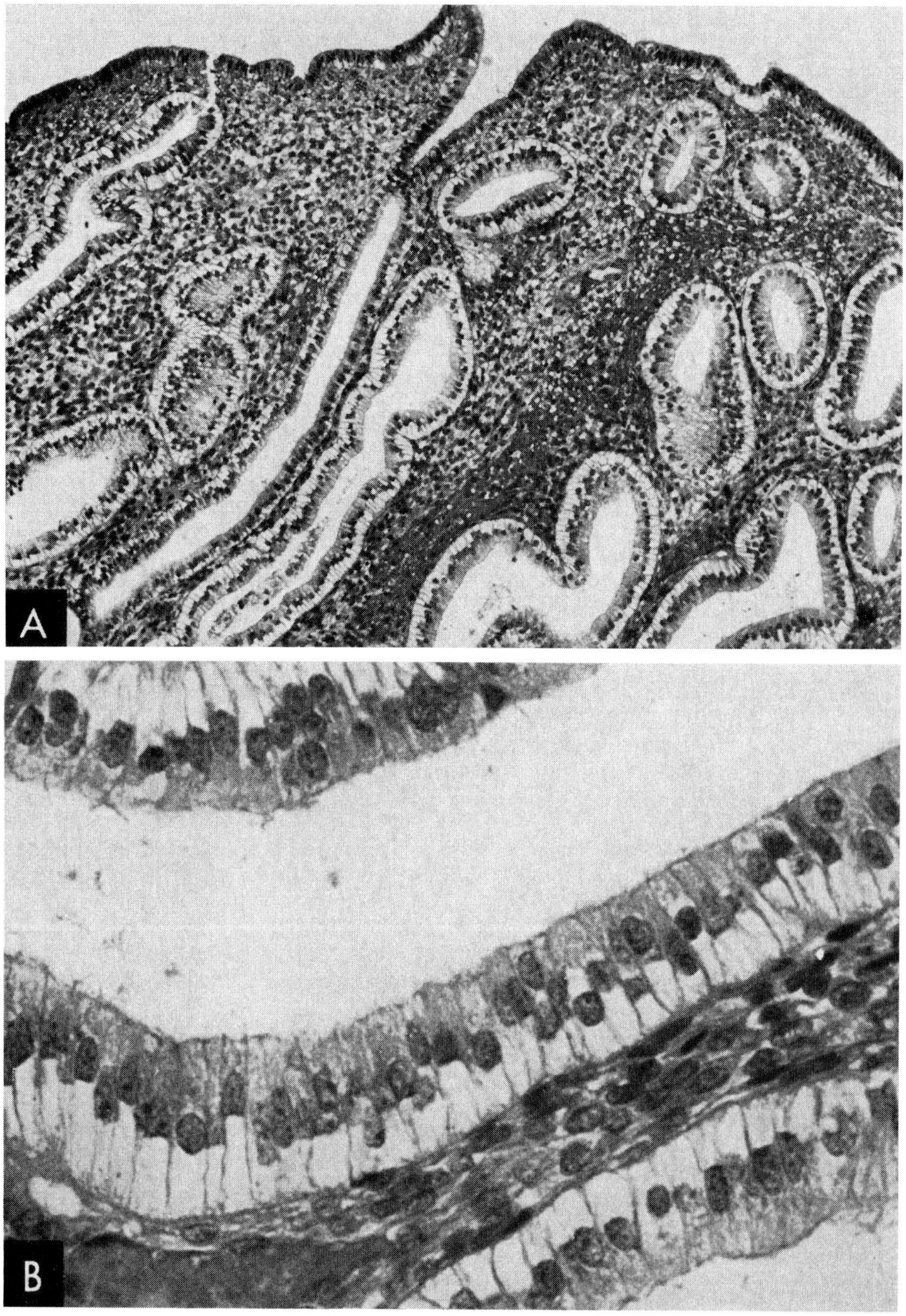

Fig. 3-15. Third postovulatory day. **A**, Gland nuclei are pushed to the center of the epithelial cells with cytoplasm above and vacuoles below them. (× 150.) **B**, Gland mitoses rare; pseudostratification decreasing. (× 400.) (From Noyes RW, Hertig AT, Rock J: Dating the endometrial biopsy, *Fertil Steril* 1:3, 1950.)

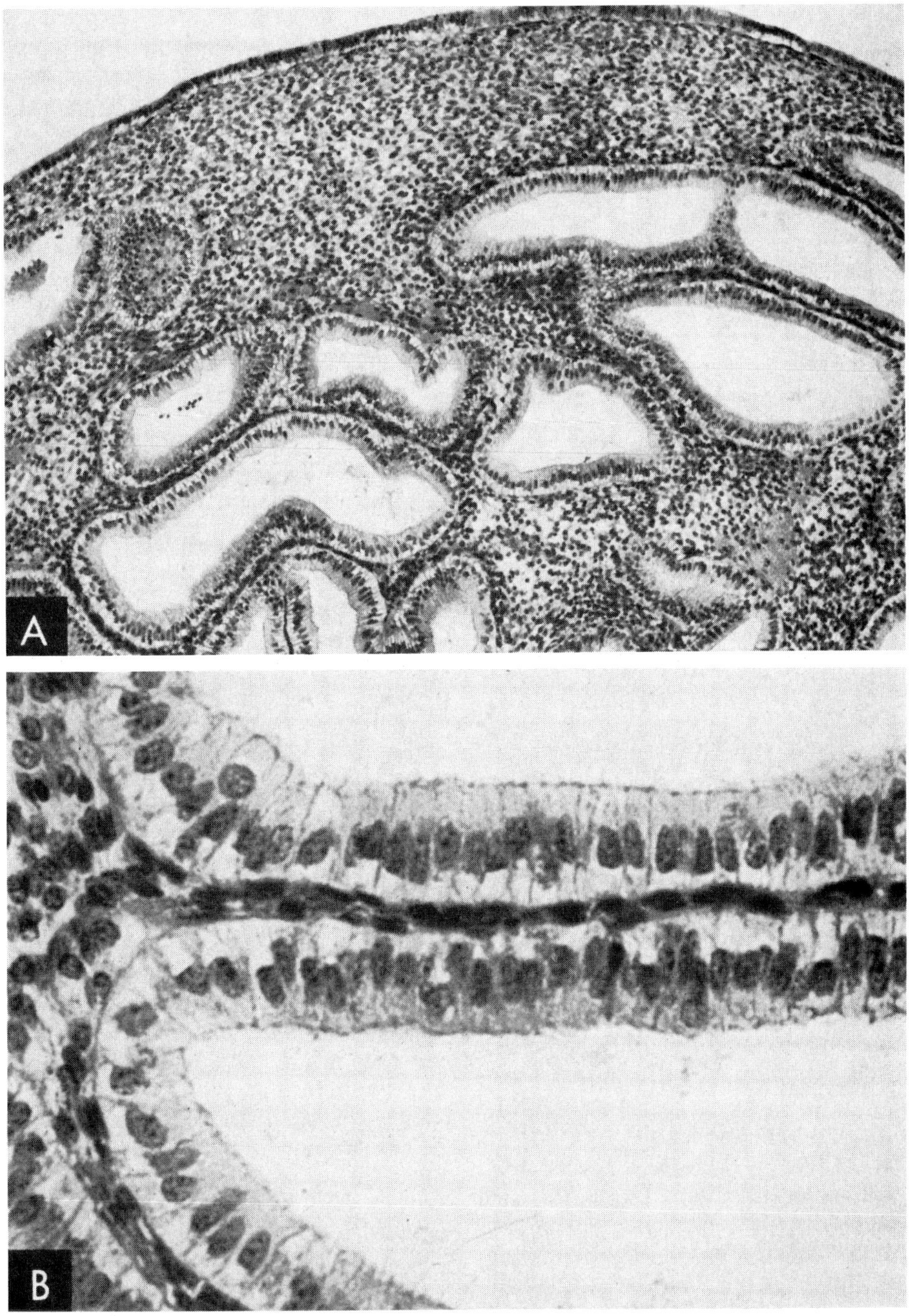

Fig. 3-16. Fourth postovulatory day. **A**, Gland nuclei are returning to base of cells. Wisps of secretory material are present in lumina. (× 150.) **B**, Some vacuoles are pushed past the nucleus on their way to empty glycogen into the lumen. Mitoses and pseudostratification of nuclei are absent. This is the stage of arrival of ovum in the uterus. (× 400.) (From Noyes RW, Hertig AT, Rock J: Dating the endometrial biopsy, *Fertil Steril* 1:3, 1950.)

but actually all cells are attached at the same level. The stroma has edema of variable degree. There are numerous mitotic figures. Scanty cytoplasm and edema give a "naked nucleus" effect. The surface epithelium is covered with columnar epithelium.

Late proliferative phase (Fig. 3-13). The glands are tortuous as a result of active growth. There are numerous mitoses and pseudostratification of the nuclei. The stroma is dense with an active growth pattern and numerous mitoses.

Secretory phase. The changes after ovulation are due to the effects of estrogen and progesterone on an endometrium previously stimulated or "primed" with estrogen. As previously mentioned, this phase lasts about 14 days: the first 7 days are characterized by typical changes in the glandular epithelium. During the last 7 days, specific stromal changes occur that may be used for dating purposes.

Day 15. Day 15 shows essentially a late proliferative pattern except for occasional vacuoles below the nuclei of the glands.

Day 16 (Fig. 3-14). Basal vacuoles are seen in most of the glands. It is the last day of pseudostratification, there are mitoses in the glands and stroma.

Day 17 (Fig. 3-15). The characteristic pattern of subnuclear glycogen vacuoles is evident, with homogeneous cytoplasm above the nuclei of the glands. The position of the nuclei is rather regular. There is a loss of pseudostratification of cells with an increase in diameter and tortuosity. Mitotic figures in the glands and the stroma are rare.

Day 18 (Fig. 3-16). Subnuclear vacuoles appear smaller as the nuclei move back toward the base of the cell. Secretion of glycogen into the lumen of the gland begins; there are no mitoses.

Day 19. Few subnuclear vacuoles are seen. It resembles the day 16 pattern except for the secretion in the lumen of the gland and the absence of pseudostratification and mitoses.

Day 20 (Fig. 3-17). Occasionally there are subnuclear vacuoles. Acidophilic secretion is prominent in the gland lumen.

Day 21. The beginning stromal effects are evident. Stroma cells have dark, dense nuclei with filamentous cytoplasm. Stromal edema is beginning.

Day 22 (Fig. 3-18). Day 22 is the maximum point of stromal edema. Thin-walled spiral arterioles may be seen. Secretion in the gland lumen is active but subsiding and undergoing inspissation.

Day 23 (Fig. 3-19). The edema of stroma persists, but a condensation of the stroma around the spiral arterioles is also characteristic. This is due to an enlargement of the stromal nuclei with an increase in the cytoplasm and is called the *predecidual change*.

Day 24 (Fig. 3-20). Predecidual collections surrounding arterioles are marked. There are active stromal mitoses, but stromal edema is lessening. The endometrium is now beginning to undergo involution unless it is maintained by pregnancy.

Day 25 (Fig. 3-21). The predecidua is forming beneath the surface epithelium, and there is some edema around the arterioles. Lymphocytic infiltration of the stroma is beginning.

Day 26. A gradual increase in predecidua is seen throughout the stroma, with infiltration of polymorphonuclear leukocytes.

Day 27. The predecidua is prominent around the blood vessels and under the surface epithelium. There is marked infiltration of polymorphonuclear leukocytes.

Day 28. There is beginning focal necrosis of the predecidua with small areas of stromal hemorrhage. Stromal cells are clumped together. There is extensive polymorphonuclear leukocytic infiltration. Tortuous glands appear to have undergone secretory "exhaustion."

Certain specific changes in glands and stroma may be considered to indicate physiologic changes occurring in the endometrium. Thus *gland mitoses* indicate active proliferation and growth and may be found from day 3 or 4 until day 16 or 17 of the cycle.

Pseudostratification of the gland nuclei begins after the postmenstrual involution and usually disappears by day 17. It is an indication of proliferative glandular growth; its appearance is due to crowding of the nuclei when the gland is sectioned transversely. *Basal vacuolation* is the earliest morphologic evidence of ovulation discernible in the endometrium. Although one may be seen occasionally in the absence of progesterone, basal vacuoles are usually identified between day 15 and day 19, the glycogen being pushed into the gland lumen about day 19 or 20. The characteristic lining up of the nuclei above the vacuoles is best seen on day 17 and is an excellent indication of recent ovulation.

The secretory function of the glands is evident from day 18 until day 22 by the appearance of loose, feathery material in the lumina. If the blastocyst implants itself on the surface of the endometrium about 6 days after ovulation, it would appear that morphology and function are well correlated, since days 20 to 22 would be critical from the standpoint of nutrient materials. The *edema* of the stroma, most striking between days 22 and 23, may represent an effort of the endometrium to simplify the implantation process by lessening tissue resistance. Periarterial *predecidual reaction* is evident, beginning about days 23 and 24 and may represent a protective mechanism against premature vascular disruption. The predecidua is looked on as providing a supporting framework for newly developed blood vessels to aid in their increased load should pregnancy supervene. These changes in morphologic features are graphically summarized in Fig. 3-10.

MENSTRUAL ABNORMALITIES

Amenorrhea and oligomenorrhea

Primary versus secondary amenorrhea. Primary amenorrhea is present when the first menses has not occurred

Text continued on p. 36.

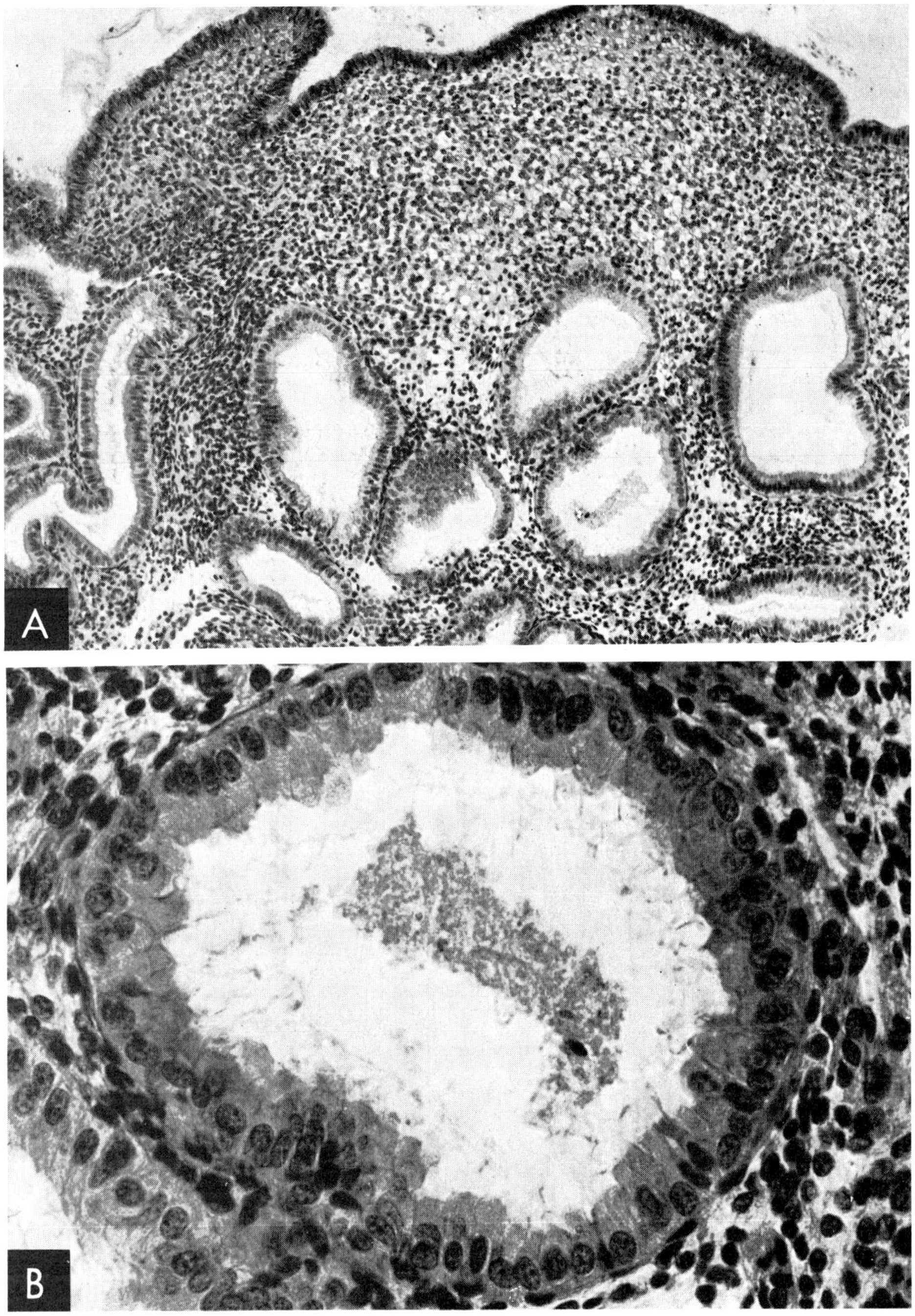

Fig. 3-17. Sixth postovulatory day, corresponding to the beginning implantation in the fertile cycle. **A**, Secretion in gland lumen at peak; beginning of accumulation of extravascular fluid in stroma. (× 150.) **B**, Subnuclear vacuoles are rare; nuclei round and basally located. (× 400.) (From Noyes RW, Hertig AT, Rock J: Dating the endometrial biopsy, *Fertil Steril* 1:3, 1950.)

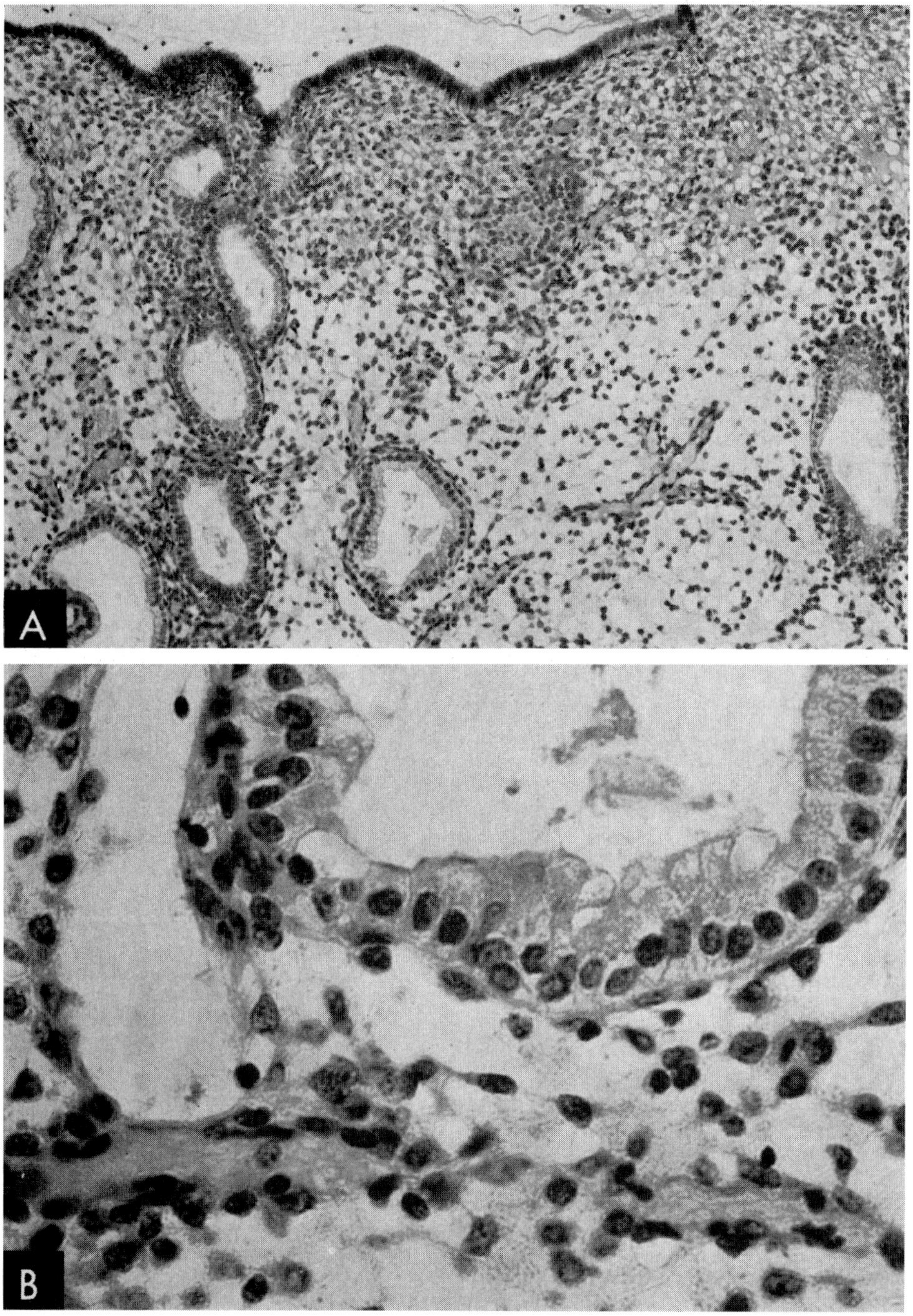

Fig. 3-18. Eighth postovulatory day. **A**, Extracellular fluid maximal. The walls of spiral arterioles are not prominent. (× 150.) **B**, Stromal cells still appear as small, dense "naked nuclei" widely separated by extracellular fluid. Glandular secretion is still active but is subsiding. (× 400.) (From Noyes RW, Hertig AT, Rock J: Dating the endometrial biopsy, *Fertil Steril* 1:3, 1950.)

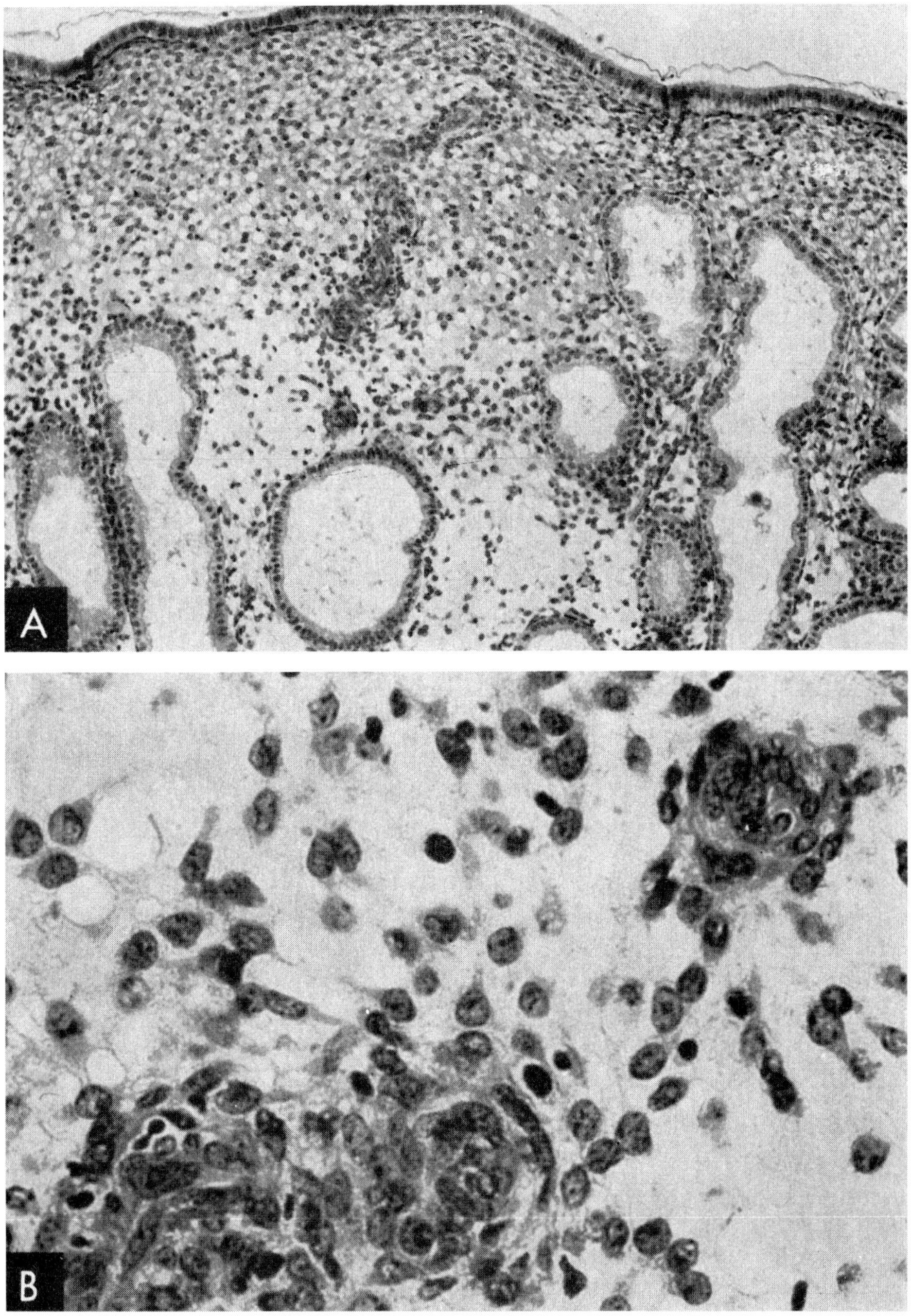

Fig. 3-19. Ninth postovulatory day. **A**, Spiral arterioles become prominent because of condensation of surrounding stroma. (× 150.) **B**, Both nuclei and cytoplasm of periarteriolar stromal cells are enlarging. This is the earliest predecidual reaction. (× 400.) (From Noyes RW, Hertig AT, Rock J: Dating the endometrial biopsy, *Fertil Steril* 1:3, 1950.)

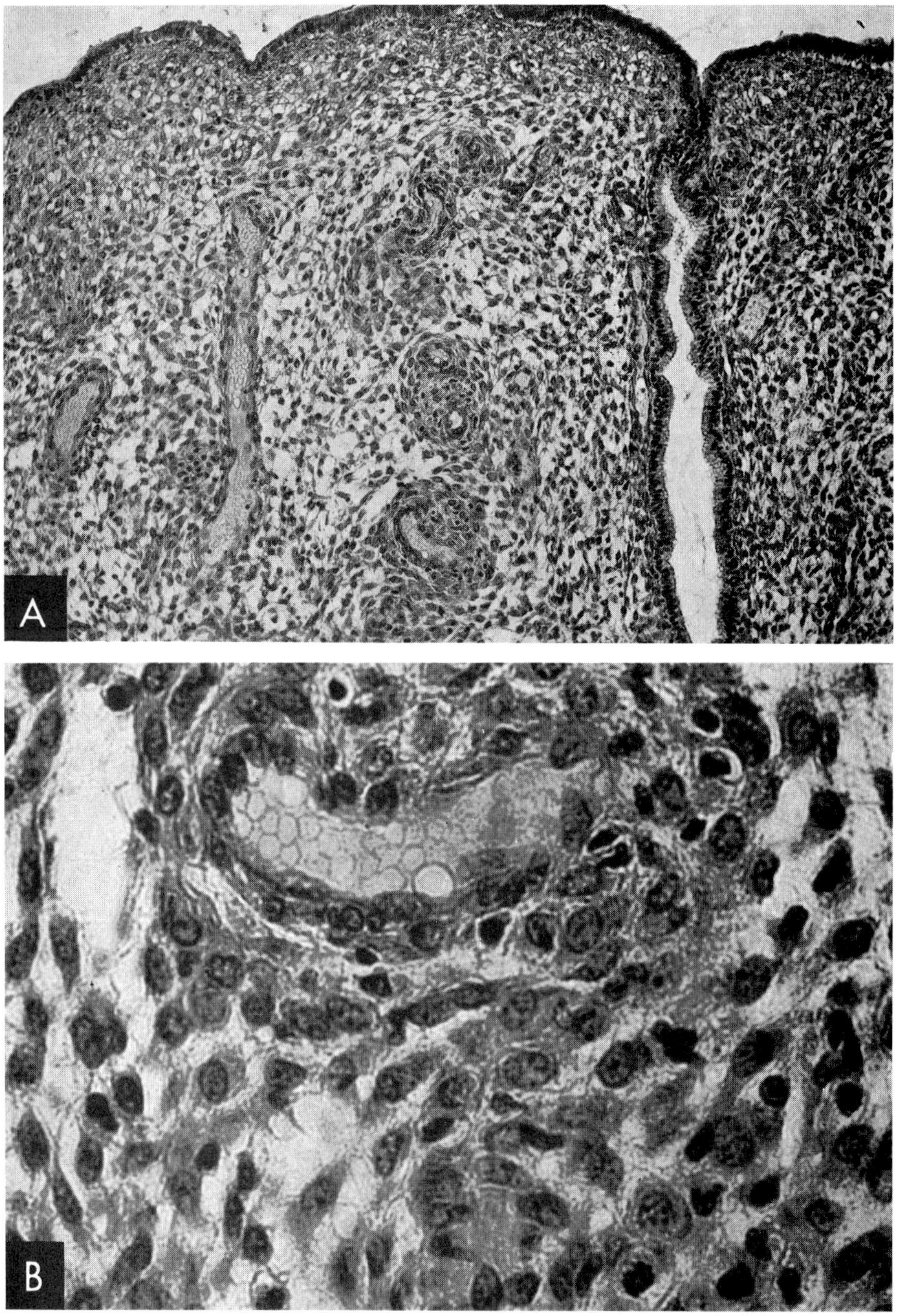

Fig. 3-20. Tenth postovulatory day. **A**, Spiral arterioles and surrounding predecidua still more prominent; extracellular fluid subsiding. (× 150.) **B**, Thickening of periarteriolar predecidual cuff; stromal mitosis evident. (× 400.) (From Noyes RW, Hertig AT, Rock J: Dating the endometrial biopsy, *Fertil Steril* 1:3, 1950.)

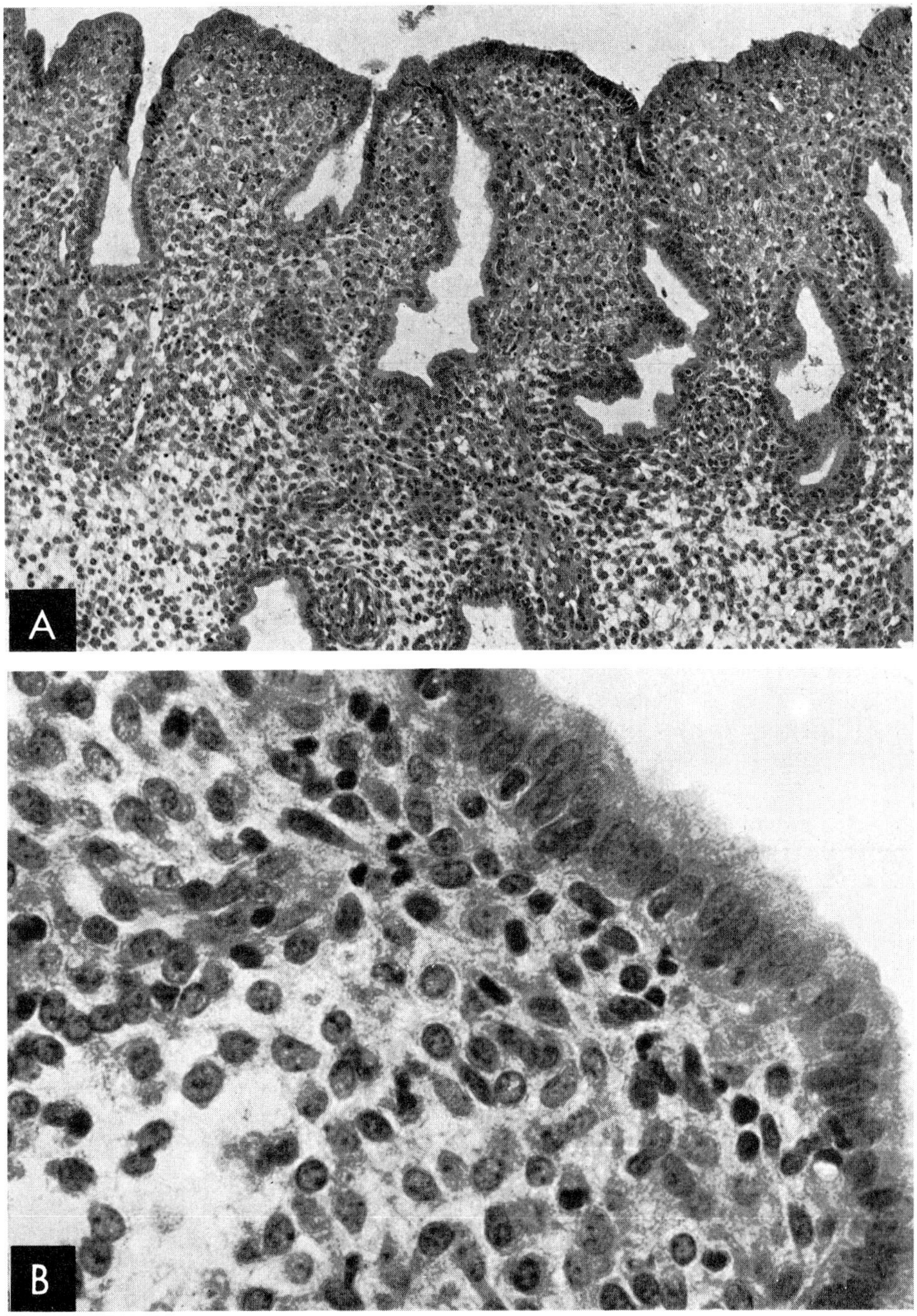

Fig. 3-21. Eleventh postovulatory day. **A**, Pseudodecidua begins to differentiate under the surface epithelium. Stroma of the stratum spongiosum still contains extracellular fluid except in areas near a spiral arteriole. (× 150.) **B**, Round-cell infiltration accompanies predecidual differentiation. Stromal cells swell to become predecidual in type. (× 400.) (From Noyes RW, Hertig AT, Rock J: Dating the endometrial biopsy, *Fertil Steril* 1:3, 1950.)

by age 16 years. Primary amenorrhea is usually due to a genetic or congenital developmental defect.[22] Primary amenorrhea is often associated with disorders of pubertal development.[39] The differential diagnosis of primary amenorrhea is presented in detail in Chapter 23. Secondary amenorrhea is present when a woman with previously regular cyclic menses has 3 or more months of amenorrhea. By necessity this definition is arbitrary. Episodes of physiologic amenorrhea (the perimenarchal period, the immediate postpartum state, and lactation) should not prompt an evaluation of secondary amenorrhea. Secondary amenorrhea is usually due to environmental effects (stress, exercise), or acquired (not congenital) disease. Oligomenorrhea is present when the interval between menstrual cycles is routinely greater than 35 days. The etiological mechanisms that cause oligomenorrhea are identical to those that cause secondary amenorrhea. Therefore the differential diagnosis, evaluation, and therapy of oligomenorrhea are similar to those for secondary amenorrhea. Secondary amenorrhea is at least 10 times more common than primary amenorrhea.

In one Swedish population cohort study, the prevalence of amenorrhea of 3 months duration was 1.8% and the prevalence of amenorrhea of 12 months duration was 1.2%.[37]

Secondary amenorrhea. As noted earlier, secondary amenorrhea is present when a woman with previously regular cyclic menses has 3 or more months of amenorrhea. The most common cause of secondary amenorrhea is pregnancy. Before a detailed workup of secondary amenorrhea is begun, pregnancy should be ruled out with a sensitive test for β-hCG. Once pregnancy is excluded, the workup of secondary amenorrhea can be organized by systematically evaluating the four major compartments necessary for reproduction: (1) hypothalamus, (2) pituitary, (3) ovary, and (4) uterus. Studies of large numbers of women with secondary amenorrhea demonstrate that the etiologic causes of secondary amenorrhea are usually distributed as follows: (1) 55% of cases are due to hypothalamic causes, (2) 20% of cases are due to pituitary diseases, (3) 20% of cases are due to ovarian dysfunction, and (4) 5% of cases are due to uterine abnormalities (Table 3-2).[14,21,40] The workup of secondary amenorrhea is outlined in Fig. 3-22.

Hypothalamic causes. The arcuate nucleus of the hypothalamus contains neurons that are neuroendocrine transducers. These neurons receive *neural inputs* from many diverse brain areas and integrate these signals into a pulsatile *endocrine output* (GnRH secretion). Maintenance of normal ovarian follicular function requires a GnRH pulse frequency of approximately one pulse every 90 minutes during the follicular phase. Marked decreases in GnRH pulse frequency (or amplitude) will prevent ovarian follicular development and can result in amenorrhea. The congenital absence of GnRH neurons produces primary amenorrhea and is often termed *Kallmann's syndrome*. As noted in Table 3-2, the most common disorders that produce marked decreases in GnRH pulse frequency (and consequently secondary amenorrhea) are (1) abnormalities of weight, (2) strenuous exercise, (3) environmental stress, and (4) infiltrative diseases of the hypothalamus. Each of these abnormalities is reviewed.

Abnormalities of weight. The onset of menarche appears to be determined in part by total body weight and body composition, especially the amount of body fat. Normal menarche requires that approximately 17% of body mass be fat. Teleologically, body fat is an important determinant of ovulation because successful pregnancy, birth, and lactation require a large amount of stored energy.

ANOREXIA NERVOSA. The extreme example of the association between weight loss and amenorrhea is the disease of anorexia nervosa. Anorexia nervosa is a major psychiatric problem present in about 0.5% of young women. The typical diagnostic features of anorexia nervosa include the following: (1) onset between ages 10 and 25 years; (2) weight more than 15% below normal; (3) distorted body image (the patient believes she is not thin, whereas objective observers are impressed by the patient's emaciation); and (4) amenorrhea, constipation, low blood pressure, hypercarotenemia, and diabetes insipidus. Anorexia nervosa is associated with numerous endocrine abnormalities, which are summarized in Table 3-3. Some patients with anorexia nervosa develop eating habits that are characterized by episodes of food gorging (bulimia) immediately followed by self-induced vomiting. Anorectic patients with the bulimia-vomiting complex are extremely difficult to treat, and as many as 5% of these women will die (usually from a combination of electrolyte imbalance, prerenal azotemia, malnutrition, and cardiac arrhythmias). Many anorectic individuals surrepti-

Table 3-2. The most common causes of secondary amenorrhea (excluding pregnancy) and their relative frequency

	Relative frequency (%)
Hypothalamus	
Abnormalities of weight (and nutrition)	25
Exercise	15
Stress	15
Infiltrative disease (craniopharyngioma, sarcoidosis)	< 1
Pituitary	
Prolactin-secreting pituitary tumors	17
Empty sella syndrome	2
Sheehan's syndrome	< 1
ACTH-secreting pituitary tumors (Cushing's disease)	< 1
Ovary	
Ovarian failure	15
Polycystic ovarian disease	5
Uterine	
Asherman's syndrome	5

Table 3-3. Neuroendocrine and endocrine abnormalities observed in women with anorexia nervosa

Hormone deficiencies	Hormone excess
Vasopressin	Cortisol
GnRH	Growth hormone
LH and FSH	Reverse T_3
Prolactin	
Total thyroxine (T_4)	
Total triiodothyronine (T_3)	
Dehydroepiandrosterone sulfate	
Estradiol	
Progesterone	

tiously use diuretics to control body weight; such use is often associated with severe electrolyte imbalance.

The cause of anorexia nervosa is unknown. Many psychiatrists believe that anorexia nervosa is a psychologic manifestation of dysfunctional family relationships. Family environments that stress perfection and overachieving may foster the development of anorexia nervosa. Anorexia nervosa causes exceedingly low GnRH pulse frequencies, which prevents ovarian follicular development and results in amenorrhea. Treating women who have anorexia nervosa with intravenous pulses of GnRH results in ovulatory menstrual cycles.

Mild cases of anorexia nervosa can often be treated with a number of counseling interventions: (1) explaining the association of weight loss and amenorrhea in a reassuring manner, (2) exploring the patient's distorted body image, (3) discussing problems of adolescent self-esteem in a supportive manner, and (4) exploring dysfunctional family relationships. Many cases of anorexia nervosa will require skilled therapy by psychiatrists and counselors experienced in this problem.

Women with secondary amenorrhea and height and weight measurements suggesting that leanness is the cause of the amenorrhea, still need a complete amenorrhea evaluation (e.g., serum prolactin level, FSH level; Fig. 3-22). Many women with pituitary tumors and hyperprolactinemia are also extremely lean. To avoid incorrect diagnoses, one must be sure that the amenorrhea evaluation is as complete as possible. For women with low body fat percentage as the cause of the amenorrhea, dietary changes can often cause the resumption of normal ovulatory menses. Simple dietary changes can include adding bread and butter to two meals per day or adding a dessert to one meal per day.

STRENUOUS EXERCISE. During the last 10 years, there has been a tremendous increase in the number of well-trained women athletes. For the majority of women who exercise at mild to moderate exertional levels for 30 to 60 minutes each day, the exercise will not usually disrupt menstrual function. For the female athlete who exercises at high intensity for 1 hour or more daily, the exercise can often cause a decrease in GnRH pulse frequency, which can cause amenorrhea. The mechanisms by which strenuous exercise decreases GnRH pulse frequency are not clear. However, weight loss, low body fat, and stress are contributing factors. Many competitive women athletes have less than 20% total body fat. This low body fat percentage is not always compatible with maintenance of normal menstruation. The stress of athletic competition may also contribute to the loss of menstrual cyclicity.

Regular exercise is an exceedingly effective way of maximizing health and appears to decrease the risk of developing fatal heart disease and certain cancers. Therefore, in general, physicians should not counsel women to abandon their exercise programs. In women of reproductive age, exercise-induced amenorrhea is associated with a decrease in bone density. The severity of the decrease in bone density and its clinical consequences appears to be partly dependent on the severity of the hypoestrogenism and the type of exercise. For example, stress fractures are uncommon in heavyweight oarswomen and swimmers. In contrast, stress fractures are common in professional dancers. The dancers are typically very lean, have marked hypoestrogenism, and stress their bones with high-impact training. Given the overwhelmingly positive health effects of exercise, we do not believe that exercise-induced amenorrhea in a woman not seeking immediate fertility necessarily requires treatment. These women should be thoroughly evaluated to exclude other causes of secondary amenorrhea, such as pituitary tumor. If osteoporosis is present or is a major concern, treatment with combined estrogen-progestogen contraceptives can increase bone density and may reduce the risk of stress fractures.

ENVIRONMENTAL STRESS. A significant percentage of high school girls who leave home to go to college develop oligomenorrhea or secondary amenorrhea. Examinations, sports competition, loss of a spouse, and other stresses can also cause secondary amenorrhea. The mechanisms by which stress causes secondary amenorrhea have not been fully elucidated. However, evidence that corticotropin-releasing factor (CRF) may be involved in stress-related amenorrhea is mounting. CRF is a hypothalamic neuroprotein that stimulates pituitary ACTH and consequently controls adrenal cortisol production. During stress, CRF may be chronically elevated. Interestingly, elevated hypothalamic concentrations of CRF inhibit GnRH pulsation. Recent experiments in primates suggest that hypothalamic opioids such as endorphin may mediate the CRF suppression of GnRH pulsatility. The decrease in GnRH pulse frequency results in amenorrhea. In general, stress-related amenorrhea requires no therapy and will spontaneously resolve once the stress ceases. Before deciding that environmental stress is the cause of amenorrhea, the physician must ensure that other possible causes (e.g., pituitary tumor, ovarian failure, anorexia nervosa) are not present.

INFILTRATIVE DISEASE OF THE HYPOTHALAMUS. Infiltrative disease of the hypothalamus is a rare cause of secondary amenorrhea. Histiocytosis X (infiltration of hypothalamus

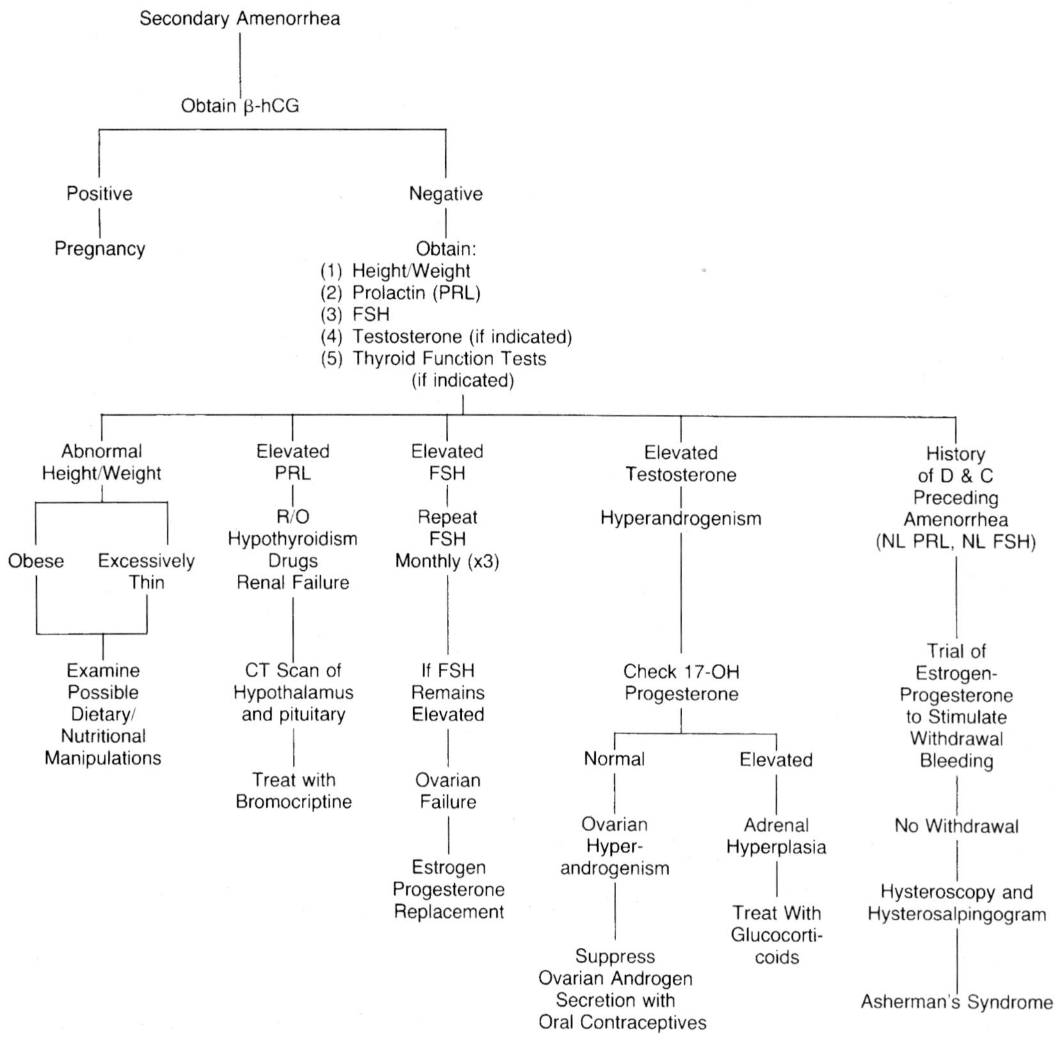

Fig. 3-22. Workup for diagnosis of secondary amenorrhea.

by lipid-laden histiocytes), sarcoidosis (infiltration of hypothalamus by granulomas), and craniopharyngiomas (tumors of Rathke pouch remnants) can all cause secondary amenorrhea. Although these diseases are rare, failure to diagnose them can have important health implications for the patient.

PITUITARY CAUSES. As noted in Table 3-2, the most common pituitary causes of secondary amenorrhea are (1) prolactin-secreting pituitary tumors, (2) empty sella syndrome, (3) Sheehan's syndrome, and (4) ACTH-secreting pituitary tumors (Cushing's disease). Prolactinomas are 10 times more common than all other pituitary causes of secondary amenorrhea and therefore will be discussed in detail.

Prolactin-secreting pituitary tumors (prolactinomas). Hyperprolactinemia is a common finding in women with secondary amenorrhea. The most common causes of hyperprolactinemia are (1) pregnancy, (2) prolactin-secreting pituitary tumors, (3) psychoactive drugs (e.g., phenothiazines), (4) renal failure, (5) hypothyroidism, and (6) infiltrative diseases of the hypothalamus. In a patient with hyperprolactinemia, pregnancy, hypothyroidism, and renal failure should be ruled out by appropriate laboratory tests (β-hCG, T_4, TSH, BUN, and creatinine levels). Drug use can be assessed by taking a detailed history. If the hyperprolactinemia can be documented on two or more occasions, a structural study of the hypothalamus and pituitary needs to be obtained. The two best methods of studying hypothalamic-pituitary structure are magnetic resonance imaging (MRI), or high-resolution x-ray computed tomography (CT) scanning. MRI has the advantage of no ionizing radiation dosage. The resolution of an MRI scan depends in part on the strength of the magnetic field. For high-resolution study of the hypothalamic-pituitary area, MRI imaging units with a field strength of at least 1 tesla should be used. Clinicians should be aware that most MRI units do not have a field strength of 1 tesla.

In patients with hyperprolactinemia, the MRI or CT scan usually reveals normal hypothalamic-pituitary anatomy (idiopathic hyperprolactinemia), or a pituitary tumor (prolactinemia). For clinical purposes, pituitary tumors are divided into two broad categories based on tumor size: microadenomas (< 1 cm) or macroadenomas (> 1 cm). Large pituitary tumors are often associated with headache and visual field changes. The mechanisms by which prolactinomas produce amenorrhea are not completely understood. Hyperprolactinemia appears to be associated with abnormalities in catecholamine metabolism in the hypothalamus. Apparently, by altering patterns of hypothalamic catecholamine metabolism, hyperprolactinemia causes a decrease in GnRH pulsation.

The four goals of treating patients with prolactinomas are the following: (1) normalization of serum prolactin levels, (2) preservation of anterior pituitary function, (3) decrease in size of the pituitary tumor, and (4) prevention of future recurrences of the tumor. The three therapeutic modalities currently available to achieve these goals are (1) bromocriptine therapy, (2) transphenoidal microsurgical resection of the pituitary tumor, and (3) radiotherapy. Radiotherapy is a poor alternative because it may take many years to produce a beneficial effect, usually results in panhypotuitarism, and can damage normal adjacent structures. Transphenoidal microsurgical resection of small pituitary tumors is successful in approximately 75% of cases. However, in more than 50% of the cases that are apparently "successfully" treated by surgery, the tumor will recur within 5 years. Because of these considerations, chronic bromocriptine therapy is the treatment of choice for prolactinomas.

Prolactin is unique among the anterior pituitary hormones because it is under tonic inhibition by hypothalamic dopamine. Normal pituitary lactotrophes and cells in prolactinomas contain high concentrations of cell surface dopamine receptors. Activation of these dopamine receptors suppresses prolactin secretion and decreases overall cellular metabolism. Bromocriptine is a dopamine agonist; it is a synthetic derivative of an ergot alkaloid with a structure resembling dopamine. Bromocriptine binds to pituitary dopamine receptors, inhibits prolactin secretion, and decreases lactotrope cellular metabolism. In patients with prolactinomas, bromocriptine therapy normalizes serum prolactin levels in 85% of cases and decreases pituitary size in 60% of cases. Unfortunately, cessation of bromocriptine therapy is usually accompanied by the return of hyperprolactinemia, return of amenorrhea, and regrowth of the tumor to pretreatment size.[2]

Bromocriptine is the agent of choice for the induction of ovulation in anovulatory, infertile women with hyperprolactinemia. There are virtually no contraindications to bromocriptine except for a previous history of sensitivity to ergot compounds. Before initiation of bromocriptine therapy, the possible adverse effects of pregnancy in a woman with a prolactin-secreting pituitary tumor need to be assessed. If the prolactin-producing tumor is small (microademona < 1 cm in diameter), a pregnancy is usually associated with less than 5% adverse clinical outcomes. However, if the prolactin-producing tumor is large (macroadenoma > 1 cm in diameter), a bromocriptine-induced pregnancy is associated with adverse clinical outcomes in approximately 40% of cases. These adverse outcomes include enlargement of the tumor, severe headaches, and visual field defects (bitemporal hemianopsia secondary to compression of the optic chiasma, cranial nerve palsies, and intrapituitary hemorrhage). Given these observations, infertile women with microprolactinomas can be treated with bromocriptine in the expectation that few problems will occur in a subsequent pregnancy. However, infertile women with macroprolactinomas should probably have a neurosurgical procedure to reduce the tumor prior to attempting pregnancy, or should be treated throughout the pregnancy with bromocriptine.

Initiation of bromocriptine therapy can be associated with nausea, vomiting, postural hypotension, and syncope. Clinical experience suggests that these side effects can best be avoided by prescribing small amounts of bromocriptine taken at bedtime and gradually increasing the dose. A standard protocol for starting bromocriptine therapy is (1) 1.25 mg (one-half tablet) of bromocriptine each night for 14 nights, then (2) 2.5 mg (one tablet) of bromocriptine each night for 14 nights, and finally (3) the standard dose of 2.5 mg of bromocriptine twice daily. In an occasional patient, bromocriptine in doses between 7.5 and 15 mg/day will be required to fully suppress prolactin overproduction. In many cases, bromocriptine in doses as low as 2.5 mg/day will normalize prolactin levels and result in ovulatory menses.

Empty sella syndrome. The roof of the pituitary gland (the diaphragm sella) is perforated by the pituitary stalk, which connects the hypothalamic median eminence to the pituitary. In cases where the perforation in the diaphragm sella is excessively large, the pia mater and accompanying cerebrospinal fluid can herniate into the pituitary fossa. Herniation of this fluid, which is under reasonably high pressure, can produce compression atrophy of the pituitary gland, resulting in hypopituitarism and amenorrhea. The empty sella syndrome can be documented by high-resolution MRI or CT scanning of the pituitary. Therapy is directed to the specific replacement of documented hormonal abnormalities.

Sheehan's syndrome. Sheehan's syndrome is the presence of hypopituitarism caused by acute pituitary necrosis occurring after a postpartum hemorrhage. During pregnancy, the pituitary gland doubles in size as a result of an increase in size and number of pituitary lactotropes. The enlarged pituitary of pregnancy is especially vulnerable to ischemia from hypotension. Severe postpartum hemorrhage and shock will often lead to acute panhypopituitarism. In milder cases, hormonal reserve of single pituitary hormones (e.g., ACTH) may be lost. In patients with suspected Sheehan's syndrome, the physician should carefully search for hypocortisolism and hypothyroidism. If gonadotropin reserve is lost, estrogen replacement therapy will be required. Patients with Sheehans' syndrome who desire a future pregnancy should be treated with exogenous gonadotropin therapy.

Cushing's disease. Cushing's disease is the presence of an ACTH-producing pituitary tumor that results in chronic hypercortisolism. The evaluation of Cushing's disease is discussed in Chapter 12.

Ovarian causes

Premature ovarian failure. Loss of all ovarian follicles results in the cessation of normal ovarian cyclicity (ovarian failure). Ovarian failure prior to age 40 years is termed premature ovarian failure. Loss of all ovarian follicles results in a marked increase in the serum FSH level secondary to a loss of estrogen and inhibin feedback inhibition of FSH. Therefore the diagnosis of ovarian failure is best made by measuring the serum FSH level. In cases of complete ovarian failure, the FSH level will usually be greater than 40 mIU/mL. In cases of incipient ovarian failure, the FSH level may be between 20 and 40 mIU/mL. In women with incipient ovarian failure, FSH levels can fluctuate markedly. Measurement of FSH and estradiol levels monthly for 3 months will often assist the physician in gauging the permanency of the ovarian failure.

The most common cause of premature ovarian failure is genetic abnormality in the sex chromosomes. Although most of these patients have ovarian failure prior to puberty, some will have a few years of normal menstrual function and then cease to menstruate. Therefore any woman with ovarian failure prior to age 30 years should be screened for chromosomal abnormalities by karyotyping, or by polymerase chain reaction screening for y-chromosome elements.

Ovarian failure can also be caused by autoimmune processes. Women with polyglandular autoimmune endocrine disease (e.g., hypoparathyroidism, Addison's disease, hypothyroidism, diabetes mellitus) can develop antiovarian antibodies and ovarian failure. One of the best studied examples of autoimmune ovarian failure occurs in women with myasthenia gravis. Women with myasthenia gravis produce antiacetylcholine receptor antibodies, which result in neuromotor abnormalities. Women with myasthenia gravis can produce anti-FSH receptor antibodies, which result in accelerated loss of developing follicles. This accelerated follicular destruction leads to premature ovarian failure.

Ovarian failure can be caused by chemotherapy (especially alkalyting agents such as cyclophosphamide), radiotherapy (as little as 500 rads to the ovaries), wedge biopsy of the ovaries, and infections.[25]

Specific therapy for ovarian failure is not available. Women with premature ovarian failure are at a high risk of developing osteoporosis and cardiovascular disease due to hypoestrogenism; estrogen replacement therapy should be offered unless specific contraindications exist. Advances in assisted reproductive technologies have now made it possible for women with ovarian failure to become pregnant using donor eggs and in vitro fertilization. In this procedure a donor egg is fertilized with sperm from the partner of the woman with ovarian failure. The patient is treated with estrogen and progesterone to prime the uterus to receive the developing embryo. The availability and success of donor egg programs suggest that in young women a conservative approach should be taken toward the removal of a normal uterus at the time of oophorectomy for adnexal pathology. For a full discussion of the benefits of hormone replacement therapy see Chapter 19.

Ovarian hyperandrogenism. Severe cases of ovarian hyperandrogenism can cause secondary amenorrhea. Ovarian hyperandrogenism is discussed in detail in Chapters 9 and 12.

Uterine causes

Asherman's syndrome. Asherman's syndrome is the presence of intrauterine scar tissue that interferes with normal endometrial growth and shedding. In Asherman's syndrome the intrauterine scar tissue usually develops after vigorous curettage of infected endometrium in a patient who has recently been pregnant. Therefore the history is an important clue to the presence of Asherman's syndrome. A commonly used endocrine manipulation to test for the presence of Asherman's syndrome is to prescribe 2.5 mg of conjugated estrogens daily for 35 days and medroxyprogesterone for the last 10 days (days 26 to 35). Failure to have a withdrawal bleed after such a challenge strongly suggests the presence of Asherman's syndrome. The diagnosis can be confirmed by a radiologic test (hysterosalpingogram) or by direct visualization of the scar tissue (hysteroscopy).

The typical treatment of Asherman's syndrome involves surgical lysis of the intrauterine adhesions (with hysteroscopy), followed by long-term stimulation of the endometrium with estrogen. Some women who become pregnant after therapy for Asherman's syndrome will develop placentation defects such as placenta accreta.

Laboratory evaluation

The goal in laboratory evaluation of secondary amenorrhea is to ensure that no serious disease process is causing the amenorrhea (e.g., hypothalamic or pituitary tumor, or premature ovarian failure). The initial step in this process is to exclude the possibility of a pregnancy. At times this can be accomplished by a history and physical examination, but a measurement of the serum or urine hCG level is a more reliable way to exclude pregnancy. Women with amenorrhea usually have serum prolactin and FSH levels measured. An elevated serum prolactin level can be the result of multiple causes (e.g., pregnancy, tumor, pituitary tumor, hypothyroidism, renal failure, or psychoactive drugs), each of which requires further evaluation. An elevated FSH level suggests the presence of ovarian failure. Some authorities recommend a progestin withdrawal test to diagnose ovarian failure. In the authors' opinion the sensitivity (less than 50%) and specificity (less than 50%) of the progestin withdrawal test for the diagnosis of ovarian failure are poor, and it is not recommended for this purpose. Two tests that may be of value in the diagnosis of secondary amenorrhea are serum testosterone and thyroid function tests. Occasionally, women with ovarian androgen overproduction will present with amenorrhea. Usually signs such as hirsutism and acne will point to this diagnosis. Women with hypothyroidism or hyperthyroidism will sometimes develop oligomenorrhea or amenorrhea. A good screening test for thyroid disease is the new immunoradiometric assay for TSH. It can be used to screen for both hyperthyroidism and hypothyroidism.

Although the progestin withdrawal test is of little value in diagnosing ovarian failure, it can be of value in evaluating hypothalamic-pituitary function in patients with secondary amenorrhea. The test consists of the administration of a progestin and monitoring the amount of uterine bleeding that occurs in the week after the progestin challenge. Prior to administration of the test, pregnancy must be excluded. The progestin can be administered orally (10 mg of medroxyprogesterone acetate/day for 5 days) or parenterally (100 mg of progesterone in oil). If the uterus is normal, bleeding in the week after the progestin challenge is a sign that significant endogenous estrogen production is present. Failure to bleed in the week after the progestin challenge suggests the presence of very low endogenous estrogen production. This is usually due to severe hypothalamic-pituitary dysfunction with very little GnRH, LH, or FSH output. Women with amenorrhea and an abnormal progestin withdrawal test result need to be evaluated carefully and followed closely. Many clinicians suggest that these women should have a structural study of the hypothalamus and pituitary. However, these amenorrheic women may occasionally have a large hypothalamic or pituitary tumor that is endocrinologically silent.

ABNORMAL AND EXCESSIVE UTERINE BLEEDING

Abnormal uterine bleeding is one of the most common clinical problems in gynecology. Uterine bleeding is abnormal if the bleeding pattern is *irregular* (polymenorrhea, less than 21 days between cycles; oligomenorrhea, more than 35 days between cycles), abnormal in *duration* (hypermenorrhea, more than 7 days of bleeding), or abnormal in *amount* (menorrhagia, more than 80 mL of blood loss during menses). Menometrorrhagia is an all-encompassing term used to describe irregular or excessive bleeding (or both) during menstruation or between menstrual cycles.

Abnormal uterine bleeding can be caused by a myriad of problems including (1) pregnancy (e.g., spontaneous abortion, ectopic pregnancy, gestational trophoblastic disease), (2) tumors of the uterus (benign and malignant), (3) infection (e.g., endometritis), (4) hormonal abnormalities (e.g., anovulation and estrogen therapy), (5) intrauterine foreign bodies (e.g., intrauterine device [IUD]), and (6) coagulopathies (Table 3-4). The differential diagnosis of abnormal uterine bleeding is complex, but a systematic approach to the patient with uterine bleeding will usually result in the diagnosis of a treatable disease process.

The endometrium is a remarkably dynamic tissue. During the follicular phase of the menstrual cycle under the stimulation of estrogen, the endometrium grows from 0.5 to 3.5 mm in thickness. Histologically, this growth is marked by many *mitoses* in the endometrial glands (proliferative phase). During the luteal phase of the menstrual cycle, the production of large amounts (25 mg/day) of progesterone by the corpus luteum causes the endometrium to stop growing and to differentiate in preparation for implantation of an embryo (secretory phase). At the end of the menstrual cycle, the programmed demise of the corpus luteum results in the withdrawal of progesterone and estrogen and sloughing of the endometrium with menstrual bleeding.

The initiation and termination of normal menstrual bleeding require the orderly interaction of hormonal and structural events. The luteal-phase endometrium consists of three zones: basalis, stratum spongiosum, and stratum compactum. The inferior-most zone is the basalis, which connects the base of the endometrium to the myometrium. The basalis is the source of endometrial regeneration after menstrual sloughing has occurred. The stratum spongiosum is the midzone of the endometrium. In the luteal phase the stratum spongiosum is the largest zone and represents 50% of total endometrial thickness. The most impressive histologic features of the stratum spongiosum is the presence of spiral or coiled arteries. These spiral arteries are very vasoactive. Just prior to the onset of menstruation, decreases in estrogen and progesterone levels and increases in prostaglandin levels cause the spiral arteries to undergo intense vasoconstriction. The vasospasm in the spiral arteries causes ischemia in the upper

Table 3-4. Differential diagnosis of abnormal uterine bleeding

- I. Pregnancy
  - A. Spontaneous abortion
  - B. Ectopic pregnancy
  - C. Gestational trophoblastic disease
- II. Tumors of the uterus
  - A. Benign
    - 1. Cervical polyps
    - 2. Endometrial polyps
    - 3. Fibroids
  - B. Malignant
    - 1. Cervical cancer
    - 2. Endometrial cancer
    - 3. Fallopian tube cancer
- III. Infection
  - A. Endometritis
  - B. Cervicitis
- IV. Hormonal abnormalities
  - A. Endogenous (anovulation dysfunctional uterine bleeding)
  - B. Exogenous (hormone administration, e.g., estrogen)
- V. Intrauterine foreign body (e.g., IUD)
- VI. Coagulopathies
  - A. Platelet disorders
  - B. Clotting factor abnormalities

zones of the endometrium and initiates menstrual sloughing of the endometrium. The superficial layer of the endometrium is the stratum compactum. The strata spongiosum and compactum comprise the "functional" zones of the endometrium, which participate in the cyclic process of menstruation.

The mechanisms by which pregnancy or tumors of the uterus cause abnormal uterine bleeding are easily understood. Implantation of the embryo involves invasion of the trophoblast into the endometrium and parasitization of the maternal blood supply. If the pregnancy should degenerate, the maternal blood supply becomes directly exposed to the uterine cavity and bleeding ensues. Tumors of the uterus can cause abnormal bleeding by disrupting the normally continuous endometrial surface. Discontinuity in the endometrial surface results in bleeding. Endometritis produces abnormal uterine bleeding by disrupting the continuity of endometrial glands and blood vessels. The first step in the normal process of clotting is formation of a platelet plug. Any disease that interferes with the formation of a platelet plug (von Willebrand's disease or thrombocytopenia), can be associated with abnormal uterine bleeding. The hormonal abnormality that is the most common cause of abnormal uterine bleeding is anovulation. Chronic exposure of the endometrium to estrogen without the stabilizing effects of progesterone produces a fragile endometrial surface that is prone to bleeding.

Diagnostic evaluation

The history should characterize the temporal pattern, the duration, and the amount of bleeding. Contraceptive and sexual practices and the use of hormonal medication need to be explored. Bleeding during previous surgery and a family history of abnormal bleeding require discussion. The physical examination focuses on a determination of intravascular volume status (e.g., orthostatic hypotension, tachycardia), a careful pelvic examination to assess whether the bleeding is vaginal or uterine, and a thorough evaluation of uterine size. Is it enlarged, irregular, or tender? Examination of the skin for ecchymoses or petechiae may provide evidence for an underlying coagulopathy.

The laboratory evaluation of abnormal uterine bleeding should include the following: (1) a complete blood cell count (CBC), (2) a Papanicolaou smear, (3) a sensitive blood pregnancy test (β-hCG), and (4) an endometrial biopsy if necessary. The CBC will provide evidence for the diagnosis of anemia or thrombocytopenia. The Papanicolaou smear provides evidence for the presence of cervical cancer and in some instances endometrial cancer. A normal β-hCG test result rules out pregnancy. The endometrial biopsy provides a direct pathologic evaluation of endometrial histology (e.g., endometrial cancer, hyperplasia, endometritis). These four tests and a complete history and physical examination will result in the diagnosis of a treatable disease in most cases of abnormal uterine bleeding.

Hormonal abnormalities causing abnormal uterine bleeding

Normal cyclic uterine bleeding requires the sequential appearance of estrogen alone, which promotes endometrial growth, followed by progesterone, which causes differentiation of the endometrium. As noted earlier the cessation of estrogen and progesterone secretion (demise of the corpus luteum) initiates menstrual sloughing of the endometrium. The key factors that ensure normal menstrual cyclicity are the sequence of estrogen stimulation of the endometrium followed by progesterone-induced differentiation. Processes that interfere with this normal sequence will often result in abnormal uterine bleeding. The most common process that interferes with this normal sequence is constant estrogen stimulation in the absence of cyclic progesterone exposure. This can occur because of endogenous hormonal abnormalities (anovulation) or exogenous administration of estrogen.

Dysfunctional uterine bleeding is the term used to describe abnormal bleeding because of hormonal abnormalities in the absence of pregnancy, tumor, infection, or coagulopathy. Most cases of dysfunctional uterine bleeding are associated with anovulation in a setting of modest ovarian estrogen production. Elite women athletes often develop anovulation and amenorrhea. In elite women athletes, low levels of GnRH result in very little ovarian estrogen production. Although many of these women are anovulatory, they do not develop abnormal uterine bleeding because their estrogen levels are too low to stimulate endometrial growth. In contrast, some women with polycystic ovary syndrome have significant amounts of continuous ovarian estrogen production but no ovulation and no progesterone production. These women have a high risk for developing dysfunctional uterine bleeding. In summary, dysfunctional uterine bleeding occurs most often in those anovulatory women who are producing significant amounts of ovarian estrogen. Anovulatory women producing no ovarian estrogen do not usually develop dysfunctional uterine bleeding.

Continuous ovarian estrogen production associated with anovulation occurs most commonly in teenage and perimenopausal women. The diagnosis of dysfunctional uterine bleeding is made most often for women in these two age groups. In teenage women the hypothalamus begins to secrete GnRH once a critical body mass (weight) is achieved. The GnRH secretion stimulates LH and FSH secretion, which causes an increase in ovarian estrogen production, but ovulation may not occur. The continuous estrogen exposure results in endometrial growth. The absence of ovulation and progesterone exposure prevents the proper maturation of the endometrium and may result in abnormal uterine bleeding. In teenage women who are not pregnant, abnormal uterine bleeding is almost always due to a hormonal abnormality (anovulation) or a coagulopathy.

Like teenage women, perimenopausal women develop dysfunctional uterine bleeding because of continuous exposure to estrogen without exposure to progesterone. In perimenopausal women the ovary becomes depleted of healthy follicles and oocytes. Due to the low number of follicles present in the ovary, FSH levels become abnormally elevated. This stimulates estrogen production from the few remaining ovarian follicles. These "aged" follicles are often unable to grow to a size that would initiate ovulation. The hormonal milieu is therefore characterized by continuous estrogen unopposed by progesterone. In contrast to teenage women, perimenopausal women frequently have endometrial hyperplasia or endometrial cancer as the cause of uterine bleeding. Therefore all perimenopausal women with abnormal uterine bleeding need to have an endometrial biopsy to ensure that endometrial cancer is not present. Perimenopausal women with abnormal uterine bleeding should not be treated with hormones until the results of the endometrial biopsy are available.

Chronic exposure to estrogen unopposed by progesterone is associated with a high risk of developing dysfunctional uterine bleeding. In most women the ovary is the major source of estrogen production. However, estrogen can also be produced in fat tissue by the extraovarian aromatization of androstenedione to estrone. In markedly obese women the excess adipose tissue results in abnormally increased extraovarian estrogen production. Since obesity is also associated with anovulation, obese women are at high risk for developing abnormal uterine bleeding.

The three groups of women who are at the greatest risk of developing dysfunctional uterine bleeding are teenage, obese, and perimenopausal women. Before making a diagnosis of dysfunctional uterine bleeding, the clinician must be sure that pregnancy, tumor, and infection are not the cause of bleeding. If chronic estrogen exposure unopposed by progesterone is the cause of bleeding, therapy is directed to replacement of adequate amounts of progesterone. The method of progesterone replacement used to treat dysfunctional uterine bleeding depends on the patient's clinical presentation. For the teenage woman , oral contraceptives provide an excellent means of replacing her progesterone deficiency. For the perimenopausal woman, administration of an oral progestogen for 10 to 14 days each month helps regulate endometrial cyclicity. Many different oral progestins can be used for this purpose. One of the most commonly used oral progestins is medroxyprogesterone acetate (10 mg/day for 10 to 14 days each month).

For the woman with anovulation and dysfunctional uterine bleeding who desires fertility, ovulation induction with clomiphene citrate or gonadotropins will cause ovulation, endogenous progesterone production, and possibly pregnancy. Many forms of progesterone replacement are available. The oral administration of "natural" progesterone results in low levels of progesterone in the blood because of intestinal and hepatic metabolism. However, natural progesterone can be given intramuscularly (100 mg each month) or intravaginally (25 mg three times daily for 10 days each month). The expense of progesterone vaginal suppositories limits the practicality of this dosage form.

Many synthetic progestins that are well absorbed via the oral route have been produced. Medroxyprogesterone acetate and megestrol acetate are two synthetic progestins that are structurally very similar to progesterone (Fig. 3-23, A and B). Typically, medroxyprogesterone is administered at a dose of 10 or 20 mg daily for 10 to 14 days. This duration of therapy is recommended because courses of progestin therapy shorter than 10 days can fail to prevent the appearance of endometrial hyperplasia. Courses of progestin therapy are repeated every month or every other month until the patient begins to ovulate spontaneously.

Norethindrone, norethindrone acetate, and norgestrel are three synthetic progestins that are structurally similar to progesterone and testosterone (Fig. 3-23, C and D). Because of the structural similarities between norethindrone, norethindrone acetate, norgestrel, and testosterone, these three synthetic progestins have androgenic actions. All three decrease HDL levels at doses commonly used. Decreased HDL levels may be associated with an increased risk of atherosclerosis. In general, medroxyprogesterone acetate and megestrol acetate are the preferred agents for the treatment of abnormal uterine bleeding. If norethindrone or norethindrone acetate are used in the treatment of dysfunctional uterine bleeding, they are usually prescribed at a dose of 5 mg daily for 10 to 14 days.

Occasionally, abnormal uterine bleeding is caused by the administration of hormones. The chronic administration of exogenous estrogen will often result in abnormal uterine bleeding (chronic estrogen unopposed by progesterone). This clinical occurrence is so widely appreciated that it is unusual to find a woman with an intact uterus who is being treated with unopposed estrogen. Approximately 20% of women receiving danazol have irregular uterine bleeding. In these women, endometrial biopsy specimens usually demonstrate atrophic endometrium.

An unusual endocrine cause of dysfunctional uterine bleeding is hyperthyroidism or hypothyroidism. Women with dysfunctional uterine bleeding who fail to respond to the standard therapy should be screened for thyroid disease by taking a detailed history, physical examination, and thyroid function tests.

Abnormal uterine bleeding due to infections

Infections of the endometrium are characterized grossly by hyperemia and microscopically by edema and white blood cell infiltration. Disruption of vascular integrity by the infection can result in abnormal uterine bleeding. Bleeding caused by endometritis is usually characterized by intermittent spotting, not severe hemorrhage.

When compared with the fallopian tube, the endometrium is relatively resistant to infection. Incomplete spontaneous or therapeutic abortion often cause endometrial infections. In this setting causative organisms include *Escherichia coli*, *enterococci*, *Pseudomonas aeruginosa*, and *Bacteroides* species. These infections are best treated by broad-spectrum antibiotic therapy and D&C. Endometritis not associated with

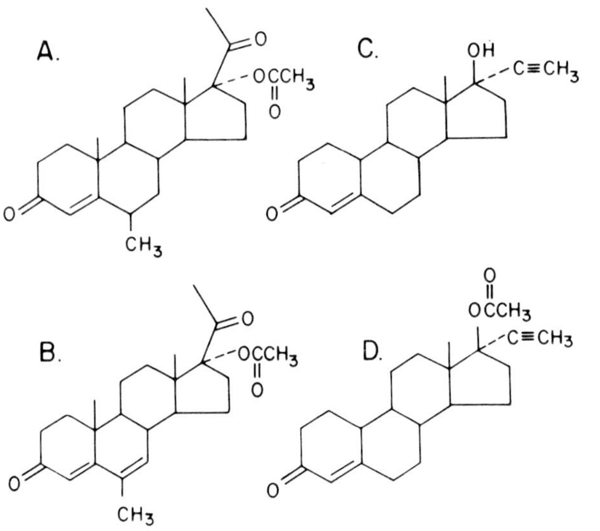

Fig. 3-23. Chemical structures of (**A**) medroxyprogesterone acetate, (**B**) megestrol acetate, (**C**) norethindrone, and (**D**) norethindrone acetate.

a recent pregnancy can be due to *Chlamydia* or *Mycoplasma* species. These patients can be treated with tetracycline (250 mg orally four times daily for 3 weeks) or doxycycline (100 mg orally twice daily for 2 to 3 weeks).

Abnormal uterine bleeding caused by coagulopathies

The initial step in clot formation is the formation of a platelet plug. Diseases that inhibit platelet aggregation or decrease platelet number can be associated with abnormal uterine bleeding. Thrombocytopenia can be caused by a variety of diseases, including acute and chronic leukemias, lymphomas, and idiopathic thrombocytopenic purpura. Currently the commonest cause of thrombocytopenia is treatment with high-dose chemotherapeutic agents such as cyclophosphamide. von Willebrand's disease is a disorder of platelet aggregation and clot formation caused by an abnormal factor VIII. Abnormal uterine bleeding caused by coagulopathies is best treated by correcting the underlying abnormality; in many cases, however, this is not possible.

An alternative approach is to produce a quiescent endometrium that is not cycling and will not undergo withdrawal bleeding. This can be accomplished by chronic GnRH agonist therapy or with combined estrogen-progestogen oral contraceptives. The GnRH agonists produce paradoxical inhibition (downregulation) of pituitary gonadotropin production and cause the cessation of ovarian estrogen production. In a hypoestrogenic environment, the endometrium becomes inactive. Another approach is to use combined estrogen-progestin oral contraceptives to prevent a menstrual bleed during an episode of thrombocytopenia. This approach is of special value for women receiving cyclic courses of chemotherapeutic agents such as cyclophosphamide. In these women the oral contraceptives can be used to prevent a menstrual bleed during the thrombocytopenic episode that follows chemotherapy. After the thrombocytopenic episode is past, the oral contraceptives can be stopped and a "normal" withdrawal bleed will be initiated.

Treatment of life-threatening uterine bleeding

Occasionally, women will come to the emergency room of a hospital with life-threatening vaginal bleeding. Rapid evaluation and therapy are required to minimize morbidity and mortality. Initial evaluation should include a CBC, coagulation studies (prothrombin time, partial thromboplastin time), a rapid, sensitive pregnancy test, and if indicated, an endometrial curettage. Coagulopathies require correction with the appropriate replacement products (platelets or fresh frozen plasma). If the uterus is structurally normal by physical examination, ultrasound, or both, the pregnancy test result is negative, and the D&C does not slow the bleeding, aggressive hormonal therapy may be required. Conjugated estrogens (25 mg intravenously every 4 hours for three doses) have been used successfully in the treatment of life-threatening uterine hemorrhage that is not due to a pregnancy or a tumor. Alternatively, large doses of a combined estrogen-progestin medication may be used. For example, 0.05 mg of ethinyl estradiol plus 0.5 mg of norgestrel (Ovral) given four times daily for up to 7 days may slow the bleeding.

In severe cases of uterine bleeding where conventional therapy has failed, angiographic embolization of the uterine arteries may help control the bleeding. In some cases hysterectomy may be required to treat episodes of life-threatening uterine bleeding.

DYSMENORRHEA

Dysmenorrhea, or painful menstruation, is one of the most common gynecologic problems. Approximately 50% of all women experience dysmenorrhea, and approximately 1% of women of reproductive age are incapacitated for 1 to 3 days each month because of severe dysmenorrhea. For clinical purposes, dysmenorrhea is often divided into two broad categories: primary and secondary. Primary dysmenorrhea is the presence of painful menstruation in the absence of demonstrable pelvic disease. Secondary dysmenorrhea is the occurrence of painful menstruation caused by pelvic pathology, such as endometriosis, chronic pelvic inflammatory disease, or uterine leiomyomas. It is often difficult to differentiate between primary and secondary dysmenorrhea based on the history and physical examination. Trials of empiric drug therapy and diagnostic laparoscopy are often necessary to discover the cause of the dysmenorrhea.

In primary dysmenorrhea the pain characteristically begins with the onset of menstruation and lasts for 12 to 72 hours. The pain is usually confined to the lower abdomen and is most intense in the midline. The pain is often described as crampy and intermittently intense. In some women, back pain and thigh pain may be severe. The abdominal pain is often accompanied by nausea, diarrhea, fatigue, headache, and a general sense of malaise. The pain is usually most severe on the first day of menstruation and gradually diminishes.

Current evidence suggests that prostaglandin $F_{2\alpha}$ ($PGF_{2\alpha}$) and prostaglandin E_2 (PGE_2) released from the endometrium at the time of menstruation cause primary dysmenorrhea.[59] Prostaglandin $F_{2\alpha}$ and PGE_2 are derivatives of the fatty acid arachidonic acid. The sequential stimulation of the endometrium by estrogen followed by progesterone results in a dramatic increase in prostaglandin production by the endometrium. At the time of menstruation the endometrial cells undergo lysis and release of $PGF_{2\alpha}$ and PGE_2. Prostaglandins induce smooth muscle contraction (or relaxation) in many diverse tissues. Uterine smooth muscle contractions induced by the prostaglandins produce the colicky, spasmodic, labor-like lower abdominal and back pain characteristic of dysmenorrhea. Prostaglandin-induced uterine contractions can last many minutes and may produce intrauterine pressures greater than 60 mm Hg. When uterine pressure exceeds mean arterial pressure for a prolonged period of time, uterine ischemia will ensue. Uterine ischemia results in the accumulation of anaerobic metabolites that can stimulate the small type-C pain neurons. In many ways, primary dysmenorrhea is like "angina" of the uterus.

Many factors can modulate prostaglandin-induced uterine contractions. For example, strenuous exercise can increase uterine tone (possibly because of decreased uterine blood flow). Many women athletes note that strenuous exercise at the time of menstruation increases the severity of their dysmenorrhea. Other women report that caffeine ingestion can decrease the severity of dysmenorrhea. Caffeine may increase uterine cyclic adenosine monophosphate levels that result in decreased uterine tone. In addition to stimulating uterine contractions, $PGF_{2\alpha}$ and PGE_2 can cause contraction of bronchial, bowel, and vascular smooth muscle that produces bronchoconstriction (asthma), diarrhea, and hypertension. As noted earlier, diarrhea is commonly associated with primary dysmenorrhea.

The hypothesis that prostaglandins released from the endometrium cause primary dysmenorrhea is supported by the observation that endometrial concentrations of PGE_2 and $PGF_{2\alpha}$ correlate with the severity of dysmenorrhea. In general, women with the highest endometrial concentrations of $PGF_{2\alpha}$ and PGE_2 have the most severe dysmenorrhea.[5] High rates of endometrial prostaglandin production require the sequential stimulation of the endometrium by estrogen followed by progesterone. Usually women who menstruate without ovulating (no progesterone) do not have primary dysmenorrhea. In most girls the menses which immediately follow menarche (approximate age 12 years) are anovulatory due to immaturity of the hypothalamic-pituitary axis. Since regular ovulatory cycles may not begin until 2 to 5 years after menarche, in many teenagers primary dysmenorrhea begins a few years after menarche.

Secondary dysmenorrhea is the occurrence of painful menstruation due to pelvic pathology such as endometriosis or chronic pelvic inflammatory disease. The major goal of the clinical evaluation of dysmenorrhea is to identify whether the process is primary or secondary. It is often difficult to differentiate between primary and secondary dysmenorrhea based on history and physical examination. However, many women with secondary dysmenorrhea will report that the dysmenorrhea (1) began after age 20 years, (2) often lasts for 5 to 7 days each month, and (3) has increased in severity. In addition, women with secondary dysmenorrhea usually report pelvic pain at times other than menses. By definition, women with primary dysmenorrhea have a normal pelvic examination. Women with secondary dysmenorrhea may also have a normal pelvic examination if the pelvic pathology cannot be palpated (e.g., stage I endometriosis, adenomyosis, pelvic adhesions). Some women with secondary dysmenorrhea have markedly abnormal pelvic examinations. If the pelvic examination is abnormal, appropriate clinical action should be immediately undertaken (e.g., ultrasound, diagnostic laparoscopy, exploratory laparotomy). For example, a woman with dysmenorrhea and a pelvic examination suggestive of severe endometriosis (cul-de-sac induration, uterosacral ligament nodularity, adnexal masses) should be scheduled for laparoscopy or laparotomy to confirm the diagnosis. In the evaluation of a woman with dysmenorrhea, pelvic ultrasound may be helpful in identifying uterine (fibroids) or adnexal masses (hydrosalpinx) that cannot be palpated on pelvic examination. In women with secondary dysmenorrhea, a CBC and erythrocyte sedimentation rate (ESR) may raise the suspicion of chronic pelvic inflammatory disease (high white blood cell count and high ESR).

Dysmenorrhea in a woman who has a history consistent with primary dysmenorrhea and a normal pelvic examination is treated as primary dysmenorrhea. If aggressive therapy for primary dysmenorrhea fails to relieve the pain, additional studies (e.g., ultrasound, laparoscopy) should be considered to determine if a cause of secondary dysmenorrhea is present. As previously noted, the cause of primary dysmenorrhea is elevated endometrial prostaglandin production. Therefore the therapy for primary dysmenorrhea should be directed at reducing endometrial prostaglandin production. Antiinflammatory agents that directly inhibit prostaglandin production or action (ibuprofen) and agents that suppress ovulation (oral contraceptives) are very effective in reducing endometrial prostaglandin production. Table 3-5 lists inhibitors of prostaglandin production that have been used successfully in the treatment of dysmenorrhea. All of these agents inhibit the cyclooxygenase enzyme. In addition to inhibiting the cyclooxygenase enzyme system, mefenamic acid also directly blocks activation of the prostaglandin receptor. The agents listed in Table 3-5 are associated with a very low incidence of serious adverse effects. In fact, ibuprofen is available without a prescription. Side effects of the prostaglandin synthesis inhibitors include gastrointestinal irritation and ulceration, nausea, prolonged bleeding time, renal papillary necrosis, and decreased renal blood flow.

In general, therapy for dysmenorrhea is initiated with ibuprofen at a dose of 400 mg orally 4 times daily. Therapy is initiated just prior to menses for women who can accurately predict when their menses begins, or when menses actually begins. Therapy usually lasts 3 to 4 days. If ibuprofen (an arylpropionic acid derivative) fails to be effective, a drug in the fenamate class (mefenamic acid) is tried. If naproxen is to be used in the treatment of primary dysmenorrhea, the sodium salt is preferred because it is more rapidly absorbed and reaches a higher peak plasma level than the acid.

Oral contraceptives contain a combination of estrogen (ethinyl estradiol) and a progestogen (19-norprogestin). Oral contraceptives suppress endometrial prostaglandin production by inhibiting ovulation (no endogenous progesterone production) and by preventing normal synchronous endometrial growth and differentiation (constant estrogen and progestogen prevents normal endometrial growth).

If 3 to 6 months of therapy fails to produce a significant decrease in dysmenorrhea, the clinician should carefully review the history and physical examination to be sure that a cause of secondary dysmenorrhea has not been overlooked. Pelvic ultrasound and diagnostic laparoscopy should be considered if the patient fails to respond to treatment with prostaglandin synthesis inhibitors. Two studies of chronic pelvic pain, one in a population of adolescent girls and one in a population of adult women, demonstrate the importance of performing diagnostic laparoscopy in women with chronic pelvic pain that fails to respond to supportive therapy.[16,26] In both studies a significant number (more than 30%) of women with chronic pelvic pain had documented pelvic abnormalities (e.g., adhesions, endometriosis, pelvic inflammatory disease) that accounted for the pain.

PREMENSTRUAL SYNDROME

Premenstrual syndrome (PMS) can be defined as the cyclic recurrence during the luteal phase of the menstrual cycle of a combination of distressing physical, psychologic, or behavioral changes that interfere with family, social, or work-related activities. Approximately 1% of women of reproductive age have such severe PMS that it threatens their work and interpersonal relationships. Premenstrual syndrome is most common in women 25 to 45 years of age. The symptoms of PMS are diverse but include the following: (1) body pain (headache, cramps, fatigue), (2) water retention (weight gain, swelling, painful breasts), (3) negative affect (depression, crying, loneliness, irritability), (4) autonomic reactions (cold sweats, dizziness, fainting), (5) behavioral changes (decreased efficiency, difficulty concentrating, lowered motor coordination), and (6) somatization (feelings of suffocation, chest pain, ringing in the ears, blind spots, blurry vision, numbness, tingling). To order these diverse symptoms and signs, Abraham devised a classification schema consisting of four categories (Table 3-6).[1] These categories are not all-inclusive, but they do help the clinician organize history taking for patients with PMS.

The first step in the diagnosis of PMS is to have the patient keep a daily symptom diary for 2 months. If examination of the daily symptom diary reveals that the symptoms are temporally clustered prior to menses (late luteal phase) and disappear 2 or 3 days after the initiation of menses, PMS should be strongly suspected. In addition to late luteal-phase symptoms, an occasional woman with PMS has periovulatory exacerbation of symptoms. If examination of the symptom diary reveals no symptom-free week in the early follicular phase, a chronic psychiatric disorder such as depression or anxiety should be strongly suspected.

Approximately 30% of women who seek treatment for PMS have a chronic psychiatric disorder. As noted above, these women can often be identified by the absence of a symptom-free week in the follicular phase of the menstrual cycle. In addition, some experienced practitioners suggest that all women with symptoms consistent with PMS complete a personality inventory such as the Minnesota Multiphasic Personality Inventory or Beck's Depression Inventory to further screen for individuals with depression or pathological anxiety. Women with symptoms of PMS and major depression or severe anxiety are best treated by referral to psychiatric or psychologic counseling. In summary, the diagnosis of PMS is a two-step process. The first step involves obtaining a daily symptom diary to assess the temporal relationship of the symptoms to menses. The second step involves screening for chronic psychiatric problems. Since there is no "blood test" for the diagnosis of PMS, the skills of each clinician are challenged in the evaluation of each woman with this disorder.[12]

The cause of PMS is not understood. Numerous theories have been proposed—estrogen excess, progesterone deficiency, fluid retention, vitamin B_6 deficiency, hyperprolactinemia, hormone allergies, and prostaglandin abnormalities—but none have been proven. Currently, a popular theory is that progesterone or metabolites of progesterone interact with neurotransmitters and ion channels in the brain. Recent experiments suggest that metabolites of progesterone

Table 3-5. Inhibitors of prostaglandin synthesis commonly used in the treatment of dysmenorrhea

Drug class	Drug	Standard dose
Fenamates	Mefenamic acid	500 mg loading dose; 250 mg 4 times daily
	Flufenamic acid	100 to 200 mg 3 times daily
	Tolfenamic acid	133 mg 3 times daily
Phenylpropionic acid	Ibuprofen	400 mg 4 times daily
	Naproxen sodium	550 mg loading dose; 275 mg 4 times daily
	Ketoprofen	50 mg 3 times daily

may modulate neural γ-aminobutyric acid receptors (a common neural ion channel). Another hypothesis is that some women develop abnormalities of endogenous neural opioid peptides and demonstrate symptoms of endogenous opioid withdrawal in the late luteal phase of the menstrual cycle. Investigators have demonstrated abnormally low levels of circulating opioid peptides in women with PMS in the late luteal phase of the menstrual cycle. The symptoms of PMS are probably due to the complex interaction of ovarian hormones, central neurotransmitters, and the autonomic nervous system.[28]

Therapy for PMS should include a comprehensive program of education, psychologic counseling and support, exercise, dietary assessment, and if necessary, pharmacologic interventions. Effective dietary considerations include minimizing daily intake of alcohol, nicotine, simple sugars, caffeine, and salt. Exercise programs and psychologic counseling can help the individual with PMS regain control of her life. Pharmacologic therapy of PMS is controversial. At least 10 different pharmacologic agents have been used in the treatment of PMS. These agents include mefanamic acid, alprazolam, fluoxetine, bromocriptine, vitamin B_6, γ-linoleic acid, GnRH agonists, progesterone, oral contraceptives, diuretics, and lithium. A major problem with pharmacologic trials for the treatment of PMS is that few have been conducted in a randomized, prospective fashion utilizing placebo controls. Since placebo therapy can cause significant improvement in PMS, controlled clinical trials are absolutely necessary before a drug can be accepted as effective.[29] Six agents of significant clinical value are mefanamic acid, γ-linoleic acid, GnRH agonists, alprazolam, fluoxetine, and diuretics. The use of each agent in the treatment of PMS will be described.

Table 3-6. Abraham's (1983) classification of premenstrual syndrome

A—Anxiety
Nervous tension
Mood swings
Irritability
Anxiety
C—Cravings
Headache
Craving for sweets
Increase appetite
Heart pounding
Fatigue
Dizziness or faintness
D—Depression
Depression
Forgetfulness
Crying
Confusion
Insomnia
H—Water-related symptoms
Weight gain
Swelling of extremities
Breast tenderness
Abdominal bloating

Mefanamic acid is a nonsteroidal agent that inhibits prostaglandin synthesis and competes for binding at the prostaglandin receptor site. In addition to its use in PMS, mefanamic acid is also of value in the treatment of moderate pain. As noted in Table 3-5, for the treatment of PMS, mefanamic acid is usually administered as a 500 mg loading dose followed by 250 mg 4 times daily for up to 7 days. Prolonged administration of mefanamic acid is not recommended since it can result in decreased renal blood flow and renal papillary necrosis. Common side effects of mefanamic acid therapy include diarrhea, nausea, vomiting, and drowsiness. Mefanamic acid is especially effective in the treatment of pain symptoms associated with PMS.

γ-Linoleic acid (evening primrose oil) is a dietary supplement especially useful in the treatment of breast symptoms, bloating, weight gain, and edema associated with PMS. γ-Linoleic acid is a precursor for prostaglandin E_1 (PGE_1) and may be effective in the treatment of PMS because it alters prostaglandin production and metabolism. A standard dose of γ-linoleic acid is 3 gm/day in the late luteal phase of the cycle. Evening primrose oil is available without a prescription in stores specializing in dietary supplements.

GnRH agonists such as nafarelin and leuprolide are especially useful in the treatment of severe PMS.[34] Synthetic changes in amino acids 6 and 10 of the hypothalamic decapeptide GnRH produce agents with long half-lives and high affinity for the pituitary GnRH receptor. Chronic administration of these compounds produces a transient stimulation of pituitary LH and FSH secretion and then paradoxically results in the complete suppression of LH and FSH secretion. Therefore chronic administration of the GnRH agonists produces an anovulatory, amenorrheic state that usually results in complete relief of the symptoms of PMS. The major side effects of the GnRH agonists are attributable to hypoestrogenism (e.g., osteoporosis, hot flushes, dry vagina). Prolonged use of GnRH agonists (greater than 6 months) has not been demonstrated to be safe. Effective doses of the GnRH agonists are 0.5 mg of leuprolide administered subcutaneously daily, 3.75 mg of depot leuprolide administered every 4 weeks, or 200 mg of nafarelin administered twice daily intranasally.

Alprazolam is a member of the benzodiazepine class of psychoactive agents. The molecular action of alprazolam is unknown, but all benzodiazepines cause a dose-related CNS depressant effect. Alprazolam is especially effective in the treatment of anxiety caused by PMS. For the treatment of PMS, alprazolam is recommended at a dose of 0.25 mg 3 times daily during the late luteal phase of the cycle. The dose can be titrated to the needs of the patient. A major side effect of alprazolam is drowsiness. In some patients discontinuance of benzodiazepines can produce withdrawal symptoms that include insomnia, dysphoria, abdominal cramps, sweating, tremors, and convulsions. When prescribing alprazolam for the treatment of PMS, the clinician must carefully screen for the occurrence of withdrawal symptoms. If withdrawal symptoms occur, the drug should be permanently discontinued.

Fluoxetine is a specific serotonin-uptake inhibitor approved for the treatment of depression. In a double-blind, placebo-controlled, crossover study, Wood et al demonstrated that daily fluoxetine (20 mg) was superior to placebo in reducing symptoms of depression, anger, and anxiety.[57] A preliminary follow-up study suggests that limiting fluoxitene therapy to the luteal phase of the cycle may be as effective in the treatment of PMS as therapy throughout the follicular and luteal phases of the cycle. The most common side effects caused by fluoxitene include nervousness, insomnia, drowsiness, nausea, and anorexia.

In women with significant premenstrual weight gain (more than 1.5 kg), short-term diuretic therapy may help relieve the symptoms of bloating, edema, and breast fullness. Metolazone (2.5 mg/day) or spironolactone (25 mg four times daily) administered during the late luteal phase of the menstrual cycle have been shown to be effective in the treatment of PMS. All diuretics can produce electrolyte imbalance, and women given diuretics for PMS should be evaluated for electrolyte abnormalities.

Three agents that have been reported to be successful in the treatment of PMS in uncontrolled trials are progesterone, oral contraceptives, and lithium. However, controlled clinical trials have failed to consistently demonstrate a beneficial effect of these agents. Until further research is completed, these agents are not recommended in the treatment of PMS.

Vitamin B_6 at doses of 500 mg daily has been demonstrated to be effective in the treatment of PMS. However, at this dose level, vitamin B_6 therapy may be associated with the onset of sensorineural deficits. Given the potentially serious side effects of high-dose vitamin B_6 therapy, its use is not recommended.

Bromocriptine is a dopamine agonist that is extremely effective in the treatment of hyperprolactinemia. The majority of controlled clinical trials do not suggest that it is of significant value in the treatment of PMS. If used in the treatment of PMS, it should probably be reserved for women with complaints isolated to the breast. It should be emphasized that pharmacologic therapy should not be an isolated intervention in the treatment of PMS. Drug therapy should be part of a comprehensive program of diet, exercise, and counseling therapy.

REFERENCES

1. Abraham GE: Nutritional factors in the etiology of the premenstrual tension syndromes, *J Reprod Med* 28:446, 1983.
2. Barbieri RL, Ryan KJ: Bromocriptine, endocrine pharmacology, and therapeutic applications, *Fertil Steril* 39:727, 1983.
3. Burgas R et al: Structure moleculair du facteur hypothalamique (LRF) d'origine ovine controlant la secretion de l'hormone gonadotrope hypophysaire de luteinisation (LH), *C R Acad Sci* 273:1611, 1971.
4. Catt KJ, Pierce JG: Gonadotropic hormones of the adenohypophysis. In Yen SSC, Jaffe RB, editors: *Reproductive endocrinology*, Philadelphia, 1986, WB Saunders.
5. Chan WY, Dawood MY, Fuchs F: Relief of dysmenorrhea with the prostaglandin synthetase inhibitor ibuprofen: effect of prostaglandin levels in menstrual fluid, *Am J Obstet Gynecol* 135:102, 1979.
6. Crowley WF et al: The physiology of gonadotropin-releasing hormone (GnRH) secretion in men and women, *Recent Prog Horm Res* 41:473, 1985.
7. Demura R et al: Human plasma free activin and inhibin levels during the menstrual cycle, *J Clin Endocrinol Metab* 76:1080, 1993.
8. DiZerga GS, Hodgen GD: Folliculogenesis in the primate ovarian cycle, *Endocr Rev* 2:27, 1981.
9. Dorrington JH, Armstrong DT: Effects of FSH on gonadal functions, *Recent Prog Horm Res* 35:301, 1979.
10. Erickson GF et al: Cyclic changes in insulin-like growth factor 4 messenger RNA in the rat ovary, *Endocrinology* 130:625, 1991.
11. Erickson GF et al: Localization of insulin-like binding protein-5 in rat ovaries during the estrous cycle, *Endocrinology* 130:1867, 1992.
12. Freeman EN et al: Evaluating premenstrual symptoms in medical practice, *Obstet Gynecol* 65:500, 1985.
13. Friedman AJ, Barbieri RL: Leuprolide acetate: applications in gynecology, *Curr Probl Obstet Gynecol Fertil* 6:209, 1988.
14. Fries H: Epidemiology of secondary amenorrhea, *Am J Obstet Gynecol* 118:473, 1974.
15. Giudice LC: Insulin-like growth factors and ovarian follicular development, *Endocr Rev* 13:641, 1991.
16. Goldstein DP et al: Laparoscopy in the diagnosis and management of pelvic pain in adolescents, *J Reprod Med* 24:251, 1980.
17. Greep RO: Gonadotropins. In McCann SM, editor: *Endocrinology, people and ideas*, Bethesda, Md, 1988, American Physiological Society.
18. Halberg L, Nilsson L: Determination of menstrual blood loss, *Scand J Clin Lab Invest* 16:244, 1964.
19. Harris GW: Humours and hormones: the Sir Henry Dale lecture for 1971, *J Endocrinol* 53:185-186, 1972.
20. Hitschmann F, Adler L: Der Bau der Uterusschleimhaut des geschlechtsreifen Weibes, mit besonderer Berücksichtigung der Menstruation, *Mschr Geburtsh Gynak* 27:1, 1908.
21. Hull MGR et al: The practical value of the progesterone challenge test in the assessment of the estrogen state and response to clomiphene in amenorrhea, *Br J Obstet Gynaecol* 86:799, 1979.
22. Joseph A, Thomas IM: Cytogenetic investigation in 150 cases with complaints of sterility or primary amenorrhea, *Hum Genet* 61:105, 1982.
23. Khoury SA et al: Diurnal patterns of pulsatile luteinizing hormone secretion in hypothalamic amenorrhea, *J Clin Endocrinol Metab* 64:755, 1987.
24. Knobil E: The neuroendocrine control of the menstrual cycle, *Recent Prog Horm Res* 36:53, 1980.
25. Koyama H: Cyclophosphamide-induced ovarian failure, *Cancer* 39:1403, 1977.
26. Kresch AJ et al: Laparoscopy in 100 women with chronic pelvic pain, *Obstet Gynecol* 64:672, 1984.
27. Landgren BM, Unden AL, Diczfalusy E: Hormonal profile of the cycle in 68 normally menstruating women, *Acta Endocrinol* 94:89, 1980.
28. Lightman A et al: The ovarian renin-angiotensin system, *Am J Obstet Gynecol* 156:808, 1987.
29. Maddocks S et al: A double-blind placebo-controlled trial of progesterone vaginal suppositories in the treatment of premenstrual syndrome, *Am J Obstet Gynecol* 154:573, 1986.
30. The Menstrual Cycle: In McCann SM, editor: *Endocrinology, people and ideas*, Bethesda, Md, 1988, American Physiological Society.
31. McCann SM, Rettori V: Physiology of luteinizing hormone-n-releasing hormone, *Semin Reprod Endocrinol* 5:33, 1987.
32. McNatty KP et al: The microenvironment of the human antral follicle, *J Clin Endocrinol Metab* 49:851, 1979.

33. Moore RY: Neuroendocrine mechanisms: cells and systems. In Yen SSC, Jaffe RB, editors: *Reproductive endocrinology*, Philadelphia, 1986, WB Saunders.
34. Muse KN et al: The premenstrual syndrome: the effects of "medical ovariectomy," *N Engl J Med* 311:1345, 1984.
35. Nakamura T et al: Activin-binding protein from rat ovary is follistatin, *Science* 247:836, 1990.
36. Noyes RW, Hertig AT, Rock J: Dating the endometrial biopsy, *Fertil Steril* 1:3, 1950.
37. Pettersson F, Fires H, Millius SJ: Epidemiology of secondary amenorrhea. I. Incidence and prevalence rates, *Am J Obstet Gynecol* 117:80, 1973.
38. Reid RL, Yen SSC: Premenstrual syndrome, *Am J Obstet Gynecol* 139:85, 1981.
39. Reindollar RH: Delayed sexual development: a study of 252 patients, *Am J Obstet Gynecol* 140:371, 1981.
40. Reindollar RH et al: Adult-onset amenorrhea: a study of 262 patients, *Am J Obstet Gynecol* 155:531, 1986.
41. Ross GT, Schreiber JR: The ovary. In Yen SSC, Jaffe RB, editors: *Reproductive endocrinology*, Philadelphia, 1986, WB Saunders.
42. Ryan KJ: Human ovarian function. In Sakamoto S, Tojo S, Nakayama T, editors: *Gynecology and obstetrics*, Proceedings of the IX World Congress of Gynecology and Obstetrics, Amsterdam, 1980, Excepta Medica.
43. Ryan KJ: The endocrine pattern and control of the ovulatory cycle. In Insler V, Lunenfeld B, editors: *Infertility: male and female*, New York, 1986, Churchill Livingstone.
44. Ryan KJ: Endocrine function of the ovary. In McCann SM, editor: *Endocrinology, people and ideas*, Bethesda, Md, 1988, American Physiological Society.
45. Ryan KJ, Makris A: Significance of angiogenic and growth factors in ovarian follicular development. In Mahesh VB et al editors: *Regulation of ovarian and testicular function*, New York, 1987, Plenum Press.
46. Ryan KJ, Petro Z, Kaiser J: Steroid formation by isolated and recombined ovarian granulosa and thecal cells, *J Clin Endocrinol Metab* 28:355, 1968.
47. Ryan KJ, Smith OW: Biogenesis of steroid hormones in the human ovary, *Recent Prog Horm Res* 21:367, 1965.
48. Savard K, Marsh JM, Rice BF: Gonadotropins and ovarian steroidogenesis, *Recent Prog Horm Res* 21:285, 1965.
49. Sawyer CH: Anterior pituitary neural control concepts. In McCann SM, editor: *Endocrinology, people and ideas*, Bethesda Md, 1988, American Physiological Society.
50. Schally AV et al: Gonadotropin-releasing hormone: one polypeptide regulates secretion of luteinizing and follicle-stimulating hormones, *Science* 173:1036, 1971.
51. Shimasaki S et al: Structural characterization of a follicle-stimulating hormone action inhibitor in porcine ovarian follicular fluid, *J Biol Chem* 265:2198, 1990.
52. Soules MR et al: Luteal phase deficiency characterization of reproductive hormones over the menstrual cycle, *J Clin Endocrinol Metab* 69.804, 1989.
53. Treloar AE et al: Variations of the human menstrual cycle through reproductive life, *Int J Fertil* 12:77, 1967.
54. Tureck RW, Strauss JF III: Progesterone synthesis by luteinized human granulosa cells in culture: the role of de novo sterol synthesis and lipoprotein-carried sterol, *J Clin Endocrinol Metab* 54:367, 1982.
55. Waldstreicher J et al: Hyperfunction of the hypothalamic-pituitary axis in women with polycystic ovarian disease, *J Clin Endocrinol Metab* 66:165, 1988.
56. Weiss G et al: Secretion of progesterone and relaxin by the human corpus luteum in midpregnancy and at term, *Obstet Gynecol* 50:679, 1977.
57. Wood SH et al: Treatment of premenstrual syndrome with fluoxetine: a double blind, placebo controlled, crossover study, *Obstet Gynecol* 80:339, 1991.
58. Yen SSC: Neuroendocrine control of hypophyseal function. In Yen SSC, Jaffe RB, editors: *Reproductive endocrinology*, Philadelphia, 1986, WB Saunders.
59. Ylikorkala O, Dawood MY: New concepts in dysmenorrhea, *Am J Obstet Gynecol* 130:833, 1978.
60. Zhou J, Bondy C: Anatomy of the human ovarian insulin-like growth factor system, *Biol Reprod* 48:467, 1993.

Chapter 4

THE VULVA

Frederick H. Sillman
Michael G. Muto

GENERAL CONSIDERATIONS

The vulva and external genitalia include the mons, labia majora and minora, clitoris, vestibule, and urethral meatus. The vulva covers and protects the entrance to the vagina, vestibule, and urethra.

Since the vulva is covered with skin, any skin disease can occur there. Its location and nature also make vulvar skin unique. Its *location* subjects it to warmth, friction, less aeration, more moisture (vulvar secretions and sweat, vaginal discharge, urine), and feces. Its dependence makes it more susceptible to edema and stasis. By *nature* it is more penetrable and sensitive than any other skin.[85] It can dehydrate easily and absorb substances more readily. It is vulnerable to maceration and loss of integrity, which can compound vulvar pathology. Medial parts have less or no protective keratin. For all these reasons the vulva is predisposed to numerous systemic and general skin diseases and in addition it is prone to infection from sexually transmitted diseases.

Vulvar hygiene is an important part of the care and cure of many diseases and syndromes. Basic hygiene includes the following: use of a mild, nondrying soap washing underwear with mild soap and rinsing well; wearing white, 100% cotton underwear, cotton skirts and dresses; and avoiding extra layers and tight slacks, all possible reactive substances (unneeded medicines, tinted toilet tissue, all "feminine hygiene" products), excessive sweating without aeration, and public pools and hot tubs. It is important to be keenly conscious of what "aggravates" vulvar skin. A dermatologic cliché is to "dry wet lesions" (soaks and compresses) and "moisturize dry lesions" (creams and ointments). Ointments are longer lasting and therefore penetrate thick plaques better. Lotions contain alcohol, which dries the skin, and generally should be avoided. After diagnosis, the prime disease as well as any compounding infection or other pathology should be treated aggressively.

Vulvar diagnoses are often delayed because of patient procrastination and embarrassment, professional omission or neglect, and medication before a correct diagnosis is made. Delay in diagnosis can influence infectious morbidity and malignant mortality. Accurate diagnosis begins with a thorough history to determine the nature, site, and duration of specific complaints, as well as general symptoms and problems. Inquiry should be made about discharge, diarrhea, topical contacts of any kind, medications, contraceptives, sexual practices, clothing, and stress or anxiety. Examination should include: oral mucosa, scalp, skin, nails, and pubic hair. It is not sufficient to allay symptoms temporarily. The cause of the disorder should be found and specific therapy instituted.

Magnification is helpful in evaluating contours (ulcers or exophytic growths) and vessels. Vessels are not as easily visualized through keratinized epithelium, but Iverson found abnormal vessels in 58% of patients with vulvar carcinoma in situ. In addition to enhancing one's choice for biopsy, magnification can be helpful in assessing lesions not requiring biopsy (e.g., the nature and shape of ulcers or finding parasites or nits). Dermatologists favor 2 to 4 fold magnification with a large illuminated lens. Gynecologists magnify 7.5 to 14 fold with a colposcope ("vulvoscope").

ANATOMY AND HISTOLOGY

Mons pubis

The mons consists of an accumulation of subcutaneous fat in a rounded pad overlying the symphysis pubis. The fat pad characteristically remains even after marked weight loss. It is covered by pubic hair and the skin is similar to that of the labia majora. The typical female escutcheon of hair over the mons is triangular and usually does not extend upward along the abdomen, although there is much variation depending on racial and familial traits.

Labia majora

The labia majora (and mons) form the outer extent of the external genitalia. The vulvar folds continue cephalad toward the lower abdomen and fuse in the midline as the mons pubis or anterior commissure. The union of the labia majora caudally is the posterior commissure and the posterior extent of the vulva (Fig. 4-1).

The covering skin contains many sebaceous, apocrine, and sweat (eccrine) glands and is covered with hair lateral to the pilosebaceous line along the crest. The pronounced glandular and adnexal development accounts for the frequency of sebaceous cysts and hair follicle infections. On the inner aspect of the labia majora, the sebaceous glands empty directly onto the skin surface and are less numerous. The skin is made up of stratified squamous epithelium with moderate keratosis and a well-vascularized dermis. Involuntary muscle fibers or dartos are present but are much less developed than in the scrotum. A large amount of fatty tissue is usually present in lobules, separated by elastic and connective tissue fibers. This elastic connective tissue forms a well-defined sac with an anterior inner opening medial to the inguinal region. This opening is where the round ligament enters the labium, its fibers dispersing into the fibroelastic sac. The round ligament is the embryologic analog of the male gubernaculum.

The blood supply of the labia majora is derived from the internal pudendal artery through the posterior labial branch and from a small branch of the obturator artery. The veins have approximately the same source but also communicate with the vesicovaginal plexus and the inferior hemorrhoidal veins.

The nerve supply is from multiple sources. The pudendal nerve, derived from the second to fourth sacral nerves, gives off the perineal branch from which the posterior labial nerve arises. The latter innervates the labia majora and the lateral portion of the urethral triangle. There is adjunctive innervation from the ilioinguinal, internal branch of the genitocrural and the genital branch of the lesser sciatic (posterior femoral cutaneous) nerves (Fig. 4-2).

Labia minora

The labia minora consist of two medial folds approximate to each other with a convex free border. They extend from the prepuce and frenulum of the clitoris to join the labia majora posteriorly as they terminate in the posterior fourchette. Between this fourchette and the hymenal ring is a curved depression, the fossa navicularis (Fig. 4-1). The

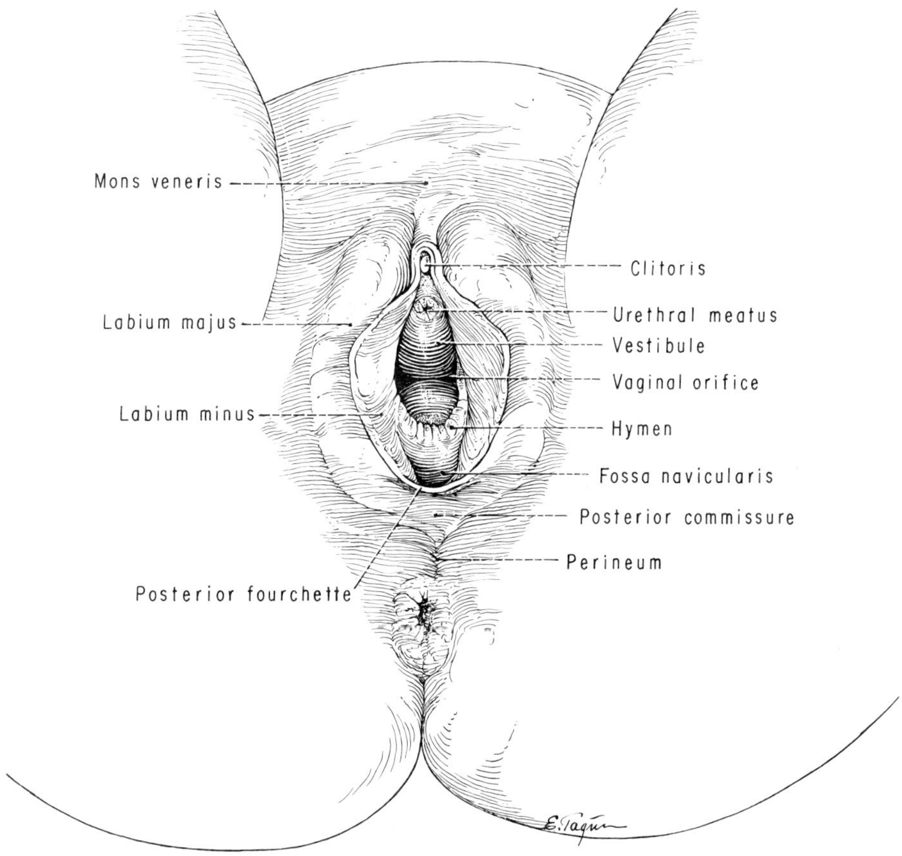

Fig. 4-1. External genitalia of the female.

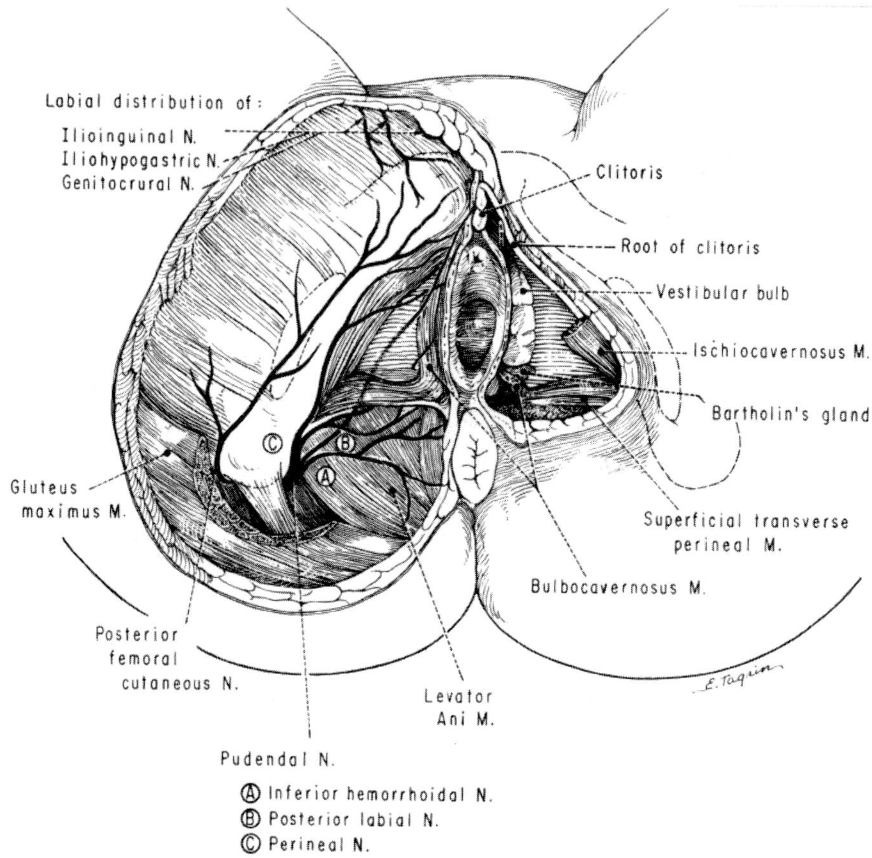

Fig. 4-2. The nerve supply of the vulva is represented at left. At right, the ischiocavernosus and bulbocavernosus muscles have been reflected to show the anatomy of the clitoris and vestibular bulbs.

labia minora are reduplications of skin and not mucosa. Although some pathologists have called the labia minora and vagina "mucous membranes", mucus is not secreted from the epithelium of either the vagina or the labia minora.

The skin of the labia minora contains abundant pigment and blood vessels. Microscopically the stratified squamous epithelium is characterized by minimal keratinization but the rete ridges are numerous and prominent. Subcutaneously there is connective tissue with numerous bundles of elastic fibers and blood vessels and wisps of smooth muscle but little fat. Sweat glands are sparse and hair follicles are absent but sebaceous glands are abundant, especially laterally. The blood supply is derived from the labial vessels and from the dorsal artery to the clitoris, which is a terminal branch of the internal pudendal artery. The nerve supply is the same as that of the labia majora. Immediately preceding and during coitus the labia become moist and lubricated with secretions from vestibular and sebaceous glands.

The labia minora have specific importance in the process of urination. Following vulvectomy, uncontrolled "spraying" is common.

Clitoris

The clitoris is composed of two roots that traverse the pubic rami to unite posterior to the symphysis in the clitoral body. The body terminates in the upper portion of the vestibule as the glans. The roots and body are covered by overlying muscle but the glans is exposed. Fig. 4-2 illustrates the relationship of the root of the clitoris to the overlying ischiocavernosus muscle. The roots, or crura, are 3 to 4 cm long in the flaccid state but in erection are 4.5 to 5.0 cm long. The body is 2.5 to 3.0 cm long and is surrounded by a connective tissue capsule of fibroelastic tissue termed the clitoridean fascia. Unlike the penis, the clitoris contains no corpus spongiosum and does not possess as much erectile tissue.

The function of the clitoris is that of a sexual "nerve center." Before contact, sexual stimulation causes vascular engorgement and enlargement, so that when the penis is inserted the clitoris becomes particularly sensitive to the motion of the shaft. Orgasm in the female may be brought about by this stimulation even in the absence of the vagina and consists of an interrelated reflex resulting in forceful contractions of voluntary and involuntary musculature of the pelvis and pelvic viscera. After orgasm has been experienced and a conditioned reflex established, the presence of the clitoris is not absolutely necessary. Women who have had vulvectomy with excision of the clitoris are capable of experiencing orgasm. However, major sexual problems are common, as they are with women who have undergone "female circumcision."

The arteries of the clitoris arise from the internal pudendal. The veins correspond to the arteries except for the large dorsal vein of the clitoris, which runs beneath the arcuate ligament of the symphysis through a small notch and communicates with the pelvic veins.

The most common abnormality of the clitoris is enlargement. This can occur idiopathically or from excess androgens (e.g., with adrenal hyperplasia or neoplasia; or Sertoli-Leydig cell tumor or hilus cell tumor of the ovary).

Vestibule

The vestibule (introitus) is an elliptical space situated just inside the labia minora. It extends from the frenulum to the posterior fourchette. The epithelium is not pigmented nor keratinized. The urethra, vagina, and eccrine gland ducts open into the vestibule. Mucus-secreting, minor vestibular glands also empty into the vestibule, mostly posteriorly, as do the ducts of the major vestibular glands of Bartholin and Skene.[132]

Bartholin's glands and ducts

Bartholin's glands are the homolog of bulbourethral glands in the male. They secrete mucus, particularly during sexual stimulation. Situated at each side of the vaginal orifice, distal to the hymen, the glands are normally small and can be palpated only in rather thin women or if enlarged by inflammation or tumor. The duct openings are in the posterolateral introitus at 5 and 7 o'clock. Rapid growth occurs at puberty and shrinkage occurs after menopause. Microscopically the glands are racemose and show a single layer of high columnar epithelium in the alveoli. The ducts are lined by transitional epithelium except for a short invagination of stratified squamous epithelium at the orifice.

Skene's periurethral glands and ducts

The periurethral ducts are the external orifices of the Skene's glands that are situated beneath the urethral floor. The duct orifices are small, usually grossly visible crypts just lateral and posterior to the urethral meatus. The glands arise from the urethral mucosa and are histologically similar. They are the rudimentary homolog of the prostate gland and are commonly invaded by lower genital organisms, such as the gonococcus. When the glands are infected, pus may be expressed from the openings. Skene's and Bartholin's ducts can harbor other infectious agents, such as human papilloma virus (HPV), making eradication difficult, since good regional and systemic therapies do not yet exist.

Vestibular bulbs

Vestibular bulbs correspond to the corpus spongiosum of the male and consist of truncated masses of erectile tissue on either side of the vaginal orifice. They are situated above the inferior fascia of the pelvic diaphragm and below the bulbocavernosus muscles (Fig. 4-2). The anterior ends taper to join the bulb of the opposite side in the pars intermedia. The posterior ends are in contact with Bartholin's glands.

Hymen

The hymen is an irregular membranous fold of varying thickness that partially occludes the vaginal orifice. It extends from the floor of the urethra to the fossa navicularis and may be complete (imperforate), absent, incomplete, or cribriform. The hymen may be avulsed by examination, trauma, surgery, or coitus. Usually irregular remnants persist, which form a fleshy fringe about the vaginal opening (the carunculae multiformes) (Fig. 4-1).

The hymen can be involved in developmental defects, often unnoticed until menarche or later. An imperforate hymen is usually noticed at menarche when menstrual blood accumulates behind the membrane with resultant hematocolpos and hematometra. Blood may rarely be forced into the peritoneal cavity, which gives rise to peritoneal signs and symptoms and later, endometriosis. The diagnosis is usually obvious by inspection—there is a bluish, bulging membrane presenting at the introitus (Fig. 4-3). Rectal examination will reveal a distended vagina and an enlarged uterus. This condition should be treated in the operating room by a generous cruciate incision or by excision of a portion of the hymen.

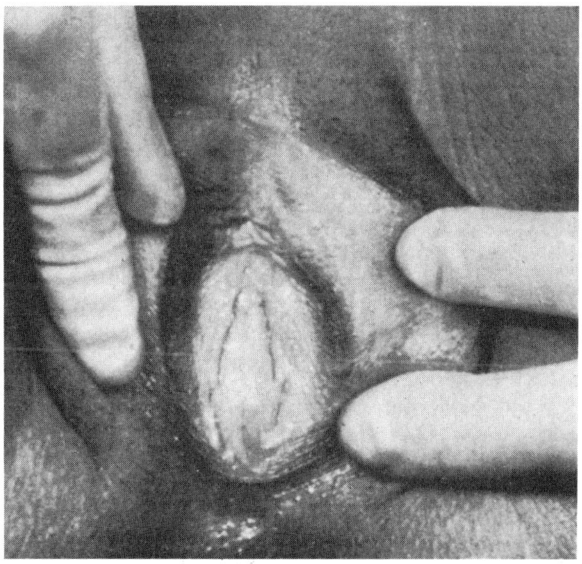

Fig. 4-3. Imperforate hymen.

A rigid hymen can cause dyspareunia. This may be due to the presence of an excess amount of tough, fibrous tissue or to the presence of multiple small orifices, none of which is large enough to admit the penis. If not helped by gradual dilatation, surgical correction is indicated. A hymenectomy is a simple procedure and the results are immediate and permanent.

Urethra

The urethral meatus is just inferior to the clitoris and may be visualized by separating the labia minora. It has a cleft-like appearance with slightly raised lateral margins and is the uppermost structure of the vestibule (Fig. 4-1).

Malformations of the urethra include stenosis, diverticula, and hypospadias. Mild degrees of stenosis are fairly common and usually cause no symptoms. In some patients there may be tenesmus and recurrent cystitis from urinary retention. Urethral dilation and treatment of the cystitis are attended by marked relief. Diverticula result from incomplete development of the urethrovaginal septum. There may be single or multiple outpouchings of the urethra along its inferior surface but without connection with the vagina. The diagnosis is made by expressing urine or pus by firm pressure on the diverticulum. Treatment is surgical excision.

INJURIES

Accidental injuries

Accidental injuries to the vulva may be from blunt or penetrating trauma. Such injuries are most common in the young and frequently result from straddle injuries. Such blows may rupture venous plexi, the vestibular bulb, or vulvar varicosities. Bleeding may result in small contusions or massive, life threatening vulvar and retroperitoneal hematomas.

As in the evaluation of any traumatic injury, the clinician should make every attempt to accurately reconstruct the accident to anticipate the possible extent of injury. For example, a vulvar hematoma resulting from riding a mechanical bull is caused by shearing forces of the labial fat against the underlying pubic bone. Tears in the periclitoral veins and superficial venous plexi can be anticipated in such an injury. On the other hand, a fall on to a tree limb or picket fence may result in both superficial and penetrating injury with arterial bleeding. High speed impact, reported in water skiing accidents, may result in pelvic fractures. When the patient is unable to report the nature of the accident, witnesses should be sought.

After determining the mechanism of injury, the physician must assess the extent. If a hematoma is present, the volume of blood contained within it should be estimated and serial examinations performed to determine if it is expanding. Small contusions are best treated with the application of cold compresses. Large hematomas, particularly those that are expanding or are associated with hypotension, should be evacuated and packed so as to control bleeding, reduce the risk of infection, and limit pressure necrosis of the overlying skin. Broad spectrum antibiotics are indicated. A Foley catheter or suprapubic tube may be required if the urethra is injured or obstructed. Careful inspection of the urethra, clitoris, vagina, perineum and anus should be performed to rule out perforating injuries. An inadequate examination of the patient while awake requires another examination under anesthesia.

Continued blood loss which is not apparent, may herald the formation of an expanding retroperitoneal hematoma. An abdominal-pelvic computed tomography (CT) scan may help detect and manage such hematomas. Injuries to the urinary tract may require gravity cystography, intravenous pyelography, or cystoscopy. Finally, in cases of high speed or violent injury, pelvic bone fractures must be ruled out.

Coital injuries

Hymeneal lacerations at the coitarche are usually minor, but may occasionally result in massive bleeding. Lacerations caused by forced entry, such as too vigorous sexual activity, rape, or sexual molestation may be far more extensive. A complete discussion of coital injuries in the young is presented in Chapter 23. As is the case with accidental injuries, a meticulous examination to assess the extent of the injury is essential. When dealing with the consequences of traumatic sexual acts, the physician must demonstrate extraordinary sensitivity and tact. If sex was consensual, the patient and her partner may be deeply embarrassed by the injury and withhold information vital to rendering appropriate care; if sexual molestation or rape is suspected, the physician must also pay strict attention to the collection of evidence as outlined in the institution's rape protocol. When dealing with self-inflicted injuries, psychiatric counseling should be obtained to establish whether the patient is a threat to herself or others.

INFECTIONS AND SEXUAL DISEASES

Syphilis, gonorrhea, herpes, and acquired immune deficiency syndrome (AIDS) are covered in detail in Chapter 21. Human papillomavirus (HPV) is covered in detail in Chapter 6. Infections that are primarily vaginal are covered in Chapter 5. This chapter focuses on infections as they pertain to the vulva.

General principles are as follows:

1. Any persistent lesion should be evaluated for its infectious and/or neoplastic etiology.
2. One sexually transmitted disease places the patient at higher risk for others; therefore, as indicated, other diseases should be tested for by wet or stained smears, cultures (especially chlamydia and gonorrhea), serologies (hepatitis B, herpes, HIV, syphilis), cytology and biopsies. The presence of one disease, especially if superficial injury is induced, can facilitate the "take" of another agent in the region, as has been suggested for HPV and HIV inoculations.

3. Any endophytic or ulcerative lesion should possibly be cultured for herpes, examined with dark field, and a biopsy should be performed. A biopsy should also be performed on any exophytic lesion unless it is an obvious condyloma or papilloma.
4. The public health is best served when partners are diagnosed and treated. There are lessons to be learned from increases in drug-resistant syphilis, tuberculosis, and the spread of AIDS.

Condyloma acuminata

Anogenital HPV and oncogenesis will be discussed in Chapter 6. This section focuses on the diagnosis and treatment of vulvar condyloma acuminata. HPV is the most prevalent and one of the most contagious genital infections, with about 40 million men and women infected and at least 1 million new infections per year in the United States.[92] These figures may be a conservative estimate because most infected individuals are asymptomatic and do not have condylomas.

Vulvar condylomas (Fig. 4-4) are part of a regional anogenital infection that must be diagnosed and treated as such. This means that patients presenting with vulvar "condylomas" require the following:

1. A definitive diagnosis (i.e., not treat undiagnosed neoplasia with medicines or destruction) (Fig. 4-5). "Typical" vulvar condylomas do not require a histologic diagnosis initially, but biopsies should be liberally done if there is any colposcopic variation from the "typical" acuminate condyloma, or the rounded, older papilloma, or if lesions persist more than two months despite treatment (Fig. 4-5).
2. The entire lower genital-anal tract should be colposcoped for occult HPV or neoplasia.
3. Other sexual diseases should be tested for (as per above). There is the belief that other infections, especially trichomonas, can enhance condylomas, possibly by creating microtrauma or other mechanisms.

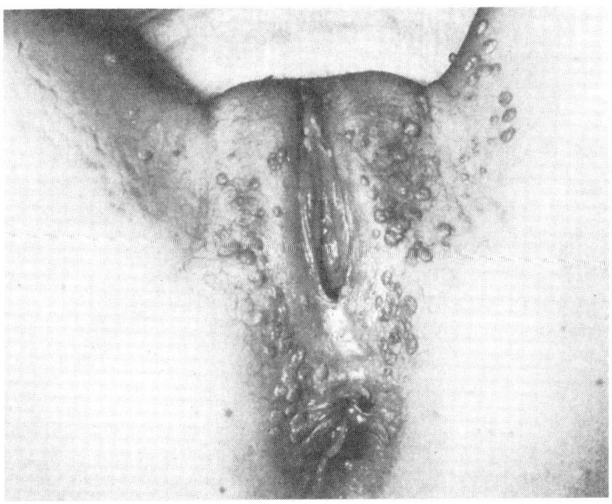

Fig. 4-4. Condylomata acuminata.

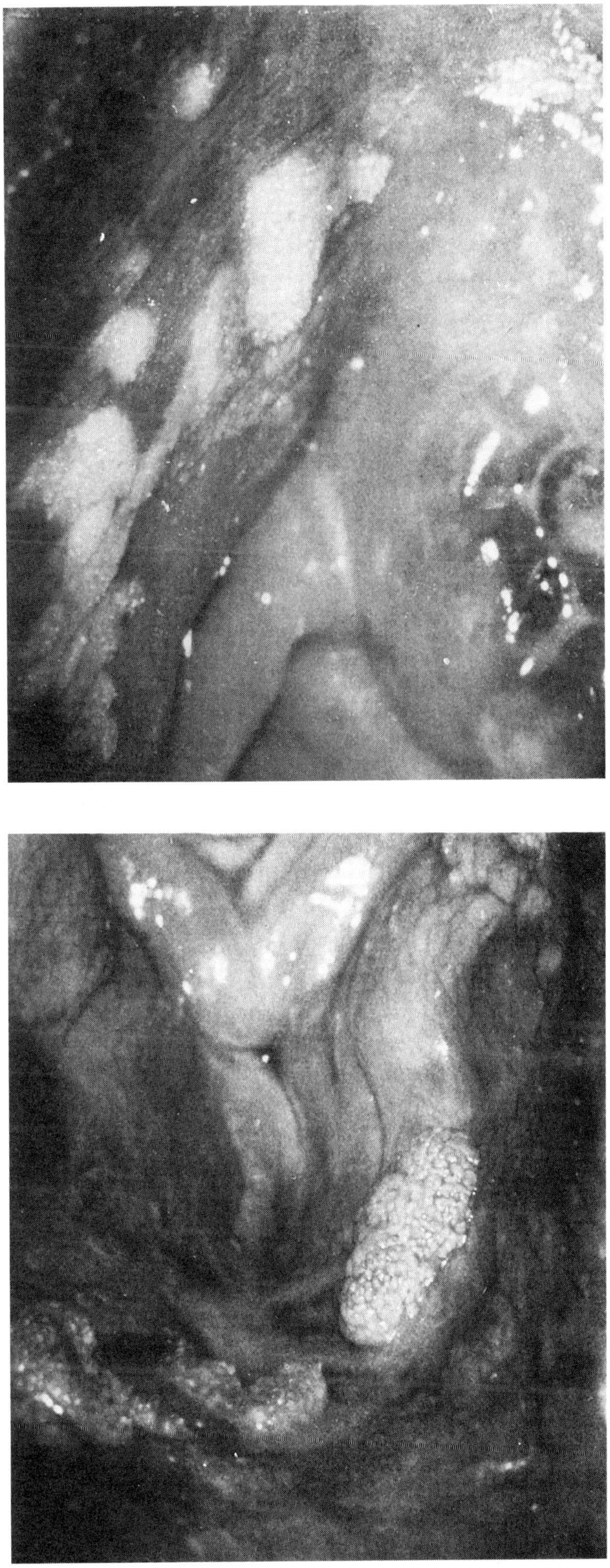

A

B

Fig. 4-5. A, HPV only at 11 o'clock. **B,** Moderate "warty" dysplasia at 5 o'clock. (From Sillman FH: *Obstet Gynecol* 58:356, 1981, and Sillman, FH: *Obstet Gynecol Clin North Am* 14:537, 1987.)

Treatment. The present missing piece is the lack of an antivirotic that will rid the patient's anogenital tract of HPV. Therefore current goals are: remove macroscopic condylomas within 6 months; reduce the patient's viral "load"; monitor for persistence, recurrence or neoplasia.

Treatment is guided by location, size, and whether condylomas are primary, persistent, or recurrent. Although 80% of vulvar condylomas are HPV types 6 or 11, the clinical usefulness of viral typing is still being investigated. Single or combination therapy might be the best for an individual patient. *Medical treatments* include: podophyllin 25% or the pure, 0.5%, self administered podofilox; bichloracetic acid; topical 5-fluorouracil (5-FU); interferon (IF); and liquid nitrogen. *Surgical options* are: removal with knife, scissors, chemosurgery, electrosurgery, ultrasonic aspirator, or laser. Treatments not recommended are: 25% podophyllin, cryosurgery, and IF. Podophyllin 25% is potentially toxic and achieves less than 50% remission.[92] Cryosurgery is not precise and condylomas are located only in the superficial epidermis. IF is health professional intensive for frequent injections, has unpleasant symptoms, and offers no special, redeeming therapeutic advantage.[98]

The surgical choices favored by the authors are laser and chemosurgery. *Laser* is so precise that when properly done there is minimal stromal injury.[93-95] *Chemosurgery* is pretreatment with topical 5-FU and then low power electrosurgical epidermal removal. Chemosurgery is virtually fail-safe from stromal injury (see section on Vulvar Intraepithelial Neoplasia). Condylomas rarely "invade" subepithelial sanctuaries,[30,93] therefore only epidermal depth should be required. Avoiding stromal injury is important because condylomas tend to recur in about 30% of patients and a surgical mode, without cumulative morbidity, is preferable.

Persistent or recurrent condylomas are challenging and the need for an effective systemic antivirotic is clear. Until one is discovered, the best regional therapy is topical 5-FU. Topical 5-FU is well tolerated if care is taken to avoid overdosing, which can result in painful chemoinflammation. Mild chemoinflammation cannot always be avoided and this risk must be acceptable to patient and physician, or 5-FU should not be used. Preoperative and postoperative 5-FU is a useful surgical adjunct for persistent or recurrent condylomas.[65] Because it appears that pregnancy and oral contraceptives may cause condylomas to proliferate, oral contraceptives should be discontinued and barrier methods used. During pregnancy, chloracetic acid (applied with a tuberculin syringe during vulvoscopy) and laser treatment can be used safely for debulking condylomas. While liberal serologic surveys and other tests are recommended initially, HIV testing is especially encouraged with persistent or recurrent condylomas.

The evaluation of partners is controversial. Past and present partners are probably infected and should have penoscopy if any macroscopic or palpable lesions are noted, or if the patient and partner want screening. Partners are also at higher risk for other sexual diseases. Patients should be encouraged to discuss their HPV infection with future partners and condom use should be encouraged.

Fungal infections

The vulvovaginal area harbors numerous fungi. Normal floral balance and cellular immunity maintain a healthy homeostasis. Lowered resistance, increased heat, friction and/or excessive perspiration can upset the normal balance and fungi may become pathogens. Predisposing causes are pregnancy, oral contraceptives, broad spectrum antibiotics, diabetes and other chronic diseases, and immunosuppression. These should be investigated when a fungal infection is diagnosed. The initial nidus is often the vagina, especially during the estrogenated, reproductive years, and the gastrointestinal tract. Occasionally, adjacent intertrigo or the vulva itself can be the initial site. The most common forms are candida and tinea.

Candida. Nine fungi have been found to cause mycotic vulvitis. The most common normal and pathogenic type is *albicans* (Monilia), which causes 66% to 75% of vulvovaginal fungal infections.[55] Infection can begin as an erythema or a reddish papule, which later becomes vesicular or pustular. After these rupture, a moist, red membrane remains. Secondary infection is common, and the vagina and vulva can become markedly edematous and tender. The vulva may be covered with a tenacious gray-white frosting (Fig. 4-6), or there may be marked inflammation due in part to repetitive scratching. The most common symptom is intense pruritus. A white, curdlike vaginal discharge may develop as the infection becomes more severe. If chafing occurs, a secondary dermatitis of the

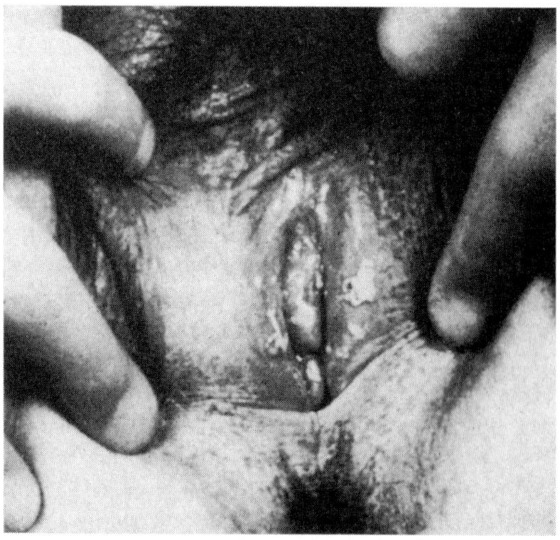

Fig. 4-6. Candidiasis of vulva.

thighs may also be present. Intercourse may be painful or impossible because of swelling, abrasion, and inflammation. Walking may be uncomfortable because of chafing.

In some patients these characteristics of *Candida* infection are so obvious that they may be identified by inspection alone. In older patients with the early stages of infection or when secondary bacterial infection is present, diagnosis is more difficult.

Diagnosis is made by seeing "budding" hyphae on wet smear, Gram stain, or culture. A dark brown or black growth occurs on Nickerson's medium in about 48 hours if *Candida* organisms are present.

Treatment. Imidazole (clotrimazole and others) creams and suppositories are effective and should be used in the vagina and on the vulva. Cool sitz baths help relieve pruritus and irritation. Hydroxyzine taken at bedtime is helpful for pruritus-induced insomnia. In patients with persistent or recurrent infections, systemic disease should be ruled out and substitution made for oral contraceptives. The patient and partner should be cultured for specific fungus and appropriate treatment instituted. A broader spectrum triazole (terconazole) might be in order.[124] Short courses of a prophylactic, postmenstrual antifungal agent might help. The gastrointestinal tract is a ready source, therefore oral nystatin (or ketoconazole) may also be added. In these patients a culture test of cure should be taken two weeks after therapy.

Tinea. Dermatophytes grow on dead, superficial, keratinized layers of the skin.[41] Tinea is well known to many parts of the body (e.g., tinea capitis, tinea corporis [ring worm], tinea pedis [athlete's foot], tinea cruris [jock itch] occurs more commonly in males).[60]

Tinea cruris is usually caused by *Epidermophyton floccosum* (or *Trichophyton rubrum*). It is characterized by superficial, pale-pink to bright-red lesions with well-defined scaly borders. Central clearing led to the term "ring worm." By a process of coalescence, the vulvar skin, thighs and pubis may become involved. Following periods of scratching or maceration, the process may resemble a "weeping" type of eczema.

Diagnosis is made by KOH, microscopic examination of scrapings showing nonbudding hyphae (spores are not seen), Gram stain, or culture on Sabouraud's maltose agar.[60] In office practice, scrapings planted on dermatophyte test medium will result in colonies that change color from yellow to red. This is in contrast *to Candida* in which color change is rare.

Treatment is with a topical imidazole and aeration to reduce warmth and humidity. For chronic, intractable tinea, after reevaluating for predisposing causes, systemic griseofulvin or ketoconazole may be a needed adjunct.

Intertrigo. This diagnosis is arrived at after excluding the following: a primary fungal infection, contact dermatitis, eczema, psoriasis, and seborrheic dermatitis. It can result from maceration in folds, where drying and corticoids can help, or it can have a superimposed fungal (or other) infection. Its clearance requires keeping the area clean and dry, and the diagnosis and treatment of fungal infection if present.

Parasites

Scabies. Millions of people are infected each year with the female itch mite, *Sarcoptes scabiei.*[28] Transmission is by close but not necessarily sexual contact. Pruritus begins about one month after initial infection. Examination reveals papular lesions on the hands, wrists, and other joints, axillae, nipples, and umbilicus, in addition to the pubis. Pruritus may be intense, and is usually nocturnal. The neck and head are seldom involved.

Diagnosis is made by finding light-gray, thread-like burrows (magnification is helpful) and obtaining eggs or a mite (dark spot at end of burrow) with a needle for microscopic examination of an oil preparation.

Treatment begins with rubbing the scabicide permethrin (or lindane) into the skin and under the fingernails. Bathe after 12 hours and change and decontaminate bedding, towels, and clothing daily until remission. Repeat medication in one week. Severe dermatitis should be treated with soothing baths, lotions, and if secondarily infected, with topical antibiotics, oral erythromycin, or dicloxacillin. Sexual partners and close contacts (including pets) should be examined and treated.[29]

Pediculosis pubis. The pubic louse (*Phthirius pubis*) infects over 1 million people each year in the United States. It pierces the skin and the "saliva" can produce a severe, allergic pruritus and erythema.[10] The disease is most easily spread by coitus, but can be spread by any contact, towels, or bedding.

Diagnosis is made by removing a hair carrying an egg-filled nit or capturing a crab-shaped ectoparasite and examining it microscopically.

Treatment is permethrin (or lindane) and should include sexual partners.[29]

Other infections

Chancroid. Chancroid is caused by *Hemophilus ducreyi*. Approximately 4000 patients are infected each year in the United States.[28] More men than women are infected (7:1) because of transmission mainly by prostitutes. The incubation period is 4 to 10 days. Infection begins as a papule which soon becomes a painful, nonindurated ("soft") ulcer, with irregular, undermined, red edges and a necrotic base, best seen with a vulvoscope. The ulcers are deeper and wider than those of syphilis and herpes. One third to one half of patients have multiple ulcers.[34,60,102]

Diagnosis is usually made clinically. Gram stain can be helpful, but the characteristic "school of fish" arrangement of the gram-negative bacilli is not specific. The organisms may be cultured from ulcers or aspirate from infected nodes. However, growth is difficult. There is no clinical serologic test. Exclusion of herpes and syphilis is supportive of the diagnosis. However, 20% of patients with chancroid have syphilis, herpes, or HIV.

Treatment is oral azithromycin 1 gm or erythromycin 500 mg for a week, or 250 mg of ceftriaxone intramuscularly. Sexual partners should be treated.[29]

Lymphogranuloma venereum. Lymphogranuloma venereum (LGV) is caused by *Chlamydia trachomatis*. It is found mainly in the tropics and there are only about 500 cases diagnosed in the United States each year.[28] Inoculation occurs only through disrupted epithelium.[34,60] After an incubation period of up to 4 weeks, a genital papule appears followed by a small ulcer that is present for only a few days and may be asymptomatic with spontaneous healing. About 2 weeks later, following prodromal systemic symptoms of fever and malaise, the infection takes hold in the principal site—the lymph nodes. Painful, suppurative, inguinal adenitis develops with subsequent necrosis, abscess formation (buboes), and later, ulcerations and draining sinuses. Fibrous bands, including Poupart's ligament, indent the buboes and form the characteristic genital-inguinal "grooves". Fibrosis and scarring are late manifestations, and lymphatic obstruction can result in marked edema of the vulva. Lymphatic extension to adjacent organs may produce abscesses around and strictures of the urethra, anus, and rectum. The late disfigurement and destruction of infected structures may raise a question of suppurative hidradenitis or Crohn's disease. Both of the latter spare the labia minora.

Diagnosis is usually made clinically and with a complement fixation test. Culture from aspirated buboes and an immunofluorescent test with monoclonal antibodies are available in certain laboratories. In the presence of hard, enlarged lymph nodes it is important to rule out carcinoma and lymphoma.

Treatment includes local cleansing. Buboes should be aspirated; incising promotes chronic fistula formation. Tetracyclines should be given for at least 3 weeks and until remission. In the chronic state, antibiotics are less effective. For severe deformities, vulvectomy or colostomy may be necessary.

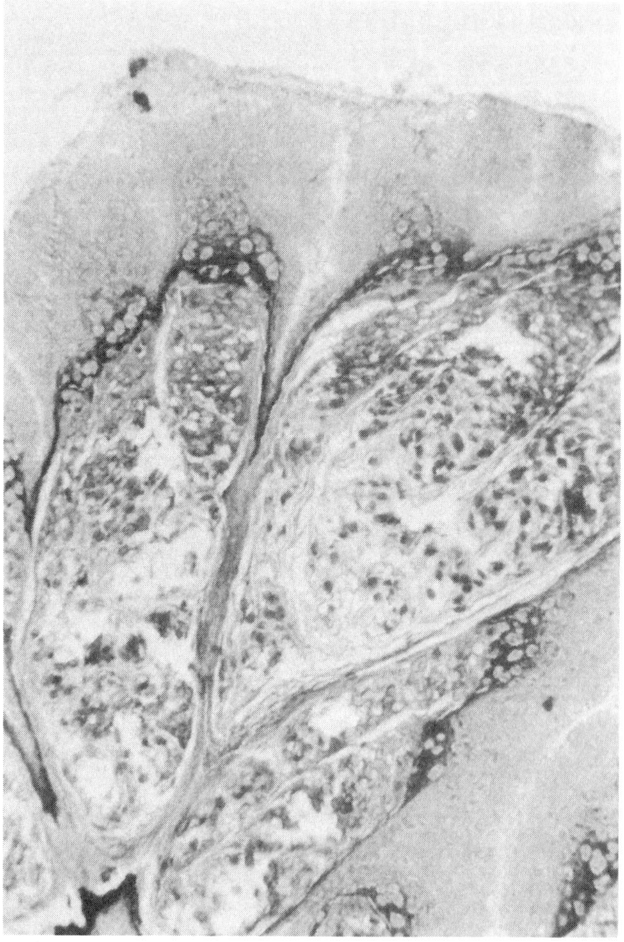

Fig. 4-8. Molluscum contagiosum with molluscum body.

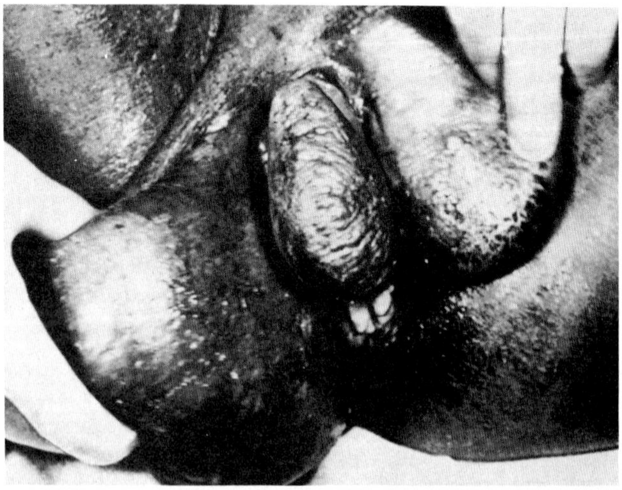

Fig. 4-7. Severe edema and vulvar distortion resulting from granuloma inguinale.

Granuloma inguinale. Granuloma inguinale is a chronic granulomatous, mainly tropical disease rarely found in the United States (less than 50 cases per year).[28] The etiologic agent is *Calymmatobacteria* (Donovania) *granulomatis*. The incubation period is 2 to 12 weeks. Transmission can occur non-sexually. The disease begins as a small, painless papule that gradually becomes a serpiginous, red, raised, irregular, velvety, friable ulcer. If not treated, subcutaneous granulomas and other ulcers develop, which become secondarily infected. Infections and granulomas can ultimately lead to scarring, edema, and tissue destruction (Fig. 4-7).[60] The carcinogenic potential of granuloma inguinale is still in doubt.

Diagnosis is established by finding Donovan bodies—groups of bacilli—in Wright stains of scrapings or biopsy.

Treatment is 1 gram of tetracycline daily for at least 2 weeks until healing occurs. Occasionally, late, marked edema and damage necessitates a vulvectomy.

Molluscum. *Molluscum contagiosum* is a pox virus that has an incubation period of about 1 month. Infection can occur from nonsexual contact. This rare, usually asymptomatic, sometimes pruritic infection is seen with increasing frequency because of AIDS and the increasing use of immunosuppressive drugs for certain diseases and transplantations. Because the lesions are asymptomatic and amorbid, national statistics are not kept.

The typical lesions are small (2 to 5 mm), dome-shaped, waxy, flesh-colored papules with a smooth surface. Mature lesions often have a central dimple.

Diagnosis is confirmed cytologically and histologically by unroofing and expressing, or curetting the waxy contents onto a slide and finding molluscum bodies—dark, intracytoplasmic inclusions within epithelial cells (Fig. 4-8).

Treatment of choice is incision with a large needle and curettage to remove the infected cells and debris. Other therapies include liquid nitrogen, chloracetic acid, or cantharidin. Gentle electrodesiccation or laser should be used with care because more than the minimal necessary surgery can cause scarring.

Folliculitis. Folliculitis may occur on the vulva, as on any hair-bearing skin surface. The initial lesion appears papular and results from obstruction and infection of the hair follicle and adjacent pilosebaceous unit. This may progress to a pustule. When fluctuant these abscesses should be drained and a wick placed to allow continued drainage. Surrounding erythema is common but cellulitis is rare. In patients who are elderly, diabetic, irradiated, or otherwise immunosuppressed, the infection may be more aggressive. When continued symptoms are present, antibiotics should be instituted and inpatient management considered.[43]

Necrotizing fasciitis. Necrotizing fasciitis and the associated progressive bacterial synergistic gangrene represent the most dangerous of all vulvar infections. Necrotizing fasciitis is a rapidly progressive, frequently fatal infection that may develop at a site of minimal trauma or prior localized infection.[22] Risk factors for the development of necrotizing fasciitis include diabetes mellitus, arteriosclerosis, prior vulvar surgery, irradiation, or immunosuppression.[99] It may also develop spontaneously in neutropenic patients and those with vulvar carcinoma.[1,52] The infection is polymicrobial and frequently associated with anaerobic streptococcus and enterococci.

In a recent study of 29 nonpregnant women with necrotizing fasciitis of the vulva, a delay in diagnosis of more than 48 hours was associated with a 78% mortality rate. Nearly all the deaths occurred in diabetics, or when the infections were clinically felt to be mild labial cellulitis.[116]

Clinical symptoms suggestive of necrotizing fasciitis include pain out of proportion to the clinical findings. Signs include: a pallor and edema of the overlying skin, paresthesia, anesthesia, and crepitance. A grey "fish water" discharge may also be noted. Finally signs of sepsis including hypotension become apparent.

Treatment must be aggressive and includes fluid resuscitation, arterial and pulmonary artery monitoring, the rapid institution of broad spectrum antibiotics, and immediate surgical debridement. It is not unusual to remove enormous areas of damaged soft tissue from the vulva, medial thigh, and anterior abdominal wall. An adequate surgical margin is achieved when pink, bleeding tissue is encountered. Frozen section analysis of margins may help to guide the limits of resection. Debrided areas should be packed, not closed, to allow for the inevitable secondary debridement procedures. Extension of the process to the endopelvic fascia is associated with a grim prognosis.

Hidradenitis suppurativa. Hidradenitis suppurativa is an infection resulting from mixtures of *Staphylococcus, Streptococcus,* and occasionally coliform organisms. The disease results from plugging of sweat glands by keratin, subsequent rupture, and secondary infection with abscess formation, which ultimately lead to the development of fistulous tracts. It is not seen before puberty. The disease affects mainly labia majora, intercrural folds, occasionally the mons, and rarely the clitoris or labia minora. Because of the cyclic nature of the disease in the early stages, it may respond favorably to the use of intermittent oral estrogens or cyclic oral contraceptives. Once the disease progresses to the suppurative phase, multiple abscesses form. These abscesses can drain spontaneously or be drained surgically. Chronic drainage leads to deep scarring. Ultimately the treatment of choice is wide surgical excision while sparing the labia minora, the clitoris, and the prepuce, followed by skin grafting.[9]

Fox-Fordyce disease. Fox-Fordyce disease is also limited to the sweat glands and is papular in appearance, secondary to plugging. It is believed that subsequent extravasation of sweat into the epidermal tissue results in the intense pruritus that accompanies the lesion. The axilla may be simultaneously involved with the same process, and there appears to be some relationship between pruritus and a particular time in the menstrual cycle. Treatment may be successful using cyclic oral contraceptives. Occasional relief using topical antibiotics has also been reported.[35]

SYSTEMIC DISEASES

Vulvar skin shares much in common with other skin and thus could merit a vulvar dermatology textbook; its unique *location* and sensitive *nature* can make it a sentinel skin site, or even a first body site, to signal a systemic or skin disease. The following common, systemic diseases affect the vulva.

Acquired immune deficiency syndrome

Patients with AIDS can suffer a host of skin diseases that can appear on the vulva. Kaposi's sarcoma may be the most specific and "AIDS ulcers" are likely to be genitally located.[21] Many infections can become florid vulvar problems: monilia, herpes, HPV, molluscum, and more. Systemic diseases that rarely appear on the vulva (e.g., tuberculosis) are more likely in immunosuppressed patients.

Blood dyscrasias

Leukemia, aplastic anemia, and agranulocytosis may cause vulvar ulceration. These ulcers are deep, well-demarcated oval lesions usually covered with a thin, gray membrane. Such lesions have also been found following administration of bone marrow depressing drugs (e.g., methotrexate). The ulcers heal spontaneously following cessation of the drug. In pernicious anemia, vulvar ulceration and hyperpigmentation may be part of the general tissue hypovitaminosis and devitalization.

Other blood diseases (anemias, polycythemia, dyscrasias) can be associated with nonspecific vulvar changes.

Circulatory disturbances

The most common disturbances are edema and varicose veins. With no muscular "pump", marked edema may be found in the presence of generalized anasarcas, lymphatic obstruction, inflammation, or pelvic tumors.

Problematic varicose veins are rare outside pregnancy. Hemorrhoids and leg varicosities are especially prominent during the last trimester. The patient may complain of burning, itching and heaviness of the vulva. Relief can come with pressure against the vulva from a sanitary napkin or foam rubber. Rest, with legs and hips elevated at or above the heart, is necessary. On rare occasion, varices may need excision. After delivery the veins become smaller and usually asymptomatic. Rarely, an angioma may produce unilateral vulvar swelling.

Diabetes

Diabetic vulvitis (usually fungal) may be the first sign of diabetes, or it may arise when known diabetes is inadequately controlled. There is acute erythema, pruritus, edema sometimes, and burning as urine strikes the inflamed vulva. Frequently there is an associated monilial vaginitis. Hyperkeratosis ensues with time. Therefore red inflamed areas appear interspersed with white opaque patches.

Control of diabetes together with antifungal agents, vaginally and on the vulva, provides improvement within one week. Low potency, topical, short term corticoids can be used, if necessary, to control severe pruritus, inflammation, and squamous hyperplasia. Meticulous skin care is essential.

Uremia

Late-stage renal disease may result in "uremic frost" of the vulva as well as mouth. Labial surfaces are covered with a gray-white-brown membrane containing urea and uric acid deposits. Treatment consists of local cleansing and correction of renal failure.

Vitamin deficiencies

In the United States, deficiencies are usually due to anorexia and malabsorptive states, debility, or chronic diseases. Deficiencies of vitamins A, B (especially niacin or riboflavin), and C can cause chronic vulvitis. The skin can be dry and scaly, or fissured and ulcerated.[60] Excess vitamin A can cause an erythematous, exudative dermatitis.

Autoimmune diseases

Crohn's disease (regional enteritis). Crohn's disease is found primarily in the ileum. Early symptoms are low-grade fever, abdominal pain, and diarrhea. On occasion this disease may present as draining sinuses or abscesses in the anogenital region. About one fifth of patients will have anogenital involvement—mainly anoperineal, rarely labia majora.[61,82] Anogenital Crohn's can be the terminus of a bowel fistula or it can be "metastatic" with no bowel connection.[68] Constitutional symptoms often include low fever, diarrhea, fatigue, and weight loss.

Diagnosis is confirmed by radiologic evidence of bowel pathology and communicating sinuses.

Differential diagnoses include: hidradenitis suppurativa, lymphogranuloma venereum, granuloma inguinale, tuberculosis, and Behcet's syndrome.

Treatment. Surgical treatment alone is usually futile; the disease may become progressively more destructive with creation of a cloaca. Treatment of the primary disease is essential and usually requires steroids plus antibiotics, and removal of involved bowel, if necessary. Biopsy of the anogenital lesions will reveal nonspecific, noncaseating, granulomatous change. Ulcers and sinus tracts should be debrided and cleansed frequently with povidone-iodine and hydrogen peroxide. Once healing has progressed, wide excision of sinus tracts may be indicated, usually with good results.

Behçet's syndrome. This syndrome is a triad of *ulcerations* of buccal and vulvar epithelium and anterior *uveitis*. There can be multiple other manifestations, particularly arthritis and vasculitis.[60] Ulcers are often small but deep, and tend to come and go spontaneously.

Diagnosis is made clinically by characteristic recurrent oral and vulvar ulcers and uveitis (and other features).

Differential diagnoses include: herpes, syphilis, lichen planus, lupus, pemphigus, and Stevens-Johnson syndrome. Biopsy of vulvar ulcers reveals nonspecific inflammation and vasculitis.

Treatment is careful cleansing; corticosteroids may be helpful. There have been reports that high estrogen oral contraceptives might help.[60] Surgery is contraindicated unless the vulvar lesions are incapacitating.

NONNEOPLASTIC EPITHELIAL DISORDERS

In 1987 the International Society for the Study of Vulvar Disease adopted the following classification[59,76] for "benign" epithelial disorders: lichen sclerosus, squamous hyperplasia, other dermatoses. While the first two are mainly vulvar, the latter are *general skin dermatoses* and are described in the following sections.

Psoriasis

Psoriasis is an incurable, inflammatory dermatosis characterized by light-red plaques covered by a silvery scale. There are about 5 million sufferers in the United States; a genetic predisposition appears to be activated by trauma, infection, and stress. For unknown reasons, keratinocyte kinetics are speeded to 28 times the normal epidermal cell production.[40]

Psoriasis may involve the vulva, although the more common sites are the scalp, nails, extensor surfaces of the elbows and knees, and sacrum[17]; the face is spared. Scratching can produce two characteristic signs. The Koebner phenomenon which is the appearance of small papules in a row of microtrauma. Scratching is a major factor in initiating new lesions and secondary infections—an important reason to break the itch/scratch cycle. Auspitz's sign is the appearance of punctate bleeding points as capillaries are disrupted.

As with all scaly dermatoses, the moist, warm, less aerated vulvar environment makes lesions less scaly and white but redder. Psoriasis has periods of exacerbation and remission.

Diagnosis can be made by inspection; biopsy is confirmatory. Microscopically there is parakeratosis, rete peg elongation with clubbing, and microabscesses in the stratum corneum.

Differential diagnoses include: seborrheic or reactive dermatitis, fungi, lymphoma, vulvar intraepithelial neoplasia or Paget's disease.

Treatment is with ultraviolet light (natural or artificial), tars, or salicylic acid (2 % to 10%) ointments. Short term, topical fluorinated corticosteroid ointments are helpful. Long term use of topical corticosteroids is best avoided to minimize fibrosis and atrophy. In severe cases methotrexate can help slow the rapid cell turnover; relieving stress might also help.

Seborrheic dermatitis

Seborrheic dermatitis is a red, scaly rash appearing in areas of skin where there is a high concentration of sebaceous glands.[60] However, it is not a disease of sebaceous glands. The skin appears oily and white-yellow-red, "greasy" plaques may occur. Common sites include the scalp ("dandruff" is often the initial site), central face and trunk, and various "folds" (including behind the ears and groin). The labia majora, mons, and perianus are rarer sites and are sometimes pruritic.

Differential diagnoses include psoriasis, fungi, reactive dermatitis, squamous hyperplasia, and Paget's disease. Asymmetry of this lesion is the exception and, in such cases, an alternative diagnosis should be considered.[42]

Diagnosis is by appearance, distribution, and elimination (e.g., negative KOH slide). Histology is nonspecific and biopsy is not usually necessary.

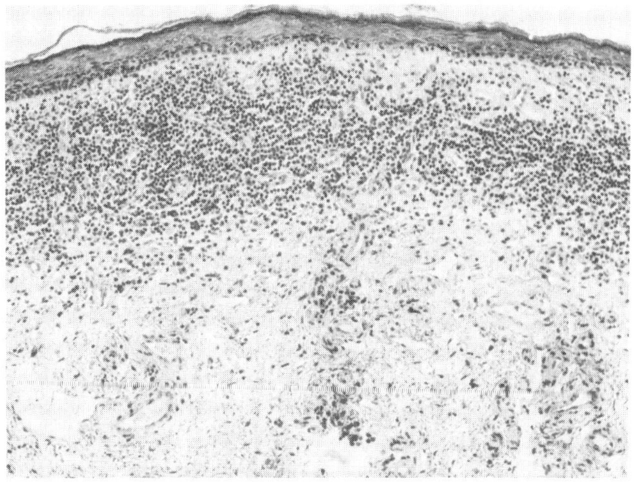

Fig. 4-9. Lichen planus.

Treatment. The disease is not curable but may be ameliorated with good hygiene, Burow's solution, and topical steroids. Topicals are best applied after a bath or shower, when there is less and softer keratin and thereby better penetration. Ketoconazole can improve the condition because of the association with *Pityrosporum*.

Lichen planus

Lichen planus is an inflammatory dermatosis of unknown origin. It is characterized by multiple, small, purple, polygonal papules that are shiny, not scaly. There are usually associated lesions elsewhere on the body, especially flexor surfaces (wrists, ankles, and thighs). Internal sites (mouth, medial vulva, and vagina), which are usually involved, have a different appearance of white, lacy lesions.[4] Lichen planus can produce an inflamed, erosive vaginitis.

Diagnosis is made by biopsy, which shows hyperkeratosis, absence of parakeratosis, "saw-toothed" rete pegs, and a characteristic band of chronic inflammatory cells in the upper dermis (Fig. 4-9). There seems to be some relation to an autoimmune cell-mediated response, since the disease is common in patients who have had bone marrow transplants with graft versus host reaction.

Differential diagnoses are psoriasis, vulvar intraepithelial neoplasia, and Kaposi's sarcoma.

Treatment with topical steroids and retin-A relieves pruritus and cutaneous lesions.[114] Vulvovaginal lesions are often refractory; vaginal stenosis and atrophy can ensue.

Reactive dermatitis

Dermatitis may be caused by direct contact with any laundering material, deodorant, toilet paper additives, "feminine hygiene" product, local contraceptives, and any skin allergens such as poison ivy or nail polish. A careful history about exposures and chronology is crucial. Contact dermatitis is confluent at the contact site.

The vulva can also be vulnerable to ingested allergens. Other skin sites may respond but be less sensitive. The initial reaction is usually pruritus followed by erythema and edema, which can become vesicular, with ulcerations and weeping when severe.[60] Later hyperkeratotic scaly whitening can ensue.

Diagnosis can be difficult when an irritant, allergen or other disease (psoriasis, seborrheic dermatitis, fungi, squamous hyperplasia) is not obvious. The reaction may not be to the main substance but to its vehicle, preservative, or other ingredient. Marren did patch testing with 78 possible allergens, but seldom found this to be of significant help.

Treatment includes elimination of the offending agent. During the acute phase, application of cool Burow's compresses, ice, corticosteroid cream, antihistamine, and short term antipruritics (hydroxyzine) are helpful.

Vulvar "dermatoses"

Lichen sclerosus. Lichen sclerosus is an atrophic, shrinking disease that usually occurs in postmenopausal women. The main symptom, if any, is pruritus. It can appear in children but remits after the menarche. The skin thins to a dry, shiny, fragile, finely wrinkled, parchment-like appearance and the external genitalia contract and lose their shape and definition. White patches fuse into a symmetric, "keyhole" pattern, often encompassing the perianus (Fig. 4-10). Telangiectasia and mid-line skin "splits" are common. Histologically the epidermis is thin with flattened rete pegs (Fig. 4-11). The dermis is edematous and hyalinized, with a loss of elastic fibers . There is a chronic inflammatory infiltrate in the lower dermis.[85]

Autoimmunity may play a role in the development. Patients with lichen sclerosus have an increased incidence of autoimmune antibodies and diseases; the main mechanism, however, may be testosterone deficiency or dysfunction. The principle trophic hormone for the ectoderm-derived skin is testosterone (versus estrogen for müllerian-derived epithelium). Friedrich suggested that reduced 5-alpha reductase activity, the enzyme that converts free testosterone to the more potent dihydrotestosterone, may contribute to the development of lichen sclerosus.[44]

In older women there is an association of lichen sclerosus with invasive cancer.[23,67] Lynch estimates that 4% of patients with lichen sclerosus will develop invasion—a ten fold increased risk. Whether lichen sclerosus plays an etiologic role in carcinogenesis is unknown.

Diagnosis can be made by inspection, but biopsy is confirmatory and will also determine if there is a hyperplastic or neoplastic component that would influence treatment.

Treatment is replacement of the deficient hormone. Testosterone propionate (2%) in petrolatum should be applied twice daily until the condition is in remission, which may not occur until after several months of use. Maintenance therapy (about twice weekly) is needed indefinitely. Android side effects such as clitoral hypertrophy, increased libido, and hirsutism merit surveillance and adjustment of dose. Estrogen is not helpful. If pruritus is severe, it is best controlled with corticoid cream. This should be used only briefly since it will compound the atrophy.

Squamous hyperplasia. Squamous hyperplasia is a chronic reactive disorder to problems such as chronic fungal vulvitis (with or without diabetes), allergies, or unknown stimuli. Pruritus and the chronic trauma of scratching play an important role in the development.

Diagnosis begins by searching for any initiating factor(s). Inflammation (Fig. 4-12), often whitening, excoriation, increased skin markings, and lichenification are present.[70] Histologically there are nonspecific changes of hyperkeratosis, lengthening of rete pegs, and chronic inflammation (Fig. 4-13).

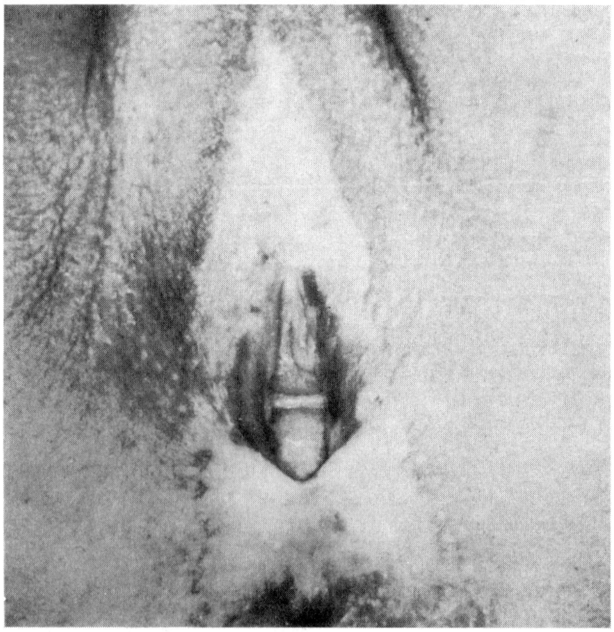

Fig. 4-10. Lichen sclerosus of vulva.

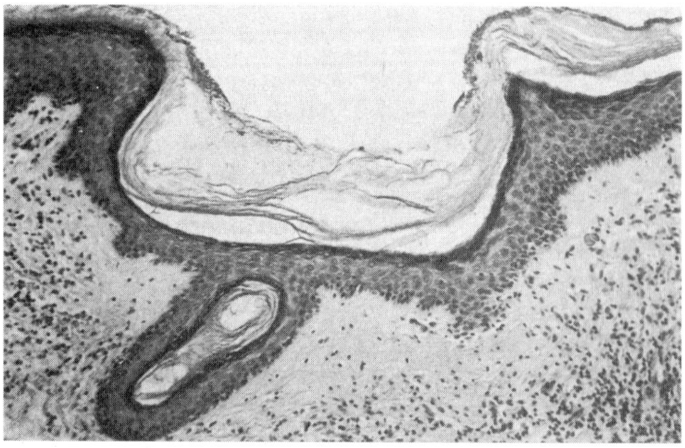

Fig. 4-11. Histologic appearance of lichen sclerosus.

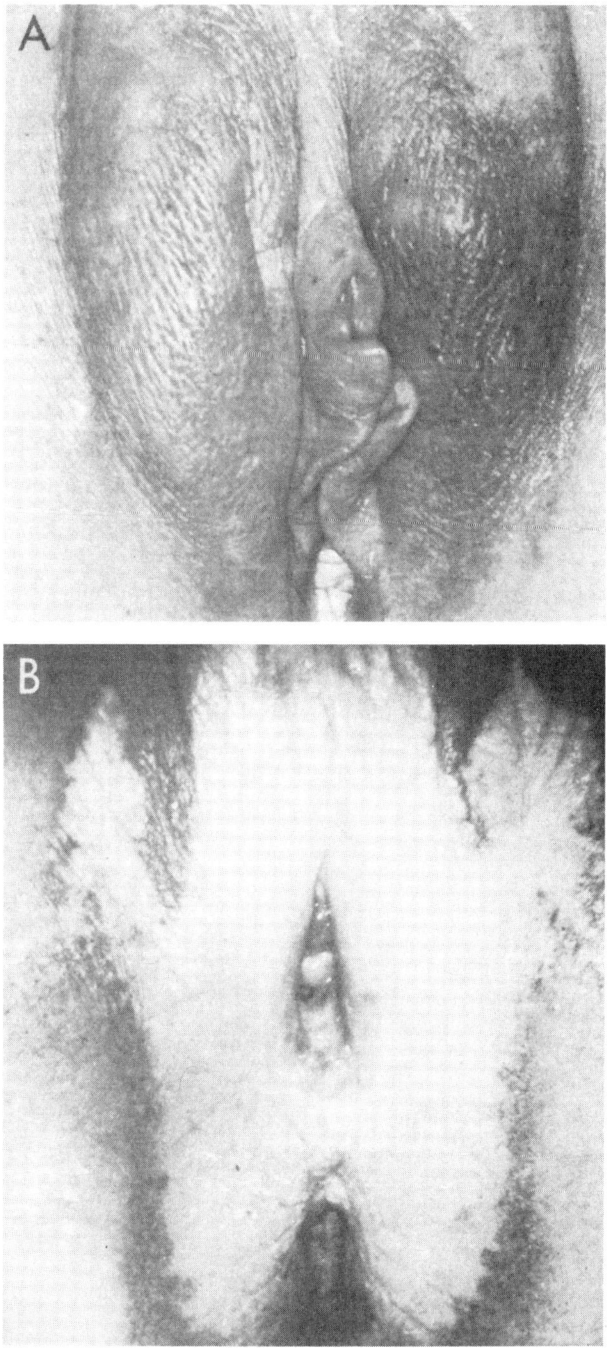

Fig. 4-12. Squamous hyperplasia. **A,** Edema and lichenification of early stage. **B,** Extensive hyperkeratosis in late stage.

Differential diagnoses are lichen sclerosus, psoriasis, seborrheic dermatitis, vitiligo, tinea, and vulvar intraepithelial neoplasia. Biopsy is essential to rule out the latter.

Treatment is most effective if an inciting cause can be found and corrected. Additional nonspecific therapy begins with potent, fluorinated corticoids (for 6 weeks or less) to relieve pruritus and reduce the hyperplasia. After relief of symptoms, lower potency, nonfluorinated corticoids should be substituted, while tapering off the dose as indicated. General hygiene and antipruritic medicines to break the itch/scratch cycle are needed.

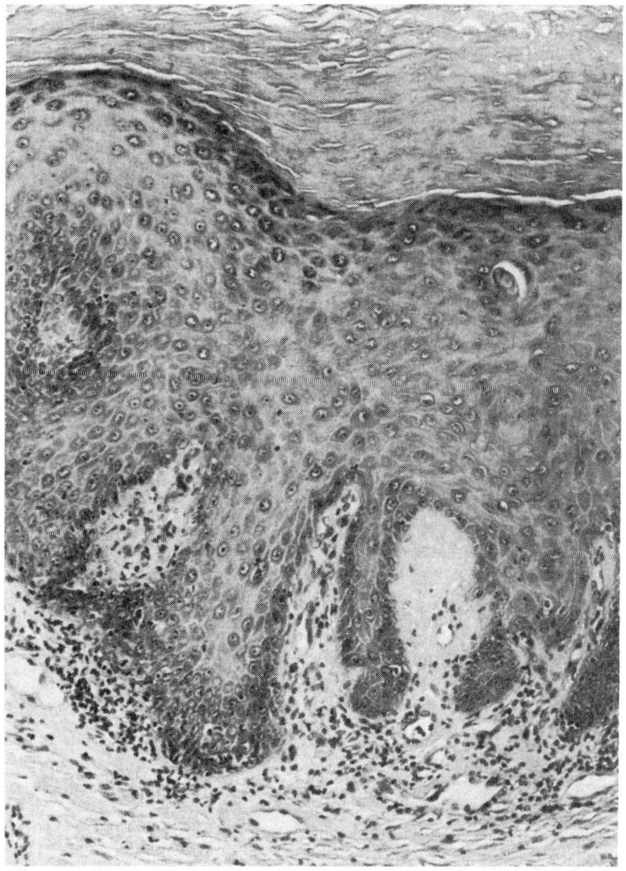

Fig. 4-13. Histologic changes in squamous hyperplasia.

LESIONS OF COLOR

Squamous neoplasia can be white, red, or dark (see vulvar intraepithelial neoplasia below).

White lesions include HPV (especially after acetic acid), lichen sclerosis, and squamous hyperplasia.

Red lesions are more likely to be on medial, less keratinized epithelium. They include vulvovaginitis, reactive vulvitis, angiomas and Paget's disease.[12] Certain red lesions (psoriasis, seborrheic dermatitis, fungi) become thicker, more scaly, and whiter on the lateral vulva.

Purple lesions include lichen planus, Kaposi's sarcoma, and hemangiomas.

Dark lesions are rare in African-American women; in Caucasian women 10% to 12% of gynecologic patients have "dark" lesions.[100] Forty percent of these lesions are lentigines, 20% nevi, and 16% vulvar intraepithelial neoplasia.

Lentigines (freckles) and melanosis

A lentigo is the most common dark lesion on the vulva and poses no danger. It is usually a variegated brown and macular (flat). Under magnification, no changes in contour or skin markings are obvious until the lesions are stretched, then normal color appears between the brown areas.

Lentigines and melanosis have increased melanin. The reason for increase in melanin is not known. Lentigines have melanin confined to the basal layer of the epidermis. Melanosis involves higher layers and is therefore darker. With melanosis there can be histologic hyperplasia, but this is not clinically apparent.

Nevi (moles)

Nevi are usually papular (raised), tan to black in color, and most are on the medial vulva. In descending order they are compound, intradermal, and junctional. The latter has neoplastic potential, as do congenital and dysplastic nevi.[60] The vulva does not have more high risk nevi than other sites, therefore it is not known why dark lesions of the vulva have a higher neoplastic risk than other skin sites. Half of melanomas arise from dysplastic nevi and half de novo.[60] The only sure way to distinguish between a benign nevus, a dysplastic nevus, and early melanoma is by biopsy.

Differential diagnoses are melanoma, basal cell carcinoma, vulvar intraepithelial neoplasia, seborrheic keratosis, "warty" papilloma, angiokeratoma, dark angiomas, hidradenoma, and accessory nipple.[119]

Because of the potential for pre-neoplasia and invasive neoplasia, all but small, flat lentigines (less than 3 mm) should be biopsied. Nevi should be excised, with at least 5 mm lateral margins and full thickness of dermis. Any change in size, contour, or color warrants immediate excision.

ULCERS

The diagnostic dichotomy is infectious versus neoplastic processes. On occasion, allergies (topical or ingestion, e.g., tetracycline) or trauma can ulcerate. Trauma includes scratching (Pruritus). One third of carcinomas ulcerate.[42] Cytology, colposcopy, and biopsy, especially of persistent lesions, are helpful in diagnosis. Since ulcers do not have a keratinized surface, smears can be particularly helpful with chancroid, herpes, syphilis (dark field), granuloma inguinale, and neoplasia. Biopsy may lead to the diagnosis of rare tumors such as basal cell carcinoma, granular cell myoblastoma, or hidradenoma.[42]

Kraus emphasizes that infectious ulcers are secondary lesions. They follow *vesicles* (herpes), *papules* (syphilis, chancroid, granuloma inguinale, LGV), or *pustules* (folliculitis). Therefore history just before ulceration, report of self-examination (preferably with a photograph), or early professional inspection are all diagnostically helpful. Ulcers from AIDS have been described in addition to increased susceptibility to other ulcerative infections. Rarely a syndrome such as Behcet's is the cause. *Solitary* ulcers suggest neoplasia, syphilis, or LGV. *Multiple* ulcers suggest herpes, chancroid, granuloma inguinale (trauma or allergy); pain and tenderness suggest herpes and chancroid. Nontender ulcers suggest neoplasia, syphilis, granuloma inguinale, or LGV.

PRURITUS, PAIN, AND TENDERNESS SYNDROMES

Relatively little is known about these syndromes, and until recently they have not received sufficient attention. *Pruritus* is the most common gynecologic complaint. *Vulvodynia* is estimated to affect about 200,000 women in the United States.[14] Goetsch, in questioning and testing 210 consecutive gynecologic patients, found 15% to have *vestibulitis*.[48]

In patients with otherwise unexplainable *vulvar pruritus*, pain, or tenderness, psychosocial-sexual-economic situations and stresses at home and work should be investigated. In addition, the patient should be asked if she has ever been threatened or abused (physically, sexually, or mentally). Are there any clues of hypersensitivity, stress, or depression?

One should not label these syndromes until all possible diseases are ruled out. There are sometimes multiple causes—organic diseases and psychosocial-sexual problems—which can be hard to quantify.[84] Sometimes the psychosocial-sexual aspects are primary or secondary, as with any chronic, unremitting condition. Anxiety, interpersonal or sexual dysfunction, and insomnia can become significant secondary compounders. One can do a disservice attributing symptoms solely to the psyche when data do not confirm this. Because psychosocial-sexual factors are often involved to some degree, emotional support, setting realistic goals (i.e., improvement versus cure),[77] and obtaining *appropriate consultations* (dermatologic, medical, neurologic, psychologic, and sexual when indicated) are helpful. Management of all these syndromes should include aggressive diagnosis, treatment, and monitoring of any lower genital infection, and basic *vulvar hygiene.* Finally, if inclined and appropriate, one might consider less "traditional" methods, such as hypnosis, biofeedback, acupuncture, and nutritional therapy.

Because of the vagaries and complexities of these syndromes, it is important to define them as specifically as possible. *Organically unexplained* pruritus, pain, and tenderness are discussed below.

Pruritus syndrome

The pathway to concluding a patient has a *pruritic syndrome* (versus a *symptom* of a *disease*) is long and varied. Many systemic, general skin, and vulva-specific diseases can be heralded or accompanied by pruritus. The list of diseases in this chapter not associated with pruritus is shorter than those that are.

Diagnosis. To avoid the maze of pruritus' differential, Bornstein[12] stresses the need for an orderly *diagnostic* pursuit:

1. Efficiency dictates a brief screening history, a general examination, and proceeding to the source. Is there a *vulvar lesion?* If so, color, vulvoscopy, and liberal biopsy can help.
2. If no obvious lesion, is there a lower genital *infection* on inspection, wet and Pap smears, and cultures, especially fungal? Lice or scabies might require careful, magnified inspection. Skin pathology can be due to a disease or to chronic scratching. The need to address all contributing factors is illustrated by diabetes, which can be pruritic or facilitate a pruritic fungal infection. The diabetes needs better control and the fungal infection needs treatment. A pruritic diabetic neuropathy might also develop. To treat the neuropathy and break the itch/scratch cycle, hydroxyzine or amitriptyline may be needed. Scratching can induce squamous hyperplasia, which is treated with corticoids. The latter can enhance fungal growth. It is important to monitor and balance the management of diabetes, candida, squamous hyperplasia, and pruritus.
3. If there is no specific vulvar lesion or lower genital pathology, one needs to work through systemic diseases by the following:
   a. A more detailed *history*—dermatologic and systemic symptoms (malaise, fever, weight loss), possible inciting medicines or products;
   b. *Examination*—with particular attention to mouth, skin, and lymph nodes;
   c. *Tests*—including hematologic and metabolic surveys, liver and renal chemistries, urinalysis.

   Vulvar pruritus can signal anemia, diabetes, drug allergies, gout, hepato biliary disease, leukemia, lymphoma, nutritional deficiency, polycythemia, renal disease, and thyroid disease.[41]
4. If no local, general dermatologic, or systemic diagnosis is found, then psychosocial-sexual problems should be considered. If no problem surfaces, one is left with a pure pruritus syndrome in need of symptomatic therapy. Vulvar findings on such a patient would be nothing specific, or squamous hyperplasia from scratching.

Treatment for all pruritic problems is to *stop the itch/scratch cycle*. Pruritus and pain are carried along the same neural pathways; converting pruritus to pain by scratching is more tolerable. This chronic trauma produces its own hyperplastic dermatopathology. Management includes the appropriate corticoid; an antipruritic (systemic—hydroxyzine or amitriptyline, particularly at bedtime to stop scratching during sleep and relieve insomnia; topical-lidocaine or crotamiton); cool compresses or ice; and general hygiene. If all fail to relieve the pruritus, then consultation or injection of triamcinolone should be tried. Kelly et al found the latter to be effective (1 or more months relief) in 78% of patients who had pruritus syndrome more than 6 months. The mean duration of relief was 6 months. Neither alcohol injections nor the Mehring denervation operation are recommended by the authors.

Pain syndrome of vulvodynia

Diagnosis. Vulvodynia (formerly "burning vulva syndrome") is defined by the International Society for the Study of Vulvar Diseases as: *"chronic vulvar discomfort, characterized by burning,* (stinging, irritation, or rawness)." There can also be tenderness and dyspareunia, but the hallmark is chronic, constant, spontaneous, unexplained pain. After neoplasia, infection, and other diseases have been ruled out by *history* (McKay uses an 80 question screen) *examination,* and *tests* (including wet smear, PH, fungal culture, Pap, vulvoscopy and biopsy—if *any* abnormality is seen), the syndrome of vulvodynia remains.

The most probable mechanism for vulvodynia appears to be neurogenic (peripheral sympathetic or central nerves), although psychosomatic factors can play a prominent role. Postherpetic or neuralgia of the pudendal nerve should be considered.[120] The possibility of a prior, occult herpetic infection is suggested by the number of patients with positive titers exceeding those with a history of herpes; a positive titer does not rule in herpetic neuralgia and rule out vulvodynia.

Treatment. When by exclusion the problem appears to be pure vulvodynia, *management* includes estrogen (if postmenopausal), hygiene, and a tricyclic antidepressant. Estrogen is empirically recommended since most sufferers are post menopausal and not using estrogen. Even with no evidence of reactive dermatitis, it cannot hurt to remove all possible causes. Low-dose amitriptyline may reduce symptoms in selected patients.[77]

There is preliminary evidence that nutritional therapy, specifically reducing levels of calcium oxalate, might help some patients.[14]

Tenderness syndrome of vestibulitis

Diagnosis. This syndrome has some specificity in terms of symptoms, signs, and histology. The prime *symptom* and *sign* is tenderness to touch—intercourse, tampons, Q-tip, and speculum. There is also *erythema,* diffuse or focal (around the openings of the major and minor vestibular ducts) and slight whitening of duct openings, because of metaplasia and/or HPV. Histology shows nonspecific, periductal, *chronic inflammatory changes*. The vestibular glands are not involved.

Erythema and histologic findings are nonspecific and variable.[66] Erythema can be minimal with this syndrome and present without tenderness. Furlonge,[46] in examining biopsies of 24 patients, and Pyka,[88] in studying 41 vestibulectomy specimens, found that the only consistent histology was chronic inflammation. Using special stains, Pyka found no evidence of specific infectious organisms or allergies. Twenty-seven percent of his patients and one third of Furlonge's patients demonstrated evidence of HPV infection. Almost one third of Goetsch's patients gave a history of HPV-related lesions.[48]

Almost half of Goetsch's patients noted tenderness before the coitarche versus 9% for Peckham.[83] Nulliparas were more likely to have vestibulitis. The median age was 34 and median duration was 10 years.

There are several diseases associated with vestibulitis which can be the prime cause (e.g., candida), or an associated condition can contribute to the syndrome, but not be causal, (such as HPV infection). Treatments for condylomas appear to have precipitated the syndrome in some patients after chloracetic acid, podophyllin, 5-FU cream, or laser. In some patients with documented HPV infection interferon provided an inconsistent benefit.[122] Additional associations are chronic or recurrent gardnerella and trichomonas infections, which irritate with infection and alkaline discharge, group B streptococcus, and other irritants and allergens.

Secor stresses the importance of prompt, effective diagnosis and treatment of any acute vestibular tenderness, which is more amenable to medical treatment than the chronic vestibulitis syndrome.[103]

Treatment. If tenderness persists after treatment of any associated diseases, symptomatic treatment can begin with lidocaine jelly prior to intercourse. Empiric antibiotics, corticoids, retinoids, chloracetic acid, IF,[122] 5-FU, and laser[104] have not proven effective. Half of Peckham's patients went into spontaneous remission. Goetsch found remissions rare unless vestibulitis developed postpartum, or treatment of an associated infection led to early relief.

When vestibulitis leads to chronic, severe sexual incapacity and the patient desires no more conservative therapy, vestibulectomy becomes the last and usually effective option. Vestibulectomy can be partial or total. Focal excision does not work well since tenderness is usually multifocal or diffuse. However, there is a predilection for the posterior vestibule; that degree of partial excision is worth considering if there is no anterior tenderness. The hymen and vestibule are removed and the distal vagina undermined and attached to the perineum. Complete or significant improvement occurs in 80% of properly chosen patients.[73] Mann attributes the improvement to removal of the tender vestibule and relaxation and enlargement of the introital outlet.[72] While vestibulectomy perineoplasty is the most effective current therapy, it is a transient technique that will be replaced by less radical therapy in the future.

TUMORS AND BENIGN GROWTHS

Vulvar tumors

Benign vulvar tumors may be cystic or solid. Cystic tumors include Bartholin's duct cyst or abscess, hydrocele, or hernia. Conditions such as endometriosis may also give rise to vulvar masses. The most common solid tumors of the vulva include lipomas, fibromas, and hidradenomas. Less common tumors include lymphangiomas, hemangiomas, and myxomas. Although these tumors are benign, they may achieve significant size and cause disability.

Bartholin's cyst and abscess

The Bartholin's gland undergoes cystic dilation when it becomes obstructed as a result of chronic inflammation. It is uncommon for a Bartholin's cyst to cause significant symptoms. It requires drainage only if it impairs walking or intercourse. The cyst becomes painful when an abscess develops. The infection tends to be polymicrobial with gonococcus involved 20% to 30% of the time.[131] Rapid amelioration of symptoms results from any abscess incision and drainage procedure (usually under local anesthesic). Every attempt should be made to incise the abscess at or behind the hymenal ring. This avoids a vulvar scar and allows packing or catheter placement within the vagina, where it is far more controllable. Placement of a WORD catheter through a 6-mm, Keyes-punched hole allows for thorough drainage and for the formation of an epithelialized tract for further cyst or duct drainage. This tiny, balloon-tipped device can be placed in the abscess cavity; the tip is then inflated with saline. The catheter is left in for three weeks and removed in an outpatient setting. Such a device is particularly suited for recurrent Bartholin's abscesses.

For recalcitrant abscesses not responsive to catheter drainage, marsupialization may be performed by surgically creating a large fenestration in the gland behind the hymenal ring. The edges of this opening are sutured to the skin to maintain patency. With the widespread use of the WORD catheter, marsupialization is required infrequently.

Uncommonly, vaginal dryness or dyspareunia may result from chronic Bartholin's abscesses and loss of lubrication. If a scar or mass exists after the acute infection has subsided, it may be necessary to excise the entire gland. This procedure involves dissection deep within the vulva in close proximity to the pudendal vessels and venous plexi of the vestibular bulb. Significant blood loss is possible. Finally, abscess formation in the postmenopausal patient may be secondary to malignancy. A biopsy of the cyst wall or cyst excision is recommended in these cases.

Hernia of the canal of Nuck

The round ligament, the anlage of the gubernaculum in the male, leaves the pelvis via the canal of Nuck and terminates in the apex of the labia majora. The ligament carries its peritoneal investments through the external inguinal ring. Hydroceles, cysts, and hernias may form along this tract and present as cystic vulvar tumors. Although sometimes confused with Bartholin's cysts, these cystic tumors are more anterior within the labia majora and frequently bilateral. Bartholin's cysts tend to split the labia minora and are unilateral. This difference in anatomic location has practical applications—attempting to incise and drain a hernia sac may lead to bowel injury. Drainage of a hydrocele or cyst will inevitably be ineffective. Repair of hernias of the canal of Nuck include dissection of the hernia sac followed by high ligation and reinforcement of the external inguinal ring.

Endometriosis

Implants of endometriosis may occur along the canal of Nuck, in the labia, or at the site of previous episiotomy scars or other surgery. These lesions may be cystic or partially solid. Inflammatory changes may be cyclic. Treatment is surgical excision and either medical or surgical management of the underlying disorder.

Lipoma

A lipoma is a benign tumor that arises from the fatty tissue of the labia majora or mons veneris and usually grows slowly. It causes no symptoms except when its size is excessive. When this occurs, the mass acquires a pedicle and hangs from the groin or vulva as a pendulum. If the pedicle is wide, it may resemble a hernia. Some lipomas have attained gigantic size, but usually they are not larger than 10 to 12 cm. The histologic appearance is that of normal fat cells with a connective tissue framework and capsule. The incidence of liposarcoma is extremely rare. Nevertheless, the lesion should be excised since difficulty in walking or coitus will eventually occur.

Fibroma

A fibroma is a lesion that usually develops as a firm nodule on the labia majora, which then enlarges and develops a pedicle that may hang down for several inches (or feet). Ulceration and necrosis of the distal portion may occur. The histologic picture is that of any dermatofibroma with a well-circumscribed lesion made up of intertwined collagen bundles and fibroblasts. In rare cases the number of nuclei is excessive, which is suspicious of fibrosarcoma. The circumscription of the lesion and absence of mitotic figures and giant cells are usually sufficient to indicate benignity. These lesions should be removed mainly for cosmetic effect.

Hidradenoma

A hidradenoma is a benign, slow-growing, sweat gland tumor, whose histology simulates that of an adenocarcinoma. It is usually about 1 to 2 cm in diameter with a slightly raised, brown surface, which may be umbilicated. As seen in Fig. 4-14, the lesion may become quite large, and cystic changes may occur. Histologically this is an adenoma of the vulvar apocrine glands. It is not connected with the epidermis and is usually well encapsulated. The basic pattern is that of cystlike spaces into which numerous interlacing villous structures project (Fig. 4-15). These structures, as

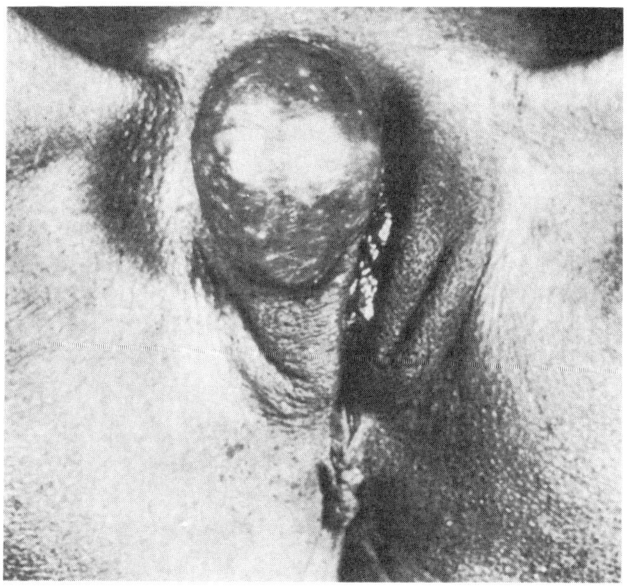

Fig. 4-14. Vulvar hidradenoma.

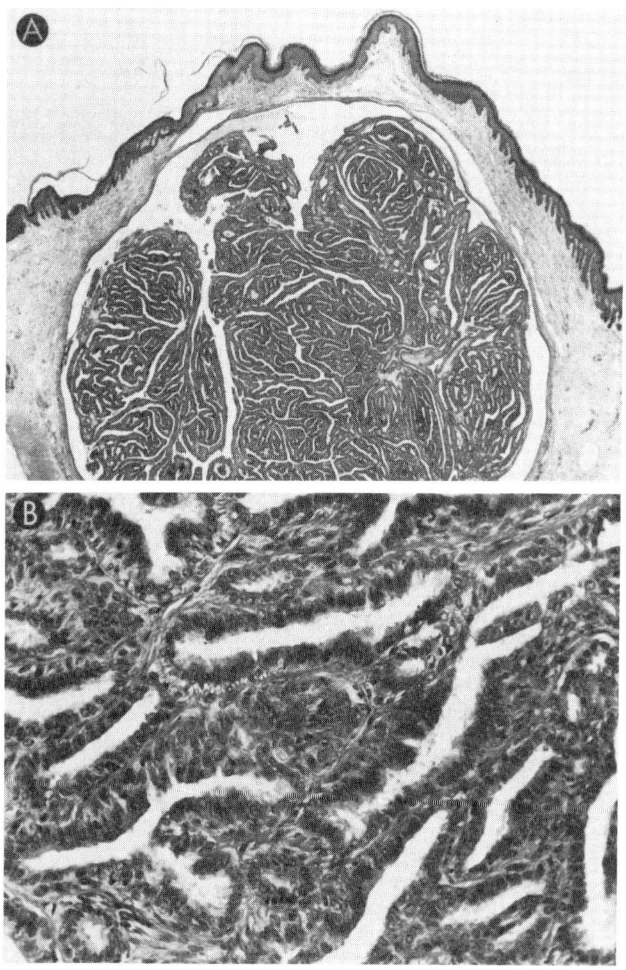

Fig. 4-15. Hidradenoma. **A,** Low power. **B,** High power, showing myoepithelial cells under the secretory cylindrical cells.

well as the wall of the cyst, are lined by a single layer of high cylindrical cells with eosinophilic cytoplasm and a large, oval, pale-staining nucleus. The cells are regular and no anaplasia is evident. Characteristic is a layer of myoepithelial cells under the secretory cylindrical cells, similar to that of apocrine tumors in the mammary gland. A rare variant is the clear cell hidradenoma. This lesion is almost always benign, but since a few hidradenocarcinomas have been reported, all should be excised and submitted to pathologic examination.[127]

VULVAR INTRAEPITHELIAL NEOPLASIA

Vulvar intraepithelial neoplasia is now diagnosed more frequently than in the past and is occurring in younger women. At John Hopkins in the first half of this century, four patients per decade were diagnosed with vulvar carcinoma in situ. In the latter 1980s the rate was five per month.[133] Patients with vulvar carcinoma in situ in their 20s are known to most large clinic centers. Increasing prevalence is probably a combination of greater incidence due to increased exposure to HPV during and after the "sexual revolution", and greater public and professional attention to preinvasive symptoms and signs, more expertise, and the use of vulvoscopy and biopsies.

While the mean age of invasive vulvar carcinoma has remained stable (early 60s), the mean age of patients with vulvar carcinoma in situ has dropped from 53 to 42 years in the past 30 years.[109,133]

The natural history of vulvar neoplasia is not as well known as that of the cervix. We do know that the mean age of patients with vulvar carcinoma in situ is 20 years younger than those with invasion. Therefore the time to progress from dysplasia to invasion is even more than 20 years. The likelihood of progression to invasion is unknown. Vulvar intraepithelial neoplasia will rarely become invasive before the sixth decade, unless the patient is immunosuppressed.[133]

Etiology

The etiology of vulvar intraepithelial neoplasia appears to be similar to other anogenital sites, with HPV a major but not the only factor. HPV 16 is the type most associated with vulvar intraepithelial neoplasia III; HPV 18 and 31 are found less often.[16,23,60] In about one fifth of patients with vulvar intraepithelial neoplasia III, there is no evidence of HPV. A review by Crum describes two groups of patients with invasive vulvar cancer. One group conforms to the HPV 16 model. The other group is older (mostly over 60), less than 15% HPV-associated, and the majority have lichen sclerosus.[23,67] The association with lichen sclerosus, and to a lesser extent squamous hyperplasia, is about twice that of prior or accompanying vulvar intraepithelial neoplasia.

Although vulvar intraepithelial neoplasia is more consistently associated with HPV 16, one wonders what are the precedents to all the "non-HPV" cancers. Do these patients have insufficient preventive care to detect vulvar intraepithelial neoplasia and HPV? Were they diagnosed so late that HPV DNA was so fully integrated into host DNA that it had lost its detectability? Or is lichen sclerosus the precursor to invasion in most older patients? While vulvar intraepithelial neoplasia does not have as well-defined a dichotomy as invasive vulvar cancer, there is a tendency for patients under age 40 to have multifocal, HPV-related vulvar intraepithelial neoplasia, and over age 50 to have unifocal, "non-HPV" vulvar intraepithelial neoplasia.

Risk factors for vulvar intraepithelial neoplasia are any sexual disease, especially HPV, any anogenital neoplasm, immunosuppression and smoking.

Diagnosis

Patients should be educated about the significance of any *symptom*—discomfort, burning, and especially pruritus —present in most patients with vulvar intraepithelial neoplasia. They should be taught genital self-examination[15] and the importance of prompt diagnosis of any *lesions* found on inspection or palpation in the shower or bath. A decade ago Bernstein[8] reported that 18% of vulvar carcinoma-in-situ patients noticed no abnormal symptoms or lesions. Today with more education and awareness, fewer patients develop vulvar carcinoma in situ without at least sensing, seeing, or feeling something abnormal.

Gynecologists and other primary care physicians need to coordinate periodic preventive examinations with their patients. Vulvar dysplasia can be very subtle.[25] Close inspection will reveal color and contour changes in the great majority of cases. Vulvar carcinoma in situ usually appears as a raised, white lesion (hyperplastic and/or increased keratin) two thirds of the time—more detectable after a 5 minute soak with 5% acetic acid; dark lesion (increased melanin) one quarter of the time; or red lesion (hypervascular and/or inflamed) one tenth of the time (usually in less keratinized, medial areas). Punctate and mosaic vessels are not as easily seen colposcopically in keratinized epithelium, but Iverson found abnormal vessels in 58% of patients with vulvar carcinoma in situ.[56]

One half of patients have vulvar intraepithelial neoplasia on more than one vulvar site. Thirty percent of patients with vulvar intraepithelial neoplasia have associated cervical neoplasia, 4% have vaginal neoplasia, 3% have both, and one fifth have associated anal neoplasia.[30,58] Patients who are immunosuppressed, and/or have an anogenital tract neoplastic syndrome, have much higher associations.[109,111] The immunosuppressed population is rising because of the increased use of suppressive medicines with various diseases, organ transplants, and the AIDS epidemic. Therefore patients with vulvar intraepithelial neoplasia need full anogenital surveillance. This surveillance includes cervical and possibly anal cytology, and colposcopy of the entire anogenital tract. Anoscopy should be included if a

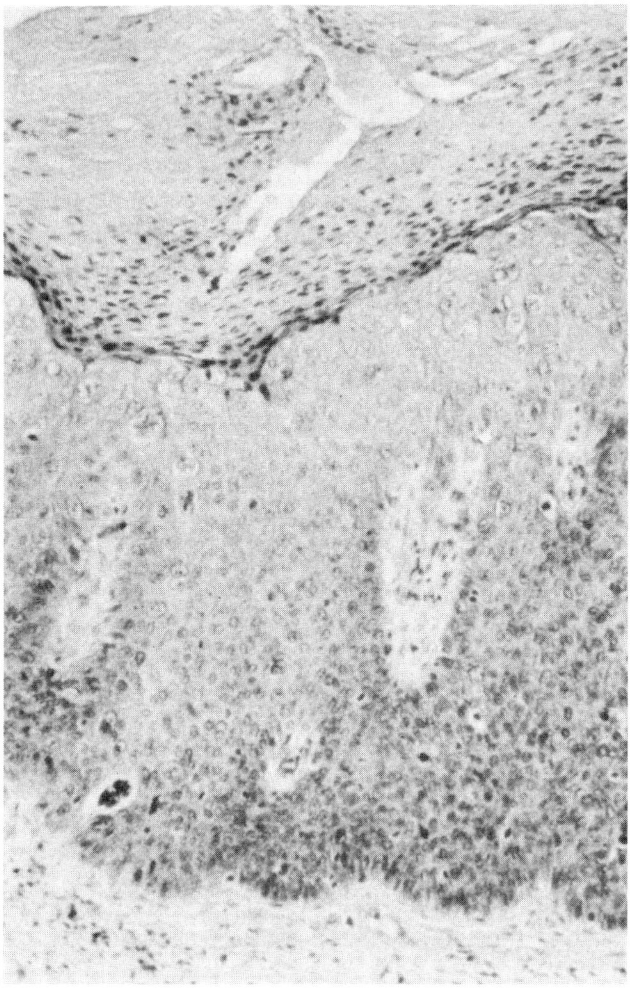

Fig. 4-16. Carcinoma in situ of the vulva beneath a thick, hyperkeratotic patch.

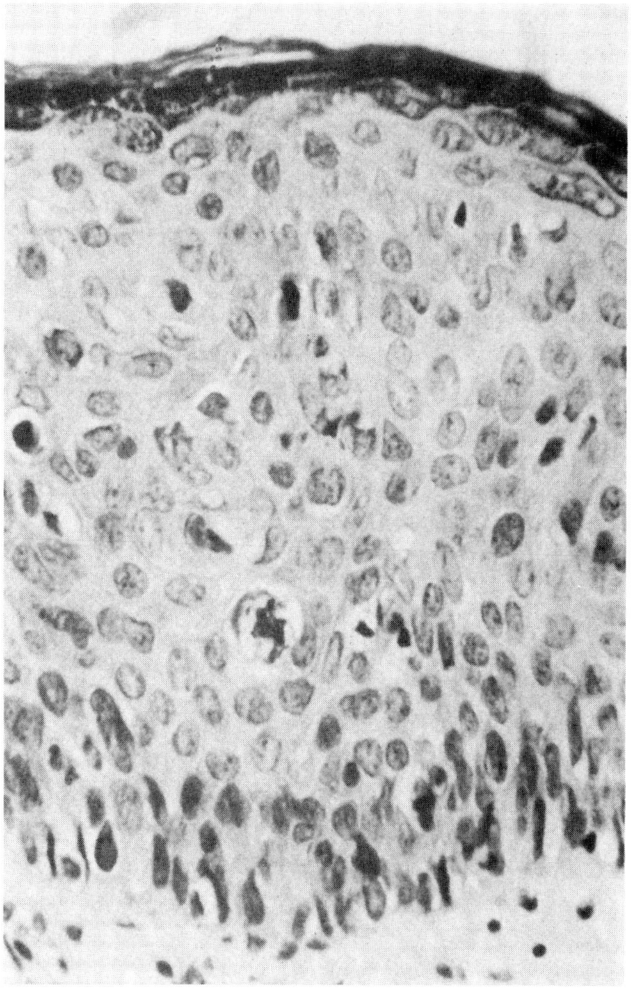

Fig. 4-17. Carcinoma in situ of the vulva. Note cellular disarray, abnormal mitoses, and dyskeratosis.

lesion is adjacent, or if the patient is immunosuppressed, or has an atypical anal Pap or a palpated irregularity.

Cytology of keratinized epithelium is underutilized.[63,115] One needs to first soak the area with saline gauze to soften the keratin. With a scalpel scrape off the keratin, then scrape cells for cytology. A cytobrush is good for anal Paps. Cytology of keratinized epithelium is no substitute for initial biopsy. However, it can help reduce repeated biopsies in patients with constant, slight acetowhitening due to persistent or recurrent HPV. If cytology shows any atypia or worse, biopsies should be performed.

A biopsy should be performed on any suspicious lesion. Adequate sampling often requires multiple biopsies. Ruling out invasion is especially important if there is to be no histology with treatment of vulvar intraepithelial neoplasia, (e.g., laser vaporization). Multiple biopsies can also define depth of subepithelial extension and thereby help define depth of surgery. Discomfort with biopsies can be minimized by first spraying the site before injecting buffered lidocaine with a size 27 to 30 needle. Keyes punches come 2 to 6 mm in diameter. The depth of biopsy is determined by clinical impression (e.g., lichen sclerosus, medial or lateral vulvar intraepithelial neoplasia, or suspicion of invasion). Except for questionable invasion, full dermal depth is not necessary. Reaching subcutaneous fat is usually too deep. If cored only to the depth needed and excised with plastic surgical forceps and scissors, under colposcopic view, an atraumatic biopsy can be taken without suturing. If necessary, Monsel's solution and a Keyes-punched piece of gelfoam can be placed in the defect.[25] A full thickness, excisional biopsy is only indicated for a pigmented nevus or suspected melanoma, or where there is ulceration, irregular contours, or atypical vessels suspicious for invasion.

Histology and topography

The degree of neoplasia and the dimensions of vulvar intraepithelial neoplasia are crucial to planning therapy. Normally there is a progressive maturation towards the surface. With neoplasia there is a loss of this progressive maturation and cellular disorganization and crowding ensues. Mitoses are seen above the basal layer. With lesser dysplasia there can be accompanying HPV koilocytic and keratotic changes. Mild dysplasia shows neoplastic abnormalities in the lower third of the epithelium. Nuclear abnormalities include varied and increasing size, multinucleation, pleomorphism, hyperchromasia with coarsening of chromatin, and atypia. As neoplasia progresses, these changes include the upper epithelium, with full thickness involvement, and more anaplastic changes indicating carcinoma in situ (Fig. 4-16). Atypical mitoses can be seen throughout the epithelium, reflecting the aneuploid cell populations (Fig. 4-17). Vulvar in situ has more variety than cervical in situ and can appear warty, classically anaplastic and undifferentiated, or rarely, deceptively differentiated. The potential for invasion cannot be predicted from the morphology of vulvar in situ.

The thickness of *normal* vulvar epithelium varies from less than 0.3 mm in the vestibule, to 0.3 mm on the labia minora, to about 0.4 mm on the labia majora.[6,7,110,134] The mean vulvar intraepithelial neoplasia thickness is 0.57 mm. Age (postmenopausal versus premenopausal), location (thinner medial versus thicker lateral neoplasia), degree of neoplasia (mild dysplasia versus in situ), and hyperkeratosis (less versus more warty) all affect thickness by about 0.1 to 0.2 mm.

The depth of vulvar intraepithelial neoplasia involves not only epithelial thickness, but possible extension into subepithelial sanctuaries such as hair follicles and ducts of vestibular, eccrine, apocrine, and sebaceous glands. Wright states that apocrine duct involvement has not been described. He found eccrine involvement in 3.6% of patients; Mene found the same in 2%; Baggish found none. Vestibular duct involvement is rare and is usually less than 1 mm. Sebaceous ducts, medial to the hair line, are rarely involved beyond 1 mm.[6,7,105] Lateral to the hair line the sebaceous ducts empty into hair follicles. Fifty-five percent of lateral vulvar intraepithelial neoplasia extends down into follicles, to a mean depth of 1.4 mm and rarely beyond 3 mm.[6,78,105,134] The uninvolved deeper parts of the follicles can extend through the full dermis and even into the subcutaneous tissues, reaching a depth of over 5 mm. The perineum (except for a few hair follicles) and anus have intraepithelial neoplasia confined essentially to the surface.

Therefore medial vulvar intraepithelial neoplasia should be treated to a depth of 1 mm or less and lateral to the hair line for 2.5 to 3 mm.[6,7,105,109,110]

Treatment

With the potential for vulvar dysplasia to progress to invasion less clear and slower than for cervical dysplasia and reports of spontaneous regression,[45] the vigor with which to treat mild dysplasia remains open to question. Moderate dysplasia and worse is considered premalignant and requires treatment, at least until viral, and molecular biologic research indicate otherwise.

The treatment of vulvar neoplasia began medicinally. In Ebers papyrus, written in 1550 BC, a mixture of garlic, horn, bile, dates, and asses milk was prescribed for what appears to have been vulvar neoplasia.[32] In the ensuing 3500 years the quest for a "magic" medicine has lead to hokums, dissolved topical mustard gas, a series of topical anticancer agents (the most popular being 5-fluorouracil 5-FU), immunotherapy with dinitrochlorobenzene, interferon, photodynamic therapy with hematoporphyrin sensitization, and more. None to date has proven sufficient alone. Adjunctive 5-FU and interferon have proven useful in some patients.[65,96] However, the main treatment is *surgical removal*.

Only 25 years ago the standard treatment for vulvar neoplasia in situ was vulvectomy. This involved removal of epidermis, dermis, and subcutaneous tissues down to the deep fascia. This was even employed for "leukoplakia" that was thought to have a 20% risk of progressing to cancer.[60] Probably much of the leukoplakia was squamous hyperplasia or dysplasia. In 1968 Rutledge and Sinclair introduced the "skinning" vulvectomy that removed only epidermis and dermis,[101] whereas DiSaia in 1981 emphasized clitoral preservation.[26] Today the most widely used methods are skinning excisions and laser. *Skinning excision* involves removing epidermis and dermis to a depth of about 5 mm. The defect needs to be closed or grafted. If the excision is not too wide, the loose tissue of the labia majora permits closure. Lateral to the hair line, vulvar intraepithelial neoplasia rarely exceeds 3 mm in depth; most patients therefore require less than full thickness skinning excision.

Laser might be the most popular method used today. It can excise but is used predominantly to vaporize. A major disadvantage is lack of tissue for pathologic examination, although wide and deep margins can be sampled with a small Keyes punch. Any stromal damage can result in scarring. However, when the deeper reticular dermis is left intact, scarring is often minimal. Surface epithelium will regenerate from epithelium in follicular depths and any remaining vellus hairs. Reid emphasizes the use of the proper power—low enough to control the depth of penetration and high enough to minimize thermal necrosis. Necrosis can extend 0.1 to 0.5 mm deeper than vulvar in situ removal.[94,95] Reid stresses knowledge of landmarks and planes. This is more important than measurement of depth which is hard to accomplish to fractions of a millimeter; different parts of the vulva and different lesions have different depths of subepithelial extension.[30] Reid states that the art of laser use is to judge the depth of penetration so that the deepest margin of thermal necrosis corresponds to the desired depth of surgery. *First plane* laser removes the epidermis and is appropriate for removal of condylomas. The *second plane* laser removes the superficial papillary dermis, needed to remove medial vulvar intraepithelial neoplasia. The *third plane* laser extends into the superficial reticular dermis, where lateral vulvar intraepithelial neoplasia can reach into hair shafts. Vulvar intraepithelial neoplasia rarely extend deeper; if so, full skinning excision with closure or grafting is necessary. By understanding depths and planes, it is possible to remove vulvar intraepithelial neoplasia, while preserving the coitally important lubricating glands and ducts and the depths of the follicles whose keratinocytes provide a source for regeneration of epithelium.

Newer techniques include loop, ultrasonic surgical aspirator, and chemosurgery. Ferenczy[37] has used a flat loop to excise vulvar intraepithelial neoplasia. Rader et al reported favorable results with ultrasonic surgical aspiration.[89]

Chemosurgery, introduced in 1977, has not been widely adopted because of discomfort from chemoinflammation from 5-FU when used alone.[107] It is a tedious microsurgical procedure, and until recently there was not a "gynecologic" instrument for use. Before the proliferation of loop generators, a "dermatologic" hyfrecator was necessary. Chemosurgery is the least traumatic technique because pretreatment with 5-FU loosens the neoplasia so that it can be easily removed with a low power (in the range of 8 to 12 units versus 40+ with loop) electrosurgical paddle blade.[108,109,110] The dermis is left intact and there is no scarring to compromise structure or function. Chemosurgery is ideal for intraepithelial neoplasia on sites where there is no or minimal sub epithelial extension (medial vulvar intraepithelial neoplasia and anal intraepithelial neoplasia). Seventy percent of patients have vulvar intraepithelial neoplasia medial to the hair line, where a surgical depth of 1 mm or less is in order.[105,134] Chemosurgery is especially helpful for patients who are immunosuppressed or have persistent or recurrent vulvar intraepithelial neoplasia.

Sometimes a combination of techniques might best serve a particular patient and lesion and cause less trauma with equivalent results.[11,60,108-110,134] Chemosurgery or superficial laser can debulk much vulvar intraepithelial neoplasia so that smaller, lateral, focal areas can be removed by skinning excision, if desirable. For immunosuppressed patients or those with an anogenital neoplastic syndrome, chemosurgery and laser "drilling" of white, suspicious hair shafts has worked well.[110] All 16 patients treated through 1992 for vulvar intraepithelial neoplasia with chemosurgery are currently in remission.

Minimal, effective treatment is the goal. One wants to minimize scarring and loss of lubrication from glands. By going too deep medially and destroying sebaceous, apocrine, eccrine, and vestibular glands and ducts, dryness and dyspareunia can result. Choice of modalities is based on the patient, invasion not being present, the location and extent of neoplasia, and prior treatments.

The overall recurrence rate for vulvar intraepithelial neoplasia is approximately 30%. It is higher in immunosuppressed patients, where retreatment is often required. Finding all sites and *gaining free margins* does more to lower persistent or recurrent rates than the "radicality" of surgery. Margins can be checked on frozen sections or after surgery; with negative margins, the persistent or recurrent rate is less than 10%[60,110]; with positive margins, the persistent or recurrent rate is over 50%. One can help assure negative margins by frozen section confirmation and removing 5 mm beyond vulvar in situ. Ferenczy found occult HPV in adjacent normal appearing skin.[38] Pretreatment with 5-FU can highlight otherwise occult vulvar intraepithelial neoplasia and can be a useful suppressive adjunct for HPV/oncogenic expression regardless of the surgical method used.

Postoperative care for all but skinning excision includes the following: sitz baths (with instant ocean or other appropriate additives, as desired); good hygiene and care so that regenerating epithelium can rapidly cover the wound; betadine/peroxide (1:3) or Burow's cleansing; short-term silver sulfadiazine (long-term leads to fungal infections); and analgesia.

MALIGNANT NEOPLASMS

Malignant neoplasms of the vulva are uncommon and represent 5% of all malignancies of the female genital tract. Ninety percent of cancers are squamous, arising on the labia majora, minora, or vestibule. Less frequently, adenocarcinomas may arise in adnexal structures, Bartholin's glands, and even ectopic breast tissue. The vulva may develop skin malignancies, including melanoma, basal cell carcinoma, and Paget's disease.

The broad spectrum of skin lesions affecting the vulva makes careful inspection an ongoing and challenging task. Vulvar neoplasms have a very wide range of presenting symptoms, colorations, and anatomic distribution. Frequently ignorance, modesty, or denial combine to cause dangerous delays before the patient reports a vulvar lesion. Once brought to the physician's attention, additional delay and ineffective topical therapy may compound the problem. It is of paramount importance for the physician to biopsy most vulvar lesions before initiating therapy.

Squamous Carcinoma

Epidemiology. Squamous carcinoma is a disease of postmenopausal women with a mean age of 61.1 years. Unlike the incidence of vulvar intraepithelial neoplasia that has doubled, the incidence of invasive carcinoma has remained constant. It may be that initiated women are not old enough to develop the invasive lesions, and the incidence will rise over the next decade. Alternatively, aggressive therapy currently employed for vulvar intraepithelial neoplasia lesions may prevent invasion; however, vulvar intraepithelial neoplasia may not always represent a continuum to invasion.[13]

Risk factors for the development of invasive squamous cancer include chronic inflammatory diseases of the vulva, such as some vulvar dystrophies, poor hygiene, and women over 70 years of age. Risk factors commonly associated with cervical cancer include the number of sexual partners, an abnormal Pap smear, any anogenital HPV/neoplasm,

Table 4-1. FIGO staging for carcinoma of the vulva

Stage 0	
Tis	Carcinoma in situ, intraepithelial carcinoma
Stage I	
T1 N0 M0	Tumor confined to the vulva and/or perineum; 2 cm or less in greatest dimension; nodes are not palpable
Stage II	
T2 N0 M0	Tumor confined to the vulva and/or perineum; more than 2 cm in greatest dimension; nodes are not palpable
Stage III	
T3 N0 M0	Tumor of any size with...
T3 N1 M0	1. adjacent spread to the lower urethra and/or the vagina, or the anus, and/or...
T1 N1 M0	2. unilateral regional lymph node metastasis
T2 N1 M0	
Stage IVA	
T1 N2 M0	Tumor invades any of the following:
T1 N2 M0	Upper uretha, bladder mucosa, rectal mucosa, pelvic bone, and/or bilateral regional node metastasis
T3 N2 M0	
T4 any N M0	
Stage IVB	
Any T	Any distant metastasis including
Any N, M1	pelvic lymph nodes

From American Joint Committee on Cancer: *Manual for staging cancer*, ed 4, Chicago, 1992, The Committee.

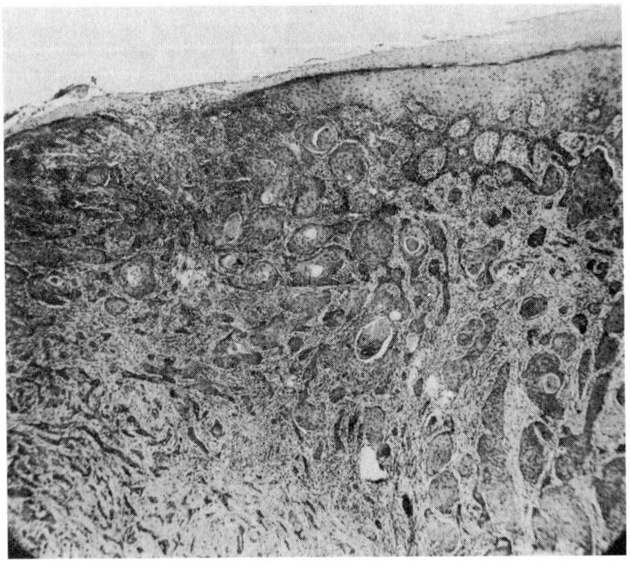

Fig. 4-18. High-power photomicrograph of carcinoma of the vulva. (Courtesy Armed Forces Institute of Pathology, no. 70121.)

smoking, and immunosuppression—all increase the risk of developing invasion. The similarity of risk factors for cervical and vulvar cancer have led some to conclude that HPV is the prime etiologic factor in the development of squamous cancer of the vulva.[23a,117a] However, there is growing support for the notion that in some invasive squamous carcinomas, HPV may not play a dominant role, as it appears to in preinvasive lesions.[2,23a]

Mode of spread. The mode of cancer spread is important in designing diagnostic and therapeutic approaches. Cancers may spread by direct extension, implantation, and lymphatic or vascular dissemination. Squamous cancers of the vulva spread predominantly by direct extension and lymphatic dissemination. Therefore knowing the lymphatic drainage of the vulva is crucial to understanding the biologic behavior of the tumor and the rationale for therapy.

Lymphatics from the external genitalia, including the labia, vestibule, and lower vagina, drain to the superficial inguinal lymph nodes. These nodes are located in the femoral triangle defined superiorly by the inguinal ligament, medially by the adductor longus, and laterally by the sartorius muscle. Clustered around the superficial saphenous vein, the nodes then drain to the deep or femoral nodes. The most superior deep femoral node, lying just beneath the inguinal ligament, is Cloquet's node. Cloquet's node was at one time felt to be a sentinel node, which when positive necessitated removal of the pelvic lymph nodes. With the introduction of pelvic radiotherapy, pelvic lymph node dissection for carcinoma of the vulva became less necessary, and the clinical importance of Cloquet's node has been diminished.

The deep femoral nodes ultimately drain to the external iliac, common iliac, and aortic nodal groups. Although some lymphatic channels from the clitoris have been shown to drain directly to the deep femoral nodes, the clinical significance of these anatomic findings is unclear.[85a]

Classification and staging. The current system for staging squamous cell carcinoma of the vulva is based on a surgical staging system. Staging reflects the known biologic behavior of the disease, its pattern of growth, and new prognostic variables, including the number and location of involved lymph nodes (Table 4-1). Establishment of an accurate surgical stage is of great value in prognosis, therapy,and the uniform reporting of data.

Histologic grade. Squamous carcinomas of the vulva are generally well- to moderately-differentiated tumors (Fig. 4-18). The degree of differentiation is important in predicting the biologic behavior of these tumors. Well-differentiated tumors are characterized by minimal cytologic atypia and a tendency toward keratinization. Frequently these tumors form epithelial "pearls" that are composed of concentric layers of squamous cells. In contrast, undifferentiated cells are characterized by scant cytoplasm and marked nuclear pleomorphism. Such anaplastic cells are frequently seen deeply invading the underlying stroma in smears or clusters. There is a lack of keratin and multiple, bizarre mitotic figures.

The grade of squamous cancers is defined by the ratio of differentiated and undifferentiated regions within the tumor. Grade 1, or well-differentiated tumors, show no regions of undifferentiation, whereas grade 3 tumors are comprised of greater than 50% undifferentiated cells. The grade of the squamous cancer is a strong predictor of biologic behavior. Increasing dedifferentiation comes with an increasing tendency for deep invasion, lymphatic or vascular space involvement, and regional nodal spread.

Treatment. Squamous carcinoma of the vulva is generally a local malignancy with a predilection for sequential nodal involvement. Distant metastases are uncommon in the absence of advanced local disease. Since the introduction of radical vulvectomy and inguinal lymphadenectomy by Taussig in 1940, the radical surgical approach has often been successful.[51a,78a,117b,126]

As more knowledge of the factors affecting outcome has been obtained, there has been an evolution toward a more tailored operation. For appropriately selected patients, this offers a less mutilating, less morbid but equally effective result. When first described by Taussig and Way, the vulva was removed in continuity with inguinal and femoral nodal tissue. To eliminate the possibility of leaving lymphatic metastases between vulva and groin, the intervening skin bridges were removed, resulting in a butterfly shaped skin defect. Understanding that the mode of metastatic spread was embolic rather than by contiguous growth allowed for the development of the 3-incision technique, which dramatically reduced overall morbidity with no impact on recurrence or survival.[50a,51a]

Recently the radical vulvectomy has been modified further for patients with small, lateral lesions. A radical wide local excision combined with an ipsilateral, superficial inguinal lymphadenectomy in selected patients now appears appropriate.

Treatment based on stage

Early stage disease. For patients with small (less than 2 cm) lateral lesions, a radical wide local excision with ipsilateral groin node dissection is an appropriate initial procedure. If at the time of frozen section of the ipsilateral nodes a positive node is detected, the contralateral inguinal nodes are explored.[15a] If surgical margins on the vulva are within 1 cm, or two or more inguinal nodes are positive for metastasis, adjuvant radiotherapy to vulva, pelvic nodes, or inguinal nodes may be required.[118a]

For patients with early but centrally located lesions, a 3-incision radical vulvectomy is preferred. Once again, adjuvant radiotherapy may be required for close vulvar margins or multiple positive inguinal nodes.

Management of advanced vulvar cancer. For patients presenting with advanced vulvar lesions involving urethra, anal sphincter, or vagina, a primary surgical approach would involve an extensive resection or possible exenteration. An alternative is the use of local radiotherapy or a combination of chemotherapy and radiation. Such neoadjuvant chemoradiation therapy has been shown to reduce dramatically tumor bulk and allow for more limited surgical resection.[83a,118b] A similar strategy may be employed for patients with fixed inguinal lymph nodes.

Treatment of microinvasive carcinoma of the vulva. There is a subset of vulvar carcinomas with virtually no risk of nodal spread. Such microinvasive lesions can be managed in a nonradical way. The initial definitions of microinvasion were defined as lesions demonstrating less than 5 mm of invasion. Given that 50% of all vulvar cancers are less than 5 mm thick and that 20% of these have metastasized, such a definition is inappropriate.

A Gynecologic Oncology Group study better defined the term microinvasive vulvar cancer, based not only on the thickness of the primary lesion but also on its size, degree of differentiation, location, presence of vascular space involvement, and clinical status of the regional lymph nodes.

It is now clear that well-differentiated squamous cancers less than 1 mm in thickness and distant from the clitoris or perineum have virtually no risk of metastasis to the ipsilateral groin nodes. This is particularly true in the absence of lymphatic or vascular space involvement, or clinically palpable lymph nodes. It is therefore appropriate to offer this subset of vulvar cancer patients a wide local excision without lymphadenectomy.[103a]

PAGET'S DISEASE

Since it was first described in 1895, the origin, biologic behavior, and optimal management of Paget's disease of the vulva have remained controversial.[31] Unlike Paget's disease of the breast, a cutaneous manifestation of underlying ductal carcinoma, vulvar Paget's is associated with underlying carcinoma only 25% of the time. This suggests a different natural history and malignant potential for vulvar Paget's when compared with breast or other extramammary sites in which the association with underlying carcinoma is high.[113]

Paget's cells may develop from an intraepithelial site such as apocrine cells.[75] Recent immunocytochemistry studies utilizing a panel of monoclonal antibodies specific for cytokeratins has added support to this hypothesis.[5] An apocrine cell of origin is consistent with the observation that Paget's disease is frequently multicentric and multifocal.[118]

The occurrence of invasive adenocarcinomas associated with Paget's disease may occur within, beneath, or distant from the epithelial lesion. There may be a coexisting underlying adenocarcinoma of the vulva, usually contiguous adnexal carcinomas, sometimes palpable beneath the epithelial changes.[62,127] There may be carcinomas distant from the site of the intraepithelial lesion, such as carcinomas of the breast, cervix, colon, and skin.[39] Paget's rarely

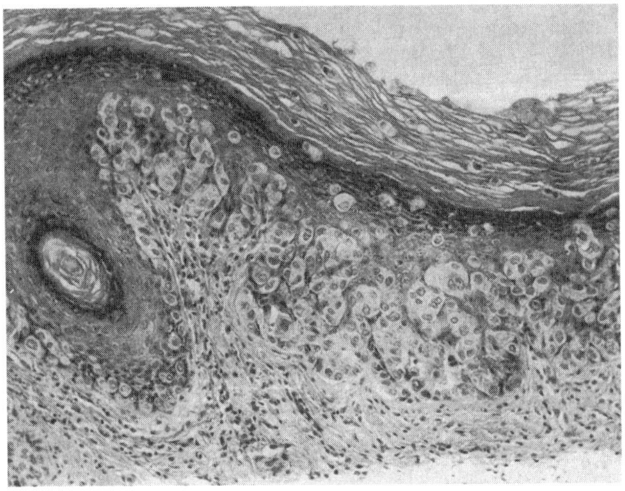

Fig. 4-19. Paget's disease of the vulva, showing marked hyperkeratosis and parakeratosis. Large, irregular cells are seen in the basal layer of the epidermis and infiltrating the upper layers as well. The Paget cells contain clear, vacuolated cytoplasm and vesicular nuclei, which vary in size, shape, and staining quality.

invades directly from its intraepithelial site but can result in metastatic Paget's disease up to 10.8 years following local resection.[51,57,81]

Paget's disease accounts for less than 1% of vulvar malignancies. It is most frequently a disease of the seventh decade of life, characterized by red raised lesions that are frequently dotted with pale white "islands" of epithelium. The lesion may occur at any site on the vulva or perineum. Cases of extension to the mons or thigh have been reported.[50] Paget's is a difficult disease to eradicate because of its propensity to recur despite free excisional margins.

As with any other vulvar lesion, directed biopsy, either excisional or with Keyes punch, is mandatory to establish the diagnosis (Fig. 4-19). Once confirmed, management must take into account the risk of malignancy within, beneath, or distant from the Paget's lesion. PAP smear, breast examination, and mammography are all critical for preoperative evaluation. A wide local excision of the lesion, including 0.5 to 1 cm of underlying fat should be performed if no vulvar mass is present. Any mass beneath the lesion should be fully excised and submitted for histopathologic evaluation to rule out an underlying malignancy.

Frozen sections of the surgical resection margins should be obtained. Although the margins of the Paget's lesion may appear clear, it is frequently the case that Pagetoid cells extend beyond the margin of the resection. Negative resection margins (wide and deep) significantly reduce the risk of local recurrence. Extensive resection may necessitate skin grafting.

The role of laser ablation of Paget's disease is controversial. Laser surgery is best suited for the treatment of recurrent disease in which underlying adenocarcinoma has already been ruled out by wide local excision. It may also be useful for cases in which grossly negative but histologically positive margins extend to areas such as paraclitoral, urethral, or anal, where delicate and precise surgical procedures are preferred.[33]

Regardless of the treatment selected, frequent follow-up is required due to the high recurrence rate.

Table 4-2. Vulvar melanoma staging

Level	Description	Corrected 5-year survival rate (%)
I	Intraepithelial	100
II	≤1 mm from granular layer	100
III	1-2 mm from granular layer	40
IV	>2 mm from granular layer	40
V	Into subcutaneous fat	20

MELANOMA

Malignant melanoma represents 2% of all vulvar malignancies. The average age at diagnosis is 57 years, but melanoma may affect women as young as 20 years of age. In a recent survey of 219 consecutive cases of malignant vulvar melanoma in Sweden, 75% of patients were over 60 years of age. Most frequently the lesions involve the clitoris and labia minora and are usually noticed by the patient due to enlargement of a preexisting mole, bleeding, or pruritus.

There are three types of melanomas. The superficial spreading and nodular melanoma account for the majority of vulvar melanomas. The superficial spreading melanoma has a protracted intraepithelial growth phase followed by stromal invasion, whereas nodular melanomas have a vertical growth resulting in rapid and deep invasion.

Because management and prognosis are based largely on the depth of invasion, the diagnosis should be made by an excisional biopsy. Vulvar melanomas are microstaged based on the depth of skin involvement. Because of variations in vulvar skin, staging utilizing the lesion's thickness correlates best with prognosis (Table 4-2).

The treatment for vulvar melanoma remains controversial largely because of the rarity of the lesion and a lack of a consistent treatment strategy. In the past radical vulvectomy with inguinal lymphadenectomy has been employed. Unfortunately a radical resection does not eliminate the risk of local recurrence, which may happen 30% to 42% of the time.[86,90] Davidson et al reviewed the outcomes of 32 patients with vulvar melanoma. They found that the five-year survival rate, local control rate, and disease-free interval were not affected by the type of surgical procedure performed, whether it was local resection, simple vulvectomy, or radical vulvectomy with inguinal lymphadenectomy.[24] Confusing the issue is the fact that the five-year survival rate for melanomas does *not* equate with cure. In one series with a ten-year follow-up, 50% of patients alive at five years were deceased by the tenth anniversary of their diagnosis. Based on these observations, regional lymph node sampling may yield important prognostic information but is unlikely to impact survival.

A prudent recommendation is to tailor the surgical resection based on thickness of the melanoma. A radical local excision with 2 cm margins should be performed for melanomas less than or equal to 1 mm from the granular layer (Chung level II) and a radical local excision with 3 cm margins should be used for more deeply invasive lesions (levels III-IV). Superficial (level I) lesions may be treated with simple excision. Although controversial, dissection of the regional nodes is recommended.[59]

Carcinoma of Bartholin's gland

Adenocarcinomas arising in Bartholin's gland are rare. A cystic mass in the lateral walls of the vestibule is far more likely to represent a benign condition than a malignancy. Bartholin's gland rarely exceeds 1 cm in size and undergoes gradual involution in women over 30 years of age. Therefore the occurrence of an enlarged vulvar mass in an older woman, particularly if she is postmenopausal, is worrisome. It is recommended that incision and drainage of a presumed Bartholin's cyst or cyst abscess in a postmenopausal woman be accompanied by a biopsy of the cyst wall.

Carcinoma of Bartholin's gland may derive from the transitional cells that line the duct, or from the mucin-secreting cells of the gland itself. Mucous-secreting tumors tend to be less aggressive than transitional-cell carcinomas.

Unfortunately, Bartholin's gland carcinomas arise deep within vulvar tissue rich with both lymphatic and vascular supply, and metastasis to inguinal and pelvic lymph nodes is common. A radical hemivulvectomy, ipsilateral inguinal lymphadenectomy, and adjuvant radiotherapy to pelvic node groups are recommended.

Basal cell carcinoma

Despite being the most common tumor of the skin, vulvar basal cell carcinoma is rare with fewer than 150 cases reported. The lesion has a characteristic pearly-grey appearance with marked telangiectasis. Brown or black pigmentation may be present and central ulceration is not uncommon. Bilateral tumors have been reported.[117]

Basal cell carcinoma is a locally aggressive epidermal tumor that rarely metastasizes. However, it is important to examine the inguinal nodes and to resect any suspicious node. When local nodes are not suspicious, a wide local excision is adequate therapy for the primary lesion. Care in obtaining histologically negative margins will dramatically reduce the risk of local recurrence. The prognosis following complete local resection is excellent.

Sarcomas

Sarcomas may arise from any connective tissue component of the vulva. Epithelioid sarcomas appear to have more aggressive behavior when occurring on the vulva. Such tumors occur in young women and may mimic a Bartholin's cyst. They are characterized by very rapid progression and death. Cases of Kaposi's sarcoma have been reported in association with acquired immunodeficiency syndrome; the tumor presents as a small vulvar papilloma. Regardless of the histologic type of sarcoma, radical surgery is ineffective and the prognosis is poor.

Verrucous carcinoma

Verrucous carcinoma of the vulva affects postmenopausal women. It is a locally invasive, slow growing tumor characterized by a cauliflower or verrucoid growth pattern. The lesion may be very large and cause severe genital itching. Histologic features include papillary bands of highly differentiated, hyperkeratotic epithelium with a very abrupt transition to normal skin. Superficial biopsies of these large lesions may be misleading. In this type of tumor, unlike benign condyloma, the fibrovascular cores so prominent in condyloma are limited to the superficial layers of the verrucous carcinoma.

Wide local excision with negative margins is an appropriate operation in the absence of clinically suspicious nodes. In case of recurrent disease, regional lymph node dissection is advocated. Local radiation therapy may cause anaplastic transformation of this tumor and is contraindicated. Once local control of the tumor is achieved the prognosis is excellent.

Acknowledgments

We gratefully acknowledge the legacy of this chapter from **Dr. Thomas Leavitt, Jr.** for his advice in the current edition and the many kind and generous hours he devoted to our training as residents and fellows.

We thank **Drs. Christopher P. Crum** and **Harley Haynes** for their expertise and help with pathology and dermatology, respectively.

REFERENCES

1. Adelson MD, Miranda FR, Strumpf KB: Necrotizing fasciitis: a complication of squamous cell carcinoma of the vulva, *Gynecol Oncol* 42:98, 1991.
2. Andersen WA et al: Vulvar squamous cell carcinoma and papilloma viruses: two separate entities? *Am J Obstet Gynecol* 165:2, 329-335, 1991.
3. Deleted in proofs.
4. Arndt KA: Lichen planus. In Fitzpatrick TB et al: *Dermatology in general medicine*, ed 4, New York, 1993, McGraw-Hill.
5. Bacchi CE et al: Paget's disease and melanoma of the vulva: use of a panel of monoclonal antibodies to identify cell type and to microscopically define adequacy of surgical margins, *Gynecol Oncol* 46:216-221, 1992.
6. Baggish MS et al: Quantitative evaluation of the skin and accessory appendages in vulvar carcinoma in situ, *Obstet Gynecol* 74:169-174, 1989.

7. Benedet JL, Wilson PS, Matisic J: Epidermal thickness and skin appendage involvement in vulvar intraepithelial neoplasia, *J Reprod Med* 36: 608-612, 1991.
8. Bernstein SG et al: Vulvar carcinoma in situ, *Obstet Gynecol* 58:304-307, 1983.
9. Bhaha NN, Bergman A, Broen EM: Advanced hidradenitis suppurativa of the vulva: a report of 3 cases, *J Reprod Med* 29:436, 1984.
10. Billstein SA: Human Lice. In Holmes KK et al: *Sexually transmitted diseases*, ed 2, New York, 1990, McGraw Hill.
11. Bornstein J, Kaufman RH: Combination of surgical excision and carbon dioxide laser vaporization for multifocal vulvar intraepithelial neoplasia, *Am J Obstet Gynecol* 158:459-464, 1988.
12. Bornstein J, Pascal B, Abramovici HZ: The common problem of vulvar pruritus, *Obstet Gynecol Surv* 48(2):111-118, 1993.
13. Brinton LA et al: Case-control study of cancer of the vulva, *Obstet Gynecol* 75:5, 859-866, 1990.
14. Brody J: A painful women's problem isn't in the mind, *New York Times*, Oct. 27, 1993:C-11.
15. Brucks JA, Jacobs EW: Practical tips for assessment and management of vulvar and vaginal human papillomavirus, *Nurse Pract Forum* 3(3):169-176, 1992.
15a. Burke TW et al: Radical wide excision and selective inguinal node dissection for squamous cell carcinoma of the vulva, *Gynecol Oncol* 38:328-332, 1990.
16. Buscema J et al: The predominance of human papilloma virus type 16 in vulvar neoplasia, *Obstet Gynecol* 71:601-606, 1988.
17. Christopher E, Sterry W: Psoriasis. In Fitzpatrick TB et al, *Dermatology in general medicine*, ed 4, New York, 1993, McGraw-Hill.
18. Chung AF, Woodruff JD, Lewis JL: Malignant melanoma of the vulva: a reprint of 44 cases, *Obstet Gynecol* 45:638, 1975.
19. Deleted in proofs.
20. Deleted in proofs.
21. Covino JM, McCormack WM: Vulvar ulcer of unknown etiology in a human immunodeficiency virus-infected woman: response to treatment with Zidovudine, *Am J Obstet Gynecol* 163: 116-118, 1990.
22. Cruikshank SH, McLauchlan L: A de novo case of vulvar synergistic necrotizing fasciitis, *Obstet Gynecol* 69:516, 1987.
23. Crum CP: Carcinoma of the vulva: epidemiology and pathogenesis, *Obstet Gynecol* 79:3, 448-454, 1992.
23a. Daling JR et al: Cigarette smoking and the risk of anogenital cancer, *Am J Epidemiol* 135:2, 180-189, 1992.
24. Davidson T, Kissin M, Westung G: Vulvovaginal melanoma—should radical surgery be abandoned? *Br J Obstet Gynecol* 94(5):473-476, 1987.
25. DiSaia PJ, Creasman WT: *Clinical Gynecologic Oncology*, ed 4, St Louis, 1993, Mosby Year Book.
26. DiSaia PJ, Rich WM: Surgical approach to multifocal carcinoma in situ of the vulva, *Am J Obstet Gynecol* 140:136-145, 1981.
27. DiSaia PJ, Rutledge F, Smith JP: Sarcoma of the vulva: report of 12 patients, *Obstet Gynecol* 38:2,180-184, 1971.
28. Division of STD/HIV Prevention: Sexually Transmitted Disease Surveillance, 1991, U.S. Department of Health and Human Services, Public Health Service. Atlanta: Centers for Disease Control, July 1992.
29. Division of STD/HIV Prevention: Sexually Transmitted Diseases Treatment Guidelines, U.S. Department of Health and Human Services, Public Health Service. Atlanta, 1993, Centers for Disease Control.
30. Dorsey JH: Understanding CO_2 laser surgery of the vulva, *Colposcopy & Gynecol Laser Surgery* 1(3):205-213, 1984.
31. Dubreuilh W: Paget's disease of the vulva, *Brit J Dermatol* 13:407-413, 1901.
32. Ebbell B: *The Papyrus Ebers*, London, 1937, Oxford University Press.
33. Ewing TL: Paget's disease of the vulva treated by combined surgery and laser, *Gynecol Oncol* 43:137-140, 1991.
34. Faro S: Lymphogranuloma venereum, chancroid, and granuloma inguinale, *Obstet Gynecol Clin North Am* 16:517-530, 1989.
35. Feldmann R et al: Fox-Fordyce disease: successful treatment with topical clindamycin in alcoholic propylene glycol solution, *Dermatology* 184:310, 1992.
36. Deleted in proofs.
37. Ferenczy A: Comparison of CO_2 laser ablation and loop electrosurgical excision procedure for the treatment of vulvar intraepithelial neoplasia, *Gynecol Oncol* 45:76, 1992 (SGO abstract).
38. Ferenczy A et al: Latent papillomavirus and recurring genital warts, *N Engl J Med* 313:784-788, 1985.
39. Feuer GA, Sheuchuk M, Calanog A: Vulvar Paget's disease: the needs to exclude an invasive lesion, *Gynecol Oncol* 38:81-89; 1990.
40. Fitzpatrick TB et al, editors: *Color atlas and synopsis of clinical dermatology*, ed 2, New York, 1992, McGraw-Hill.
41. Fitzpatrick TB et al, editors: *Dermatology in general medicine*, ed 4, New York, 1993, McGraw-Hill.
42. Friedrich EG Jr: *Vulvar disease*, ed 2, Philadelphia, 1983, WB Saunders.
43. Friedrich EG Jr: Vulvar disease. In *Major Problems in Obstetrics and Gynecology vol. 9*, edition 2, Philadelphia, 1983, WB Saunders.
44. Friedrich EG Jr, Kalra PS: Serum levels of sex hormones in vulvar lichen sclerosus and the effect of topical testosterone, *N Engl J Med* 310(8):488-491, 1984.
45. Friedrich EG, Wilkinson EJ, Fu YS: Carcinoma in situ of the vulva: a continuing challenge, *Am J Obstet Gynecol* 136:830, 1980.
46. Furlonge CB et al: Vulvar vestibulitis syndrome: a clinico-pathological study, *Br J Obstet Gynecol* 98(7):703-706, 1991.
47. Gianini GD, Method MW, Christman JE: Traumatic vulvar hematomas: assessing and treating non-obstetric patients, *Postgrad Med* 89:115, 1991.
48. Goetsch MF: Vulvar vestibulitis: prevalence and historic features in a general gynecologic practice population, *Am J Obstet Gynecol* 164:1609-1614, 1991.
49. Deleted in proofs.
50. Gunn RA, Gallager HS: Vulvar Paget's disease: a topographic study, *Cancer* 46:590-594, 1980.
50a. Hacken NF et al: Radical vulvectomy and bilateral inguinal lymphadenectomy through separate groin incisions, *Obstet Gynecol* 58:574-579, 1981.
51. Hart W, Millman J: Progression of intraepithelial Paget's disease of the vulva to invasive carcinoma, *Cancer* 40:2333-2337, 1977.
51a. Heaps JM et al: Surgical-pathologic variables predictive of local recurrence in squamous carcinoma of the vulva, *Gynecol Oncol* 38:309-314, 1990.
52. Hoffman MS, Turnquist D: Necrotizing fasciitis of the vulva during chemotherapy, *Obstet Gynecol* 74:483, 1989.
53. Holmes KK, Sparling PF et al: *Sexually transmitted diseases*, ed 2, New York, 1990, McGraw Hill.
54. Horowitz BJ: Interferon therapy for condylomatous vulvitis, *Obstet Gynecol* 73:446-448, 1989.
55. Horowitz BJ: Mycotic vulvovaginitis, *Am J Obstet Gynecol* 165:1188-1192, 1991.
56. Iverson T, Abeler V, Kolstad P: Squamous carcinoma in situ of the vulva; a clinical and histopathologic study, *Gynecol Oncol* 11:224, 1981.
57. Jones R, Austin C, Ackerman A: Extramammary Paget's disease: a critical re-examination, *Amer J Dermopathol* 1:101-132, 1979.
58. Kaplan AL et al: Intraepithelial carcinoma of the vulva with extension to the anal canal, *Obstet Gynecol* 58:368-371, 1981.
59. Kaufman RH: Vulvar dystrophies, *ACOG Technical Bulletin*, no.139, January 1990.
60. Kaufman RH, Friedrich EG Jr, Gardner HL: *Benign disease of the vulva and vagina*, ed 3, Chicago, 1989, Year Book Medical Publishers.
61. Kim NI et al: Crohn's disease of the vulva, *J A Acad Dermatol* 27:764-765, 1992.
62. Koss L, Ladinsky S, Brockunier A: Paget's disease of the vulva: report of 10 cases, *Obstet Gynecol* 31:513-525, 1968.

63. Koss LG: *Diagnostic cytology and its histopathologic bases,* ed 4, Philadelphia, 1992, JB Lippincott.
64. Kraus SJ: Diagnosis and management of acute genital ulcers in sexually active patients, *Semin in Dermatol* 9:160-166, 1990.
65. Krebs HB: Prophylactic topical 5-fluorouracil following treatment of human papilloma-associated lesions of the vulva and vagina, *Obstet Gynecol* 68:837-841, 1986.
66. Vulvar Vestibulitis, *Lancet* 338:729-730, 1991 (editorial).
67. Leibowitch M et al: The epithelial changes associated with squamous cell carcinoma of the vulva: a review of the clinical, histologic, and viral findings in 78 women, *Br J Obstet Gynaecol* 97:1135-1139, 1990.
68. Levine EM, Barton JJ, Grier EA: Metatastic Crohn's disease of the vulva, *Obstet Gynecol* 60:395-397, 1982.
69. Deleted in proofs.
70. Lynch PJ: Vulvar dystrophies and intraepithelial neoplasias, *Dermatol Clin* 5:789-799, 1987.
71. Mandell GL, Douglas RG Jr, Bennett JE, editors: *Principles and practice of infectious diseases*, ed 3, New York, 1990, Churchill Livingstone.
72. Mann MS et al: Vulvar vestibulitis: significant clinical variables and treatment outcome, *Obstet Gynecol* 79(1):122-125, 1992.
73. Marinoff SC, Turner MLC: Vulvar vestibulitis syndrome: an overview, *Am J Obstet Gynecol* 165:1228-1233, 1991.
74. Marren P, Wojnarowska F, Powell S: Allergic contact dermatitis and vulvar dermatoses, *Br J Dermatol* 126(1):52-56, 1992.
75. Mazoujian G, Pinkus GS, Mangensen DE: Extramammary Paget's disease: evidence of an apocrine origin, *Am J Surg Pathol* 8:43-50, 1984.
76. McKay M: Vulvitis and vulvovaginitis: cutaneous considerations, *Am J Obstet Gynecol* 165(4)pt. 2:1176-1182, 1991.
77. McKay M: Vulvodynia: diagnostic patterns, *Dermatol Clin* 10(2):423-433, 1992.
78. Mene A, Buckley CH: Involvement of the vulva skin appendages by intraepithelial neoplasia, *Br J Obstet Gynaecol* 92:634-638, 1985.
78a. Morley GW: Infiltrative carcinoma of the vulva: results of surgical treatment, *Am J Obstet Gynecol* 124:847-884, 1976.
79. Morrow CP, Pisaia PJ: Malignant melanoma of the female genitalia: a clinical analysis, *Obstet Gynecol Surv* 31:233-271, 1976.
80. Pack GT, Oropeza R: A comparative study of melanomas and epidermoid carcinomas of the vulva, *Rev Surg* 24:305-324, 1967.
81. Parmley T, Woodruff J, Julian C: Invasive vulvar Paget's disease, *Obstet Gynecol* 46:341-346, 1975.
82. Patton LW, Elgart ML, Williams CM: Extraintestinal Crohn's disease of the vulva, *Arch Dermatol* 126(10):1351-1354, 1990.
83. Peckam BM et al: Focal vulvitis: a characteristic syndrome and cause of dyspareunia, *Am J Obstet Gynecol* 154(4):855-864, 1986.
83a. Perez CA et al: Radiation therapy in the management of carcinoma of the vulva with emphasis on conservative therapy, *Cancer* 71 (11):3707-3716, 1993.
84. Pincus SH: Vulvar dermatoses and pruritus vulvae, *Dermatol Clin* 10(2):297-308, 1992.
85. Pincus SH, McKay M: Disorders of the female genitalia. In Fitzpatrick TB et al: *Dermatology in general medicine*, 1463-1481, 1993.
85a. Plentl AA, Friedman EA: *Lymphatic system of the female genitalia*, Philadelphia, 1971, W.B. Saunders.
86. Podratz KC et al: Melanoma of the vulva: an update, *Gynecol Oncol* 16:153-168, 1983.
87. Deleted in proofs..
88. Pyka RE et al: The histopathology of vulvar vestibulitis syndrome, *Int J Gynecol Pathol* 7:249-257, 1988.
89. Rader JS et al: Ultrasonic surgical aspiration in the treatment of vulvar disease, *Obstet Gynecol* 77:573-576, 1991.
90. Ragnansson-Olding B et al: Malignant melanoma of the vulva and vagina: trends in incidence, age distribution, and long term survival among 245 consecutive cases in Sweden 1960-1984, *Cancer* 71(5):1893-1897, 1993.
91. Deleted in proofs.
92. Reichman RC, Bonnez W: Papillomaviruses. In Mandell GL et al: *Principles and practice of infectious diseases*, ed 3, New York, 1990, Churchill Livingstone.
93. Reid R: Superficial laser vulvectomy. I. The efficacy of extended superficial ablation for refractory and very extensive condylomas, *Am J Obstet Gynecol* 151(8):1047-1052, 1985.
94. Reid R et al: Superficial laser vulvectomy. II. The anatomic and biophysical principles permitting accurate control over the depth of dermal destruction with the carbon dioxide laser, *Am J Obstet Gynecol* 152(3):261-271, 1985.
95. Reid R: Superficial laser vulvectomy. III. A new surgical technique for appendage-conserving ablation of refractory condylomas and vulvar intraepithelial neoplasia, *Am J Obstet Gynecol* 152(5):504-509, 1985.
96. Reid R et al: Superficial laser vulvectomy. IV. Extended laser vaporization and adjunctive 5-fluorouracil therapy of human papillomavirus-associated vular disease, *Obstet Gynecol* 76(3):439-448, 1990.
97. Reid R: Laser surgery of the vulva, *Obstet Gynecol Clin North Am* 18:491-510, 1991.
98. Reid R, Greenberg MD: Human papillomavirus-related diseases of the vulva, *Clin Obstet Gynecol* 34(3):630-650, 1991.
99. Roberts DB: Necrotizing fasciitis of the vulva, *Am J Obstet Gynecol* 157:568, 1987.
100. Rock B: Pigmented lesions of the vulva, *Dermatol Clin* 10:361-370, 1992.
101. Rutledge F, Sinclair M: Treatment of intraepithelial carcinoma of the vulva by skin excision and graft, *Am J Obstet Gynecol* 102:806, 1968.
102. Schmid GP: Chancroid. In Evans AS, Brachmen PS, editors: *Bacterial infection of humans: epidemiology and control*, ed 2, New York, 1991, Plenum Medical Book.
103. Secor RM, Fertitta L: Vulvar vestibulitis syndrome, *Nurse Pract Forum* 3(3):161-168, 1992.
103a. Sedlis A et al: Positive groin lymph nodes in superficial squamous cell vulvar cancer: A Gynecologic Oncology Group Study, *Am J Obstet Gynecol* 156 (5):1159-1164, 1987.
104. Shafi MI et al: Carbon dioxide laser treatment for vulval papillomatosis (vulvodynia), *Br J Obstet Gynaecol* 97(12):1148-1150, 1990.
105. Shatz P et al: Vulvar intraepithelial neoplasia and skin appendage involvement, *Obstet Gynecol* 74:769-774, 1989.
106. Deleted in proofs.
107. Sillman FH et al: 5-fluorouracil/chemosurgery in the treatment of intraepithelial neoplasia of the lower genital tract, *Obstet Gynecol* 58:356-360, 1981.
108. Sillman FH, Sedlis A, Boyce J: 5-FU/chemosurgery for difficult lower genital intraepithelial neoplasia, *Contemp Obstet Gynecol* 27:79-101, 1985.
109. Sillman FH, Sedlis A, Boyce J: A review of lower genital intraepithelial neoplasia and the use of topical 5-fluorouracil, *Obstet Gynecol Surv* 40:190-220, 1985.
110. Sillman FH, Sedlis A: 5-FU/chemosurgery in the treatment of vulvar intraepithelial neoplasia, *Colposcopy and Gynecologic Laser Surgery* 4:171-185, 1988.
111. Sillman FH, Sedlis A: Anogenital HPV/neoplasia in immunosuppressed women: an update, *Dermatol Clin North Am* 9:353-369, 1991.
112. Simonsen E et al: Basal cell carcinoma of the vulva, *Ac Obstet Scand* 64(3):231-234, 1985.
113. Sitakalin C, Ackerman AB: Mammary and extramammary Paget's disease, *Amer J Dermatopathol* 7(33):340, 1985.

114. Soper DE et al: Lichen planus of the vulva, *Obstet Gynecol* 72(1):74-76, 1988.
115. Sorensen K, Somrak TM: Vulva and vagina. In Bibbo M: *Comprehensive cytopathology,* Philadelphia, 1991, WB Saunders.
116. Stephenson H et al: Necrotizing fasciitis of the vulva, *Am J Obstet Gynecol* 166:1324, 1992.
117. Stiller M et al: Bilateral vulvar basal cell carcinomata, *J Am Acad Dermatol* 28: 836-838, 1993.
117a. Sturgeon SR et al: In situ and invasive vulvar cancer incidence trends (1973-1987), *Am J Obstet Gynecol* 166:5, 1482-1485, 1992.
117b. Taussig FJ: *Cancer of the vulva,* Am J Obstet Gynecol 40:764-767, 1940.
118. Taylor PT, Stenwig JT, Klausen H: Paget's disease of the vulva, *Gynecol Oncol* 3:46-60, 1975.
118a. Thomas GM et al: Changing concepts in the management of vulvar cancer, *Gynecol Oncol* 42:9-12, 1991.
118b. Thomas G et al: Concurrent radiation and chemotherapy in vulvar carcinoma, *Gynecol Oncol* 34:263-267, 1987.
119. Tovell HMM, Young AW Jr: *Diseases of the vulva in clinical practice,* New York, 1991, Elsevier.
120. Turner MLC, Marinoff SC: Pudendal neuralgia, *Am J Obstet Gynecol* 165:1233-1235, 1991.
121. Ulbright TM et al: Epithelioid sarcoma of the vulva: evidence suggesting a more aggressive behaviour than extragenital epithelioid sarcoma, *Cancer* 52(8):1462-1469, 1983.
122. Umpierre SA et al: Human papillomavirus DNA in tissue biopsy specimens of vulvar vestibulitis patients treated with interferon, *Obstet Gynecol* 78(4):693-695, 1991.
123. Deleted in proofs.
124. Van Cutsem J: The in vitro activity of terconazole against yeasts:its topical long-acting therapeutic efficacy in experimental vaginal candidiasis in rats, *Am J OG,* 165:1200-1206, 1991.
125. Vermesh M, Deppe G, Zbella E: Non-puerperal traumatic vulvar hematoma, *J Gynaecol Obstet* 22:217, 1984.
126. Way S: Carcinoma of the vulva, *Am J Obstet Gynecol* 79:692-697, 1960.
127. Wick M et al: Vulvar sweat gland carcinomas, *Arch Pathol Lab Med* 109:43-47, 1985.
128. Wilkinson EJ, editor: *Pathology of the vulva and vagina,* New York, 1987, Churchill Livingstone.
129. Wilkinson EJ, Freidrich EG Jr: Diseases of the vulva. In Kurman RJ, editor: *Blaustein's pathology of the female genital tract,* ed 3, New York, 1987, Springer.
130. Winkelmann SE, Llorens AS: Metastatic basal cell carcinoma of the vulva, *Gynecol Oncol* 38(1):138-140, 1990.
131. Woodruff JD: The vulva. In Rosenwaks Z, Benjamin F, Stone ML, editors: *Gynecology principles and practice,* New York, 1987, Macmillan Publishing.
132. Woodruff JD, Friedrich EG Jr: The vestibule, *Clin Obstet Gynecol* 28(1):134-141, 1985.
133. Woodruff JD: Carcinoma in situ of the vulva, *Clin Obstet Gynecol* 34:669-676, 1991.
134. Wright VC, Chapman WB: Colposcopy of intraepithelial neoplasia of the vulva and adjacent sites, *Obstet Gynecol Clin* 20:231-255, 1993.

Chapter 5

THE VAGINA

Joan M. Bengtson

The vagina is a tubular, fibromuscular structure that extends from the vestibule to the uterus. It is the interface between the environment and the generative tract. Its functions are to provide an outflow duct for menstrual discharge, to receive the penis during intercourse, and to form the lowermost part of the birth canal. Clinically it provides access to upper genital tract structures.

EMBRYOLOGY

The embryology of the vagina remains controversial, despite extensive historic interest in the topic and recently renewed interest stimulated by diethylstilbestrol (DES)-associated pathology. While certain events are well established, the histogenesis of the vaginal epithelium is uncertain. One theory favors a dual origin such that the upper vagina derives from the mesodermal müllerian ducts and the lower vagina from the endodermal urogenital sinus. Another proposes that the entire vagina originates in the urogenital sinus.

Development is identical in male and female fetuses until the seventh week. Two sets of genital ducts develop, the mesonephric (or wolffian) and the paramesonephric (or müllerian). In males the presence of the Y chromosome directs the development of testes. The indifferent stage ends when the developing testes begin producing androgenic steroids.[100] Androgens stimulate development of the mesonephric duct system into the epididymis, vas deferens, and seminal vesicles. In addition, a polypeptide, müllerian inhibiting factor (MIF) is produced and acts to suppress growth and induce resorption of the müllerian ducts. In females the absence of androgens and MIF permits further development of the müllerian structures and regression of the mesonephric ducts.

The müllerian ducts develop in the embryos of both sexes during the sixth week (11 mm stage).[42] They form as bilateral longitudinal evaginations of the coelomic epithelium into the mesonephric ridge ventrolateral to the mesonephric duct. Tubular structures result as the process of evagination is completed. Each müllerian duct remains open to the coelomic cavity at its cephalic end via an ostium. Caudally the duct initially runs parallel and lateral to the mesonephric duct. It then crosses ventral to the mesonephric duct to meet the contralateral müllerian duct in the midline (Fig. 5-1). The ducts fuse forming the primordial uterovaginal canal (30 mm embryo). This structure initially contains a longitudinal septum. The septum usually disappears by the eleventh week (56 mm embryo). The cranial segment of each müllerian duct ultimately forms a fallopian tube, its ostium becoming the fimbriated extremity. As the midline septum resorbs from the fused middle segment, the uterine corpus and cervix form. The caudal end of the fused müllerian ducts joins the urogenital sinus.

The attachment of the distal, fused müllerian ducts to the urogenital sinus stimulates a proliferation of cells in its dorsal wall. A prominence called the müllerian tubercle is formed.[42] The adjacent urogenital sinus epithelium also proliferates bilaterally forming the sinovaginal bulbs (63 mm embryo). Further proliferation results in the formation of a solid midline cord of cells called the vaginal plate (120 mm embryo). Growth and elongation of the vaginal plate increases the distance between the uterocervical canal and the urogenital sinus (Fig. 5-2). The vaginal plate also divides the urogenital sinus into an upper portion that develops into the bladder and urethra (the vesicourethral canal) and a lower portion that forms the definitive urogenital sinus and ultimately the vestibule.

Canalization of the vaginal plate occurs as the central cells degenerate. This begins at the urogenital sinus and proceeds cranially to form the vault. The process is completed by approximately the fifth month. The lumen of the vagina remains separated from the lumen of the urogenital sinus by

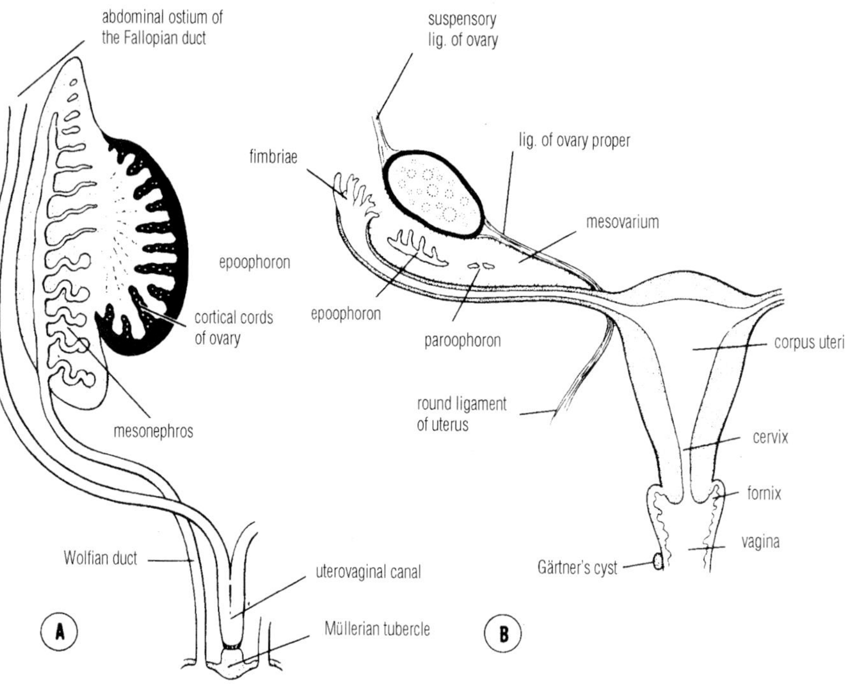

Fig. 5-1. **A**, Schematic drawing of the genital ducts in the female at the end of the second month of development. Note the müllerian tubercle and the formation of the uterovaginal canal. **B**, The genital ducts after descent of the ovary. The only parts remaining of the mesonephric system are the epoophoron, paroophoron, and Gartner's cyst. Note the suspensory ligament of the ovary, the ligament of the ovary proper, and the round ligament of the uterus. (From Saddler TW: *Langman's medical embryology*, ed 5, Baltimore, 1985, Williams & Wilkins.)

the formation of the hymen. The hymen usually develops at least a partial opening sometime later.

The ultimate derivation of the vaginal squamous epithelium is disputed.[26] The theory of dual origin suggests that the caudal end of the müllerian uterovaginal canal forms the upper four fifths of the vagina while the lower one fifth derives from the endodermal urogenital sinus. The hymen demarcates the junction. After canalization occurs, the müllerian columnar epithelium undergoes metaplasia to form a squamous epithelium that joins the epithelium derived from the urogenital sinus.[12] Another theory suggests that the vaginal plate is derived from proliferation of the sinovaginal bulbs, and thus the entire vagina is of urogenital sinus origin.[13] It is likely that a normal interaction of both müllerian and urogenital sinus tissue is necessary for normal vaginal development.

ANATOMY AND HISTOLOGY

The vagina is a compressed but distensible musculomembranous canal extending from the vulva to the uterine cervix (Fig. 5-3). It is directed cephalad and posterior from the vestibule toward the sacral promontory. Anteriorly the vagina is closely related to the bladder and urethra. The trigone lies against the upper third of the vagina. The urethra courses inferiorly apposed to the anterior vaginal wall. The tissue between these structures, the vesicovaginal septum and the urethrovaginal septum, consists of supporting fibrous tissue of the endopelvic fascia and a potential avascular space.

The posterior vaginal wall is related to the peritoneal cul-de-sac of Douglas at its upper third, the ampulla of the rectum at its middle third, and the perineal body at its lower third. The relationship to the cul-de-sac of Douglas is clinically important because it provides an easy route of access to the peritoneal cavity through the vagina. The rectovaginal septum, like its anterior counterpart, has a potential avascular plane between supporting layers of endopelvic fascia. Though the vagina and rectum are closely apposed in the region of the septum, their orifices are more widely separated by the perineal body. The perineal body is an important structure that provides a central area of insertion for the supporting musculature of the urogenital diaphragm and pelvic floor.

The lateral relations of the vagina include the parametrial tissues at its superior extent. The ureters pass through this tissue 1 to 2 cm lateral to the vagina as they course toward the trigone, an important relationship to consider when vaginal surgery is performed. At the junction of the middle and lower third of the vagina, the pubococcygeal portion of the

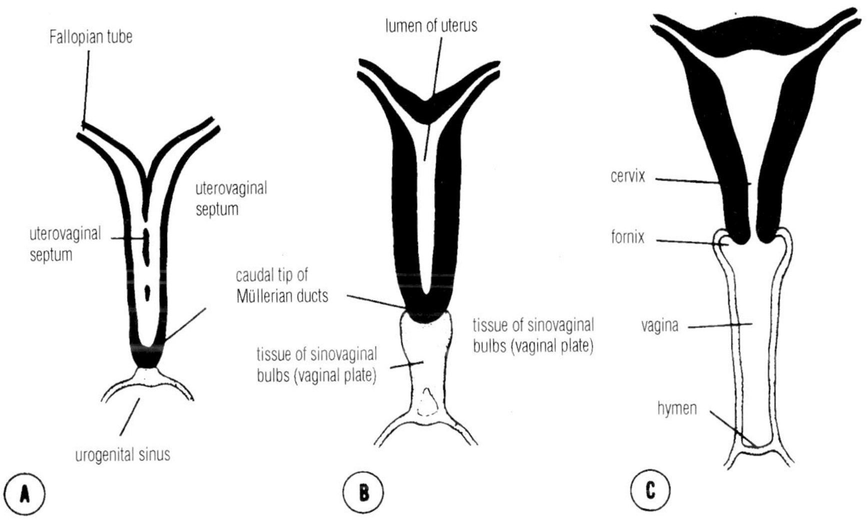

Fig. 5-2. Schematic drawing showing the formation of the uterus and vagina. **A**, At 9 weeks. Note the disappearance of the uterovaginal septum. **B**, At the end of the third month. Note the tissue of the sinovaginal bulbs, extending between the uterus and the urogenital sinus. **C**, Newborn. The vagina and the fornices are formed by vacuolization of the tissue of the sinovaginal bulbs. (From Sadler TW: *Langman's medical embryology*, ed 5, Baltimore, 1985, Williams & Wilkins.)

levator ani muscle forms a hiatus through which the vagina passes. At the introitus the vagina is related laterally to the bulbocavernosus muscles. Posterolateral to these muscles is the ischiorectal fossa.

Superiorly the uterine cervix projects into the vagina through its anterior wall. The axis of the vagina forms an angle of approximately 90 degrees with the axis of the cervical canal. The posterior wall of the vagina is longer than the anterior wall by approximately 3 cm due to the anterior attachment of the cervix. The recesses of the vaginal vault above the cervix are called the fornices, the deepest being the posterior fornix.

The vaginal length is variable but usually ranges from 8 to 10 cm. The perineal muscles cause a relative constriction of the outlet diameter. The midportion is flattened when relaxed, which creates only a potential space, but it has a remarkable ability to distend. This is demonstrated at the time of parturition when the vault must accommodate passage of the fetus. Stretching is allowed by the presence of multiple circumferential folds or rugae in the vaginal wall. The rugae becomes less prominent after menopause.

The hymen is a thin membranous fold at the vaginal orifice. It is variable in appearance and may form a complete membrane occluding the vagina, an incomplete membrane, or assume a cribriform appearance. If it is ruptured, irregular fragments may persist as the carunculae hymenales.

The blood supply to the upper vagina is by the vaginal artery that usually arises directly from the internal iliac artery. Alternatively it may be a branch of the uterine artery. The internal pudendal artery, a terminal branch of the internal iliac artery, supplies the lower vagina as well as the vulva and perineum. Venous drainage is through an extensive plexus running along the lateral margins of the vagina. The channels coalesce to empty into the internal iliac vein.

The lymphatic drainage is complex. In general the upper vagina drains into the interiliac lymph nodes similar to the cervical drainage, and the lower vagina tends to follow the course of vulvar drainage into the femoral and inguinal lymph nodes.[7]

Vaginal innervation is by the pudendal nerve with distal fibers coursing with the blood and lymphatic vessels. In marked contrast to the nearby vulvar skin, the vagina has few sensory nerve endings and therefore is relatively asensory.

Histologically, three layers can be distinguished in the vagina: (1) mucous membrane, (2) muscularis, and (3) adventitia.[75] The mucous membrane is composed of a nonkeratinized, stratified squamous epithelium and a lamina propria (Fig. 5-4). The epithelium is several cell layers thick. Cells of the basal layers are cylindrical with rounded, dark nuclei; intermediate layers are comprised of larger cells with more elliptical nuclei; and the superficial layers consist of flattened cells with smaller nuclei. The thickness of the epithelium is influenced by estrogen and progesterone levels.[81] The epithelium is continuous onto the cervical portio, but is distinguished from cervical epithelium by the formation of undulating papillae projecting into the lamina propia. The lamina propria is a dense layer of fibroelastic tissue generously supplied with blood vessels and lymphatics. It functions as erectile tissue during sexual arousal. The mucosa has no glandular elements or hair follicles.

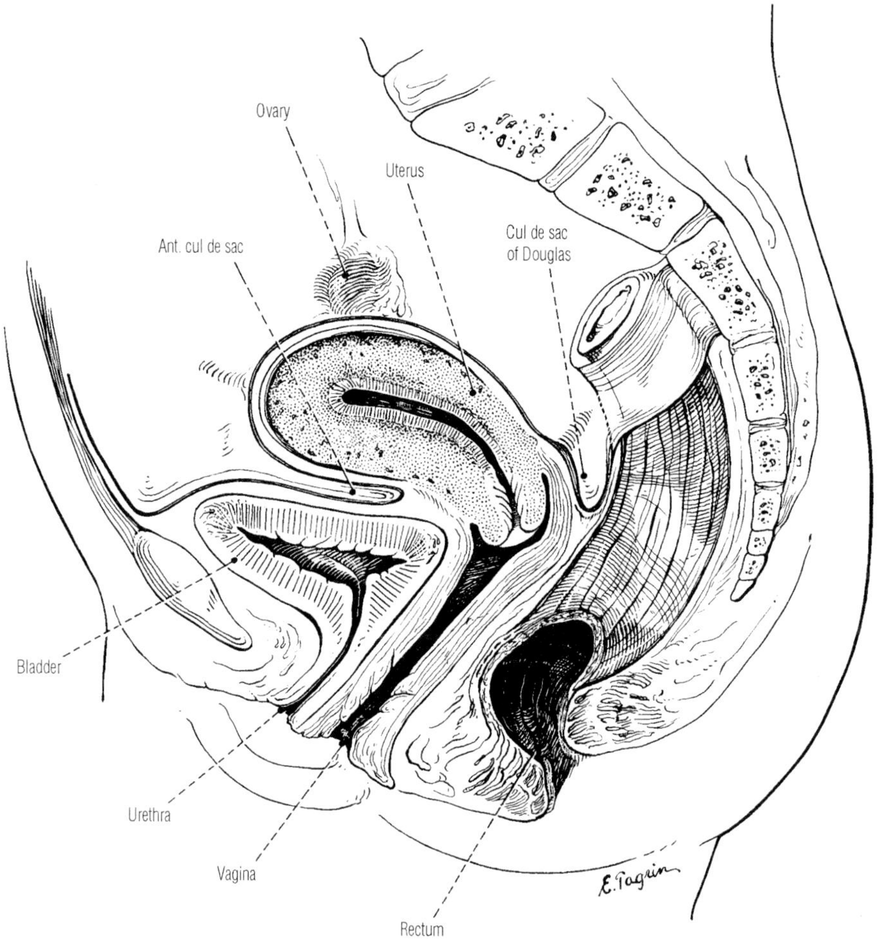

Fig. 5-3. Sagittal section of the human female pelvis showing the vagina and related structures.

Deep to the mucous membrane is the muscularis that consists of an inner circular and outer longitudinal layer of smooth muscle. The layers are not distinguished by interposed fascial fibers. The adventitial layer consists of dense connective tissue, nerves, and blood vessels. It is continuous with the endopelvic fascia, the supportive connective tissue layer investing all the pelvic viscera and muscles.

PHYSIOLOGIC ALTERATIONS

Vaginal physiology depends on an appropriate hormonal and bacteriologic milieu. The vagina is a target organ for ovarian estrogen. Estrogen induces proliferation and maturation of the stratified squamous epithelium, causes glycogen storage in the superficial and intermediate cells, and increases blood flow through the paravaginal tissues. The increased thickness of the epithelium and enriched blood supply act to create an effective mechanical barrier between the vagina and the environment. The stored glycogen participates in the formation of chemical and microbiologic barriers.

The vaginal squamous epithelium consists of several layers of cells that demonstrate progressive maturation as they are displaced upward by proliferation of the basal stratum germinativum.[11] Three cell types are seen:

1. *Parabasal cells* originate just above the stratum germinativum and are small round cells with a high nuclear to cytoplasmic ratio.
2. *Intermediate cells* are larger and polygonal. The nuclear to cytoplasmic ratio is less than for parabasal cells but a definite nuclear chromatin pattern is observed.
3. *Superficial cells* are large, polyhedral, flat cells with small, pyknotic nuclei.

Cells desquamate and may be collected for cytologic evaluation. The appearance will reflect the influence of estrogen on epithelial growth. The sample should be obtained by scraping the lateral wall of the upper third of the vagina with a spatula. The sample is smeared thinly on a slide, fixed, and submitted for cytologic study. The estrogen effect is expressed as a maturation index reported as the ratio of superficial to intermediate to parabasal cells. Estrogen stimulation results in a predominance of the more mature superficial cells. An absolute lack of estrogen, or a hormonal environment marked by a relative decrease in the estrogen/progesterone ratio, favors desquamation of parabasal cells.

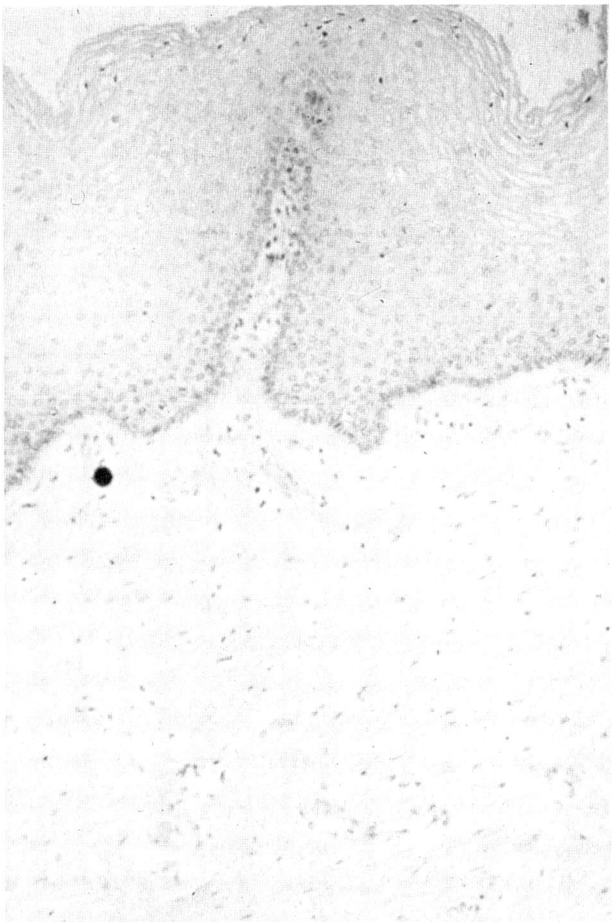

Fig. 5-4. Photomicrograph showing normal vaginal mucosa.

A wide variety of bacteria can be cultured from the normal vagina.[45] The number and type depend in part on the culture medium used. *Lactobacillus*, *Staphylococcus epidermidis*, diphtheroids, and aerobic and anaerobic streptococci are most frequently isolated. Competition for nutrients is an important mechanism that normally keeps pathologic organisms present in numbers insufficient to cause clinical infection.

The normal vaginal environment is acidic. Glycogen stored in the intermediate and superficial cells serves as a substrate for carbohydrate metabolism by the bacterium *Lactobacillus vaginalis*. The product of fermentation is lactic acid which maintains the low vaginal pH (normal 3.5 to 4.5). The acidity in turn favors continued growth of the nonpathogenic *Lactobacillus* and inhibits colonization by more virulent organisms.

Atrophic vaginitis

Clinically, hypoestrogenism is associated with atrophic vaginitis. Symptoms include painful intercourse (dyspareunia), dryness, pruritus, and abnormal bleeding. The mucous membrane is thin and thus subject to traumatic injury. Physiologic vaginal fluids are produced primarily by transudation across the epithelium with a smaller contribution from cervical and vestibular gland secretions. The amount and composition are influenced by the hormonal status and by the presence of erotic stimuli. Estrogen deprivation causes a decrease in blood flow to the paravaginal tissues that reduces tissue turgor and depresses production of vaginal fluids in basal and aroused states. While these changes are typically seen in postmenopausal states (absolute lack of estrogen), they may also occur in pregnancy, lactation, and other progesterone dominant states. Atrophic vaginitis is treated with local or systemic estrogens.[76] Symptomatic treatment with vaginal lubricants is available to women who cannot or will not use estrogen.

Vaginismus

Dyspareunia has a variety of etiologies. Some of the structural or organic causes include atrophic vaginitis, infectious vaginitis, congenital defects, endometriosis, pelvic inflammatory disease, cystitis, urethritis, fistula, vulvar vestibulitis, and fibrosis due to poor healing of a laceration or episiotomy.

When the anatomic findings are normal and there is no other evidence of organic disease, vaginismus should be considered. Vaginismus is the involuntary spasm of the vaginal constrictor and/or levator ani muscles occurring during attempted penetration of the vaginal vault. The condition is thought to be psychologically mediated through the mechanisms of fear of injury, guilt about sexuality, or dissatisfaction with the relationship.[73]

Evaluation of the patient with dyspareunia begins with a careful history. Often patients will not spontaneously complain of dyspareunia and it must be gently elicited by the clinician. Important characteristics of the pain are its chronicity, location (superficial versus deep), and associated symptoms. The physical examination must be done with great care and is directed toward identifying structural causes. Palpation of tender, contracted constrictor muscles helps to determine vaginismus as an etiology.

Treatment of dyspareunia depends on its cause. Pain secondary to an organic condition is best managed by treating the underlying disease. Vaginismus is managed by desensitization techniques performed in a supportive setting. Gradual self-dilation of the vault that reinforces the patient's control is effective treatment in most cases. Sets of soft rubber vaginal dilators of increasing size are available to assist the process. Often it is appropriate to combine their use with psychotherapy.

MALFORMATIONS

Vaginal anomalies are rare and they may be classified as follows: (1) absence, (2) failure of lateral fusion, and (3) failure of canalization.

Congenital absence of the vagina (the Rokitansky-Kuster-Hauser syndrome), which results from müllerian duct agenesis, occurs with an incidence of one in 4000 to 5000 female births.[31] The embryologic defect affects development of a variable portion of the fused, caudal end of the müllerian (paramesonephric) duct. The etiology is not known, but does not appear to be the result of a single gene defect or known teratogenic effect.[23] It is usually associated with uterine agenesis, but in approximately 8% of patients a rudimentary bipartite uterus with a functional endometrium is present.[101]

The clinical presentation depends on the absence or presence of a functioning uterus. The typical patient is a teenager and complains of primary amenorrhea. Vaginal agenesis is the second most common cause of primary amenorrhea and accounts for about 15% of cases.[68] Only gonadal dysgenesis is found more frequently. Alternatively, if endometrial tissue is present, she may present with cyclic pain. Ovarian function is normal and may induce cyclic shedding of the endometrium. However, since there is no outflow tract, the menstrual products are retained and cause symptoms. If retrograde flow of the menstrual endometrium occurs, endometriosis may result.

Patients display normal growth and normal development of secondary sexual characteristics. The external genitalia are normal. Examination of the vaginal area reveals a mucosal wall beyond the introitus. A vaginal dimple may be present. Rectal examination usually demonstrates the absence of a uterus, although ultrasonography should be performed to confirm the diagnosis. Renal and skeletal anomalies are frequently associated and should be diagnosed by appropriate imaging techniques.[31]

The differential diagnosis includes imperforate hymen and testicular feminization (androgen insensitivity) syndrome. In the former a uterus is present and can usually be detected by physical examination or imaging studies. Patients with congenital absence of the vagina are distinguished from patients with testicular feminization by their normal female karyotype and normal female serum testosterone levels.

Menstrual and reproductive function are not possible in most cases. The goal of treatment is to create a vaginal vault adequate for sexual function. Both surgical and nonsurgical approaches are reported. The Frank nonsurgical method for formation of a vagina involves the application of vaginal dilators to the introital region. Intermittent pressure is applied with progressively longer and wider dilators. The technique requires considerable patient cooperation and diligence but is reported to achieve good results without complications.[94] The McIndoe vaginoplasty involves surgical dissection of the areolar tissues in the potential vaginal space followed by placement of a split-thickness skin graft to achieve epithelialization. Other surgical methods include creation of musculocutaneous flaps and use of intestinal grafts.

If symptoms arise from a rudimentary uterine anlage, it should be surgically removed. The possibility of pregnancy exists only for rare patients with an intact uterus. A surgical approach that incorporates uterine conservation is preferred in this group.[6]

Failure of lateral fusion of the paramesonephric ducts results in longitudinal septae. As with agenesis, the extent of the developmental abnormality can be variable. There may be only a partial, distal fibromuscular band in the sagittal plane of the vagina. In the extreme situation, there may be duplication of all the müllerian derivatives—the patient has two uterine horns, cervices, and vaginas.[15] Cases are classified as obstructive or nonobstructive. If the hemivagina created by the septum does not communicate with the introitus, there is obstruction of the ipsilateral uterine horn. If the uterus has functioning endometrium, a painful hematocolpos and hematometra may occur with menstruation. Since the contralateral horn continues to discharge its menstrual effluent normally, the diagnosis may not be considered unless a tender mass is found on careful physical examination.

Treatment is individualized and is based on the lesion and symptoms. Obstructive lesions require surgical resection of the septum to resolve the hematocolpos and prevent endometriosis. Surgery is also indicated for dyspareunia. Asymptomatic septae do not require treatment.

Failure of canalization of the vaginal plate results in transverse septae. The incidence is reported as 1 in 30,000 to 80,000 females.[72] They may occur at any level of the vagina, and occasionally more than one may be present. The septum consists of a fibromuscular membrane covered with squamous epithelium. The septum may be partial forming a constricting band, or complete, which results in obstruction.

The diagnosis usually is made at menarche when cyclic abdominal pain from retained menstrual blood prompts an evaluation. Preoperative evaluation should include pelvic ultrasonography to delineate the septal thickness and to demonstrate a normal uterus and ovaries. An intravenous pyelogram is done to exclude renal anomalies and ureteral obstruction. Treatment requires surgical resection of the septum and reanastomosis of the upper and lower vaginal vaults.

The hymen probably forms at the junction of the vaginal plate and the urogenital sinus. If it fails to develop its normal lumen and remains imperforate, retained menstrual blood and/or dyspareunia can result. Treatment is accomplished surgically by performing a cruciate incision in the membrane followed by resection of the resulting triangular membranous flaps. The subject of imperforate hymen is discussed in further detail in Chapter 23, Pediatric and Adolescent Gynecology.

VAGINITIS

Vaginitis is one of the most common gynecologic diagnoses and is responsible for a substantial percentage of ambulatory visits annually. Patients with vaginitis present with a variety of symptoms and signs, which depend on the etiology (Table 5-1). The usual manifestations, which occur singly or in combination, are an abnormal vaginal discharge, vaginal discomfort, pruritus, and an abnormal odor.

Approximately 95% of cases result from an infection involving one of three organisms: *Candida albicans*, *Trichomonas vaginalis*, and *Gardnerella vaginalis*. In a typical

Table 5-1. Differential diagnosis of vaginal infections

	Bacterial vaginosis	**Candida vulvovaginitis**	**Trichomonas vaginitis**
Primary symptom	Odor	Pruritus	Discharge
Gross appearance of discharge	Thin, homogenous, grey, moderate amount	White, "curd-like" adherent to sidewalls	Copious, frothy yellow-green
pH	> 4.5	$\leq$ 4.0	$\geq$ 4.5
Whiff test	Positive	Negative	$\pm$
Microscopy	Clue cells, few WBCs	Budding hyphae spores	Motile trichomonads, numerous WBCs

population of reproductive-aged women, *candida* and *trichomonas* infections each account for about 25% of cases, while *gardnerella*-associated bacterial vaginosis accounts for the rest. Noninfectious vaginitis occurs much less frequently as a result of a localized allergic reaction, a reaction to a foreign body, nonspecific inflammation, or due to senescent changes in the vaginal mucosa. Cervicitis or lower urinary tract infection can mimic the symptoms of vaginitis and should be distinguished from a primary pathologic process of the vaginal mucosa.

The pathophysiology of vaginitis is best understood by considering the vagina to be a complex ecosystem. Vaginitis results from a perturbation of the system.[45] The components of the ecosystem are the mucosa and the normally colonizing microbes that are its inhabitants. The status of the mucosa is influenced primarily by hormonal factors. The composition of the populating organisms is determined by the environment and by complex interactions with each other.

Establishing the correct diagnosis is paramount for the successful treatment of vaginitis and requires a logical, comprehensive approach. The evaluation should begin with an accurate history. The symptoms should be elucidated in detail. The presence of a discharge and its specific characteristics are important. Associated symptoms of pruritus, pain, and dysuria should be noted.

Risk factors that can lead to vaginitis by altering normal vaginal physiology should be identified. Absolute or relative hypoestrogenism of menopause, pregnancy, lactation, or the use of oral contraceptives may contribute. Use of systemic antibiotics may suppress the growth of *Lactobacillus* and other normal inhabitants and create an environment favoring growth of pathogens. Sexual activity may cause symptoms due to exposure to sexually transmitted diseases or the basic pH of seminal fluid. Comorbid diseases causing immunocompromise (such as infection with HIV), or the use of corticosteroids may impede the normal immune mechanism of the vagina. Alteration in carbohydrate metabolism, as in diabetes mellitus, is also a consideration.

The physical examination provides the next opportunity to gather information leading to an accurate diagnosis. Often vaginitis becomes symptomatic only after it spreads to the very sensitive vulvar skin. This should be inspected for evidence of a rash, erythema, excoriation, or edema. The gross appearance of the vaginal mucosa should be assessed. Thin, pale mucosa lacking rugae suggests relative or absolute estrogen deprivation. Erythema, increased vascularity, mucosal ulcerations, or other lesions are noted. The status of the cervical portio is likewise evaluated. If a discharge is present, its specific characteristics will be helpful in establishing the diagnosis; the amount, color, consistency, odor, and pH should be assessed.

The most useful clinical tool for diagnosis is the microscopic appearance of the vaginal discharge. Two preparations are used. In one the vaginal secretions are suspended in isotonic saline and a coverslip is applied. The slide is observed for the presence of the motile protozoan *Trichomonas*, for "clue cells," and for leukocytes. Clue cells are desquamated vaginal mucosal cells with a dense-stippled appearance due to attached *Gardnerella vaginalis* organisms (Fig. 5-5). The second preparation is a suspension of the vaginal discharge in 10% potassium hydroxide. The cellular elements present on the slide are lysed by the KOH, which leaves the mycelia of *C. albicans* unobscured. If the diagnosis remains doubtful despite the "wet preps", then gram stains and cultures will help establish the diagnosis.

Gardnerella-associated bacterial vaginosis

Gardnerella vaginalis is an aerobic, pleomorphic coccobacillus and part of the normal vaginal bacterial flora. It is responsible for infection under certain circumstances when it proliferates and interacts with various anaerobic bacteria to produce symptoms.[10] The term "nonspecific vaginitis"

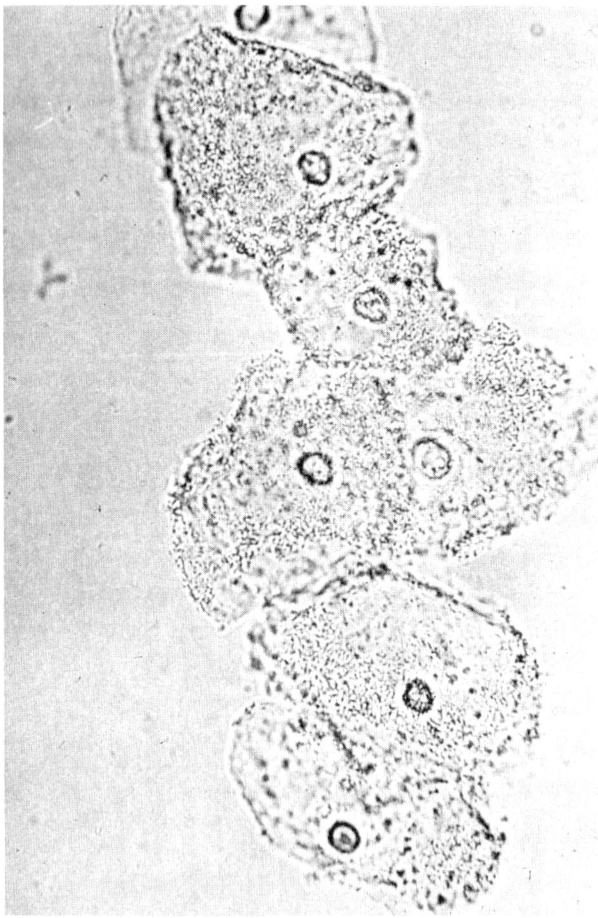

Fig. 5-5. Saline wet preparation showing clue cells.

was applied to this condition in the past. As the role of *G. vaginalis* as an etiologic agent has become better defined, the term is less appropriate. However, the nature of the complex interaction between *G. vaginalis* and the anaerobes that ultimately cause infection remains incompletely understood. This uncertainty continues to be reflected in the current terminology whereby the condition is called *Gardnerella*-associated bacterial vaginosis.

G. vaginalis can be recovered from the vaginas of asymptomatic women about 30% of the time. In contrast it is present in at least 90% of women with bacterial vaginosis. A quantitative difference is also seen between patients and unaffected individuals. Approximately 10^5 bacteria/gm of secretion are recovered from normal women, while about 10^{11} bacteria/gm of secretion are found in women with bacterial vaginosis.[93] The cause of these changes is not certain. In particular it is difficult to know whether to consider it a sexually-transmitted infection. Bacterial vaginosis is rare in women who are not sexually active. *G. vaginalis* is frequently recovered from the urethras of male partners of affected women.

The predominant symptom of bacterial vaginosis is an unpleasant "fishy" odor usually associated with a vaginal discharge. Irritative symptoms such as dysuria and dyspareunia are not typical. On physical examination the vulva and vagina appear normal except for the presence of the discharge. The discharge is homogeneous, thin, grey-white, and present in moderate quantity.

The diagnosis is based on the clinical evaluation of the discharge. Three of four criteria must be present to confirm bacterial vaginosis:

1. A homogeneous discharge that adheres to the walls of the vagina but is easily wiped away
2. Elevated vaginal pH (> 4.5)
3. Clue cells detected on saline wet preparation of the vaginal discharge
4. Positive "whiff test"

The pH is elevated above 4.5 in virtually all cases and is usually between 5.0 and 5.5. Clue cells are best identified from the obscuring of cell borders by the adherent bacterial clusters and a clean background appearance on the slide. The wet preparation is also notable for the absence of neutrophils. The characteristic fishy odor of the discharge is often readily detected. If not, it can be demonstrated by adding 10% KOH to a drop of the discharge on a microscope slide. Alkalinization volatizes the two main amines, putrescine and cadaverine, which produce the odor and are the basis for the so-called "whiff test."[25] Bacterial cultures should not be relied upon to establish the diagnosis because of a lack of specificity.[41]

The recommended treatment is metronidazole 500 mg by mouth 2 times per day for 7 days. Patients should be warned to avoid alcohol consumption during treatment, as a reaction similar to that produced by disulfiram (Antabuse) may occur. Clindamycin 300 mg by mouth 2 times per day for 7 days is also effective. Both drugs are active against anaerobes and have minimal impact on the normal vaginal flora. A single dose regimen has been proposed but may be associated with higher rates of relapse and is therefore not recommended.[50,90] Topical preparations of metronidazole and clindamycin are available and have been shown to be effective.[9,48] The metronidazole preparation is a 0.75% gel used intravaginally twice daily for 5 days, and the clindamycin preparation is a 2% cream used intravaginally once per day for 7 days.

Treatment of asymptomatic bacterial vaginosis is controversial. Infectious sequelae have been associated with it in postoperative and obstetric settings.[87,99] Although unproven, treatment has been recommended prior to invasive pelvic procedures.[93] There is no uniform recommendation for treatment of asymptomatic pregnant women.

Gardnerella-associated bacterial vaginosis is a disease of sexually active women, but it has not been demonstrated that treatment of the male partner reduces the risk of recurrence.[98] However, it may be helpful in particularly difficult cases, in conjunction with the use of intravaginal acidifying agents.[22]

Candida vulvovaginitis

Vaginal fungal infections are caused by *Candida albicans* in 85% to 95% of patients while *C. glabrata* and *C. tropicalis* account for most of the rest. *C. albicans* is a ubiquitous saprophyte that may be isolated from the vagina in up to 20% of asymptomatic women.[56] Treatment is not indicated unless symptoms are present. Clinical infections result from overgrowth due to alterations in either host-related or pathogen-related factors.

Factors associated with candidiasis include systemic antibiotics, pregnancy, diabetes mellitus, and immunosuppressants. Antibiotic use may predispose to yeast infections by suppressing the vaginal flora that normally inhibit the growth of *Candida* through competition for nutrients.[86] The effect is seen most commonly with broad spectrum antibiotics, such as the tetracyclines, and probably depends on suppression of growth of the *Lactobacillus*. The mechanism by which pregnancy predisposes to vaginal candidiasis is not known, but the rate of infection may be doubled in gravidas. An alteration in glycogen metabolism and depression of local cell mediated immunity have been proposed as mechanisms through which other factors may operate.[91] It is important to note, however, that most cases of candidiasis occur in patients with no identified risk factors.

The usual clinical presentation for a patient with candidiasis is the complaint of vulvovaginal pruritus. The itching is usually intense and may be accompanied by dysuria and dyspareunia. The onset of symptoms may coincide with menses or with intercourse. The patient may notice a thick, white discharge, but often this is not a prominent feature of the history. Candidiasis is not associated with a foul odor.

On physical examination extensive involvement of the vulva may be apparent. The skin will demonstrate well-demarcated erythematous areas with scaling, edema, and excoriations. Often the crural and labial folds are affected. The vaginal mucosa may also be inflamed and edematous. The classic finding, however, is a white, thick, curd-like discharge forming patches adherent to the vaginal walls. The pH of the discharge is usually < 4.0.

The diagnosis is confirmed by identifying budding pseudohyphae or spores on a wet preparation of the vaginal discharge suspended in 10% KOH under light microscopy. False-negative results are obtained in about 25% of cases. If yeast is suspected, vaginal cultures on selective media are used to establish the diagnosis. Nickerson's medium or Sabaroud's agar are most often used to isolate fungi in these more difficult cases.[22]

Treatment of candidiasis is accomplished by the topical application of antifungal agents. Several preparations are available. Imidazole agents (clotrimazole, butoconazole, and miconazole) have been shown to have higher initial cure rates and require shorter durations of treatment than nystatin.[37] Administration is by vaginal suppository or cream. The choice of formulation is dictated by patient preference. Suppositories are less messy, while creams offer the advantage of application directly to the vulvar skin for more immediate relief. Most nonpregnant patients respond to 3 days of therapy with 200 mg suppositories or a 1% to 2% cream. Seven days of therapy are required for persistent infection and in pregnancy. Persistent infection is also an indication for newer, more potent agents such as terconazole.

Another effective therapy is boric acid.[97] A gelatin capsule containing 600 to 650 mg of boric acid powder is inserted intravaginally daily for 14 days. Results compared with nystatin indicate that this is an effective and inexpensive alternative. Boric acid suppositories may be especially useful in managing patients with chronic symptoms. Patients may establish an intermittent dosing schedule that keeps their symptoms controlled. No serious side effects have been reported with its use, but it should be avoided in pregnancy.

Approximately 10% of cases will not respond to initial therapy. Persistent or frequently recurrent vaginal candidiasis is a difficult problem to treat. The clinician should consider host-related and pathogen-related contributing factors. Host factors such as poor diabetes control, immune compromise, and hygienic factors should be addressed. Cultures are obtained to exclude infection with a more resistant *Candida* species such as *C. glabrata* or *tropicalis*. These species may require much higher doses of antifungal agents, and it is possible that the recent trend to shorter treatment regimens is another reason for selecting them.

Prolonging treatment up to 14 days may cure some patients with recurrent or persistent disease. Chronic suppression for 6 to 12 months with vaginal acidifying agents may be added. Also it has been suggested that some patients are chronically infected because of gastrointestinal colonization with *C. albicans*.[54] Oral therapy directed at eliminating this reservoir has been advocated. Ketoconazole is an effective oral therapy available for treatment of *Candida*. It is well absorbed from the gastrointestinal tract, but whether its efficacy is due to a systemic or local action is not known. Hepatotoxicity is the main side effect of the drug. Recurrence rates are high after ketoconazole is discontinued. A newer oral agent, fluconazole, lacks liver toxicity and may be helpful in suppressive doses given once per month.[85] Additional measures such as avoidance of harsh soaps in the genital area, eliminating restrictive synthetic underwear, and prolonged air drying of the genital area after washing are also recommended to the patient. Treatment of sexual partners and dietary modifications are probably not effective.

Trichomonas vaginitis

Trichomonas vaginalis is a flagellate, motile protozoan capable of causing vaginitis. Its growth is enhanced by a moist, anaerobic environment in which the pH is somewhat more alkaline (5.5 to 6.5) than the normal vagina. Trichomonads are not part of the normal vaginal flora. When present in the vaginal vault, the organisms can usually be recovered from the urethra and cervix as well. Infection is usually transmitted through sexual contact. However, viable organisms have been recovered from swimming pools and fomites such as moist towels, which suggest nonsexual transmission is also possible.[67] Trichomoniasis is frequently associated with other sexually transmitted diseases.[57] Patients should be screened for gonorrhea and chlamydia when the diagnosis of trichomoniasis is made.

The clinical manifestations of trichomoniasis vary from asymptomatic infection to an intense local inflammatory response. Systemic infection does not occur. Some studies show that up to 50% of infected women are asymptomatic.[102] When symptoms exist the patient complains primarily of a profuse vaginal discharge. The discharge may cause vulvovaginal discomfort and irritation. Pruritus and odor are less common complaints. Dysuria and dyspareunia are occasionally noted and if severe inflammation is present, vaginal spotting may occur.

The vulvar examination is often normal, but may demonstrate erythema and excoriations. Erythema of the vaginal epithelium may also be noted. A classic description of severe inflammation is the "strawberry cervix," which consists of tiny, punctate hemorrhages grossly visible on the mucosa but it is only seen in a small minority of cases. The vaginal discharge is the most striking feature of the examination. The discharge is copious, opaque, grey to yellow-green, and malodorous. Occasionally, small bubbles are present giving the discharge a frothy appearance. The pH of the discharge is usually 5.0 to 6.5 and reflects the growth requirement of the parasite for a more alkaline environment.

Trichomoniasis is diagnosed by direct identification of the motile organism by microscopy. A wet mount is prepared by suspending a small amount of the discharge in a drop of saline on a microscope slide. A coverslip is applied and the preparation is examined. The organisms are slightly larger than leukocytes, which are usually abundant in the smear due to the inflammatory response. *T. vaginalis* is pear-shaped with visible flagellae and moves with a characteristic jittery motion. Cultures with specialized media are available and may improve the diagnostic accuracy if a particular patient presents a diagnostic dilemma.[32] The diagnosis can also be made by identifying the parasites on a Papanicolaou smear. Notwithstanding, this diagnosis should not be relied on since false-negative findings are reported in up to 48% of patients.[60]

Trichomoniasis is treated with systemic metronidazole, a derivative of 5-nitroimidazole. Topical therapy is inadequate; colonization in the bladder and urethra will not be affected by vaginal application and is a source of reinfection. As trichomoniasis is usually a sexually transmitted disease, the sexual partner must also be treated to avoid reinfection. Metronidazole is taken orally either as a 2 g single dose, or 250 mg dose 3 times daily for 7 days. The cure rates for the two regimens are comparable.[44] Single dose therapy offers the advantages of lower cost, lower total drug dose, and increased patient compliance. Patients should be advised to avoid alcohol consumption during and for 48 hours after treatment with metronidazole to prevent severe nausea and vomiting. Other side effects include a metallic aftertaste, headaches, and rarely, peripheral neuropathies after prolonged therapy. The drug probably should not be given in early pregnancy. There are experimental data in animals suggesting a carcinogenic or mutagenic potential, although no clinical studies have demonstrated an increased risk.[22] Infected pregnant women may obtain symptomatic relief with clotrimazole, but a cure is unlikely.

A 5% to 10% failure rate is reported following a single course of therapy with metronidazole. Most often this is due to poor compliance or failure to treat the patient's sexual partner. Resistant strains of *Trichomonas vaginalis* have been reported and may require more intensive systemic therapy combined with topical application.[49] No other effective treatments have been reported.

DISORDERS OF PELVIC SUPPORT

The vagina is a potential space in the pelvic floor through which the pelvic organs may descend under the influence of gravity if they are not properly supported. Normally the axis of the vaginal lumen assumes a 45° angle from the vertical in an erect posture. Therefore gravitational forces are not applied directly parallel to the vaginal tube toward the introitus, but rather are absorbed along its length by various muscular, fascial, and ligamentous supports. The important muscular structures of the pelvic floor that contribute support include the pelvic diaphragm, the urogenital diaphragm, and the perineal body.

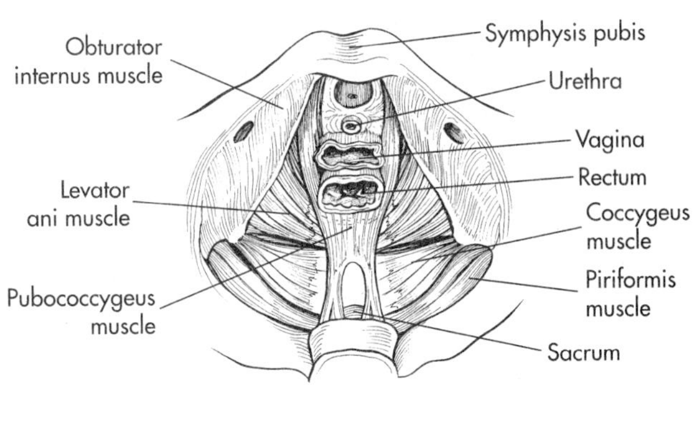

Fig. 5-6. View of the pelvic floor from above showing the anatomy of the levator ani and coccygeus muscles. (From Mattingly RF: *Telinde's operative gynecology,* ed 5, Philadelphia, 1977, JB Lippincott, p 31.)

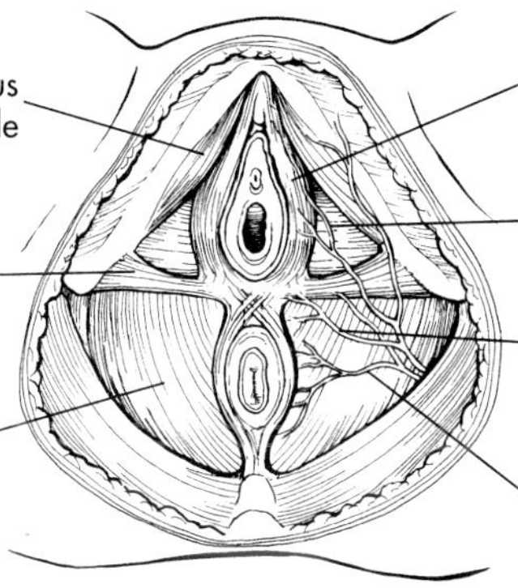

Fig. 5-7. View of the pelvic floor from below showing the anatomy of the perineum. (From Mattingly RF: *Telinde's operative gynecology,* ed 5, Philadelphia, 1977, JB Lippincott, p 41.)

The pelvic diaphragm is the most superior layer of the pelvic floor and is formed from the components of the levator ani and coccygeus muscles (Fig. 5-6). The levator ani orginates at the pubic and ileal bones and sweeps across the hollow of the pelvis to insert into the ischium and coccyx. From lateral to medial, three muscle components are identified by their origins and insertions: the ileococcygeus, the pubococcygeus, and the puborectalis. The puborectalis is interrupted by the lumens of the urethra, vagina, and rectum. As it encircles and invests these organs, it contributes skeletal muscle support. The function of the levator ani is to draw the hollow viscera forward toward the pubic bone and act as a valve to close off the pelvic floor. The coccygeus muscle completes the posterolateral aspect of the pelvic diaphragm, which originates at the ischial spine and inserts into the sacrum.

Inferior to the pelvic diaphragm and covering the anterior half of the pelvic outlet is the urogenital diaphragm. This layer is also interrupted by the hollow openings of the urethra and vagina. Because of the angular course of the tubular structures, however, the defects in this layer are not aligned vertically with the corresponding defects in the pelvic diaphragm. This is an important mechanism of pelvic support.

The urogenital diaphragm is divided into deep and superficial compartments. The muscular components of the deep compartment of the urogenital diaphragm are the deep transverse perineal muscle and the striated sphincter urethrae muscle. These muscles originate along the ischiopubic rami, course medially, and terminate as fibers blending into the submucosal tissues of the vagina and urethra respectively. The most posterior fibers of the deep transverse perineal muscles meet their contralateral counterpart in the midline and insert into the perineal body. A fascial layer separates the deep muscles from the superficial compartment of the urogenital diaphragm. Three paired muscles define this triangular area of the perineum (Fig. 5-7). They are the bulbocavernosus muscles that surround the vaginal introitus and cover the erectile tissue of the vestibular bulbs; the ischiocavernosus muscles that originate at the ischial tuberosities and insert over the crura of the clitoris; and the superficial transverse perineal muscles.

The perineal body comprises the fibrous central point of insertion of the muscles of the pelvic diaphragm, the urogenital diaphragm, and the external rectal sphincter muscle. Thus fibers from the levator ani, the deep transverse perineal muscles, the superficial transverse perineal muscles, and the bulbocavernosus muscles comprise the perineal body and form the major posterior support for the vagina. As the vagina courses posteriorly toward the hollow of the sacrum from the introitus, it rests upon the perineal body.

The next component contributing to the support of the pelvic structures is the endopelvic fascia. The muscular arrangement of the pelvic floor and the positions of the pelvic organs are sustained by this ubiquitous layer of connective tissue. It binds the muscles to each other, to the pelvic viscera, and ultimately to the fixed support of the bony pelvis. Endopelvic fascia forms a connective tissue continuum enveloping all the muscles described above, and covers their superior and inferior surfaces. In addition, it is continuous onto the bladder, vagina, rectum, and uterus, interdigitating with and becoming indistinct from their adventitial layers at the points where these organs pierce the pelvic floor. The endopelvic fascia adds strength to the pelvic floor and allows it to resist gravity and maintain the positions of the pelvic viscera. It also adds strength to the walls of the hollow pelvic organs so that they can resist the potentially high intraluminal pressures that develop within them. Weakness of the endopelvic fascia is a major cause of pelvic support disorders.

In certain locations the fibers of the endopelvic fascia layer condense to form recognizable ligamentous structures that suspend the uterus and vagina within the pelvis (Fig. 5-8). The cardinal ligaments extend from the lateral cervix and upper vagina to the pelvic sidewalls. Posteriorly the uterosacral ligaments run from the cervix around the rectum to the sacrum. The peritoneal pouch, or cul-de-sac of Douglas, lies between these ligaments. It separates the rectum from the cervix and posterior vaginal fornix and is a potential weak spot in the floor of the pelvis. Anteriorly, less well defined fibers called the pubocervical fascia extend from the pubic bone to support the urethra and vagina. Extensions of endopelvic fascia along the vagina form part of the

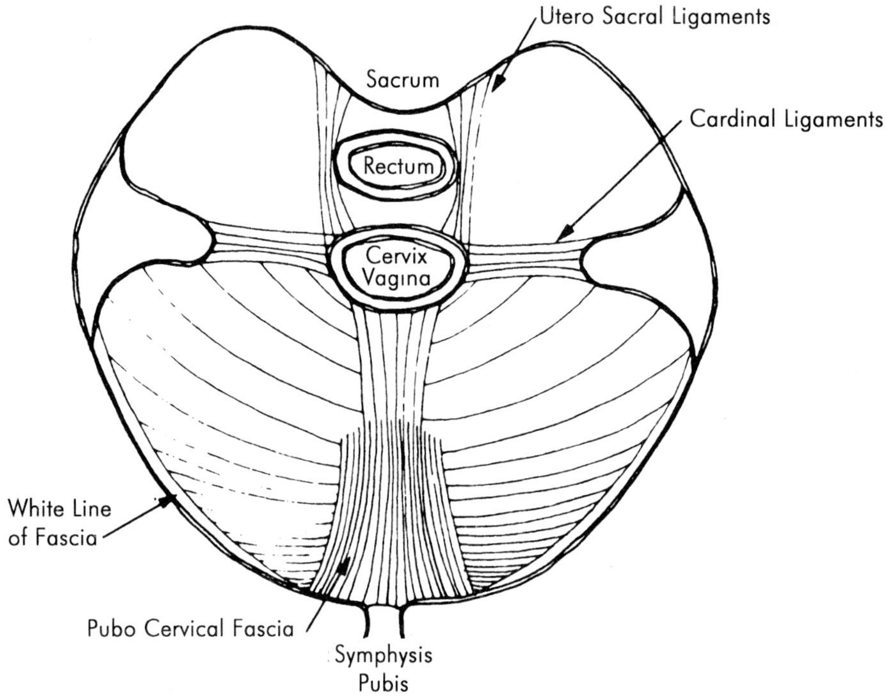

Fig. 5-8. Pelvic fascial supports (plane of midpelvis). Diagrammatic representation of the fascial supports that "suspend" the vaginal vault and cervix in the midpelvic plane. The bladder and urethra are supported by the floor of fascia comprised of the dense midline pubocervical fascia and its extensions to the white line of fascia laterally and the cardinal ligaments posteriorly. This fascia is less dense in its lateral and posterior aspects, as shown. (From Beck RP: *Principles and practice of clinical gynecology*, New York, 1983, John Wiley.)

vesicovaginal septum anteriorly and the rectovaginal septum posteriorly.

The midportion of the vagina is attached laterally to the pelvic sidewall by dense connective tissue fibers that insert into the arcus tendineus fasciae pelvis.[19] The arcus tendineus fasciae pelvis or "white line" lies on the superior surface of the pelvic diaphragm between the lower portion of the pubic bone and the ischial spine. It is also the site of lateral attachment of the bladder.

Classification

Disorders of pelvic support are the pathologic conditions caused by failure of the muscular, fascial, and ligamentous supporting structures just described. The result is descent or prolapse of one or more of the pelvic viscera through a defect in the pelvic floor. When the defect involves the cul-de-sac of Douglas, a true hernia may form as a pouch of peritoneum extends into the rectovaginal septum. In addition, the connective tissues that maintain the integrity of the walls of the bladder, vagina, and rectum can be weakened and result in overdistention of these hollow viscera. Sometimes the structural problems result in functional derangements as well. Pelvic relaxation is classified by the organ or organs involved. Usually a combination of defects occur together.

Each site of potential prolapse is individually assessed and graded for severity. Severity is determined in the lithotomy position with the patient at rest and then straining. The following scale is used[80]:

0 – no prolapse
1 – site descends past the midvaginal axis
2 – site descends to the hymenal ring
3 – site descends beyond the hymenal ring
4 – site is fully outside the hymenal ring

Uterine prolapse exists when the cervix and fundus descend into the vaginal vault as a result of attenuation and lengthening of the uterosacral and cardinal ligaments. Following hysterectomy, it is possible for the apex of the vaginal pouch to undergo similar descent by eversion. This is called a vaginal-vault prolapse.

A cystocele results from the descent of the bladder into the anterior vagina (Fig. 5-9). It is caused by either one of two defects in the supporting tissues of the bladder. Midline defects in the endopelvic fascia of the vesicovaginal septum result in a bulging of the dilated bladder base into the anterior wall of the vagina. A second type of cystocele is due to the detachment of the lateral supports of the bladder from the arcus tendineus fasciae pelvis.[69] The term urethrocele has been applied when the lower anterior vaginal wall is involved.

This is a misnomer as no dilation of the urethral wall is demonstrated. Rather, in this case there is a posterior rotational descent of the upper urethra from its normally firm attachment to the posterior surface of the pubic bone. It results from a weakening of the fibers of the pubocervical fascia. Prolapse of the upper urethra is believed to be the important mechanism of urinary stress incontinence.

Prolapse involving the posterior vaginal wall may represent either a rectocele or an enterocele. A rectocele is a prolapse of the anterior wall of the rectum into the vagina through the weakened endopelvic fascia of the rectovaginal septum. It usually involves the lower half of the vagina and helps to distinguish it from an enterocele that usually involves the upper posterior wall of the vagina. An enterocele is a herniation of the posterior peritoneal cul-de-sac between the uterosacral ligaments into the upper posterior vagina. The sac dissects along the rectovaginal septum. The herniated peritoneal sac may or may not contain loops of bowel. Even if small bowel is present in the sac, incarceration is very rare. Enterocoeles are probably more common than is appreciated because of the inherent weakness of the cul-de-sac and its dependent position in the pelvis. Failure to identify and

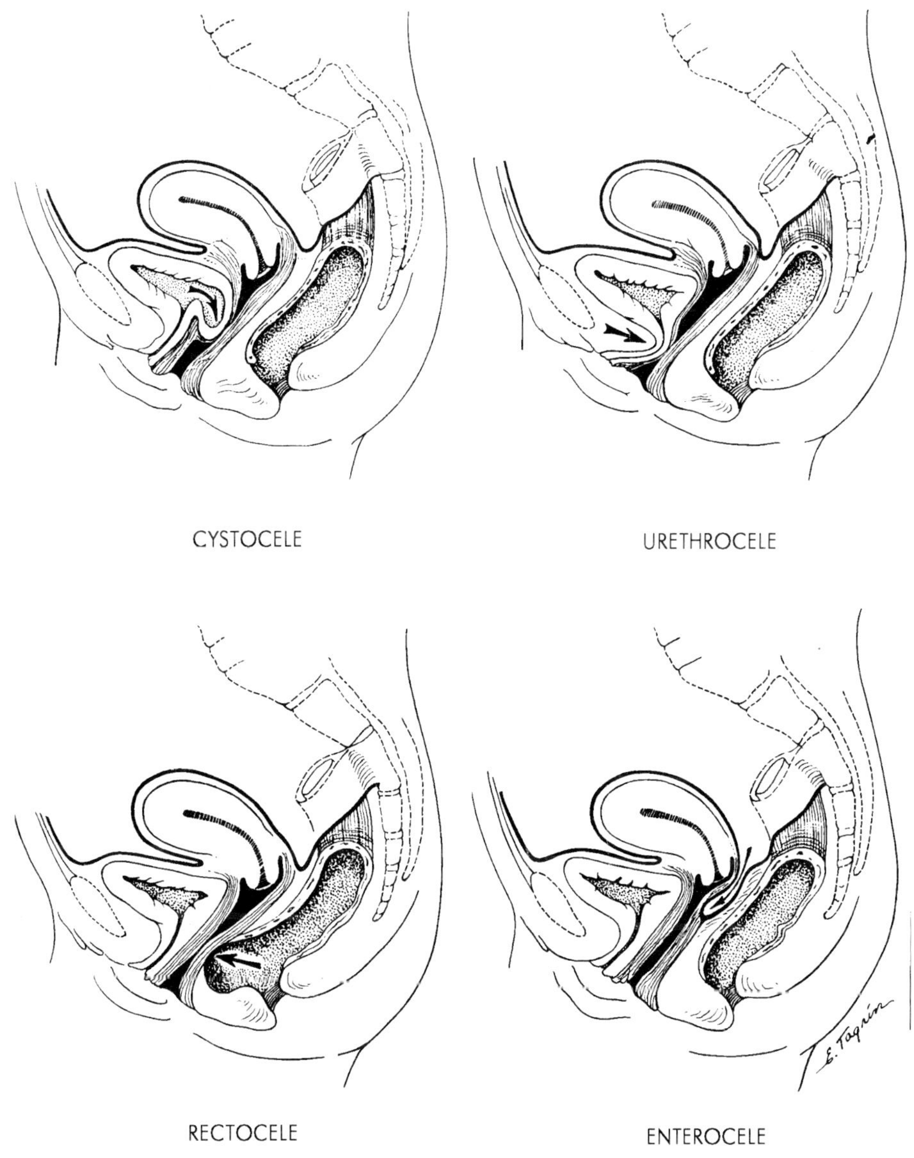

Fig. 5-9. Diagrammatic representation of the four commonest types of pelvic floor relaxation: cystocele, urethrocele, retrocele, and enterocele. Arrows depict the sites of maximum protrusion.

repair a small enterocele is a major cause of failure in surgical procedures to correct pelvic relaxation.[66]

Perineal relaxation refers to weakening of the musculofascial components of the perineal body. It may result only in a gaping of the introitus at the posterior fourchette. However, if the rectal sphincter is involved, functional aberrations with fecal incontinence may occur.

Etiology

Genital prolapse is a consequence of the bipedal condition. Gravity exerts a constant pull on the pelvic organs through the hollow pelvic outlet and is resisted by musculofascial supports, not the fixed bony structures. In addition, pressure within the abdominal cavity tends to exert a constant push toward the pelvic floor. Nonetheless, only a small proportion of women ever develop symptomatic prolapse. Several predisposing factors have been identified. Age is the most important factor associated with prolapse. Pelvic support problems are rarely seen in young women; the effects on the tissues accumulate slowly over time. Menopause may accelerate the process. Estrogen helps to maintain adequate blood flow to the pelvic organs and paravaginal tissues. Estrogen deprivation results in atrophic changes that render the tissues more subject to prolapse.

Childbearing is another risk factor for both immediate and delayed pelvic floor dysfunction. The injury may be pelvic nerve damage leading to functional derangements such as urinary and anal incontinence or muscle and connective tissue disruption, which contribute to the structural problems of prolapse. Vaginal delivery results in demonstrable nerve damage in 30% to 40% of parturients.[84] Denervation injury alone may contribute significantly to loss of pelvic floor support and result in prolapse.[82]

The use of obstetrical interventions such as episiotomy and forceps delivery to minimize pelvic floor damage is controversial. Although the length of the second stage of labor is decreased, a beneficial effect has not been demonstrated.[3] Most studies, including a recent one that assessed both apparent and occult anal sphincter damage, show an increased risk with use of episiotomy and forceps.[89] However, no study has adequately controlled for all confounding factors such as infant size and weight. Episiotomy and forceps therefore cannot be claimed to be clearly beneficial in preventing pelvic floor damage.

Racial and genetic factors that determine the intrinsic strength of the connective tissues may influence the incidence of prolapse.[96] Also connective tissue diseases such as Marfan's syndrome may predispose affected women to support disorders.

Conditions that result in chronic increases in intraabdominal pressure are thought to render women more susceptible to pelvic relaxation. Patients should be screened for chronic cough, chronic constipation, and repetitive heavy lifting. Pelvic masses, ascites, and obesity are also included in this group.

Signs and symptoms

Mild degrees of pelvic relaxation may be asymptomatic. More severe forms usually cause the patient to complain of a sagging or "dropping" sensation in the pelvis. It may be accompanied by a mild lower back ache. Often symptoms are worse at the end of the day and are relieved by lying down. Some patients will note a bulge or lump protruding from the vagina. The exteriorized mucosa may become irritated and cause pain, ulceration, or bleeding. Occasionally patients will complain that the presence of the abnormal bulge causes discomfort with sexual intercourse.

In addition to the anatomic changes, relaxation of the anterior vaginal wall may disturb the function of the bladder and urethra and result in specific urinary symptoms. A common misconception is that a cystocele causes stress incontinence. In fact the herniated bladder wall may actually kink the bladder outlet and cause urinary retention.[14] Some patients are able to void only after manually reducing the bulging bladder back to a position superior to the bladder outlet. A cystocele may also prevent complete bladder emptying, and the residual urine may predispose to cystitis.

Stress incontinence is also a consequence of pelvic relaxation that results from loss of support to the proximal urethra, not the bladder. Disruption of the normal urethral supports allows excessive mobility of the bladder outlet during episodes of increased intraabdominal pressure (stress). The hypermobile urethra may fail to maintain a water-tight closure with stress and incontinence results. The subject of urinary stress incontinence is discussed in further detail in Chapter 18.

Posterior vaginal wall relaxation may cause difficulty with defecation. Again reduction of the bulge by manual pressure may be required to effect a bowel movement. Fecal incontinence occasionally results from severe relaxation involving the rectal sphincter muscle. Usually this occurs only if the sphincter has been completely avulsed. This symptom is rare and should prompt a search for other causes such as a fistula or a neurologic deficit. Perineal relaxation may cause a patient to complain of unsatisfactory sensations with sexual intercourse.

Physical examination

The diagnosis of pelvic relaxation is established by physical examination. The challenge is to carefully assess each of the various organs and their supporting structures, determine which have become lax, and plan effective therapy on an individual basis. The vaginal introitus and vault are conveniently examined in the lithotomy position. However, prolapse may be prominent only while the patient is standing; therefore an examination should be performed in this position as well.

The mucosa is inspected for evidence of atrophy. Estrogen-deprived epithelium will be thin, friable, pale, and lacking in rugae. Prolonged eversion of the vaginal epithelium may result in traumatic lesions, secondary infection, or hyperkeratosis. The support of the vaginal walls is assessed sequentially using a Sims retractor or the disarticulated posterior blade of a Graves' speculum. The anterior vaginal wall is evaluated by retracting the posterior wall with the single speculum blade and asking the patient to bear down. The posterior wall is then evaluated by repositioning the speculum to retract the anterior wall. The degree of cervical descent may be further evaluated by applying gentle traction to the cervix with a tenaculum.

A bimanual examination permits an assessment of the size of the pelvic organs and determines the presence of any abnormal pelvic masses. The rectovaginal examination is essential for differentiating a rectocele from an enterocele. A rectocele is demonstrated by manually pushing the bulging tissues of the weakened rectovaginal septum into the vagina. An enterocele is diagnosed by palpating the slippery herniated peritoneal sac within the rectovaginal septum high in the vaginal vault.

The degree of descent of the bladder neck may be demonstrated by the "Q-tip test." A sterile lubricated cotton tip applicator is placed in the urethra at the urethrovesical junction. In the dorsal lithotomy position the applicator will assume a 0° angle with the horizontal. If the bladder neck is well supported, then this angle will change only slightly with straining and should remain less than 20°. If the support of the bladder neck is lax, then straining results in downward hypermobility of the proximal urethra and forces the distal end of the applicator upward to an angle of more than 30°. If functional problems such as incontinence are present, additional urodynamic testing may be indicated.

Treatment

The approach to treatment of pelvic relaxation depends on the following variables: severity of prolapse, age and general health of the patient, desire for future fertility, sexual activity, and associated pelvic pathology. Mild asymptomatic prolapse does not require any therapy. Patients who wish to avoid surgery or for whom surgery is considered too risky may benefit from nonoperative management. However, the approach will usually be surgical repair of the lax support structures by a plastic procedure.

Nonoperative management includes measures to avoid progression of symptoms, pelvic floor exercises, treatment of mucosal alterations, and use of vaginal pessaries. Situations that cause sudden, substantial increases in intra-abdominal pressure should be prevented. Patients should be instructed to avoid heavy lifting and high impact exercises. Constipation should be treated by dietary modification and stool softeners. Conditions associated with chronic coughing should also be promptly treated.

The purpose of pelvic floor exercises (also called Kegel exercises) is to strengthen the pubococcygeal muscle of the levator ani. The patient is instructed to identify the muscle by supervised palpation within the vaginal vault. Once identified, the patient practices tightening the muscle for 3 to 5 seconds in sets of 10 throughout the day. The number of sets is progressively increased until results are appreciated. Pelvic floor exercises are particularly useful to restore vaginal tone in the postpartum state, but they are of limited benefit in cases of severe prolapse.

Restoration of mucosal integrity is important for patient comfort but should also precede any contemplated surgery. Healing of the thickened or ulcerated mucosa requires replacement of the everted vagina to its normal internal position. Often the temporary use of a pessary is required, although tampons lubricated with glycerine may be effective. Dilute vinegar or iodine douches may help treat an associated bacterial infection. Local or systemic estrogen therapy improves blood supply and is trophic for the vaginal mucosa.

Pessaries, available in a variety of shapes and sizes (Fig. 5-10), are rubber or plastic devices fitted to the vault. They are worn to elevate the vagina and maintain normal anatomic relations by supporting the prolapsing structures against the

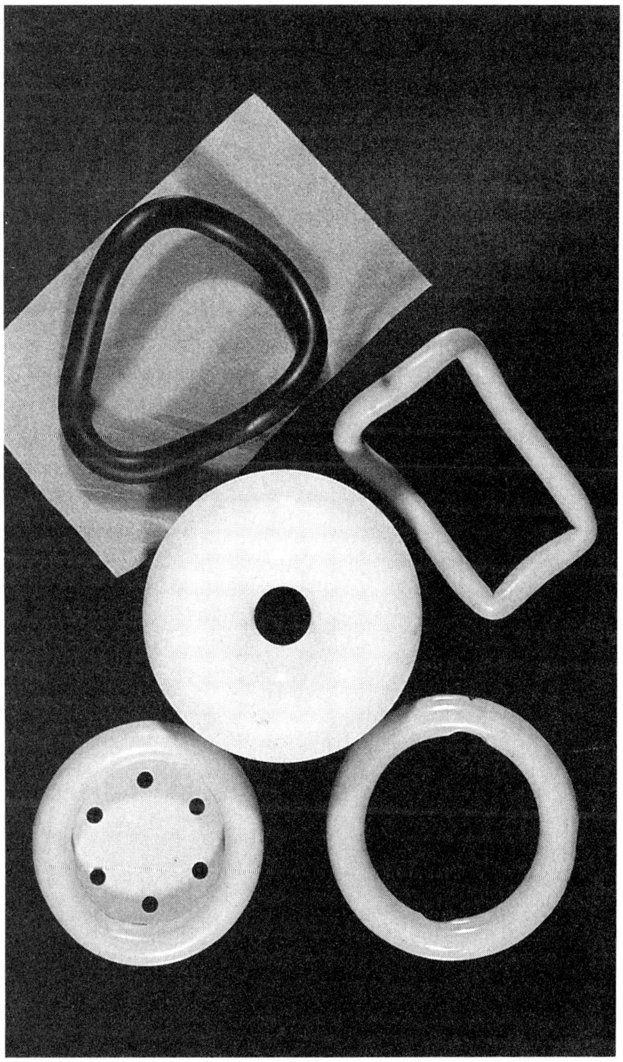

Fig. 5-10. Vaginal pessaries. (Courtesy Dr. Rapin Osathanondh.)

perineal body or the pubic bone. A pessary may be used temporarily in patients with prolapse as a diagnostic tool that simulates the results of surgery and assesses the impact on symptoms. Alternatively, some patients are satisfactorily managed over the long run with a pessary and thus never require operative intervention. Such patients do require close follow-up, however. They must be seen at least every 2 to 3 months so the pessary can be removed and cleaned, and so the mucosa can be inspected for pressure ulcers or infection.

Surgical treatment of genital prolapse is designed to address the specific defects present in an individual patient. The goals are the relief of symptoms, the restoration of normal vaginal anatomy, and the preservation of function. Ideally they are accomplished by repairing the weakened muscular, fascial, and ligamentous supports. If repair is not possible, then suspension procedures utilizing nonanatomic structures are performed so that symptoms are relieved and normal function is achieved. Occasionally, when surgical options are limited by the severity of the condition or the poor health of the patient, function must be compromised to obtain relief of symptoms.

Uterine prolapse is best treated by a vaginal hysterectomy. This requires completion of child-bearing, the absence of pelvic pathology, such as ovarian enlargement or large fibroids that are more appropriately managed by laparotomy, and adequate health to tolerate a major surgical procedure. Following removal of the uterus, the stretched uterosacral and cardinal ligaments are foreshortened by plication and sutured to the vaginal vault to suspend it.[17] Care is taken to avoid foreshortening the vagina or altering its normal axis of inclination in order to prevent subsequent vault prolapse. Plication of the uterosacral ligaments also helps to obliterate the cul-de-sac and is important in preventing subsequent enterocele formation.[30]

Older women who are no longer sexually active may be treated for uterine prolapse by a colpocleisis.[2] The uterus is left in situ, but the vaginal space is obliterated surgically by approximating the anterior and posterior walls. It is less satisfying than a procedure that attempts a more anatomically correct repair. However, it is quick and can be performed under local anesthesia, which makes it applicable to frail women in whom a vaginal hysterectomy may be poorly tolerated. It is very difficult to assess the health of the uterus and cervix following colpocleisis—any suspicion of pathology in these organs contraindicates the procedure.

Prolapse of the vaginal vault following hysterectomy presents a surgical challenge. The normal support structures, the cardinal and uterosacral ligaments, cannot be isolated for repair nor relied upon to provide adequate support to the vault. Two approaches to the problem have been described. The sacrospinous ligament suspension is a vaginal approach involving dissection of the pararectal space to the sacrospinous ligament.[55] The upper aspect of the vaginal vault is then suspended from the ligament by permanent sutures. Alternatively, an abdominal approach may be used; the vault is suspended from the periosteum of the sacral promontory by way of an interposed bridge of synthetic mesh.[1] The abdominal sacral colpopexy is preferred if other pelvic pathology dictates the need for laparotomy.

Repair of a cystocele due to a midline defect in the bladder endopelvic fascia is accomplished by anterior colporrhaphy. The vaginal mucosa is dissected from the bladder and redundant mucosa is excised. Submucosally the endopelvic fascia investing the bladder is dissected laterally until healthy fascia is identified. It is then plicated across the midline to reduce the bulging bladder tissues and re-create normal support. The plication may also be carried out near the bladder neck and elevates and fixes a hypermobile proximal urethra. This restores the vesicourethral angle to its normal anatomic position and corrects bladder neck prolapse. The procedure is called a Kelly plication and is applied to correct stress incontinence. Other procedures to restore bladder neck anatomy for the treatment of urinary incontinence are discussed in Chapter 18.

Cystoceles resulting from disruption of the attachment of the lateral vagina and bladder to the arcus tendineus fasciae pelvis are corrected by the paravaginal repair. The retropubic space is entered via a low transverse abdominal incision. The defect is repaired by suturing the vagina and its investing layer of endopelvic fascia to the pelvic sidewall at the level of the white line.[79]

A rectocele is repaired by posterior colporrhaphy. The posterior vaginal wall is incised and dissected laterally off the underlying perirectal endopelvic fascia. The endopelvic fascia investing the rectum is plicated across the attenuated defect in the midline thus reducing the prolapse. Usually this procedure is combined with a perineorrhaphy to correct associated perineal relaxation. The frequently used term "posterior repair" is not specific but typically refers to the combined posterior colporrhaphy and perineorrhaphy. A perineorrhaphy approximates the fascia of the perineal muscles (levator ani, deep and superficial transverse perineal, and bulbocavernosus) in the midline to re-create a strong perineal body.

An enterocele is a true herniation of a sac of peritoneum along the rectovaginal septum. A vaginal approach is often used for the repair. The posterior vaginal mucosa is opened and the dissection carried out cephalad along the rectovaginal septum until the enterocele sac is identified. The sac must be isolated from the rectum and vagina, opened, ligated high on its neck, and excised. The uterosacral ligaments are plicated across the midline to prevent recurrence (the McCall culdoplasty). Alternatively, an enterocele may be repaired abdominally by obliterating the cul-de-sac with concentric purse-string stitches placed in the peritoneum. This approach is called the Moschcowitz procedure.

BENIGN CONDITIONS OF THE VAGINA

The vagina is an uncommon site for the development of benign tumors. When they occur they are often asymptomatic and are detected only on pelvic examination. Benign tumors of the vagina may be either solid masses or cystic in nature. Small, asymptomatic cysts do not require treatment. Larger masses may occlude the vault and cause dyspareunia or pelvic pressure. Surgical excision is then indicated. Solid tumors should be excised to establish a histologic diagnosis and to exclude malignancy.

Vaginal cysts may form from remnants of the mesonephric duct or arise as epithelial inclusion cysts. The mesonephric ducts course laterally to the fused müllerian ducts during vaginal development. Normally they undergo degeneration due to a lack of androgenic support. When remnants persist, it is called Gartner's duct. Foci of cells of Gartner's duct may be located anywhere along the lateral walls of the vagina in the submucosal tissues and also may occur within the leaves of the broad ligament and mesosalpinx. The epithelium may actively secrete a mucinous material that is retained and forms a Gartner's duct cyst. Histologically the cysts are lined by a single layer of cuboidal or columnar cells. Occasionally a cyst may dissect deeply into the paravaginal tissues making excision difficult and bloody. Incision, drainage, and marsupialization of the cyst wall is preferred in this situation. The differential diagnosis includes epithelial inclusion cysts and suburethral diverticulum. Diverticuli are located along the course of the urethra and usually present in the 12 o'clock position when examining the patient in the lithotomy position.

Epithelial inclusion cysts arise from vaginal epithelium buried under the mucosa during healing from a traumatic injury. Obstetric laceration and episiotomy are common antecedents. The vaginal mucosa is not secretory. However, if the tissue remains viable, cell turnover and desquamation will occur. Subsequent degeneration of the cellular material results in the accumulation of a thick cheesy substance. These cysts are distinguished from Gartner's duct cysts on the basis of their contents, histology (stratified squamous epithelium), and location.[75] They usually occur in the lower third of the vagina on the posterior or posterolateral wall.

Solid tumors are more rare and arise from the connective tissue elements of the vagina. Clinically they present as polypoid growths or as firm nontender masses, often within the rectovaginal septum.[71] Histologic examination usually reveals smooth muscle elements (leiomyoma), fibrous tissue (fibromyoma), or a mixed pattern. Rarely, skeletal muscle elements (rhabdomyoma) are identified. Surgical excision to exclude malignancy is the appropriate management.[92]

The vagina is a relatively common site for extraperitoneal endometriosis, though overall the incidence of vaginal occurrence is low.[65] Patients may complain of cyclic pain and dyspareunia. The implants often form small cysts that on gross inspection are a dark blue color. They may be tender on palpation. The diagnosis is established by biopsy and treatment is by surgical excision or hormonal therapy.

The squamous epithelium of the vagina may become infected with certain types of the human papilloma virus resulting in condylomas. The soft, verrucous tumors may occur singly, in small clusters, or as confluent growths. Vaginal condylomas may be accompanied by lesions on the cervix, vulva, and perianal skin, and treatment may be difficult. Podophyllin, a cytotoxic agent widely used to treat vulvar condyloma, is not recommended for vaginal therapy. Excessive absorption may occur and result in neurotoxicity. Chemical cauterization with bichloracetic acid and trichloroacetic acid may be used. Other therapies include laser ablation, cryocautery, and interferon.[83]

CLEAR CELL ADENOCARCINOMA

In 1971 Herbst and coworkers described an increased risk of clear cell adenocarcinoma of the vagina in young women with in utero exposure to diethylstilbestrol.[34] DES, a synthetic estrogen, was administered in the mid-1940s to some women with high risk pregnancies to prevent miscarriage. Prior to 1970 only rare cases of clear cell adenocarcinoma had been reported. Following the recognition of the relationship with DES, a registry was established that now contains over 500 cases of clear cell adenocarcinoma of the vagina and cervix.[52] Exposure to DES during gestation has been confirmed in up to 88% of cases, although maternal recall of the exposure is not very reliable.[78]

The risk of developing clear cell adenocarcinoma among exposed females is approximately 1 in 1000.[33] The risk increases inversely with gestational age at exposure but is not clearly associated with total dose. Occurrence of the cancers appears to be age related. The median age at diagnosis is 19 years and more than 90% of cases have occurred when these women were between 15 and 27 years. The prognosis for survival is related to the extent of disease at the time of diagnosis. Tumors confined to the vaginal wall (stage I) are associated with a 5-year survival rate of about 90%.[71] Therapeutic modalities used in the treatment of these patients have included surgery, radiation, chemotherapy, and combined approaches.

Clear cell adenocarcinoma of the vagina is not the only DES-related abnormality of the genital tract. Vaginal adenosis and structural anomalies of the genital tract occur more frequently in this group of patients than the nonexposed controls.[40,77] Vaginal adenosis is the presence of glandular-columnar epithelium and its mucinous secretory products in the vagina. The prevalence of this condition is over 90% in DES-exposed women. The strong association between adenosis and prenatal DES exposure suggests the drug interferes with normal vaginal development. The precise mechanism is unknown; the replacement of müllerian columnar epithelium may be impeded by upward growing squamous epithelium from the urogenital sinus.[95]

Adenosis is most often encountered on the upper, anterior vaginal wall and may be continuous onto the cervical portio that forms a cervical ectropion. Clinically it has a granular, red appearance compared with the smooth, pink squamous mucosa. Sometimes it is submucosal and then detected only by careful palpation of the vaginal walls. Vaginal adenosis is usually asymptomatic, but it may cause excessive vaginal secretions. Over time it may regress as the columnar epithelium is converted to a squamous-type by metaplasia. It is usually found in association with clear cell adenocarcinomas, but progression of adenosis to cancer has not been documented.[29] Adenosis should be followed carefully by cytologic and clinical examination, and treatment reserved only for symptoms.

DES-related structural anomalies have been described for the vagina, cervix, uterus, and fallopian tubes. The vagina and cervix may develop a transverse ridge of tissue usually on the anterior portion that in extreme cases may be circumferential. They have been variably referred to as hoods, collars, and cockscomb cervices. A pseudopolyp may develop on the exocervix. The polypoid appearance results from a thick constricting stromal groove encircling the exocervix and causing protrusion of the endocervical tissue. The cervix may be hypoplastic and the vaginal fornices may be absent or poorly developed. Changes in the endometrial cavity include a small cavity, a T-shaped cavity, and constrictions. They occur more frequently in women with cervical abnormalities.[40] Fallopian tube abnormalities include a withered, foreshortened, and convoluted appearance. The clinical implication of these structural changes is an adverse effect on reproductive potential. Fertility rates may be decreased in this group of women; following conception they are also at increased risk for spontaneous abortion, ectopic pregnancy, and preterm delivery.[77]

Women with in utero DES exposure may have an increased risk of cervical intraepithelial neoplasia (CIN) and vaginal intraepithelial neoplasia (VaIN).[70] The hypothesized reason for this is the more extensive transformation zone occurring on the cervices of DES-exposed women. The transformation zone is an area of active metaplastic growth and is a site for CIN. Thus far no increase in squamous cell carcinomas has been documented.[24] However, as these patients grow older and approach the age of peak incidence of invasive carcinoma, close follow-up will be required to exclude a higher risk.

VAGINAL INTRAEPITHELIAL NEOPLASIA

Vaginal intraepithelial neoplasia is an uncommon pathologic entity. However, in recent decades it has been diagnosed with increased frequency, probably because of more extensive cytologic screening even in women who have undergone hysterectomy. The incidence of vaginal carcinoma in situ is approximately 0.2 to 0.3 cases per 100,000 women,[16] which is only about one third the rate for invasive lesions. Patients range in age from 25 to 80 years, with a mean age of 50 to 55 years.

A striking association in reported series of patients with VaIN is the occurrence of neoplasia at another genital tract site. Evidence of another genital tract neoplasm occurs in 50% to 75% of patients.[8,35,46] Most of the prior or concomitant neoplastic lesions are squamous and involve the cervix or vulva. This is cited as support for the hypothesized "field response" of the squamous epithelium of the lower genital tract.[51] According to this theory, tissues with a common embryonic origin share susceptibility to common carcinogens. The urogenital sinus is the ultimate source of the epithelium of the vulva, vagina, and cervix. Under appropriate conditions, neoplasms developing in these tissues may arise as multicentric lesions instead of originating with neoplastic transformation of a single cell. This may explain the clinical observation; there is an alternative explanation, however.

Lower genital tract neoplasms often grow by contiguous spread. Extension of a single lesion to a neighboring tissue may occur without recognition. Incomplete removal or treatment may result. Thus failure to initially diagnose the true extent of a single neoplasm might result in a misdiagnosis of independent development of two separate lesions. Regardless of etiology, the important clinical implication is the need for careful evaluation and follow-up of the entire lower genital tract whenever a patient presents with a neoplasm involving the vulva, vagina, or cervix. The carcinogenic agents responsible for squamous cell neoplasms of the lower genital tract are not known. Factors that have been implicated include infection with human papilloma virus (HPV) and exposure to radiation.[4]

Vaginal intraepithelial neoplasia is asymptomatic except in occasional patients with postcoital staining or a vaginal discharge. In some cases an astute examiner will detect a mucosal lesion on physical examination; most patients, however, will have abnormal Papanicolaou smears, which prompt the diagnostic evaluation.

The diagnosis is established by colposcopically directed biopsies. Colposcopic examination of the vagina is difficult; a vaginal speculum must be repositioned enough times to visualize the entire mucosal surface. The lesions of VaIN tend to be multifocal and most commonly occur in the upper third of the vagina. The colposcopic findings are similar to those seen in CIN and include white epithelium, punctuation, and mosaicism. White lesions may become more obvious after application of 3% acetic acid solution to the mucosa. An iodine stain, such as Schiller's solution, may also be used to demonstrate abnormal areas. Normal vaginal epithelial cells stain brown due to the high glycogen content. Dysplastic cells often contain less glycogen and therefore do not take up the dye.

The histologic findings of VaIN are similar to CIN. The abnormalities are confined to the surface epithelial cells. Neoplastic changes include the presence of abnormal mitotic figures, nuclear pleomorphism, and loss of polarity. The degree of severity is determined by the depth of epithelial involvement. If only the lower third of the cell layers of the squamous epithelium is affected, it is graded VaIN I or mild; involvement of the middle third is graded VaIN II or moderate; and involvement of the upper third is graded VaIN III or severe. Involvement of the full thickness of the epithelium is called vaginal carcinoma in situ.

Vaginal intraepithelial neoplasia is considered a premalignant lesion analogous to CIN. However, because of its lower incidence, much less information regarding the magnitude of its premalignant potential, transition times from premalignant to malignant, and factors influencing the transition is available. Once diagnosed, treatment is indicated to prevent progression (Fig. 5-11). Several treatment options exist. The rationale for all modalities is to excise or destroy the dysplastic cells and cause minimal damage to normal epithelium and submucosa. In the healing process, dysplastic cells are then replaced by normal squamous epithelium. The age of the patient, the desire for future sexual function, and the extent of disease will determine the choice of treatment.

Surgical excision has been the traditional therapy. This may involve a wide local excision with primary repair for an isolated lesion or a total vaginectomy if the disease is widespread.[38,58] Repair following a vaginectomy may be by colpocleisis in a woman no longer sexually active. Otherwise repair necessitates formation of a neovagina using a split-thickness skin graft. Surgical treatment is successful in more than 80% of cases, but recurrences have been reported even involving the skin grafts.[27]

Chemotherapy with topical 5-fluorouracil (5-FU) is effective in treating a majority of in situ lesions. It offers the advantage of treating the entire epithelial surface at risk in this potentially multifocal disease. It is a pyrimidine analog that blocks DNA synthesis, especially in rapidly

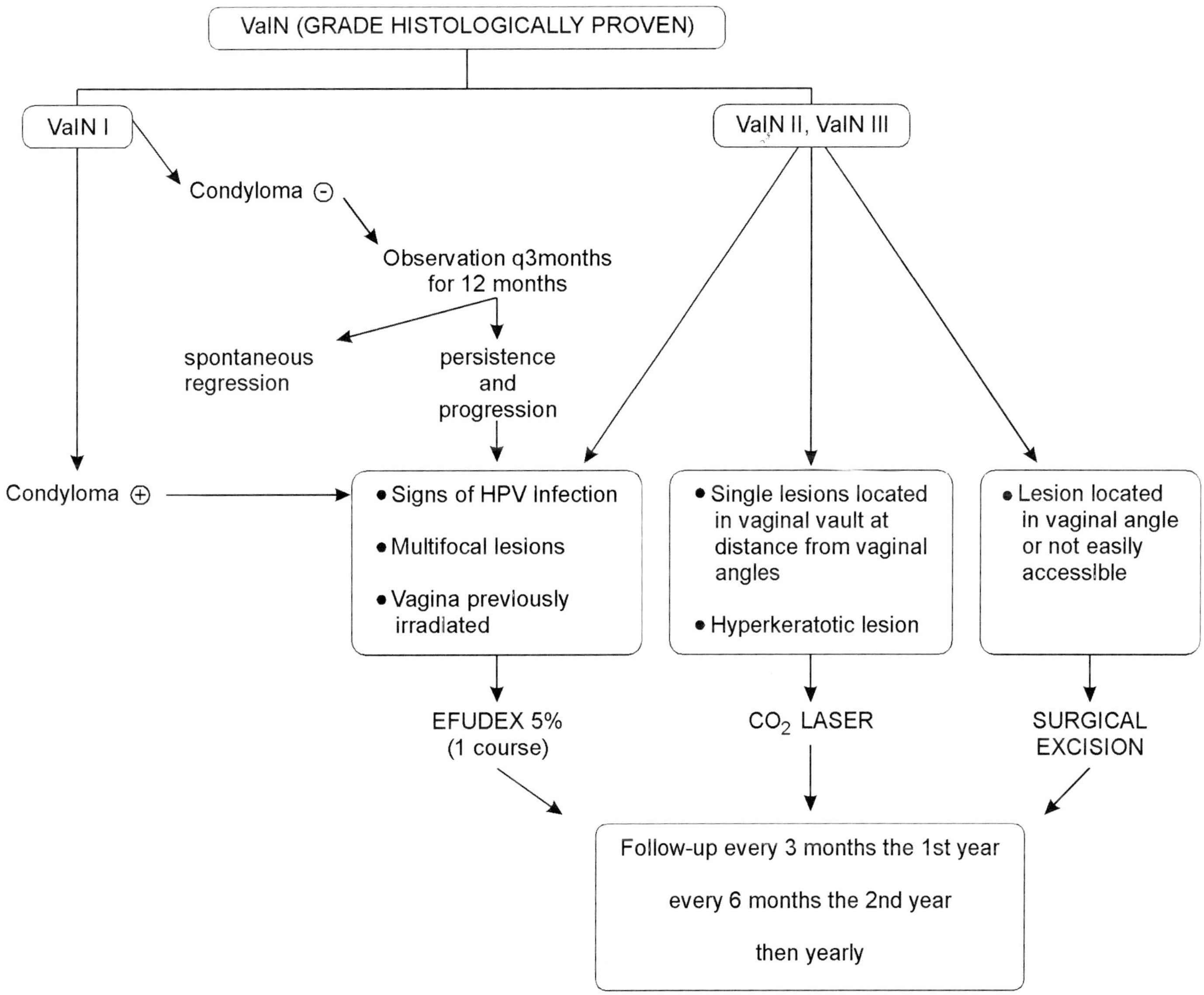

Fig. 5-11. Algorithm for the treatment of vaginal intraepithelial neoplasia. (From Audet-Lapointe P et al: Vaginal intraepithelial neoplasia, *Gynecol Oncol* 36:232, 1990.)

proliferating tissues. Its effect occurs locally by ulceration and erosion followed by reepithelialization. Side effects include pain, vulvar irritation, and dysuria. A disadvantage compared with surgery is the lack of availability of a histologic specimen to exclude concomitant invasive disease. However, the reported results with 5-FU suggest remission rates of 80%, a value that compares favorably with those obtained surgically.[43]

Another approach to the treatment of VaIN utilizes the carbon dioxide laser, which was used initially to ablate isolated lesions. If the entire mucosa is vaporized, success rates are reported to be comparable with those achieved with 5-FU.[39] The technique avoids the problem of vulvitis associated with 5-FU, and excellent functional results are reported. As with 5-FU therapy, no histology is available after treatment. Therefore laser treatment requires an exhaustive pretreatment colposcopic examination to exclude invasive cancer.

Other therapies for VaIN have included radiation therapy and cryocautery. Tissue damage is harder to control with these modalities. As a result, higher failure rates and unacceptable complications because of damage to adjacent organs have occurred; they are not currently recommended.

MALIGNANT NEOPLASMS

Primary malignant tumors are rare in the vagina. Only 1% to 2% of genital tract cancers originate in the vaginal tissues; the majority are squamous cell carcinomas. Other primary cancers include melanoma, sarcoma, adenocarcinoma, and endodermal sinus tumors. Most malignant vaginal lesions are secondary. They occur as extensions of cervical or vulvar carcinoma, or as metastatic cancers usually arising in the bladder, rectum, uterus, or ovary.

Squamous cell carcinoma

Squamous cell carcinomas account for about 90% of primary vaginal cancers. Patients range in age from 30 to 90 years with an average age at diagnosis of approximately 60 years. The etiology of this tumor is not known. One theory suggests prolonged exposure of the mucosa to irritants has a causative role.[74] Most cancers are located near the posterior fornix, which suggests a pooling phenomenon. No data are available to substantiate such a relationship, however nor is there a proven relationship of vaginal cancer to pessary use or prolapse, or other potential chronic irritants. Other factors implicated are pelvic radiation and viral infections.[53]

The symptoms most often attributed to vaginal cancer are abnormal bleeding or a blood-tinged discharge. Bleeding may occur only with intercourse or douching. Anterior wall lesions may cause urinary symptoms such as frequency, dysuria, and hematuria. Rectal involvement from a posterior wall tumor may manifest as tenesmus, melena, or pain. Many patients report no symptoms and the diagnosis is then established by pelvic examination. It is essential that the entire mucosal surface be visualized (by rotating the speculum blades) and be palpated during the pelvic examination. Occasionally small lesions are detected colposcopically in response to an abnormal cytologic smear. The vaginal vault is highly distensible and can accommodate a relatively large mass lesion before the onset of symptoms. For this reason, and because many older patients avoid seeking medical care despite symptoms, diagnosis is often delayed.[7] This is unfortunate since vaginal cancer occurs in a clinically accessible site and thus the opportunity for early diagnosis and treatment exists.

The diagnosis of vaginal carcinoma is confirmed by biopsy of a visible or palpable vaginal lesion. Gross lesions vary in appearance. They may present as exophytic growths, superficial plaques, or as ulcerative lesions. Histologically, neoplastic epidermoid cells are identified invading the submucous tissues as well as the vascular and lymphatic spaces. There is usually an associated inflammatory infiltrate. The histologic appearance may be graded based on its degree of differentiation, but this does not give reliable prognostic information.[20]

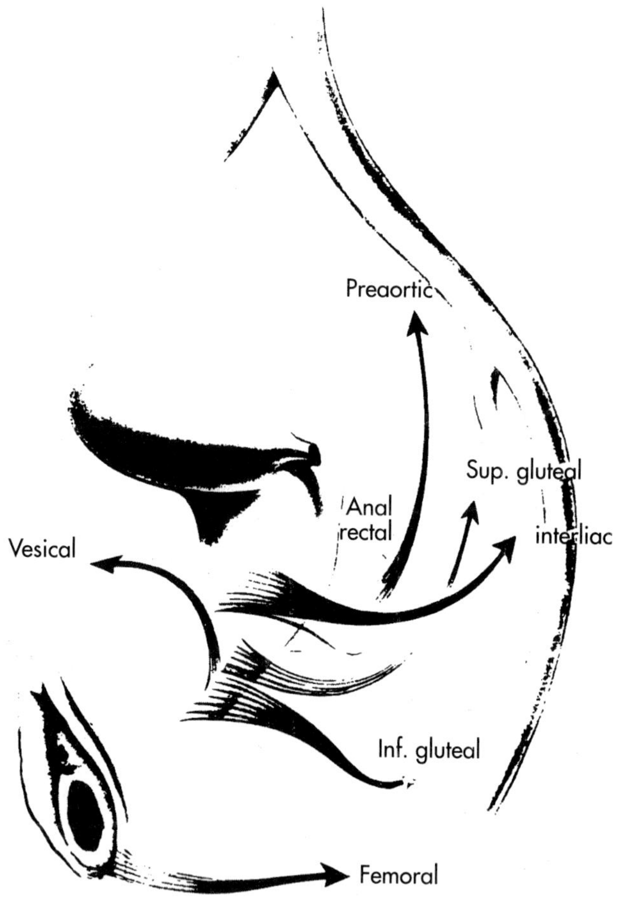

Fig. 5-12. Lymphatic drainage of the vagina. The upper vagina follows the cervical drainage pattern to the pelvic lymph nodes. The lower vagina follows the vulvar drainage pattern to the femoral lymph nodes. (From Plentl AA, Friedman EA: *Lymphatic system of the female genitalia: the morphologic basis of oncologic diagnosis and therapy*, Philadelphia, 1971, WB Saunders, p 55.)

Vaginal squamous cell carcinoma spreads by contiguous growth and by the lymphatic vasculature. Local growth occurs initially in the submucous layers with gradual extension to the paracolpos, bladder, and rectum. Growth may involve the cervix or the vulva; by convention a squamous tumor that involves both the vagina and one of the adjacent genital organs at the time of diagnosis is considered to be a primary cancer of either the cervix or the vulva.

Metastatic spread via the lymphatics follows a pattern that depends on the location of the primary lesion (Fig. 5-12). Tumors located in the upper vagina tend to spread into the pelvic lymph nodes (the iliac, hypogastric, and obturator groups), similar to cervical cancer. Tumors arising in the lower vagina often metastasize first to the femoral and inguinal lymph nodes as do the vulvar cancers. Lymphatic involvement is present about one fourth of the time at diagnosis.[75]

Staging is based on a careful history and clinical examination. In addition, a chest x-ray, intravenous pyelogram, barium enema, cystoscopy, and proctosigmoidoscopy are performed to determine local or distant spread. The staging system is based on the recommendations of the International Federation of Gynecology and Obstetrics (FIGO; Table 5-2). The distribution of patients among the stages varies with the different series reported. Typically 30% to 40% of patients will have stage III or stage IV disease.[5,21,61]

The treatment of vaginal squamous cell carcinoma has been by radiation therapy primarily, though in some cases surgery may be an option. The therapeutic plan should be individualized according to the following factors: the extent of disease, the patient's general health, the desire for vaginal function, and the childbearing status. In addition, the proximity of the vagina to the bladder and rectum must be recognized, to minimize complications.

Surgical excision as primary therapy applies only to small localized tumors in the upper third of the vagina. Tumors arising on the posterior vaginal wall are more easily resected than those occurring anteriorly near the more intimate attachment of the bladder. Treatments reported consist of radical hysterectomy with vaginectomy and excision of the pelvic lymph nodes, radical vaginectomy, and wide local excision.[5] The surgical approach may be used adjunctively to treat advanced disease or recurrences following radiation therapy.

Radiation therapy has become the main treatment modality for vaginal cancer in most patients.[61] A combined approach using both external radiation therapy and local implants is applied. A dose of 4000 to 5000 rads of whole pelvis radiation may be administered first to initiate shrinkage of a large tumor and render local therapy more effective. Radium or cesium implants are then placed intravaginally to deliver an additional 3000 to 4000 rads directly to the tumor. This may be impossible to carry out with very large tumors; additional therapy by external beam may be administered.

The normal vaginal mucosa is relatively radioresistant. However, the proximity of the radiosensitive bladder and rectal tissues results in radiation complications in approximately 15% to 25% of patients.[28,59,62] Complications include proctitis, rectovaginal and vesicovaginal fistulae, and strictures. They occur more frequently in patients with advanced disease who receive higher doses of radiation.

Table 5-2. International Federation of Gynecology and Obstetrics—classification of vaginal cancer

Stage 0	Carcinoma in situ
Stage I	Carcinoma limited to the vaginal wall
Stage II	Carcinoma involving the subvaginal tissues but not extending to the pelvic wall
Stage III	Carcinoma extending to the pelvic wall
Stage IV	Carcinoma extending beyond the true pelvis or involving the mucosa of the bladder or rectum. (Bullous edema alone does not permit allotment of a case to stage IV)
Stage IVA	Involvement of adjacent organs (bladder, rectum)
Stage IVB	Involvement of distant organs

The prognosis for patients with vaginal squamous cell carcinoma depends primarily on the extent of disease at the time of diagnosis.[7] Stage I disease treated with radiation therapy results in 5-year survival rates of 80% to 90%. Five-year survival rates for higher stages are 45% to 58% for stage II, 25% to 40% for stage III, and up to 10% for stage IV. The overall 5-year survival rate is approximately 45%.

Recurrences often occur locally and are more common in higher stages. Distant metastases occur later and usually involve the lung and bone. Radical surgery may be attempted in selected cases of isolated, local recurrence. Chemotherapy is being evaluated for a possible role in cases with systemic recurrence.

Malignant melanoma

Malignant melanomas may arise from vaginal melanocytes. They are rare tumors and comprise less than 1% of all melanomas in women.[64] Patients may be asymptomatic or present with a mass, discharge, or vaginal bleeding. The gross appearance of the tumors is variable and ranges from a flat, spreading lesion to a heaped up, polypoid mass. Most lesions are pigmented, but others are not. The diagnosis must be confirmed by histologic evaluation of a biopsy specimen.

The prognosis for patients with vaginal melanoma is poor. The disease is often well advanced when diagnosed. The tumors are not responsive to radiation therapy, and effective chemotherapeutic agents have not been identified. Radical surgical therapy, which includes lymph node dissection if the primary tumor is more than superficially invasive, is currently the most recommended treatment.[47]

Adenocarcinoma

Adenocarcinoma of the vagina associated with in utero DES-exposure has previously been discussed. A much rarer type of vaginal adenocarcinoma is the endodermal sinus tumor.[103] It occurs exclusively in infants, usually under two years old. The tumor probably arises from extragonadal germ cells. Endodermal sinus tumors occurring in the vagina may secrete alpha-fetoprotein like their ovarian counterparts. This is a useful marker to monitor disease activity in patients undergoing treatment. Combination therapy consisting of surgery and chemotherapy, has resulted in several long term survivors. The most commonly used chemotherapeutic agents are vincristine, actinomycin D, and cyclophosphamide.

Vaginal sarcoma

Sarcomas are extremely rare and comprise less than 2% of vaginal malignancies. They tend to occur as one of two types based on their age predilection.[88] Sarcoma botryoides (embryonal rhabdomyosarcoma) usually afflicts children less than 2 years old. The tumors form friable clusters of polypoid masses that protrude from the vagina. They are frequently multicentric and appear to arise from the vaginal subepithelium. Histologically there is diffuse proliferation of spindled neoplastic cells mixed with embryonic striated muscle cells. Clinically they are aggressive tumors with a poor prognosis. The traditional therapy has been radical surgery. However, a multimodal approach combining less radical surgery with chemotherapy or radiation may offer equal efficacy with less morbidity.[36]

Vaginal sarcomas in adults are represented by a varied group of histologic types. The commonest is the smooth muscle tumor, leiomyosarcoma. Others are classified as fibrosarcomas, reticulum cell sarcomas, malignant schwannomas, müllerian stromal sarcomas, and mixed cell types; they all have a poor prognosis. One series reported a 5-year survival of 23%.[18] The extreme rarity of these tumors makes evaluation of treatment regimens difficult. Treatment is usually radical surgical excision supplemented by radiation therapy to control local disease.

Secondary carcinoma

In the vagina metastatic cancer occurs more frequently than primary disease. Contiguous spread from the uterine cervix accounts for most. Other sites of primary malignancy that may involve the vagina include the vulva, endometrium, ovary, bladder, urethra, kidney, rectum, and malignant trophoblastic disease.

REFERENCES

1. Addison WA et al: Abdominal sacral colpopexy with Mersilene mesh in the retroperitoneal position in the management of post-hysterectomy vaginal vault prolapse and enterocele, *Am J Obstet Gynecol* 153:140-146,1985.
2. Ahranjani M et al: Neugebauer-LeFort operation for vaginal prolapse: a review of 38 cases, *J Reprod Med* 37:959-964, 1992.
3. Allen RE et al: Pelvic floor damage and childbirth: a neurophysiologic study, *Br J Obstet Gynaecol* 97:770-779, 1990.
4. Audet-Lapoint P et al: Vaginal intraepithelial neoplasia, *Gynecol Oncol* 36:232-239, 1990.
5. Ball HG, Berman ML: Management of primary vaginal carcinoma, *Gynecol Oncol* 14:154-163, 1982.
6. Bates GW, Wiser WL: A technique for uterine conservation in adolescents with vaginal agenesis and a functional uterus, *Obstet Gynecol* 66:290-294, 1985.
7. Benedet JL: Vaginal malignancy: curr opinion, *Obstet Gynecol* 3:73-77, 1991.
8. Benedet JL, Sanders BH: Carcinoma in situ of the vagina, *Am J Obstet Gynecol* 148:695-700, 1984.
9. Bistolleti P et al: Comparison of oral and vaginal metronidazole therapy for nonspecific bacterial vaginosis, *Gynecol Obstet Invest* 21:144-149, 1986.
10. Biswas MK: Bacterial vaginosis, *Clin Obstet Gynecol* 36:66-76, 1993.
11. Blaustein RL: Cytology of the female genital tract. In Kurman RJ, editor: *Blaustein's pathology of the female genital tract*, New York, 1987, Springer-Verlag.
12. Boutin EL, Battle E, Cunha GR: The response of female urogenital tract epithelia to mesenchymal inductors is restricted by the germ layer origin of the epithelium: prostatic inductions, *Differentiation* 48:99-105, 1991.
13. Bulmer D: The development of the human vagina, *J Anat* 91:490-508, 1957.
14. Bump RC, Fantl JA, Hurt WG: The mechanism of urinary continence in women with severe uterovaginal prolapse: results of barrier studies, *Obstet Gynecol* 72:291-295, 1988.
15. Buttram VC: Müllerian anomalies and their management, *Fertil Steril* 40:159-163, 1983.
16. Cramer DW, Cutler SJ: Incidence and histopathology of malignancies of the female genital organs in the United States, *Am J Obstet Gynecol* 118:443-460, 1974.
17. Cruickshank SH: Preventing post hysterectomy vaginal vault prolapse and enterocele during vaginal hysterectomy, *Am J Obstet Gynecol* 156:1433-1440, 1987.
18. Davos I, Abell MR: Sarcomas of the vagina, *Obstet Gynecol* 47:342-350, 1975.
19. DeLancey JOL: Anatomic aspects of vaginal eversion after hysterectomy, *Am J Obstet Gynecol* 166:1717-1728, 1992.
20. Dixit S, Singhal S, Baboo HA: Squamous cell carcinoma of the vagina: a review of 70 cases, *Gynecol Oncol* 48:80-87, 1993.
21. Eddy GL et al: Primary invasive vaginal carcinoma, *Am J Obstet Gynecol* 165:292-298, 1991.
22. Eschenbach DA: Vaginal infection, *Clin Obstet Gynecol* 26:186-202, 1983.
23. Evans TN, Poland ML, Boving RL: Vaginal malformations, *Am J Obstet Gynecol* 141:910-917, 1991.
24. Faber K, Jones M, Tarraza HM: Invasive squamous cell carcinoma of the vagina in a diethylstilbestrol-exposed woman, *Gynecol Oncol* 37:125-128, 1990.
25. Fleury FJ: Adult vaginitis, *Clin Obstet Gynecol* 24:407-438, 1981.
26. Forsberg JG: Cervicovaginal epithelium: its origin and development, *Am J Obstet Gynecol* 115:1025-1043, 1973.
27. Gallup DG, Castle CA, Stock RJ: Recurrent carcinoma in situ of the vagina following split-thickness skin graft vaginoplasty, *Gynecol Oncol* 26:98-102, 1987a.
28. Gallup DG et al: Invasive squamous cell carcinoma of the vagina: a fourteen year study, *Obstet Gynecol* 69:782-785, 1987b.
29. Ghosh TK, Cera PJ: Transition of benign vaginal adenosis to clear cell carcinoma, *Obstet Gynecol* 61:126-130, 1983.
30. Given FT: Posterior culdoplasty: revisited, *Am J Obstet Gynecol* 153:135-139, 1985.
31. Griffin JE et al: Congenital absence of the vagina: the Mayer-Rokitansky-Kuster-Hauser syndrome, *Ann Int Med* 85:224-236, 1976.
32. Heine P, McGregor JA: Trichomonas vaginalis: a re-emerging pathogen, *Clin Obstet Gynecol* 36:137-144, 1993.

33. Herbst AL, Anderson D: Clear cell adenocarcinoma of the vagina and cervix secondary to intrauterine exposure to diethylstilbestrol, *Semin Surg Oncol* 6:343-346, 1990.
34. Herbst AL, Ulfelder H, Poskanzer DC: Adenocarcinoma of the vagina: association of material stilbestrol therapy with tumor appearance in young women, *N Engl J Med* 284:878-881, 1971.
35. Hernandez-Linares W et al: Carcinoma in situ of the vagina: past and present management, *Obstet Gynecol* 56:356-360, 1980.
36. Hicks ML, Piver MS: Conservative surgery plus adjuvant therapy for vulvovaginal rhabdomyosarcoma, diethylstilbestrol clear cell adenocarcinoma of the vagina, and unilateral germ cell tumors of the ovary, *Pediatr Adolesc Gynecol* 19:219-233, 1992.
37. Higton BK: A trial of clotrimazole and nystatin in vaginal moniliasis, *Br J Obstet Gynecol* 80:992-995, 1973.
38. Hoffman MS et al: Upper vaginectomy for in situ and occult, superficially invasive carcinoma of the vagina, *Am J Obstet Gynecol* 166:30-33, 1992.
39. Jobson VW, Homesley HD: Treatment of vaginal intraepithelial neoplasia with the carbon dioxide laser, *Obstet Gynecol* 62:90-93, 1983.
40. Kaufman RH et al: Upper genital tract changes associated with exposure in utero to diethylstilbestrol, *Am J Obstet Gynecol* 128:51-56, 1977.
41. Kempers RD: Vaginitis, *Postgrad Obstet Gynecol* 5:1-6, 1985.
42. Koff AK: Development of the vagina in the human fetus, *Contrib Embryol* 24:61-90, 1933.
43. Krebs HB: Treatment of vaginal intraepithelial neoplasia with laser and topical 5-fluorouracil. *Obstet Gynecol* 73:657-660, 1989.
44. Landers DV: The treatment of vaginitis: trichomonas, yeast, and bacterial vaginosis, *Clin Obstet Gynecol* 31:473-479, 1988.
45. Larsen B: Vaginal flora in health and disease, *Clin Obstet Gynecol* 36:107-121, 1993.
46. Lenehan PM, Meffe F, Lickrish GM: Vaginal intraepithelial neoplasia: biologic aspects and management, *Obstet Gynecol* 68:333-337, 1986.
47. Liu LY, Hou YJ, Li JZ: Primary malignant melanoma of the vagina: a report of seven cases, *Obstet Gynecol* 70:569-572, 1987.
48. Livengood CH, Thomason JL, Hill GB: Bacterial vaginosis: treatment with topical intravaginal clindamycin phosphate, *Obstet Gynecol* 76:118-123, 1990.
49. Lossick JG, Muller M, Gorrell TE: In vitro drug susceptibility and doses of metronidazole required for cure in cases of refractory vaginal trichomoniasis, *J Infect Dis* 153:948-955, 1986.
50. Lugo-Miro VL, Green M, Mazur L: Comparison of different metronidazole therapeutic regimens for bacterial vaginosis, *JAMA* 268:92-95, 1992.
51. Marcus SL: Multiple squamous cell carcinomas involving the cervix, vagina and vulva: the theory of multicentric origin, *Am J Obstet Gynecol* 80:802-812, 1960.
52. Melnick S et al: Rates and risks of diethylstilbestrol-related clear-cell adenocarcinoma of the vagina and cervix, *N Engl J Med* 316:514-516, 1987.
53. Merino MJ: Vaginal cancer: the role of infectious and environmental factors, *Am J Obstet Gynecol* 165:1255-1262, 1991.
54. Miles MR, Olsen L, Rogers A: Recurrent vaginal candidiasis: importance of an intestinal reservoir, *JAMA* 238:1836-1837, 1977.
55. Nichols DH: Sacrospinous fixation for massive eversion of the vagina, *Am J Obstet Gynecol* 142:901-904, 1982.
56. Oriel JD et al: Genital yeast infections, *Br Med J* 4:761-764, 1972.
57. Osborne NG, Grubin L, Pratson L: Vaginitis in sexually active women: relationship to nine sexually transmitted organisms, *Am J Obstet Gynecol* 142:962-967, 1982.
58. Patsner B: Treatment of vaginal dysplasia with loop excision: report of five cases, *Am J Obstet Gynecol* 169:179-180, 1993.
59. Perez CA, Camel HM: Long term follow-up in radiation therapy of carcinoma of the vagina, *Cancer* 49:1308-1315, 1982.
60. Perl G: Errors in the diagnosis of trichomonas vaginalis infection as observed among 1199 patients, *Obstet Gynecol* 39:7-9, 1972.
61. Podczaski E, Herbst AL: Cancer of the vagina and fallopian tube. In Knapp RC, Berkowitz RS, editors: *Gynecologic oncology*, ed 2, New York, 1993, McGraw-Hill
62. Pride GL et al: Primary invasive squamous carcinoma of the vagina, *Obstet Gynecol* 53:218-225, 1979.
63. Pritchard JA, MacDonald PC, Gant NF: *Williams obstetrics*, ed 17, Norwalk Conn, 1985, Appleton Century Crofts.
64. Ragnarsson-Olding B et al: Malignant melanoma of the vulva and vagina, *Cancer* 71:1893-1897, 1993.
65. Ranney B: Endometriosis: pathogenesis, symptoms, and findings, *Clin Obstet Gynecol* 23:865-874, 1980.
66. Ranney B: Enterocele, vaginal prolapse, pelvic hernia: recognition and treatment, *Am J Obstet Gynecol* 140:53-57, 1981.
67. Rein MF, Muller M: Trichomonas vaginalis. In Holmes KK et al, editors: *Sexually transmitted diseases*, New York, 1984, McGraw-Hill.
68. Reindollar RH, Byrd JR, McDonough PG: Delayed sexual development: a study of 252 patients, *Am J Obstet Gynecol* 140:371-380, 1981.
69. Richardson AC, Lyon JB, Williams NL: A new look at pelvic relaxation, *Am J Obstet Gynecol* 126:568-571, 1976.
70. Robboy SJ et al: Increased incidence of cervical and vaginal dysplasia in 3980 diethylstilbestrol-exposed young women, *JAMA* 252:2979-2983, 1984.
71. Robboy SJ, Welch WR: Selected topics in the pathology of the vagina, *Hum Path* 22:868-876, 1991.
72. Rock JA, Azziz R: Genital anomalies in childhood, *Clin Obstet Gynecol* 30:682-696, 1987.
73. Scholl GM: Prognostic variables in treating vaginismus, *Obstet Gynecol* 72:231-235, 1988.
74. Schraub S et al: Cervical and vaginal cancer associated with pessary use, *Cancer* 69:2505-2509, 1992.
75. Sedlis A, Robby SJ: Diseases of the vagina. In Kurman RJ, editor: *Blaustein's pathology of the female genital tract*, New York, 1987, Springer-Verlag.
76. Semmens JP et al: Effects of estrogen therapy on vaginal physiology during menopause, *Obstet Gynecol* 66:15-18, 1985.
77. Senekjian EK et al: Infertility among daughters either exposed or not exposed to diethylstilbestrol, *Am J Obstet Gynecol* 158:493-498, 1988.
78. Sharp GB et al: Clear cell adenocarcinoma of the lower genital tract: correlation of mother's recall of diethylstilbestrol history with obstetrical records, *Cancer* 66:2215-2220, 1990.
79. Shull BL, Baden WF: A six-year experience with paravaginal defect repair for stress urinary incontinence, *Am J Obstet Gynecol* 160:1432-1439, 1989.
80. Shull BL et al: Preoperative and postoperative analysis of site-specific pelvic support defects in 81 women treated with sacrospinous ligament suspension and pelvic reconstruction, *Am J Obstet Gynecol* 166:1764-1771, 1992.
81. Sjoberg I: The vagina: morphological, functional and ecological aspects, *Acta Obstet Gynecol Scan* 71:84-85, 1992.
82. Smith ARB, Hosker GL, Warrell DW: The role of partial denervation of the pelvic floor in the aetiology of genitourinary prolapse and stress incontinence of urine: a neurophysiologic study, *Br J Obstet Gynaecol* 96:24-28, 1989.
83. Smotkin D: Human papillomavirus infection of the vagina, *Clin Obstet Gynecol* 36:188-194, 1993.
84. Snooks SJ et al: Injury to innervation of pelvic floor sphincter musculature in childbirth, *Lancet* 2:546-550, 1984.
85. Sobel JD: Pathogenesis and treatment of recurrent vulvovaginal candidiasis, *Clin Infect Dis* 14(S1):S148-153, 1992.
86. Sobel JD: Candidal vulvovaginitis, *Clin Obstet Gyencol* 36:153-165, 1993.

87. Soper DE, Bump RC, Hurt WG: Bacterial vaginosis and trichomonas vaginitis are risk factors for cuff cellulitis after abdominal hysterectomy, *Am J Obstet Gynecol* 163:1016-1023, 1990.
88. Sulak P et al: Nonsquamous cancer of the vagina, *Gynecol Oncol* 29:309-320, 1988.
89. Sultan AH et al: Anal-sphincter disruption during vaginal delivery, *N Engl J Med* 329:1905-1911, 1993.
90. Swedberg J, Steiner JF, Deiss F: Comparison of single dose vs one week course of metronidazole for symptomatic bacterial vaginosis, *JAMA* 254:1046-1049, 1985.
91. Syverson RE et al: Cellular and humoral immune status in women with chronic candida vaginitis, *Am J Obstet Gynecol* 134:624-627, 1979.
92. Tavossoli FA, Norris HJ: Smooth muscle tumors of the vagina, *Obstet Gynecol* 53:689-693, 1979.
93. Thomason JL, Gelbart SM, Scaglione NJ: Bacterial vaginosis: current review with indications for asymptomatic therapy, *Am J Obstet Gynecol* 165:1210-1217, 1991.
94. Tollhurst DE, van der Helm TWJS: The treatment of vaginal atresia, *Surg Gynecol Obstet* 172:407-414, 1991.
95. Ulfelder H, Robboy SJ: The embryologic development of the human vagina, *Am J Obstet Gynecol* 126:769-776, 1976.
96. Ulmsten V et al: Different biochemical composition of connective tissue in continent and stress incontinent women, *Acta Obstet Gynecol Scand* 66:455-457, 1987.
97. Van Slyke KT, Michel VP, Rein MF: Treatment of vulvovaginal candidiasis with boric acid powder, *Am J Obstet Gynecol* 141:145-148, 1981.
98. Vejtorp M et al: Bacterial vaginosis: a double blind randomized trial of the effect of treatment of the sexual partner, *Br J Obstet Gynaecol* 95:920-926, 1988.
99. Watts DH et al: Bacterial vaginosis as a risk factor for post cesarean endometritis, *Obstet Gynecol* 75:52-58, 1990.
100. Wilson JD, George FW, Griffin JE: The hormonal control of sexual development, *Science* 211:1278-1284, 1981.
101. Wiser WL, Bates GW: Management of agenesis of the vagina, *Surg Obstet Gynecol* 159:108-112, 1984.
102. Wolner-Hanssen P et al: Clinical manifestations of vaginal trichomoniasis, *JAMA* 261:571-576, 1989.
103. Young RH, Scully RE: Endodermal sinus tumor of the vagina: a report of nine cases and review of the literature, *Gynecol Oncol* 18:380-392, 1984.

Chapter 6

THE CERVIX

Ellen E. Sheets
Howard M. Goodman

EMBRYOLOGY

The cervix as an embryologic entity does not begin to develop until the early fetal period at about 12 weeks' gestation, yet its origin is intimately associated with the earlier development of the entire müllerian system. The müllerian (paramesonephric) duct system begins to develop in the fourth week as an invagination of the coelomic epithelium lateral to the wolffian (mesonephric) duct. Initially these paired ducts run caudally, but at 6 weeks' gestation they turn medially to meet in the midline, after which they again run caudally to reach the urogenital sinus at approximately 8 weeks' gestation (Fig. 6-1). The point of contact between the now-fused müllerian ducts and the urogenital sinus enlarges to form the müllerian tubercle, and the wolffian ducts now enter the sinus immediately lateral to the tubercle.

Evagination of the sinus between the wolffian ducts and the müllerian tubercle produces the sinovaginal bulbs, which proliferate to form the vaginal plate or vaginal cord. This solid plate advances in a caudal-cranial direction and obliterates the fused müllerian ducts (vaginal canal) as the müllerian epithelium degenerates. At 11 weeks' gestation, cavitation commences in a caudal-cranial direction again and the vaginal lumen is created At the same time a constriction appears between the developing corpus and cervix, and the cervix is identified by a fusiform thickening of the surrounding mesenchyme (Fig. 6-2). Cranial proliferation of the vaginal plate around the developing cervix forms the vaginal fornices, which are well delineated by the 21st week.[37,70]

Just prior to the time of proliferation of the vaginal plate, the original müllerian epithelium of the vaginal canal is replaced by a pseudostratified epithelium of müllerian origin. Canalization of the vagina results in a stratified squamous epithelium, the origin of which remains in dispute. Koff suggested that the lower fifth of the vaginal epithelium is derived from the urogenital sinus and the remainder from transformed müllerian epithelium,[65] whereas Bulmer proposed that the sinus and müllerian epithelium are histologically distinct and that the vaginal epithelium is derived completely from sinus epithelium.[22] Forsberg, using histochemical methods, postulated a wolffian origin for the vaginal lining.[41] Forsberg later showed in animals that inhibiting stratification of the original müllerian epithelium by estrogens caused heterotopic columnar epithelium to form in the adult vagina—

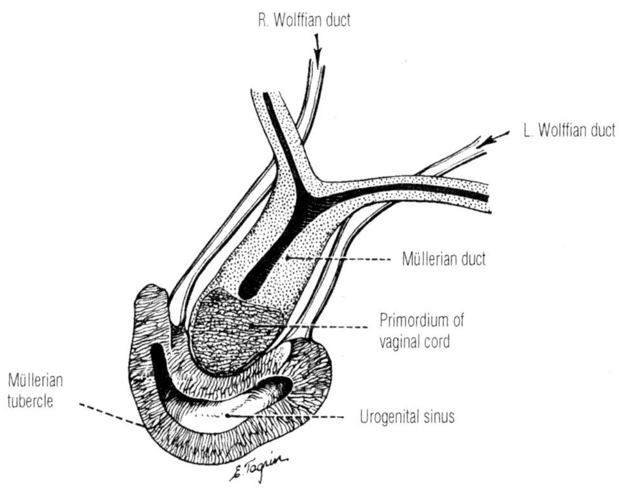

Fig. 6-1. Formation of the lower portion of the vagina. The müllerian tubercle is formed as the terminal ends of the müllerian ducts impinge on the urogenital sinus. Thus the vagina has a double origin: from the müllerian tubercle and from outgrowths of the urogenital sinus.

a response highly suggestive of the adenosis associated with diethylstilbestrol (DES) exposure.[42] The origin of the adult vaginal epithelium would seem to play no part in this presumed mechanism of stilbestrol teratogenesis.

The origin of the endocervical mucosa is likewise controversial. Fluhmann postulated that the upward growth of the vaginal squamous epithelium that he believed was of sinus origin, extended into the endocervix with subsequent columnar transformation.[40] Most authors favor a müllerian origin for the endocervical mucosa.

Abnormalities in the development or fusion of one or both müllerian ducts may result in malformations of the cervix. These include a double cervix with a septate or bicornuate uterus in conjunction with a normal or double vagina; a double cervix with uterus didelphys; or rarely, complete atresia of the cervix (Fig. 6-3).

In any discussion of the embryology of the cervix, mention should be made of the importance of *mesonephric remnants*. Characteristically these structures are found as minute tubules or canaliculi in the lateral cervical wall. They are lined with nonciliated simple columnar or cuboidal cells that have translucent cytoplasm and large, round nuclei.[54] Bizarre tumors, both benign and malignant, may arise from these remnants and may prove to be histogenetically confusing if their origin is not appreciated.

ANATOMY

The cervix ("neck" in Latin) is the narrowed, most caudad portion of the uterus (Fig. 6-4). Somewhat conical, it has a truncated apex that is directed downward and backward. It measures approximately 2.5 to 3.0 cm in the adult nulligravida and is contiguous with the inferior aspect of the uterine

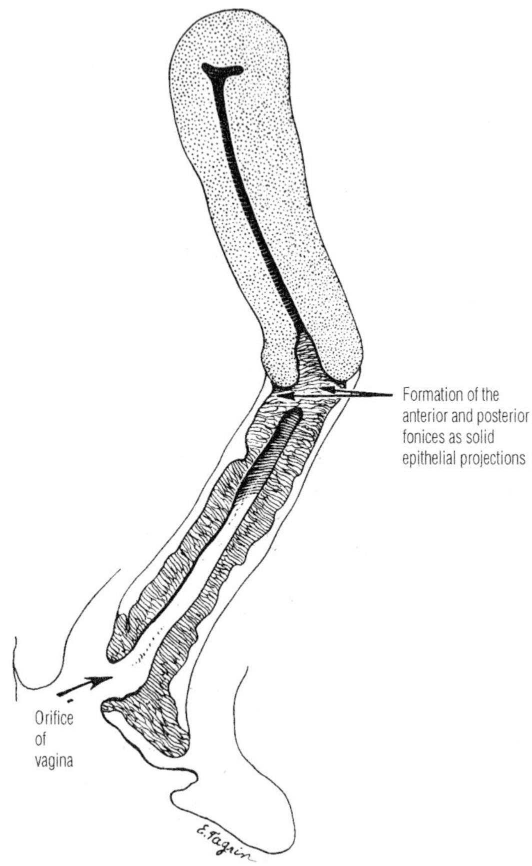

Fig. 6-2. Formation of the upper portion of the vagina in the 151-mm embryo. At this stage the cranial end of the vagina contains two solid epithelial projections that become the anterior and posterior fornices.

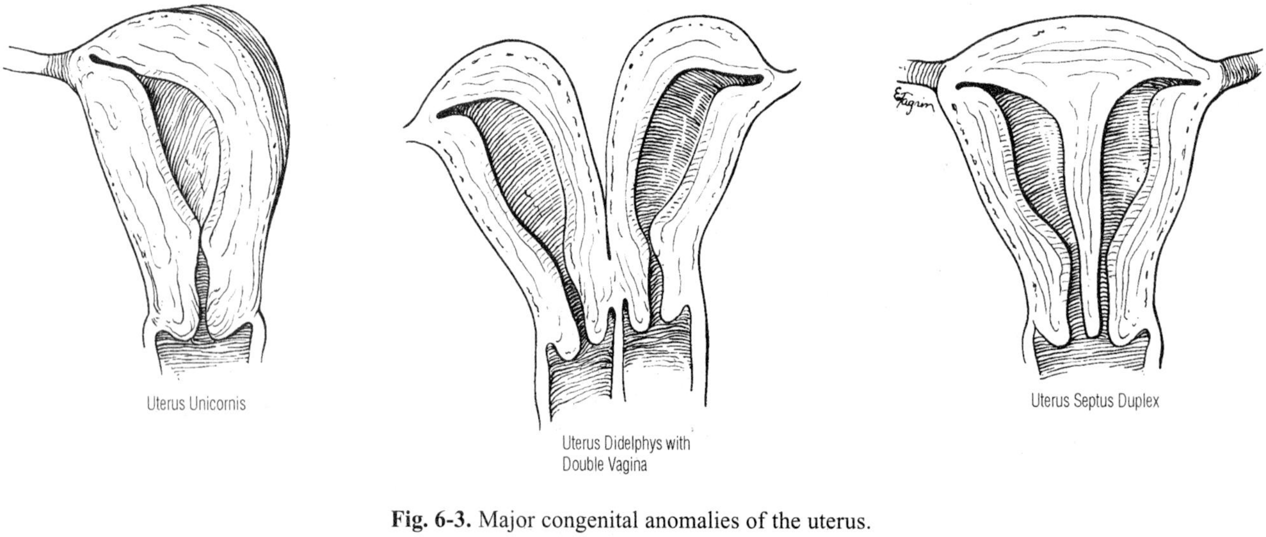

Fig. 6-3. Major congenital anomalies of the uterus.

corpus; the point of juncture is known as the isthmus. The vagina is attached obliquely around the center of the cervical periphery and divides the cervix into two segments—an upper, supravaginal portion and a lower, vaginal portion. The cervix enters the vagina at an angle through the anterior vaginal wall, and in most women its vaginal portion is in contact with the posterior vaginal wall. The supravaginal segment of the cervix is separated anteriorly from the bladder by a layer of endopelvic fascia, the pubovesicocervical fascia. Laterally at the same level, the cervix is in continuity with the paracervical ligaments or cardinal ligaments of Mackenrodt, which contain the uterine blood vessels. Posteriorly the supravaginal cervix is covered by peritoneum as it reflects off the uterosacral ligaments downward toward the vaginal apex.

The vaginal portion *(portio vaginalis, exocervix, ectocervix,* or *anatomical portio)* projects into the upper portion of the vagina, between the anterior and posterior fornices, as a convex prominence of elliptical shape. A small aperture, usually round or slit-like in the nullipara, is in the center of the projection and constitutes the external os. This orifice joins the uterine cavity with the vagina and is surrounded by the anterior and posterior lips. The cervical canal extends from the external os to the anatomic internal os, where it connects with the uterine cavity. It is somewhat fusiform or spindle-shaped and measures approximately 8 mm at its greatest width.

The isthmus is defined as that area of the uterus that lies between the anatomic internal os above and the histologic internal os below. The latter is defined as the area of transition from the endometrial to the endocervical glands. The isthmic musculature is somewhat thinner than that of the corpus and thereby facilitates effacement and dilation during labor. This area is frequently referred to as the lower uterine segment during pregnancy and labor.

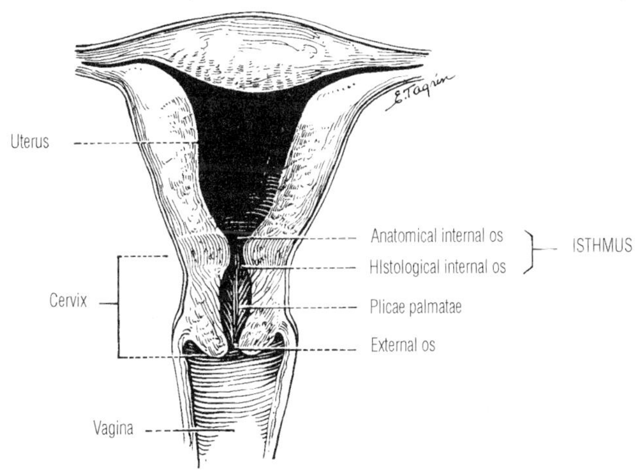

Fig. 6-4. Frontal section of the uterine cervix and corpus.

The uterine artery constitutes the major blood supply to the cervix and reaches its lateral walls within the cardinal ligaments (as noted previously). The venous drainage mirrors the arterial system. The cervical lymphatics, described in greater detail later, drain primarily lateral to the hypogastric obturator and external iliac nodes, but also anterior to the posterior bladder wall nodes, and posterior to the presacral nodes. Innervation of the cervix arises from the superior, middle, and inferior hypogastric plexuses and is primarily limited to the endocervix and the deeper areas of the exocervix. This accounts for the relative insensitivity to pain of the exocervix.[37]

PHYSIOLOGY

The cervix functions passively as a segment of the birth canal and as a channel for menstrual discharge. Its primary physiologic function is the secretion of mucus, which facilitates the transport of spermatozoa and subsequently acts as a plug to seal off the gravid uterine cavity from the external environment.

This cervical mucus is subject to profound cyclic changes in relation to the levels of circulating ovarian hormones. In the immediate postmenstrual phase when the circulatory level of estrogen is low, and in the postovulatory period under the influence of progesterone, the cervical mucus is sparse, thick, and viscid. If it is allowed to dry on a slide, abundant vaginal and cervical cells, leukocytes, and mucous particles can be seen. From the eighth day of the cycle until ovulation, under the stimulation of rising levels of estrogen, the amount of mucus increases, its viscosity decreases, and it becomes highly permeable to spermatozoa. Just prior to ovulation the mucus is glassy, transparent, and highly elastic. The term *spinnbarkeit* is applied to this characteristic elasticity. If allowed to dry on a slide, the mucus assumes the form of fern or palm leaves with a few notable cellular elements (Fig. 6-5).

Fern test technique

The specimen of mucus should be aspirated from the external os after initial dry cleansing. The mucus is permitted to air dry and is then examined under a magnification of approximately 100 power. False-positive fern test results are possible if (1) the aspirating tube is wet, (2) salt solution rather than distilled water is used for cleaning or sterilizing the tube, or (3) excessive blood is mixed with the mucus.

Mucous secretions and most body fluids show the phenomenon of ferning, or arborization, in the dried state. This seems to represent a special form of crystallization of sodium chloride in the medium of drying cervical mucus. Although ferning is a nonspecific process, its occurrence in cervical mucus does depend on adequate estrogenic stimulation.

From a clinical point of view, the examination of cervical mucus is a simple test of ovarian function. When no ovarian function occurs, small amounts of exogenous estrogen will cause arborization, whereas progesterone modifies this

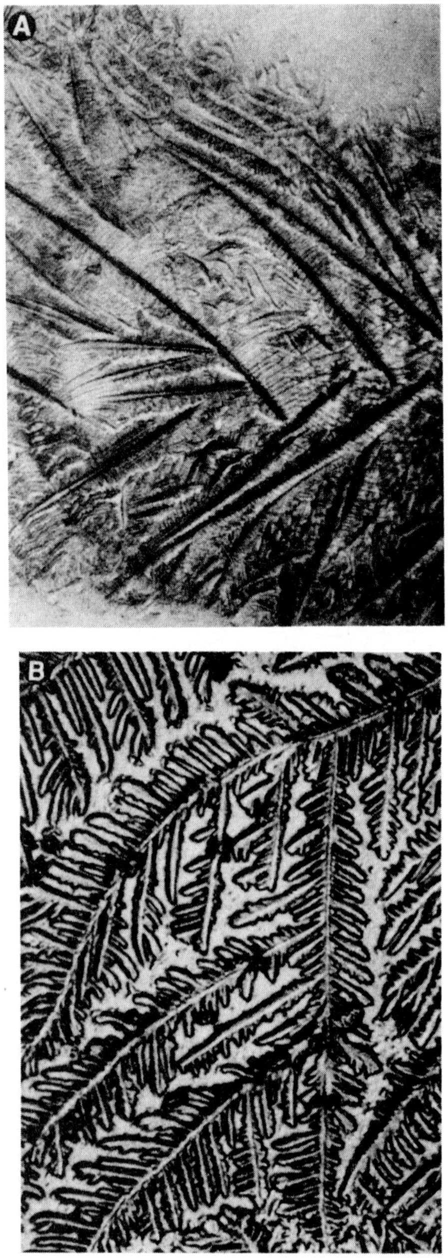

Fig. 6-5. Fern phenomenon in cervical mucus during the normal menstrual cycle between days 12 and 16. **A,** Low power. **B,** High power. (Courtesy Dr. Maxwell Roland.)

action of estrogen. In patients who are amenorrheic, a persistently normal fern test suggests insufficient estrogenic stimulation.[115]

PHYSIOLOGIC ALTERATIONS

Changes in endocervical mucosa

With the advent of colposcopy, many of the gross and microscopic variations previously considered to be pathologic are now regarded as normal physiologic alterations. Prominent among these is the growth of endocervical mucosa onto the anatomic portio, which was believed to be a prolapse of that mucosa. The popular term for this physiologic alteration was "cervical erosion," which incorrectly implied that the epithelium was denuded. The proper term now is *eversion* or *ectropion.* This normal physiologic growth alteration appears to be related to age, the first pregnancy, and estrogenic stimulation.

During the childbearing years, endocervical glands are found just below the internal os and extend to just below the external os (i.e., onto the anatomic portio), which creates this so-called cervical erosion. After 40 years of age, as a result of waning ovarian activity, the endocervical mucosa ascends the canal so that during the menopausal years the lowest glands, the original squamocolumnar junction, and the transformation zone are at or above the anatomic external os. Coppleson and Reid[32] and Song[114] attribute the downward shift and eversion of the endocervix to an increase in mucosal volume during the years when estrogen stimulation was maximal. This explains the increase in eversions noted after the first pregnancy (Fig. 6-6).

During the latter part of intrauterine development, when growth of the cervix is accelerated as a result of high levels of circulating estrogens, such growth is not shared by the corpus. At birth the cervix/corpus ratio may approach 3:1. After birth there is a rapid regression in cervical length, which returns to the more normal cervix/corpus ratio seen in the adult. During the third trimester the endocervical cells change from cuboidal to tall columnar with evidence of mucin secretion, and the mucosa deeply infolds into the stroma to form clefts or glands. This excessive *proliferation of endocervical mucosa* after the 28th week produces the congenital eversion seen in 50% of female neonates. In contrast, the endometrium is incompletely developed, usually inactive, and presents only a few tubular glands. Squamous cells of the exocervix in the newborn are likewise affected by maternal estrogens, since they are well stratified and contain abundant glycogen. At puberty, with the stimulation of estrogen from the developing ovarian follicles, these changes presumably occur again, although adequate morphologic studies in this age group are lacking.[70]

HISTOLOGY

A careful consideration of cervical histology will allow us to understand how and where benign, precancerous, and cancerous lesions of the cervix occur. The cervix is essentially composed of two different types of epithelium: squamous and columnar. The area of transition between these two epithelial types gives rise to the three histologic zones: (1) the histologic portio, (2) the transitional or transformation zone, and (3) the histologic endocervix. Further, it is in the transition from columnar to squamous epithelium that precancerous and cancerous lesions can arise.

Histologic portio

The histologic portio is defined as a cervical stroma devoid of glands and covered by stratified squamous epithelium

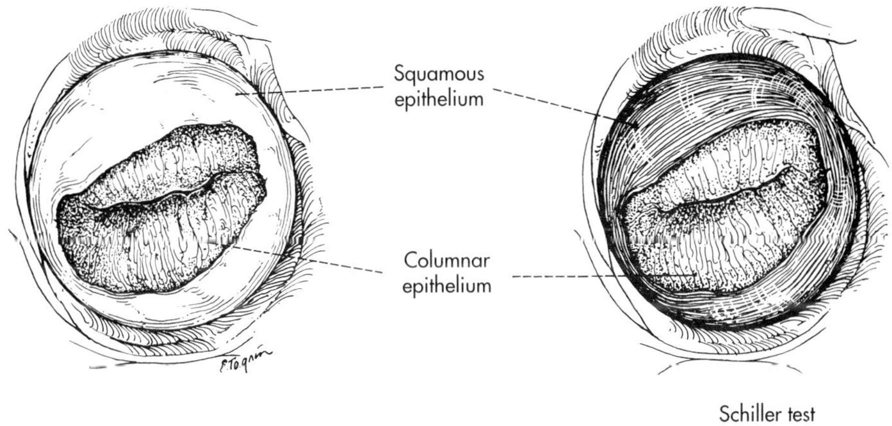

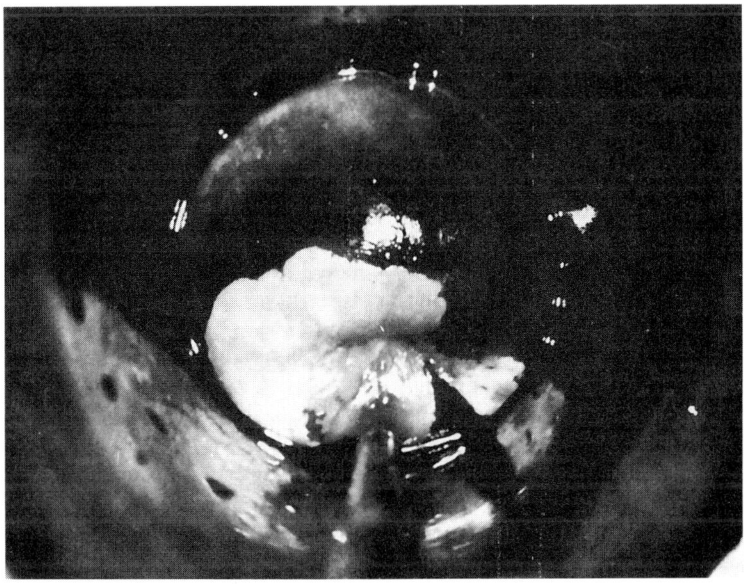

Fig. 6-6. Application of Schiller's solution will stain the normal squamous epithelium dark brown. Endocervical epithelium does not stain.

(Fig. 6-7). This epithelium is 15 to 20 cells thick and demonstrates a progressive and orderly maturation from the lowest basal layer through the prickle cell layer to the superficial zone, where cornification occurs under estrogenic stimulation.

The basal layer (stratum germinativum), responsible for epithelial regeneration, consists of a single row of small cylindrical cells with large nuclei and scanty cytoplasm. Mitotic figures may occasionally be seen. Above the basal cells is a layer of larger polyhedral cells, 4 to 10 cells thick, arranged in an irregular mosaic pattern and interconnected by numerous tonofilament-desmosomal complexes. These characteristic intercellular bridges have led to the designation *prickle cells*, and their location has led to the designation *parabasal cells*. The cytoplasmic basophilia seen in these first two cell types is attributed to their RNA content. The beginning of cytoplasmic glycogenolysis is seen in the parabasal layer.

Above the prickle cells is a layer of larger oval or navicular cells with relatively small nuclei. These cells are involved in ascending maturation during which nuclear size remains constant while cytoplasmic volume gradually increases. This layer is called the intermediate, clear cell, or *navicular zone*. The most superficial layer or stratum corneum consists of flattened, elongated cells with small pyknotic nuclei. These are the cornified cells or squames seen in cytologic smears. The superficial and intermediate cells are rich in glycogen but appear clear in histologic sections, since the glycogen is washed out during fixation.

The basal layer is usually quite regular and does not show the rete peg formation seen in the vulva and vagina. The cervical squamous epithelium rests on a basement membrane that is inconsistently seen under the light microscope and appears to consist of condensed stromal collagen. The underlying fibrous connective tissue stroma contains a lush capillary network at the epithelial junction, with scattered papillae extending upward into the epithelium.[41]

Transformation zone

The transformation zone lies between the histologic portio and the endocervical mucosa and consists of endocervical stroma and glands covered by squamous epithelium. The squamous epithelium comes to lie on the endocervical stroma as a result of several physiologic or pathologic processes. Although these processes cause upward displacement of the squamocolumnar junction, the junction between the histologic portio and the transformation zone can be termed the *original squamocolumnar junction.* The anatomic location of the transformation zone is dependent on age, estrogen influence, and previous trauma or surgery on the cervix. With Fig. 6-4 as a guide, the transformation zone may be located on the vaginal portion of the cervix, at the external os, or above the external os within the cervical canal. Therefore one should not equate the location of the histologic transformation zone with the location of the anatomic external os. The importance of the location of this zone will become apparent in the section on colposcopy.

Histologic endocervix

The histologic endocervix is lined by a single layer of tall columnar epithelial cells characterized by dense, basal nuclei and pale pink-staining cytoplasm in standard hematoxylin-eosin preparations (Fig. 6-8). Two cell types are present in this epithelium: the more prevalent mucus-secreting cells and scattered ciliated cells located in patches within the cervical canal and in gland orifices. The slight variation in height of these cells gives the appearance of a picket fence in histologic sections. These endocervical glands are actually formed by complex, cleft-like infoldings of the epithelium, which appear as simple glandular units in histologic section.[37,40] Although this concept renders the term "gland" a misnomer, reference to endocervical glands will most likely persist. The cleft arrangement increases the surface area of the endocervical mucosa and permits the increased production of mucus that is dependent on estrogen. Maximal production and secretion of mucus occurs prior to ovulation, and in certain patients true mucorrhea exists.

For some years the location of cervical lesions, particularly those of a neoplastic nature, has been a matter of controversy between clinicians and pathologists. This again

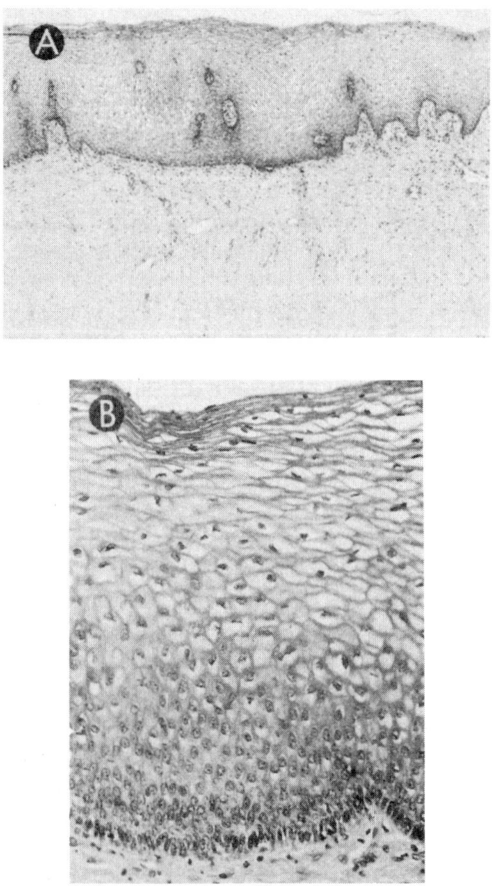

Fig. 6-7. A, Normal exocervix. (× 50.) **B,** High-power magnification (× 150) to show process of stratification and cornification.

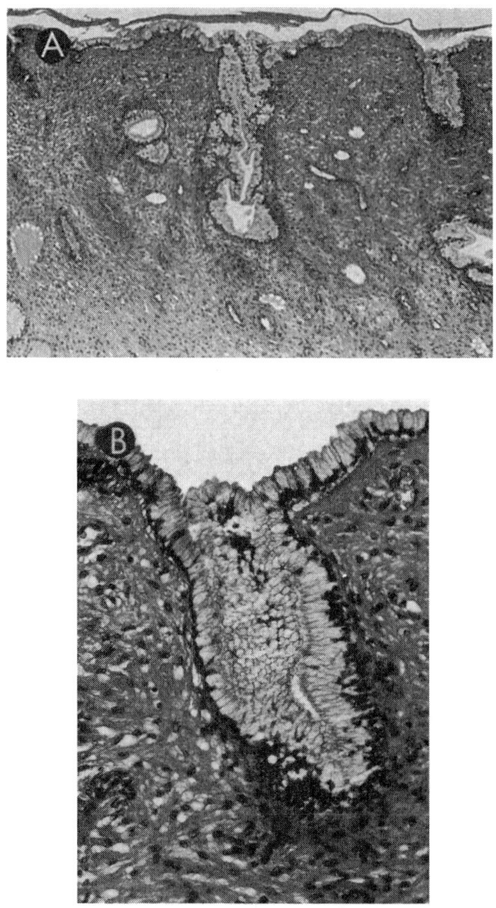

Fig. 6-8. A, Normal endocervix. (× 50.) **B,** High-power magnification (× 150) to show typical high columnar epithelium.

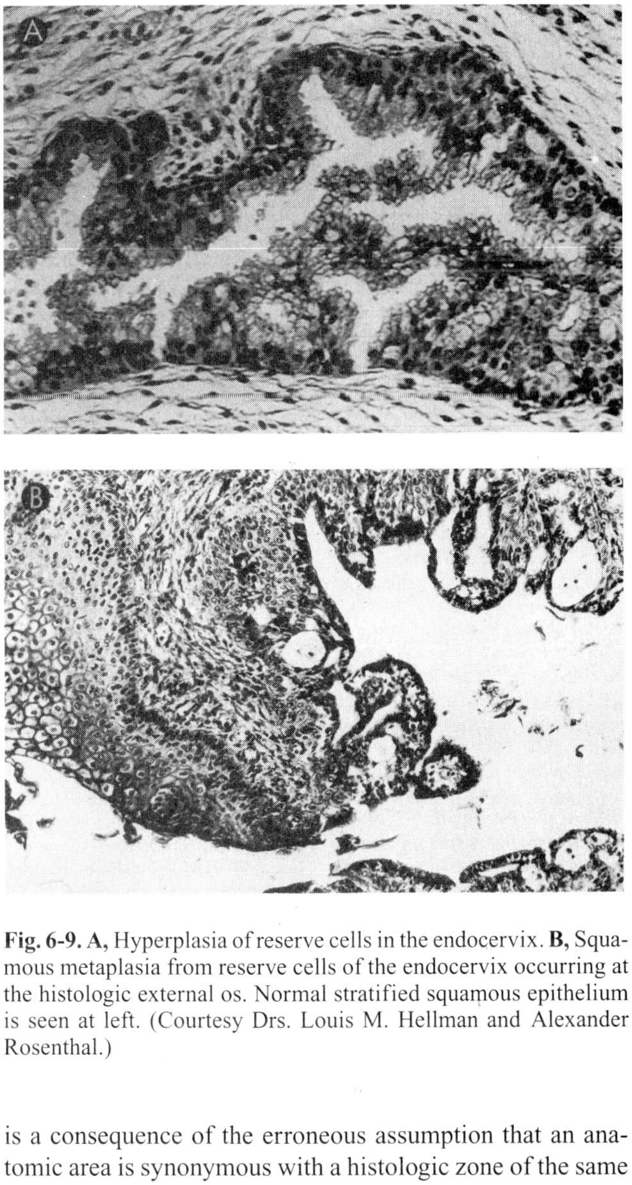

Fig. 6-9. A, Hyperplasia of reserve cells in the endocervix. **B,** Squamous metaplasia from reserve cells of the endocervix occurring at the histologic external os. Normal stratified squamous epithelium is seen at left. (Courtesy Drs. Louis M. Hellman and Alexander Rosenthal.)

is a consequence of the erroneous assumption that an anatomic area is synonymous with a histologic zone of the same designation. For example, the clinician defines a lesion of the portio as one existing on that area of the cervix that can be visualized with a speculum; whereas the pathologist defines a lesion of the portio as one arising in the squamous epithelium of the histologic portio. A lesion arising in the transformation zone (overlying endocervical glands) or in the columnar epithelium may thus be classified pathologically as endocervical even though it is located on the anatomic portio. Obviously the anatomic location of a lesion must be clearly distinguished from its histologic location.

The majority of early neoplastic cervical lesions in women of childbearing age occur on the anatomic portio, where they are readily available for biopsy. Histopathologic reports indicating that the majority of these lesions occur in the endocervix refer only to their histologic position.

From the anatomic and histologic characteristics described earlier, it is obvious that the cervix differs from the corpus in several important ways:

1. The cervix has only a small surface covered by peritoneum.
2. Approximately 85% of the cervix is made up of fibrous connective tissue.
3. There are no cervical venous sinuses.
4. Cervical mucosa does not undergo marked menstrual change as does the endometrium, although there are some cyclic changes dependent on estrogen and progesterone.
5. The vaginal cervix is covered by stratified squamous epithelium.

Squamous metaplasia and epithelialization

After menarche and through the reproductive period, the previously described cervical ectropion essentially disappears, and the squamocolumnar junction moves out of view within the cervical canal. Two mechanisms for replacement of the endocervical eversion by squamous epithelium have been proposed as the histogenesis of the transformation zone. Since virtually all cases of cervical squamous neoplasia originate in the transformation zone, its histogenesis provides insight into the oncogenesis of cervical neoplasia.

The first mechanism, termed squamous metaplasia, is the result of a process known as subcolumnar reserve cell metaplasia. These reserve cells are undifferentiated, spherical, or polygonal cells with plump, centrally placed, dark-staining nuclei, and scant cytoplasm. They come to lie beneath the columnar epithelium, and their origin is controversial. It has been proposed that they are derived from (1) embryonal rests of urogenital sinus epithelium, (2) direct or indirect metaplasia of columnar cells, (3) basal cells of the portio, or (4) stromal cells. Coppleson and Reid suggest that the metaplastic process is initiated by the exposure of the endocervical mucosa to the lower pH of the vagina, and that estrogen plays a crucial role by promoting endocervical hyperplasia and prolapse and acidifying the vaginal environment.[32] In support of this mechanism, Hellman et al found a striking increase in reserve cell hyperplasia and metaplasia after the administration of large doses of estrogen to postmenopausal women.[51]

The probable sequence of events in the metaplastic process is outlined as follows:

1. Endocervical eversion
2. Reserve cell hyperplasia (Fig. 6-9, *A*)
3. Reserve cell metaplasia and stratification (Fig. 6-9, *B*)
4. Overlying columnar epithelium sloughs off
5. Differentiation into a multilayered, immature, squamous epithelium
6. Differentiation into a mature, stratified, squamous epithelium

The end point of the metaplastic process is the differentiation into squamous epithelium that is indistinguishable from native squamous epithelium. The more commonly seen immature metaplastic epithelium is characterized by a lack of surface maturation and glycogen and is usually sharply

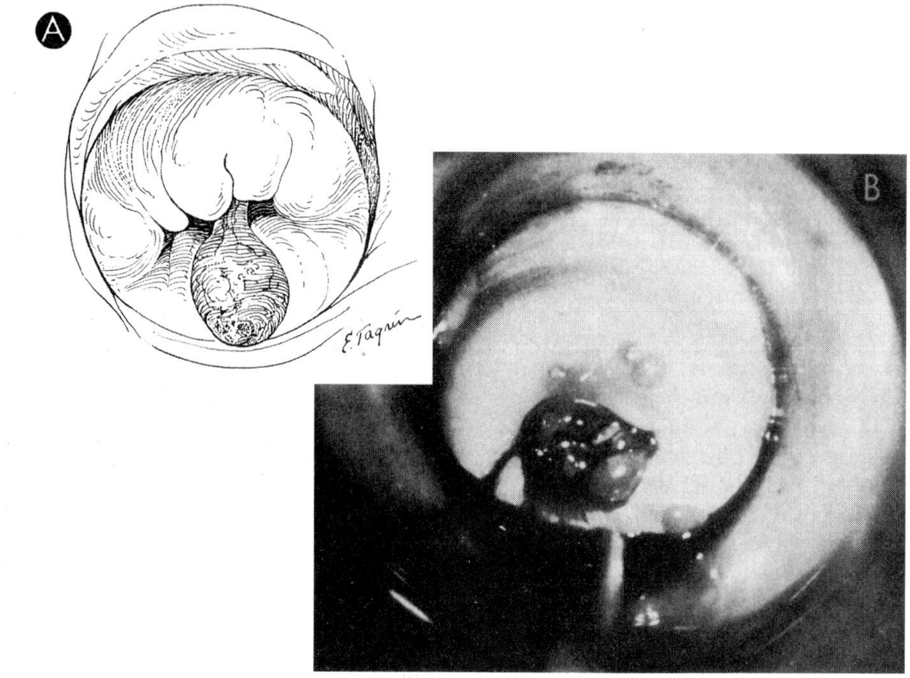

Fig. 6-10. Endocervical polyps. **A,** A solitary polyp protruding through the external os. **B,** Several endocervical polyps occluding the exocervix. Several nabothian (mucous) cysts are seen on the portio epithelium.

demarcated from the adjacent portio. Particularly active squamous metaplasia filling multiple glands may be confused with carcinoma in situ, although hyperchromatism, nuclear atypia, and abnormal mitotic activity are not present.

The second mechanism by which squamous epithelium comes to overlie endocervical stroma is termed squamous epithelialization.[58] The initiating event may be a true pathologic erosion of the distal endocervix followed by an ingrowth or over-glide of portio squamous cells. In the early stages of this process, the squamous epithelium may be seen as a tenuous strand of immature squamous cells, gradually decreasing in height as they are stretched over an otherwise denuded and inflamed stroma. Others have shown that the squamous epithelium of the portio may grow beneath the adjacent, intact, endocervical epithelium, with loss of the overlying columnar cells on maturation and stratification of the squamous elements.[37,58] As with many reparative and regenerative processes, mitotic activity with associated basal cell hyperplasia may be considerable, although the atypia of malignancy is absent. The extension of the new epithelium over the mouth of the endocervical gland may result in occlusion and the formation of mucinous retention (nabothian) cysts. These are grossly visible on the portio as spherical elevations or small cysts 2 to 10 mm in diameter (Fig. 6-10). Microscopically the cystic space is seen to be lined with low cuboidal or flattened endocervical cells.

BENIGN CERVICAL LESIONS

Cervical polyps

Cervical polyps are usually derived from the endocervix as a result of a chronic papillary endocervicitis and present as soft, spherical, glistening red masses several millimeters to several centimeters in size (Fig. 6-10). They are frequently quite friable and may be associated with profuse leukorrhea secondary to the underlying endocervicitis. Histologically they are composed of endocervical epithelium with a fibrovascular stalk. The differential diagnosis includes (1) polypoid fragments of endocervical carcinoma or carcinosarcoma protruding through the os; (2) retained products of conception; (3) the grape-like swellings of sarcoma botryoides that occasionally originate in the cervix; and (4) prolapsing submucous fibroids or endometrial polyps. Most cervical polyps can be grasped with a clamp and twisted free, and the base cauterized for hemostasis. Certainly all cervical polyps should be submitted for pathologic evaluation, although malignancy is extremely rare.

Leiomyomas

Leiomyomas or fibroids are the most common uterine tumors. Cervical involvement occurs in as many as 8% of cases. Cervical leiomyomas are grossly and histologically identical to those found in the corpus. Although they are frequently incidental findings on physical examination, with excessive growth they may cause bowel or bladder symptoms, dyspareunia, or dystocia in labor. The treatment for symptomatic fibroids is either myomectomy or hysterectomy.

Endometriosis

Endometriosis of the cervix presents as red or reddish-blue vesicular lesions evident on the exocervix. They are usually asymptomatic but may cause dysmenorrhea or dyspareunia, which is most evident premenstrually. Biopsy specimens are best taken at this time for adequate pathologic interpretation. This pattern of endometriosis is frequently seen several months after cervical biopsy, cauterization, or trachelorrhaphy in menstruating women and thus suggests implantation as its etiology. However, areas of decidual reaction may occasionally be seen in the cervices of pregnant women who have not undergone any cervical procedures. This suggests that multi-potential cells capable of responding to estrogen and progesterone are present in the cervical stroma.

Infertility is associated with extensive cervical endometriosis and is probably due to destruction of endocervical glands and decreased mucous production. After biopsy confirmation, the treatment should consist of hormonal therapy and potentially deep cauterization, excision, or laser vaporization. Other less common benign tumors that may involve the cervix include hemangiomas, adenomyomas, fibroadenomas, fibromas, and lipomas.

Keratinization

Since keratinization is not a physiologic property of cervical squamous epithelium, any tendency in this direction must be considered abnormal, although some degree of focal keratinization may occasionally be observed in the absence of other abnormalities. Hyperkeratosis and parakeratosis usually appear grossly visible as white, raised plaques (leukoplakia) on the portio. Microscopically, hyperkeratosis exhibits a thickened layer of keratin, scant intraepithelial glycogen, and no cytologic atypia. It is not commonly seen except in cases of procidentia. Parakeratosis, the most common abnormality presenting as a white cervical lesion, exhibits similar features but with the retention of pyknotic nuclei in the keratin layer (Fig. 6-11). There is no evidence to indicate that either hyperkeratosis or parakeratosis is premalignant; however, these histologic features may be associated with cervical neoplasia. Therefore all white lesions of the cervix deserve biopsy for tissue diagnosis.

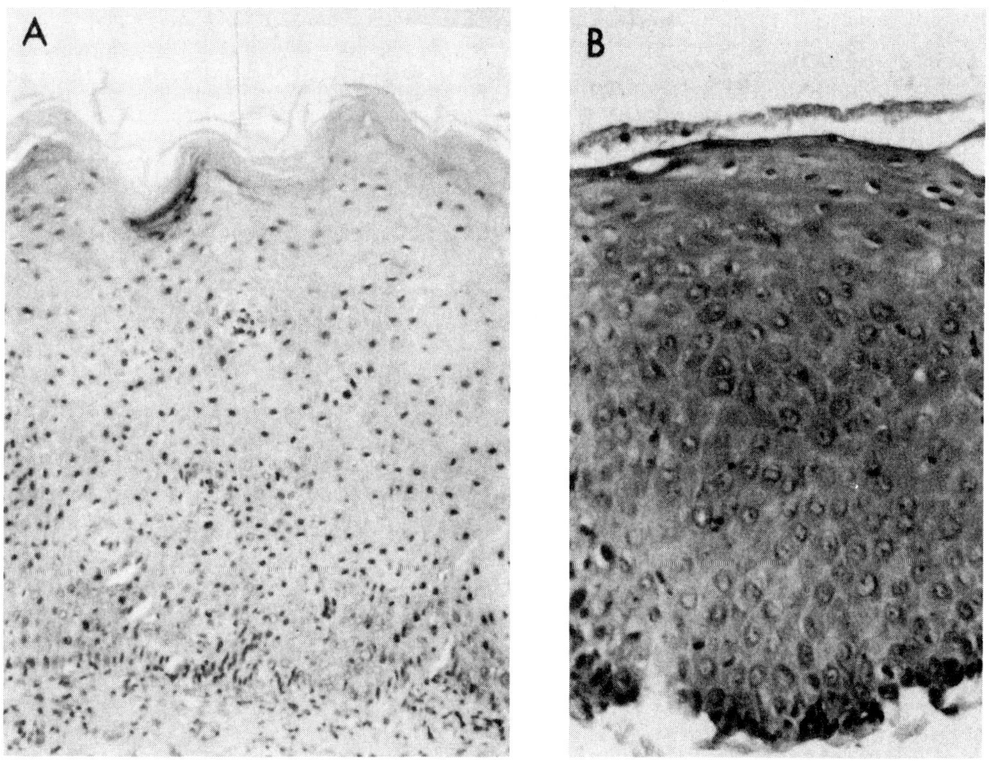

Fig. 6-11. A, Hyperkeratosis (× 120): normal ascending cellular maturation with a thickened keratin layer can be seen. **B,** Parakeratosis (× 200): pyknotic nuclei are evident within the keratin layer. (× 200.) (Courtesy Dr. Robert Ehrmann and the Division of Women's and Perinatal Pathology, Brigham and Women's Hospital, Boston.)

Mucopurulent cervicitis

From the time of the earliest clinical and microscopic descriptions of cervical disease, cervicitis has been implicated in the pathogenesis of cervical eversion, squamous metaplasia, basal cell hyperplasia, leukoplakia, polyps, and carcinoma. In the past a distinction was made between acute and chronic cervicitis. Although clinically difficult to distinguish, histology can be used to discern between the two entities. In chronic cervicitis, a neutrophilic infiltration with epithelial necrosis is found; whereas in acute cervicitis, stromal edema with a polymorphonuclear infiltrate and mucosal ulceration is seen.[101,114]

Clinically the presenting symptoms are a purulent discharge and postcoital or postdouche vaginal spotting or bleeding. On physical examination, a reddened, often friable cervix covered with thick, tenacious, yellowish-white discharge is found. The inflammation or infection can be confined to the cervix or extend to the paracervical tissues, which gives the picture of pelvic inflammatory disease. A culture of the cervix can be done and the most common result is *Chlamydia trachomatis*. Other organisms can be cultured and in descending order of frequency after *Chlamydia* include the following: *Neisseria gonorrhoeae*, *Trichomonas vaginalis*, *Candida*, group B *Streptococcus*, *Gardnerella vaginalis*, *Mycoplasma hominis*, and *Ureaplasma urealyticum*. Not all cases will be culture positive and an association between mucopurulent cervicitis and bacterial vaginosis, the use of oral contraceptives, and sexual contact with men who have nongonococcal urethritis increase the chance of similar symptoms occurring.[132]

A tentative diagnosis can be made on inspection; biopsy and tissue diagnosis are mandatory, however, to rule out a cervical neoplasia that can present with a similar clinical picture. The inflammation and bleeding associated with chronic cervicitis render Papanicolaou (Pap) smears unreliable in excluding carcinoma. Conversely those patients whose Pap smears reveal inflammation have the same chance of having a positive cervical culture as do patients whose smears do not reveal inflammation. Therefore Pap smears with inflammatory changes do not necessarily represent cervicitis.[88]

Once carcinoma is excluded, treatment can be offered. Those patients with a culture-proven organism can be treated by using the appropriate antibiotics. Patients for whom the culture is not positive can receive an empiric treatment course of antibiotics. If their cervicitis does not respond, other treatment methods that denude the epithelium can be used such as cryosurgery or laser.[107] Due to the excessive vaginal discharge that accompanies this problem, patients often prefer empiric treatment.

The role of *C. trachomatis* in the pathogenesis of genital tract disease has become well established. As many as 66% of women seen at venereal disease clinics may harbor *Chlamydia* in their cervices. Infection may be asymptomatic and limited to the cervix, or may ascend and cause pelvic inflammatory disease. A diagnosis requires culture techniques

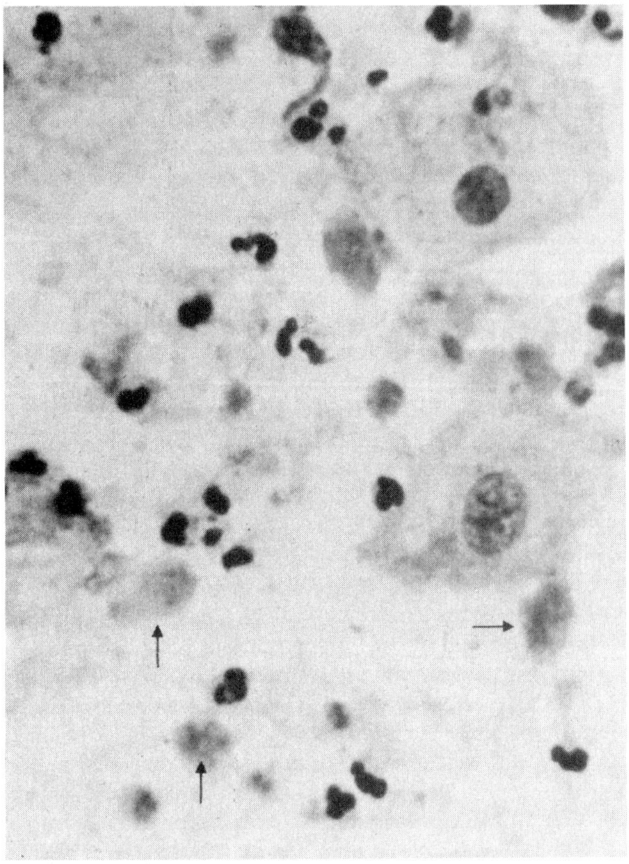

Fig. 6-12. Papanicolaou smear demonstrating *T. vaginalis*. (× 800.) The characteristic pear-shaped protozoans with eccentrically placed, spindle-shaped nuclei are shown (*arrows*). The flagella are usually not well demonstrated on Papanicolaou smears. (Courtesy Dr. Robert Ehrmann and the Division of Women's and Perinatal Pathology, Brigham and Women's Hospital, Boston.)

or the presence of the characteristic intracytoplasmic inclusion bodies as seen on Giemsa stains of cervical smears. Although several authors have reported an increased rate of cervical neoplasia in cervices harboring *Chlamydia*,[73,85] a more recent study that controlled for the presence of human papillomavirus infection did not reveal any significant increase in preinvasive disease.[56] In fact low-grade, squamous intraepithelial lesions and atypia are not uncommon in the face of a chlamydial infection, and treatment must be completed before repeating the cervical smear.[77]

Trichomonas vaginalis is a flagellated protozoan that attacks the squamous epithelium of the vagina and cervix and destroys the epithelial cells on contact. In response there is an outpouring of polymorphonuclear leukocytes and a marked proliferation of small blood vessels that yield the characteristic colposcopic appearance of looped or hairpin capillaries. Although this infection may be asymptomatic, the classic presentation is a profuse, greenish-gray, frothy, vaginal discharge with pruritus, dysuria, and occasionally vaginal bleeding. Diagnosis is easily made from the presence of the flagellate on microscopic examination of the discharge diluted in normal saline (Fig. 6-12). A culture may be required as wet mounts miss approximately 30% of infected women. The pH of the vagina is frequently alkaline in the presence of *T. vaginalis.* The association of abnormal Pap smears with trichomonal infections is well described. Cytologic and colposcopic abnormalities revert to normal with appropriate treatment.[18]

Tuberculous cervicitis is seen in approximately 3% to 5% of all cases of genital tuberculosis. The affected cervix may appear entirely normal, exhibit erythema with a mucopurulent discharge, or be invaded by a fungating mass suggestive of carcinoma. Histologically, caseating or noncaseating granulomas may be seen. Diagnosis requires the demonstration of acid-fast bacilli by suitable staining techniques or by culture. The differential diagnosis of granulomatous cervicitis includes syphilis, lymphogranuloma venereum, granuloma inguinale, chancroid, sarcoid, schistosomiasis, and pinworm.

Viral cervicitis

Herpes simplex virus. *Herpesvirus hominis* types 1 and 2, the etiologic agents of genital herpes, belong to the group of herpes viruses that are found in almost every animal species studied. These are large DNA viruses with five members associated with disease in humans: herpes simplex virus (HSV) types 1 and 2, varicella-zoster virus, cytomegalovirus, and Epstein-Barr virus. Infection requires direct contact followed by an incubation period of 1 to 45 days and averaging 6 days. Clinically, herpes genitalis may be conveniently divided into either primary or recurrent infection, the former reserved for infection resulting from the first exposure to either HSV type 1 or 2 and the latter for any subsequent infection.

Multiple painful vesicles, usually 1 to 2 mm, appear on an erythematous background; these rapidly erode and coalesce to form larger ulcers. Cervical involvement occurs in 80% of primary infections and presents as a nonspecific inflammation, vesicles, ulcers, or occasionally as a fungating mass indistinguishable from invasive carcinoma. Symptoms include vulvar and pelvic pain, dysuria, and vaginal discharge, the last especially with cervical involvement. Complete healing requires several weeks as the symptoms and lesions slowly resolve. Recurrent pelvic infections involve the cervix less commonly than in primary infections. The clinical impression may be confirmed by tissue culture. Serologic conversion will occur after the initial infection. Therefore serology after an initial infection will not help confirm subsequent cervical infections. Cervical cytology, which is less sensitive than tissue culture, may demonstrate multinucleated giant cells or intranuclear viral inclusion bodies (Fig. 6-13).

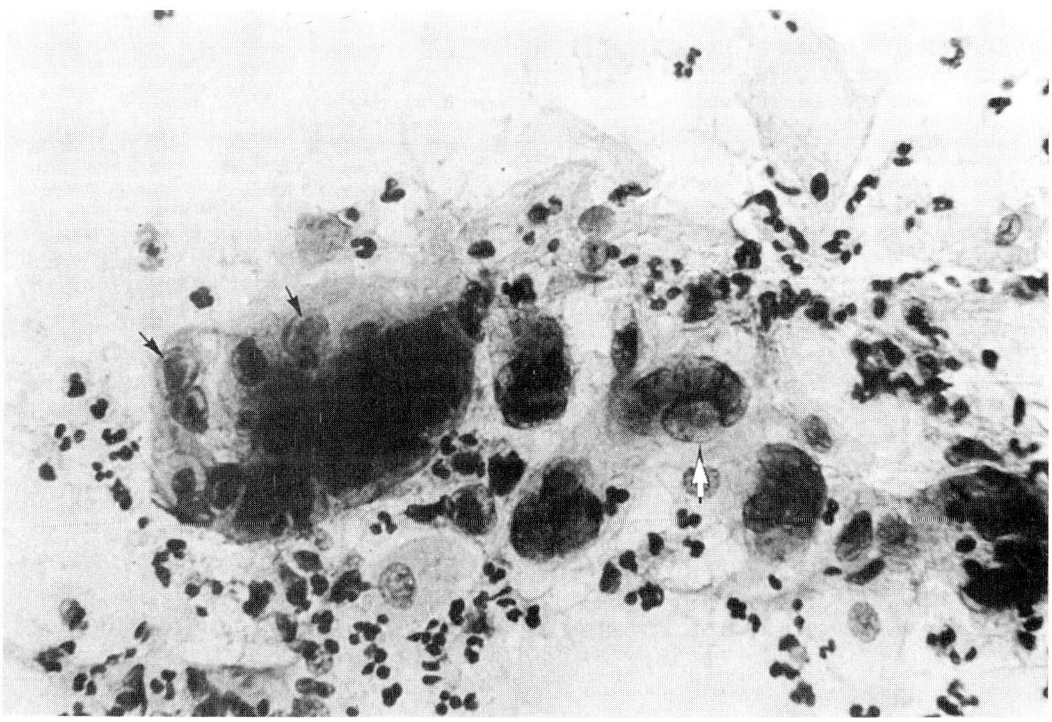

Fig. 6-13. Pap smear exhibiting the characteristic features of herpesvirus infection. (× 530.) Intranuclear inclusions (*small arrows*) that may represent virus particles and multinucleated giant cells are evident. Enlarged, ground-glass-appearing nuclei can also be seen (*large arrow*). (Courtesy Dr. Robert Ehrmann and the Division of Women's and Perinatal Pathology, Brigham and Women's Hospital, Boston.)

Human papillomavirus. Although human papillomavirus (HPV) does not cause a mucopurulent cervicitis, it is the most common cervical viral infection. The clinical manifestations of HPV infection can be divided into two types: the classic exophytic wart, or the changes that are associated with cervical neoplasia. The classic infection, described since the Roman-Hellenistic era, consists of an exophytic, grape-like lesion that is visible to the naked eye and is rarely found on the cervix (Fig. 6-14). Only 254 cases of cervical warts were reported in the literature through 1974.[119] In contrast, cervical neoplasia is considered to be epidemic with up to 600,000 cases identified yearly in the United States.[36]

The papovaviridae family is composed of two branches: simian virus 40 and polyomavirus make up one side and the papilloma viruses the other. HPVs are 8000-kilobase DNA viruses composed of many different subtypes. Each subtype represents a virus that has less than 50% DNA base sequence homology with other types. Currently there are more than 60 types of HPVs and each type appears to have a preference for a certain epithelial surface. For example, HPV type 1 is involved in plantar warts, whereas HPV types 5 and 14 are involved in a rare external skin disease, epidermodysplasia verruciformis. HPV types 6, 11, 16, 18, 31, 35, and some types in the 50s are found in genital epithelial surfaces.

Our understanding of HPV infections is greatly hampered by the lack of a culture system for the virus. For reasons yet unknown, the mature viral particle for HPV requires the permissive environment of a mature keratinocyte to form and replicate. This has required investigators to use various detection techniques, such as producing antibodies against the viral capsule proteins. The antibodies are then detected by immunoperoxidase staining. Other detection methods include characteristic histologic changes, and sophisticated DNA hybridization.

Microscopically the classic wart is characterized by papillomatosis, acanthosis, lengthening and thickening of the rete pegs, submucosal capillary proliferation, and the presence of koilocytes. Koilocytes, first described by Koss and Durfee in 1956, exhibit hyperchromasia, multinucleation, and perinuclear cytoplasmic vacuolization (Fig. 6-15).[67] Initially, koilocytes were believed to be pathognomonic of HPV infections, but as understanding of HPV expanded via DNA hybridization, this constant association was called into doubt. Further, long-term epidemiologic studies with extensive follow-up will be necessary before we can define more clearly the cytologic finding of koilocytosis.

In 1977 Meisels et al described two cervical lesions with koilocytotic atypia and other features suggestive of condylomata but without the typical gross papillary features.[79] The "flat condyloma" is a flattened area of acanthosis with mild accentuation of the rete pegs and koilocytotic changes. They pointed out the striking contrast between the essentially normal-appearing, deeper layers of the epithelium and the superficial areas that exhibit the koilocytosis. The second lesion they described is the endophytic or inverted condyloma that demonstrates gland involvement and may be mistaken for invasive carcinoma. Usually not visible without the colposcope, these lesions exhibit fine punctuation on a white background.

Meisels et al reviewed 152 cervical smears diagnosed as mild dysplasia and found that 70% were suggestive of HPV infection.[79] This finding led the authors to consider koilocytotic atypia as an early phase in the natural history of cervical neoplasia. The relationship between condylomata and cervical carcinoma will be more fully discussed later. Condylomatous cervicitis is a very common disease with 1% to 3% of all Pap smears exhibiting koilocytotic changes. When DNA hybridization techniques are used on Pap smears, the incidence of HPV is tenfold higher and represents 10% to 20% of all smears.[9,72] If the polymerase chain reaction (PCR) is used as the basis of detection, the incidence of HPV infection varies from 2% to 80%. The variance is typically ascribed to differences in laboratory technique and in the population evaluated.[120,124,125]

The treatment of cervical condylomata depends on several factors, the most important of which are histology and

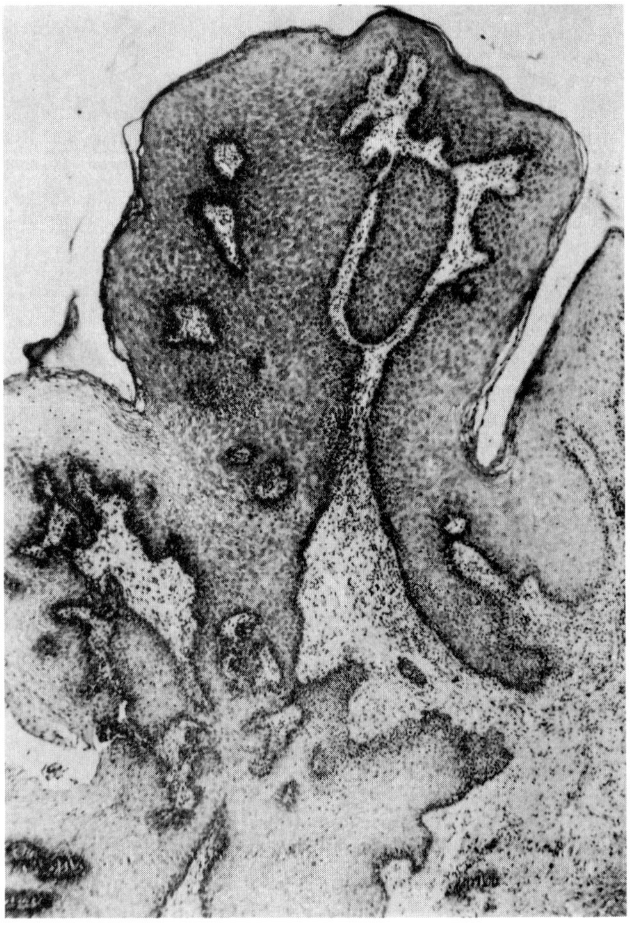

Fig. 6-14. Condyloma acuminatum of cervix. (From Kistner RW, Hertig AT: *Obstet Gynecol* 6:147, 1955.)

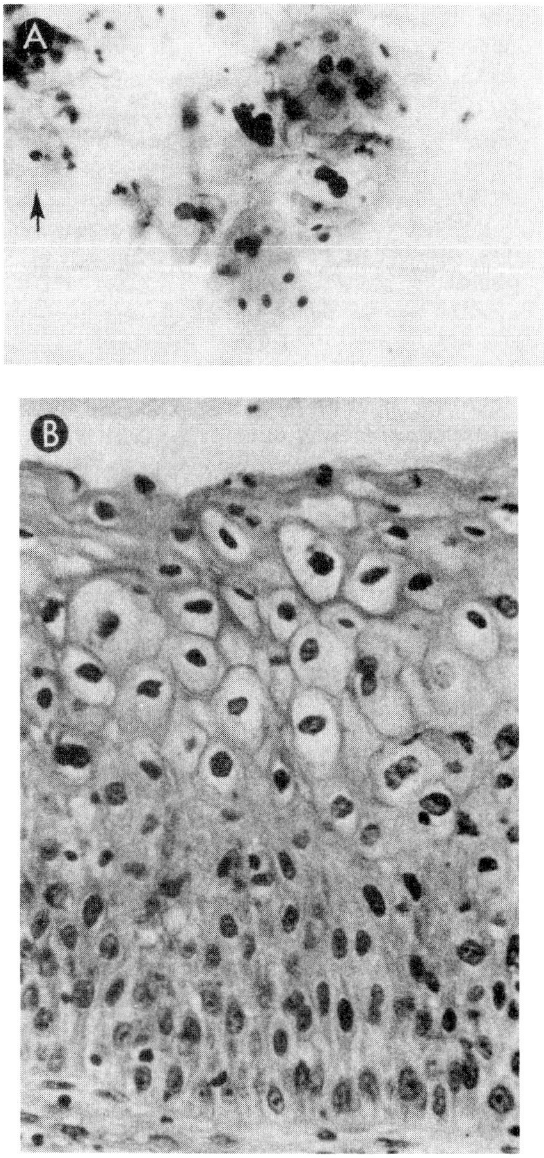

Fig. 6-15. A, Koilocytes on a Papanicolaou smear. (× 320.) The nuclei are hyperchromatic with characteristic, perinuclear, cytoplasmic vacuolization. Multinucleated forms are evident. A normal, superficial cell is shown for comparison (*arrow*). B, Flat condyloma. (× 530.) Koilocytotic changes can be seen in the superficial layers. (Courtesy Dr. Robert Ehrmann and the Division of Women's and Perinatal Pathology, Brigham and Women's Hospital, Boston.)

patient preference. If the histology identifies only condylomata and contains no cytologic atypia or dysplasia, the lesion can be closely observed or treated with topical therapy. Topical therapy such as trichloroacetic acid or 5-FU causes exfoliation of the epithelium. If cytologic atypia or dysplasia is present, ablative therapy such as cryocautery or laser should be strongly recommended. Since treatment of a single clinical lesion will not necessarily eradicate the patient's HPV infection, she should be well informed of the potential risks and benefits of treatment and the need for careful, long-term screening. Treatment methods will be more thoroughly discussed in the section under cervical intraepithelial neoplasia.

CERVICAL NEOPLASIA

Cervical neoplasia represents a neoplastic alteration of a normal physiologic change that occurs in the cervical epithelium (i.e., metaplasia). This alteration ranges from minor changes in the epithelium (i.e., low-grade, cervical, intraepithelial neoplasia), to full-thickness involvement of the epithelium (i.e., cervical carcinoma in situ), to invasive cervical cancer. Many investigators feel that cervical neoplasia represents a continuum of disease and that lesions that are preinvasive (i.e., confined to the epithelium), can either spontaneously regress to normal epithelium or progress to invasive cancer.

Epidemiology

The earliest epidemiologic studies of cervical neoplasia were conducted in 1842 by Rigoni-Stern. He showed that the incidence of cervical carcinoma was higher in married and widowed women and lower in never-married women and among nuns in certain religious orders.[104] Since then numerous epidemiologic studies have looked at the association between cancer of the cervix and *coitus*. Handley looked at the role of circumcision in relation to cervical cancer.[49] He found a lower incidence of cervical cancer among subsets of ethnic groups that practiced circumcision in comparison to those who did not. The concept of a "high-risk male" was furthered by Kessler. Compared to a control population, he found a several-fold increase in risk for the development of cervical carcinoma among women whose husbands were previously married to women with cervical carcinoma.[61,62]

The relationship between *HSV infections* and cervical cancer was noted by Josey et al[59] and Rawls et al.[98] Their serologic data revealed a significantly higher frequency and titer of HSV type 2 antibodies in patients with cervical carcinoma compared with the controls. Criticisms of these studies included the lack of controls adequately matched for sexual history and the technical difficulty in 1968 of differentiating HSV type 1 exposure from HSV type 2 exposure.

Further studies on HSV have revolved around locating its DNA, RNA, or related proteins within preinvasive and invasive cancers. No constant relationship has been found between cervical neoplasia and HSV on this molecular level, which makes it unlikely that HSV alone is responsible for cervical neoplasia. A possible role for HSV remains, since investigators have demonstrated that HSV infection can induce chromosomal breaks in the host cell DNA. This and other data such as HSV's ability to mutate certain genes support the fact that HSV is oncogenic. In fact some investigators believe that these properties of HSV are consistent with an initiator's role in the two-step theory of the development of cancer; therefore, HSV DNA or HSV RNA do not have to be present to support the role of HSV in the development of cervical neoplasia.[44,82,137]

As evaluation of HSV progressed, it became obvious that HPV-related lesions were also present in cervical neoplasia. HPV research took a giant step forward in 1980 when Gissmann and zur Hausen isolated HPV DNA from a genital condyloma.[46] This HPV DNA was designated HPV type 6. With the use of elegant DNA hybridization techniques and HPV type 6 as the initial probe, our understanding of HPV's intimate role in the development of intraepithelial neoplasia and invasive cancers of the cervix exploded.

Since 1980 data have shown that HPV DNA is present in all exophytic condylomata and in the vast majority of precancerous and cancerous changes of the cervix. In addition, the oncogenic potential of HPV was proven. Basically HPV types are broken down into two groups: those with low oncogenic potential (HPV types 6, 11, 35) and those with high oncogenic potential (HPV types 16, 18, 31, some 50s) Low-risk HPVs are associated with condylomata and low grade precancers. High-risk HPVs are associated with high grade precancers and invasive cancer. Although the vast majority of these lesions seem to stick to one HPV type and follow these general trends, this is not an absolute. Therefore cancerous lesions can have more than one HPV type present or could be associated with HPV type 6 or 11 and vice versa.[11] This ability of HPV types to be present in all facets of clinical lesions leads to difficulty in predicting which patient will be at risk for a serious clinical problem, when relying solely on HPV type. Adding to this dilemma is the well-known fact that HPV can remain dormant in normal-appearing skin,[38] which further decreases the predictive value of screening women for HPV types.[48] Readers interested in further detail are referred to appropriate reviews.[53,136]

Although how HPV DNA causes precancerous and cancerous changes in cervical epithelium is not known, it is no longer disputed that it does. Overwhelming epidemiologic data support a causative role for HPV. Hopefully its mechanism of action, either alone or with other co-factors, will be defined soon. Even when all other risk factors are considered, the presence of HPV infection is the leading risk factor for the development of cervical cancer and its precursors.[109]

When evaluating nonsexual factors that could enhance the occurrence of cervical neoplasia, sexual factors have to be controlled. The most commonly considered nonsexual risk factors are cigarette smoking, diet, and use of oral contraceptives. Even though the exact mechanism remains undefined, epidemiologic data leave little doubt that cigarette smoking is a risk factor for cervical neoplasia. Overall relative risk for precancerous and cancerous change is between 1.5 to 2.0 and the change appears to be dose related. The more cigarettes smoked, the greater the relative risk.[47]

The mechanism underlying the increased risk does not appear to be related to increased levels of mutagens in cervical mucus.[52] Although nicotine in cervical mucus is present in large amounts when comparing active smokers with those passively exposed or to nonsmokers, mutagenicity tests do not parallel.[75] A recent study looked at the relative risk of becoming infected with high-risk HPV types and cigarette smoking, when sexual factors are controlled. It appears that the more one smokes, the greater the chance of becoming infected with a high-risk HPV type. These findings will require further evaluation.[23]

Although dietary factors were not as extensively studied as other risk factors, there appears to be a trend; when controlled for confounding factors, it appears that those women whose diet is deficient in vitamin A or C are at a greater risk for cervical cancer. Recent data also support folate deficiency as a risk factor. These factors might explain the regional variation in cervical cancer incidence.[100,126]

As a result of confounding factors beyond the traditional sexual risks, the role that oral contraceptives may play in the development of cervical neoplasia is difficult to evaluate.

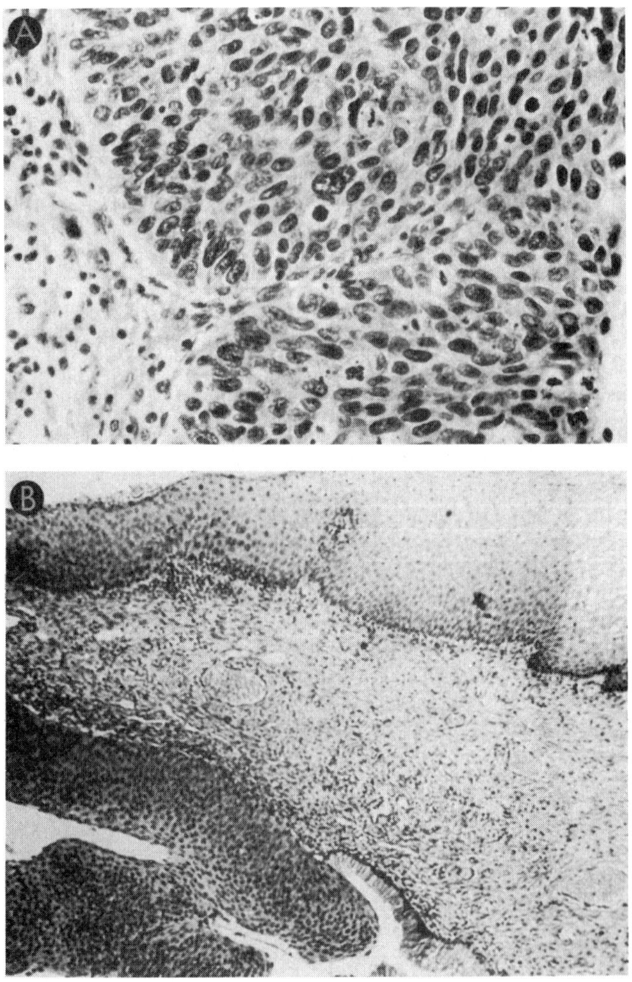

Fig. 6-16. A, Carcinoma in situ (CIS) of cervix. (From Hertig AT, Gore HM: Tumors of the female sex organs, fasc 33, *Atlas of tumor pathology.* Washington, DC, 1960, Armed Forces Institute of Pathology.) **B,** CIS of cervix with gland involvement. An area of parakeratosis is seen at the upper right.

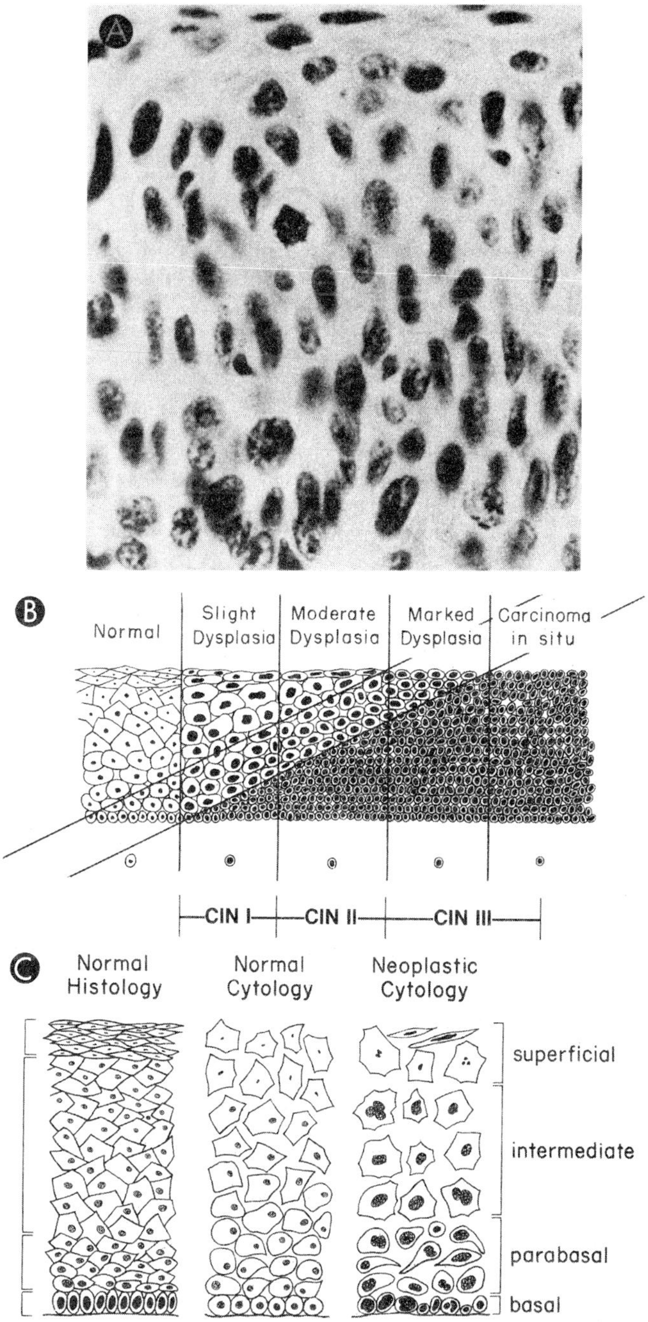

Fig. 6-17. A, High-power magnification of CIS of cervix. **B,** Diagrammatic representation of changes in cellular morphology from slight dysplasia to CIS. Nuclear/cytoplasmic ratios are shown at the bottom. **C,** Diagrammatic representation of exfoliated cells from the normal cervix compared with variations of exfoliated cells from the neoplastic cervix. (**B** and **C** courtesy Dr. Paul A. Younge.)

Not only do the traditional risk factors require control, but also with whom the cases are compared. Women who use barrier contraceptives may have some degree of protection over those who do not. Studies that control for all of these factors indicate that the longer a woman uses the pill, the greater her risk of developing cervical cancer. For example, an overall relative adjusted risk of 1.3 comes from the World Health Organization (WHO) Collaborative Study of Neoplasia and Steroid Contraceptives for pill users; the same group found a 1.5 relative adjusted risk when the pill was used for 5 or more years.[7]

Cervical intraepithelial neoplasia

Carcinoma in situ (CIS) may be defined as an intraepithelial lesion with cytologic atypia similar to that seen in invasive carcinoma but without evidence of invasion into the stroma (Fig. 6-16). These atypical cells extend through the entire thickness of the epithelium and have enlarged, pleomorphic nuclei with dense, coarse chromatin, and scant cytoplasm. The polarity of the cells as well as the polarity of the epithelium (i.e., the normal surface maturation and differentiation) are lost. Various degrees of parakeratosis may be seen.

Lesions composed of similar atypical cells that retain some degree of surface maturation have been referred to as "dysplasias" by Reagan et al.[99] Dysplastic epithelium spans a range of severity from a mild loss of polarity with a high degree of cellular differentiation and few mitoses (mild dysplasia), to a lesion resembling CIS. The latter shows marked cytologic and nuclear atypia and increased mitotic activity but retains some degree of epithelial polarization (severe dysplasia); (Fig. 6-17). In many cases pathologic differentiation of CIS from severe dysplasia may be very difficult and may hinge on minimal cellular flattening in the most superficial cell layers of the epithelium.

The major significance of CIS lies in its role as a precursor to invasive cancer. In a multiple series of untreated patients with CIS (diagnosed on biopsy) who were followed conservatively, the progression to invasive carcinoma occurred in as many as 70% of the cases.[66,116] More controversial is whether or not cervical dysplasia should be considered premalignant. Observed progression of dysplasia to CIS has been reported in 5% to 60% of cases, and this variation in percentages appears to result from differences in the criteria used to define each lesion and varying periods of follow-up.[26,103]

These reports also suggest that dysplastic lesions regress in as many as 50% of cases. It has been shown that biopsy may remove the dysplastic lesion entirely or that the inflammatory process accompanying repair at the biopsy site may destroy remaining areas of atypicality, thereby giving the false clinical impression of regression. More recent studies in which patients were diagnosed cytologically and then followed cytologically and colposcopically (thereby eliminating the "biopsy effect"), confirm the progression of dysplasia to CIS in 40% to 60% of cases, and spontaneous regression rates as high as 30% for mild or moderate dysplasia. The more severe the dysplasia, the higher the rate and speed of progression toward CIS and the lower the rate of regression. The average age of patients with dysplasia is consistently 5 to 10 years younger than that of patients with CIS, which runs 10 to 15 years behind the average age of patients with invasive squamous cell carcinoma.[76]

The suggestion that these lesions represent a continuum of change that begins with mild dysplasia and advances through CIS, led Richart to introduce the concept of cervical intraepithelial neoplasia (CIN) and the following classification: CIN I indicates mild dysplasia, CIN II indicates moderate dysplasia, and CIN III indicates severe dysplasia and carcinoma in situ.[103] Evidence in support of Richart's classification comes from the finding of aneuploid changes in the nuclei of dysplastic cells—the same chromosomal changes usually found associated with malignant tumors but not with benign tumors. Autoradiographic studies have demonstrated a steady increase in the mitotic activity of these lesions that corresponds exactly to the degree of histologic dedifferentiation and maturation present[102]; this is consistent with the postulate that CIN represents stages in a continuum of disease.

Histologic and colposcopic observations have established the transformation zone as the origin of virtually all CIN. These lesions are thought to arise from the basal cell of the transformation zone. If progression occurs, this can result in large-cell nonkeratinizing squamous cell carcinoma. Small-cell carcinoma is thought to arise from the subcolumnar reserve cells of the endocervical canal, whereas large-cell keratinizing carcinoma is thought to arise from the basal cells of the native squamous epithelium. Large-cell nonkeratinizing squamous carcinoma is by far the most common histologic type seen, which supports the observation that the majority of CIN originates in the transformation zone.

Although in a small percentage of cases CIN lesions will regress spontaneously or after biopsy, a finite percentage will progress to invasion. Until we can accurately predict when CIN will progress, regress, or remain stable, these lesions must be considered premalignant, and the patient must be evaluated, treated, and followed up appropriately. At the same time each case must be individualized to take into account age, desire for fertility, and the presence or absence of other pelvic disease.

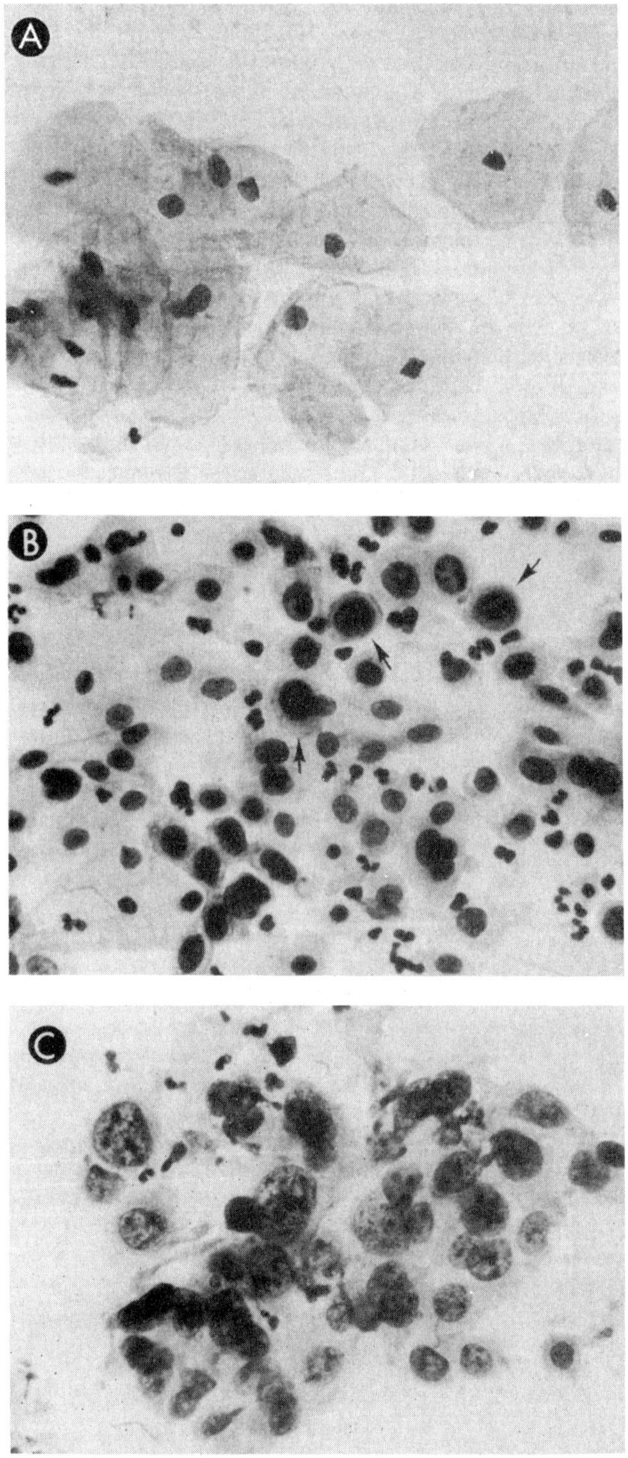

Fig. 6-18. A, Class I Pap smear, benign. (× 320.) Normal superficial cell, polygonal in shape with small pyknotic nuclei. **B,** Class IV Pap smear, CIS. (× 320.) Neoplastic cells are large and uniform in size, with hyperplastic nuclei and an increased nuclear/cytoplasmic ratio (*arrows*). **C,** Class V Pap smear, invasive cancer. (× 320.) The nuclei exhibit coarse, clumped chromatin and may contain multiple nucleoli. Marked pleomorphism and atypical mitotic figures may be seen. (Courtesy Dr. Robert Ehrmann and the Division of Women's and Perinatal Pathology, Brigham and Women's Hospital, Boston.)

Diagnosis of cervical neoplasia

Cytology. The contribution of the late George Papanicolaou to the field of cancer detection was outstanding. In studying cells exfoliated from the female genital tract in the late 1920s, Papanicolaou noted characteristic cellular changes associated with cervical carcinoma. These cellular abnormalities included anomalies of staining reaction, pleomorphism, nuclear irregularity, hyperchromasia, the presence of multiple nucleoli, and an increased nuclear/cytoplasmic ratio

Table 6-1. Comparison of the cervical intraepithelial neoplasia (CIN) Pap smear classification and the Bethesda system

Modern classification	Bethesda system
Squamous lesions	**Squamous lesions**
No evidence of malignant cells	No evidence of malignant cells
Atypical cells, possibly inflammatory	Atypical cells of undetermined significance; this term should not include inflammatory cells
HPV effect, cervical intraepithelial neoplasia grade I	Squamous intraepithelial lesion (SIL), low grade
CIN grade II/III, CIS	SIL, high grade
Squamous cell cancer	Squamous cell cancer

(Fig. 6-18). As with so many important discoveries, fully 20 years elapsed before Papanicolaou's cytologic technique (the *Papanicolaou test)* was accepted as a cancer screening measure.

Initially the Papanicolaou test (Pap smear) was used to detect women with invasive asymptomatic cervical cancer. As the concept of preinvasive cancer was recognized, the Pap smear classification system was revised to reflect the preinvasive disease diagnoses. Recently the criteria for different categories of preinvasive disease were strengthened by the Bethesda system. This system represents an effort on the part of cytologists, pathologists, and clinicians to tighten the criteria for preinvasive disease (Table 6-1). Although developed with the Pap smear in mind, histology is supposed to report preinvasive disease along the same guidelines.[13]

The earliest technique used for collecting cytologic material was aspiration from the posterior vaginal fornix via a glass pipette. Using this technique, various series reported failure rates of up to 60% in detecting documented CIN, and failure rates of 45% in identifying CIS. In 1947 Ayre devised a wooden spatula with which a "scrape biopsy" of the cervical epithelial cells could be carried out.[8] He quoted a 95% accuracy in screening for cervical neoplasms when this technique was used in conjunction with endocervical sampling.

Despite the overall success of exfoliative cytology, there is a significant incidence of *false-negative smears*. Although numerous subsequent reports in the literature confirm a false-negative rate of 15% to 20% for cervical cytologic diagnosis, increasing the frequency of screening (i.e., decreasing the interval between smears) will have an impact on the rate of diagnostic failure to the individual patient.[9]

Technique of obtaining vaginal and cervical smears. The following equipment is needed:

1. Clean glass (microscope) slides; those with frosted ends permit easy labeling in pencil with the patient's name and also identify the "right side," or smeared side of the slide
2. A cotton swab moistened with normal saline solution or an endocervical brush
3. Spatula to be used for cervical scrapings and to prepare smear
4. A fixative; any one of several dehydrating agents can be used:
   a. Half-and-half mixture of 95% ethyl alcohol and ether
   b. Plain 95% alcohol or lesser dilutions to 75%
   c. 75% to 95% methyl alcohol
   d. 75% to 95% isopropyl alcohol or commercially available cytologic fixatives

Smears are obtained prior to digital examination with the patient in the lithotomy position; lubricants, which spoil the staining characteristics of the cells are not used. Douches dilute and wet the cells; therefore a satisfactory smear cannot be obtained within 12 to 24 hours after douching. The endocervix is sampled first and then the portio is scraped with a spatula. In a two-slide technique the sample is immediately plated and the slide fixed. If one wishes to use a one-slide technique, the endocervix should be sampled and smeared before the cervical scrape is taken. The moisture inherent in the endocervical sample is believed to keep the drying artifact to a minimum, prior to fixation of the one slide. Fixation is complete in 15 to 30 minutes if an immersion dehydrating agent is used or immediately if a cytologic fixative is used. In either case the air-drying artifact is the most common error in a Pap smear technique and should be kept in mind when a fixation is performed.

Some authors believe that a greater yield of endocervical cells is obtained by the using the brush over the swab; this method decreases the number of Pap smears that are inadequate because of a lack of endocervical cells.[122,129] The importance of endocervical sampling cannot be over emphasized; it at least doubles the detection rate of abnormal cytology.[45]

The diagnosis rendered by the cytopathologist can be no better than an accurate interpretation of the cytologic abnormality present on the slide. Certainly the clinician can help to limit the number of false-negative smears by obtaining a proper smear from the area of the transformation zone, by obtaining an adequate endocervical sample, and by assuring rapid fixation to give the examiner the best chance to provide an accurate diagnosis.

The effects of Pap smear screening have been well documented. It is estimated that screening every 3 years for women who are between the ages of 20 and 65 years will decrease the incidence and mortality of invasive cervical cancer by approximately 90%.[36] Factors that will affect the mortality from cervical cancer include the population's natural incidence of the disease, the preclinical stage duration, the sensitivity and specificity of the screening process, and the quality of treatment available for preinvasive and invasive diagnoses.[60] Studies have evaluated the age at which screening should start, how frequently it should be done, at what age screening should cease, and who should perform the screening examination.

There seems to be little debate about when a woman should start to undergo periodic screening. Most would agree that once regular intercourse has started, the risk for developing preinvasive disease is present. How often a Pap smear should be done after initiation of periodic screening is not clear. In 1988 the American College of Obstetrics and Gynecology, in conjunction with the American Cancer Society and several other cancer organizations, agreed on recommendations for Pap smear screening intervals.[3] They believe that every woman should have a Pap smear annually after age 18 years or after the onset of sexual activity. If three consecutive Pap smears and pelvic examinations 1 year apart are entirely normal, the screening interval can be lengthened at the discretion of the physician. They do not recommend lengthening the interval if the patient or her sexual partner has had more than one other sexual partner. These recommendations do not apply to women being followed for abnormal Pap smears or after treatment of such. All clinicians need to stress the importance of screening and pelvic examinations since other reproductive tract cancers may be found.

There has been much debate as to the cost-effectiveness of this approach.[4] Eddy's data indicate that screening every 1 to 2 years as compared to every 3 years increases the effectiveness by less than 5%.[36] His data clearly show that as screening becomes more frequent, the cost and inconvenience due to unnecessary diagnostic procedures grows.

Biopsy and histologic diagnosis. Clinicians have depended on the Pap smear as a screening method for detection of cervical neoplasia. Serial sampling over time provides a longitudinal look at the cervix, which decreases the impact of isolated false-negative smears. The Pap smear, however, must remain a *screening* technique. Biopsy and histologic diagnosis remain the cornerstones in the management of cervical neoplasia.

A biopsy must be performed on every abnormal, visible cervical lesion. The literature is replete with cases in which a gross cervical abnormality was followed conservatively because multiple Pap smears were falsely negative or exhibited inflammatory changes only.[42a]

Random cervical biopsies were first used to obtain histologic material from cervices determined to be abnormal by Pap smear, in an attempt to obviate conization in all patients with abnormal smears. This technique lead to a low rate of diagnosis. A targeting technique developed by Schiller in 1938 (now known as the *Schiller test*) may be used to highlight cervical abnormalities and make them visible for biopsy (Fig. 6-6). A solution of sodium iodide and iodine is painted onto the cervix. The iodine reacts with glycogen to stain the normal squamous epithelium of the cervix and vagina dark brown. Nonstaining or Schiller-positive areas stand out from the dark background and represent surfaces lacking glycogen; these include columnar epithelium, true pathologic erosions, immature metaplastic epithelium, and neoplastic lesions. Due to the relatively nonspecific staining patterns, this test is generally reserved for usage at the time of cervical conization.

Colposcopy has superseded Schiller's technique as the initial step in evaluating abnormal Pap smears.[128] Hinselman developed the colposcope in 1925 in an attempt to localize small ulcerations that he theorized represented small cervical neoplasms. He found, however, that the low-power magnification of the colposcope (×6 to ×40) revealed not the neoplastic cervical epithelium but alterations of the underlying stromal vasculature. These alterations from the neoplastic process could then be visualized through the thin epithelial layer. The degree of alteration in vascular pattern, in intercapillary distance, and in surface color and texture was found to correlate well with the severity of the neoplastic process. These patterns are enhanced by applications of 3% acetic acid to the cervical epithelium. Use of 3% acetic acid not only cleanses the epithelium but tends to precipitate out nucleic proteins in the superficial layers. This gives rise to the classic aceto-white epithelium that is one of the features of abnormal epithelium. (For a detailed review of colposcopy, the reader is referred to a standard colposcopic atlas.)

Adequate colposcopic evaluation requires complete visualization of the transformation zone and the lesion in question, as well as correlation between the cytologic and histologic diagnoses and the clinical impression of the colposcopist. Endocervical curettage should be performed as part of every colposcopic examination. Almost 90% of women with abnormal cytologic findings may be adequately evaluated with colposcopy.

Colposcopy and cervical biopsy. Cervical biopsy is perhaps the most frequent minor surgical procedure performed by the gynecologist. Simple and relatively painless, it may be performed as part of the routine office examination. Contraindications to cervical biopsy are limited to acute pelvic inflammatory disease and acute cervicitis. Certainly patients with coagulopathies should be managed in a hospital setting. Pregnancy is not a contraindication to biopsy.

Technique. The cervix is visualized with a speculum and adequately illuminated. A Pap smear is repeated at the start of the examination for later correlation with the histology obtained on biopsy. Then the cervix is carefully cleaned and soaked with 3% acetic acid. It is generally believed that the most commot error in colposcopy is not keeping the cervix adequately soaked with acetic acid, such that the abnormal areas are missed. The endocervical curettage is obtained prior to biopsies on the cervical portio to reduce the number of curettages contaminated by detached fragments of cervical epithelium. A rectangular biopsy specimen is obtained using a Kevorkian or Younge biopsy punch and is then immediately fixed. Postbiopsy bleeding may be controlled by pressure, cauterizing with silver nitrate or ferrous subsulfate (Monsel's solution), packing with oxidized regenerated cellulose, or suturing as required. The patient is instructed to avoid douching, the use of tampons, and intercourse for 2 weeks after biopsy.

Therapy for cervical intraepithelial neoplasia. The type of therapy for preinvasive cervical disease depends on the results of the colposcopy and biopsy:

1. Lesions identified colposcopically must be seen entirely. If they extend to the endocervical canal, their uppermost extent must be seen.
2. The entire transformation zone must be visualized (often termed an *adequate* or *satisfactory* examination).
3. Results of endocervical curettage must be negative for neoplasia.
4. Biopsies and cytologic examination must reveal intraepithelial disease only.
5. Cytologic and histologic diagnoses must correlate.

Perhaps 85% to 90% of all patients with CIN may have lesions limited to the portio and at the same time fulfill all the criteria obviating conization.

The approach to treatment of preinvasive cervical neoplasia has undergone dramatic changes over the past several decades as the pathogenesis of cervical neoplasia has become better understood. Treatment in general has become less aggressive, and preinvasive disease is rarely treated with removal of the uterus. Most clinicians favor ablative procedures such as laser therapy or cryosurgery if the criteria listed above are met. For excisional procedures, the laser excisional cone was very popular until the advent of the simple-loop excision of the transformation zone. Cold-knife cervical conization has become reserved for ruling out invasive disease in unsatisfactory colposcopy patients when adenocarcinoma in situ is found or when the pap smear indicates a possible invasion. Hysterectomy still plays a role in treatment but is reserved for patients who have completed childbearing and have severe precancerous lesions, or repetitive treatment failures, or deep margins of conization with lesions.

Some clinicians feel that the grade of the lesion, whether or not it involves endocervical glands, and the size of the lesion should dictate what type of therapy is performed. The data surrounding these issues are difficult to interpret. When the majority of confounding factors are removed, it appears that the most important issue for patients in whom the transformation zone is seen and the lesion documented is where the lesion is found on the ectocervix.[39] If the area of neoplasia is close to the endocervical os and does not exceed 3 cm in diameter, then either cryosurgery or laser can be used. If the neoplasia involves the endocervical os but is entirely seen, or if it is greater than 3 cm in diameter, then cryosurgery becomes less effective.

Cryocauterization. This technique appears to be the simplest and safest outpatient modality developed. This technique uses a cryoprobe cooled by carbon dioxide or freon to necrose the surface epithelium that it contacts. Probes of various shapes are available for different cervices. After treatment a watery discharge is common but resolves in several weeks. Reepithelialization begins immediately and is virtually complete in 6 weeks.[34] The most common technique for cryosurgery is to freeze the cervix for 3 minutes, allow the cervix to thaw for 5 minutes, and resume a second freeze for 3 minutes. It is well shown that when properly performed cryocautery produces necrosis to a depth of 5 to 6 mm, which should theoretically destroy more than 99% of the involved glands.[5]

Criticism of cryocauterization has resulted from reports of invasive carcinoma developing after the procedure. This implies that residual neoplasia had been buried during the reparative process and had progressed to invasion while undetectable by cytologic or colposcopic techniques. Sevin et al reviewed eight such cases and found that seven of these patients had not undergone a pretreatment endocervical curettage, five had not undergone biopsy, one biopsy was misinterpreted and actually represented invasive carcinoma, and only three patients underwent a colposcopic examination.[111] This implies that these failures were due to inadequate initial evaluation rather than a consequence of cryocauterization.

Laser therapy. Laser light is generated by electricity running through gas, generally CO_2 gas for lower genital tract lesions. This device produces a coherent or in-phase parallel beam of light of very high energy that is capable of instantantly boiling water and thus vaporizing cells. Originally the laser was used to eradicate the lesion itself, which spared the remaining cervix. However, failure rates averaged 10% to 30%, and it became clear that the entire transformation zone could be vaporized safely to a depth of 5 to 7 mm to yield cure rates exceeding 90%.[123] The major drawbacks of this technique are the cost of the laser apparatus and the greater skill required when compared with cryocauterization. Proponents cite less cervical scarring than with cryocauterization. The major benefit from less scarring is the ability to achieve adequate colposcopic evaluation after laser therapy. In younger childbearing women, the need for conization is reduced by the necessity to repeat colposcopy in the future should an abnormal cytologic smear be obtained.

Large-loop excision of the transformation zone. In the late 1980s Prendiville et al[95,96] and others[81] described the results of excising the cervical transformation zone using a thin wire loop and a blended form of electrocautery.[81,95,96] The advantages of this technique are that a further histologic specimen is obtained, and it can be performed in the office under local anesthesia. Wright et al were responsible for popularizing this technique in the United States in the early 1990s.[134]

Technique. Although often performed in Western Europe as a "see-and-treat" procedure, where the patient is colposcoped for an abnormal Pap smear, cervical lesions are identified, and loop excision of the transformation zone is immediately performed, this approach has not been as popular in the United States.[81] Most clinicians feel it is important to make sure that the patient fits the same criteria as any other patient they wish to treat with outpatient ablative therapy. When one follows the same pattern as expected for ablative therapy, large-loop excision results in a success rate of greater than 90%.

In the office the patient is placed in the dorsal lithotomy position and grounded for electrocautery. A speculum that has been insulated for electrical current is used to visualize the cervix. The margins of excision are usually delineated by iodine staining although colposcopy can be used. Local anesthetic with 1:100,000 epinephrine is placed into the cervical stroma. A wire loop that is large enough to remove at least the disease located on a single lip of the cervix is used. Preferably a single pass technique can be used. The specimen is sent to pathology for further evaluation.

Difficulty can be encountered in interpreting the margins of resection either due to lack of orientation or thermal damage. Unless invasive cancer is identified, most clinicians have adopted a policy of follow-up, even for margins felt to be involved with preinvasive disease. The patient will be evaluated at 4 months after the procedure by Pap smear, colposcopy, endocervical curettage, and cervical biopsy when appropriate. If that assessment is normal, then careful follow-up with Pap smears is done on a 4-month basis for a year. If all results are normal, then a 6-month follow-up and eventually a yearly follow-up is recommended.[81,134]

Cervical conization. Cervical conization remains the standard against which all outpatient evaluation techniques must be weighed. A properly performed conization removes the entire transformation zone and virtually the entire endocervical canal and provides the pathologist with the maximum amount of tissue to rule out invasive carcinoma. Drawbacks of this procedure include the need for anesthetic, a complication rate approaching 10% (primarily postoperative hemorrhage), and possible adverse effects on fertility.

Technique. Using adequate general or regional anesthetic, the patient is placed in the dorsal lithotomy position. The vagina and perineum are prepared with povidone-iodine (Betadine) with care to avoid traumatizing the delicate cervical mucosa. A pelvic examination is performed and a weighted retractor is placed in the posterior fornix; a Sims retractor is placed anteriorly and the cervix is visualized. A colposcopy or Schiller's test is performed to delineate the extent of disease on the portio. Lateral-angle sutures are placed into the stroma of the cervix at the 3 and 9 o'clock positions to ligate the descending branches of the uterine artery. These sutures are left long (for tying at the end of the procedure). Some clinicians infiltrate the cervix with dilute solutions of 20 units of vasopressin in 20 mL of normal saline or bupivacaine (Marcaine) hydrochloride with epinephrine 1:200,000 to aid hemostasis.

The mucosa is incised circumferentially while a margin of 2 to 3 mm is maintained beyond the lesions (as delineated via colposcopy or Schiller's staining). A cone-shaped specimen to a length of 1.5 to 1.8 cm is excised encircling the endocervical canal. A uterine sound may be placed within the canal to aid in the dissection. Once the specimen is removed, a suture is placed at the 12 o'clock position in the stroma of the specimen to aid in pathologic orientation. The uterus is then sounded and dilated, and an endometrial sample is taken as desired.

Bleeding is usually minimal with this technique. Bleeding points may be electrocauterized or ligated with size 0 chromic sutures in a figure-of-eight pattern. The canal is then packed with Surgicel, which is gently tied into place with the long ends of the lateral sutures. Generally, conization is an outpatient surgery; the patient is observed until the anesthetic has worn off. The patient is then discharged with instructions to avoid douching, use of tampons, and intercourse for 3 weeks.

Conization for any degree of CIN has a cure rate of 98% when surgical margins are normal and thus requires no further therapy. Close follow-up is suggested and includes Pap smears every 3 months for 1 year and every 6 months thereafter. Given the 70% to 80% cure rate reported after conization with abnormal margins, conservative management with serial endocervical sampling, colposcopy, and cytology is acceptable if patient compliance can be expected. Otherwise reconization or hysterectomy is indicated. When the upper vagina is shown to be normal preoperatively with colposcopy or Schiller's staining, there is no need for a wide vaginal cuff.

INVASIVE CANCER

Fifty years ago carcinoma of the cervix was the leading cause of death from malignant disease in American women. Since 1940, however, the mortality rate from cervical carcinoma has declined by more than 50%. Yet it still ranks sixth in cancer mortality with estimates of 4500 deaths each year in the United States. Each year in the United States there are 12,500 new cases of invasive cervical carcinoma with the peak incidence between ages 45 to 55 years, and more than 44,000 new cases of in situ cervical carcinoma discovered. Despite the recognition of a significant preinvasive phase and the availability of screening methods, cervical neoplasia remains a major health problem.[17,36,100]

The incidence of cervical cancer varies according to geographic area and race. Cervical cancer is the leading cause of cancer death among women in underdeveloped countries. In the United States the incidence rate for African-Americans, Hispanics, and Native Americans is approximately two times higher than it is for Caucasians. The risk for Orientals is similar to those for Caucasians.[36] Interestingly, results from the 1987 U.S. National Health Interview Survey indicate that African-Americans are screened at comparable or higher rates than Caucasians through age 69. Hispanics had a decreased screening rate compared to Caucasians. Why African-Americans have a higher incidence rate is unknown.[50]

Symptoms and diagnosis

There are no specific symptoms that characterize cervical cancer especially in its early stages. Irregular vaginal bleeding, postcoital bleeding, or both may be noted, or there may be only a pink discharge that is occasionally odorous. Abnormal vaginal bleeding may first be noted as a prolonged menstrual period or as profuse flow at the time of a normal period. As the disease progresses, an initially scant serosanguineous discharge may become grossly hemorrhagic. A common complaint is the daily appearance of a little blood, usually noted after voiding. In advanced cancer a characteristic bloody, malodorous discharge together with pain from either fistula formation or nerve irritation may be present. Pain is a late symptom and is typical of a sciatic distribution that radiates down the back of the buttock, thigh, and knee. Endophytic tumors may cause little or no bleeding or discharge; however, the cancer may spread rapidly to the sacral plexus and produce severe pain. These symptoms, if a result of cervical cancer, will become manifest when lesions are of moderate size.

The patient should be advised to visit her physician for proper diagnostic procedures at least once yearly. As noted earlier, CIS presents no characteristic gross lesion and is detectable only by the judicious use of cervical cytologic studies and adequate biopsies. Similarly in early invasive carcinoma, the cervix may appear normal or may exhibit what seems to be an erosion. A biopsy of any suspect lesion on the cervix should always be taken. It should not be necessary to emphasize the importance of a digital and speculum examination in women in all age groups. No patient should be advised to take douches for abnormal discharges or bleeding without having a pelvic examination.

The gross clinical appearance of invasive cervical lesions is generally of two types: *exophytic* (proliferative) and *endophytic* (ulcerating). The exophytic lesion may involve the entire cervix and have a cauliflower-like appearance, whereas the endophytic lesion has a predilection to invade upward into the endocervical canal, often expanding the lower uterine segment and giving rise to the so-called barrel-shaped cervix. Although an endophytic lesion may infiltrate the tissue adjacent to the cervix earlier than an exophytic tumor, either type may extend into the parametrium and involve the uterosacral ligaments or may spread into the vaginal mucosa and down the vaginal canal. This spread causes the tissues to feel firm and nodular. The rectum and bladder may likewise be infiltrated by tumor. Spread towards the bladder usually involves the vesicovaginal septum and formation of bullous edema of the bladder prior to actual involvement of the bladder mucosa. Posterior spread involves the rectovaginal septum, and only late in the disease is there involvement of the rectal mucosa.

Differential diagnosis

The lesions most commonly confused with cervical cancer are eversions, polyps, papillary endocervicitis, and papillomas. Tuberculosis, syphilitic chancres, and granuloma inguinale rarely involve the cervix, although it may be impossible to differentiate these benign lesions from early invasive cancer by any method other than biopsy. In many cases repeat or multiple biopsies are necessary before a final diagnosis can be made. This has been particularly true in papillomas of the cervix, which are frequently difficult to distinguish from low-grade papillary carcinomas.

Secondary carcinoma of the cervix may occur by direct extension from the corpus or vagina. Metastatic ovarian, bladder, and breast carcinomas have also been reported, although breast cancer may first spread to the ovary and then to the cervix. Lymphomas, particularly histiocytic lymphoma, may present as a cervical tumor.

Pathology

Squamous cell carcinoma accounts for 80% of invasive cervical cancer. *Adenocarcinoma* accounts for approximately 10% to 15%, and the remainder are sarcomas and primary or secondary lymphomas. The incidence of adenocarcinoma has been reported as 25% in women younger than 35 years.[12]

Wentz and Reagan divided squamous cell carcinoma into three types: keratinizing, nonkeratinizing, and small-cell.[130] Keratinizing cells show foci of keratinization with cornified "pearls." Nonkeratinizing cells have well-demarcated tumor-stromal borders, but no evidence of keratinization or cornified pearls. The small-cell type consists of small, round, or spindle-shaped cells with poorly defined tumor-stromal borders. Although they account for only 1% to 2% of all cervical cancers, small-cell cervical cancers should be recognized as a group that covers a wide variety of subtle, histologically different cancers that manifest markedly different clinical outcomes.

The significant features differentiating invasive cancer from CIS are the breakdown of the basement membrane and involvement of the stroma. Nests and clusters of epithelial cells can be seen scattered in an irregular pattern within a stroma infiltrated by inflammatory cells (Fig. 6-19, A). Individual cells of invasive squamous cell carcinoma show the same characteristics described for in situ cancer, namely, loss

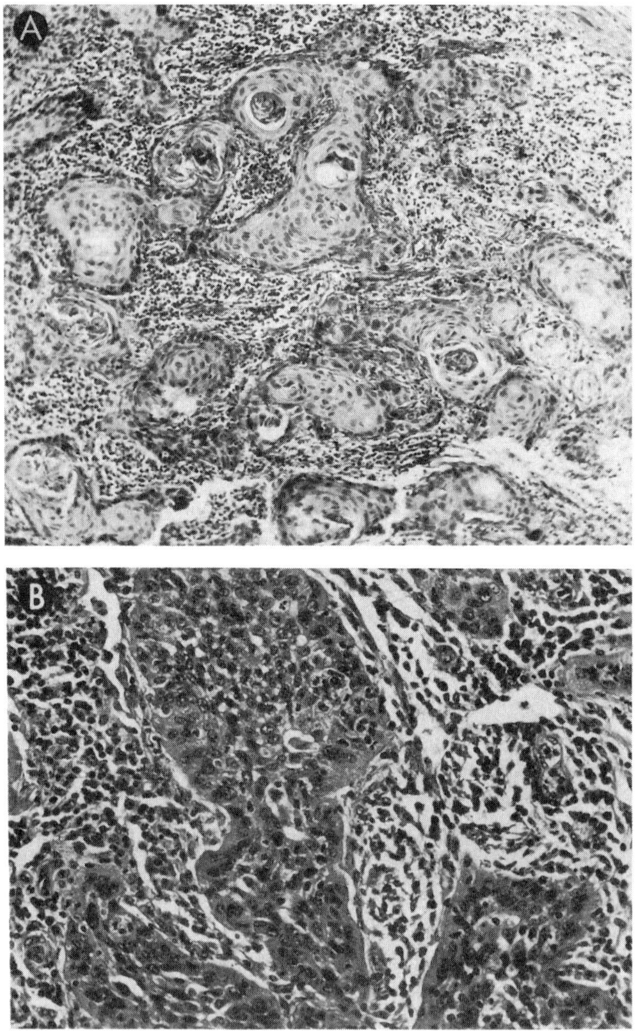

Fig. 6-19. A, Typical grade 1 squamous cell carcinoma of the cervix. There is extensive keratinization with "pearl" formation and lymphocytic infiltration of the stroma. (From Hertig AT, Gore HM: Tumors of the female sex organs, fasc 33, *Atlas of tumor pathology*, Washington, DC, 1960, Armed Forces Institute of Pathology.) **B**, Grade 2 squamous cell carcinoma of the cervix. Several nests of malignant cells show pleomorphism, nuclear hyperchromatism, and atypical mitotic figures.

of stratification and polarity with numerous atypical mitotic figures, pleomorphism, nuclear hyperchromatism (Fig. 6-19, B), and dyskaryosis. Tumor giant cells may be found along with areas of necrosis and cellular degeneration.

The typical appearance of cervical adenocarcinoma is shown in Fig. 6-20. Adenocarcinoma arises from the columnar cells lining the endocervical canal and glands. The number of glandular elements is greatly increased, and they show a marked variation in size and shape. Cellular pleomorphism, nuclear enlargement and hyperchromatism, and increased mitotic activity with areas of necrosis and degeneration are seen.

Adenosquamous carcinoma consists of intermingled malignant epithelial cell cores and malignant glandular structures. If the squamous component appears benign, the tumor is referred to as an *adenoacanthoma*. The *glassy cell carcinoma* is a mixed carcinoma consisting of a poorly differentiated adenocarcinoma and squamous carcinoma. It is such a rare entity that Maier and Norris question whether it indeed represents a distinct clinical and pathologic entity.[74] Although this tumor is believed to respond poorly to therapy, the number of reported cases is too small to allow any conclusions about survival rates.

Histologic grading of cervical cancer

The degree of cervical cancer differentiation as viewed under high power magnification determines its histologic grade. The grade classification most generally accepted is that of Broders. In 1926 he divided tumors into differentiated and undifferentiated groups and then assigned one of three grades depending on the relative amount of cellular differentiation present.[19] Keratinization was used as an index of differentiation. By this scheme, grade 1 would be the most differentiated and grade 3 the least differentiated or most anaplastic. Since this original report, numerous publications concerning histological grading and survival have appeared. Most of these reviews do not consider the risk factors that may influence prognosis, other than histologic grading. Chung et al evaluated histologic grade and prognosis and noted that the more undifferentiated the tumor, the higher the incidence of pelvic node metastases.[27] But they also noted that these less differentiated tumors tended to be larger than the more differentiated lesions. They concluded that the poor prognosis may depend more on the size and ultimately the stage of the lesion than on the degree of histologic differentiation.

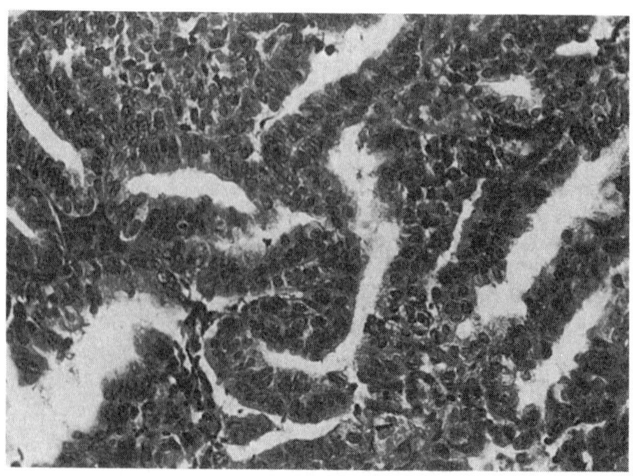

Fig. 6-20. Adenocarcinoma of the cervix. The malignant cells are arranged in a glandular pattern. The typical columnar appearance of the cell has been lost, and numerous cells show atypical mitoses.

Mode of spread of cervical cancer

Carcinoma of the cervix spreads principally by direct local invasion and via the lymphatics. The number of tumors with a biologic propensity for hematogenous spread totals no more than 5%, but this may result in distant extra pelvic metastatic foci in spite of limited pelvic disease. Tumor growth commonly occurs by contiguous spread to the vagina, uterine cavity, and laterally through the cardinal and uterosacral ligaments. Lateral spread may occur within the substance of the ligaments or in the areolar tissue adjacent to them. Laterally extending carcinoma may encompass and obstruct the ureters as they traverse the paracervical region and ultimately cause hydroureter, hydronephrosis, and eventual loss of kidney function. This may lead to uremia and ultimately death. The cancer may traverse the paravaginal fascia with extension into the bladder or bowel and can result in vesicovaginal or rectovaginal fistulas.

Plentl and Friedman evaluated pelvic node metastases in cervical cancer by stage and found 15.4% abnormal nodes in stage I, 28.6% abnormal nodes in stage II, and 47% abnormal nodes in stage III.[93] They further noted that the preferential metastatic spread is to the external iliac, hypogastric, and obturator lymph nodes. The next most commonly involved groups of nodes are the common iliac, parametrial, and paracervical. Therefore the lymphatic trunks leaving the cervix within the base of the broad ligament tend to be the preferred channels for lymphatic embolization. The posterior channels that drain to the sacral and then periaortic nodes are less frequently used pathways for tumor dissemination. It appears that the parametrial and paracervical nodes are frequently skipped in the transit of tumor emboli to the more preferred distal sites.

Pretreatment laparotomy has defined the spread of cervical carcinoma beyond the pelvis. The incidence of periaortic node metastases is about 6% in stage IB, 14% in stage IIA, 22% in stage IIB, and 33% in stage IIIB.[69] Buchsbaum reported 23 patients with abnormal aortic nodes who underwent left scalene node biopsies of which 8 (34.8%) were abnormal.[20] The sites of distant organ metastases in order of frequency are lung, liver, and bone.

Clinical staging of cervical cancer

Clinical staging remains the most important prognostic criterion in determining the patient's response to therapy. The staging process includes a pelvic and rectal examination under anesthesia, chest x-ray, routine liver function tests, and evaluation of the urinary tract by intravenous dye and x-ray studies. Proctoscopy and cystoscopy are reserved for advanced disease or those patients for whom radiation therapy is planned. Contiguous spread of cervical cancer into the vagina, adjacent parametrium, and pelvic organs is a rather characteristic course in the natural history of this disease and forms the basis for clinical staging. All of these studies are generally available worldwide and represent a standard approach to staging.

Once all the data is obtained, they are used to assign a clinical stage of disease as outlined by the International Federation of Gynecologists and Obstetricians (FIGO; Table 6-2). Often a computed tomography (CT) with intravenous contrast is used in lieu of an intravenous pyelogram in the United States. Information obtained on intraabdominal or lymph node status cannot be used in the clinical staging. However, this data could alter clinical management, and therefore any abnormalities or lymph node enlargements should be sampled by external CT guided biopsies. *The final staging cannot be changed once therapy has begun.*

Certain difficulties and misinterpretations are unavoidable in clinical staging. On occasion the examiner may interpret pelvic inflammatory processes or scarring resulting from endometriosis as a tumor, thereby "overstaging" the disease. Conversely the lateral pelvis may be soft when palpated but abnormal lymph nodes may be found surgically. Staging will

Table 6-2. International Federation of Gynecologists and Obstetricians—clinical staging of invasive cervical cancer

Stage 0	CIS, intraepithelial carcinoma
Stage I	Carcinoma is confined to the cervix
Stage IA	Preclinical carcinoma; those diagnosed only by microscopy
Stage IA-1	Minimal microscopically evident stromal invasion
Stage IA-2	Lesions detected microscopically that can be measured. Depth of invasion from the base of epithelium not more than 5 mm, horizontal spread not greater than 7 mm
Stage IB	All other stage 1 lesions. Occult cancer should be marked "occ"
Stage II	Carcinoma extends beyond the cervix but has not extended to the pelvic wall. It involves the vagina but not the lower third
Stage IIA	No obvious parametrial involvement
Stage IIB	Obvious parametrial involvement
Stage III	Carcinoma has extended to the pelvic wall. On rectal examination there is no cancer-free space between the tumor and the pelvic wall. The tumor involves the lower third of the vagina. All cases with hydronephrosis or nonfunctioning kidney
Stage IV	Carcinoma has extended beyond the true pelvis or has clinically involved the mucosa of the bladder or rectum. A bullous edema is not classified as stage IV
Stage IVA	Spread of the growth to adjacent organs
Stage IVB	Spread to distant organs

thus vary somewhat with the experience of the examiner. Discrepancies between the clinical staging and the surgical pathologic findings have been reported in as many as 25% to 40% of cases.[90]

It is for this reason that some investigators have elected to perform laparotomy prior to instituting therapy, to determine the presence of metastases to the aortic nodes or other sites beyond the pelvis. Extending the field of treatment to include involved nodal groups is then performed in the hope of improving survival. Although the complication rates have been minimized by extraperitoneal approaches, pretreatment laparotomy has not been shown to increase the survival of these patients. More recently with advances in operative laparoscopy, these same nodal dissections may be performed as a day surgical procedure. It remains to be seen whether these staging lymphadenectomies will impact on overall survival.

Treatment

Conventionally, cervical cancer has been treated with either radical surgery (i.e., radical hysterectomy with pelvic lymph node dissection) or radiation therapy. In certain instances, hysterectomy is performed after radiation therapy. This approach is used when bulky central pelvic disease is present, since radiation therapy is somewhat compromised in sterilizing such disease. These situations include cervical adenocarcinomas that have a propensity to endophytic growth and enlargement of the lower uterine segment, and the so-called barrel-shaped cervix that similarly exhibits infiltration and expansion of the lower uterine segment.

Because of the success in managing head and neck squamous cell cancer, a neoadjuvant approach to the management of bulky squamous cervical tumors is employed in many centers. Tumor cytoreduction via cytotoxic chemotherapy is accomplished prior to definitive therapy with radiation therapy or radical surgery. Chemotherapeutic agents may additionally be employed as radiation sensitizers to enhance response in patients with advanced disease.

Radical surgery. The surgical approach for invasive cervical cancer was first popularized by Wertheim of Vienna in the late 1800s. Because of the inherent morbidity and mortality of surgery in that era (18.9% mortality in Wertheim's first 500 cases reported in 1907),[131] and with the discovery of radium by the Curies and its tissue effects by Bequerel, radiation therapy became the standard treatment modality for invasive cervical cancer. The radical surgical approach, however, was kept alive and refined by centers in Japan, Germany, Austria, and England. The radical vaginal hysterectomy was introduced in 1901 by Schauta in an attempt to minimize the morbidity and mortality associated with the abdominal radical or Wertheim hysterectomy.[108a] This procedure permitted the wide excision of the parametrial tissues but was limited by the obvious inability to perform a lymph node dissection. Joseph Meigs reintroduced and popularized the radical hysterectomy in the United States.[78] By 1955 Liu and Meigs reported a mortality rate of 1.7% in their first 500 cases.[71] With the development of laparoscopic lymphadenectomy, several European centers are "rediscovering" the radical vaginal hysterectomy.

Radical hysterectomy. Radical hysterectomy requires removal of the uterus, cervix, parametrial tissues, and upper vagina in conjunction with a pelvic lymphadenectomy from the bifurcation of the iliac vessels to approximately the level of the inguinal ligament. The higher chains, common iliacs, and paraaortic may be sampled at the discretion of the operating surgeon. As cervical cancer rarely metastasizes to the ovaries, they may be preserved in the younger patient to avoid the need for replacement therapy. The difficulty in this operation revolves around the need to preserve the integrity and function of the adjacent structures—sidewall vessels, bladder, rectum, and ureters, and at the same time remove enough tissue to assure clearance of the cancer.

Prophylactic antibiotics and pneumatic calf-compression boots are used routinely. The surgery may be performed through either a low midline or a low transverse muscle splitting incision. The latter incision provides excellent exposure to the pelvic sidewalls and permits the common iliac nodes to be dissected as well as the low paraaortic chain. The abdomen and pelvis are carefully explored to exclude the presence of metastatic disease. Suspicious lymph nodes in the common iliac or aortic chains are sampled and sent for frozen section evaluation. Metastatic disease in these areas should be marked with clips for assistance in radiation therapy planning and the planned surgery terminated. The parametrial (cardinal and uterosacral ligaments), vesicouterine, and rectouterine tissues should similarly be carefully evaluated. Extension to these areas would suggest the need for primary radiation therapy. If the patient is considered a surgical candidate, the radical hysterectomy proceeds as follows:

1. The retroperitoneum of the pelvic sidewalls is opened by suture-ligating and dividing of the round ligaments and the peritoneum. The ureter is identified and the infundibulapelvic ligament or uteroovarian pedicle (depending on whether the ovaries are to be preserved or removed) are ligated. The pararectal and paravesical spaces may now be fully developed, providing access to the parametrial tissues. The paravesical space is bordered medially by the bladder, laterally by the obturator internus muscle, inferiorly by the external iliac vein, posteriorly by the cardinal ligament, and anteriorly by the pubic symphysis. The pararectal space is bordered medially by the rectum, laterally by the internal iliac artery and vein, posteriorly by the sacrum, and anteriorly by the cardinal ligament. In some centers the lymphadenectomy is performed at this point. Others prefer to sample only suspicious nodes and reserve the complete lymph node dissection to the end of the procedure.
2. The uterine artery is identified at its origin from the hypogastric artery, divided, and brought medially over

the ureter by dividing the lateral attachments with clips or cautery. The peritoneum covering the anterior aspect of the uterus is divided above the bladder and carefully dissected from cervix and upper vagina.

3. The ureter is then freed from its peritoneal attachments and followed to the cervical area. The tissue overlying the ureter at that point is the anterior parametrium. Keeping the ureter in clear view, right angle clamps are used to divide the anterior portion of the parametrial tunnel above the ureter, which is then ligated. Additional bladder dissection may be required at this time to provide access to the portion of vagina planned for resection.
4. Next the cul-de-sac peritoneum is incised to provide access to the rectovaginal septum. The rectum is bluntly moved away from the vagina and uterosacral ligaments. Care is taken to avoid injury to the underlying rectum. The uterosacral ligaments are isolated, divided, and ligated. The ureter must be kept in view throughout this procedure to avoid injury.
5. The residual uterosacral ligaments and parametrial and paravaginal tissues are clamped adjacent to the vagina and suture-ligated. The vagina may then be transected at a level that will ensure removal of the upper one third of the vagina, and the specimen is excised. The vagina is then closed with hemostatic, absorbable sutures.
6. The pelvic lymphadenectomy is now completed. Nodal tissue is removed from the common iliac artery and vein proximal to the bifurcation to the deep circumflex iliac vein distally. Care is taken to avoid injury to the genitofemoral nerve. The proximal and distal pedicles are ligated with either clips or sutures to aid in prevention of lymphocyst formation. The areolar tissue beneath the external iliac vein is dissected to provide access to the obturator space. Nodal tissue above the obturator nerve is dissected from the nerve. Hemoclips or ties are again placed at the distal and proximal limits of the dissection. Ten percent of patients will have an aberrant obturator vein draining into the external iliac vein. Closed suction drains are generally used to drain the pelvis and are removed after the removal of the Foley catheter.
7. If the ovaries have been preserved, they may be suspended above the pelvic brim to protect them in the event that postoperative radiation therapy is required. Alternatively the ovaries can be stabilized with several interrupted sutures to the lateral peritoneum to minimize the risk of torsion.
8. The bladder can be drained postoperatively with the urethral Foley or via a suprapubic Foley catheter placed at the time of surgery. A voiding trial is performed generally 4 to 7 days postoperatively. With demonstration of adequate bladder capacity (greater than 200 cc total volume) and low postvoid residual (less than 100 cc), the patient is usually discharged. Failure of the voiding trial may be treated by a repeated trial in several days or by discharge with a suprapubic or urethral catheter in place, followed by subsequent attempts to void in the outpatient setting. Bladder care should emphasize prevention of overdistention as this may compromise the bladder and ureters.

The operative mortality associated with radical hysterectomy is 1% or less in appropriately skilled hands; otherwise the morbidity rate may approach 30%. The complications associated with radical hysterectomy are in great part due to the extent of dissection required. Bladder dysfunction may be seen in 10% to 20% of patients because of denervation injury. Although usually transient, urinary stasis may result in chronic cystitis, ureteritis, and pyelonephritis. A rare patient may suffer permanent bladder paralysis but can learn to control micturition by developing a semiautomatic bladder that will empty itself with the aid of voluntary abdominal pressure. Urinary tract fistulas, either ureteral or vesicle, are a result of vascular compromise and may occur in 1% to 2% of cases. Thromboembolic sequelae are in great part avoided by pneumatic compression boots. Subcutaneous low-dose heparin is not as effective as compression boots and may increase the risk of lymphocysts following the pelvic lymph node dissection.

Radiation therapy. Radiation therapy is administered in most clinics in two forms: external beam whole pelvic radiation and transvaginal intracavitary cesium. The ability to cure cervical cancer with an acceptable level of complication is contingent upon intracavitary or interstitial techniques that permit high-dose delivery to the cervix and vagina, while at the same time minimizing the dose to the bladder or rectum.

External beam whole pelvic radiation is generally delivered to the patient in divided doses over the course of 4 to 5 weeks in an outpatient setting. The current dose convention for external radiation was defined by the international system of weights and measures (SI). In the past, radiation doses were defined by the rad, the *radiation absorbed dose*. More recently the SI designated the term *Gray* (Gy) to represent the absorbed dose and is equivalent to 100 rads. Therefore 1 rad equals 1 cGy. Most centers will give a single dose of 180 to 200 cGy each weekday until an accumulative dose of 4500 to 5000 cGy to the pelvis is achieved.

Transvaginal applicators allow significantly larger doses of radiation to be given to the surface of the cervix. Most applicators are placed into the vagina at the time of an examination using anesthetic. The cervix is dilated and a hollow tube (*tandem*) is placed into the endocervical canal to the fundus. Two small hollow round applicators (*ovoids*) are placed externally to the cervix in the side vaginal fornices. The bladder and rectum are packed away from the applicators using gauze.

While external beam therapy is limited to 4500 to 5000 cGy due to the tolerance of other pelvic organs, the surface of the cervix and vagina can tolerate up to 15,000 to 20,000 cGy. Typically, between 4000 to 8000 additional cGy can be given to the cervix by transvaginal application. This represents a total cervical tumor dose that is between 10,000 to 15,000 cGy. It is estimated that 10,000 cGy or more is necessary to sterilize a squamous cell tumor. Therefore the unique accessibility of the cervix for radiation therapy makes it one of the few internal cancers that can be cured by radiation therapy alone. Generally, tumors deep in the body cannot be treated adequately enough for a cure without risking serious complications to the surrounding organs. An example would be a tumor located in proximity to the small intestine. The small bowel can only tolerate a dose of 4000 to 4200 cGy without suffering serious damage.

Radiation therapy is not without moderate incidence of complications because of either inherent sensitivity or improper application. The most common difficulties following radiation treatment are cystitis and proctitis. Cystitis is usually delayed 1 year or more after treatment and is characterized by marked frequency, urgency with occasional incontinence, nocturia, dysuria, and hematuria. Results of urine specimens and cultures are usually normal, but the cystoscopic examination is diagnostic. The bladder mucosa is pale and smooth, blood vessels appear constricted, and there is a loss of normal elasticity resulting in diminished bladder capacity. The entire process is due to the late effects of radiation, namely, a gradual obliteration of capillaries and scarring of supportive tissues. Treatment is frequently unsatisfactory and protracted, but some relief may be obtained with antispasmodics and with bladder irrigations using dilute silver nitrate or analgesic oily solutions.

Proctitis usually occurs shortly after radium administration but is transient in most cases. Symptoms include diarrhea, tenesmus, and painful defecation. Relief is obtained with a preparation of diphenoxylate hydrochloride and atropine sulfate (Lomotil) or with paregoric. Analgesic rectal suppositories are useful if tenesmus persists, and some patients benefit from steroid enemas. In a few patients the radiation reaction may be delayed 1 year or more, and in these cases there may be constipation, diarrhea, and rectal bleeding. Extensive fibrosis may seriously diminish the caliber of the rectosigmoid region so that colostomy is occasionally necessary. This condition is because of a combined effect of intracavitary treatment and x-rays.

Vesicovaginal and rectovaginal fistulas are only rarely a result of radiation therapy. Usually these are due to tumor or the destruction of tumor areas by irradiation. However, poor positioning of the intracavitary applicator or overdose may result in a fistula in the absence of cancer. This is not the fault of the methods but of the technique.[118]

Pelvic inflammatory disease contraindicates the use of either intracavitary cesium or external radiation; the disease may be markedly activated or aggravated and lead to tuboovarian abscesses, septicemia, and occasionally death. If pyometra is found at the time of uterine curettage, it should be drained and antibiotics given until evidence of infection has subsided. If inflammatory tuboovarian masses are present, a preliminary salpingo-oophorectomy should be carried out prior to radiation therapy.

Vaginal stenosis may develop after radiation treatment. This may be prevented in younger women by frequent examinations and by breaking up the thin synechiae as they develop. Coitus will aid in keeping the vagina of normal size, and local application of an estrogen cream will prevent bleeding resulting from the changes that are inevitable with senescence. In older women the vagina usually closes off so that the cervix is no longer available for inspection or cytologic examination. This may restrict vaginal sexual activity and it prevents adequate follow-up by means of vaginal smears. Many of these problems may be minimized or prevented by routine use of vaginal dilators in patients treated by radiation therapy.

External radiation can cause nausea and vomiting (radiation sickness) and depression of the bone marrow with subsequent mild leukopenia. A complete blood count should be performed once weekly during the period of therapy. Similarly if severe nausea or vomiting develops during treatment, hospitalization is recommended. Phenothiazines and intravenous fluids are given. Skin hyperemia is an occasional result of external therapy, and in some individuals with fair skin, blistering and ulceration may develop. Cessation of treatment for a few days and the use of a soothing ointment will usually permit adequate healing. The skin in these areas remains "tanned" for months, after which there is a gradual whitening with dilation of capillaries and extensive telangiectasia may be evident. The use of the supervoltage technique has minimized this complication.

Other effects of radiation therapy include late small bowel obstruction and perforation and loss of ovarian function if premenopausal. Loss of hormonal function typically occurs at 1000 cGy or higher and can result in decreased libido and menopausal symptoms. Bowel obstruction or perforation may occur as late as 10 years after therapy. More often the patient may note vague lower abdominal crampy pain, irregular bowel habits, and blood in the stool. Roentgenograms may give entirely normal findings, but exploration will reveal multiple loops of small bowel adherent to each other and to adjacent structures. In the more severe forms, arteriolar occlusion may result in localized areas of necrosis with perforation. It is well to remember this possible complication of radiation therapy in the differential diagnosis of an acute abdomen.

Hot flashes and sweats typical of the artificially induced menopause may be troublesome in some patients. Estrogen replacement therapy is recommended for most patients undergoing radiation therapy for cervical cancer. This is not considered to be a hormonally responsive tumor, and there is no evidence that such therapy will bring about a recurrence of cervical cancer.

Neoadjuvant chemotherapy. In the past, chemotherapy has been used as a salvage modality in patients with recurrent disease not amenable to surgical resection or radiotherapy. Although this type of treatment had some success, a cure was rarely if ever achieved. These results led to a general disbelief that chemotherapy could play an effective role in primary cervical cancer treatment.

Based on the experiences gained from the successful use of neoadjuvant therapy in the management of squamous head and neck and anal cancers, and the fact that bulky squamous cervical disease of any stage had an elevated risk of recurrence, neoadjuvant (primary) chemotherapy has recently attracted wide usage. There are clear theoretic advantages:

1. Drug delivery should be enhanced prior to vascular compromise induced by radiotherapy or radical surgery.
2. Optimal dosing may be achieved before radiation compromise of the bone marrow or to renal compromise from fibrosis or tumor.
3. Chemo-induced cytoreduction may render some patients operable, and in others permit delivery of radiotherapy in the face of smaller volume disease.
4. Micrometastases may be treated.
5. The radiation-sensitizing effects of some chemotherapeutic agents (platinum, 5-FU) may enhance the results achieved with conventional radiation therapy.[16]

Although the concept of neoadjuvant chemotherapy (NAC) is not new in the world of oncology, its application to cervical cancer has been relatively recent. Initial studies were started in the late 1980s and early 1990s, which means 5-year survival data are not yet available. Most studies evaluate initial tumor response, and some add 2- to 3-year follow-up data while others project 5-year survival using statistic methods. Recent data indicate a mixed report on response to initial chemotherapy ranging from essentially no responses to high levels of complete or partial responses. NAC protocols include initial treatment with cisplatin in combination with bleomycin, vincristine, or methotrexate. Three to four cycles of combination chemotherapy are given and tumor response is evaluated clinically. Response rates vary from a low of 23% partial response to a high of 15% complete response and a 68% partial response.[97]

In reviewing the NAC literature, one can conclude the following:

1. Small squamous cell cervical tumors (less than 4 cm) do not benefit from primary chemotherapy if survival is the endpoint assessed.[25] Bulky squamous cell cervical cancers (greater than IIA disease) may have good clinical response to NAC, but the results after radical surgery have not been durable.[97,108,135]
2. Some questions have arisen regarding cancer cell cycle time. Resistance may occur quickly. A few preliminary studies with intensive initial chemotherapy and subsequent radiotherapy have had good responses.[87]
3. When comparing studies that used radiotherapy and not surgery for secondary treatment, radiotherapy appears to obtain a better, more durable response.[63]
4. The Society of Gynecologic Oncologists has reported, as well as others, that combination chemotherapy is no better than single agent platinum for advanced (stage IIB) squamous cell disease.[28,86]

Appropriate therapy based on clinical staging. Management of invasive cervical cancer is to a certain degree stage dependent. Stage I/IIA disease allows for the option of surgical management or radiation therapy where traditionally disease at stage IIB and beyond requires treatment with radiation. Within stage I disease, it is important to realize that surgery and radiation have the same chance for cure. How to decide which to use depends on: the age of patient (less than 65 years have surgery; greater than 65 years have radiation only), body habitus (obesity can preclude surgery), hormonal function (surgery can preserve function), and underlying medical problems.

Stage IA. The concept of minimally invasive or microinvasive cervical carcinoma was first suggested by Mestwerdt in 1947. He suggested that patients with minimal degrees of invasion (3 to 5 mm below the basement membrane) are at virtually no risk for either parametrial spread or lymph node involvement and could be treated with simple hysterectomy (Fig. 6-21). The critical issue is to identify which group of patients would benefit from more conservative therapy. The Society of Gynecologic Oncologists (SGO) has proposed the following definition: a microinvasive lesion should be defined as one in which neoplastic epithelium invades the stroma in one or more places to a depth of 3 mm or less below the base of the epithelium and in which lymphatic or vascular involvement is not demonstrated. When this definition of microinvasive cervical cancer is used, the risk of lymph node involvement is less than 1%,[110] and in most centers a total extrafascial hysterectomy performed either abdominally or vaginally without lymph node dissection may be considered adequate treatment.

In 1985 the Staging Committee of FIGO developed specific criteria for defining minimally invasive or microinvasive cervical carcinoma (Table 6-2). Stage IA-2 was defined as a preclinical cancer with a maximum depth of invasion from the basement membrane of 5 mm and maximum lateral spread of 7 mm. This depth of invasion is certainly more than the SGO definition accepts. Although stage assignment must be made according to the FIGO system, patient management in this country is based on the SGO definition.

Preliminary data indicate that cone biopsy alone may be adequate therapy for patients who fulfill the SGO definition. This should only be considered in patients desirous of retaining fertility, when cone margins are free of disease, when patient compliance for Pap smear follow-up is expected, and after appropriate counseling and informed consent.[31] Microinvasive carcinoma may also be treated with intracavitary radioactive sources alone (7000 to 9000 cGy in one or two insertions). However, since many of these patients are young, surgical treatment is preferable since it preserves normal ovarian function.

Stages IB and IIA. Patients with stages IB or IIA (confined to upper vagina) may be treated with either radical

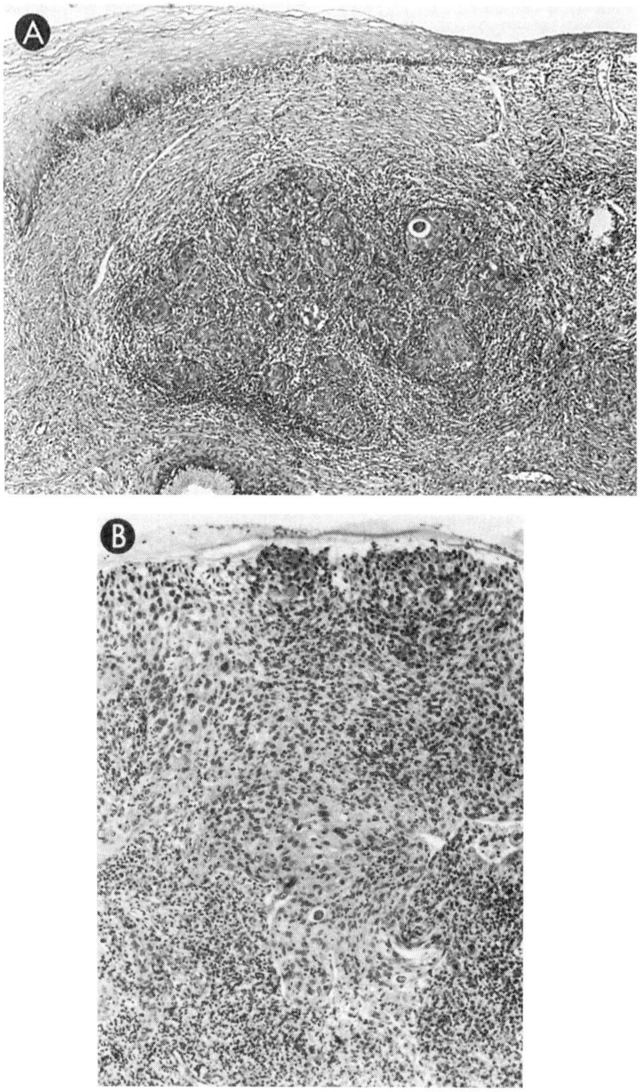

Fig. 6-21. A, Microinvasive carcinoma underlying normal portio epithelium. No other areas of invasion could be found in this cervix. CIS from which this miniature cancer must have arisen was found in the endocervix. **B,** Late stromal invasion characterized by a confluence of invasive buds into an inflamed stroma. The surface epithelium is absent on the right, but overlying CIS is visible on the left.

surgery or radiation therapy. Overall the survival for stage IB cervical cancer treated with either radiation therapy or radical surgery is approximately 85% at 5 years. For stage IIA, survival with either modality approaches 75%. Patients with extensive stage IIA disease are routinely treated with radiation therapy. Patients with involvement of the pelvic nodes diagnosed from radical hysterectomy and node dissection are often treated with postoperative pelvic radiation therapy, although there is little evidence that this approach improves survival rates. It does appear to increase the likelihood of pelvic control.[112]

Within the stage IB grouping, lesion size must be taken into consideration when deciding on treatment. In one large series of women treated by radical hysterectomy, Piver and Chung reported a 5-year survival of 85% for stage IB lesions up to 3 cm in diameter but only a 66% survival for tumors 4 to 5 cm in diameter.[91] In a later study Van Nagell et al found that for stage I lesions of more than 2 to 5 cm in diameter, the failure rate was 24% for surgery and only 11% for radiation.[127] These studies suggest that stage I lesions larger than 3 cm are best treated with radiation therapy, although it has been shown that increasing tumor size may be associated with reduced survival rates in patients treated with radiation therapy as well.[89,117] Based on these data and because of the technical difficulties in radically excising large lesions patients with tumors greater than 3 cm are usually treated with radiation therapy.

Recently, Bloss et al at the University of California, Irvine Medical Center reported that patients with a bulky cervical carcinoma of greater than 4 cm, were treated with radical hysterectomy and node dissection.[15] Adjuvant radiotherapy was tailored to the clinical picture based on such variables as nodal involvement, deep invasion, or close margins. Morbidity was adjudged similar to their experience with radical hysterectomy for smaller lesions: 50% of the patients received radiotherapy and 70% of those had a 5-year survival rate.

Patients with stage IB or IIA disease not amenable to radical surgery are usually treated with radiation therapy. If the initial bulk of disease is minimal, the tandem and ovoid can be utilized first, which decreases the amount of external beam therapy. If the initial bulk of disease is large, then external beam therapy is delivered in an attempt to achieve maximum tumor shrinkage in preparation for brachytherapy. A neoadjuvant approach may also be considered for these patients. Based on tumor size, many patients will become operable after chemo-cytoreduction.

Barrel-shaped cervix. In patients treated with a single therapy, the probability of pelvic failure increases with increasing tumor size. In surgery the risk of nodal involvement increases with increasing bulk. For radiation therapy this is due to the inability of radiation to sterilize bulky tumor masses, that likely contain hypoxic (radiation-resistant) areas. Reports suggest that conservative hysterectomy following radiation therapy to remove the bulky, central stage I disease may improve local control and increase survival.[43] This technique is frequently employed in the management of endocervical adenocarcinoma that has a propensity for endophytic growth with upward involvement and expansion of the lower uterine segment.

Stages IIB, III, and IVA. Patients with these stages of cervical carcinoma are best treated with radiation therapy techniques, since adequate dissection beyond the boundaries of the tumor is not technically feasible. External-beam therapy is expanded to encompass the common iliac nodes, the upper half of the vagina, as well as the central pelvis. Stage IIB may be treated with 4000 cGy to the pelvis, plus an additional parametrial boost to

1000 cGy delivered either before or after the intracavitary treatment. This results in a slightly higher dose to the medial parametria/lateral cervix. The 5-year survival for stage IIB treated in this fashion is 60% to 65%.

The treatment of patients with stage III disease requires a higher dose provided by external therapy. For example, 5000 cGy to the whole pelvis with an additional parametrial boost of 1000 to 1500 cGy to the involved sides may be prescribed. This would be followed by one intracavitary treatment providing a total dose to the nodal areas of 6500 to 7000 cGy and to the medial parametria/lateral cervix of 8500 to 9500 cGy. In all circumstances the higher the dose that can be provided by intracavitary therapy, the lower the dose delivered to the bladder and rectum. The 5-year survival for stage III ranges from 25% to 40%. Patients with stage IVA (bladder or rectum) can be treated with either high-dose radiation therapy or exenterative surgery. A neoadjuvant approach may be considered for patients with advanced stage disease.

Stage IVB. Patients diagnosed with distant metastases at initial presentation are rarely cured, given the limitations of conventional treatment modalities. The exception is the occasional patient with disease spread to an area that can be aggressively irradiated. For example, patients with extrapelvic disease limited to the paraaortic chain may receive extended field radiotherapy with cure rates in the 20% to 30% range at 5 years.[94] Morbidity and mortality of extended field radiation therapy following paraaortic dissection is high, usually as a result of GI dysfunction. The typical patient with stage IVB disease will receive systemic cytotoxic chemotherapy. Although the anecdotal patient may do well, the prognosis for this stage is dismal.

Recurrent cervical carcinoma. When cancer of the cervix recurs, it is usually within 2 to 3 years of primary treatment. Symptoms may include vaginal bleeding, bloody discharge, hematuria, dysuria, constipation, melena, pelvic and leg pain, edema of the leg, and fistulas. If sacral backache or pain of sciatic distribution occurs, it is invariably due to tumors of the sacral plexus.

Costovertebral angle and flank pain may herald the development of ureteral obstruction and pyelonephritis. There is usually associated lassitude, anorexia, weight loss, and anemia. Diagnosis may be simplified by routine cytologic studies on follow-up examination, since tumor cells may be detected before symptoms develop. This is applicable to recurrence in the vagina and cervix only, since a tumor in the pelvic nodes or broad ligament will not exfoliate tumor cells into the vaginal vault. In most cases the diagnosis depends on an evaluation of symptoms and a careful pelvic examination. Progressive firm nodularity in the paracervical and uterosacral area, felt best on rectal examination, is usually pathognomonic of a viable tumor.

Cervical or vaginal vault (central) recurrences should always be confirmed by biopsy. Computed axial tomography is useful for defining a tumor in enlarged lymph nodes and distant metastases. Abnormalities on the excretory urogram, such as the development of hydroureter and hydronephrosis, suggest periureteral compression by tumor—although radiation fibrosis may produce the same condition and be amenable to surgical correction by ureteral implantation or urinary diversion.

The anatomic sites of treatment failure correlate closely with tumor stage and volume. With adequate local resection or satisfactory dosimetry, any recurrences are rare in small volume stage I or IIA disease. Patients with more extensive pelvic disease generally experience treatment failure and recurrence because of the difficulty of controlling a bulky tumor with radiation therapy alone. Improved radiotherapy techniques have improved our ability to attain local control in recent years. However, because of the high incidence of failure in patients with advanced stage disease, effective systemic therapy is needed to impact on long-term survival.

Patients with recurrent cervical cancer may be treated for cure only if the disease is confined to the pelvis. Patients with central recurrence following radical hysterectomy are in general treated with radiation therapy. This combines external beam therapy with an intracavitary or interstitial approach. Salvage rates approaching 50% have been reported, although patients with massive central recurrence may be difficult to salvage with radiotherapy alone.[35] Neoadjuvant chemotherapy may be considered.

Patients who have previously been treated with radiotherapy may be treated for cure only by radical pelvic surgery. Patients with minimal disease may be considered for radical hysterectomy, although the complication rate related to fistula formation may be as high as 50% and requires permanent diversion for correction. The majority of patients, however, require ultraradical, multivisceral pelvic resection, or pelvic exenteration. This procedure entails resection of the bladder, distal ureters, rectum, vagina, internal genitalia, and parametrial tissues, and diversion of the urinary stream to a permanent conduit and the fecal stream to a colostomy. Vaginal reconstruction may be performed at the time of exenteration. Similarly, low rectal anastomosis and/or construction of a continent urinary conduit may make this procedure more acceptable to the patient. As a result of the extensive nature of this surgery and the permanent changes in organ function and body image, exenteration should be performed for cure. Patients with extra pelvic disease or with extension to the pelvic sidewalls or lymph nodes should be considered inoperable as the prognosis is dismal. Morley reported on the use of pelvic exenteration for treating recurrent cervical cancer.[80] Of more than 90 patients, 75% were treated with total pelvic exenteration; based on the location of the tumor, the remainder were treated with either resection of the bladder anteriorly or excision of the bowel posteriorly. The 5-year survival rate for recurrent carcinoma of the cervix in his series was 63%.

Ureteral compression either in the pelvis or near the kidney, with uremia, pyelonephritis, or both is a major cause of death and is found in about 50% of patients. Other causes of death are infection (peritonitis, pelvic abscess, septicemia), uncontrolled hemorrhage, and extra pelvic metastases. Patients treated for cardiac failure will sometimes have severe pulmonary edema together with edema of the arms and neck. Usually there is a redness of the face and neck. This entity is due to superior vena caval obstruction from metastatic cervical cancer.

In 13% of deaths from cancer of the cervix, the cause was gastrointestinal tract involvement that usually manifests itself as a large bowel obstruction at the rectosigmoid level. Occasionally, perforation of the large or small bowel results in fatal peritonitis. Jaundice caused by extensive hepatic metastases may be noted terminally.

Chemotherapy. A variety of single agents have been employed in the treatment of women with recurrent squamous cell carcinoma of the cervix, with cisplatin uniformly yielding response rates of 25% to 30%. Other active agents include 5-FU, mitomycin, ifosfamide, adriamycin, vincristine, and bleomycin. In general the response rates with combination therapy have been higher, although at the expense of increased toxicity.[57] The majority of combinations have included platinum with frequent response rates of 50% to 70%.[2,68,106] Although these would appear to be acceptable results, the durations of response have been dismally short, 4 to 6 months in most series with only the occasional patient reaching a complete response. Several factors contribute to these poor results:

1. Pelvic radiation therapy compromises bone marrow reserve.
2. Renal insufficiency secondary to tumor recurrence or radiation fibrosis limits adequate drug dosing.
3. Radiation fibrosis or vascular distortion associated with radical surgery may impair drug delivery.

In an attempt to bypass these issues, upfront chemotherapy used neoadjuvantly or as a radiation sensitizer, is gaining widespread acceptance. Additionally there are reports of using chemotherapy either with or without radiation therapy in patients found to be node positive following radical hysterectomy and node dissection.[121]

Carcinoma of the cervix in pregnancy

Carcinoma of the cervix complicates pregnancy in approximately 0.01% of patients. Therapeutic decisions are based on the stage of the cancer, pregnancy trimester, and the wishes of the pregnant woman. Although pregnancy does not appear to have a detrimental effect on the course of the disease, it is essential that the diagnosis be made promptly since delay in treatment can alter prognosis. Vaginal delivery does not affect prognosis either.

Prior to the third trimester, treatment for the malignancy is carried out according to the stage of disease. For stage I and IIA lesions, radical hysterectomy with pelvic lymph node dissection is acceptable therapy. If radiation therapy is planned, the uterus may be evacuated at the time of the first radium application or whole-pelvis irradiation may be started. If abortion does not occur, surgical evacuation of the uterus follows the completion of external irradiation at the time of radium application.

For patients in the late second trimester, therapy may be delayed until fetal viability is assured. For stage I and IIA lesions, a classic cesarean section is performed, followed immediately by radical hysterectomy and pelvic lymph node dissection. In more advanced stages, external radiation is delivered after cesarean section. This usually requires a delay of 7 to 10 days until the abdominal incision has healed. After completion of the radiation therapy, intracavitary radiation is employed as outlined earlier for the appropriate stage.

Clear cell adenocarcinoma of the cervix

The incidence of clear cell adenocarcinoma in women exposed in utero to diethylstilbestrol (DES) is 1:1000 of women exposed. This low-risk level indicates that DES is not a complete carcinogen but requires some other factor in order to induce cancer. Cases have occurred in women as young as 16- to 27-years old with a median age of 19 years. Follow-up of the DES-exposed women consists of annual Pap smears from the cervix and vaginal walls and careful palpation of the vaginal walls for evidence of adenosis or masses.[30]

There remains some controversy over whether DES-exposed women are more likely to develop intraepithelial neoplasia of the vagina and/or cervix compared to non-exposed women. Since there is no conclusive evidence either way, yearly Pap smears are recommended with referral for colposcopy when any abnormality appears.[30] In mothers who took DES during pregnancy, there appears to be an increased rate of breast cancer of 1.35. This risk does not appear to increase with age.[29]

Treatment for cervical clear cell adenocarcinoma is similar to that outlined for squamous cell carcinoma of the cervix. However, because of the young age of these women the preferred therapy is radical hysterectomy and pelvic lymph node dissection in patients with stage I and IIA disease. Ovarian conservation is maintained; if the vagina is involved, a vaginectomy followed by reconstruction is performed, which provides excellent functional results.

The overall survival for women with DES-associated clear cell carcinoma is 80%. In cases of stage I disease, the 5-year survival exceeds 90%.

Although most DES-related clear cell carcinomas appear to recur within 3 years of the initial treatment, late recurrences have been reported. Burks et al reported the longest interval to recurrence was 17 years after initial therapy; they recommended long-term yearly follow-up with periodic chest x-rays.[24] Pulmonary and supraclavicular nodal metastases are more frequent when compared with squamous cell carcinoma of either the cervix or the vagina. If there is local recurrence without side wall involvement, pelvic exenteration may be considered. If either aortic or pelvic nodes are involved, exenteration is contraindicated.[64]

Carcinoma of the cervical stump

In the past decades subtotal hysterectomy has become somewhat unusual and accounts for a decreased incidence of cervical stump cancers. Recently, with increased interest in minimally invasive surgery and attempts to preserve sexual function, there may be an increase in the incidence of stump cancers.

Carcinoma of the cervical stump poses special challenges to the treating physician, both from a surgical and a radiotherapeutic standpoint. Radical cervicectomy and pelvic lymph node dissection may be performed. However, the prior surgery may have introduced fibrosis and scarring to the retroperitoneum, significantly increasing the difficulty of the ureteral dissections. Morbidity and outcome, however, have been similar to that reported for treatment by radical hysterectomy.[33]

Radiotherapy may be compromised by the inability to employ a uterine tandem, which is critical in dosing the central tumor and medial parametria. Transvaginal or interstitial therapy is commonly used when a tandem cannot be employed, and in most circumstances the dose administered via external beam to the pelvis must be increased. These changes in dose as well as the likelihood of adhesions to the bowel at the vaginal apex suggest that survival may be compromised by increased complications. Survival in most series, however, is similar to that seen in patients treated with an intact uterus, although the complication rate may be modestly increased.[83,133]

Incidental invasive cervical carcinoma found at conservative hysterectomy

Invasive carcinoma may be discovered following a hysterectomy performed for benign indications. This may occur when emergent surgery precludes complete cervical evaluation, or as a result of inadequate evaluation prior to elective surgery, or when a hysterectomy is performed following a false-negative Pap test. Prognosis is related to the extent of tumor present. Patients with apparently minimal disease confined to the cervix do well. In contrast, patients with more extensive disease with tumors do poorly.[6] Patients treated with radiation therapy may have similar problems to those encountered when treating stump cancers, or with exploration, radical parametrectomy, and node dissection that obviate the increased complication rate associated with radical radiotherapy.[84]

Cervical adenocarcinoma

In the past, cervical adenocarcinomas accounted for perhaps 5% of the total number of invasive cervical cancers treated in the United States. More recently this relative proportion has increased, with glandular tumors accounting for 10% to 20% of the total. This in part arises from an absolute decrease in the number of squamous cell carcinomas as well as a probable absolute increase in the number of adenocarcinomas. From a diagnostic standpoint, early diagnosis is difficult. The false-negative rate of Pap testing may be as high as 80% despite occult cervical adenocarcinoma. Many patients are diagnosed once symptoms of bleeding or discharge are noted.[55]

These lesions arise from the endocervical epithelium and have a propensity for endophytic growth and upward spread to the lower uterine segment. Frequently this gives rise to bulky tumors in a barrel-shaped distribution. The pattern of spread is otherwise similar to that seen with squamous tumors. A higher local failure rate for these tumors when treated with radiation therapy suggests that these are relatively radiation-resistant when compared to the squamous lesions. However, the higher local failure rate is probably because of higher tumor volume secondary to its distinctive pattern of spread. As a result, many investigators have recommended a combined modality approach with radiotherapy followed by simple hysterectomy, similar to that recommended for patients with barrel-shaped squamous cell carcinoma of the cervix.[10] Radical hysterectomy and node dissection remains an excellent treatment option for these patients. This treatment obviates the issues surrounding extensive central uterine disease. Patients with recurrent disease are treated in a manner similar to that employed for the squamous tumors. The role of chemotherapy, however, is yet to be defined as the agents now available have little effect on these lesions.

Unusual histologies and cancer metastatic to the uterine cervix

Sarcoma. Sarcomas account for approximately 0.5% of all cervical cancers.[105] Histologically these tumors are classified in a manner similar to other uterine sarcomas—heterologous and homologous. These tumors are exceedingly uncommon and hence must be differentiated from corpus primaries by the following criteria[1]:

1. The uterus must be available for examination with the neoplasm confined to the cervix and the corpus histologically uninvolved.
2. The tumor must appear to arise from the cervix, and the endometrial curettings must be histologically negative with no enlargement of the corpus.
3. If the tumor arises from a cervical stump, the previous subtotal hysterectomy specimen must be examined to exclude the presence of a corpus primary.

Therapy usually entails total hysterectomy with consideration of adjunctive radiation or chemotherapy.

Small cell and neuroendocrine small cell carcinoma. Small cell carcinomas of the cervix account for 1% to 6% of all cervical cancers. Further classification by the pathologist is small cell squamous cell carcinoma, which is managed in a manner similar to that for other cervical squamous cancers, and neuroendocrine small cell carcinoma, which requires more aggressive therapy and carries a dismal prognosis. These latter tumors may arise from either the argyrophil cells of the cervix (part of the APUD system) or from subcolumnar reserve cells and are histologically identical to oat cell carcinoma of the lung. These tumors have a high propensity for early lymphatic and systemic spread and are currently treated aggressively with a combined modality approach including surgery, radiation, and chemotherapy.[113]

Verrucous carcinoma. Verrucous carcinoma is a rare, extremely well-differentiated, squamous cell carcinoma that grows in a papillary pattern, mimicking the growth pattern of condylomata. These tumors demonstrate only an occasional mitosis, and only minimal cytologic atypia is noted. A pushing rather than an infiltrative border is seen, and the adjacent tissues show a marked inflammatory response. This inflammatory response may initially suggest the diagnosis. Clinically these tumors exhibit slow growth and limited potential for distal spread. Surgical resection is recommended as radiation therapy has little effect on these lesions and in fact may induce anaplastic transformation.

Others. Lymphoma, melanoma, and carcinoid tumors rarely arise in the cervix. The reader is referred to a gynecologic oncology text for more information regarding these lesions.

Cancer metastatic to the uterine cervix. A variety of tumors may metastasize to the cervix, and cervical cytology may be the first indication of a malignancy. Endometrial, bladder, and rectal cancer may spread directly to the cervix. Intraabdominal cancers may involve the cervix as a sequelae of extensive pelvic involvement and extension via the vagina, uterus, or uterosacral ligaments. On occasion, hematogenous spread may occur to the uterus or cervix from such sites as the breast or lung. Therapy is aimed at the primary site of origin.

REFERENCES

1. Abell MR, Ramirez JA: Sarcomas and carcinomas of the uterine cervix, *Cancer* 31:1176-1180, 1973.
2. Alberts DS, Mason-Liddil N: The role of cisplatin in the management of advanced squamous cell cancer of the cervix, *Semin Oncol* (Suppl 6), 16:66-78, 1989.
3. Am Coll Obstet Gynecol Newslett: ACOG and other organizations draw closer on frequency of Pap smears, *ACOG Newsletter* 32:1, 1988.
4. American College of Obstetrics and Gynecology Committee Opinion: *Report of the task force on routine cancer screening*, Washington DC, *ACOG Committee Opinion* 68:1, 1989.
5. Anderson MD, Hartley RB: Cervical crypt involvement by intraepithelial neoplasia, *Obstet Gynecol* 55:546, 1980.
6. Andras EJ, Fletcher GH: Radiotherapy of carcinoma of the cervix following simple hysterectomy, *Am J Obstet Gynecol* 115:647-651, 1973.
7. Anonymous: Invasive squamous-cell cervical carcinoma and combined oral contraceptives: results from a multinational study, WHO collaborative study of neoplasia and steroid contraceptives, *Int J Cancer* 55(2):228-236, 1993.
8. Ayre JE: Selective cytology smear for diagnosis of cancer, *Am J Obstet Gynecol* 53:604, 1947.
9. Bearman DM et al: Papanicolaou smear history of patients developing cervical cancer: an assessment of screening protocols, *Obstet Gynecol* 69:151, 1987.
10. Berek JS, Castaldo TW: Adenocarcinoma of the uterine cervix, *Cancer* 48:2734-2741, 1981.
11. Bergeron C et al: Multicentric human papillomavirus infections of the female genital tract: correlation of viral types with abnormal mitotic figures, colposcopic presentation and location, *Obstet Gynecol* 69:736, 1987.
12. Berkowitz RS et al: Invasive cervical cancer in young women, *Gynecol Oncol* 8:311, 1979.
13. 1988 Bethesda System for reporting cervical/vaginal cytologic diagnoses, *JAMA* 262(7):931-934, 1989.
14. Blaustein A, editor: *Pathology of the female genital tract*, ed 2, New York, 1982, Springer-Verlag.
15. Bloss JD et al: Bulky stage IB cervical carcinoma managed by primary radical hysterectomy followed by tailored radiotherapy, *Gynecol Oncol* 47:21-27, 1992.
16. Bonomi P, Blessing J: A phase II evaluation of cisplatin and 5-fluorouracil in patients with advanced squamous cell carcinoma of the cervix: a gynecologic oncology group study, *Gynecol Oncol* 34:357-359, 1989.
17. Boring CC, Squires TS, Tong T: Cancer statistics, 1993, *CA Cancer J Clin* 43(1):7-26, 1993.
18. Borken M, Friedman EA: Duration of colposcopic changes associated with *Trichomonas vaginitis*, *Obstet Gynecol* 51:111, 1979.
19. Broders AC: Carcinoma grading and practical application, *Arch Pathol* 2:376, 1926.
20. Buchsbaum HJ: Extrapelvic lymph node metastases in cervical carcinoma, *Am J Obstet Gynecol* 133:814, 1979.
21. Buckley CH et al: Cervical intraepithelial neoplasia, *J Clin Pathol* 35:1, 1982.
22. Bulmer D: The development of the human vagina, *J Anat* 91:490, 1957.
23. Burger MP et al: Cigarette smoking and human papillomavirus in patients with reported cervical cytological abnormality, *BMJ* 306(6880):749-752, 1993.
24. Burks RT et al: Late recurrence of clear-cell adenocarcinoma of the cervix: case report, *Obstet Gynecol* 76(3 Pt 2):525-527, 1990.
25. Chang HC et al: Neoadjuvant chemotherapy with cisplatin, vincristine, and bleomycin and radical surgery in early-stage bulky cervical carcinoma, *Cancer Chemother Pharmacol* 30(4):281-285, 1992.
26. Christopherson WM, Gray LA: Dysplasia and preclinical carcinoma of the uterine cervix: diagnosis and management, *Semin Oncol* 9:265, 1982.
27. Chung CK et al: Histologic grade and prognosis of carcinoma of the cervix, *Obstet Gynecol* 57:636, 1981.
28. Coleman RE et al: A phase II study of ifosfamide and cisplatin chemotherapy for metastatic or relapsed carcinoma of the cervix, *Cancer Chemother Pharmacol* 27:52-54, 1990.
29. Colton T et al: Breast cancer in mothers prescribed diethylstilbestrol in pregnancy: further follow-up, *JAMA* 269(16):2096-2100, 1993.
30. Committee on Gynecologic Practice: Diethylstilbestrol, *ACOG Committee Opinion* 131:1, 1993.
31. Copeland LJ, Silva EG: Superficially invasive squamous cell carcinoma of the cervix, *Gynecol Oncol* 45:307-312, 1992.
32. Coppleson M, Reid BL: *Preclinical carcinoma of the cervix uteri*, New York, 1967, Pergamon Press.
33. Creadick RN: Carcinoma of the cervical stump, *Am J Obstet Gynecol* 75:564-567, 1958.
34. Creasman WT et al: Results of outpatient therapy of cervical intraepithelial neoplasia, *Obstet Gynecol* 12:5306, 1981.
35. Deutsch M, Parsons JA: Radiotherapy for carcinoma of the cervix recurrent after surgery, *Cancer* 34:205, 1974.
36. Eddy DM: Screening for cervical cancer, *Ann Intern Med* 113:214-226, 1990.
37. Ferenczy A: Anatomy and histology of the cervix. In Blaustein A, editor: *Pathology of the female genital tract*, ed 2, New York, 1982, Springer-Verlag.

38. Ferenczy A: Comparison of cryo- and carbon dioxide laser therapy for cervical intraepithelial neoplasia, *Obstet Gynecol* 66:793-797, 1985.
39. Ferenczy A et al: Latent papillomavirus and recurring genital warts, *N Engl J Med* 313:784, 1985.
40. Fluhmann CF: Developmental anatomy of the cervix uteri, *Obstet Gynecol* 15:62, 1960.
41. Forsberg JG: Origin of vaginal epithelium, *Obstet Gynecol* 25:787, 1965.
42. Forsberg JG: Estrogen, vaginal cancer, and vaginal development, *Am J Obstet Gynecol* 113:83, 1972.
42a. Frisch LE: Inflammatory atypia and the false-negative smear in cervical intraepithelial neoplasia, *Acta Cytol* 31:873-7, 1987.
43. Gallion HH: Combined radiation therapy and extrafascial hysterectomy in the treatment of stage IB barrel-shaped cervical cancer, *Cancer* 56:262, 1985.
44. Galloway DA, McDougall JK: The oncogenic potential of herpes simplex viruses: evidence for a "hit and run" mechanism, *Nature* 302:22, 1983.
45. Garite TJ, Feldman MJ: An evaluation of cytologic sampling techniques: a comparative study, *Acta Cytol* 22:13, 1978.
46. Gissmann L, zur Hausen H: Partial characterization of viral DNA from human genital warts (condylomata acuminata), *Int J Cancer* 25:605, 1980.
47. Gram IT, Austin H, Stalsberg H: Cigarette smoking and the incidence of cervical intraepithelial neoplasia, grade III, and cancer of the cervix uteri, *Am J Epidemiol* 135(4):341-346, 1992.
48. Grunebaum AN et al: Association of human papillomavirus infection with cervical intraepithelial neoplasia, *Obstet Gynecol* 62:448, 1983.
49. Handley WS: The prevention of cancer, *Lancet* 1:987, 1936.
50. Harlan LC, Bernstein AM, Kessler LG: Cervical cancer screening: who is not screened and why? *Am J Public Health* 81:885-890, 1991.
51. Hellman LM et al: Some factors influencing the proliferation of the reserve cells in the human cervix, *Am J Obstet Gynecol* 67:899, 1954.
52. Holly EA et al: Detection of mutagens in cervical mucus in smokers and nonsmokers, *Cancer Epidemiol Biomarkers Prev* 2(3):223-228, 1993.
53. Howley PM: Role of the human papillomaviruses in human cancer, *Cancer Res* 51:5019s-5022s, 1991.
54. Huffman J: Mesonephric remnants in the cervix, *Am J Obstet Gynecol* 56:233, 1948.
55. Hurt GW et al: Adenocarcinoma of the cervix: histologic and clinical features, *Am J Obstet Gynecol* 129:304, 1977.
56. Jha PK et al: Antibodies to human papillomavirus and to other genital infectious agents and invasive cervical cancer risk, *Lancet* 341(8853):1116-1118, 1993.
57. Jobson VW et al: Chemotherapy of advanced carcinoma of the cervix with cyclophosphamide and cis-platinum, *Proc Am Soc Clin Oncol* 22:475, 1981.
58. Johnson LD et al: The histogenesis of carcinoma in situ of the uterine cervix: a preliminary report of the origin of carcinoma in situ in subcylindrical cell anaplasia, *Cancer* 17:213, 1964.
59. Josey WE et al: Genital infection with type II herpesvirus hominis, *Am J Obstet Gynecol* 101:718, 1968.
60. Klassen AC, Celentano DD, Brookmeyer R: Variation in the duration of protection given by screening using the Pap test for cervical cancer, *J Clin Epidemiol* 42:1003-1011, 1989.
61. Kessler II: Human cervical cancer as a venereal disease, *Cancer Res* 36:783, 1976.
62. Kessler II: Etiological concepts in cervical carcinogenesis, *Gynecol Oncol* 12:57, 1981.
63. Killackey MA, Boardman L, Carroll DS: Adjuvant chemotherapy and radiation in patients with poor prognostic stage IB/IIA cervical cancer, *Gynecol Oncol* 49:377-379, 1993.
64. Knapp RC: Clear cell carcinoma of the vagina. In Heintz APM, Griffiths CT, Trimbos JB, editors: *Surgery in gynecological oncology*, The Hague, 1984, Martinus Nijhoff.
65. Koff AK: Development of the vagina in the human fetus, *Contrib Embryol Carnegie Inst* 24:54, 1993.
66. Kolstad P, Klem V: Long term follow-up of 1121 cases of carcinoma in situ, *Obstet Gynecol* 48:125, 1976.
67. Koss LG, Durfee GR: Unusual patterns of squamous epithelium of uterine cervix: cytologic and pathologic study of koilocytotic atypia, *Ann NY Acad Sci* 63:1235, 1956.
68. Kumar L, Bhargava VL: Chemotherapy in recurrent and advanced cervical cancer, *Gynecol Oncol* 40:107-111, 1991.
69. Lagasse LD: Results and complications of operative staging in cervical cancer: experience of the Gynecologic Oncology Group, *Gynecol Oncol* 9:90, 1980.
70. Langman J: *Medical embryology*, Baltimore, 1981, Williams & Wilkins.
71. Liu W, Meigs JV: Radical hysterectomy and pelvic lymphadenectomy, *Am J Obstet Gynecol* 69:1, 1955.
72. Lorincz AT et al: Characterization of human papillomaviruses in cervical neoplasias and their detection in routine clinical screening. In Peto R, zur Hausen H, editors: *Viral etiology of cervical cancer*, Banbury Report 21, New York, 1986, Cold Spring Harbor Laboratory.
73. MacDonald-Burns DC: *Chlamydia* and other genital pathogens, *Clin Obstet Gynecol* 8:215, 1981.
74. Maier RC, Norris HJ: Glassy cell carcinoma of the cervix, *Obstet Gynecol* 60:219, 1982.
75. McCann MF et al: Nicotine and cotinine in the cervical mucus of smokers, passive smokers, and nonsmokers, *Cancer Epidemiol Biomarkers Prev* 1(2):125-129, 1992.
76. Meanwell CA: The epidemiology of human papillomavirus infection in relation to cervical cancer, *Cancer Sur* 7:481-497, 1988.
77. Mecsie R et al: Genital *Chlamydia trachomatis* infections in patients with abnormal cervical smears: effect of tetracycline treatment on cell changes, *Obstet Gynecol* 73:317-321, 1989.
78. Meigs JV: Carcinoma of the cervix: the Wertheim operation, *Surg Gynecol Obstet* 78:1, 1944.
79. Meisels A et al: Condylomatous lesions of the cervix. II. Cytologic, colposcopic, and histopathologic study, *Acta Cytol* 21:379, 1977.
80. Morley GW: Pelvic exenteration in the treatment of recurrent cervical cancer. In Heintz APM, Griffiths CT, Trimbos JB, editors: *Surgery in gynecologic oncology*, The Hague, 1984, Martinus Nijhoff.
81. Murdoch JB et al: Histological incomplete excision of CIN after large-loop excision of the transformation zone (LLETZ) merits careful follow up, not retreatment, *Br J Obstet Gynaecol* 99:990-993, 1992.
82. Nahmias AJ, Sawanabani S: The genital herpes-cervical cancer hypothesis—10 years later, *Prog Exp Tumor Res* 21:117, 1978.
83. Oats JJ: Carcinoma of the cervical stump, *Br J Obstet Gynecol* 83:896-900, 1976.
84. Orr JW: Surgical treatment of women found to have invasive cervical cancer at the time of total hysterectomy, *Obstet Gynecol* 68:353-355, 1986.
85. Paavonen J: Colposcopic and histologic findings in cervical *Chlamydia* infection, *Obstet Gynecol* 59:712, 1982.
86. Park RC, Thigpen JT: Chemotherapy in advanced and recurrent cervical cancer: a review, *Cancer* 71:1446-1450, 1993.
87. Park TK et al: Role of induction chemotherapy in invasive cervical cancer, *Gynecol Oncol* 41:107-112, 1991.
88. Parsons WL et al: Prevalence of cervical pathogens in women with and without inflammatory changes on smear testing, *BMJ* 306(6886):1173-1174, 1993.
89. Patanaphan V, Poussin-Rusillo H: Cancer of uterine cervix stage IB treatment results and prognostic factors, *Cancer* 57:866-870, 1986.
90. Piver MS, Barlow JJ: Paraaortic lymphadenectomy in staging patients with advanced local cervical cancer, *Obstet Gynecol* 43:544, 1974.

91. Piver MS, Chung WS: Prognostic significance of cervical lesion size and pelvic node metastases in cervical carcinoma, *Obstet Gynecol* 46:507, 1975.
92. Piver MS et al: Hydroxyurea and radiation therapy in advanced cervical cancer, *Am J Obstet Gynecol* 120:969, 1974.
93. Plentl AA, Friedman EA: Clinical significance of cervical lymphatics. In *Lymphatic systems of the female genitalia,* Philadelphia, 1971, WB Saunders.
94. Potish RA et al: The utility and limitations of decision theory in the utilization of surgical staging and extended field radiotherapy in cervical cancer, *Obstet Gynecol Surv* 39:555, 1984.
95. Prendiville W, Cullimore J, Norman S: Large-loop excision of the transformation zone (LLETZ): a new method of management for women with cervical intraepithelial neoplasia, *Br J Obstet Gynecol* 96:1054-1060, 1989.
96. Prendiville W, Davies R, Berry PJ: A low voltage diathermy loop for taking cervical biopsies: a qualitative comparison with punch biopsy forceps, *Br J Obstet Gynaecol* 93:773-776, 1986.
97. Rabinovich MG et al: Neo-adjuvant chemotherapy for cervical carcinoma, *Obstet Gynecol* 78:685, 1991.
98. Rawls WE et al: Herpes virus type II: association with carcinoma of the cervix, *Science* 161:1255, 1968.
99. Reagan JW et al: Concepts of genesis and development in early cervical neoplasia, *Obstet Gynecol Surv* 24:860, 1969.
100. Reeves WC, Rawls WE, Brinton LA: Epidemiology of genital papillomaviruses and cervical cancer, *Rev Infect Dis* 11:426-435, 1989.
101. Rein M, Hart G: Gonococcal infection. In Top FH, Wehrle PF, editors: *Communicable and infectious diseases,* St Louis, 1976, CV Mosby.
102. Richart RM: A radioautographic analysis of cellular proliferation in dysplasia and carcinoma in situ of the uterine cervix, *Am J Obstet Gynecol* 86:925, 1963.
103. Richart RM: Influence of diagnostic and therapeutic procedures in the distribution of cervical intraepithelial neoplasia, *Cancer* 19:1635, 1966.
104. Rigoni-Stern: In The Walton report, *Can Med Assoc J* 114:2, 1976.
105. Rotmensch J: Cervical sarcoma: a review, *Obstet Gynecol Surv* 38:456-465, 1983.
106. Rotmensch J, Senekjian EK: Evaluation of bolus cis-platinum and continuous 5-fluorouracil infusion for metastatic and recurrent squamous cell carcinoma of the cervix, *Gynecol Oncol* 29:76-81, 1988.
107. Rubinstein E: CO_2 laser vaporization for chronic cervicitis, *Lasers Surg Med* 5(6):563-569, 1985.
108. Sardi J et al: Results of a prospective randomized trial with neoadjuvant chemotherapy in stage IB, bulky, squamous carcinoma of the cervix, *Gynecol Oncol* 49:156-165, 1993.
108a. Schauta F: Die operation des Gebarmutterkrebes mittels des Schuchardt'schen paravaginalschnittes, *Montasschr. Geburtsh. u. Gynäk*, 15:133, 1902.
109. Schiffman MH et al: Epidemiologic evidence showing that human papillomavirus infection causes most cervical intraepithelial neoplasia, *J Nat Cancer Instit* 12:958-963, 1993.
110. Seski JC et al: Microinvasive squamous carcinoma of the cervix, *Obstet Gynecol* 50:410, 1977.
111. Sevin BU et al: Invasive cancer of the cervix after cryosurgery: pitfalls of conservative management, *Obstet Gynecol* 53:465, 1979.
112. SGO Panel Report: Is pelvic radiation beneficial in the postoperative management of stage IB squamous cell carcinoma of the cervix with pelvic node metastasis treated by radical hysterectomy and pelvic lymphadenectomy? *Gynecol Oncol* 10:105, 1980.
113. Sheets EE et al: Surgically treated early-stage neuroendocrine small-cell cervical carcinoma, *Obstet Gynecol* 71:1-10, 1988.
114. Song J: *The human uterus: morphogenesis and embryological basis for cancer,* Springfield, Ill, 1964, Charles C Thomas.
115. Speroff L, Glass RH, Kase N: *Clinical gynecologic endocrinology and infertility,* Baltimore, 1985, Williams & Wilkins.
116. Spriggs AI, Boddington MM: Progression and regression of cervical lesions: review of smears from women followed without initial biopsy or treatment, *J Clin Pathol* 33:517, 1980.
117. Stehman FB, Bundy BN: Carcinoma of the cervix treated with radiation therapy I, *Cancer* 67:2776-2785, 1991.
118. Stryker JA et al: Bladder and rectal complications following radiotherapy for cervical cancer, *Gynecol Oncol* 29:1, 1988.
119. Syrjanen KJ: Current concepts of human papillomavirus infections in the genital tract and the relationship to intraepithelial neoplasia and squamous cell carcinoma, *Obstet Gynecol Surv* 39:252, 1984.
120. Syrjanen K, Syrjanen S: Epidemiology of human papillomavirus infections and genital neoplasia, *Scand J Infect Dis Suppl* 69:7-17, 1990.
121. Tattersall MHN, Ramirez C: A randomized trial of adjuvant chemotherapy after radical hysterectomy in stage IB-IIA cervical cancer patients with pelvic lymph node metastases, *Gynecol Oncol* 46:176-181, 1992.
122. Taylor PT et al: The screening Papanicolaou smear: contribution of the endocervical brush, *Obstet Gynecol* 70:734, 1987.
123. Townsend DE, Richart RM: Cryotherapy and carbon dioxide laser management of cervical intraepithelial neoplasia: a controlled comparison, *Obstet Gynecol* 61:75, 1983.
124. Van Den Brule AJ et al: Difference in prevalence of human papillomavirus genotypes in cytomorphologically normal cervical smears is associated with a history of cervical intraepithelial neoplasia, *Int J Cancer* 48(3):404-408, 1991.
125. Van Doornum GJ et al: Prevalence of human papillomavirus infections among heterosexual men and women with multiple sexual partners, *J Med Virol* 37(1):13-21, 1992.
126. VanEenwyk J, Davis FG, Colman N: Folate, vitamin C, and cervical intraepithelial neoplasia, *Cancer Epidemiol Biomarkers Prev* 1(2):119-124, 1992.
127. Van Nagell JR et al: Therapeutic implications for patterns of recurrence in cancer of the uterine cervix, *Cancer* 44:2354, 1979.
128. Wagner AC, McElin TW: Colposcopy. In Sciarra JT, editor: *Gynecology and obstetrics*, vol 1, New York, 1984, Harper & Row.
129. Weitzman GA et al: Endocervical brush cytology, an alternative to endocervical curettage? *J Reprod Med* 33:677, 1988.
130. Wentz WB, Reagan JW: Survival in cervical cancer with respect to cell type, *Cancer* 12:384, 1959.
131. Wertheim E: The radical abdominal operation in carcinoma of the cervix uteri, *Surg Gynecol Obstet* 4:1, 1907.
132. Willmott FE: Mucopurulent cervicitis: a clinical entity? *Genitourin Med* 64(3):169-171, 1988.
133. Wimbush PR, Fletcher GH: Radiation therapy of carcinoma of the cervical stump, *Radiology* 93:655-659, 1969.
134. Wright TC Jr. et al: Treatment of cervical intraepithelial neoplasia using the loop electrosurgical excision procedure, *Obstet Gynecol* 79:173-178, 1992.
135. Zanetta G et al: Three-year results after neoadjuvant chemotherapy, radical surgery, and radiotherapy in locally advanced cervical carcinoma, *Obstet Gynecol* 82:447-450, 1993.
136. zur Hausen H: Papillomaviruses in human cancers, *Mol Carcinog* 1:147-150, 1988.
137. zur Hausen H et al: Viruses and the etiology of human genital cancer, *Prog Med Virol* 30:170, 1984.

Chapter 7

THE UTERINE CORPUS

Michael G. Muto
Andrew J. Friedman

GENERAL CONSIDERATIONS

The principal function of the uterine corpus is to allow for normal childbearing. The corpus is uniquely designed to sustain, protect, and ultimately deliver the fetus. Menstruation occurs only when the process of ovulation is not followed by successful fertilization and should not be regarded as a primary function.

The uterus consists of two portions, the corpus and the cervix. The uterine corpus, the focus of this chapter, consists of the thick muscular myometrium and the thin lining epithelium, the endometrium. The myometrium gives rise to the most common solid tumor in women, the leiomyoma. Leiomyomas are present in up to one third of all women in their reproductive years and are a major indication for hysterectomy. The endometrial cavity is frequently the site of both hyperplasia and neoplasia. These conditions frequently result in irregular bleeding. Because the uterine cavity is readily available for thorough investigation by endometrial biopsy, such premalignant or malignant conditions lend themselves to early diagnosis. Effective therapy has led to excellent outcomes for women with endometrial carcinoma.

An understanding of the anatomy of the uterine corpus, developmental anomalies, and benign, premalignant and malignant conditions are essential for the student of obstetrics and gynecology.

ANATOMY

The uterus (Fig. 7-1) is a muscular, hollow organ that lies in the true pelvis between the bladder and rectum. The cephalic portion of the corpus is known as the fundus and is characterized by lateral flarings known as the *cornua*. The fallopian tubes enter the fundus in the region of these cornua and demarcate the fundus from the main body of the uterus. As the corpus approaches the cervix, it becomes narrowed. This constricted area separates the corpus from the cervix and is known as the *isthmus*. The cavity of the corpus is continuous with that of the endocervix and vagina; it has an average depth of about 6 cm and a capacity of 3 to 8 mL.

The corpus possesses anterior and posterior surfaces, which are covered by visceral peritoneum. The anterior surface lies in contact with the most cephalad portion of the urinary bladder. As the uterine peritoneum approaches the region of the isthmus on the anterior uterine wall, it is reflected ventrally onto the bladder and then continues as the parietal layer. The narrow space between these layers of reflected peritoneum is known as the anterior cul-de-sac. A

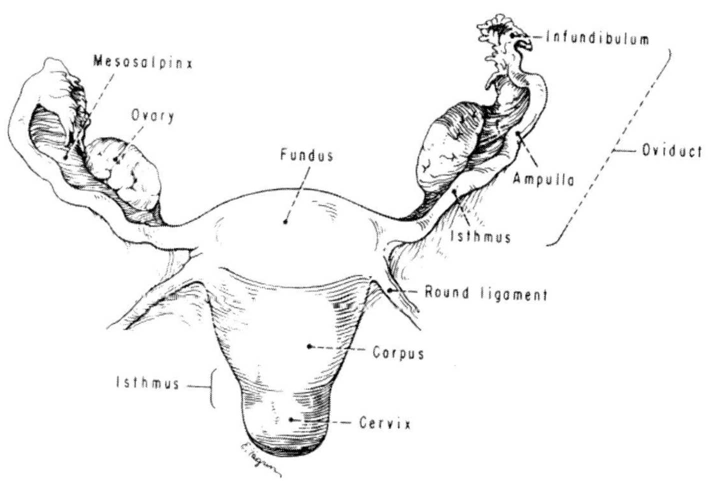

Fig. 7-1. Anterior view of uterus.

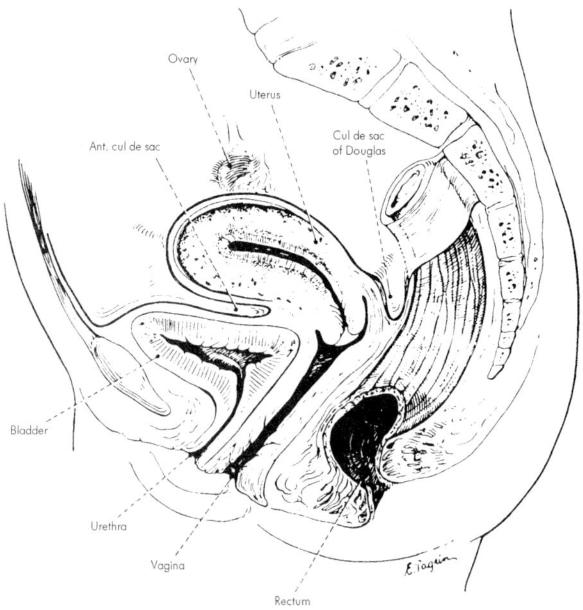

Fig. 7-2. Sagittal section through pelvis.

sagittal section through the normal female pelvis (Fig. 7-2) shows that the anterior surface of the uterine isthmus is not covered by peritoneum. The posterior surface of the corpus is completely invested with a peritoneal covering. Caudally this peritoneal envelope is continued over the uterosacral ligaments, cervix, and upper portion of the posterior vaginal wall and is then reflected dorsally and cephalad over the rectum and lower sigmoid colon. The space between the reflected layers of peritoneum is known as the *pouch of Douglas,* or the *posterior cul-de-sac*.

The anterior and posterior peritoneal coverings of the corpus join at the lateral uterine margin and form the leaves of the broad ligament (Fig. 7-3). The peritoneal surfaces are in close proximity except where they diverge slightly to invest the round and infundibulopelvic ligaments. The broad ligament is therefore a double layer of peritoneum that extends from the lateral surface of the uterus outward to the pelvic wall. Its upper border consists of the peritoneal fold over the fallopian tube and the lateral extension from the ovary encircling the infundibulopelvic vessels. The midportion encompasses the round ligament. The most inferior portion is thickened and contains a condensation of connective tissue and muscle fibers called the *cardinal ligament* or the *transverse cervical ligament of Mackenrodt*. The uterine vessels approach the lateral aspect of the cervix in the cardinal ligament, an anatomical point of importance in total hysterectomy.

The portion of the broad ligament between the ovary and the fallopian tube contains many small blood vessels and is termed the *mesosalpinx* or the *tubal mesentery*. Vestigial remnants of the mesonephric tubules and duct are located within the leaves of the mesentery and are known as the *epoophoron* (i.e., lateral portion of the tubules) and the *paraoophoron* (i.e., medial portion of the tubules). All of these vestigial tubules are connected with the remnants of the mesonephric duct (Gartner's duct). The blind upper extremity of the duct is occasionally dilated into one or more cystic structures known as the *hydatids of Morgagni*. Cysts may develop from the main duct or from one of the smaller tubules and may be confused with ovarian cysts during a pelvic examination.

The round ligaments, embryologic anlages of the gubernaculum in the male, consist principally of bands of muscle tissue that extend laterally from the anterolateral aspect of the fundus. They leave the peritoneal cavity through the internal inguinal ring, traverse the inguinal canal to the labia majora, and terminate by the dissemination of fibers into the surrounding tissue. The short tubular process into the inguinal canal (canal of Nuck) is generally obliterated in the adult. Occasionally it may persist and be the source of benign cystic structures that are frequently mistaken for hernias. The ligaments were formerly believed to play a major part in uterine support, particularly the maintenance of the normal anterior position. Numerous ineffective operations were devised to shorten these ligaments in the hope that this shortening would hold the fundus forward. The ligaments hypertrophy during pregnancy and may be the source of localized lower quadrant pain.

The uterosacral ligaments arise from the posterior wall of the uterus at the level of the internal cervical os. They are made up of connective tissue and involuntary muscle, and contain blood vessels, lymphatics, and nerve filaments of the parasympathetic and sympathetic systems. Each ligament passes dorsally around the rectosigmoid and inserts on the sacral wall at the level of the second and third sacral vertebrae. The function of these ligaments is to exert tension on the cervix in a dorsal direction, keeping the corpus anterior and the axis of the corpus and cervix at a right angle to the vagina. This prevents the uterus from assuming a position

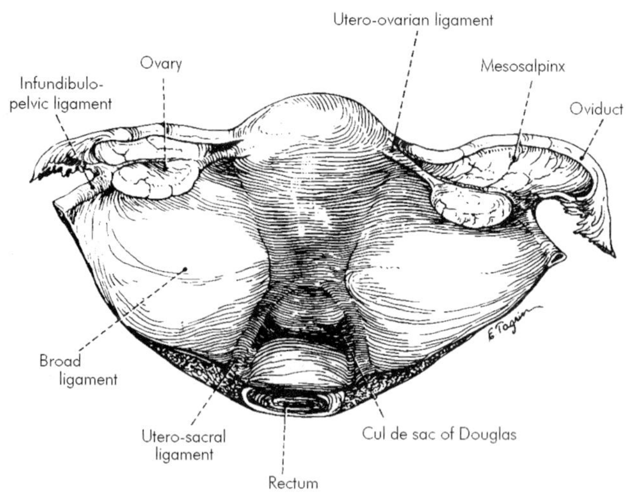

Fig. 7-3. Posterior view of uterus.

that would be in the axis of, and in direct line with, the vagina—a situation that is almost always associated with uterine prolapse.

As mentioned previously, the cardinal or transverse cervical ligaments (of Mackenrodt) form the inferior aspect or the base of the broad ligament. They offer the chief support for the cervix and the upper portion of the vagina. They do this by integrating posteriorly with the uterosacral ligaments and anteriorly with the cervicovaginal portion of the endopelvic fascia. As they fan out laterally, the tissues of the ligaments insert into the fascia overlying the obturator muscles and the muscles of the pelvic diaphragm. As pointed out by Anson and Curtis, they follow the course of the major vessels as a supporting framework.[5]

The uteroovarian ligament (i.e., suspensory ligament of the ovary) extends from the lateral aspect of the uterus (i.e., between the round ligament and fallopian tube) to the inferior pole of the ovary. It consists of connective tissue and smooth muscle in a rounded cord and is ensheathed between layers of the broad ligament.

Uterine structure

The uterus is composed of three separate and distinct layers: (1) the serosa, an outer peritoneal covering; (2) the myometrium, an inner layer of smooth muscle; and (3) the endometrium, the mucous membrane lining the cavity (Fig. 7-4). The uterine serosa is continued laterally as the leaves of the broad ligament and is continued anteriorly and posteriorly as bladder and rectal reflections. The myometrium is composed of three rather indistinct layers of smooth muscle fibers. In each layer there is an interlacing and intermixture of the nonstriated muscle cells. These are held in juxtaposition by a connective tissue rich in elastic fibers. The outer muscular layer (i.e., stratum supravasculare) is chiefly longitudinal and is continuous with fibers entering the broad and round ligaments. The middle layer is thicker and presents fibers in a circular arrangement. The middle layer makes up the major portion of the myometrium and contains many blood vessels that are located between muscle bands (i.e., stratum vasculare). The inner layer represents an exaggerated muscularis mucosae and is composed of thin muscle strands arranged obliquely and longitudinally. The arrangement of the blood vessels between muscle bundles affords an ideal method for hemostasis following delivery. This is borne out clinically by patients whose uteri are atonic and who often hemorrhage following parturition.

The endometrium is a soft inner layer of variable thickness made up of simple tubular glands, a stroma of resting cells in fine connective tissue mesh, and a sensitive vasculature. The histology and physiological variations of this layer are considered in Chapter 3.

Blood supply

Uterus. To understand the blood supply to the uterus, it is necessary to understand the blood supply and collateral circulation in the pelvis. The abdominal aorta bifurcates at the L-4 level directly beneath the umbilicus. Before bifurcating, however, the aorta gives off major branches two of which are the ovarian arteries and the inferior mesenteric artery. Although the course of the right and left ovarian arteries differ somewhat, they both enter the infundibulopelvic ligament to supply the ovary and communicate with an arcade that anastomoses with uterine artery branches.

The common iliac arteries bifurcate into external and hypogastric (i.e., internal iliac) arteries. The hypogastric artery provides the major blood supply to the pelvis and continues through the ischiorectal fossa as the internal pudendal artery. The hypogastric artery is usually divided into an anterior and posterior trunk. The posterior trunk divides to give off the iliolumbar, lateral sacral, and superior gluteal arteries. The anterior trunk provides both visceral and parietal branches (Table 7-1). The uterus possesses a dual blood

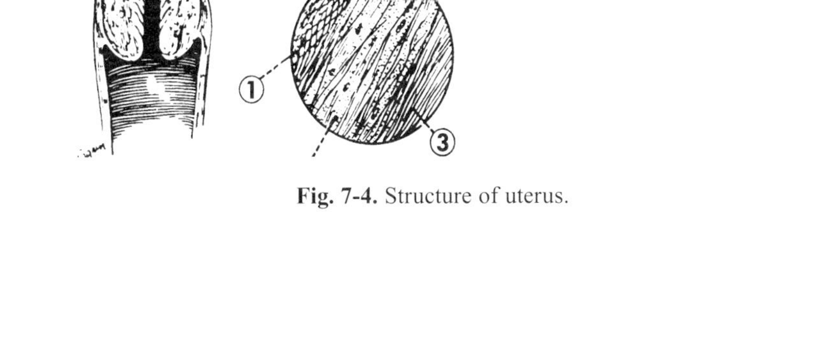

Fig. 7-4. Structure of uterus.

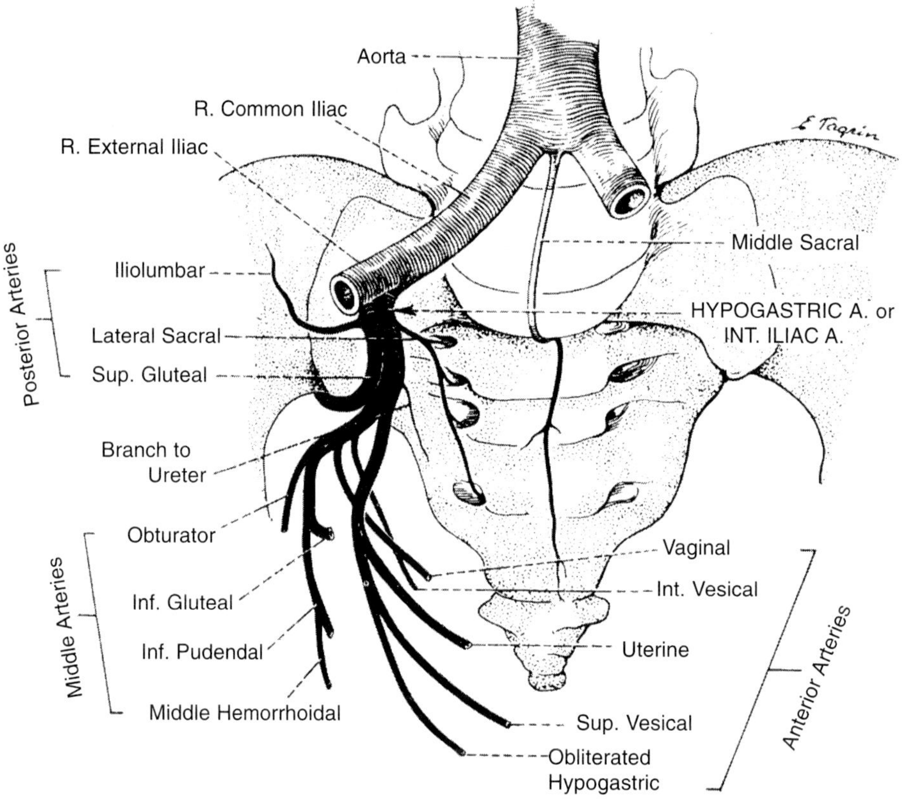

Fig. 7-5. Division of the hypogastric artery.

supply, receiving branches from both the uterine and ovarian arteries. The uterine artery is derived from the hypogastric anterior trunk (Fig. 7-5). It crosses over the ureter at the level of the internal os of the cervix and divides into ascending and descending limbs. The former runs tortuously upward between the leaves of the broad ligament and gives horizontal anterior and posterior branches to the cervix and corpus. As it reaches the cornu, a branch (i.e., artery of Samson) is sent to the round ligament and then is projected along the oviduct to anastomose with the ovarian vessels in the mesosalpinx. The descending branch of the uterine artery turns inferiorly and supplies the vagina from the lateral aspect. It anastomoses freely with the vaginal artery along its course.

The collecting veins from the corpus flow into two longitudinal trunks, which are usually distinct. The anterior surface is drained by the anterior uterine vein situated anterior to the ureter and lateral to the uterine artery. This vein empties into the hypogastric vein. The posterior uterine surfaces, however, drain into a short and long trunk that pass posterior to the uterus and inferior to the uterine artery before joining either the hypogastric or obturator vein.

The collateral circulation of the pelvis includes arterial supply from the aorta, the femoral artery, and the external iliac artery that communicates with branches of the hypogastric artery (Table 7-2). Ligation of the hypogastric artery has controlled pelvic hemorrhage. The main effect is to reduce the arterial pulse pressure to the anterior division of the hypogastric artery.

Endometrium. The processes of menstruation and pregnancy give singular importance to an understanding of the anatomical vascular pattern of the endometrium. As previously mentioned, a series of radial arteries are given off at right angles from the uterine artery as it courses along the corpus (Fig. 7-6). These radial arteries branch in the inner third of the myometrium into straight and spiral (coiled) vessels. The straight arteries pass only as far as the basal layer of the endometrium and terminate in capillaries. The spiral arteries, however, follow a coiled course throughout the thickness of the endometrium, give off a few branches in the endometrium, then fork and give rise to superficial capillaries just below the surface epithelium. These capillaries form plexuses in the stroma and a meshwork around the glands. In the superficial layer of the endometrium, the capillaries form sinuslike dilations known as *lakes*. The blood is returned via small veins that drain these vascular lakes and capillary plexuses. It should be remembered that the vascular pattern is a dynamic one, with constant proliferation and regression. The specific morphologic details are considered in the section on menstruation.

Table 7-1. Branches of the hypogastric artery

Anterior division	Posterior division
Visceral	Iliolumbar
Uterine	Lateral sacral
Superior vesical	Superior gluteal
Middle vesical	
Inferior vesical	
Middle hemorrhoidal	
Inferior hemorrhoidal	
Vaginal	
Parietal	
Obturator	
Inferior gluteal	
Internal pudendal	

Table 7-2. Collateral circulation of pelvis

Extrapelvic source	Hypogastric branch
Aorta	Uterine artery
Ovarian artery	Middle and inferior hemorrhoidal arteries
Inferior mesenteric artery (superior hemorrhoidal)	Iliolumbar artery
Lumbar and vertebral arteries	
Middle sacral artery	Lateral sacral artery
External iliac artery	Iliolumbar and superior gluteal arteries
Iliac circumflex artery	
Inferior epigastric gives rise to obturator in 25%	

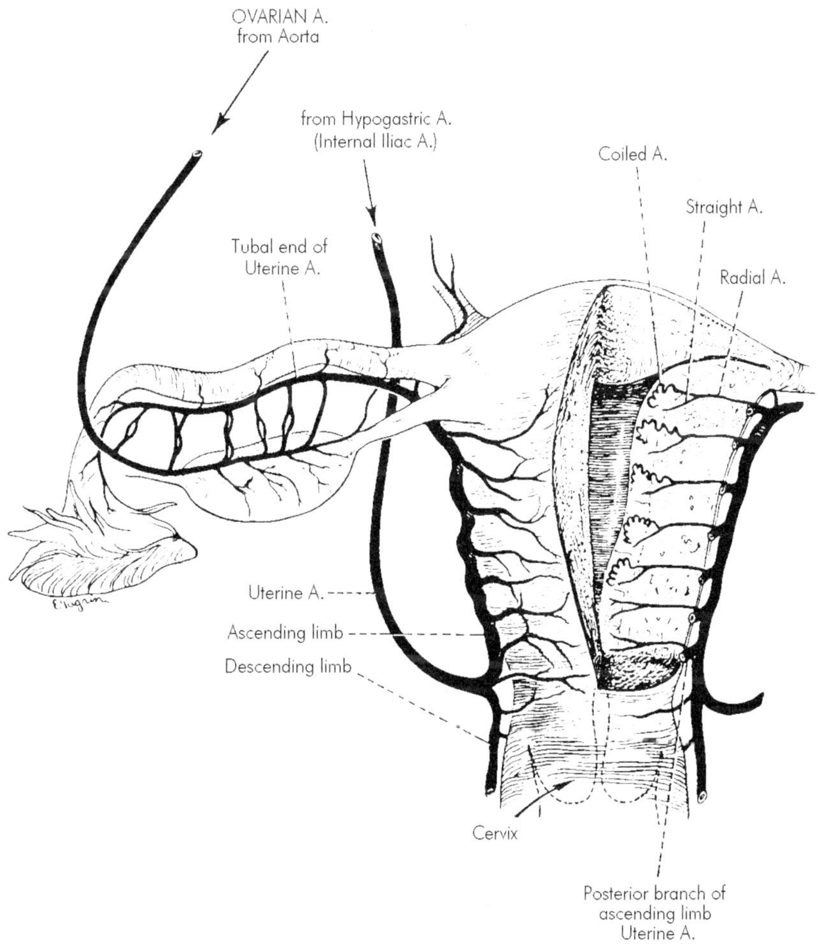

Fig. 7-6. Blood supply to the uterus.

Although the prime function of the straight arteries is to supply the basal endometrium, they may also support regeneration of the lower portion of the functional layer. The coiled arteries alone supply blood to the superficial third of the endometrium and most of the blood to the middle third. Some straight arteries may be converted into coiled ones and then later to the straight type. Thus it is possible that the blood supply of the endometrium could regenerate and develop specificity of function even after complete curettage.

The importance of the coiled arteries is not completely known. It should be pointed out, however, that they are absent or not fully developed in areas where extensive cyclic variations do not occur. Thus in the lower uterine segment and lateral recesses of the endometrium, the vascular supply is mostly through straight arteries.

Nerve supply

The uterine extrinsic nerve supply is derived from the following three sources (Fig. 7-7):

1. Motor fibers from the upper sympathetic thoracic ganglia course through the aortic plexus and the celiac ganglion to the superior hypogastric plexus. The fibers then diverge as they pass caudally to form the inferior hypogastric plexus. They then pass forward over the lateral surface of the rectal ampulla to join the pelvic plexus or cervical ganglion of Frankenhauser. From this plexus, fibers pass along the uterosacral ligament to the smooth muscle of the uterus. Clinical evidence indicates that the motor fibers to the uterus leave the spinal cord at levels higher than the 10th thoracic nerve.
2. Sensory fibers are special visceral afferents that run through the hypogastric and aortic plexuses, through the 11th and 12th sympathetic ganglia without synapse, into the dorsal spinal root ganglia of these segments, then up the dorsolateral fasciculus to the thalamus. The sensory supply to the cervix travels through the sacral parasympathetic chain and communicates with the second, third, and fourth sacral nerves.
3. Sensory and motor fibers to the lower uterine segment and cervix are found in the sympathetic and parasympathetic plexuses. These fibers communicate with the second, third, and fourth sacral nerves. Visceral efferent fibers that are believed to be motor to the longitudinal muscle of the lower uterine segment and to the circular fibers of the cervix, and possibly inhibitory to the uterine fundus, travel in the parasympathetic chain.

It should be remembered that although the sensory nerve fibers course through pelvic, hypogastric, and aortic plexuses before reaching the 11th and 12th thoracic nerves, they are functionally independent of the autonomic system. Although the sensory supply to the cervix, traverses the sacral parasympathetics, it is also functionally independent of the autonomic system.

Lymphatic supply

The lymphatics of the uterine corpus proceed in four or five channels through the broad ligament just below the oviducts, then upward along the ovarian vessels. In the course of their passage through the parametrium and ovarian ligament, they communicate with the ovarian lymphatics to terminate in the lumbar lymph nodes found in front of the aorta from its bifurcation to the diaphragm. The lymphatics from the lower uterine segment anastomose with adjacent lymph channels from the cervix and drain to the obturator, iliac, hypogastric, and sacral nodes. A third route of lymphatic drainage, especially from the fundal area, is via the round ligament to the superficial inguinal nodes.

Uterine anomalies

Uterine anomalies may be congenital or acquired following infection or mechanical trauma. They may lead to reproductive or menstrual dysfunction. An understanding of the association between altered uterine structure and impaired function is essential for the gynecologist in order to select an appropriate therapy.

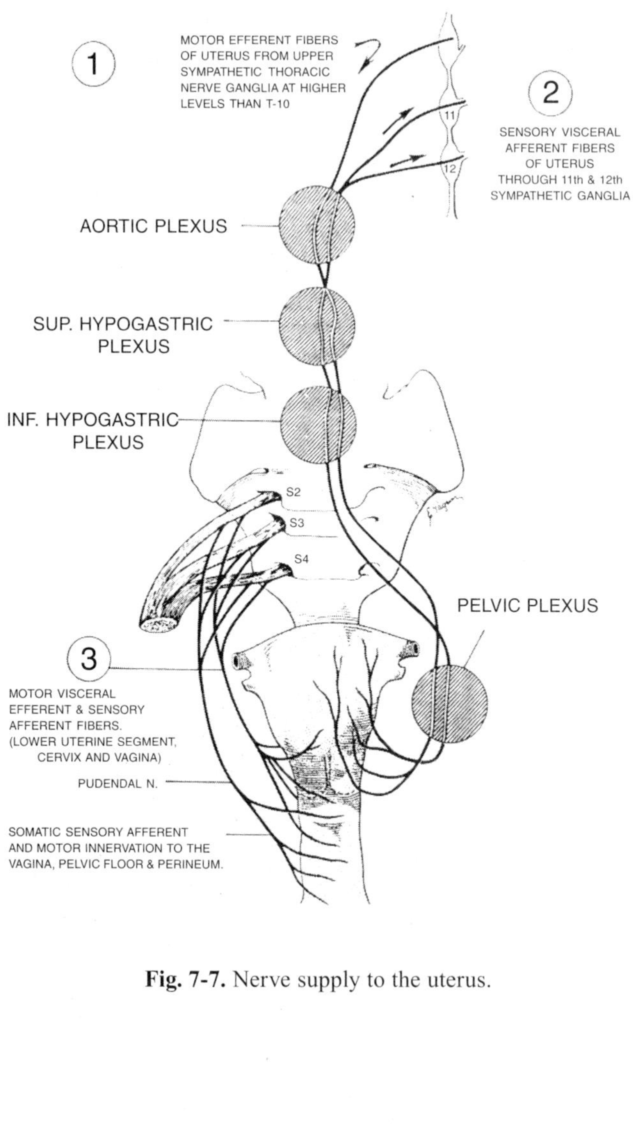

Fig. 7-7. Nerve supply to the uterus.

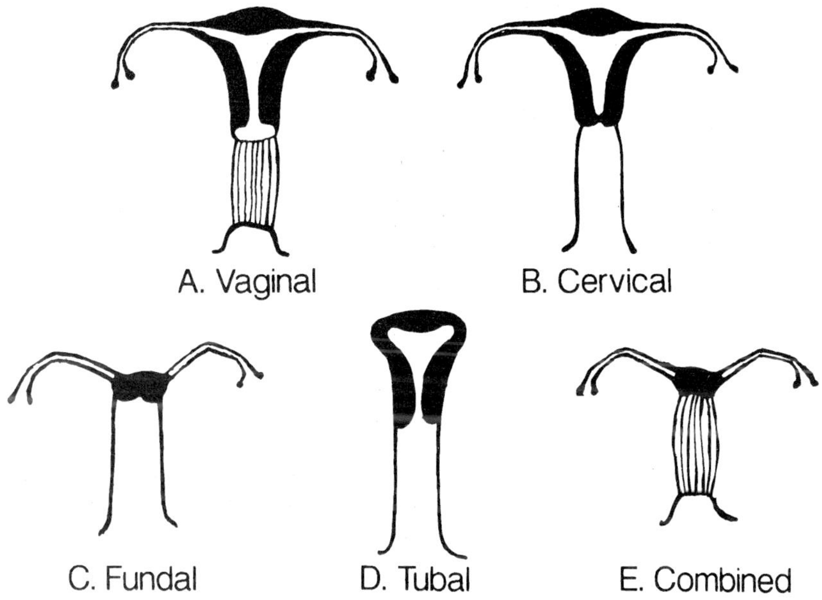

Fig. 7-8. A-E, Congenital uterine anomalies. Class I: Hypoplasia/Agenesis (From the American Fertility Society: The American Fertility Society classifications of adnexal adhesions, distal occlusion, tubal occlusion secondary to tubal ligation, tubal pregnancies, müllerian anomalies and intrauterine adhesions, *Fertil Steril* 49:944, 1988.)

Congenital anomalies. Müllerian anomalies result from defective fusion or absorption of the female reproductive system during embryonic life. Their incidence is difficult to estimate because the majority of congenital anomalies do not result in clinical manifestations.[161] Patients with symptomatic müllerian anomalies usually have signs of obstruction or reproductive dysfunction. Diagnostic methods for determining the exact nature of a müllerian anomaly have evolved from bimanual examination, postpartum manual exploration, and dilation and curettage (D & C), to the more sophisticated techniques of hysterography, laparoscopy, hysteroscopy, ultrasonography, and magnetic resonance imaging (MRI). The increased capacity of the latter techniques to yield complete information will undoubtedly be reflected in a higher reported incidence of the more subtle anomalies.

When reviewing the literature on reproductive tract anomalies, the clinician is often confused and frustrated by the lack of uniformity in the classification and reporting of müllerian anomalies. A classification scheme has been adopted by the American Fertility Society to enhance uniformity.[3] Figs. 7-8 through 7-14 depict the seven müllerian anomalies according to this classification system. This section discusses the effects of each of these anomalies on reproductive outcome and the treatment. Retrospective studies have revealed that approximately 25% of women with congenital uterine anomalies encounter reproductive difficulties, although conception rates are not different from women in control groups.[1,4,83] Spontaneous abortions, premature births, and fetal malpresentations are common in the presence of congenital uterine anomalies. For a discussion on the treatment of obstructing congenital anomalies, the reader is referred to Chapter 23.

In a review of 554 patients with class I müllerian anomalies (Fig. 7-8), 8% had isolated vaginal agenesis (class IA), 83% had vaginal-cervical-fundal agenesis (class IE, often referred to as the Mayer-Rokitansky-Kuster-Hauser syndrome), and 9% exhibited androgen insensitivity syndrome (often referred to as testicular feminization syndrome).[22] The incidence of the class IA anomaly and the androgen insensitivity syndrome are estimated at 1 in 75,000 and 1 in 50,000 phenotypic-appearing females respectively.

Although rare, patients with class IA anomalies may be treated by the creation of an artificial vagina (i.e., the McIndoe procedure). The rate of success is good in restoring menses and in achieving pregnancy.[121] However, most patients with suspected class IA anomalies also have associated uterine or cervical abnormalities.

Patients with class IE anomalies comprise the second largest subpopulation presenting with primary amenorrhea. (Gonadal dysgenesis is the most common cause.) Although fertility is not possible for this group of patients, sexual intercourse may be possible if an artificial vagina is created by dilator therapy,[61] vaginal reconstruction (the McIndoe procedure), or Williams vulvovaginoplasty.[25] Pure cases of cervical agenesis (class IB), fundal agenesis (class IC), and tubal agenesis (class ID) are exceedingly rare.

In a review of the literature published since 1959 on class II anomalies (i.e., unicornuate uterus; Fig. 7-9), Buttram reported a spontaneous abortion rate of 33%, a premature delivery rate of 29%, and a live birth rate of 66%.[22] However, some patients in these reviewed series may actually have had class III anomalies (i.e., uterus didelphys). In a review of 31 patients with true class II anomalies experiencing 60 pregnancies, there were 40% live births, 17% premature deliveries, and 48% spontaneous pregnancy losses during the first and second trimesters.[22]

Resection of a noncommunicating horn-containing endometrium (i.e., a class IIA1b anomaly) is recommended to prevent the development or spread of endometriosis. Patients with communicating horns (class IIA1a) may benefit from uterine unification (i.e., the Strassmann procedure),[76] excision of the horn, or expectant management. The best choice depends upon the size of the horn and the associated symptoms. Ectopic pregnancies resulting from transperitoneal migration of sperm or fertilized ova in patients with noncommunicating uterine horns (classes IIA1b and IIA2) have been reported and have frequently resulted in catastrophic rupture of the rudimentary uterine horn.[144]

Although limited data are available, it appears that the reproductive outcome for patients with uterus didelphys (class III; Fig. 7-10) is similar to that for patients with unicornuate uteri (class II). In a series of 124 pregnancies, the live birth rate was 55%, the abortion rate was 43% and the premature delivery rate was 45%.[22] Because of the "acceptable" rate of fetal salvage and the difficulty of uteroplasty, surgical therapy is rarely performed. Therapeutic modalities that have been suggested for this anomaly (without documentation of their efficacy) include a modified Strassmann procedure and a cervical cerclage.[80,177] Of note, sagittal vaginal septa appear concurrently with uterus didelphys approximately 75% of the time.

The bicornuate uterus (classes IVA and IVB; Fig. 7-11) is impossible to distinguish from the septate uterus (classes VA and VB; Fig. 7-12) by hysterography. Unless two distinct horns can be palpated at pelvic examination, laparoscopy, or occasionally ultrasonography or MRI is necessary to distinguish these two classes of müllerian anomalies.[56,198] Unfortunately, many older series of cases group bicornuate and septate uteri together when reproductive outcome is discussed. In a review of 110 patients with known bicornuate uteri, 57% of pregnancies resulted in live births, 35% ended in spontaneous abortion, and 23% culminated in premature delivery. The Strassmann procedure constitutes appropriate treatment for symptomatic patients with bicornuate uteri. Vaginal septa are seen in fewer than 5% of patients with bicornuate uteri.

The arcuate uterus (class VI; Fig. 7-13), defined as a small convex indentation of the upper uterine cavity with or without an indented external uterine contour, is considered a variant of a normal uterus. The true arcuate uterus is not associated with infertility or pregnancy loss and thus should not be subjected to surgery.

Except for anomalies associated with in utero exposure to diethylstilbestrol (DES; Fig. 7-14), septate uteri (class V) are the most frequent müllerian anomalies. The rate of pregnancy loss is extremely high among women with class V anomalies and is approximately double that for class IV patients. In combined series of class V anomalies, approximately two thirds of conceptions terminated in abortion, one third in premature delivery, and 28% in live births.[22] It has been hypothesized that poor blood supply to the uterine septum may be the cause of such a high abortion rate. Accordingly, the chance of reproductive failure is higher the more complete the septum. Approximately 25% of patients with septate uteri have associated sagittal vaginal septa.

Fortunately, rates of fetal salvage range between 70% and 90% among patients surgically treated.[22,122] The Tompkins metroplasty, the Jones wedge procedure, and more recently, hysteroscopic division of the uterine septum are appropriate surgical treatments for patients with symptomatic septate uteri.[41,44,151,187] In properly selected patients, hysteroscopic

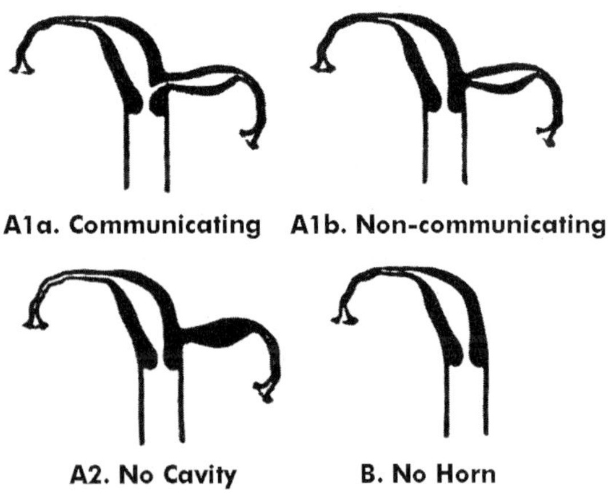

Fig. 7-9. A-D, Congenital uterine anomalies. Class II: Unicornuate. (From the American Fertility Society: The American Fertility Society classifications of adnexal adhesions, distal occlusion, tubal occlusion secondary to tubal ligation, tubal pregnancies, müllerian anomalies, and intrauterine adhesions, *Fertil Steril* 49:944, 1988.)

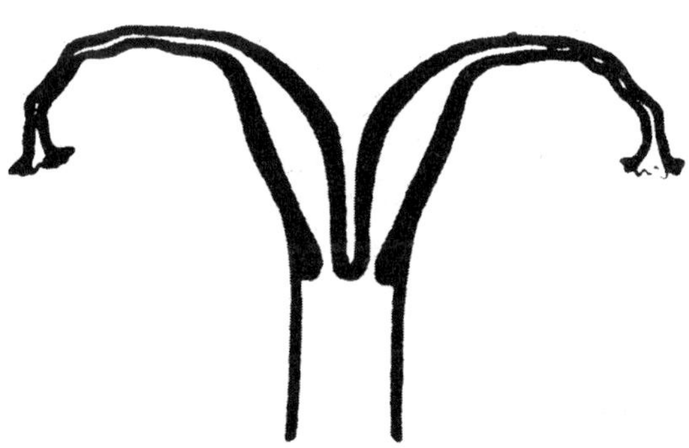

Fig. 7-10. Congenital uterine anomalies. Class III: Didelphys. (From the American Fertility Society: The American Fertility Society classifications of adnexal adhesions, distal occlusion, tubal occlusion secondary to tubal ligation, tubal pregnancies, müllerian anomalies, and intrauterine adhesions, *Fertil Steril* 49:944, 1988.)

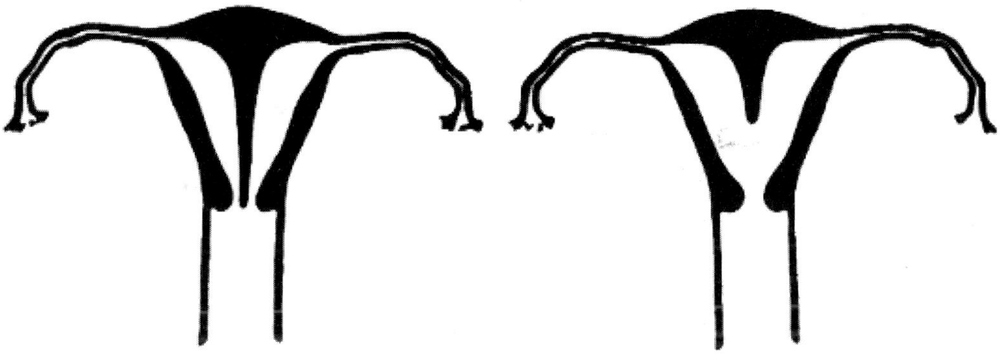

Fig. 7-11. A, B, congenital uterine anomalies. Class IV: Bicornuate (From the American Fertility Society: The American Fertility Society classifications of adnexal adhesions, distal occlusion, tubal occlusion secondary to tubal ligation, tubal pregnancies, müllerian anomalies and intrauterine adhesions, *Fertil Steril* 49:944, 1988.)

metroplasty, as opposed to abdominal metroplasty (i.e., the Tompkins or Jones procedure), is a shorter, simpler operation. There is less trauma, lower morbidity, a shorter recovery time, a lower cost, and a greater opportunity for subsequent vaginal delivery.[54]

Of 144 patients with müllerian anomalies of classes I to V, 31% had abnormalities detectable by intravenous pyelography (IVP).[23] The most frequent abnormality was unilateral renal agenesis, usually found on the ipsilateral side of the associated müllerian agenesis or hypoplasia. There appears to be no increase in the frequency of structural urological abnormalities detected by IVP in patients with septate uteri relative to the frequency of abnormalities noted in women with normally shaped uteri.

Between the late 1940s and 1970, 2 to 3 million women received DES during pregnancy; as a consequence, 1 to 1.5 million female offspring were exposed to the drug in utero.[174] The degree of reproductive failure in such in uteroexposed females is directly correlated with the dosage of DES used during the mother's pregnancy.[12] In a series of 267 DES-exposed women undergoing hysterosalpingography (HSG), 69% had demonstrable abnormalities of the upper genital tract.[98] A significant relationship was found between abnormal HSG findings and structural abnormalities of the cervix and vaginal epithelium. Of all women with abnormalities in uterine contour, 31% had small T-shaped cavities, 13% had small cavities ("hypoplastic uterus"), 6% had T-shaped cavities with constriction, 5% had small cavities with constriction, 4% had constriction alone, and 8% had other assorted anomalies.[98]

The viable birth rate was significantly lower among DES-exposed women with abnormal uterine contours

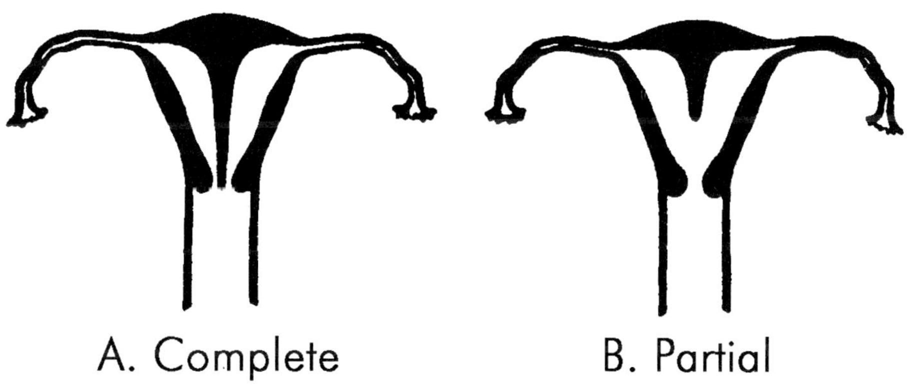

Fig. 7-12. A, B, congenital uterine anomalies. Class V: Septate. (From the American Fertility Society: the American Fertility Society classifications of adnexal adhesions, distal occlusion, tubal occlusion secondary to tubal ligation, tubal pregnancies, müllerian anomalies, and intrauterine adhesions, *Fertil Steril* 49:944, 1988.)

detectable by HSG than among those with normal-appearing uterine cavities.[98] In addition, women with abnormal HSG findings had a higher incidence of ectopic pregnancy, spontaneous abortion, and premature delivery than women with normal findings. In a combined series including a total of 579 pregnancies among DES-exposed women, the ectopic pregnancy rate was 5.4%, the spontaneous abortion rate was 27%, the premature delivery rate was 28%, and the viable birth rate was 63%. Considerable debate continues as to whether or not DES-exposed women have—in addition to an increased incidence of poor pregnancy outcome—a higher rate of both primary and secondary infertility than unexposed controls.

The incidence of second-trimester abortions is higher among DES-exposed women than among those with müllerian anomalies of other etiologies. Kaufman et al reported abortion rates of 19% in the first trimester and 12% in the second trimester among DES-exposed patients.[98] Such rates suggest that prophylactic cervical cerclage may be efficacious in women with DES-associated changes. Currently, no surgical procedure can restore the normal uterine contour in DES-exposed women with an abnormal uterine shape.

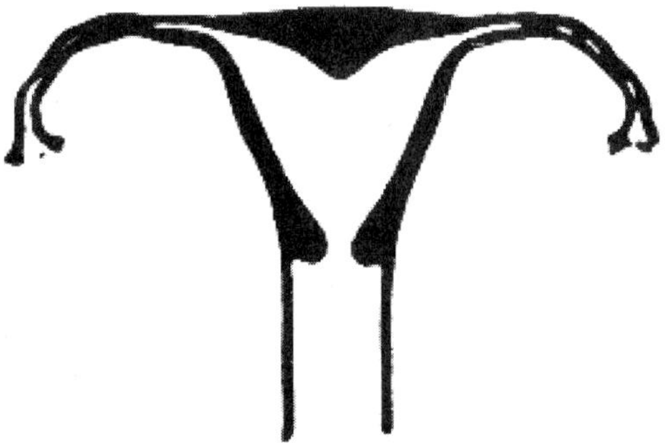

Fig. 7-13. Congenital uterine anomalies. Class VI: arcuate. (From the American Fertility Society: The American Fertility Society classifications of adnexal adhesions, distal occlusion, tubal occlusion secondary to tubal ligation, tubal pregnancies, müllerian anomalies, and intrauterine adhesions, *Fertil Steril* 49:944, 1988.)

Asherman's syndrome. Asherman's syndrome is the partial or complete obliteration of the uterine cavity by adherence of the uterine walls from scarring. It is often associated with menstrual and/or reproductive abnormalities, particularly amenorrhea or hypomenorrhea, dysmenorrhea, infertility, and recurrent abortion. Although first described in 1894 by Heinrich Fritsch in a patient who developed secondary amenorrhea after curettage for delayed postpartum hemorrhage,[71] the syndrome acquired worldwide attention only after Asherman's original publication in 1948.[9]

The incidence of Asherman's syndrome is difficult to determine. It has been estimated to be involved in 1.7% of all cases of secondary amenorrhea.[95] The diagnosis is frequently based on HSG findings (Fig. 7-15), but hysteroscopy is the most accurate method of detection.[117]

Curettage of a gravid or recently gravid uterus is the most common cause of Asherman's syndrome. In a combined series evaluating predisposing factors in patients with intrauterine adhesions, 91% of cases were associated with pregnancy-related curettage. Asherman's syndrome developed in 67% of cases after postabortion curettage, 22% after postpartum curettage, 2% after cesarean section, and in fewer than 1% after evacuation of a hydatidiform mole.[165] Many investigators have hypothesized that gestational changes soften the uterus, making it more difficult to gauge the depth of curettage. The resultant denudation of the basalis layer favors the formation of adhesions over sites of endometrial regeneration. Other rare causes of Asherman's syndrome include infection (i.e., genital tuberculosis), myomectomy, metroplasty, and curettage of a nonpregnant uterus.

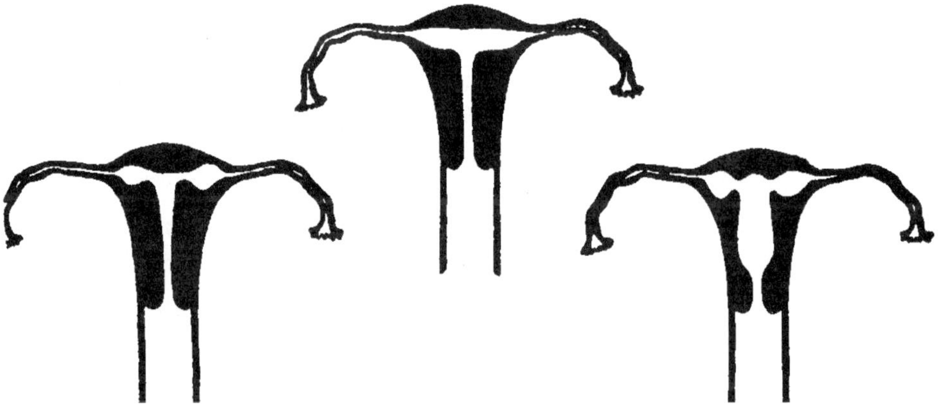

Fig. 7-14. Congenital uterine anomalies. Class VII: DES drug related. (From the American Fertility Society: The American Fertility Society classifications of adnexal adhesions, distal occlusion, tubal occlusion secondary to tubal ligation, tubal pregnancies, müllerian anomalies, and intrauterine adhesions, *Fertil Steril* 1988; 49:944.)

Symptoms of Asherman's syndrome include menstrual and fertility dysfunction. Amenorrhea, documented in 37% of patients, may result when adhesions occlude the cervix or obliterate the entire uterine cavity.[165] Hypomenorrhea, reported by 31% of patients, may occur with partial cervical or cavitary obliteration. Dysmenorrhea and menometrorrhagia are also occasionally noted.[165] Only 6% of patients with diagnosed Asherman's syndrome have normal menses. Infertility is the most common presenting symptom in this syndrome and is seen in 43% of cases of intrauterine syncchiac.[165] Infertility secondary to Asherman's syndrome is frequently accompanied by menstrual abnormalities. The two factors most commonly thought to account for infertility resulting from intrauterine adhesions are interference with sperm transport and embryo implantation.

Approximately 14% of patients presenting with Asherman's syndrome have had repeated pregnancy losses.[165] These repeated abortions have been attributed to defective endometrial vascularization and growth near the site of nidation and to decreased size of the uterine cavity.

Among patients with Asherman's syndrome who conceive, there is a high incidence of complications. Premature labor, placenta accreta, placenta previa, and postpartum hemorrhage are common in patients who have undergone treatment for intrauterine synechiae.[65,93] Placenta accreta is thought to occur when—because of the original endometrial insult as well as the treatment—a defective basalis allows abnormal trophoblastic penetration. The incidence of gravid hysterectomies is high in patients who exhibit abnormal placentation and postpartum hemorrhage.

Asherman's syndrome may be diagnosed by hysterography or hysteroscopy (Fig. 7-15). Many investigators believe that hysterography can only suggest the diagnosis and that hysteroscopy is essential for confirmation.

Treatment of Asherman's syndrome requires surgical removal of intrauterine adhesions with simultaneous prevention of the formation of new adhesions. Methods of adhesion removal include abdominal hysterotomy, hysteroscopic lysis of adhesions, and D&C. If possible, hysteroscopic treatment is preferable because it is associated with lower morbidity and is less costly than the abdominal approach. Because of the high risk of uterine perforation during a vaginal procedure, concurrent laparoscopy is recommended.

After the removal of intrauterine adhesions, many surgeons insert an intrauterine stent (i.e., intrauterine device or Foley catheter) that separates the uterine walls in an effort to prevent the formation of new adhesions. Also postoperative treatment with high-dose estrogen, followed by progestin withdrawal, is often used to facilitate endometrial proliferation over previously scarred areas. Antibiotics and steroids are less consistently employed in the prevention of postoperative intrauterine synechiae. To date, the efficacy of these postoperative adjunctive measures has not been evaluated in a randomized series.

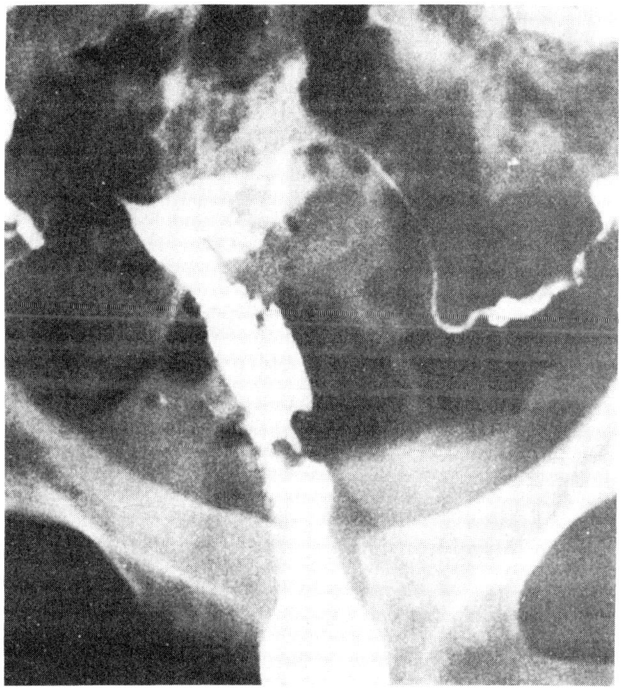

Fig. 7-15. Severe Asherman's syndrome noted on hysterosalpingogram. (From Toaff R, Ballas S: Traumatic hypomenorrhea-amenorrhea [Asherman's syndrome], *Fertil Steril* 30:379, 1978.)

The results of surgical therapy are excellent in terms of the restoration of normal menstrual function and are good in terms of reversing infertility. In a combined series, including 1586 patients treated for Asherman's syndrome, 84% of women had normal menses restored, 11% had hypomenorrhea, and 5% suffered from amenorrhea.[165] Of patients presenting with infertility, 51% conceived. Term births resulted in 55% of cases, premature deliveries in 9%, abortions in 25%, and ongoing pregnancy in 9% at the time of the report.[165] Placenta accreta was documented in 9% of deliveries, with other severe complications in 3% of treated patients.[65,93] The prognosis of Asherman's syndrome is related to the degree of endometrial obliteration. With extensive intrauterine synechiae, the restoration of fertility and normal menstrual function is more difficult.

Leiomyomas

Uterine leiomyomas, commonly known as fibroids, are well-circumscribed, nonencapsulated benign tumors. They are composed of both smooth muscle and extracellular matrix (i.e., collagen, proteoglycan, fibronectin). Synonyms for these tumors include fibromyomas, fibromas, myofibromas, and myomas.

Incidence and etiology. Leiomyomas are the most common solid pelvic tumors in women, developing in 20% to 25% of women during the reproductive years.[142,159] In fact, leiomyomas arise in humans only during the reproductive years; de novo formation of these tumors is seldom, if ever, reported before puberty or after menopause. It is currently accepted that leiomyomas are unicellular in origin.[184] Factors responsible for the initial neoplastic transformation of a myometrial cell are not well understood. However, clinical observations and data from studies in animals suggest that an estrogenic milieu may be necessary. In a guinea pig model, multiple leiomyomas may be produced after prolonged estrogenic stimulation.[107,133]

Chromosomal studies of uterine leiomyomas have revealed nonrandom, tumor-specific cytogenetic abnormalities in approximately 25% to 50% of specimens. At least six cytogenetically abnormal subgroups have been identified: (1) reciprocal translocations of a segment of the long arms of chromosomes 12 and 14; (2) other rearrangements of the long arm of chromosome 12; (3) a deletion of a portion of the long arm of chromosome 7; (4) trisomy 7; (5) trisomy 12; and (6) rearrangements of the short arm of chromosome 6.[135] The lack of clonal chromosomal rearrangements in 50% to 75% of leiomyoma specimens may be explained by the inability of conventional cytogenetic techniques to detect point mutations, cryptic deletions, or low levels of mosaicism. Alternatively, cell culture techniques used to grow leiomyoma cells may preferentially select normal cells.

Once leiomyomatous neoplastic change has taken place, various hormones may apparently affect the growth of the tumor. Estrogenic effects have been most extensively studied. It is common to note the growth of these tumors during pregnancy and their regression after menopause. Several investigators have demonstrated higher estrogen levels within the myoma than in the myometrium of the same uterus.[53,145,155,173,197] Although the role of progesterone in the development and growth of uterine leiomyomas remains unclear, the majority of clinical evidence suggests that progestins may stimulate leiomyoma growth. This contention is supported by histologic evidence of increased mitotic activity in leiomyomas during the luteal phase of the menstrual cycle[99] and after treatment with medroxyprogesterone acetate alone.[183] Data on the relation of other hormones (e.g., prolactin, growth hormone, human placental lactogen, androgens) to the pathogenesis of leiomyoma are scant and inconclusive. Hormonal stimulation of leiomyoma growth probably involves growth factors (e.g., epidermal, insulin-like, or platelet-derived), although more research is needed to clarify this point.

Leiomyomas are characterized by their location in the uterus (Fig. 7-16). Subserosal leiomyomas are located just under the uterine serosa and may be attached to the corpus by a narrow or broad base. Intramural leiomyomas are found predominantly within the thick myometrium but may distort the cavity or cause an irregular external uterine contour. Submucous leiomyomas are located just under the uterine mucosa (endometrium); they also may be attached to the uterine corpus by a narrow or broad base. Although this classification scheme is used widely, it suffers from the limitation that few leiomyomas are actually of a single "pure" type. Most leiomyomas span more than one anatomic location and thus are hybrids (e.g., a predominantly intramural leiomyoma with a submucous component). Other types of leiomyomas include "parasitic" myomas, which receive their blood supply from structures other than the uterus (e.g., the omentum), and seedling myomas, whose greatest diameter is less than or equal to 4 mm.

Tumors in subserosal and intramural locations comprise the majority of all leiomyomas; submucous leiomyomas make up only 5% of the total number.

Pathology. The gross appearance of a leiomyoma is somewhat variable, but in general the tumor is circumscribed and well demarcated from the surrounding muscle. A pseudocapsule—flattened uterine muscle that has become compressed as the size of the tumor increases—is present. The

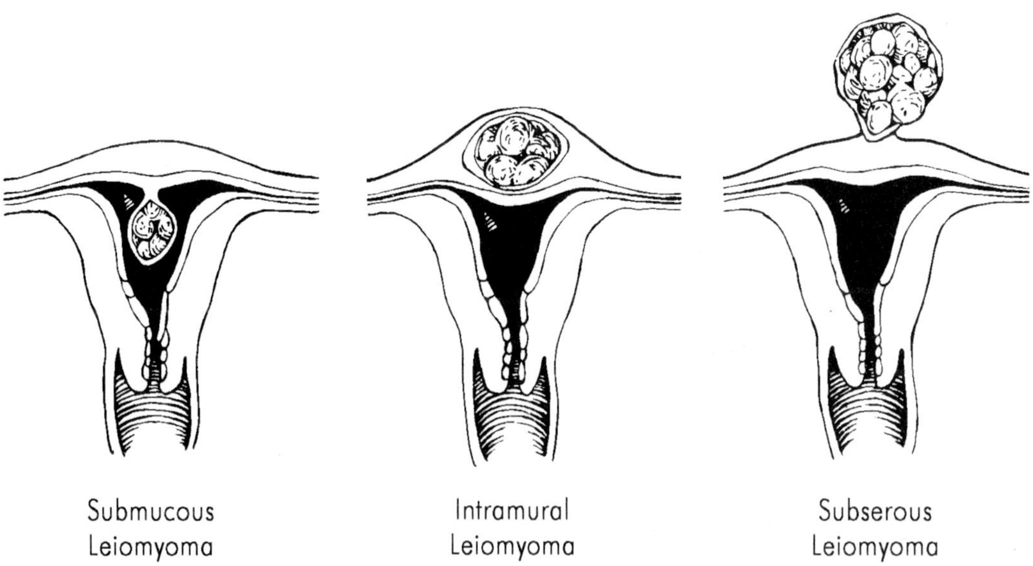

Fig. 7-16. Leiomyomas classified according to their location in the uterus.

consistency is usually firm or even hard except when degeneration or hemorrhage has occurred. The color is light gray or pinkish white, depending on the degree of vascularity. When the leiomyoma is cut across, the tissue usually projects above the level of the surrounding myometrium. When viewed in the fresh state, the smooth-muscle bundles can usually be identified in an intertwining pattern or a whorl-like arrangement.

The microscopic appearance of a leiomyoma is usually characteristic in that the nonstriated muscle fibers are arranged in bundles of various sizes that run in multiple directions (Fig. 7-17) and give the same intertwining pattern noted on gross examination. High-power microscopic examination reveals that the spindle-shaped cells have elongated nuclei, generally of uniform size and staining quality. Connective-tissue elements in varying amounts may be noted between the muscle cells. In certain tumors the amount of connective tissue is unusually large; in such cases the term "fibromyoma" may be more descriptive.

The most frequent degenerative changes are hyalinization and cyst formation. These changes result from the diminished vascularity of the connective-tissue element, so that the detail of connective-tissue fibers is lost. The hyaline material presents no cellular detail, stains deeply with eosin, and may include remnants of muscle bundles interspersed with the homogeneous matrix. If the hyalinized connective tissue undergoes liquefaction necrosis, cystic degeneration takes place. The cysts may then become filled with a gelatinous material that oozes forth when the tumor is cut across. This stage may be followed, especially in long-standing cases, by the development of focal areas of calcification. In postmenopausal women these calcified leiomyomas may be evident on radiographic examination. Another type of degeneration, "acute red degeneration," is occasionally seen as a complication of pregnancy. In this situation the cut surface resembles raw meat—a carneous change due to hemorrhage into a partially hyalinized leiomyoma. This hemorrhagic complication is the result of the accumulation of blood in the tumor because of venous obstruction and may occur during the rapid growth associated with pregnancy or during the immediate postpartum period. Acute red degeneration of leiomyomas has also been reported in association with the use of massive doses of medroxyprogesterone acetate in the treatment of endometriosis.

Symptoms. It is estimated that between 20% and 50% of women with leiomyomas experience tumor-related symptoms.[10,88,90] Menorrhagia is a common symptom, occurring in approximately 30% of women undergoing myomectomy.[24] Menorrhagia is frequently, but not always present in women with submucous leiomyomas.[115,162]

Approximately 34% of patients in a combined series evaluated for symptoms preceding myomectomy experienced pelvic pain or pressure.[19,33,59,108,119,126,130,158] Most patients with leiomyomas who experience pelvic pain also have some other pelvic disease; salpingitis, endometriosis, adenomyosis, diverticulosis, or ovarian carcinoma. Pelvic pain may occur in pregnancy if leiomyomas undergo degeneration. Pelvic pressure may be accompanied by urinary frequency and less commonly by constipation.

A review of reported cases of myomectomy, in which preoperative abortion rates were recorded, revealed that 441 (41%) of 1063 pregnancies ended in spontaneous abortion.[24] Although these statistics describe a selected population, it is likely that leiomyomas are generally associated with a significantly increased risk of abortion.

Leiomyomas are also associated with other kinds of reproductive dysfunction. Although leiomyomas are present in approximately 10% of women with infertility, it is estimated that these tumors are only responsible for infertility in 2% to 3% of cases.[24] Pregnant women with leiomyomas are more likely than pregnant women without leiomyomas to develop pain, tumor degeneration, bleeding, premature labor, fetal malpresentation, abruption, need for operative delivery, retained placenta, and postpartum hemorrhage.

Polycythemia has been reported in a patient with autonomous production of erythropoietin by a leiomyoma.[191] Ascites, hydronephrosis, and bowel obstruction resulting from the impingement of leiomyomas on pelvic and abdominal structures have also been reported.[24]

Sarcomatous transformation of uterine leiomyomas is a rare but potentially lethal complication. It is estimated to occur in approximately 0.1% of women with leiomyomas.[24] It is reportedly more frequent with large or rapidly growing tumors.[11,82,142]

Diagnosis. The diagnosis of leiomyomas is usually determined easily by bimanual examination. The uterus is enlarged, is often irregular, and may be palpated abdominally above the symphysis. Ultrasonography, MRI, and computed tomography may be useful in confirming the diagnosis, although these modalities may not distinguish between leiomyomas and adenomyomas. In patients experiencing menorrhagia or recurrent pregnancy losses, hysterography—with both anteroposterior and cross-table lateral views—may be useful. Finally, laparoscopy and hysteroscopy can aid in definitive diagnosis.

Treatment. The primary therapeutic approach in patients with large or symptomatic leiomyomas is surgical. Hysterectomy is the most frequent operative technique used to treat this disorder. In the United States approximately 175,000 hysterectomies are performed yearly for leiomyomas; a diagnosis of leiomyomas is the most common indication for this procedure.[48] Hysterectomy, the only true "cure" for leiomyomas, is often recommended when a patient presents with a uterus of greater than 12 weeks' gestational size. However, it is important to individualize the choice of therapy.[66]

When women wish to preserve childbearing potential, a myomectomy may be performed. Approximately 18,000 myomectomies are performed yearly in the United States.[132] Myomectomy diminishes menorrhagia in roughly 80% of patients presenting with this symptom.[24] It is essential to

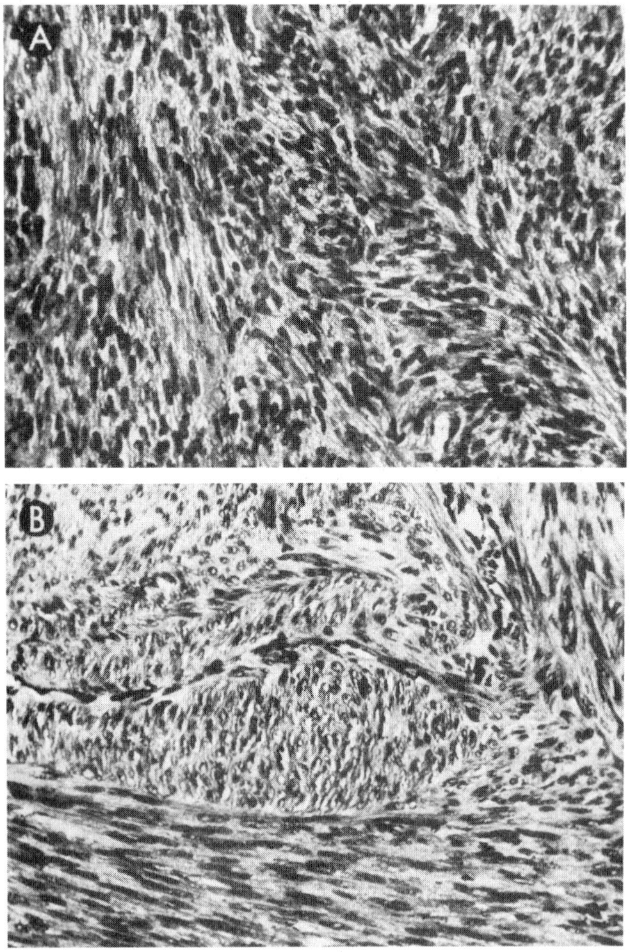

Fig. 7-17. **A**, High-power view of leiomyomas, showing typical structure. The tumor is composed of groups of smooth muscle cells arranged in twists and whorls in an interlacing pattern. It is relatively avascular. **B**, Higher power shows cellular detail. The smooth muscle fibers in the central portion have been cut across their long axes. Note uniform appearance and lack of mitoses.

inform patients undergoing myomectomy that there is a significant risk of recurrence of leiomyomas after surgery. A combined series, in which bimanual examination was used to estimate the rate of recurrence, indicated that 15% of patients develop symptomatic fibroids after myomectomy and 10% require a second major operative procedure (i.e., another myomectomy or a hysterectomy).[24] However, more recent studies using ultrasonography to assess recurrence have reported rates of 25% for women with three or fewer leiomyomas resected and 90% for women with four or more leiomyomas resected.[64] Approximately 18% of women undergoing myomectomy require blood transfusion.[15] The likelihood that transfusion will be needed is greater among women with large fibroids than among those with smaller tumors.

GnRH agonists, which induce a hypoestrogenic pseudomenopausal state, represent a recent development in the medical treatment of leiomyomas. Because fibroids are dependent on estrogen for their development and growth, induction of a hypoestrogenic state causes shrinkage of these tumors and of myometrial mass. Uterine volume has been shown to decrease 40% to 50% after 3 months of GnRH agonist therapy.[62,63,67,68] In addition, treatment with a GnRH agonist induces amenorrhea, allowing women with menorrhagia-induced anemia to increase iron stores and hemoglobin concentrations significantly.[63] However, cessation of GnRH agonist treatment is followed within 3 to 6 months by a regrowth of leiomyomas and the uterus to pretreatment volume in the majority of cases.[62,63,67,68] Currently, GnRH agonist treatment is not recommended for longer than 6 months because of the potential consequent development of osteoporosis.

Thus GnRH agonists may be useful preoperatively when it is important to decrease uterine and fibroid size and to induce amenorrhea.[69] The increase of hemoglobin concentrations in previously anemic women may allow some women to donate autologous blood for possible intraoperative or postoperative transfusion. The combination medical and surgical approach to leiomyomas is relatively new and requires further study.

The combination of GnRH agonists plus low doses of steroid hormones (i.e., "add-back" regimens) has been employed in some clinical trials in an attempt to extend the maximal duration of GnRH agonist therapy safely without sacrificing efficacy.[66,67,69] Preliminary trials have demonstrated that some patients may be successfully treated for up to 2 years with this combination. However, before this medical strategy can be employed to substitute or delay definitive surgery, the optimal steroid add-back regimen and the most cost-effective way to monitor these patients must be defined.

Androgenic agents (e.g., danazol, gestrinone) and progestins (e.g., medroxyprogesterone acetate, depomedroxyprogesterone acetate, norethindrone) have also been used to control menorrhagia in women with leiomyomas.[34,35] However, these medications do not consistently decrease uterine or fibroid volume.

Adenomyosis

Adenomyosis is a benign uterine disease in which endometrial glands and stroma are found within the myometrium. This invasion by the endometrium induces hypertrophy and hyperplasia of the myometrium and produces a diffusely enlarged uterus.

Incidence and etiology. The diagnosis of adenomyosis can be made only by microscopic examination of a specimen obtained at hysterectomy. For this reason, the exact incidence is not known. It is generally estimated that 20% of women have adenomyosis. However, careful analysis of multiple myometrial sections may reveal an incidence as high as 65%.[120]

Adenomyosis is associated with childbearing. It is estimated that at least 80% of women with this disorder are parous.[91,120,128,190] However, the incidence of adenomyosis is not correlated with increasing parity. Adenomyosis most commonly produces symptoms in women between the ages of 40 and 50 years.[120]

Although the exact cause is unknown, the most widely accepted theory of histogenesis was proposed by Meyer in 1900.[125] Meyer postulated that the normal barrier between the endometrium and myometrium, which prevents intrusion of endometrial glands and stroma, is somehow attenuated. After alteration of this barrier, the myometrium is invaded under the influence of estrogen stimulation.

More than 80% of women with adenomyosis have another pathologic process in the uterus; 50% of patients have associated leiomyomas, approximately 11% have endometriosis, and 7% have endometrial polyps.[16] The symptoms of the associated condition often obscure the diagnosis of adenomyosis.

Pathology. The typical uterus with adenomyosis is boggy and uniformly enlarged. Approximately 80% of uteri with adenomyosis weigh more than 80 gm, but it is unusual for a uterus with adenomyosis as the only pathologic process to exceed 200 gm.

When incised, the uterus with adenomyosis bulges and assumes a convex configuration. The thickening of the uterine wall is made up of coarsely trabeculated areas, stippled or granular in appearance, with small yellow or darker cystic

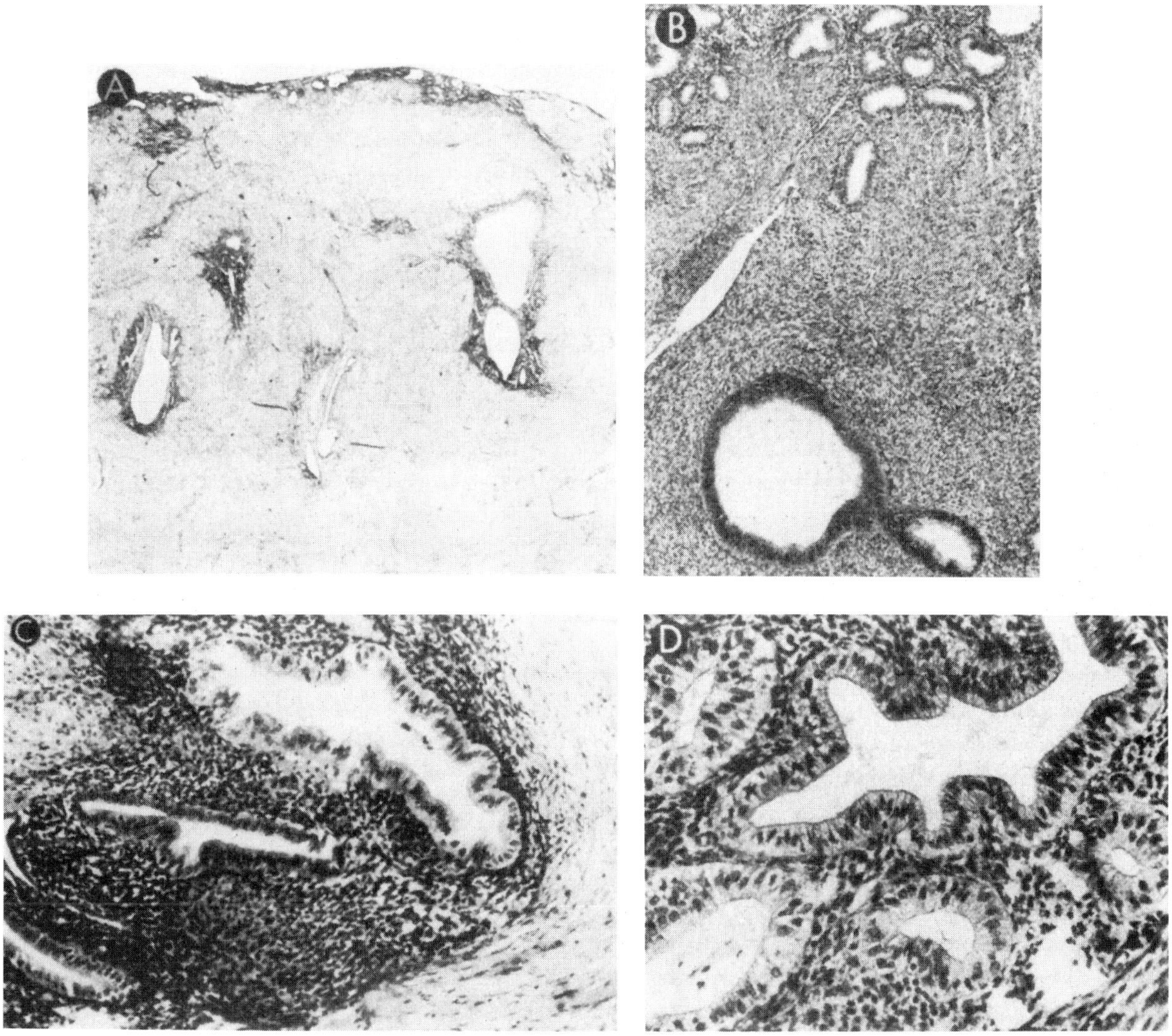

Fig. 7-18. A, Typical adenomyosis in the wall of the uterus. Foci of basal type endometrium are located deep in the myometrium. The myometrium surrounding the areas of adenomyosis shows a whorled appearance similar to that seen in leiomyoma. (From Hertig AT, Gore HM: Tumors of the vulva, vagina and uterus. In *Tumors of the female sex organs*, part 2, section 9, fasc 33, *Atlas of tumor pathology*, Washington, DC, Armed Forces Institute of Pathology, 1960.) **B**, Higher power of an area of adenomyosis showing cystic dilatation. The basal endometrium is at the top. **C**, Adenomyosis in which the glandular element at the top right has undergone anaplasia. The glands are surrounded by typical endometrial stroma. **D**, Adenomyosis showing secretory effect.

points that may contain serous fluid or old blood. Close inspection of the cut surface frequently reveals an irregularity of the endomyometrial junction with foci of down-dipping basalis. Although the pathologist usually has no difficulty diagnosing adenomyosis by gross examination of the cut specimen, the surgeon cannot approach this degree of accuracy with the uterus in situ. However, the disease may be suspected if a focal area of adenomyosis is mistaken for a leiomyoma and myomectomy is attempted. Areas of adenomyosis do not lend themselves to easy excision.

Microscopic appearance. The pathognomonic feature of adenomyosis is the presence of endometrial tissue, glands, and stroma within the myometrium (Fig. 7-18), in at least one low-power field (some authorities insist on two) from the endomyometrial junction. The misplaced endometrial tissue is similar to that of the basalis of the endometrial cavity and therefore does not always respond to hormonal stimulation. Occasionally, secretory change may be noted, or cystic or adenomatous hyperplasia may be documented. In several studies a functional response in the aberrant endometrium was found in only about 50% of the cases in which the normally located endometrium was functional. Decidual changes in the stroma of adenomyotic areas have been noted during pregnancy, and spontaneous ruptures of these areas have been reported. Symptoms of dysmenorrhea or of constant pelvic pain may be anticipated if areas of adenomyosis exhibit functional capacity, with edema and bleeding. The cause of symptoms in patients without apparent functioning areas of adenomyosis in the uterus is unknown.

Malignant neoplasia occurs rarely in the glands and/or stroma; about 30 malignant adenomyomas have been reported. These tumors may be in the form of adenocarcinomas, sarcomas, or carcinosarcomas.

The myometrium is usually altered in uteri with extensive adenomyosis so that a surrounding zone of hypertrophy/hyperplasia is usually recognizable. Phagocytized hemosiderin, indicating previous extravasation of blood, may be seen deep in the myometrium.

If adenomyosis extends into the cornua of the uterus and then laterally into the isthmic portion of the oviduct, a process may develop that is only distinguishable from salpingitis isthmica nodosa by the usual presence of inflammatory cells in the latter condition.

Symptoms. As mentioned earlier, adenomyosis most commonly produces symptoms in women between the ages of 40 and 50 years. Approximately 60% of women experience abnormal uterine bleeding, 50% develop hypermenorrhea, and 25% manifest metrorrhagia. Controversy exists as to whether deep penetration of endometrial glands and stroma into the myometrium is correlated with the occurrence of hypermenorrhea. Some authors report no correlation,[17] others have found a significant correlation.[118] However, hypermenorrhea is common among women in whose myometrium an increased density of endometrial elements is noted on microscopic examination.

Dysmenorrhea is the second most frequent symptom in patients with adenomyosis, occurring in 25% of cases.[16] Dysmenorrhea is correlated with deep penetration and with a high density of endometrial elements within the myometrium.[137]

Diagnosis. A review of the literature demonstrates that only 15% of cases of adenomyosis are correctly diagnosed preoperatively. The reasons for this low percentage are twofold: (1) many if not most patients with adenomyosis only are asymptomatic; and (2) the presence of adenomyosis is often overshadowed by associated pathology (e.g., leiomyomas, endometriosis).

D&C does not aid in diagnosis. Pelvic ultrasonography may be suggestive but is not definitive.[55] The role of MRI has not yet been defined.

Treatment. The only definitive treatment for adenomyosis is total hysterectomy, with or without ovarian conservation. Synthetic progestins are not helpful and may actually increase the level of pelvic pain in some patients. GnRH agonists have been used in a few cases, resulting in a transient decrease in uterine size, in amenorrhea, and even in the ability to conceive. Unfortunately, regrowth of the uterus and recurrence of symptoms are usually documented within 6 months of cessation of therapy.

ENDOMETRIAL POLYPS

Endometrial polyps are hyperplastic overgrowths of glands and stroma that are rather localized and form a projection above the surface. Such polyps may be sessile or pedunculated and rarely include foci of neoplastic growth.

The prevalence of polyps has been estimated at 10% to 24% among women undergoing endometrial biopsy or hysterectomy.[188] Endometrial polyps are rare among women younger than 20 years of age. The incidence of these polyps rises steadily with increasing age, peaks in the fifth decade of life, and gradually declines after menopause.

The most frequent symptom in women with endometrial polyps is metrorrhagia, reported in 50% of symptomatic cases. Postmenstrual spotting is also common. Less frequent symptoms include menorrhagia, postmenopausal bleeding, and breakthrough bleeding during hormonal therapy. Overall, endometrial polyps account for 25% of abnormal bleeding in both premenopausal and postmenopausal women.[188]

Endometrial polyps are often diagnosed by microscopic examination of a specimen obtained after a D&C. Hysterography is rarely helpful when polyps are small but may yield suggestive findings (e.g., a smooth space-occupying lesion) when the polyp is large. Hysteroscopy with directed biopsy is particularly helpful in the diagnosis of small intracavitary polyps.

The most common histologic finding in endometrial polyps is proliferative endometrium, which is seen in 44% of cases.[188] Secretory endometrium when present is frequently out of phase. Adenomatous hyperplasia and adenocarcinoma have been reported in 0.6% of cases of endometrial polyps.[188]

The majority of cases of endometrial polyps are cured by thorough curettage. This technique is especially successful in the postmenopausal age group. Therapy must be guided by the histologic pattern of the polyp and of the endometrium. Hysterectomy must be performed if adenocarcinoma is noted, but progestin therapy may be useful in patients who have only adenomatous hyperplasia or proliferative endometrium. Finally, the use of estrogen-progestin combinations is often successful and may be the treatment of choice for younger women.

Endometrial hyperplasia

Endometrial hyperplasia is an overgrowth of endometrial glands and stroma characterized by a proliferative glandular pattern with varying degrees of architectural and cytologic atypia (Fig. 7-19).[194] Some forms of endometrial hyperplasia have little or no malignant potential. Other forms, notably those demonstrating cytologic atypia, may develop into or co-exist with invasive endometrial cancer.[103] All endometrial hyperplasias, regardless of their malignant potential, may cause significant blood loss through heavy and irregular vaginal bleeding. They are associated with chronic anovulatory states, estrogen-secreting ovarian tumors, and unopposed exogenous estrogen use. Appropriate medical or surgical management depends on the degree of hyperplasia and on the age and reproductive wishes of the patient. A timely and accurate diagnosis is paramount to successful therapy.

Etiology. Risk factors for the development of endometrial hyperplasia are similar to those for endometrial cancer and include pathophysiologic states of relative estrogen excess in the face of relative progesterone deficiency. In premenopausal women, anovulatory states such as polycystic ovarian syndrome may result in continuous estrogen-induced endometrial proliferation. Progesterone, a potent antagonist to estrogen, is produced by the corpus luteum. Therefore in anovulatory women, hyperplasia is the predictable result of unopposed endogenous estrogen action on a normally responsive endometrium.

In perimenopausal or postmenopausal women, continued though waning estrogen production in the absence of ovulation has the same effect. This estrogen-dominant state is particularly pronounced in obese women who have higher circulating levels of the weak estrogen estrone produced by the peripheral conversion of androstenedione in muscle and fat cells. Unopposed exogenous estrogens may cause iatrogenic hyperplasia. Tamoxifen, a mixed estrogen-agonist/antagonist, has also been associated with endometrial hyperplasia and adenocarcinoma in women being treated for breast cancer.[31]

Estrogen-secreting ovarian tumors may induce endometrial hyperplasia. Although stromal tumors, like the granulosa cell tumor, are frequently estrogen-secreting, it is important to keep in mind that any epithelial neoplasm may cause ovarian stromal hyperplasia and produce estrogen.

Malignant potential. In classifying hyperplastic lesions, there are two histologic levels at which atypia can be described; the architectural and the cytologic. Architectural atypia is present when there is an abnormality in the number, size, or complexity of the glandular elements in the lesion. Cytologic atypia refers to the abnormal morphology of the individual cells lining the glands. It is the degree of cytologic atypia which defines the malignant potential of endometrial hyperplasia. This was demonstrated by Kurman et al who showed that non-atypical hyperplasias with cytologic atypia progressed to adenocarcinoma 29% of the time.[103]

Unfortunately, a seemingly endless proliferation of classification schemes has been developed for endometrial hyperplasias. Terms such as adenomatous hyperplasia, cystic hyperplasia, and adenocarcinoma-in-situ do not adequately describe the malignant potential of these lesions. Clinicians should understand the classification scheme used in their institutions and, in most circumstances, should review the histopathology before instituting therapy. The overriding principle, regardless of the descriptive terminology, is that the

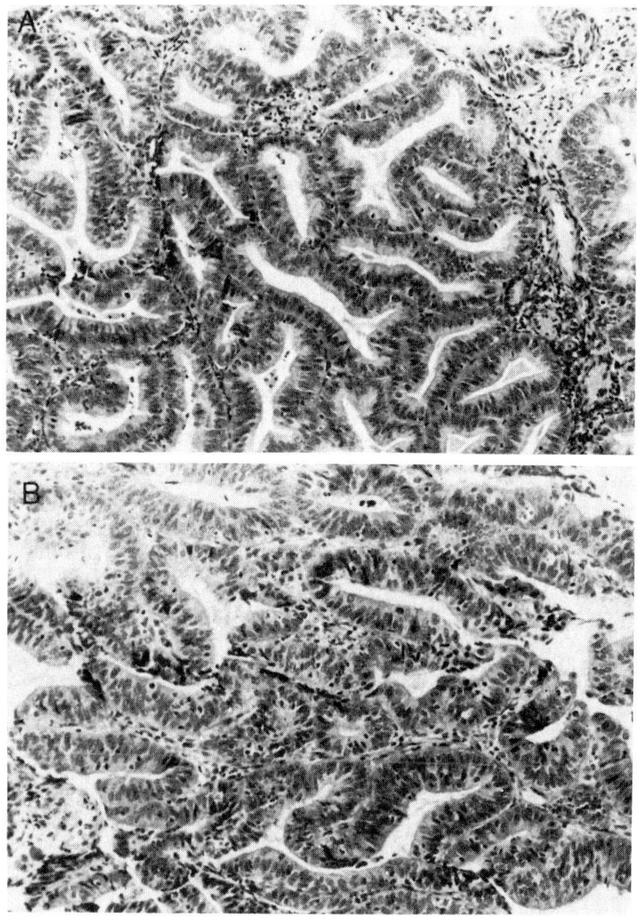

Fig. 7-19. A, Endometrial hyperplasia demonstrating architectural abnormalities without cytologic atypia. **B**, Endometrial hyperplasia with both architectural and cytologic atypia. (Courtesy Drs. W. Welch and J. Semple.)

degree of cytologic atypia determines the malignant potential of the hyperplasia, and that hyperplasias in the absence of atypia do not represent premalignant lesions.[58]

Finally, up to 25% of perimenopausal or postmenopausal women with atypical hyperplasia will have co-existing endometrial cancer. Such information must be taken into account when designing an appropriate therapeutic approach for the patient with endometrial hyperplasia.

Diagnosis. The diagnosis of endometrial hyperplasia is made by endometrial biopsy. Office biopsy methods that utilize both suction and sharp curettage (e.g., Pipelle, Vabra, Karmen) have diagnostic accuracy similar to D&C.[175] These procedures are well tolerated, require no anesthesia, and are cost effective when compared to an outpatient surgical procedure. When an inadequate sample is obtained, D&C may be required.

Treatment. The treatment of endometrial hyperplasia must be tailored to the patient's age, reproductive wishes, menopausal status, general medical health, and grade of hyperplasia. Treatment may be either medical or surgical. Medical therapy is directed toward reestablishing the equilibrium between estrogen and progesterone by stimulating the production of endogenous progestins through ovulation induction or by administering pharmacologic doses of exogenous progestins.

Among premenopausal women who desire immediate fertility, a nonatypical hyperplasia may be treated with cyclic medroxyprogesterone for 3 months in doses of 10 mg for 14 days per month. If a follow-up endometrial biopsy reveals a secretory endometrium without evidence of hyperplasia or neoplasia, ovulation induction may proceed. If an atypical hyperplasia is present, continuous megestrol acetate at doses ranging from 40 mg twice daily to 80 mg three times daily may be employed for up to 3 months.[72] If a follow-up biopsy shows persistent atypical hyperplasia, an additional cycle of therapy may be warranted at a higher daily dose. Since it is unusual for such lesions to persist after progestin therapy, patient compliance must be carefully assessed in all treatment failures. If there is a question of compliance, depot forms of progestin (e.g., depot MPA) may be administered via intramuscular injection. In women wishing to retain fertility, but delay pregnancy, low dose combination oral contraceptives are very effective in preventing recurrent hyperplasia. Among premenopausal women with atypical hyperplasia who do not desire fertility, hysterectomy is a reasonable option. For the majority of premenopausal patients, medical management will effectively reverse atypical hyperplasia. However, continued cyclic progestin therapy may be required to prevent recurrences.

Among postmenopausal patients, hyperplasia without atypia should be treated with continuous progestin therapy for a period of 3 months. If the lesion persists, hysterectomy is advisable if concurrent medical conditions like diabetes, hypertension, or morbid obesity do not preclude surgical management. Finally, postmenopausal women with atypical hyperplasia and no medical contraindication to surgery should undergo hysterectomy. The uterus should be grossly inspected for evidence of invasive carcinoma. If present, a full staging operation should be performed.

Continuous progestin therapy is generally well tolerated but may cause weight gain, mood swings, and depression.[196] There is no evidence to suggest that progestin therapy increases the likelihood of developing deep venous thrombosis, and so progestins may be used in patients with a prior thrombolic event. A far more complex problem is the impact of long-term progestin therapy on the risk of cardiovascular disease. Synthetic progestins may have a deleterious effect on lipoprotein levels by decreasing cardioprotective high-density lipoprotein cholesterol concentrations. This may in turn increase the risk of coronary artery disease and cerebral vascular accidents. Alternatives to progestins include danazol and cyproterone acetate.[92,180] Response rates are similar to those reported with progestins, but experience is limited.

Endometrial cancer

Endometrial carcinoma is the most common gynecologic malignancy, with 33,000 new cases reported in 1991.[2] The disease affects predominantly perimenopausal and postmenopausal patients with a median age at diagnosis of 61 years. Only 5% of cases occur in women under 40 years of age. It is twice as common as ovarian cancer and three times more common than invasive carcinoma of the cervix. Following a decade of increasing incidence, with a peak of 39,000 reported cases in 1979, the number of endometrial cancer cases has gradually declined. Variations in the incidence of this malignancy have been attributed to the increasing age of the population, more refined histopathologic criteria for the diagnosis of the lesion, and a changing pattern in the use of hormone replacement therapy and the oral contraceptive pill.

Despite the transient increase in incidence through 1979, the overall mortality from endometrial cancer has continued to decline and is now responsible for fewer than 4000 cancer deaths per year. This has given the false impression that endometrial cancer is an indolent disease, whereas in fact stage for stage it is just as deadly as ovarian cancer. However, unlike ovarian cancer, endometrial cancer has a hallmark early symptom—perimenopausal or postmenopausal bleeding—which prompts the physician to perform an endometrial biopsy. This biopsy leads to a diagnosis at a favorable stage in the majority of cases.

Risk factors. Most endometrial cancers arise from a background of endometrial hyperplasia and are the consequence of unopposed endogenous or exogenous estrogen on a hormonally responsive endometrium.

Endogenous estrogen excess. The most important risk factor associated with the development of endometrial cancer is obesity.[42] Women, overweight by up to 22.7 kg, have a threefold increased risk of developing this malignancy. The risk jumps to ninefold for women overweight by more than

22.7 kg. Obesity increases the risk by increasing estrogen production and bioavailability. In postmenopausal women, the ovaries and adrenals secrete negligible amounts of estrogen. The majority of estrogen is in the form of estrone, which is produced in the peripheral conversion of androstenedione in muscle and adipose tissue. Increased production of estrone has been documented in obese women.[96] In addition, obese women have lower levels of sex-hormone-binding globulin, accounting for increased bioavailability of circulating estrogen.[73] Total intake of calories derived from saturated or unsaturated fats is a risk factor independent of body weight. Women reporting a high intake of animal fat and fried food have a 2.1-fold increased risk of developing endometrial carcinoma. Women with a high intake of complex carbohydrates, predominantly breads and cereals, have a decreased risk (RR=0.6) after controlling for body mass.[156]

Other risk factors for endometrial cancer include a history of infertility, nulliparity, early menarche, and late menopause.[52,100] Hypertension and diabetes mellitus are frequently associated with obesity, but may also represent independent risk factors. Chronic anovulatory states, such as polycystic ovarian syndrome, substantially increase endometrial cancer risk. Functional ovarian neoplasms, such as certain epithelial ovarian cancers and granulosa cell tumors, may also increase risk by the endogenous production of unopposed estrogen.

Exogenous estrogen excess. Many studies have demonstrated an association between unopposed estrogen replacement therapy and the development of endometrial cancer.[111,193] The risk increases with the dose of estrogen and the duration of use. The widespread use of unopposed estrogen in the 1960s may have been responsible for the temporal rise in the endometrial cancer rate that peaked in 1979. The risk of endometrial cancer can be effectively eliminated with the addition of a progestin. Progesterone reduces estrogen receptor synthesis and increases the conversion of estradiol to the less potent metabolite estrone. Women on both estrogen and progestin replacement therapy actually have a lower risk of endometrial cancer than untreated patients.

Recent information regarding the negative impact of progestins on lipoprotein profiles has led to a resurgence of interest in the use of unopposed or minimally opposed estrogen replacement regimens. Given the indolent nature of "iatrogenic" endometrial cancer and improved biopsy and imaging techniques, the issue of low-dose estrogen replacement deserves further study. However, without a prospective trial comparing the morbidity of unopposed estrogen and periodic endometrial surveillance with estrogen-progesterone replacement therapy, the use of unopposed estrogen cannot be recommended.

Tamoxifen has been used extensively in the treatment of estrogen-receptor positive breast cancer in postmenopausal women. While on tamoxifen, these women had a reduction in new malignancies forming in the contralateral breast. This observation resulted in the use of tamoxifen in a national breast cancer chemoprevention trial. Tamoxifen has both antiestrogenic and estrogenic properties. It has been shown to reduce the risk of osteoporosis while increasing rates of both endometrial hyperplasia and neoplasia. With a trend toward more widespread use of this drug, an increase in endometrial cancer may be anticipated.

The risk of endometrial cancer is reduced by half in patients using the combination oral contraceptive pill. Most modern preparations are progestin-dominant, and the degree of risk reduction is related both to duration of use and total progestin dose. The protective effect may be greatest in nonobese nulliparous women.

Women who smoke have reduced risk of developing endometrial cancer. Smoking has been shown to increase concentrations of sex-hormone-binding globulin, thereby lowering levels of bioavailable estrogen. In addition, smoking has been linked to early menopause. Such benefits of smoking are clearly outweighed by the marked increase in risk of lung cancer and cardiovascular disease.[70]

The association between alcohol consumption and endometrial cancer is confusing despite data from breast cancer cases. These data suggest that alcohol consumption is an independent risk factor, perhaps mediated through altered estrogen metabolism.[75]

Other risk factors. Not all endometrial adenocarcinomas arise as a result of physiologic conditions of relative estrogen excess. There is a subset of adenocarcinomas that arise in women with no identifiable risk factors. These tumors may be of high grade and of unfavorable histologic type (e.g., papillary serous, clear cell, or adenosquamous variants). They arise de novo, not in an environment of endometrial hyperplasia, and are frequently aggressive tumors. In addition, there are certain rare hereditary forms of endometrial cancer, including the Lynch II family cancer syndrome. This syndrome includes nonpolyposis colorectal cancer, ovarian, and endometrial cancer.[110] A careful family history should always be obtained from cancer patients.

Diagnosis. The most common presenting symptom in endometrial cancer, abnormal vaginal bleeding, occurs in over 80% of cases. When this hallmark symptom occurs in postmenopausal women, it is dramatic, disturbing, and likely to prompt an immediate response from both patient and physician. Recent reports suggest that a subset of postmenopausal bleeding may be managed conservatively.[57] However the current standard of care is an office endometrial biopsy or D&C.

Office endometrial biopsy techniques combine suction with sharp curettage and have a sensitivity similar to that of dilation and sharp curettage. A biopsy is therefore the diagnostic modality of choice in women with abnormal uterine bleeding. These procedures are performed in an office setting, frequently without the need for local anesthetic. If an office biopsy yields an inadequate sample, D&C should be performed. A fractional dilation and curettage includes an endocervical curettage followed by uterine sounding, dilation, and endometrial curettage. Although no longer required for staging, this procedure may yield useful information regarding the site of the malignancy. There is no evidence that hysteroscopic evaluation of the endometrium improves the diagnostic accuracy of office biopsy techniques. When positive, office biopsy techniques are highly accurate.[175] However, if the tissue obtained is of insufficient quantity for diagnosis, a D&C is mandatory.

Up to 50% of patients with endometrial cancer will have an abnormal Pap smear. This makes the test unsatisfactory for screening. However, among postmenopausal women with normal endocervical cells on a routine Pap smear, 6% will have endometrial cancer, and 13% will have endometrial hyperplasia. If these endometrial cells are atypical, up to 25% will have endometrial cancer. Therefore the detection of endocervical cells on a postmenopausal Pap smear is an indication for endometrial biopsy.[202] Evaluation of endometrial cytologic preparations has not gained broad acceptance because of difficulty in interpretation.[123]

The role of ultrasonography in the diagnosis of endometrial cancer has recently been described. Granberg et al demonstrated by endometrial biopsy that among 205 postmenopausal patients with vaginal bleeding, the mean endometrial thickness was 3.4 ± 1.2 mm in patients with atrophic changes.[78] Among women with endometrial cancer, the mean endometrial thickness was 18.2 ± 6.2 mm. Using a cutoff of 5 mm, Granberg et al reported a positive predictive value for hyperplasia or neoplasia of 87.3%. These findings have been reported by other investigators as well.[97,171] The clinical utility of this observation is unclear. Among postmenopausal women with bleeding, the risk of neoplasia is sufficient to warrant an endometrial biopsy regardless of the endometrial thickness. In addition, there is no published normative data evaluating variations in endometrial thickness in a randomly selected group of asymptomatic postmenopausal patients. Until such normative data have been collected, it will remain difficult to interpret the incidental finding of a thickened endometrial stripe in an otherwise asymptomatic patient.

Is the risk of endometrial hyperplasia or neoplasia so high in some patient groups that screening by ultrasound or endometrial biopsy is warranted? Gronroos et al addressed this question by instituting mass screening of 597 women, 45 to 69 years old, with diabetes mellitus and hypertension.[79] Among women with diabetes, 6.3% were found to have neoplasia. Among women with hypertension, 1.3% were found to have neoplasia. It is unclear how many of these women would have developed bleeding spontaneously and would have reduced mortality from the disease as a result of the screening.

Women on tamoxifen for breast cancer have an increased risk of developing endometrial neoplasms. This increased risk is partly a result of the estrogen agonist effects of tamoxifen on the endometrium. However, women with a personal history of breast cancer are also at increased risk for developing ovarian or endometrial cancer, regardless of tamoxifen use. In addition, some studies have reported an excess number of poor prognosis malignancies, including clear cell and papillary serous carcinomas, in women taking tamoxifen.[31,113] Given these findings, yearly endometrial biopsies, or intermittent progesterone treatment in patients on long-term tamoxifen therapy, is recommended.

Pathology. The vast majority of carcinomas arising in the endometrium are adenocarcinomas. There are distinct histopathologic types with very different biologic behaviors. Endometrioid adenocarcinomas are the most common. These lesions may be papillary, secretory, or ciliated. Squamous differentiation is a common feature. When the tumor is malignant, it is designated as an adenosquamous variant. Other carcinomas have also been described in addition to endometrioid carcinomas: mucinous, clear cell, and pure squamous.

Histologically, endometrial carcinomas contain back-to-back glands or a cribriform pattern that gives rise to a gland-within-gland appearance (Fig. 7-20). Cytologically, mitoses are almost always present. Epithelial stratification is present

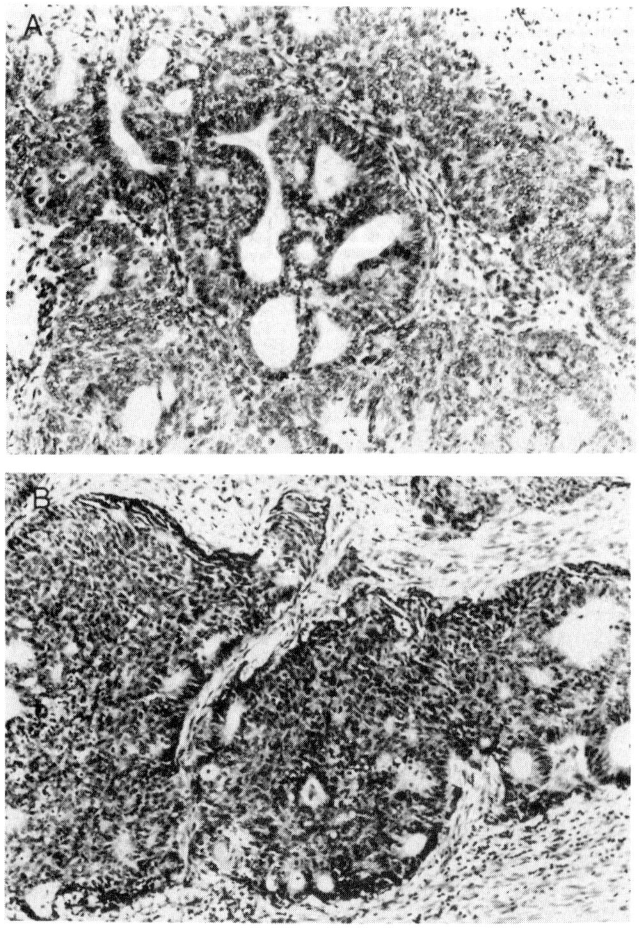

Fig. 7-20. **A**, Endometrial adenocarcinoma, well-differentiated (grade 1). **B**, Endometrial adenocarcinoma, poorly-differentiated (grade 3), demonstrating sheets of malignant cells without identifiable gland formation. (Courtesy Drs. W. Welch and J. Semple.)

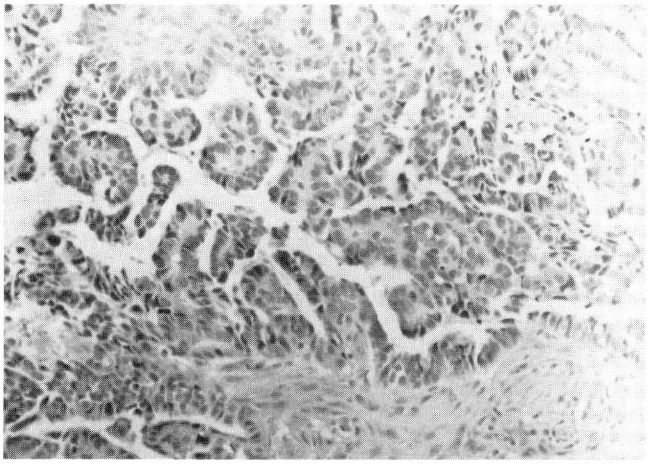

Fig. 7-21. Papillary serous carcinoma of the endometrium displaying papillary tufts of stratified, malignant epithelium histologically similar to ovarian papillary carcinoma. (Courtesy Dr. D. Genest.)

and connective tissue between glands is absent. The cells are characterized by prominent nucleoli and by an eosinophilic, granular cytoplasm. Although atypical hyperplasias may focally demonstrate similar changes, the changes are not as extensive.

The degree of differentiation of a carcinoma may be based upon cytologic or architectural criteria. For endometrial carcinomas, FIGO has established architectural criteria that may be applied to most cell types. A grade 1 tumor is defined as a tumor with less than 10% undifferentiated areas. A grade 3 tumor is more than 50% undifferentiated. Tumor grade predicts the biologic behavior of endometrial cancers. Well-differentiated lesions tend to be associated with superficial invasion and have little propensity to nodal spread. Poorly-differentiated lesions are frequently deeply invasive and metastatic.

There are three variants of endometrial adenocarcinoma that bear mentioning: the clear cell carcinoma, the papillary serous carcinoma, and the adenosquamous carcinoma. Clear cell carcinomas represent fewer than 4% of uterine carcinomas, tend to arise in older women, and have a virulent behavior.[104] Papillary serous carcinoma of the endometrium, like its ovarian counterpart, has a capacity for early intraperitoneal dissemination (Fig. 7-21). It represents less than 10% of all endometrial cancers and has a very poor prognosis.[29] Finally, adenocarcinomas that contain regions of squamous differentiation are designated adenocarcinoma with squamous metaplasia. When a poorly differentiated lesion contains a squamous component resembling a squamous cell carcinoma, the term adenosquamous carcinoma is used. Such lesions have a poor prognosis, but it is unclear whether dedifferentiation of the squamous component or the glandular component overall determines prognosis.[85,164]

It should be noted that approximately 10% of endometrial carcinomas are associated with the production of mucus, a feature frequently seen in adenocarcinomas of the cervix. Mucin production does not appear to influence biologic behavior but may make it difficult to distinguish between an endometrial and endocervical primary.

Pretreatment evaluation. Once the diagnosis of endometrial cancer has been confirmed, a complete history and physical examination should be performed. Frequently, patients with endometrial cancer are obese, hypertensive, or diabetic and may have significant intercurrent medical problems. A complete blood count to rule out anemia secondary to vaginal bleeding should be performed. Abnormal liver function tests may suggest occult metastatic disease. A chest x-ray is mandatory to rule out pulmonary metastases. Intravenous pyelography, gastrointestinal series, or barium enema are not required in asymptomatic patients. A bone scan adds little to initial evaluation.

MRI has proven to be accurate in the evaluation of myometrial invasion and in lymph node involvement.[200] Transvaginal sonography has been used to assess myometrial invasion but with somewhat less success.[199] These modalities are expensive and less accurate than data derived from surgical staging. They may be helpful in evaluating patients in whom comorbid disease precludes surgical staging but are not required for surgical staging.

Although originally described as a tumor marker for ovarian cancer, serum levels of CA-125 have been shown to be elevated in endometrial cancer.[136] It is unusual for early stage disease to cause an abnormal level. In most studies, over 80% of patients with an elevated CA-125 were found to have extrauterine disease at the time of exploratory laparotomy.[148] A role for this tumor marker in monitoring patients for tumor response or recurrence is currently under investigation.

Endometrial cancer is a surgically-staged disease. Therefore, imaging to assess the depth of myometrial invasion, and tumor markers that may suggest disseminated disease are not required before exploration. These studies, however, can be helpful in identifying a group of patients who are at high risk for advanced disease and for whom consultation with a gynecologic oncologist should be obtained to help coordinate both operative and postoperative management. This is particularly true for women with unfavorable histologic types or high-grade lesions. A coordinated team approach to the patient with advanced endometrial cancer is the goal of state-of-the-art cancer care.

Staging. The surgical staging of corpus cancer is outlined in Table 7-3. In 1988 FIGO abandoned the clinical staging system following the completion of prospective surgical staging trials.[18,40] These studies established the importance of cell type, histologic grade, depth of myometrial invasion, and nodal, adnexal, or peritoneal spread as prognostic variables. The previous clinical staging system, which determined uterine size and endocervical involvement at a fractional D&C, is now used only in patients treated with primary radiation therapy.

Surgical staging begins with an adequate abdominal incision. Any collection of free pelvic fluid should be aspirated for cytologic evaluation. If no fluid is present, saline washings should be obtained. A thorough exploration of the abdomen, including palpation of the diaphragm, bowel mesentery, and paraaortic nodal groups is essential. Any suspicious areas should be biopsied. A total extrafascial hysterectomy and adnexectomy is then performed. In selected cases, paraaortic or pelvic lymph nodes may be sampled. Any enlarged lymph nodes must be removed. An omentectomy or omental biopsy is indicated in patients with the papillary serous variant.

Paraaortic or pelvic lymph node sampling is a potentially morbid procedure and may be technically difficult in an obese patient. The risk of nodal involvement is predictable based on the histologic cell type, grade of tumor, and depth of myometrial invasion. Stage I grade 1 lesions with superficial invasion rarely metastasize to the pelvic or paraaortic nodes, whereas up to 45% of women with deeply invasive grade 3 lesions will have nodal metastasis. Therefore in patients with presumed stage I endometrial cancer, a gross or frozen section evaluation of the depth of myometrial invasion at the time of hysterectomy is invaluable in guiding intraoperative decision-making. Lymph node sampling should be strongly considered in patients with presumed stage I grade 3 lesions or of lesions of any grade with significant myometrial invasion. Patients with stage II or III disease or with an unfavorable histologic type should also have their paraaortic and pelvic lymph nodes sampled. A more complete list of risk factors for nodal involvement is summarized in Table 7-4.

Vaginal hysterectomy remains an appropriate alternative to abdominal surgery in stage I grade 1 endometrial cancer. Recent advances in operative laparoscopy have led to innovative approaches to the surgical staging of endometrial cancer. Childers and Surwitt recently published their experience with laparoscopically-assisted surgical staging of endometrial cancer.[28] This includes laparoscopic nodal sampling and vaginal hysterectomy. Preliminary data suggest that this investigational technique is well tolerated and significantly reduces hospital stay. Laparoscopy allows for upper abdominal exploration, node biopsy, and salpingo-oophorectomy. These procedures are not possible using a purely vaginal approach.

Postoperative care. Following primary therapy, endometrial cancer patients should be examined at regular intervals with a complete physical, Pap smear, and chest X-ray. The frequency of visits and duration of follow-up must be based on the patient's likelihood of developing recurrent disease. Among women with stage IA grade 1 endometrial cancer, hormone replacement therapy may be initiated after informed consent. In such patients, the risk of tumor recurrence is less than 1%, and the benefits of replacement therapy far outweigh the risks.[105] Estrogen replacement therapy is contraindicated in advanced stage, high-grade lesions.

Adjuvant therapy. Following surgical staging and treatment, adjuvant therapy may be required for patients at significant risk for pelvic or abdominal recurrence. Patients

Table 7-3. Staging of cancer of the uterine corpus

Stage	
Stage IA G123	Tumor limited to endometrium
IB G123	Invasion to < 1/2 myometrium
IC G123	Invasion to > 1/2 myometrium
IIA G123	Endocervical glandular involvement only
IIB G123	Cervical stromal invasion
IIIA G123	Tumor invades serosa and/or adnexa and/or positive peritoneal cytology
IIIB G123	Vaginal metastases
IIIC G123	Metastases to pelvic and/or paraaortic lymph nodes
IVA G123	Tumor invasion of bladder and/or bowel mucosa
IVB	Distant metastases including intraabdominal and/or inguinal nodes

Table 7-4. Frequency of nodal metastasis among risk factors

Risk factor	No. of patients	Pelvic no. (%)	Aortic no. (%)
Histology			
Endometroid			
Adenocarcinoma	599	56 (9)	30 (5)
Others	22	2 (9)	4 (18)
Grade			
1 Well	180	5 (3)	3 (2)
2 Moderate	288	25 (9)	14 (5)
3 Poor	153	28 (18)	17 (11)
Myometrial invasion			
Endometrial	87	1 (1)	1 (1)
Superficial	279	15 (5)	8 (3)
Middle	116	7 (6)	1 (1)
Deep	139	35 (25)	24 (17)
Site of tumor location			
Fundus	524	42 (8)	20 (4)
Isthmus-cervix	97	16 (16)	14 (14)
Capillary-like space involvement			
Negative	528	37 (7)	19 (9)
Positive	93	2 (27)	15 (19)
Adnexal involvement			
Negative	587	47 (8)	27 (5)
Positive	34	11 (32)	7 (20)
Other extrauterine metastasis			
Negative	586	40 (7)	26 (4)
Positive	35	18 (51)	8 (23)
Peritoneal cytology*			
Negative	537	38 (7)	20 (4)
Positive	75	19 (25)	14 (19)

From Creasman et al: Surgical pathologic spread patterns of endometrial cancer: a Gynecologic Oncology Group study, *Cancer* 60:2035, 1987.
*Nine patients did not have cytology reported.

are at high risk if they have been found to have paraaortic lymph node metastasis or adnexal or peritoneal spread. Postoperative radiation to the pelvis and aortic area may cure up to one half of patients with advanced disease.[157] Radiation treatment of only the pelvis remains controversial. Most studies show a reduction in local recurrences but no significant impact on survival.

Prognosis. Overall, 72% of women with stage I adenocarcinoma of the endometrium will survive at least 5 years. The 5-year survival rate falls to 56% for stage II disease, and 30% for stage III disease. Unfortunately, only 10% of women with stage IV lesions will survive at least 5 years.[152]

Recurrence. Endometrial cancer may metastasize intraabdominally, hematologically, or via lymphatics. The most common site of local recurrence is the vaginal cuff. Distant metastasis may be seen in lung, liver, or abdomen. Most recurrences develop within three years of initial diagnosis. Distant metastasis is associated with a grim prognosis because of a lack of effective systemic hormonal therapy or chemotherapy. However, an isolated vaginal recurrence, without pelvic extension, may be effectively treated with surgical excision or local irradiation. Up to 45% of women with this recurrence will survive 10 years.[150]

Treatment of recurrent endometrial cancer. The treatment of patients with distant recurrences of endometrial cancer is challenging and rarely results in cure. The use of local irradiation may control pain or disability from focal metastases. In order to control systemic disease, progestational agents or cytotoxic chemotherapy may be used. Response rates to progestin therapy may be as high as 15% to 20%, particularly in well-differentiated cancers that are more likely to be estrogen-receptor and progesterone-receptor positive.

The role of cytotoxic chemotherapy in the treatment of endometrial cancer is limited. The reported complete clinical response rate is only 15%. Regimens that contain platinum or adriamycin have the highest overall response rates, but these responses tend to be short lived, and survival is not prolonged.[147]

Given the toxicity associated with cytotoxic chemotherapy, progestin treatment is a rational first step in treating recurrent disease. Progestins have some desirable secondary effects, particularly as appetite stimulants, and have minimal toxicity. If a patient fails to respond to progestins, cytotoxic therapy may be considered.

Other uterine malignancies

Uterine sarcomas. Uterine sarcomas represent only 2% of all uterine malignancies, with an incidence of 2.3 in 100,000 in the United States.[84] Unlike endometrial adenocarcinoma, uterine sarcoma is more common among African-American women. The only known risk factor for the development of gynecologic sarcomas is prior radiation therapy.[7,124] This disease occurs an average of 16 years after radiation exposure.[47]

Controversy exists as to the proper classification of uterine sarcomas.[101,140,141] Table 7-5 displays an accepted classification scheme. These tumors are generally divided into pure sarcomas, mixed sarcomas, and malignant mixed müllerian tumors. Within each group, subdivisions are made for homologous elements (i.e., tumors containing cell types normally seen in the uterus) or heterologous elements (i.e., cell types not normally seen in the uterus). Overall, mixed müllerian sarcomas are the most common, followed by leiomyosarcoma and endometrial stromal sarcoma.[163] The remaining tumors are exceedingly rare.

Regardless of the histologic type, all sarcomas of the uterus have the potential for aggressive biologic behavior. Low grade leiomyosarcomas and endometrial stromal sarcomas are indolent tumors associated with excellent long term survival. Unfortunately, most of these tumors are of high grade and tend to spread by both lymphatic and hematogenous routes. At the time of diagnosis, many are systemic diseases for which there is limited effective systemic therapy.

Leiomyosarcoma. Leiomyosarcomas represent 25% of all uterine sarcomas. Although frequently arising in myomatous uteri, they are rarely found within their benign counterpart. These sarcomas most likely arise de novo and are not the consequence of malignant degeneration of a leiomyoma.

The rapid enlargement of a solitary uterine mass is a hallmark of leiomyosarcoma. This is particularly true when rapid growth occurs after menopause. Frequently these lesions are found incidentally. The gross appearance of a leiomyosarcoma differs from that of a leiomyoma; the sarcomas tend to contain extensive areas of necrosis and hemorrhage. Because histologic diagnosis requires counting mitoses per multiple high power field (HPF), frozen section diagnosis is usually limited.

Table 7-5. Classification of uterine sarcomas*

Classification
Pure homologous
Leiomyosarcoma
Endometrial stromal sarcoma
Endolymphatic stromal meiosis
Angiosarcoma
Fibrosarcoma
Pure heterologous
Rhabdomyosarcoma
Chondrosarcoma
Osteosarcoma
Liposarcoma
Mixed sarcomas
Mixed homologous
Mixed heterologous
Malignant mixed müllerian tumors
Homologous type
Heterologous type

*From Antman KH: Malignancy of the uterine corpus. In Knapp RC, Berkowitz RS, editors: *Gynecologic oncology*, New York, 1986, Macmillan Publishing.

The leiomyosarcoma may display a wide spectrum of biologic behaviors based upon the number of mitoses per 10 HPFs, the degree of cytologic atypia, and hypercellularity present. These behaviors range from a smooth muscle tumor of uncertain malignant potential to highly virulent forms with marked atypia and high mitotic counts. Because of difficulties in diagnosis and in classification of the tumors, it is vital for the pathologist and gynecologist to review the histology together and to obtain consultation from oncology specialists. Microscopically, leiomyosarcomas have a characteristic appearance with spindle, round, or giant cell types. Pleomorphism and multinucleated giant cells may be seen (Fig. 7-22).

The treatment of leiomyosarcoma is total abdominal hysterectomy and bilateral salpingo-oophorectomy. A thorough staging procedure, including lymph node biopsies, is not necessary. These lesions will frequently spread by both lymphatic and hematogenous routes, and distant metastasis is common. Rarely, a leiomyosarcoma will be detected after myomectomy. If it is high grade, with at least 10 mitoses per 10 HPFs, a hysterectomy should subsequently be performed. If the lesion is low grade, with 5 to 9 mitoses per 10 HPFs, myomectomy may be an adequate treatment.[14,143]

Other lesions that must be distinguished from leiomyosarcomas include leiomyoma of uncertain malignant potential, benign metastasizing leiomyoma, intravenous leiomyomatosis, and cellular leiomyomas. Intravenous leiomyomatosis is an interesting benign tumor with a potentially fatal outcome. These tumors arise in the uterus or its blood vessels. The tumor may extend into the vena cava and the right atrium and may obstruct venous return.[182]

Endometrial stromal sarcomas. Stromal tumors of the endometrium are divided into low-grade and high-grade lesions. A low-grade endometrial stromal sarcoma (e.g., endometrial stromal myosis) is an indolent sarcoma occurring in younger women. Recurrences or metastases are infrequent and may occur many years after primary therapy. The lesion may be hormonally dependent; oophorectomy and progestin therapy have caused tumor regression.[76] These lesions have fewer than 10 mitoses per 10 HPFs. High grade endometrial stromal sarcoma, however, is a biologically virulent tumor that metastasizes quickly and is commonly fatal with high mitotic counts (i.e., more than 10 mitoses per 10 HPFs).[140,141] These tumors may be polypoid and fleshy. Microscopically, they are composed of spindle-shaped cells with varying amounts of cytoplasm. Tumor giant cells may also be seen (Fig. 7-23).

Mixed müllerian sarcomas. Mixed müllerian sarcoma is the most common uterine sarcoma and appears to arise from the endometrial stroma or from undifferentiated cell rests. Survival is related to the degree of invasion. There are few survivors if the tumor deeply invades the uterus or the outside of the uterus.[6] Microscopically these tumors are made up of carcinomatous and sarcomatous elements of either heterologous or homologous type (Fig. 7-24). The only proven therapy for the lesion is hysterectomy and bilateral salpingo-oophorectomy.

Treatment of carcinosarcoma. The optimal treatment for uterine carcinosarcomas depends upon the stage of disease. In general, patients with tumors that are confined to the uterus, and that minimally invade the uterus, do well with hysterectomy and bilateral salpingo-oophorectomy. The role of adjuvant radiotherapy and chemotherapy is difficult to establish. Radiation therapy offers no improvement in survival rate over surgery alone in patients with stage I disease.[163] However, pelvic irradiation reduces the incidence of pelvic recurrence.[86]

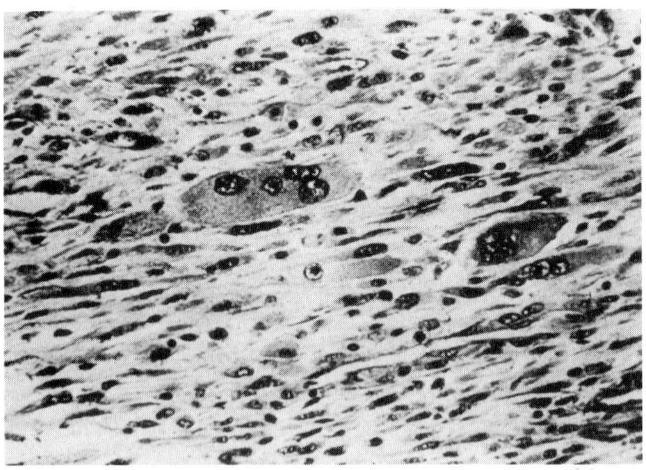

Fig. 7-22. Leiomyosarcoma demonstrating pleomorphism of muscle cells and multinucleated giant cells.

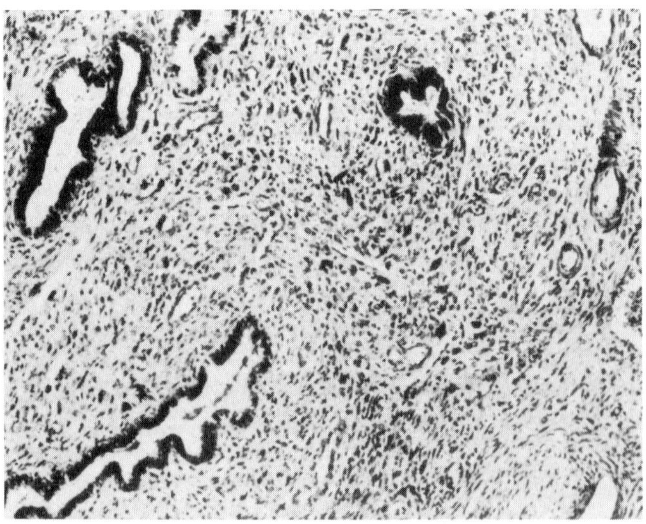

Fig. 7-23. Endometrial stromal sarcoma with neoplastic endometrial stroma and pleomorphic, giant cells scattered about proliferative glands.

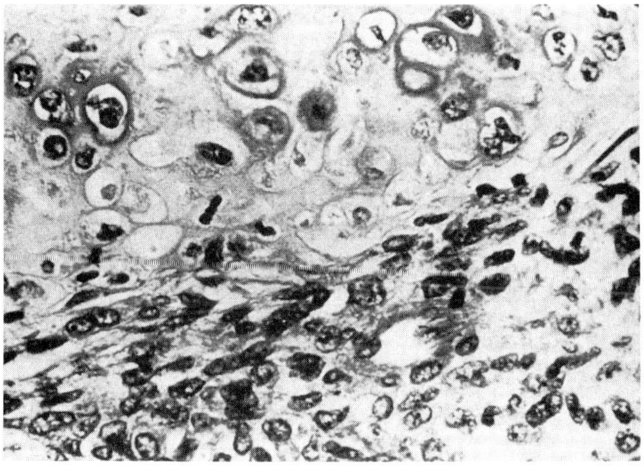

Fig. 7-24. Mixed mesodermal sarcoma of the uterus showing tendency of the tumor to form cartilage.

Chemotherapy for uterine sarcomas results in a reported combined response rate of up to 50% but in no prolongation of survival. Currently, the most active combination of drugs includes doxorubicin and dacarbazine.[50a] Ifosfamide may be considered for patients not responding to combination therapy; multiinstitutional trials are being conducted under the auspices of the Gynecologic Oncology Group.[6]

Natural history. Sarcomas may recur locally or at distant sites, and patients should be carefully followed. Uterine sarcomas tend to progress rapidly; 90% of recurrences occur within the first two years of diagnosis, and more than 90% appear outside the pelvis. The treatment of metastatic sarcoma should be palliative and should use doxorubicin, the most effective single agent. The use of progestational agents should be considered, particularly if the sarcoma has measurable steroid receptor content. However, despite earlier enthusiasm over hormonal manipulation of sarcomas, recent studies suggest that receptor status does not correlate with prognosis or disease-free survival in patients with uterine sarcomas.[172]

REFERENCES

1. Abramovici H, Faktor JH, Pascal B: Congenital uterine malformations as indication for cervical suture (cerclage) in habitual abortion and premature delivery, *Int J Fertil* 28:161-164, 1983.
2. American Cancer Society, *Cancer* 41:1, 1991
3. The American Fertility Society: Classifications of adnexal adhesions, distal tubal occlusion, tubal occlusion secondary to tubal ligation, tubal pregnancies, müllerian anomalies and intrauterine adhesions, *Fertil Steril* 49:944-955, 1988.
4. Ansbacher R: Uterine anomalies and future pregnancies, *Clin Perinatol* 10:295-304, 1983.
5. Anson BJ, Curtis AH: Anatomy of the female pelvis and perineum. In Curtis AH, editor: *Textbook of gynecology*, Philadelphia, 1946, WB Saunders.
6. Antman KH: Uterine sarcomas. In Knapp RC, Berkowitz RS, editors: *Gynecologic oncology*, New York, 1993, McGraw-Hill.
7. Antman KH et al: Preliminary results of a randomized trial of adjuvant Adriamycin for sarcomas, *J Clin Oncol* 2:601, 1984.
8. Antunes CMF et al: Endometrial cancer and estrogen use, *N Engl J Med* 300:9-13, 1979.
9. Asherman JG: Amenorrhoea traumatica (Atretica), *J Obstet Gynaecol Br Emp* 55:23-25, 1948.
10. Babaknia A, Rock JA, Jones HW Jr: Pregnancy success following abdominal myomectomy for infertility, *Fertil Steril* 30:644-647, 1978.
11. Baggish MS: Mesenchymal tumors of the uterus, *Clin Obstet Gynecol* 17:51-88, 1974.
12. Barnes AB et al: Fertility and outcome of pregnancy in women exposed in utero to diethylstilbestrol, *N Engl J Med* 302:609-613, 1980.
13. Bean HA et al: Carcinoma of the endometrium in Saskatchewan: 1966-1971, *Gynecol Oncol* 6:503-514, 1978.
14. Berchuck A et al: Treatment of uterine leiomyosarcoma, *Obstet Gynecol* 71:845-850, 1988.
15. Berkeley AS, DeCherney AH, Polan ML: Abdominal myomectomy and subsequent fertility, *Surg Gynecol Obstet* 156:319-322, 1983.
16. Bird CC, McElin TW: Adenomyosis and other benign diffuse enlargements of the uterus. In Sciarra JJ, editor: *Gynecology and obstetrics*, vol 1, New York, 1981, Harper & Row.
17. Bird CC, McElin TW, Manalo-Estrella P: The elusive adenomyosis of the uterus- revisited, *Am J Obstet Gynecol* 112:583-593, 1972.
18. Boronow RC et al: Surgical staging in endometrial cancer: clinical-pathologic findings of a prospective study, *Obstet Gynecol* 63:825-832, 1984.
19. Brown JM, Malkasian GD Jr, Symmonds RE: Abdominal myomectomy, *Am J Obstet Gynecol* 99:126-129, 1967.
20. Bruckman JE et al: Stage III adenocarcinoma of the endometrium: two prognostic groups, *Gynecol Oncol* 9:12-17, 1980.
21. Burrell MO, Franklin EW III, Powell JL: Endometrial cancer: evaluation of spread and follow-up in one hundred eighty-nine patients with stage I or stage II disease, *Am J Obstet Gynecol* 144:181-185, 1982.
22. Buttram VC Jr: Müllerian anomalies and their management, *Fertil Steril* 40:159-163, 1983.
23. Buttram VC Jr, Gibbons WE: Müllerian anomalies: a proposed classification (an analysis of 144 cases), *Fertil Steril* 32:40-46, 1979.
24. Buttram VC Jr, Reiter RC: Uterine leiomyomata: etiology, symptomatology, and management, *Fertil Steril* 36:433-445, 1981.
25. Capraro VJ, Gallego MB: Vaginal agenesis, *Am J Obstet Gynecol* 124:98-107, 1976.
26. Chambers JT et al: Uterine papillary serous carcinoma, *Obstet Gynecol* 69:109-113, 1987.
27. Cheon HK: Prognosis of endometrial carcinoma, *Obstet Gynecol* 34:680-684, 1969.
28. Childers JM et al: Laparoscopically assisted surgical staging (LASS), *J Endomet Cancer* 51:33, 1993.
29. Christopherson WM, Alberhasky RC, Connelly PJ: Carcinoma of the endometrium. II. Papillary adenocarcinoma—a clinical pathological study of 46 cases, *Am J Clin Pathol* 77:534-540, 1982.
30. Chu J, Schweid AI, Weiss NS: Survival among women with endometrial cancer: a comparison of estrogen users and nonusers, *Am J Obstet Gynecol* 143:569-573, 1982.
31. Cohen I et al: Ultrasonographic evaluation of the endometrium and correlation with endometrial sampling in postmenopausal patients treated with tamoxifen, *J Ultrasound Med* 12:275-280, 1993.
32. Coulam CB, Annegers JF, Kranz JS: Chronic anovulation syndrome and associated neoplasia, *Obstet Gynecol* 61:403-407, 1983.
33. Counseller VS, Bedard RE: Uterine myomectomy, *JAMA* 111: 675-678, 1937.
34. Coutinho EM, Boulanger GA, Goncalves MT: Regression of uterine leiomyomas after treatment with gestrinone, an antiestrogen, antiprogesterone, *Am J Obstet Gynecol* 155:761-767, 1986.
35. Coutinho EM, Goncalves MT: Long-term treatment of leiomyomas with gestrinone, *Fertil Steril* 51:939-946, 1989.
36. Cramer DW, Cutler SJ, Christine B: Trends in the incidence of endometrial cancer in the United States, *Gynecol Oncol* 2:130-143, 1974.

37. Cramer DW, Knapp RC: Review of epidemiologic studies of endometrial cancer and exogenous estrogen, *Obstet Gynecol* 54:521-526, 1979.
38. Creasman WT et al: Prognostic significance of peritoneal cytology in patients with endometrial cancer and preliminary data concerning therapy with intraperitoneal radiopharmaceuticals, *Am J Obstet Gynecol* 141:921-929, 1981.
39. Creasman WT et al: Clinical correlates of estrogen- and progesterone-binding proteins in human endometrial adenocarcinoma, *Obstet Gynecol* 55:363-370, 1980.
40. Creasman WT et al: Surgical pathologic spread patterns of endometrial cancer: a Gynecologic Oncology Group study, *Cancer* 60: 2035-2041, 1987.
41. Daly DC et al: Hysteroscopic metroplasty: surgical technique and obstetric outcome, *Fertil Steril* 39:623-628, 1983.
42. Davies JL et al: A review of the risk factors for endometrial carcinoma, *Obstet Gynecol Surv* 36:107-116, 1981.
43. Davis EW: Carcinoma of the corpus uteri: a study of 525 cases at the New York Hospital (1932-1961), *Am J Obstet Gynecol* 88:163, 1964.
44. DeCherney AH et al: Resectoscopic management of müllerian fusion defects, *Fertil Steril* 45:726-728, 1986.
45. Deppe G et al: Chemotherapy of advanced and recurrent endometrial carcinoma with cyclophosphamide, doxorubicin, 5-fluorouracil, and megestrol acetate, *Am J Obstet Gynecol* 140:313-316, 1981.
46. DeVore GR, Schwartz PE, Morris JM: Hysterography: a 5-year follow-up in patients with endometrial carcinoma, *Obstet Gynecol* 60:369-372, 1982.
47. Doss LL, Llorens AS, Henriquez FM: Carcinosarcoma of the uterus: a 40-year experience from the state of Missouri, *Gynecol Oncol* 18:43-53, 1984.
48. Easterday CL, Grimes DA, Riggs JA: Hysterectomy in the United States, *Obstet Gynecol* 62:203-212, 1983.
49. Ehrlich CE et al: Steroid receptors and clinical outcome in patients with adenocarcinoma of the endometrium, *Am J Obstet Gynecol* 158:796-807, 1988.
50. Eifel PJ et al: Adenocarcinoma of the endometrium: analysis of 256 cases with disease limited to the uterine corpus: treatment comparisons, *Cancer* 52:1026-1031, 1983.
51. Elwood JM, Boyes DA: Clinical and pathologic features and survival of endometrial cancer patients in relation to prior use of estrogens, *Gynecol Oncol* 10:173-187, 1980.
52. Elwood JM et al: Epidemiology of endometrial cancer, *J Natl Cancer Inst* 59:1055-1060, 1977.
53. Farber M et al: Estradiol binding by fibroid tumors and normal myometrium, *Obstet Gynecol* 40:479-486, 1972.
54. Fayez JA: Comparison between abdominal and hysteroscopic metroplasty, *Obstet Gynecol* 68:399-403, 1986.
55. Fedele L et al: Magnetic resonance evaluation of double uteri, *Obstet Gynecol* 74:844-847, 1989.
56. Fedele L et al: Transvaginal ultrasonography in the diagnosis of diffuse adenomyosis, *Fertil Steril* 58:94-97, 1992.
57. Feldman S, Berkowitz RS, Tosteson AN: Cost-effectiveness of strategies to evaluate postmenopausal bleeding, *Obstet Gynecol* 81:968-975, 1993.
58. Ferenczy A, Gelfand M: The biologic significance of cytologic atypia in progestogen-treated endometrial hyperplasia, *Am J Obstet Gynecol* 160:126-131, 1989.
59. Finn WF, Muller PF: Abdominal myomectomy: special reference to subsequent pregnancy and to the reappearance of fibromyomas of the uterus, *Am J Obstet Gynecol* 60:109-114, 1950.
60. Forney JP, Buschbaum HJ: Classifying, staging, and treating uterine sarcomas, *Contemp Ob Gyn* 18:47, 50, 55-56, 61-62, 64, 69, 1981.
61. Frank RT: The formation of an artificial vagina without operation, *Am J Obstet Gynecol* 35:1053-1059, 1938.
62. Friedman AJ et al: Treatment of leiomyomata with intranasal or subcutaneous leuprolide, a gonadotropin-releasing hormone agonist, *Fertil Steril* 48:560-564, 1987a.
63. Friedman AJ et al: A randomized, double-blind trial of a gonadotropin-releasing hormone agonist (leuprolide) with or without medroxyprogesterone acetate in the treatment of leiomyomata uteri, *Fertil Steril* 49:404-409, 1988.
64. Friedman AJ et al: Recurrence of myomas following myomectomy in women treated with a gonadotropin-releasing hormone agonist, *Fertil Steril* 58:205-208, 1992.
65. Friedman A, DeFazio J, DeCherney A: Severe obstetric complications after aggressive treatment of Asherman's syndrome, *Obstet Gynecol* 67:864-867, 1986.
66. Friedman AJ, Haas ST: Should uterine size be an indication for surgery for women with leiomyomas? *Am J Obstet Gynecol* 168:751-755, 1993.
67. Friedman AJ et al: A randomized, placebo-controlled, double-blind study evaluating the efficacy of leuprolide acetate depot in the treatment of uterine leiomyomata, *Fertil Steril* 51:251-256, 1989.
68. Friedman AJ et al: Treatment of leiomyomata uteri with leuprolide acetate depot: a double-blind, placebo-controlled, multicenter study, *Obstet Gynecol* 77:720-725, 1991.
69. Friedman AJ et al: Efficacy and safety considerations in women with uterine leiomyomata treated with gonadotropin-releasing hormone agonists: the estrogen threshold hypothesis, *Am J Obstet Gynecol* 163:1114-1119, 1990.
70. Friedman AJ, Ravnikar VA, Barbieri RL: Serum steroid hormone profiles in postmenopausal smokers and nonsmokers, *Fertil Steril* 47:398-401, 1987b.
71. Fritsch H: Ein Fall von volligem Schwund der Gebarmutterhohle nach Auskratzung, *Zentralbl Gynaekol* 18:1337-1341, 1984.
72. Gal D: Hormonal therapy for lesions of the endometrium, *Semin Oncol* 13(Suppl 4):33-36, 1986.
73. Gambone JC et al: In vivo availability of circulating estradiol in postmenopausal women with and without endometrial cancer, *Obstet Gynecol* 59:416-421, 1982.
74. Gambrell RD Jr: The prevention of endometrial cancer in postmenopausal women with progestogens, *Maturitas* 1:107-112, 1978.
75. Gapstur SM et al: Alcohol consumption and postmenopausal endometrial cancer: results from the Iowa Women's Health Study, *Cancer Causes Control* 4:323-329, 1993.
76. Gloor E et al: Endolymphatic stromal meiosis. Surgical and hormonal treatment of extensive adbominal recurrence 20 years after hysterectomy, *Cancer* 50:1888-1893, 1982.
77. Godsoe A et al: Cardiopulmonary changes with intermittent endotoxin administration in sheep. *Circ Shock* 25:61-74, 1988.
78. Granberg S et al: Endometrial thickness as measured by endovaginal ultrasonography for identifying endometrial abnormality, *Am J Obstet Gynecol* 164:47-52, 1991.
79. Gronroos M et al: Mass screening for endometrial cancer directed in risk groups of patients with diabetes and patients with hypertension, *Cancer* 71:1279-1282, 1993.
80. Gros A, David A, Serr DM: Management of congenital malformations of the uterus: fetal salvage, *Acta Eur Fertil* 5:301-304, 1974.
81. Gurpide E: Hormone receptors in endometrial cancer, *Cancer* 48:638-641, 1981.
82. Hannigan EV, Gomez LG: Uterine leiomyosarcoma: a review of prognostic clinical and pathologic features, *Am J Obstet Gynecol* 134:557-564, 1979.
83. Harger JH et al: Etiology of recurrent pregnancy losses and outcome of subsequent pregnancies, *Obstet Gynecol* 62:574-581, 1983.
84. Harlow BL, Weiss NS, Lofton S: The epidemiology of sarcomas of the uterus, *J Natl Cancer Inst* 76:399-402, 1986.

85. Hendrickson MR et al: Adenocarcinoma of the endometrium. Analysis of 256 cases with carcinoma limited to the uterine corpus: pathology review and analysis of prognostic variables, *Gynecol Oncol* 13:373-392, 1982.
86. Hornback NB, Omura G, Major FJ: Observations on the use of adjuvant radiation therapy in patients with stage I and II uterine sarcoma, *Int J Radiat Oncol Biol Phys* 12:2127-2130, 1986.
87. Hulka BS et al: Protection against endometrial carcinoma by combination-product oral contraceptives, *JAMA* 247:475, 1982.
88. Hunt JE, Wallach EE: Uterine factors in infertility—an overview, *Clin Obstet Gynecol* 17:44-64, 1974.
89. Imachi M et al: Peritoneal cytology in patients with endometrial carcinoma, *Gynecol Oncol* 30:76-86, 1988.
90. Ingersoll FM: Fertility following myomectomy, *Fertil Steril* 14:596-601, 1963.
91. Israel SL, Woutersz TB: Adenomyosis: a neglected diagnosis, *Obstet Gynecol* 14:168-174, 1959.
92. Jasonni VM et al: Treatment of endometrial hyperplasia with cyproterone acetate: histological and hormonal aspects, *Acta Obstet Gynecol Scand* 65:685-687, 1986.
93. Jewelewicz R et al: Obstetric complications after treatment of intrauterine synechiae (Asherman's syndrome), *Obstet Gynecol* 47:701-705, 1976.
94. Jick H et al: Replacement estrogens and endometrial cancer, *N Engl J Med* 300:218-222, 1979.
95. Jones WE: Traumatic intrauterine adhesions: a report of 8 cases with emphasis on therapy, *Am J Obstet Gynecol* 89:304-309, 1964.
96. Judd HL et al: Serum androgens and estrogens in postmenopausal women with and without endometrial cancer, *Am J Obstet Gynecol* 136:859-871, 1980.
97. Karlsson B et al: Endovaginal scanning of the endometrium compared to cytology and histology in women with postmenopausal bleeding, *Gynecol Oncol* 50:173-178, 1933.
98. Kaufman RH et al: Upper genital tract changes and pregnancy outcome in offspring exposed in utero to diethylstilbestrol, *Am J Obstet Gynecol* 137:299-308, 1980.
99. Kawaguchi K et al: Mitotic activity in uterine leiomyomas during the menstrual cycle, *Am J Obstet Gynecol* 160:637-641, 1989.
100. Kelsey JL et al: A case-control study of cancer of the endometrium, *Am J Epidemiol* 116:333-342, 1982.
101. Kempson RL, Bari W: Uterine sarcomas: classification, diagnosis, and prognosis, *Hum Pathol* 1:331-349, 1970.
102. Kinsella TJ et al: Stage II endometrial carcinoma: 10-year follow-up of combined radiation and surgical treatment, *Gynecol Oncol* 10:290-297, 1980.
103. Kurman RJ, Kaminski PF, Norris HJ: The behavior of endometrial hyperplasia: a long-term study of "untreated" hyperplasia in 170 patients, *Cancer* 56:403-412, 1985.
104. Kurman RJ, Scully RE: Clear cell carcinoma of the endometrium: an analysis of 21 cases, *Cancer* 37:872-882, 1976.
105. Lee RB, Burke TW, Park RC: Estrogen replacement therapy following treatment for stage I endometrial carcinoma, *Gynecol Oncol* 36:189-191, 1990.
106. Leibel SA, Wharam MD: Vaginal and paraaortic lymph node metastases in carcinoma of the endometrium, *Int J Radiat Oncol Biol Phys* 6:893-896, 1980.
107. Lipshultz A: Experimental fibroids and the antifibromatogenic action of steroid hormones, *JAMA* 120:173, 1942.
108. Loeffler FE, Noble AD: Myomectomy at the Chelsea Hospital for Women, *J Obstet Gynaecol Br Commonw* 77:167-170, 1970.
109. Lucas WE, Yen SS: A study of endocrine and metabolic variables in postmenopausal women with endometrial carcinoma, *Am J Obstet Gynecol* 134:180-186, 1979.
110. Lynch HT et al: Adenocarcinoma of the small bowel in Lynch syndrome II, *Cancer* 64:2178-2183, 1989.
111. Mack TM et al: Estrogens and endometrial cancer in a retirement community, *N Engl J Med* 294:1262-1267, 1976.
112. MacMahon B: Risk factors for endometrial cancer, *Gynecol Oncol* 2:122-129, 1974.
113. Magriples U et al: High-grade endometrial carcinoma in tamoxifen-treated breast cancer patients, *J Clin Oncol* 11:485-490, 1993.
114. Maheux R et al: Luteinizing hormone-releasing hormone agonist and uterine leiomyoma: a pilot study, *Am J Obstet Gynecol* 152:1034-1038, 1985.
115. Malone LJ, Ingersoll FM: Myomectomy in infertility. In Behrman SJ, Kistner RW, editors: *Progress in infertility*, Boston, 1975, Little, Brown.
116. Malviya VK et al: Reliability of frozen section examination in identifying poor prognostic indicators in stage I endometrial adenocarcinoma, *Gynecol Oncol* 34:299-304, 1989.
117. March CM, Israel R, March AD: Hysteroscopic management of intrauterine adhesions, *Am J Obstet Gynecol* 130:653-657, 1978.
118. McCausland AM: Hysteroscopic myometrial biopsy: its use in diagnosing adenomyosis and its clinical application, *Am J Obstet Gynecol* 166:1619-1628, 1992.
119. McCormick TA: Myomectomy with subsequent pregnancy, *Am J Obstet Gynecol* 75:1128-1133, 1958.
120. McElin TW, Bird CC: Adenomyosis of the uterus, *Obstet Gynecol Annu* 3:425-441, 1974.
121. McIndoe AH: The treatment of congenital absence and obliterative conditions of the vagina, *Br J Plastic Surg* 2:254-263, 1950.
122. McShane PM, Reilly RJ, Schiff I: Pregnancy outcomes following Tompkins metroplasty, *Fertil Steril* 40:190-194, 1983.
123. Meisels A, Jolicoeur C: Criteria for the cytologic assessment of hyperplasias in endometrial samples obtained by the Endopap Endometrial Sampler, *Acta Cytol* 29:297-302, 1985.
124. Meredith RF et al: An excess of uterine sarcomas after pelvic irradiation, *Cancer* 58:2003-2007, 1986.
125. Meyer R: Uber Drusen, Cyste und Adenom in Myometrium bei er Wachsen, *Z Geburtshilfe Gynaekol* 43:130-138, 1900.
126. Miller H, Tyrone C: A survey of a series of myomectomies with a follow-up, *Am J Obstet Gynecol* 26:575-581, 1933.
127. Misch KA et al: Tuberculosis of the cervix: cytology as an aid to diagnosis, *J Clin Pathol* 29:313-316, 1976.
128. Molitor JJ: Adenomyosis: a clinical and pathologic appraisal, *Am J Obstet Gynecol* 110:275-284, 1971.
129. Mortel R, Zaino R, Satyaswaroop PG: Modulation of growth and sex steroid receptor concentrations by tamoxifen in human endometrial carcinoma transplanted into nude mice, *Proc Soc Gynecol Oncol* 19:23, 1983.
130. Munnell EW, Martin FW: Abdominal myomectomy, advantages and disadvantages, *Am J Obstet Gynecol* 62:109-114, 1951.
131. Nasri MN et al: The role of vaginal scan in measurement of endometrial thickness in postmenopausal women, *Br J Obstet Gynaecol* 98:470-475, 1991.
132. National Center for Health Statistics: Hysterectomies in the United States 1965-84, *Vital and Health Statistics,* Series 13, No 92, Bethesda, Maryland Pub Co 88-1753, 1987.
133. Nelson WO: Endometrial and myometrial changes including fibromyomatous nodules induced in the guinea pig by oestrogen, *Anat Rec* 68:99, 1937.
134. Neuwirth RS, Friedman EA: Septic abortion: changing concept of management, *Am J Obstet Gynecol* 85:24, 1963.
135. Nilbert M, Heim S: Uterine leiomyoma cytogenetics, *Genes, Chromosome Cancer* 2:3-13, 1990.
136. Niloff JM et al: Elevation of serum CA-125 in carcinomas of the fallopian tube, endometrium, and endocervix, *Am J Obstet Gynecol* 148:1057-1058, 1984.
137. Nishida M: Relationship between the onset of dysmenorrhea and histologic findings in adenomyosis, *Am J Obstet Gynecol* 165:229-231, 1991.

138. Nishijima MK et al: Effect of naloxone and ibuprofen on organ blood flow during endotoxic shock in pig, *Am J Physiol* 255:H177-184, 1988.
139. Ng AB et al: Significance of endometrial cells in the detection of endometrial carcinoma and its precursors, *Acta Cytol* 18: 356-361, 1974.
140. Norris HJ, Taylor HB: Mesenchymal tumors of the uterus: I. A clinical and pathologic study of 53 endometrial stromal tumors, *Cancer* 19:755-766, 1966.
141. Norris HJ, Taylor HB: Mesenchymal tumors of the uterus: III. A clinical and pathologic study of 31 carcinosarcomas, *Cancer* 19:1459-1465, 1966.
142. Novak ER, Woodruff JD: Myoma and other benign tumors of the uterus. In *Gynecologic and obstetric pathology*, ed 8, Philadelphia, London, Toronto, 1979, WB Saunders.
143. O'Connor DM, Norris HJ: Mitotically active leiomyomas of the uterus, *Hum Pathol* 21:223-227, 1990.
144. O'Leary JL, O'Leary JA: Rudimentary horn pregnancy, *Obstet Gynecol* 22:371-377, 1963.
145. Otubu JA et al: Unconjugated steroids in leiomyomas and tumor-bearing myometrium, *Am J Obstet Gynecol* 143:130-133, 1982.
146. Padubidri V et al: The detection of endometrial tuberculosis in cases of infertility by uterine aspiration cytology, *Acta Cytol* 24:319-324, 1980.
147. Park RC et al: Corpus: epithelial tumors. In *Principles and practice of gynecologic oncology*, Philadelphia, 1992, JB Lippincott.
148. Pastner B, Mann WJ: Use of serum CA-125 in monitoring patients with uterine sarcoma: a preliminary report, *Cancer* 62:1355-1358, 1988.
149. Patsner B et al: Predictive value of preoperative serum CA-125 levels in clinically localized and advanced endometrial carcinoma, *Am J Obstet Gynecol* 158:399-402, 1988.
150. Paulsen MG, Roberts SJ: The salvage of recurrent endometrial carcinoma in the vagina and pelvis, *Int J Radiat Oncol Biol Phys* 15:809-813, 1988.
151. Perino A et al: Hysteroscopy for metroplasty of uterine septa: report of 24 cases, *Fertil Steril* 48:321-323, 1987.
152. Pettersson F, editor: *Annual report on the results of treatment in gynecologic cancer*, vol 20, International Federation of Gynecology and Obstetrics, Stockholm, 1988.
153. Piver MS et al: Paraaortic lymph node evaluation in stage I endometrial carcinoma, *Obstet Gynecol* 59:97-100, 1982.
154. Plentl AA, Friedman EA: Lymphatic system of the female genitalia. In *The morphologic basis of oncologic diagnosis and therapy*, Philadelphia, 1971, WB Saunders.
155. Pollow K et al: In vitro conversion of estradiol-17 beta into estrone in normal human myometrium and leiomyoma, *J Clin Chem Clin Biochem* 16:493-502, 1978.
156. Potischman N et al: Dietary associations in a case-control study of endometrial cancer, *Cancer Causes Control* 4:239-250, 1993.
157. Potish RA et al: Paraaortic lymph node radiotherapy in cancer of the uterine corpus, *Obstet Gynecol* 65:251-256, 1985.
158. Ranney B, Frederick I: The occasional need for myomectomy, *Obstet Gynecol* 53:437-441, 1979.
159. Robbins SL, Cotran RS: Leiomyoma (fibromyoma). In *The pathogenic basis of disease,* ed 2, Philadelphia, London, Toronto, 1979, WB Saunders.
160. Roberts DE et al: Effects of prolonged naloxone infusion in septic shock, *Lancet* 2:699-702, 1988.
161. Rock JA, Jones HW Jr: The clinical management of the double uterus, *Fertil Steril* 28:798-806, 1977.
162. Rubin A, Ford JA: Uterine fibromyomata in urban Blacks: a preliminary survey of the relationship between symptomatology, blood pressure and haemoglobin levels, *S Afr Med J* 48:2060-2062, 1974.
163. Salazar OM et al: Uterine sarcomas: natural history, treatment and prognosis, *Cancer* 42:1152-1160, 1978.
164. Salazar OM et al: Adenosquamous carcinoma of the endometrium: an entity with an inherent poor prognosis? *Cancer* 40:119-130, 1977.
165. Schenker JG, Margalioth EJ: Intrauterine adhesions: an updated appraisal, *Fertil Steril* 37:593-610, 1982.
166. Schumer W: Steroids in the treatment of clinical septic shock, *Ann Surg* 184:333-341, 1976.
167. Shah CA, Green TH Jr: Evaluation of current management of endometrial carcinoma, *Obstet Gynecol* 39:500-509, 1972.
168. Silverberg E, Lubera JA: Cancer statistics, 1988, *CA Cancer J Clin* 38:5-22, 1988.
169. Skowronski GA: The pathophysiology of shock, *Med J Aust* 148:576-579, 582-583, 1988.
170. Smith DC et al: Association of exogenous estrogen and endometrial carcinoma, *N Engl J Med* 293:1164-1167, 1975.
171. Smith P et al: Transvaginal ultrasound for identifying endometrial abnormality, *Acta Obstet Gynecol Scand* 70:591-594, 1991.
172. Soper JT et al: Cytoplasmic estrogen and progesterone receptor content of uterine sarcomas, *Am J Obstet Gynecol* 150:342-348, 1984.
173. Soules MR, McCarty KS Jr: Leiomyomas: steroid receptor content: variation within normal menstrual cycles, *Am J Obstet Gynecol* 143:6-11, 1982.
174. Stillman RJ: In utero exposure to diethylstilbestrol: adverse effects on the reproductive tract and reproductive performance in male and female offspring, *Am J Obstet Gynecol* 142:905-921, 1982.
175. Stovall TG, Solomon SK, Ling FW: Endometrial sampling prior to hysterectomy, *Obstet Gynecol* 73:405-409, 1989.
176. Strassmann EO: Operations for double uterus and endometrial atresia. *Clin Obstet Gynecol* 4:240-251, 1961.
177. Strassmann EO: Fertility and unification of double uterus, *Fertil Steril* 17:165-176, 1966.
178. Sutherland AM: Laparoscopy in diagnosis of pelvic tuberculosis, *Lancet* 2:95, 1979.
179. Sutherland AM: Gynaecologic tuberculosis: analysis of a personal series of 710 cases, *Aust N Z J Obstet Gynaecol* 25:203-207, 1985.
180. Terakawa N et al: Preliminary report on the use of danazol in the treatment of endometrial adenomatous hyperplasia, *Cancer* 62: 2618-2621, 1988.
181. Thigpen JT et al: Phase II trial of adriamycin in the treatment of advanced or recurrent endometrial carcinoma: a Gynecologic Oncology Group study, *Cancer Treat Rep* 63:21-27, 1979.
182. Tierney WM et al: Intravenous leiomyomatosis of the uterus with extension into the heart, *Am J Med* 69:471-475, 1980.
183. Tiltman AJ: The effect of progestins on the mitotic activity of uterine fibromyomas, *Int J Gynecol Pathol* 4:89-96, 1985.
184. Townsend DE et al: Unicellular histogenesis of uterine leiomyomas as determined by electrophoresis by glucose-6-phosphate dehydrogenase, *Am J Obstet Gynecol* 107:1168-1173, 1970.
185. Underwood PB et al: Endometrial carcinoma: the effect of estrogens, *Gynecol Oncol* 8:60-73, 1979.
186. Vadas P et al: Pathogenesis of hypotension in septic shock: correlation of circulating phospholipase A2 levels with circulatory collapse, *Crit Care Med* 16:1-7, 1988.
187. Valle RF, Sciarra JJ: Hysteroscopic treatment of the septate uterus, *Obstet Gynecol* 67:253-257, 1986.
188. Van Bogaert LJ: Clinicopathologic findings in endometrial polyps, *Obstet Gynecol* 71:771-773, 1988.
189. van Nagell JR Jr et al: Adjuvant vincristine, dactinomycin and cyclophosphamide therapy in stage I uterine sarcomas: a pilot study, *Cancer* 57:1451-1457, 1986.
190. Weed JC, Bryan AC: Adenomyosis: twenty years' experience, *J Med Assoc State Ala* 32:327-334, 1963.
191. Weiss DB, Aldor A, Aboulafia Y: Erythrocytosis due to erythropoietin-producing uterine fibromyoma, *Am J Obstet Gynecol* 122:358-360, 1975.
192. Weiss NS, Sayvetz TA: Incidence of endometrial cancer in relation to the use of oral contraceptives, *N Engl J Med* 302:551-554, 1980.

193. Weiss NS et al: Endometrial cancer in relation to patterns of menopausal estrogen use, *JAMA* 242:261-264, 1979.
194. Welch WR, Scully RE: Precancerous lesions of the endometrium, *Hum Pathol* 8:503-512, 1977.
195. Wentz WB: Progestin therapy in endometrial hyperplasia, *Gynecol Oncol* 2:362-367, 1974.
196. Wentz WB: Progestin therapy in lesions of the endometrium, *Semin Oncol* 12:23-27, 1985.
197. Wilson EA, Yang F, Rees ED: Estradiol and progesterone binding in uterine leiomyomata and in normal uterine tissues, *Obstet Gynecol* 55:20-24, 1980.
198. Worthen NJ, Gonzalez F: Septate uterus: sonographic diagnosis and obstetric complications, *Obstet Gynecol* 64:34S-38S, 1984.
199. Yamashita Y et al: Assessment of myometrial invasion by endometrial carcinoma: transvaginal sonography vs contrast-enhanced MR imaging, *AJR Am J Roentgenol* 16:595-599, 1993.
200. Yazigi R et al: Magnetic resonance imaging determination of myometrial invasion in endometrial carcinoma, *Gynecol Oncol* 34:94-97, 1989.
201. Yazigi R, Piver MS, Blumenson L: Malignant peritoneal cytology as prognostic indicator in stage I endometrial cancer, *Obstet Gynecol* 62:359-362, 1983.
202. Zucker PK, Kasdon EJ, Feldstein ML: The validity of Pap smear parameters as predictors of endometrial pathology in menopausal women, *Cancer* 56:2256-2263, 1985.

Chapter 8

THE FALLOPIAN TUBES AND ECTOPIC PREGNANCY

Elizabeth A. Stewart
John Yeh

ANATOMY AND HISTOLOGY

The fallopian tubes (oviducts) are paired muscular canals that extend from the uterus to the ovaries, each measuring about 12 cm in length. These structures transport the ova into the uterine cavity. As in most mammalian species, the fallopian tube is not in continuity with the ovary—it is only in apposition with it. Both tubes are covered with peritoneum and lined with epithelium, and, except for a short intrauterine portion, are enveloped in the free margin of the broad ligament known as the mesosalpinx.

The fallopian tube emerges from the uterine wall at the junction of the corpus and fundus. The proximal segment arches laterally and posteriorly, adjacent to the lower pole of the ovary. It then assumes a tortuous course along the mesovarial border of the ovary to the fimbriated end. At this point the tube is in direct relation to the medial ovarian surface. Normal variations from this description are common.

Four subdivisions of the fallopian tube are described as follows (Fig. 8-1):

1. The *interstitial* portion is short and begins at the superior angle of the uterine cavity; it connects with the uterine cavity by a 1-mm ostium. It extends through the thickness of the myometrium, angulates through the fundus, and exits at the uterine cornu just superior to the attachments of the round and uteroovarian ligaments. It may have a tortuous course.[86]
2. The *isthmic* portion is relatively straight, narrow, and thick-walled. It gradually increases in luminal diameter and shows a diminution in thickness of the wall as it progresses laterally.
3. The *ampullar* portion is the longest segment of the fallopian tube (approximately 6 cm). In its normal state it is slightly convoluted and has a relatively thin, dilatable muscular wall.
4. The *infundibular* portion is the trumpet-shaped terminal portion of the fallopian tube. It is divided into numerous delicate folds or fimbriae that appear fringed. One of these folds is prolonged and is attached to the mesosalpinx (fimbria ovarica). Frequently it lies in apposition to the tubal pole of the ovary.

The wall of the fallopian tube consists of three layers: an external or serous, an intermediate muscular, and an internal mucous layer. The serous covering is an extension of the broad ligament peritoneum and invests the tube completely except for the attachment of the mesosalpinx and the intrauterine portion. Beneath the mesothelial cells of the serosa is a connective tissue layer containing mostly blood vessels and nerves that intermingle with the subjacent muscular layer. The outer layer of the muscularis is arranged longitudinally, whereas the inner layer is arranged circularly. The mucous membrane lining presents a characteristic folded, somewhat arborescent pattern that is most pronounced toward the fimbriated portion (plicae tubariae). These longitudinal folds begin as four duplications of the mucosa in the interstitial portion of the tube, enclosing a small lumen. The lumen of the fallopian tube becomes larger as it approaches the fimbriated portion. It thus affords added space for increased mucosal folding. As the ampullary portion of the tube is reached, the plicae are extremely complicated and present numerous reduplications and outpouchings (Fig. 8-2). The mucosa is lined with a columnar epithelium containing

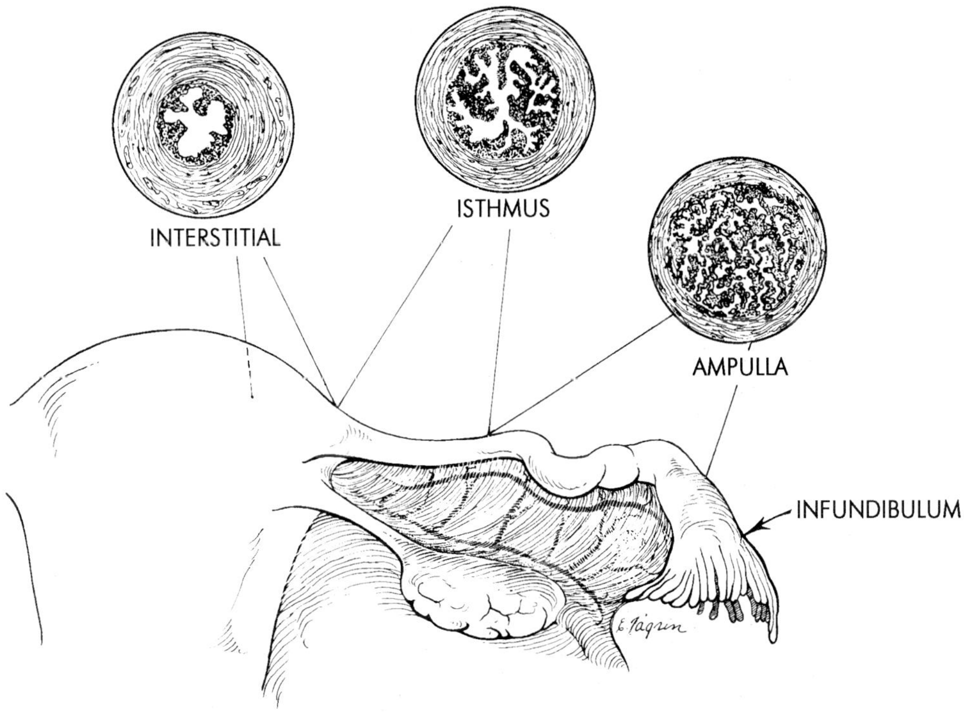

Fig. 8-1. Anatomical divisions of the oviduct.

ciliated and nonciliated or "secretory" cells. Intercalary or "peg" cells are most easily identified in the premenstrual and menstrual period. The endosalpinx, like the endometrium, exhibits a cyclic morphological variation depending on hormonal stimulation.[40,62] During the proliferative phase of estrogen stimulation, the epithelium is uniformly tall with prominent ciliated cells and narrow nonciliated cells. During the late secretory phase, the ciliated cells are much lower and the secretory cells are quite prominent, giving a rather uneven surface to the mucosa. The epithelium is rather low during the menstrual phase because the secretory cells have depleted their cytoplasm. Intercalary cells are numerous during the menstrual phase, and their appearance at this time suggests that they may be remnants of emptied secretory cells. The immediate postmenstrual phase presents a low epithelial surface in the fallopian tube, but regeneration is rapid during the proliferative phase. It is likely that estrogen is responsible for ciliogenesis and that progesterone causes deciliation under some conditions.[63]

The epithelium is low and flat during the postmenopausal period. The tubal folds become rounded and fibrous. Their cilia disappear but may be restored by estrogen replacement.

The tubal epithelium in patients with endometrial hyperplasia is usually high, with uniform, narrow cells, most of which are ciliated. This represents the effects of persistent estrogen stimulation without the normal cyclic intervention of progesterone. The hormonal effect is even more evident during pregnancy when a decidual reaction in the stromal cells may be extensive. Tubal infections cause morphological changes in tubal epithelium, especially loss of ciliated cells.

The arterial blood supply to the fallopian tube is generous, as it anastomoses from two sources, the ovary and the uterus. A tubal branch of the uterine artery passes through the mesosalpinx to join the branches of the ovarian artery. The venous drainage similarly occurs through the branches of the uterine and ovarian veins.

Lymphatic drainage follows the ovarian vessels, with drainage into lumbar or paraaortic nodes in the area of the renal vein and inferior vena cava on the right, and into the nodes between the ovarian vein and renal vein on the left.

Both sympathetic and parasympathetic nerve fibers are found. Sympathetic fibers arise from T10 through L2, synapse in numerous plexuses, and ultimately provide adrenergic innervation to the tubal musculature. Parasympathetic nerves arise from the vagus nerve and from S2 to S4 through the pelvic nerve. Sensory fibers end in T10 and T4, and referred pain may be experienced in these dermatomes.

EMBRYOLOGY

The fallopian tubes are formed by differentiation of the unfused paramesonephric ducts. (The fused portions form the uterus and a significant portion of the vagina.) Early in the seventh week, the paramesonephric (müllerian) ducts arise lateral and parallel to the mesonephric duct by a process of

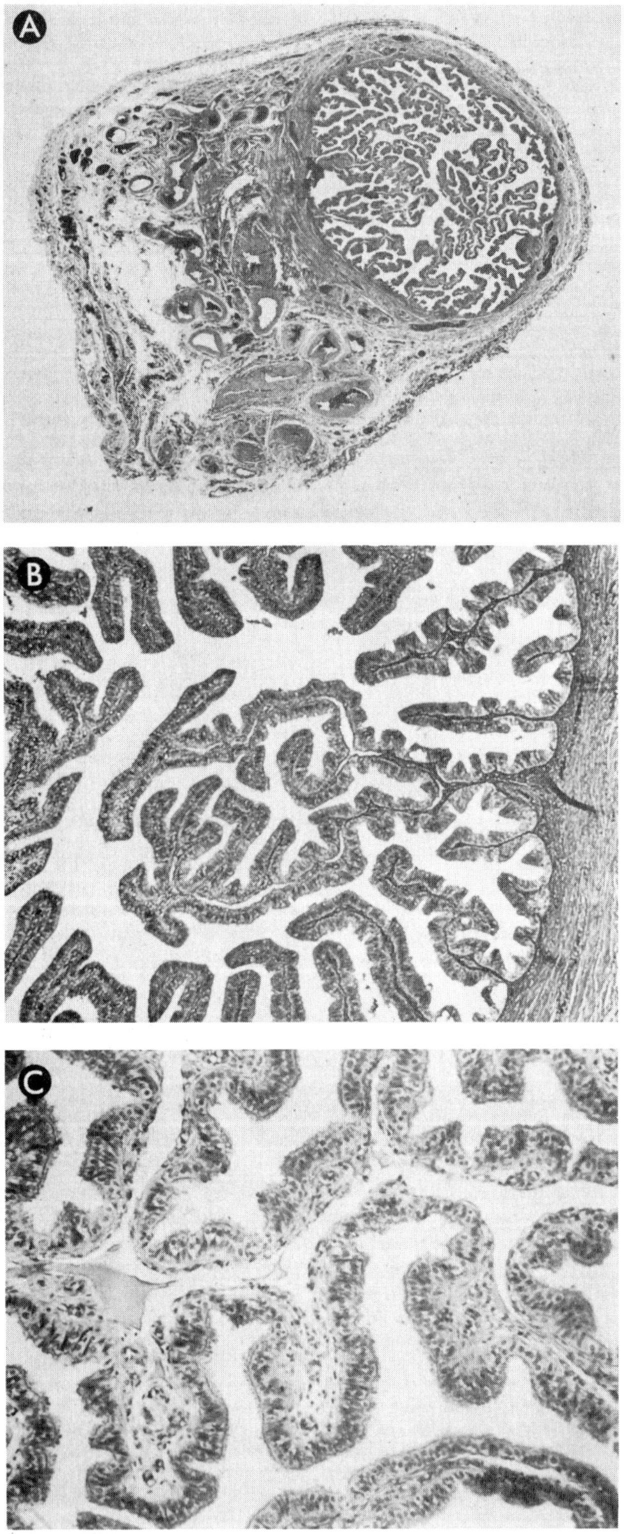

Fig. 8-2. A, Normal oviduct *(ampullary portion).* **B,** Higher power to show epithelium in proliferative phase. **C,** Higher power to show epithelium in secretory phase. (From Hall JE: *Applied gynecologic pathology,* New York, 1963, Appleton-Century-Crofts, p 197.)

invagination of the coelomic epithelium opposite the cranial end of the mesonephros. The solid portions of the ducts extend caudally through primitive mesenchyme and cross the mesonephric duct anteriorly at the level of the caudal end of the mesonephros.

The most common type of congenital anomaly of the fallopian tube is a rudimentary or absent ampullary portion. This probably occurs because of torsion and subsequent ischemic atrophy. Supernumerary fallopian tubes are rare, but duplication of the ampullary region and accessory tubal ostia are relatively common.[29] Accessory tubes that arise along the course of the fallopian tube never communicate with the lumen, but the accessory ostia located near the main ostium always do. Unilateral absence of the fallopian tube is uncommon and is associated with ureteral and renal abnormalities on the involved side.[142] Bilateral tubal absence is rare and is usually associated with uterine and vaginal agenesis. In such cases there may be normal ovaries that are attached laterally to the free edge of the empty broad ligament. Absence of one or both tubes may be secondary to autoamputation. Segmental atresia and persistence of the coiled fetal pattern are rare anomalies but may occur when large numbers of laparotomies are done for "idiopathic" infertility. Women exposed to diethylstilbestrol (DES) prenatally have a variety of malformations of their müllerian structures, including the fallopian tube.

TUBAL PHYSIOLOGY

The major physiological functions of the tube are reproductive: passage of spermatozoa, ovum pickup, provision of an adequate site for fertilization and early embryonic development, and transport of the conceptus to the uterus. Whether the fallopian tube has a significant immunologic or antibacterial function is not well established, although immunologically competent cells are present in the tube.

The mechanism of capture of the oocyte by the fallopian tube varies among mammalian species. Some species exhibit a periovarian sac that isolates the ovary from the peritoneal cavity and presumably assures capture by the fallopian tube.[13] In the human there is no anatomically isolated site, but the well-developed fimbriae reach almost any point on the ovary and allow efficient capture. Anatomical features, such as the multitude of epithelial folds with their predominance of ciliated cells that beat in the direction of the uterus, are undoubtedly important.[14] Also, the ligaments that surround the tube and the ovaries exhibit contractions that may be influenced by epinephrine, norepinephrine, prostaglandins, and other substances.[63]

The relative importance of the fimbriae, ligamentous movements, and ciliary mechanisms are unclear. Redundancy in the ovum pickup mechanism seems likely, since fertility may occur in the absence of fimbria[65,87] or following surgical reversal of fimbriectomy,[92] in women with abnormal tubo-ovarian anatomical relationships and disorders of ciliary motion (e.g., Kartagener's syndrome).[15,84]

The cumulus mass of the oocyte itself is probably critical for both ovum pickup and transport, since rabbits' eggs denuded of their covering of sticky granulosa cells do not transport normally.[14]

Ovum transport within the fallopian tube has been extensively studied in animals, but only a few thorough investigations have been accomplished in women. At least three factors seem to be involved in tubal transport: ciliary action, muscle contractions, and changes in viscosity of tubal fluid. Ciliary activity in the human fallopian tube actively transports particles, even in the absence of muscle contractions.[49] Larger particles (e.g., the ovum) permanently in contact with the mucosal cells effect a steady movement toward the ampullary-isthmic junction. An increase in muscular activity occurs during the ovulatory phase of the menstrual cycle. Slower, more uniform contractions occur during the premenstrual phase.[125] These muscular contractions begin at the ampulla and proceed to the isthmus. In addition, the frequency of the ampullary contractions is higher than those found in the isthmus. In all probability the action of the cilia provides the primary mechanism for ovum transport within the tube, aided and abetted by the muscular contractions.

It is known from the pioneering studies of Croxatto et al that the fertilized ovum resides within the fallopian tube for approximately 3 days.[27] The ovum remains in the ampulla for about 72 hours and then rapidly traverses the isthmus.[27] The reason for this delay in transit is unknown. Although fertilized ova are retained in the ampullary portion of the tube in the rabbit, this is accomplished by a physiologic closure of the isthmus. There is no evidence of a similar mechanism in the human female.

One possible mechanism of the delay of the oocyte or conceptus at the ampullary isthmic junction is the presence of a tenacious column of mucus in the isthmus at the time of ovulation.[63] A decrease in this secretion and an apparent increase in cilia become evident by scanning electron microscopy several days after ovulation. Tubal secretion appears to be under endocrine control.[72]

Attempts to alter ovum transport in women through excision or transposition of tubal segments and with gonadal steroids or neuroactive drugs have failed to elucidate completely the mechanisms of passage.[57] It is conceivable that failure of precision in the process of ovum transport is a cause of infertility in some individuals.

The delay in the fallopian tube is probably related to maturation of the ovum. Chang demonstrated a definite relation between the age of the ovum and the ability to implant.[23] If rabbit ova transfer from the fallopian tube to the uterus within 24 hours of fertilization, implantation does not occur. A small number of implantations occur after 48 hours, but the majority implant after 3 days. This observation may influence the future practice of in vitro fertilization (IVF), since the current practice is to replace the embryos in the uterine cavity at 48 hours.

The role of the fallopian tube in sperm transport is speculative. It has been known for many years that sperm can be found in the ampulla of the fallopian tube within minutes of insemination.[110] Although intrinsic sperm motility and uterine contractions resulting from intercourse and seminal plasma may play a role, inert particles deposited at the cervix also gain entry to the peritoneal cavity via the uterus and fallopian tubes. This seems contrary to the prevailing ciliary and muscular transport activity.[119]

A concentration gradient of sperm has been observed in the female reproductive tract. The cervix probably acts as both a barrier and a reservoir of sperm. The next significant anatomic barrier is thought to be the isthmus of the tube, possibly effected by its tenacious mucus. Screening out of abnormal forms is thought to occur at each site.

The role of the fallopian tube fluid in sperm capacitation is not known. In animal experiments sperm must reside a number of hours within reproductive tract fluids in order for fertilization to occur. Capacitation is the process of membrane changes that are necessary for fertilization.

Tubal fluid results from transudation and secretion.[72] Tubal fluid volume increases with estrogen stimulation and decreases with progesterone stimulation. Principal components include electrolytes with a high concentration of potassium, metabolic substrates, and bicarbonate. Albumin and immunoglobin G are the most abundant proteins. At the time of ovulation and for several days thereafter, unique proteins found in the fluid suggest a role in fertilization and in early zygote development.[73] The ability to accomplish IVF and pregnancy in the absence of these unique proteins suggests that they might enhance the efficiency of this process but may not be required for the early events.

Present evidence strongly suggests that the fallopian tube functions as more than a simple conduit for ova and sperm. The changes in tubal morphology and fluid accumulation are obviously under hormonal regulation. The formation and elaboration of specific substances needed for growth and development of the fertilized ovum are similarly controlled by estrogen, progesterone, and other factors.

ECTOPIC PREGNANCY

Ectopic pregnancy continues to be a major diagnostic problem and is responsible for approximately 15% of all obstetrically caused maternal deaths in the United States each year.[4] Ectopic pregnancy has a major economic impact, with a cost of $1.1 billion in 1990.[137] The declining case fatality rate has been offset by the fourfold increase in incidence since 1970. Most maternal deaths are attributed to hemorrhage and are thought to be preventable.[42] The incidence of ectopic pregnancy is variable, depending upon the type of hospital reporting the data, but current studies suggest that approximately 2% of all pregnancies are ectopic.[22]

Technologic advances in the past decade have changed the diagnosis and treatment of ectopic pregnancy. The use of sensitive blood and urine pregnancy tests and transvaginal ultrasound scanning have improved early diagnosis. Operative laparoscopy and methotrexate chemotherapy have increased treatment options.

Antibiotic use and conservative treatment of pelvic inflammatory disease (PID) have undoubtedly increased the incidence of tubal gestation,[138] although no evidence of salpingitis can be found in 50% to 75% of cases.[102,136] Studies in Sweden and in the United States found serologic evidence of prior chlamydial infection in more than 50% of women with ectopic pregnancies, whereas only 20% of matched controls had antibodies positive for *Chlamydia*.[19,123] A history of clinical PID is known to be a risk factor.[19,78] Gross anatomic alterations, such as adherence of mucosal folds and ultrastructural findings of deciliation and denuding of epithelium related to chronic salpingitis, may be implicated. Infertility itself is associated with an increased risk of ectopic pregnancy even after controlling for PID.[78,141] Clomiphene citrate and other hormonal therapies may be etiologic.[79,141] The first IVF pregnancy was tubal, and ectopic pregnancies continue to comprise approximately 1% to 2% of pregnancies that use assisted reproductive technologies.[114]

Strong risk factors are current use of intrauterine devices and prior tubal sterilization, especially with coagulation.[81,82,118] Tubal reconstructive surgery carries a risk of ectopic pregnancy ranging from 3% to 10%, depending principally upon the degree of intrinsic tubal damage.[71] Women with one prior ectopic pregnancy have a 10% risk of a repeat, whether or not the tube was removed.[71] DES daughters experience approximately 5% ectopic pregnancies.[26]

Clinicians caring for patients with any of these risk factors should inform their patients of the increased risk. Early surveillance of pregnancies may lead to prompt diagnosis and reduced intervention.

Practices such as smoking[25] and douching[24] are associated with an increased risk of tubal pregnancy. Fortunately, induced abortion has not been shown to increase the risk.[28,78]

Diagnosis

Presenting signs and symptoms

Pain. Pain is the most common and consistent symptom associated with ectopic pregnancy, but the type is variable, depending upon the duration and location of the gestation.[91] Most patients with an ectopic pregnancy complain of cramplike pelvic or lower abdominal pain on the affected side early in the gestation. This pain may be a result of uterine contractions and distention of the tubal serosa.

Sharp, tearing, pelvic pain associated with fainting is frequently seen in patients with acute rupture of an ectopic pregnancy. Dull, aching pain occurs with an organized hematoma around an unruptured ectopic pregnancy. About 10% of the patients have shoulder pain in addition to pelvic pain, an almost certain indication of intraperitoneal spill of blood and diaphragmatic irritation.

Abnormal vaginal bleeding. An accurate history of recent menstrual periods is of extreme importance in diagnosis. Frequently it will be discovered that the most recent bleeding did not occur at the expected time in the cycle and that it was slightly diminished in amount. In approximately 50% of patients the menstrual history will be normal. Most of these patients, however, note spotting or intermittent slight vaginal bleeding since the last normal menstrual period, and in about 10% of patients the bleeding begins simultaneously with the onset of pain. Profuse bleeding with passage of large clots is not a common symptom. Continued diminished bleeding and the absence of large clots is more characteristic of ectopic pregnancy than threatened or incomplete abortion. Amenorrhea lasting 2 or 3 months may be associated with an ectopic pregnancy in the interstitial portion of the fallopian tube or in a rudimentary uterine horn, since rupture in these areas is delayed.

Pregnancy signs and symptoms. Nausea, vomiting, and breast engorgement are uncommon. They may be present in later pregnancies that occur in the uterine cornua or in interstitial portion of the fallopian tube.

Pulse rate. The pulse rate is characteristically rapid when the ectopic pregnancy has ruptured but otherwise is normal.

Blood pressure. The blood pressure reflects both the acuteness of the process and the degree of blood loss. The blood pressure is normal in patients with unruptured ectopic pregnancies or slowly leaking ruptures with hematoma formation. Systolic pressure of less than 80 mm Hg is seen in only about 10% of patients. Pulse and blood pressure should be taken with the patient in the recumbent position and then immediately after the patient sits upright. A significant increase in pulse and decrease in blood pressure would indicate substantial compensated hemorrhage.

Temperature. A ruptured ectopic pregnancy, even with a large pelvic hematoma, causes only a slight elevation in temperature. In patients with an acute rupture, the temperature is frequently subnormal or rarely higher than 38.3°C. This characteristic of the temperature to remain subnormal or only slightly elevated is a valuable sign in differentiating an ectopic pregnancy from PID and septic abortion.

Abdomen. Examination of the abdomen usually yields negative findings in patients with an unruptured or locally confined process. There may be lower quadrant tenderness or guarding if intraperitoneal bleeding has occurred. In the presence of massive intraperitoneal bleeding, the abdomen is diffusely tender and presents typical muscular rigidity.

Pelvic examination. Findings are highly variable, depending on the duration of the pregnancy and the amount of intraperitoneal bleeding. The cervix and uterus are usually of normal size and consistency. Manipulation of the cervix usually causes pelvic pain if there is leakage of blood or rupture of the tube. In early unruptured tubal pregnancy the tubal enlargement may be too slight to be detected by bimanual examination and is frequently missed. If the adnexa on the opposite side are normal to palpation, the chances of tubal pregnancy are greater. Because chronic salpingitis is a predisposing factor to the development of ectopic pregnancy, the finding of contralateral disease does not eliminate the possibility.

After tubal abortion or rupture, the adnexal area is exquisitely tender. If the tube has ruptured, it may be less markedly enlarged than after a tubal abortion. Liquid blood in the cul-de-sac produces a doughy or full feeling, although frequently both adnexal areas feel normal even when bathed in liquid blood. After the blood has clotted, it is easily felt as a soft, somewhat indefinite, tender mass in the cul-de-sac or adnexal region. It is important to limit bimanual examinations and observe extreme gentleness doing this procedure.

Laboratory and other diagnostic procedures

hCG pregnancy testing. Blood tests specific for human chorionic gonadotropin (hCG) and urinary assays that use monoclonal antibodies have resulted in earlier diagnosis of many ectopic pregnancies. It is imperative to know the sensitivity of the pregnancy test, since low levels of hCG can be missed by less sensitive tests. However, most ectopic pregnancies manifest positive pregnancy tests.

A single hCG test result does not distinguish a normal intrauterine pregnancy from a threatened abortion or ectopic pregnancy. The combination of an hCG test and an assessment of the clinical dating of the pregnancy helps to distinguish a normal pregnancy from an abnormal one and provides guidance regarding the interpretation of ultrasound findings.

Although the absolute level of hCG is not predictive of outcome in early pregnancy, serial hCG levels can distinguish normal pregnancies from abnormal gestations with a high degree of sensitivity, because abnormal gestations produce less hCG.[7] In early pregnancy, before detectability by ultrasound, the hCG level should double approximately every 2 days. Failure to show an increased hCG level of at least 66% in a 48 hour time interval suggests either an ectopic pregnancy or an abnormal intrauterine pregnancy.[64]

Ultrasound. Using the transabdominal ultrasound technique, a uterine sac may be detectable when the hCG level is approximately 6500 mIU/mL, or about 2 weeks after missed menses.[108] The transvaginal probe is better able to detect early pregnancies because of higher resolution and anatomic proximity; intrauterine pregnancy can be detected with the hCG at about 1500 mIU/mL. Vaginal ultrasound is able to image adnexal masses, often including the demonstration of an empty uterus and an adnexal sac with a positive fetal heart motion (Fig. 8-3).[112] However, each institution may have a different threshold value of discriminating levels of hCG.

Progesterone. Studies suggest that the combination use of hCG titers and progesterone levels may aid in the diagnosis of ectopic pregnancy.[20,54] Generally, a low level of progesterone suggests a nonviable pregnancy. However, as progesterone levels do not differentiate ectopic pregnancies from early nonviable pregnancies, serial hCG values are needed for differentiation. A larger series is required to determine if obtaining progesterone levels is a cost-effective addition to hCG monitoring.

Blood examination. The hematocrit reflects the extent of bleeding, but the initial determination is modified by preexisting anemia and by the state of hydration. Of more importance than the initial count are *sequential* determinations of the hematocrit. A gradual decrease is frequently associated with persistent leakage of blood into a peritubal hematoma.

Determination of the leukocyte count is not particularly helpful. A leukocytosis exceeding 20,000/mm^3 has been noted in only about 10% of patients, and a persistent leukocytosis of this degree favors a diagnosis of PID.

Determination of Rh blood type should also be done when an ectopic pregnancy is suspected. Rh negative women should receive Rh immune globulin after treatment of ectopic pregnancy.

Culdocentesis. Culdocentesis is of particular value if the cul-de-sac is bulging. It may be performed using a long 15- to 18-gauge needle on a 10- or 20-mL syringe. A dry tap is unusual and should warrant another attempt. The fluid obtained may suggest the following: (1) a normal pelvis, if it is

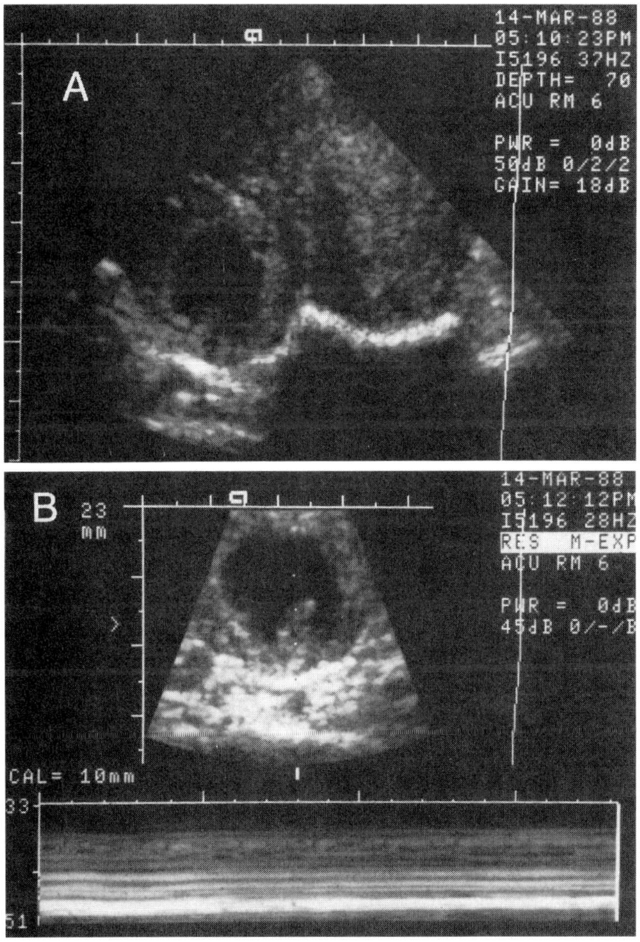

Fig. 8-3. A, Tubal ectopic pregnancy by vaginal ultrasound scan. Gestational sac with fetal pole, situated next to empty uterus. **B,** Fetal heart beat demonstrated by M-mode vaginal ultrasound. (Courtesy Dr. Peter M. Doubilet, Brigham and Women's Hospital, Harvard Medical School, Boston.)

clear, serous, and straw colored; (2) PID, if it is turbid but serous; (3) ruptured ovarian cysts, ovulation bleeding, or occasionally PID, if it is blood tinged and serous; and (4) a recently bleeding corpus luteum, a recently ruptured ectopic pregnancy with fresh bleeding, or a traumatic cul-de-sac aspiration, if it is bright red and grossly bloody.

Romero et al studied 158 women with nonclotting blood on culdocentesis; 84% had ectopic pregnancies, of which more than one half were unruptured.[107] A normal culdocentesis with a normal hCG test result was 99% predictive of not having an ectopic pregnancy. However, 16% of women with ectopic pregnancy had a nondiagnostic culdocentesis.

Uterine curettage. Because the findings from curettage are equivocal in so many patients and a normal intrauterine pregnancy may be interrupted, this procedure is not advised as a routine diagnostic procedure.

If placental tissue is found either grossly or microscopically, the presence of an intrauterine pregnancy is obvious. The rare combination of intrauterine and extrauterine pregnancy (heterotopic pregnancy), however, is still a possibility. If the curettings show only decidua, a diagnosis of ectopic pregnancy must be considered. It is possible, however, to curet a pregnant uterus and miss the pregnancy so that only decidual tissue is obtained. Similarly a decidual reaction in the endometrial stroma may result from a corpus luteum cyst, a luteinized follicular cyst, a granulosa cell tumor, or the administration of potent synthetic progestational agents.

Specific morphologic changes in the epithelium of the endometrium have been described in association with either intrauterine or extrauterine pregnancy. The presence of this *Arias-Stella reaction*, an anaplasia of pregnancy, should alert the clinician to the possibility of an ectopic pregnancy. This morphologic pattern has not been described in the endometrium of patients receiving synthetic progestational agents for pseudopregnancy.

Treatment

The traditional treatment for ectopic pregnancy is laparotomy with salpingostomy or salpingectomy. However, the advent of medical therapy for ectopic pregnancy and advanced laparoscopic techniques have expanded the options for treatment of ectopic pregnancy.

Ruptured tubal pregnancy. Ruptured tubal pregnancy remains a major cause of maternal mortality. In a patient who is hemodynamically unstable the treatment of choice remains laparotomy with removal of the ruptured fallopian tube. Before surgical resection, digital compression of the mesosalpinx vessels may aid in hemostasis. Packed red blood cells must be available for patients in shock, and if blood loss is excessive, the surgeon should watch for evidence of disseminated intravascular coagulation.

In a hemodynamically stable patient without massive intraperitoneal hemorrhage, a laparoscopic approach may be possible. A skilled laparoscopic surgeon and proper equipment are prerequisites. Either salpingectomy or segmental resection of the fallopian tube is appropriate for ruptured ectopic pregnancies. If ongoing blood loss is significant or a laparoscopic approach is difficult, rapid conversion of the procedure to a laparotomy may be necessary.

Unruptured tubal pregnancy. The goal of the surgical treatment of unruptured ectopic pregnancy has been preservation of the fallopian tube. Increasingly, tubal pregnancies are being resected at the time of laparoscopy.

A variety of techniques is available for performing linear salpingostomies by a laparoscopic approach.[18,31,43] Generally a linear incision is made along the antimesenteric border of the fallopian tube using scissors, cautery, or laser. In addition, segmental resection can also be accomplished laparoscopically. This may be the optimal therapy for unruptured isthmic pregnancies, because ectopic pregnancies may invade and destroy the musculature of the narrow isthmic segment.[30,102]

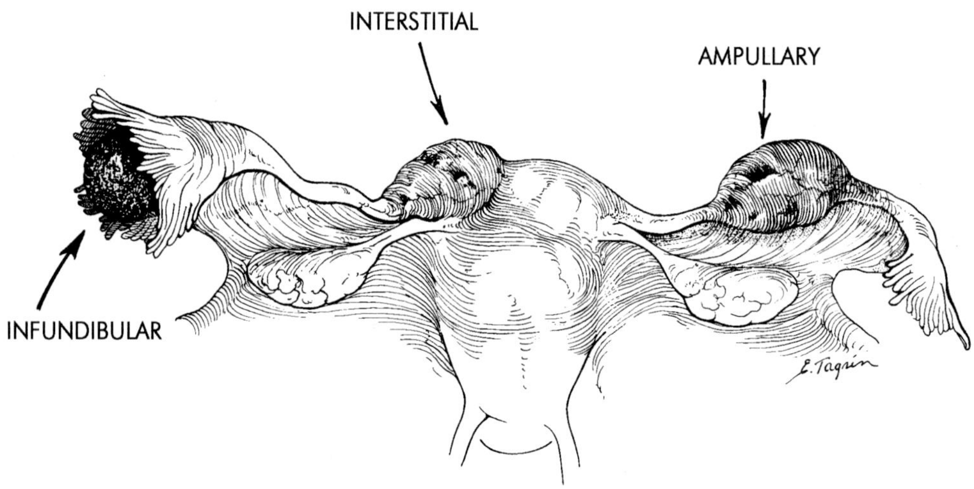

Fig. 8-4. Anatomic sites of tubal ectopic pregnancies.

When the ectopic gestation involves the fimbriated portion of the tube or even the ampulla (Fig. 8-4), particularly in a patient who has been infertile, conservative procedures may help preserve the childbearing potential.[55,115,116] Both lateral incisions of the tubes and salpingostomy with or without primary closure are methods of tubal preservation.

"Milking" or fimbrial expression of a distal ampullary pregnancy appears safe and effective, if it is accomplished without undue force or bleeding.[113]

If a patient has had conservative treatment, either by laparotomy or laparoscopy, the hCG titer must be followed to zero to determine completeness of the procedure,[66] since a significant minority of patients have evidence of persistent trophoblast.[38,135] Recurrent ectopic pregnancy in a blind ampullary segment is another potential complication of conservative therapy.[21]

Expectant management of an ectopic pregnancy may be an option when hCG values are spontaneously declining.[47,50] Generally an initial hCG of less than 1000 mIU is required, and the patient must be reliable.

MEDICAL THERAPY OF ECTOPIC PREGNANCY

Methotrexate

Interest in a nonsurgical approach in stable patients with ectopic pregnancy has recently increased. The primary agent investigated for this purpose is methotrexate, a drug used for treatment of gestational trophoblastic neoplasms. Methotrexate is a folic acid analog that inhibits purine metabolism by blocking the enzyme dihydrofolate reductase. It is thus selective for rapidly dividing cells. Methotrexate is renally excreted, therefore renal function should be addressed before treatment. The toxicity of methotrexate is reduced following high-dose treatment with a citrovorum factor (calcium leukovorum), which acts as a folate agonist to "rescue" normal cells. Citrovorum factor is not usually used with methotrexate doses of less than 50 mg/m^2.

A variety of protocols exists for using methotrexate, including intravenous, intramuscular, and oral administration (Table 8-1).[51] Although originally used as an adjunct to surgery (i.e., for the treatment of persistent postoperative ectopic pregnancy or for presumed ectopic pregnancies that could not be visualized at the time of surgery), primary treatment of ectopic pregnancy has gained acceptance in recent years. There are multiple case reports of direct injection of methotrexate. However, in the only reported randomized study of this method, three of seven patients required reoperation; thus the study was prematurely terminated.[88] Therefore this more invasive regimen cannot be recommended without further study.

Various selection criteria are used for medical therapy. Generally, only ectopic pregnancies of less than 3 to 4 cm, with no detectable fetal cardiac activity, are considered amenable to chemotherapy.[2,20] A pretreatment medical workup should consist of at least a quantitative hCG, SGOT, BUN, creatinine, CBC with platelets, and an ultrasound examination. A biweekly follow-up of hCG levels is required, with a drop in titers expected after approximately 7 to 10 days. Contraindications to methotrexate therapy include an unstable or noncompliant patient, a history of renal or hepatic disease, current thrombocytopenia or leucopenia, and the presence of fetal cardiac activity.

Late rupture can occur even with declining hCG levels, and careful follow-up of all patients is required. Initial follow-up regarding fertility suggests tubal patency is equivalent to surgical management.

SPECIAL CASES

Cervical pregnancy

Cervical pregnancy is a rare but potentially serious form of ectopic pregnancy, since trophoblast erosion into the uterine vessels is possible. Classical criteria for a true cervical pregnancy include (1) the presence of cervical glands opposite the site of placental implantation, and (2) the placenta below the level of the entrance of the uterine vessels or below the sites of peritoneal reflection. Vaginal bleeding is the chief complaint, and the risk of profuse vaginal hemorrhage can make therapy difficult.

Traditional therapy dictated hysterectomy. However, a number of new therapies have been aimed at uterine preservation. Approaches include methotrexate chemotherapy,[45] tamponade with a Foley catheter balloon, and placement of a cerclage before surgical evacuation.[11,128] In addition, radiologic embolization of either uterine or internal iliac arteries may be useful as preoperative management.[75]

Interstitial or cornual pregnancy

Classically, interstitial or cornual pregnancies present later in gestation, since the gestational sac is surrounded by the thicker myometrial walls rather than the thin-walled fallopian tube. If rupture occurs, the area is so well vascularized that hemorrhage can be profound. Traditional therapy advocates hysterectomy or cornual resection as the treatment of choice. However, improved detection of interstitial

Table 8-1. Regimens for methotrexate

Author	Mode	Dose	Citrovorum factor
Stovall et al[120]	IM	1.0 mg/kg qod days 1, 3, 5, 7 until 15% decrease in titer, or 8 days and then weekly	0.1 mg/kg IM qod days 2, 4, 6, 8*
Stovall et al[121]	IM	50 mg/m^2	None
Patsner and Keningsberg[98]	PO	0.4 mg/kg/day for 5 days	None

*Citrovorum factor can also be given orally

pregnancies plus the desire to preserve fertility potential has resulted in the use of newer methods of therapy earlier in gestation. Methotrexate by either systemic administration or by local injection has been reported as successful.[126] In addition, local injection of potassium chloride has been reported.[94]

Heterotopic pregnancy

Spontaneous heterotopic pregnancy (concomitant intrauterine and ectopic pregnancies) is rare, with an incidence of 1 in 30,000 pregnancies. However, the increasing use of ovulation induction drugs and the replacement of multiple gametes or embryos during assisted reproductive technologies have led to an increased incidence of heterotopic pregnancies. This rate appears to approach 1%.[10,41]

The diagnosis of heterotopic pregnancies is difficult. Normally rising hCG profiles are often present since multiple embryos produce combined serum levels. Also, the sonographic detection of an intrauterine pregnancy does not exclude a concomitant ectopic pregnancy. Close clinical follow-up and laparoscopy for pain are the mainstay of diagnosis. Dilatation and curettage for diagnosis is not an option for a desired pregnancy. Treatment is thus surgical to resect the ectopic pregnancy and to allow the intrauterine pregnancy to continue.

Ovarian pregnancy

True ovarian pregnancy occurs when fertilization and implantation occur within the follicle. Spiegelberg defined the classic criteria for ovarian pregnancy: (1) the fallopian tubes must be normal; (2) the pregnancy must be in the normal anatomic location of the ovary; (3) the pregnancy must be connected to the uterus by the uteroovarian ligament; and (4) ovarian and placental tissue must be present histologically.

Clinically, ovarian pregnancies tend to have a more acute presentation with sudden pain and often present with rupture and intraperitoneal hemorrhage. It is difficult to differentiate between a ruptured hemorrhagic corpus luteum and a ruptured ectopic pregnancy. Preservation of ovarian tissue is the clinical goal of treatment, which has primarily been surgical. However, there is a report of successful treatment with methotrexate.[111]

Fertility after ectopic pregnancy

Studies suggest that women with a prior ectopic pregnancy have a 50% to 79% likelihood of having a live birth.[129,133] The risk of a repeat ectopic pregnancy appears to be between 13% and 28%.[129,133]

After a second ectopic pregnancy, women have approximately a 30% chance of a third ectopic pregnancy and a 50% chance of a term delivery; thus a conservative approach is warranted.[30,132] Tubal conservation is also warranted when a pregnancy occurs in the woman's only remaining tube; about 50% of these patients will successfully deliver, although at least 20% can be expected to have another ectopic pregnancy.[33,96]

Pregnancy rates do not appear to differ between patients undergoing laparotomy or laparoscopy for resection of ectopic pregnancy.[76,97,133] A history of infertility appears to be the most important determinant of fertility after resection of ectopic pregnancy.[97] The follow-up of patients undergoing methotrexate chemotherapy for ectopic pregnancy suggests that subsequent reproductive performance is not impaired, compared to surgical management.[46]

SALPINGITIS ISTHMICA NODOSA

Salpingitis isthmica nodosa is a disease process of unknown etiology, characterized by nodular thickenings in the intramural and isthmic portions of the fallopian tube. Microscopically the nodules are noted to be in the muscular wall of the tube and to contain nests of glandlike tissue. Frequently the lumina of these glands are connected to the central tubal lumen. This disease process is also known as diverticulosis adenomyosis of the tube, adenosalpingitis, and endosalpingiosis. The incidence is variable and depends on the detailed examination of the pathologist and the number of microscopic sections taken through this portion of the fallopian tube. The disease occurs most frequently between the ages of 25 and 50 years, with the average age being 35 years. It is more common among African-Americans than among Caucasians.

The pathogenesis of this disease is controversial, but several theories have been advanced about its origin. One theory suggests that this disease is the sequel of a gonorrheal or tuberculous inflammation, because associated inflammation is found in 75% to 80% of cases. Bilateral lesions are also quite common.

The islands of glandular tissue theoretically may form as a result of an extension of the mucosa during the acute inflammatory process. Thus minute intraluminal abscesses may rupture or dissect into the softened muscularis. Against this theory is evidence that salpingitis isthmica nodosa is often contralateral to the classic inflammatory process.[9]

In several reports of patients with salpingitis isthmica nodosa, fewer than 50% had an associated inflammatory process. In such patients the lesion was thought to be of

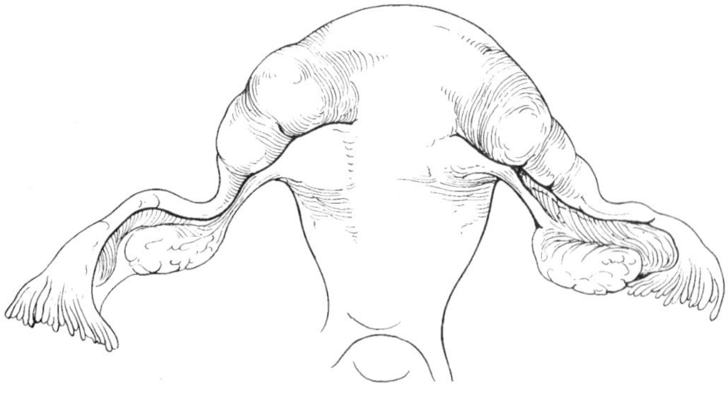

Fig. 8-5. Salpingitis isthmica nodosa.

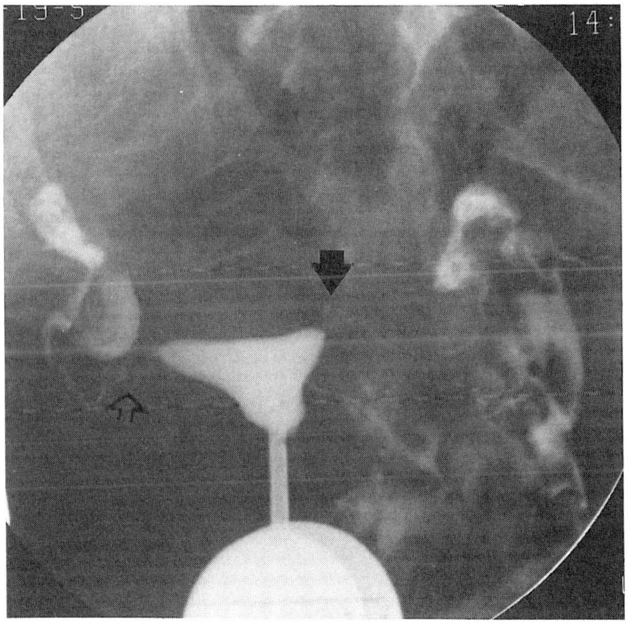

Fig. 8-6. Salpingitis isthmica nodosa as demonstrated by hysterosalpingography. Bilateral disease is present (*arrows*) although the disease is more prominent on the right (*solid arrow*).

noninflammatory origin. It was suggested that the process arose from a proliferation or hyperplasia of the epithelial lining cells of the isthmus or possibly by a contiguous spread of uterine adenomyosis.[140]

The gross appearance of salpingitis isthmica nodosa (Fig. 8-5) is characteristic. The lesions are bilateral in about 35% of patients. Usually the nodules are multiple, irregularly distributed, and present a beaded appearance. The nodules vary from a few millimeters to 2.5 cm in diameter and are frequently sharply circumscribed, firm, and irregular but with a smooth surface. These nodules can also be seen on a hysterosalpingogram (Fig. 8-6).

The microscopic appearance of salpingitis isthmica nodosa is variable. In its simplest form, there is a simple outpocketing of the tubal mucosa into the musculature. In its fully developed state, glandlike spaces are scattered throughout the myosalpinx and are associated with hyperplasia and hypertrophy of the muscle fibers. In cystically dilated glands there is a flattening of the epithelium; whereas in the smaller glandular spaces the epithelium is a mixture of that seen in the tube and the endometrium. There is a surrounding stroma of collagenous fibrous connective tissue, which is usually infiltrated with plasma cells, leukocytes, or eosinophils.

Diagnosis and treatment

The diagnosis of salpingitis isthmica nodosa is usually made at the time of the hysterosalpingogram. Tubal diverticulosis must be differentiated from tubal tuberculosis. In the latter condition, the fallopian tubes are usually rigid, devoid of peristalsis, and are often occluded at the proximal end of the ampulla.

Except for a possible association with ectopic pregnancy, the lesions are innocuous and require no specific treatment.[44,60] The lesion is not considered to be premalignant. If tubal diverticulosis is discovered as an incidental finding at laparotomy and the tubes are grossly normal, nothing needs to be done. A patient with a long-standing history of infertility, however, who has bilateral isthmic occlusion as a result of diverticulosis could be considered a candidate for assisted reproductive technology.

NONTUBERCULOUS GRANULOMATOUS SALPINGITIS

Nontuberculous granulomatous salpingitis may be a sequela of hysterosalpingograms, performed with iodine-oil preparations. The granulomatous lesion produced by the deposition of this oil in the tubal mucosa may simulate tuberculosis. The tubercle, however, is atypical; organisms are not identified by proper staining, and cultures are negative. Furthermore, caseation necrosis is not seen.

Deposition of talc granules into the peritoneal cavity at the time of surgery may cause a similar granulomatous salpingitis. Apparently the talc granules enter by the fimbriated portion of the fallopian tube and become embedded in the endosalpinx. These are most commonly seen in the fimbriated and ampullary portion of the tube. Systemic diseases, including Crohn's disease and infections such as actinomycosis and schistosomiasis, may occasionally give rise to a granulomatous salpingitis, that may be confused with tuberculosis.

Physiological salpingitis

In the course of routine examination of fallopian tubes removed during hysterectomy, salpingitis associated with menstrual endometrium has been encountered. Although the inflammatory reaction was acute and associated with an infiltration of polymorphonuclear leukocytes, it did not have the precise pathologic appearance of acute salpingitis that had resulted from bacterial infection.[90]

MICROSURGERY OF THE FALLOPIAN TUBES

The microscope has been used in operations of the pelvis for the last 30 years. In gynecology, microscopic surgery has become important because of the increase in the incidence of PID, with its consequent pelvic adhesion formation, and the desire of a number of women who have had tubal ligations to reverse their surgery. In addition, there is a subgroup of infertile women who would have a higher pregnancy rate than is currently possible with IVF, with properly selected and performed microsurgery. This section describes the principles of microsurgery techniques, the adjuvants used with microsurgical techniques to try to prevent postoperative adhesions, and the indications and reported outcomes of the gynecologic procedures in which microsurgical techniques are used.

Techniques

Adherence to the principles of microsurgical techniques is probably the paramount surgical factor that contributes to the successful outcome of the surgery. Adequate magnification of the surgical field is significant, but adherence to microsurgical principles helps the patient the most.

Principles. The key principles of microsurgical technique include gentle handling of tissue, precise hemostasis, meticulous tissue dissection, and careful approximation of tissue.[53,139] Gomel counsels that successful microsurgery is the result of adherence to these principles.[53] Gentle handling of tissue is required to minimize intraperitoneal trauma and to decrease postoperative adhesions. Precise hemostasis allows improved visualization of the operating area and should be achieved by microdiathermy needle to cauterize the exact area of bleeding. Desiccation of exposed tissue should be avoided. This is achieved by keeping the operative field constantly irrigated with heparinized Ringer's lactate solution. The heparin is intended to help prevent fibrin deposition and adhesion formation. Meticulous dissection allows complete removal of the abnormal tissues. In addition, meticulous dissection decreases the potential damage from the surgery and allows the careful reapproximation of tissue at the end of surgery. Fine, nonabsorbable suture material should be used. Catgut should be avoided because it could cause significant inflammatory reactions. Finally, care should be taken to avoid the contamination of the pelvis with foreign material, such as talc from gloves, because these materials may provoke an inflammatory response.

The skill and experience of the surgeon also contribute to the successful outcome of microsurgery. Using rabbits, Oelsner et al showed a correlation between the number of reanastomoses the surgeon has performed and outcome such as pregnancy rate.[95] This finding suggests that microscopic surgery should be performed by those who have been adequately exposed to its principles.

Microscope. Swolin was the first to report the use of the operating microscope for surgery of the pelvis.[124] In a study by Hedon et al a comparison was made between the use of loupes and microscope for tubal anastomosis in rabbits.[56] The number of rabbits achieving pregnancy was nearly 30% higher in the group in which the operating microscope was used; although (1) the time needed for the procedure was similar with both instruments, (2) the surgeons assessment of the anastomosis after the procedure was similar in both groups, and (3) the patency assessment after the surgery was similar in the two groups, the number of rabbits achieving pregnancy was nearly 30% higher in the group in which the operating microscope was used. Thus it appears that the operating microscope provides better results than loupes in the most important outcome criterion.

Surgical adjuvants

The most important factor determining successful outcome from microsurgery is good microsurgical technique. However, surgical adjuvants are commonly used to attempt to improve postoperative pregnancy rates. In particular, surgical adjuvants are used to try to decrease the postoperative incidence of adhesion formation and postoperative infections. As pointed out by Diamond et al, when a second-look laparoscopy is performed after surgery for lysis of adhesions, pelvic adhesions are again observed: new adhesions develop in a majority of the women who had the original surgery.[37] The laser has been considered as an alternative technique to decrease the rate of postoperative adhesions. However, as has been shown by Barbot et al and Tulandi, the use of laser in lysis of adhesions is no more efficacious than standard techniques in decreasing postoperative adhesions.[5,131] Thus there is a strong need for more effective prevention of postoperative adhesion formation.

Antibiotics. Holtz, in a survey of the charter members of the Society of Reproductive Surgeons of the American Fertility Society (AFS), showed that the most commonly used surgical adjuvant by pelvic surgeons is antibiotic prophylaxis.[58] He found that 73% of his respondents used antibiotics in all surgical cases, whereas 18% used antibiotics only in cases of distal tubal disease. Thus 91% of the gynecologic surgeons used some form of antibiotic prophylaxis. The most common antibiotics used were first-generation cephalosporins and doxycycline and second- or third-generation cephalosporins, in descending order.

Dextran 70. Dextran 70 is a branched polysaccharide of glucose made from sugar beets, hydrolyzed to an average molecular weight of 70 kilodaltons (kD). It is a clear, viscous fluid with the dextran dissolved in 10% dextrose. The presumed benefits of this agent, when instilled intraperitoneally, are that it (1) creates an osmotically induced transudate intraperitoneally and (2) covers all intraperitoneal surfaces with a thin film; both of which may prevent adhesion formation. Using female rabbits, Holtz et al studied the prevention of adhesion formation and reformation by dextran 70.[59] They reported a reduction in adhesion formation when dextran 70 was used after the initial injury. However, there was no decrease in re-formation of adhesions when dextran 70 was used after lysis of adhesions was performed. Even in animal studies therefore, dextran 70 may be beneficial only in circumstances in which pelvic insult occurs for the first time. As a prophylaxis against anaphylactic reactions, dextran 1 is given intravenously. This eliminates the large immune complexes required for anaphylaxis.[74]

Steroids. In the past, steroid regimens after surgery were popular with pelvic surgeons because of the potential antiinflammatory effects of the steroids. In animal studies the antiinflammatory effects appear to be a result of antagonistic reactions to histamine. However, Pfeffer et al showed in microsurgical anastomosis in rabbits that the use of steroids was of no benefit in reducing adhesions.[103] Steroid use involves risks to the patient, including psychiatric disturbance, musculoskeletal pain, edema, and infection.

THE AMERICAN FERTILITY SOCIETY CLASSIFICATION OF ADNEXAL ADHESIONS

Patient's name____________ Date ______ Chart #______

Age ____ G ____ P ____ Sp Ab ____ VTP ____ Ectopic ____ Infertile Yes ____ No ____

Other significant history (i.e. surgery, infection, etc.) ____________

HSG ____ Sonography ____ Photography ____ Laparoscopy ____ Laparotomy ____

	ADHESIONS	<1/3 Enclosure	1/3 - 2/3 Enclosure	>2/3 Enclosure
OVARY	R Filmy	1	2	4
	Dense	4	8	16
	L Filmy	1	2	4
	Dense	4	8	16
TUBE	R Filmy	1	2	4
	Dense	4*	8*	16
	L Filmy	1	2	4
	Dense	4*	8*	16

*If the fimbriated end of the fallopian tube is completely enclosed, change the point assignment to 16.

Prognostic classification for adnexal adhesions

	LEFT		RIGHT
A. Minimal	____	0-5	____
B. Mild	____	6-10	____
C. Moderate	____	11-20	____
D. Severe	____	21-32	____

Treatment (surgical procedures): ____________

Prognosis for conception & subsequent viable infant**

____ Excellent (> 75%)

____ Good (50%-75%)

____ Fair (25%-50%)

____ Poor (< 25%)

**Physician's judgment based upon adnexa with least amount of pathology.

Recommended followup treatment: ____________

Additional findings: ____________

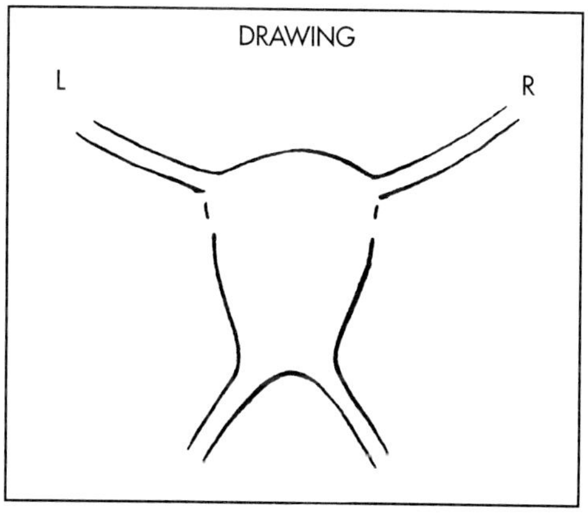

Property of
The American Fertility Society

For additional supply write to:
The American Fertility Society
2140 11th Avenue, South
Suite 200
Birmingham, Alabama 35205

Fig. 8-7. The AFS classification of adnexal adhesions. (From the American Fertility Society: The American Fertility Society classifications of adnexal adhesions, distal tubal occlusion, tubal pregnancies, müllerian anomalies and intrauterine adhesions, *Fertil Steril* 49:944, 1988.)

Hydrotubation. Hydrotubation is a technique used immediately postoperative, in which lactated Ringer's solution is instilled into the cervix to try to keep the tubes patent. In a large, prospective, randomized multicenter study, this procedure did not result in a statistically significant increase in the pregnancy rate.[106]

Other Adjuvants. Recently new techniques have been proposed to reduce the rate of postoperative pelvic adhesions. Among them is the study of Boyers et al, who tested Gore-Tex surgical membrane in rabbits.[17] Their study of the extent, type, and tenacity of adhesions after a second look at the pelvis, revealed that the Gore-Tex membrane reduced the experimental adhesion score by more than half. Calcium channel blockers are another modality reported to reduce adhesions. Steinleitner et al measured the effects of subcutaneous injections of nifedipine, a calcium channel blocker, on postoperative adhesion formation in golden hamsters.[117] The calcium channel blocker apparently decreased adhesion formation. More research is needed to determine the best ways of decreasing postoperative adhesions in microsurgical operations.

Classification and outcomes of microsurgical procedures

Because the sole purpose of pelvic microsurgery is to help the patient have a successful pregnancy, it is important to determine the most effective surgical regimens. In other words, what are the rates of spontaneous abortions, ectopic pregnancies, and live births associated with the surgical procedures? In published studies the most important criteria for determining the potential pregnancy rate include the length of follow-up, the severity of disease, the use of adjuvants, and the expression of data.[6] Because of this potential for variation in the reporting of the surgical data, major differences in results are published, along with differences in methods for classifying the surgical procedures.

In 1988 the AFS made a major advance in tubal microsurgery by publishing staging systems for adnexal adhesions, distal tubal occlusion, and tubal occlusion secondary to tubal ligation.[3] The classification schemes for these problems are important because they allow (1) the results of different studies to be compared on a similar basis, (2) the proper documentation of the severity of the disease, and (3) the formulation of an adequate prognosis for the patient.

Adnexal adhesions. The AFS classification (Fig. 8-7) divides adnexal adhesions into four categories: minimal, mild, moderate, and severe. The classification scheme emphasizes (1) that the prognosis for the patient is determined by the side with the least adhesions, (2) that the fimbriated end is of critical importance for the patient's prognosis, and (3) that filmy adhesions will have a different outcome than dense adhesions.

Salpingolysis involves the lysis of adhesions in the peritubal regions (Fig. 8-8). Though the published results are for surgery performed under a variety of circumstances, the results are encouraging. As shown in Table 8-2, in the studies published since 1980 the average rate of pregnancy after salpingolysis is 56%. For this procedure therefore the potential for successful outcome is excellent and should be offered as a potential treatment for patients with only adnexal adhesions.

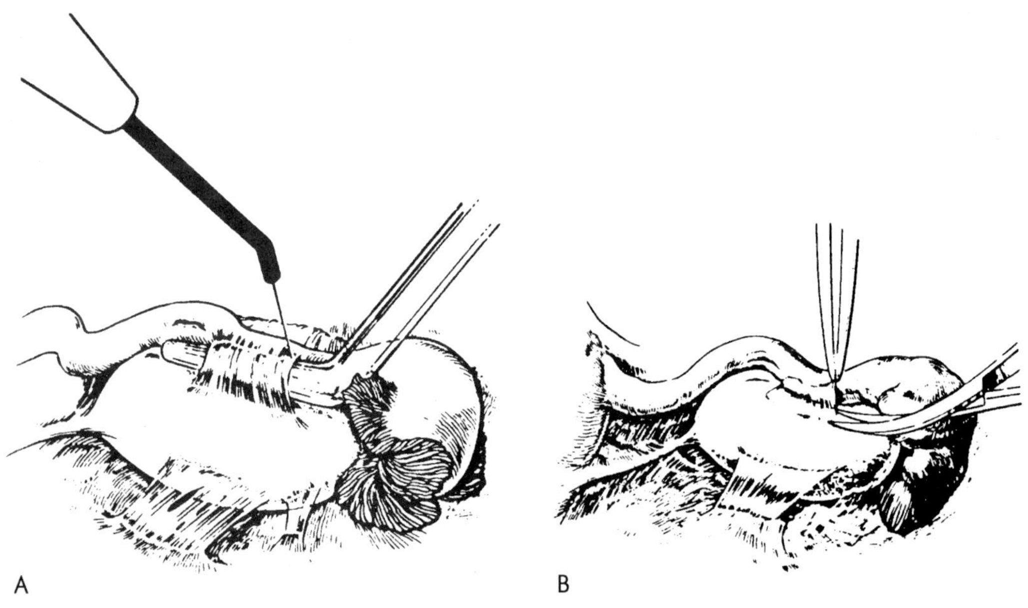

Fig. 8-8. A and **B,** Lysis of peritubal adhesions with microsurgical instruments. (From Patton GW Jr: Microsurgical reconstruction of the oviduct. In Behrman SJ, Kistner RW, Patton GW Jr, editors: *Progress in Infertility*, ed 3.)

Table 8-2. Results of lysis of adhesions by microsurgical techniques published since 1980

Author(s)	Yr	Patients (n)	Pregnancies (n) (%)
Betz et al[12]	1980	29	20 (69)
Patton[99]	1982	35	22 (63)
Frantzen and Schlösser[48]	1982	49	20 (41)
Donnez and Casanas-Roux[39]	1986	42	27 (64)
Tulandi[130]	1986	33	17 (52)
TOTAL		188	106 (56)

Table 8-3. Results of salpingostomy by microsurgical techniques published since 1980

Author(s)	Yr	Patients (n)	Pregnancies (n) (%)
DeCherney and Kase[32]	1981	54	14 (26)
Frantzen and Schlösser[48]	1982	85	12 (14)
Larsson[68]	1982	54	21 (39)
Mage and Bruhat[77]	1983	30	5 (17)
Verhoeven et al[134]	1983	82	28 (34)
Boer-Meisel et al[16]	1986	108	22 (20)
Donnez and Casanas-Roux[39]	1986	83	26 (31)
Kitchin et al[67]	1986	102	26 (25)
TOTAL		598	154 (26)

Distal tube disease. The AFS scheme for distal tubal occlusion is based on the International Federation of Fertility and Sterility classification on salpingostomy and is presented in Fig. 8-9. As Gomel has pointed out, the most important factors determining outcome after surgical correction are the condition of the endosalpinx, the amount of ampullary dilation, the condition of the tubal wall, and the presence and type of pelvic adhesions.[53] The AFS classification scheme is based on these prognostic factors.

Salpingostomy is the term used to describe the procedure in which the terminal end of the fallopian tube is reconstructed. The most common reason for performing this procedure is hydrosalpinx resulting from PID. Another cause of pelvic adhesions is previous appendicitis. Occasionally the obstructed distal tube is completely adherent to the ovary. The advantages of microsurgery in salpingostomy, as delineated by Gomel, are that precise dissection could be performed to separate the tube from the ovary, that the whole tube could be conserved, that ampullary folds could be reconstructed in their physiologic position, and that a more complete hemostasis could be achieved.[53] As shown in Table 8-3, eight papers published since 1980 have enough patients for adequate review; the average pregnancy rate after salpingostomy is 26%. For those patients who have had previous salpingostomies, the success rate after repeat salpingostomies is very low.[69] These patients should be offered assisted reproductive technologies.

Midsegment reconstruction. Midsegment reconstruction of the fallopian tube is most commonly performed for reversal of sterilization and reanastomosis of a partial salpingectomy performed for a tubal ectopic pregnancy. The AFS scheme for classification of tubal obstruction after tubal ligation is for the purposes of comparing the results of different studies and to give patients a more precise prognosis. According to the AFS scheme, the factors considered to be most important for surgical prognosis are the segmental lengths after repair and the type of anastomosis that is performed. Table 8-4 is a review of the studies published since 1980 of the success rates of microsurgical tubal anastomosis. This table is a summary of the results of different populations and different types of procedures. The average success rate in terms of pregnancy is 56%. The overall success rate of midsegment reconstruction is high enough to be offered to patients with tubal ligation as a firstline treatment.

Proximal tubal disease. For proximal tubal disease, the available operations could be divided into three categories: cornual implantation, noncornual implantation, and microsurgical anastomosis.[89] Microsurgical tubocornual anastomosis is associated with an acceptable success rate. McComb reported on a series of patients who had microsurgical tubocornual anastomosis for proximal tubal disease; they had a 57% pregnancy rate.[83] Patton et al studied patients who had primary anastomosis performed for proximal tubal occlusion and with minimal or no distal disease; the pregnancy rate for the microsurgical anastomosis was 69% after 3 years.[100] It appears that the treatment of proximal disease with anastomosis could be as successful as for those patients who undergo midsegment reconstruction. However, if the patient has combined proximal and distal disease, the prognosis is so poor that the patient should be referred for IVF.[101]

Alternative procedures

In patients with severe pelvic adhesions, missing fimbria, poor semen characteristics, or other poor prognostic factors, IVF could be considered as the first choice treatment for the infertile couple. However, alternative procedures are being developed to treat selected patients.

Novy et al reviewed a series of 28 patients who had interstitial fallopian tube obstruction diagnosed by hysterosalpingogram or by diagnostic laparoscopy, and in whom transcervical cannulation of the proximal fallopian tube was performed.[93] In patients who had hysteroscopic cannulation,

THE AMERICAN FERTILITY SOCIETY CLASSIFICATION OF DISTAL TUBAL OCCLUSION

Patient's name__________ Date ______ Chart # ______

Age ____ G ____ P ____ Sp Ab ____ VTP ____ Ectopic ____ Infertile Yes ____ No ____

Other significant history (i.e. surgery, infection, etc.) __________

HSG ____ Sonography ____ Photography ____ Laparoscopy ____ Laparotomy ____

Distal ampullary diameter		**<3 cm**	**3-5 cm**	**>5 cm**
	L	1	4	6
	R	1	4	6
Tubal wall thickness		Normal/thin	Moderately thickened or edematous	Thick & rigid
	L	1	4	6
	R	1	4	6
Mucosal folds at neostomy site		Normal/ >75% preserved	35% to 75% Preserved	<35% Preserved adherent mucosal fold
	L	1	4	6
	R	1	4	6
Extent of adhesions		None/minimal/mild	Moderate	Extensive
	L	1	3	6
	R	1	3	6
Type of adhesions		None/filmy	Moderately dense (or vascular)	Dense
	L	1	2	4
	R	1	2	4

Prognostic classification for terminal salpingostomy (salpingoneostomy)

	LEFT		RIGHT
A. Mild	____	1-3	____
B. Moderate	____	9-10	____
C. Severe	____	>10	____

Treatment (surgical procedures):

Salpingostomy	L	R
A. Terminal	____	____
B. Ampullary	____	____

Other: __________

Prognosis for conception & subsequent viable infant*

____ Excellent (> 75%)

____ Good (50%-75%)

____ Fair (25%-50%)

____ Poor (< 25%)

*Physician's judgment based upon adnexa with least amount of pathology.

Recommended followup treatment: __________

Additional findings: __________

DRAWING

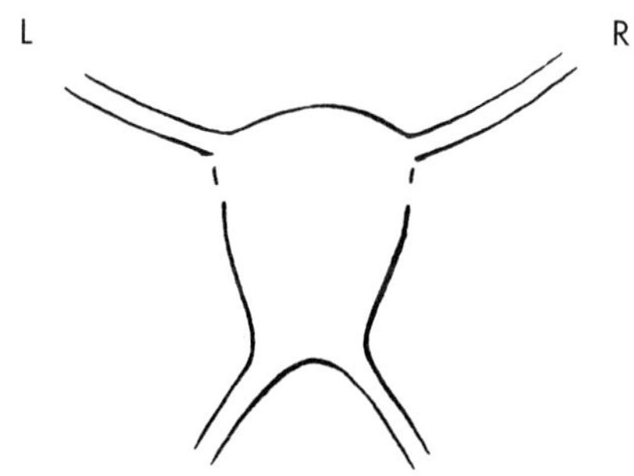

For additional supply write to:
The American Fertility Society
2140 11th Avenue, South
Suite 200
Birmingham, Alabama 35205

Property of
The American Fertility Society

Fig. 8-9. The AFS classification of distal tubal occlusion. (From the American Fertility Society: The American Fertility Society classifications of adnexal adhesions, distal tubal occlusion, tubal pregnancies, müllerian anomalies and intrauterine adhesions, *Fertil Steril* 49:944, 1988.)

Table 8-4. Results of tubal reanastomosis by microsurgical techniques published since 1980

Author(s)	Yr	Patients (n)	Pregnancies (n) (%)
Gomel[52]	1980	118	76 (64)
Meldrum[85]	1980	32	16 (50)
Diamond et al[36]	1982	46	25 (54)
Frantzen and Schlösser[48]	1982	28	12 (43)
DeCherney et al[34]	1983	129	73 (57)
Donnez and Casanas-Roux[39]	1986	82	36 (44)
Lavy et al[70]	1986	25	9 (36)
Rock et al[105]	1987	80	58 (73)
TOTAL		540	305 (56)

92% of the tubes became patent. Although previously the prognosis was poor, this technique offers hope to those patients diagnosed with interstitial tubal disease. These results should be considered in light of the findings by Sulak et al; 11 of 18 patients who had tubal resection for presumed proximal tubal disease, had no histologic evidence for proximal disease.[122]

What is the incidence of ectopic pregnancy after pelvic microsurgery, a complication that may lead to the loss of the fallopian tube and even threaten the life of the patient? Lavy et al reviewed the literature concerning the ectopic pregnancy rate after microscopic tubal surgery.[71] As would be expected, the rate of ectopic pregnancy depended on the type of surgery performed: for patients who have had lysis of adhesions, the ectopic pregnancy rate was 3.5% of the subsequent pregnancies; for salpingostomy, 28%; and for midsegment tubal anastomosis, 3.7%. Thus the rate of ectopic pregnancies is dependent on the type of procedure. This needs to be kept in mind when discussing the proposed operation with the patient.

BENIGN NEOPLASMS

Benign tumors of the fallopian tube are rare entities, yet a large variety of neoplasms have been reported as having originated in the fallopian tube. Tumors may be located in the wall, within the lumen, or occasionally may be pedunculated and project from the fimbriated portion of the tube. In a consideration of benign tumors of the fallopian tube, lesions such as salpingitis isthmica nodosa, endometriosis, and adenomyosis should be excluded. Similarly the hydatids of Morgagni are so commonplace that they should not be considered as a tumor mass. The following benign tumors have been reported in the literature: cystic and solid teratomas, papilloma, fibroadenoma, fibroma, leiomyoma, lipoma, hemangioma, lymphangioma, mesothelioma, and mesonephroma.

Somewhat more common is the adenomatoid tumor (Fig. 8-10), sometimes called an angiomyoma, mesothelioma, or a reticuloendothelioma. This is a small circumscribed tumor of the tube usually confined to the muscle wall and found incidentally at the time of laparotomy. It has a characteristic

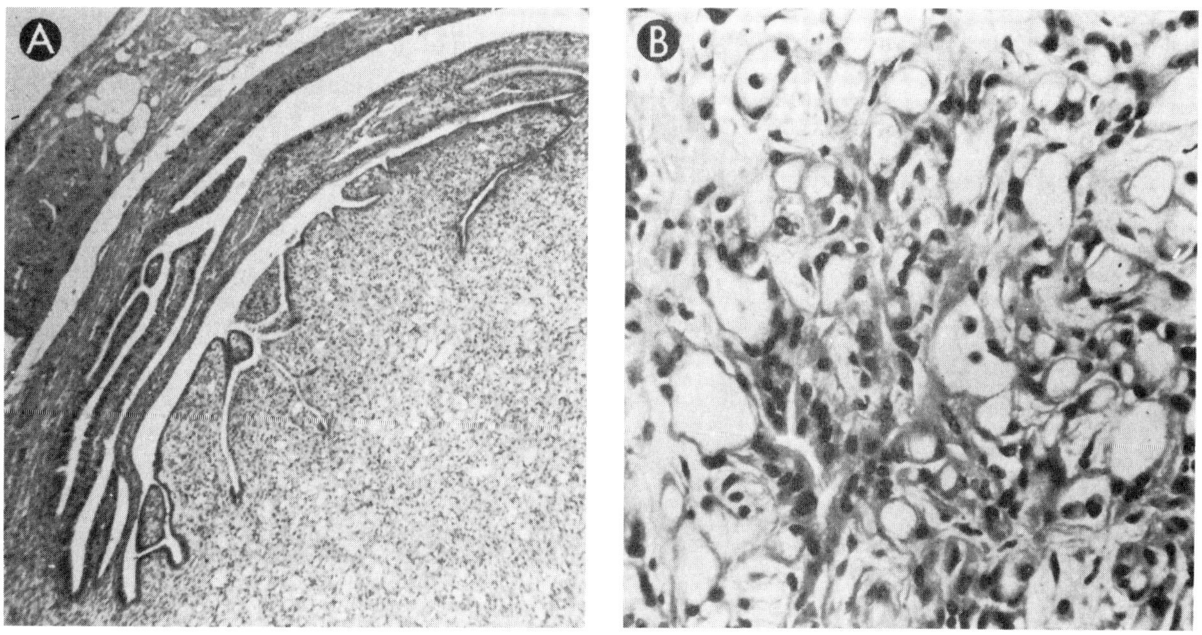

Fig. 8-10. Adenomatoid tumor. **A,** Low power. **B,** Higher power.

microscopic appearance, being composed of small glandlike spaces lined by cells of mesothelial, endothelial, or even epithelial appearance. The tumors appear as gray, gray-white, or yellow discrete nodules occupying the muscularis and rarely exceeding 3 cm in diameter. Because of the glandular arrangements of the cells, the microscopic picture has occasionally been confused with a low-grade adenocarcinoma. The histogenesis of these tumors is not clearly defined, but electron microscopic studies support its origin from mesothelial cells.[127] It is not believed that these adenomatoid tumors possess malignant potential.

Leiomyomas of the tube are usually asymptomatic lesions that are discovered during a laparotomy performed for another indication. Occasionally they have enlarged and produced acute torsion of the fallopian tube; degenerative changes similar to those occurring in uterine leiomyomas have been reported.

MALIGNANT NEOPLASMS

Primary carcinoma

The rarest carcinoma of the female genital tract is primary carcinoma of the fallopian tube. Since the report of the first patient in 1888, approximately 1400 cases of this entity have been documented.[104] The incidence of tubal carcinoma varies from 0.1% to 0.5% of all female genital cancers. Metastatic disease is much more common, accounting for 80% to 90% of fallopian tube malignancies.

The age incidence has varied from 18 to 80 years, but most patients have been between 40 and 65 years, with the mean age in the sixth decade.

Low parity has been a common finding in patients with tubal carcinoma. Salpingitis may be a causative factor in the infertility of these patients. However, salpingitis is common and malignancy is rare. In all probability the tumor itself produces a chronic inflammatory reaction, which eventually seals off the fimbriated portion of the tube and may simulate a hydrosalpinx.

Diagnosis. Because it is a rare disease with sometimes subtle or nonspecific symptoms, the diagnosis of primary carcinoma is rarely made before surgery. Although there are no distinctive symptoms that might be called pathognomonic, the most consistent sign is a watery and frequently blood-tinged vaginal discharge. Intermittent or colicky, low abdominal pain associated with abnormal bleeding may also be present. The latter may be manifested as irregular bleeding or spotting during the postmenopausal era and as menstrual irregularities during the childbearing period. Occasionally the discharge may be profuse, although the occurrence of intermittent hydrosalpinx (*hydrops tubae profluens*) as a characteristic symptom is quite rare. The latter may occur with the release of a watery or blood-tinged fluid from a hydrosalpinx through the uterus and vagina, regardless of whether or not it is associated with a tubal carcinoma.

The physical findings include an abdominal enlargement, if ascites is present and a palpable abdominal mass, or more commonly, a palpable, firm mass, found during pelvic examination. The finding of a tubal carcinoma is so rare that it is only occasionally listed as the primary preoperative diagnosis.

In postmenopausal patients the usual diagnosis is ovarian tumor. In premenopausal patients the most common diagnoses are leiomyomas and PID. If there is recurrent bleeding, or a bloody, watery discharge in a postmenopausal patient in whom biopsies of the cervix and endometrial curettage have given normal findings, the suspicion of tubal cancer should be strongly entertained. Vaginal smears may disclose neoplastic cells characteristic of tubal cancer, particularly when there is a loss of fluid from the uterus, but only a minority of patients will have abnormal cytology results.

Culdocentesis may also reveal suspicious or definite malignant elements. Occasionally hysterosalpingography has suggested a cancer of the tube, and endoscopy or culdotomy may verify the diagnosis. A dilation and curettage may reveal tubal cancer metastatic to the endometrial cavity.

Pathology. The lesion is usually unilateral; only about 30% of the patients have bilateral tumors. If the fimbriated portion of the tube is closed, the gross appearance (Fig. 8-11) of the mass may simulate that of a hydrosalpinx or pyosalpinx. If a tube with this appearance is removed during surgery, it should be opened intraoperatively to ensure the necessary surgical staging and treatment.

The serosal surface is frequently roughened and adherent to the large and small intestines. Lesions have been described as large as 17 cm in diameter, although the association of a hydrosalpinx or pyosalpinx may make the gross appearance much larger. The cross-section of the tumor reveals granular tissue that is gray or yellow-tan with a marked tendency to friability. The lesion is usually situated in the distal third of the tube, from where it may extend through the fimbriated

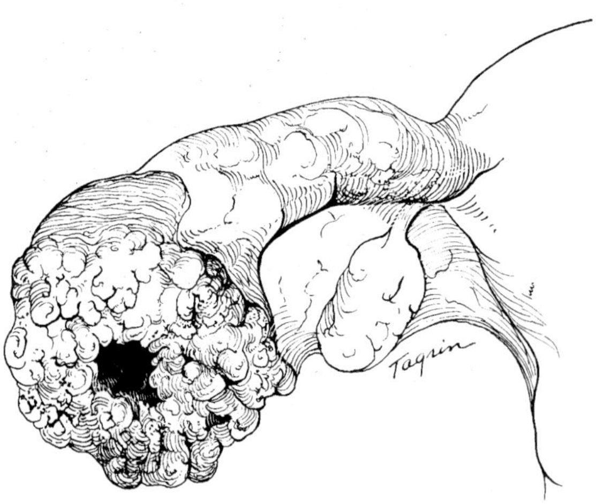

Fig. 8-11. Typical gross appearance of carcinoma of the oviduct.

portion. The tubal lumen is usually distended with fluid, and a papillary mass of friable or hemorrhagic tumor lines the mucosal surface.

For a pathologic diagnosis of primary carcinoma of the fallopian tube, the tumor must arise from the endosalpinx. The criteria suggested by Hu et al for differentiating between primary and metastatic tumors are as follows:[61]

1. Grossly the main tumor is in the tube.
2. Microscopically the mucosa should be chiefly involved and should show a papillary pattern.
3. If the tubal wall is involved to a great extent, the transition between benign and malignant tubal epithelium should be demonstrated.

The microscopic appearance of tubal carcinomas includes papillary medullary growth patterns that are variously differentiated (Fig. 8-12).

The usual method of spread of tubal carcinoma is via the lymphatics, but tumor growth may occur via the tubal lumen along the mucosal surface. Generalized peritoneal implants are uncommon, probably a result of closure of the fimbriated portion of the tube.

Metastases are found in about one third of patients.[109] The iliac, lumbar, and preaortic nodes may be involved by lymphatic permeation. Occasionally, dissemination via the round ligament to the inguinal nodes may occur. Hematogenous spread accounts for metastases to the liver and lungs. The ovary, uterine corpus, and vagina may be involved by direct extension.

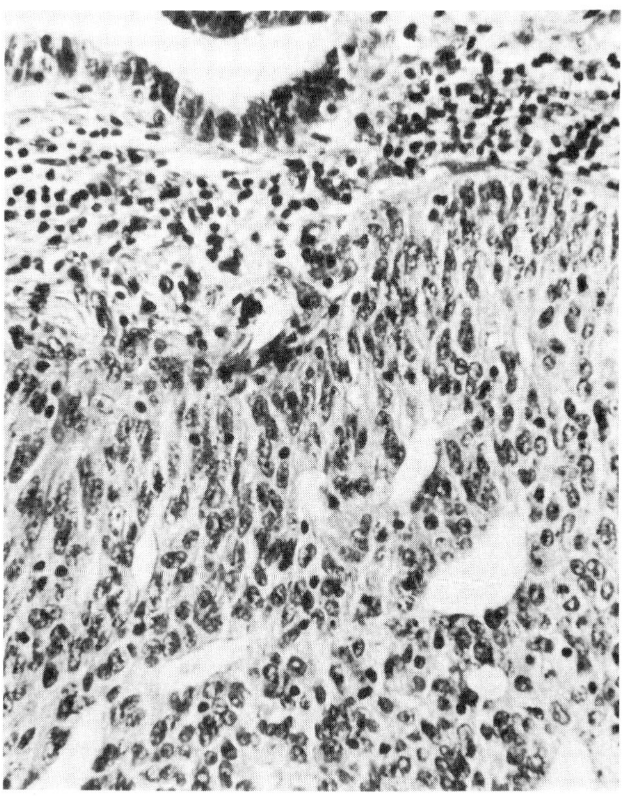

Fig. 8-12. Typical papillary carcinoma of oviduct.

FIGO does not have staging for tubal carcinoma. The clinical staging of carcinoma of the tube is a modification of the FIGO ovarian staging (Table 8-5).

Treatment. The initial method of treatment is total hysterectomy with bilateral salpingo-oophorectomy. If there is extension to the endocervix or upper portion of the vagina, a radical hysterectomy and pelvic lymphadenectomy is advisable.

Debulking should be performed for disease outside the extirpated pelvic organs. Intraoperative staging is important and includes omental biopsy, peritoneal cytology, and paraaortic node sampling.

Additional therapy should be considered if the disease has spread beyond the tubal serosa. Although external radiation therapy was used in more than half of the reported cases, a variety of treatment protocols were used; the value of each treatment was difficult to prove, however.[104]

Intraperitoneal chromic phosphate (phosphorus 32) was used in cases with no gross residual disease after surgery in an attempt to control peritoneal dissemination. Thus far the experience has been too limited to establish efficacy.[8] Various forms of chemotherapy have also been tried with some reports of regression of advanced disease, especially with multiple agents.[104] Cisplatin in combination with other agents has resulted in good 5-year survivals in some series.[80]

Prognosis is based primarily on stage rather than tumor grade, but in general is considered to be poor. The 5-year survival rate has been reported as 38%.[109] However, if a primary cancer of the tube is discovered early and removed promptly, the prognosis is good. Alertness to the possibility of tubal cancer, prompt intervention, and adequate treatment may improve the survival rate.

Table 8-5. Clinical staging for fallopian tube carcinoma*

Stage I: Growth limited to the tube
Stage IA: Growth limited to one tube, no ascites
Stage IB: Growth limited in two tubes, no ascites
Stage IC: Growth limited to one or both tubes, ascites present with malignant cells in fluid
Stage II: Growth involving one or both tubes with pelvic extension
Stage IIA: Extension and/or metastases to the uterus or ovary
Stage IIB: Extension to other pelvic tissues
Stage III: Growth involving one or both tubes with widespread intraperitoneal metastases to abdomen
Stage IV: Growth involving one or both tubes with distant metastases extraperitoneally

*From Turunen A: Carcinoma of fallopian tube, *Int J Obstet* 7:24, 1969.

Sarcoma

Sarcomas are extremely rare tumors with less than 30 cases reported in the literature.[104] The age incidence and clinical picture are similar to those in carcinoma of the tube. If the disease is extensive, the most common symptoms are pelvic pain, abdominal enlargement, and malaise. Physical examination may reveal abdominal distention, a pelvic mass, and emaciation. The tubal tumor varies from 2 to 20 cm in diameter, and the cross-section reveals a soft, papillary, or pulpy intraluminal mass. Microscopically, spindle-cell is the most common sarcoma, but other variations such as round cell, myosarcoma, myxosarcoma, perithelioma, and endothelioma have been described.

This most malignant tumor may spread via the bloodstream, the lymphatics, or direct extension to adjacent pelvic organs. The optimum method of treatment is total hysterectomy with bilateral salpingo-oophorectomy followed by radiation therapy or chemotherapy. The prognosis is poor, and it is doubtful whether therapy of any type retards the eventual outcome in advanced cases.

Carcinoma metastatic to the fallopian tube

The two organs responsible for most metastatic lesions in the fallopian tube are the ovary and the endometrium. The method of spread may be either by direct extension or via the lymphatics. Carcinoma of the stomach and pancreas may also metastasize to the tube. The lesions may be unilateral or bilateral, and there is no characteristic gross appearance. Histologically the tumors are identical with the primary tumor, and in contrast to primary carcinoma of the tube, the serosa of the fallopian tubes as well as the lymphatics of the muscularis and mesosalpinx are usually involved. The treatment is the same as for the primary disease, usually complete hysterectomy and bilateral salpingo-oophorectomy and postoperative adjuvant therapy.

REFERENCES

1. American College of Obstetricians and Gynecologists: Technical Bulletin, *Prevention of D Isoimmunization* 147:1, 1990a.
2. American College of Obstetricians and Gynecologists: Technical Bulletin, *Ectopic Pregnancy* 150:1, 1990b.
3. American Fertility Society: The American Fertility Society classifications of adnexal adhesions, distal tubal occlusion, tubal pregnancies, müllerian anomalies and intrauterine adhesions, *Fertil Steril* 49:944, 1988.
4. Atrash HK, Friede A, Hogue CJR: Ectopic pregnancy mortality in the United States, 1970-1983, *Obstet Gynecol* 70:817-822, 1987.
5. Barbot J et al: A clinical study of the CO_2 laser and electrosurgery for adhesiolysis in 172 cases followed by early second-look laparoscopy, *Fertil Steril* 48:140, 1987.
6. Bateman BG, Nunley WC, Kitchin JD: Surgical management of distal tubal obstructions—are we making progress? *Fertil Steril* 48:523, 1987.
7. Batzer FR, Corson SL: Diagnostic techniques used for ectopic pregnancy, *J Reprod Med* 31:86-93, 1986.
8. Benedet JL et al: Adenocarcinoma of the fallopian tube, *Obstet Gynecol* 50:654-657, 1977.
9. Benjamin CL, Beaver DC: Pathogenesis of salpingitis isthmica nodosa, *Am J Clin Pathol* 21:212, 1951.
10. Berger MJ, Taymor ML: Simultaneous intrauterine and tubal pregnancies following ovulation induction, *Am J Obstet Gynecol* 113:812, 1972.
11. Bernstein D et al: Conservative treatment of cervical pregnancy, *Obstet Gynecol* 58:741, 1981.
12. Betz G, Engel T, Penny LL: Tuboplasty—comparison of the methodology, *Fertil Steril* 34:534, 1980.
13. Beyth Y: Ovum pick up mechanism, a reappraisal, *Curr Probl Obstet Gynecol Fertil* 9:83, 1986.
14. Blandau RJ: Gamete transport; comparative aspects. In Hafey ESE, Blandau RJ, editors: *The mammalian oviduct*, Chicago, 1969, University of Chicago Press.
15. Bleau G, Richer CL, Bousquet D: Absence of dynein arms in cilia of endocervical cells in a fertile woman, *Fertil Steril* 30:362, 1978.
16. Boer-Meisel ME et al: Predicting the pregnancy outcome in patients treated for hydrosalpinx: a prospective study, *Fertil Steril* 45:23, 1986.
17. Boyers SP, Diamond MP, DeCherney AH: Reduction of postoperative pelvic adhesions in the rabbit with gore-tex surgical membrane, *Fertil Steril* 49:1066, 1988.
18. Bruhat MA et al: Treatment of ectopic pregnancy by means of laparoscopy, *Fertil Steril* 33:411, 1980.
19. Brunham RC et al: *Chlamydia trachomatis* infection in women with ectopic pregnancy, *Obstet Gynecol* 67:722, 1986.
20. Carson SA, Buster JE: Ectopic pregnancy, *N Engl J Med* 329:1174, 1993.
21. Cartwright PS, Entman SS: Repeat ipsilateral tubal pregnancy allowing partial salpingectomy: a case report, *Fertil Steril* 42:647, 1984.
22. Centers for Disease Control: Ectopic pregnancy—United States, 1986, *MMWR* 38:481, 1989.
23. Chang MC: Development and fate of transferred rabbit ova or blastocysts in relation to the ovulation time of recipients, *J Exp Zool* 114:197, 1950.
24. Chow W et al: Vaginal douching as a potential risk factor for tubal ectopic pregnancy, *Am J Obstet Gynecol* 153:727-729, 1985.
25. Chow W et al: Maternal cigarette smoking and tubal pregnancy, *Obstet Gynecol* 71:167-170, 1988.
26. Corson SL, Batzer FR: Ectopic pregnancy, a review of the etiologic factors, *J Reprod Med* 31:78-85, 1986.
27. Croxatto HB et al: Studies on the duration of egg transport by the human oviduct: ovum location at various intervals following LH peak, *Am J Obstet Gynecol* 132:7, 1978.
28. Daling JR et al: Ectopic pregnancy in relation to previous induced abortion, *JAMA* 253:1005-1008, 1985.
29. Daw E: Duplication of the uterine tube, *Obstet Gynecol* 42:137-138, 1973.
30. DeCherney AH, Boyers SP: Isthmic ectopic pregnancy: segmental resection as the treatment of choice, *Fertil Steril* 44:307-312, 1985.
31. DeCherney AH, Diamond MP: Laparoscopic salpingostomy for ectopic pregnancy, *Obstet Gynecol* 70:948-950, 1987.
32. DeCherney AH, Kase N: A comparison of treatment for bilateral fimbrial occlusion, *Fertil Steril* 35:162, 1981.
33. DeCherney AH, Maheaux R, Naftolin F: Salpingostomy for ectopic pregnancy in the sole patent oviduct: reproductive outcome, *Fertil Steril* 37:617-622, 1982.
34. DeCherney AH, Mezer HC, Naftolin F: Analysis of failure of microsurgical anastomosis after midsegment, noncoagulation tubal ligation, *Fertil Steril* 39:618, 1983.
35. DeCherney AH et al: Reproductive outcome following two ectopic pregnancies, *Fertil Steril* 43:82-86, 1985.
36. Diamond MP, Christianson CD, Daniell JF: Microsurgical reanastomosis of the fallopian tube: increasingly successful outcome for reversal of previous sterilization procedures, *South Med J* 75:443, 1982.
37. Diamond MP et al: Adhesion reformation and de novo adhesion formation after reproductive pelvic surgery, *Fertil Steril* 47:864, 1987.

38. DiMarchi JM et al: Persistent ectopic pregnancy, *Obstet Gynecol* 70:555-558, 1987.
39. Donnez J, Casanas-Roux F: Prognostic factors of fimbrial microsurgery, *Fertil Steril* 46:200, 1986.
40. Donnez J et al: Cyclic changes in ciliation, cell height, and mitotic activity in human tubal epithelium during reproductive life, *Fertil Steril* 43:554, 1985.
41. Dor J et al: The incidence of combined intrauterine and extrauterine pregnancy after in vitro fertilization and embryo transfer, *Fertil Steril* 55:833, 1991.
42. Dorfman SF et al: Ectopic pregnancy mortality, United States, 1979 to 1980: clinical aspects, *Obstet Gynecol* 64:386, 1984.
43. Dubuisson JB, Aubriot FX, Cardone V: Laparoscopic salpingectomy for tubal pregnancy, *Fertil Steril* 47:225, 1987.
44. Dubuisson JB et al: Tubal causes of ectopic pregnancy, *Fertil Steril* 46:970, 1986.
45. Faribow W et al: Cervical pregnancy treated with methotrexate, *NC Med J* 44:91, 1983.
46. Fernandez H et al: Return of reproductive performance after expectant management and local treatment for ectopic pregnancy, *Hum Reprod* 6:1474, 1991.
47. Fernandez H et al: Spontaneous resolution of ectopic pregnancy, *Obstet Gynecol* 71:171, 1988.
48. Frantzen C, Schlösser H-W: Microsurgery and postinfectious tubal infertility, *Fertil Steril* 38:397, 1982.
49. Gaddum-Rosse P, Blandau RJ, Thiersch JB: Ciliary activity in the human and Macaca nemestrina oviduct, *Am J Anat* 138:269, 1973.
50. Garcia AJ et al: Expectant management of presumed ectopic pregnancies, *Fertil Steril* 48:395, 1987.
51. Goldenberg M et al: Methotrexate therapy of tubal pregnancy, *Hum Reprod* 8:660, 1993.
52. Gomel V: Microsurgical reversal of female sterilization: a reappraisal, *Fertil Steril* 33:587, 1980.
53. Gomel V: An odyssey through the oviduct, *Fertil Steril* 39:144, 1983.
54. Hahlin M, Sjoblom P, Lindblom B: Combined use of progesterone and human chorionic gonadotropin determinations for differential diagnosis of very early pregnancy, *Fertil Steril* 55:492, 1991.
55. Hallatt JG: Tubal conservation in ectopic pregnancy: a study of 200 cases, *Obstet Gynecol* 154:1216, 1986.
56. Hedon B, Wineman M, Winston RML: Loupes or microscope for tubal anastomosis? An experimental study, *Fertil Steril* 34:264, 1980.
57. Hoffman JJ: The fallopian tube: an upsurge of interest, *Curr Probl Obstet Gynecol* 3:5, 1980.
58. Holtz G: Current use of ancillary modalities for adhesion prevention, *Fertil Steril* 44:174, 1985.
59. Holtz G, Baker E, Tsai C: Effect of thirty-two percent dextran 70 on peritoneal adhesion formation and reformation after lysis, *Fertil Steril* 33:660, 1980.
60. Homm RJ, Holtz G, Garvin AJ: Isthmic ectopic pregnancy and salpingitis isthmica nodosa, *Fertil Steril* 48:756-758, 1987.
61. Hu CY, Taymor ML, Hertig AT: Primary carcinoma of the fallopian tube, *Am J Obstet Gynecol* 59:58, 1950.
62. Jansen RPS: Cyclic changes in the human fallopian tube isthmus and their functional importance, *Am J Obstet Gynecol* 136:292-308, 1980.
63. Jansen RPS: Endocrine response in the fallopian tube, *Endocr Rev (Baltimore)* 5:525-542, 1984.
64. Kadar N, DeVore G, Romero R: Discriminatory hCG zone: its use in the sonographic evaluation for ectopic pregnancy, *Obstet Gynecol* 58:156, 1981.
65. Kamrava MM et al: Intrauterine pregnancy following transperitoneal migration of the ovum, *Obstet Gynecol* 60:391, 1982.
66. Kamrava MM et al: Disappearance of human chorionic gonadotropin following removal of ectopic pregnancy, *Obstet Gynecol* 62:486, 1983.
67. Kitchin JD III et al: Surgical management of distal tubal occlusion, *Am J Obstet Gynecol* 155:524, 1986.
68. Larsson B: Late results of salpingostomy combined with salpingolysis and ovariolysis by electromicrosurgery in 54 women, *Fertil Steril* 37:156, 1982.
69. Lauritsen JG et al: Results of repeated tuboplasties, *Fertil Steril* 37:68, 1982.
70. Lavy G, Diamond MP, DeCherney AH: Pregnancy following tubocornual anastomosis, *Fertil Steril* 46:21, 1986.
71. Lavy G, Diamond MP, DeCherney AH: Ectopic pregnancy: its relationship to tubal reconstructive surgery, *Fertil Steril* 47:543, 1987.
72. Leese H: The formation and function of oviduct fluid, *J Reprod Fert* 82:843, 1988.
73. Lippe J et al: Human oviductal fluid proteins, *Fertil Steril* 36:623, 1981.
74. Ljungstrom KG et al: Hapten inhibition and dextran anaphylaxis, *Anaesthesia* 43:729, 1988.
75. Lobel SM et al: Preoperative angiographic uterine artery embolization in the management of cervical pregnancy, *Obstet Gynecol* 76:938, 1990.
76. Lundorff P, Thorburn J, Lindblom B: Fertility outcome after conservative surgical treatment of ectopic pregnancy evaluated in a randomized trial, *Fertil Steril* 57:998, 1992.
77. Mage G, Bruhat MA: Pregnancy following salpingostomy: comparison between CO_2 laser and electrosurgery procedures, *Fertil Steril* 40:472, 1983.
78. Marchbanks PA et al: Risk factors for ectopic pregnancy, *JAMA* 259:1823, 1988.
79. Marchbanks PA, Coulam CB, Annegers JF: An association between clomiphene citrate and ectopic pregnancy: a preliminary report, *Fertil Steril* 44:268, 1985.
80. Maxson WZ et al: Primary carcinoma of the fallopian tube: evidence for activity of cisplatin combination therapy, *Gynecol Oncol* 26:305, 1987.
81. McCausland A: High rate of ectopic pregnancy following laparoscopic tubal coagulation failures, *Obstet Gynecol* 136:97, 1980.
82. McCausland A: Endosalpingosis ("endosalpingoblastosis") following laparoscopic tubal coagulation as an etiologic factor of ectopic pregnancy, *Obstet Gynecol* 143:12, 1982.
83. McComb P: Microsurgical tubocornual anastomosis for occlusive cornual disease: reproducible results without the need for tubouterine implantation, *Fertil Steril* 46:571, 1986.
84. McComb P et al: The oviductal cilia and Kartagener's syndrome, *Fertil Steril* 46:412, 1986.
85. Meldrum DR: Microsurgical tubal reanastomosis—the role of splints, *Obstet Gynecol* 57:613, 1981.
86. Merchant RN, Prabhu SR, Chougale A: Uterotubal junction—morphology and clinical aspects, *Int J Fertil* 28:199, 1983.
87. Metz KGP: Failures following fimbriectomy, *Fertil Steril* 28:66, 1977.
88. Mottla GL, Rulin MC, Guzick DS: Lack of resolution of ectopic pregnancy by intratubal injection of methotrexate, *Fertil Steril* 57:685, 1992.
89. Musich JR, Behrman SJ: Surgical management of tubal obstruction at the uterotubal junction, *Fertil Steril* 40:423, 1983.
90. Nassberg S, McKay DG, Hertig AT: Physiologic salpingitis, *Am J Obstet Gynecol* 67:130, 1954.
91. Newton J: Ectopic pregnancy, *Br Med J (Clin Res)* 297:633, 1988.
92. Novy MJ: Reversal of Kroener fimbriectomy sterilization, *J Obstet Gynecol* 137:198, 1980.
93. Novy MJ et al: Diagnosis of cornual obstruction by transcervical fallopian tube cannulation, *Fertil Steril* 50:434, 1988.
94. Oelsner G et al: A new approach for the treatment of interstitial pregnancy, *Fertil Steril* 59:924, 1993.
95. Oelsner G et al: The effect of training in microsurgery, *Am J Obstet Gynecol* 152:1054, 1985.
96. Oelsner G et al: Reproductive outcome after microsurgical treatment of tubal pregnancy in women with a single fallopian tube, *J Reprod Med* 31:483, 1986.

97. Ory SJ et al: Fertility after ectopic pregnancy, *Fertil Steril* 60:231, 1993.
98. Patsner B, Keningsberg D: Successful treatment of persistent ectopic pregnancy with oral methotrexate therapy, *Fertil Steril* 50:982, 1989.
99. Patton GW Jr: Pregnancy outcome following microsurgical fimbrioplasty, *Fertil Steril* 37:150, 1982.
100. Patton PE, Williams TJ, Coulam CB: Microsurgical reconstruction of the proximal oviduct, *Fertil Steril* 47:35, 1987a.
101. Patton PE, Williams TJ, Coulam CB: Results of microsurgical reconstruction in patients with combined proximal and distal tubal occlusion: double obstruction, *Fertil Steril* 48:670, 1987b.
102. Pauerstein CJ et al: Anatomy and pathology of tubal pregnancy, *Obstet Gynecol* 67:301, 1986.
103. Pfeffer WH et al: The effect of dexamethasone and promethazine administration on adhesion formation, tubal function, and ultrastructure following microsurgical anastomosis of rabbit oviducts, *Fertil Steril* 34:162, 1980.
104. Podczaski E, Herbst AL: Cancer of the vagina and fallopian tube. In Knapp RC, Berkowitz RS, editors: *Gynecologic oncology*, New York, 1993, Macmillan Publishing.
105. Rock JA et al: Tubal anastomosis: pregnancy success following reversal of Falope ring or monopolar cautery sterilization, *Fertil Steril* 48:13, 1987.
106. Rock JA et al: The efficacy of postoperative hydrotubation: a randomized prospective multicenter clinical trial, *Fertil Steril* 42:373, 1984.
107. Romero R et al: Value of culdocentesis in the diagnosis of ectopic pregnancy, *Obstet Gynecol* 65:519, 1985a.
108. Romero R et al: Diagnosis of ectopic pregnancy: value of the discriminatory human chorionic gonadotropin zone, *Obstet Gynecol* 66:357, 1985b.
109. Sedlis A: A carcinoma of the fallopian tube, *Surg Clin North Am* 58:121, 1978.
110. Settlage DSF, Motoshima M, Tredway DR: Sperm transport from the external cervical os to the fallopian tubes in women: a time and quantitation study, *Fertil Steril* 24:655, 1973.
111. Shamma FN, Schwartz LB: Primary pregnancy successfully treated with methotrexate, *Am J Obstet Gynecol* 167:1307, 1992.
112. Shapiro BS et al: Transvaginal ultrasonography for the diagnosis of ectopic pregnancy, *Fertil Steril* 50:425, 1988.
113. Sherman D et al: Reproductive outcome after fimbrial evacuation of tubal pregnancy, *Fertil Steril* 47:420, 1987.
114. Society for Assisted Reproductive Technology, The American Fertility Society. Assisted reproductive technology in the United States and Canada: 1991 results from the Society for Assisted Reproductive Technology generated from The American Fertility Society Registry, *Fertil Steril* 59:956, 1993.
115. Stangel J: Conservative surgical procedures for tubal pregnancy, *J Reprod Med* 31:103, 1986.
116. Stangel J, Gomel V: Techniques in conservative surgery for tubal gestation, *Clin Obstet Gynecol* 23:1221, 1980.
117. Steinleitner A et al: The use of calcium channel blockade for the prevention of postoperative adhesion formation, *Fertil Steril* 50:818, 1988.
118. Stock RJ, Nelson KJ: Ectopic pregnancy subsequent to sterilization: histologic evaluation and clinical implications, *Fertil Steril* 42:211, 1984.
119. Stone SC et al: Radionuclide evaluation of tubal function, *Fertil Steril* 43:757, 1985.
120. Stovall TG, Ling FW, Gray LA: Single-dose methotrexate for treatment of ectopic pregnancy, *Obstet Gynecol* 77:754, 1991a.
121. Stovall TG et al: Methotrexate treatment of unruptured ectopic pregnancy: a report of 100 cases, *Obstet Gynecol* 77:749, 1991b.
122. Sulak PJ et al: Histology of proximal tubal occlusion, *Fertil Steril* 48:437, 1987.
123. Svensson L et al: Ectopic pregnancy and antibodies to Chlamydia trachomatis, *Fertil Steril* 44:313, 1985.
124. Swolin K: Fifty fertility operations: literature and methods, *Acta Obstet Gynecol Scand* 46:234, 1967.
125. Talo A, Pulkkinen MO: Electrical activity in the human oviduct during menstrual cycle, *Am J Obstet Gynecol* 142:135, 1982.
126. Tanaka T et al: Treatment of interstitial ectopic pregnancy with methotrexate: report of a successful case, *Fertil Steril* 37:851, 1982.
127. Taxy JB, Battifora H, Oyasu R: Adenomatoid tumors: a light microscopic, histochemical and ultrastructural study, *Cancer* 34:306, 1974.
128. Thomas R, Gingold BR, Gallagher MW: Cervical pregnancy: a report of two cases, *J Reprod Med* 36:459, 1991.
129. Thorburn J, Philipson M, Lindblom B: Fertility after ectopic pregnancy in relation to background factors and surgical treatment, *Fertil Steril* 49:595, 1988.
130. Tulandi T: Salpingo-ovariolysis: a comparison between laser surgery and electrosurgery, *Fertil Steril* 45:489, 1986.
131. Tulandi T: Adhesion reformation after reproductive surgery with and without the carbon dioxide laser, *Fertil Steril* 47:704, 1987.
132. Tulandi T: Reproductive performance of women after two tubal ectopic pregnancies, *Fertil Steril* 50:164, 1988.
133. Tuomivaara L, Kauppila A: Radical or conservative surgery for ectopic pregnancy? A follow-up study of fertility of 323 patients, *Fertil Steril* 50:580, 1988.
134. Verhoeven HC, Berry H et al: Surgical treatment of distal tubal occlusion: a review of 167 cases, *J Reprod Med* 28:293, 1983.
135. Vermesh M, Silva P, Sauer M: Persistent tubal ectopic gestation: patterns of circulating B-human chorionic gonadotropin and progesterone, and management options, *Fertil Steril* 50:584, 1988.
136. Walters MD, Carlton E, Pauerstein CJ: The contralateral corpus luteum and tubal pregnancy, *Obstet Gynecol* 70:823, 1987.
137. Washington AE, Katz P: Ectopic pregnancy in the United States: economic consequences and payment source trends, *Obstet Gynecol* 81:287, 1993.
138. Westrom L, Bengtsson LPH, Mardh PA: Incidence, trends, and risks of ectopic pregnancy in a population of women, *Br Med J (Clin Res)* 282:15, 1981.
139. Winston RML: Microsurgery of the fallopian tube: from fantasy to reality, *Fertil Steril* 34:521, 1980.
140. Wrork DH, Broders AC: Adenomyosis of the fallopian tube, *Am J Obstet Gynecol* 44:412, 1942.
141. Yang C et al: Does prior infertility increase the risk of tubal pregnancy? *Fertil Steril* 48:62, 1987.
142. Zaitoon MM, Florentin H: Crossed renal ectopia with unilateral agenesis of fallopian tube and ovary, *J Urol* 128:111, 1982.

Chapter 9

THE OVARY

Laurel W. Rice
Robert L. Barbieri

The ovary is a complex organ that combines both gametogenic and endocrine functions. The estradiol and progesterone produced by the adult ovary are the primary hormonal regulators of the breast, uterus, and fallopian tubes. In fact the ovary is the master gland in gynecology. In the adult ovary, gametogenic and endocrine functions are integrated to produce the repetitive process of follicular development, ovulation, corpus luteum formation, and if pregnancy does not occur, corpus luteum regression. The repetitive growth and regression of intraovarian structures appear to predispose this major organ of reproduction to the development of multiple abnormalities of structure and function.

EMBRYOLOGY

The development of the ovary requires the coordinated assembly of three distinct embryonic tissues: (1) the primordial germ cells, (2) the coelomic epithelium of the urogenital ridge, and (3) the ovarian mesenchyme. The primordial germ cells will differentiate into oocytes. The granulosa cells and surface epithelium of the ovary will develop from the coelomic epithelium, and the ovarian mesenchyme will give rise to the stroma and theca.

Four weeks after conception, the genital ridge develops medial to the mesonephric ridge. The initial ridge consists of an inner core of mesenchyme and a thick outer layer of proliferating coelomic epithelium. In the mesenchyme are cellular condensations called the primitive sex cords, which lay at right angles to the coelomic epithelium.

A single gene, the sex-determining region Y (SRY) gene on the distal arm of the Y chromosome, causes the indifferent gonad to become a testis.[192] The SRY gene codes for a DNA-binding protein, which regulates the transcription of many other genes. In the presence of SRY the indifferent gonad becomes a testis, and in the absence of SRY the indifferent gonad becomes an ovary. Interestingly, SRY appears to regulate the transcription of genes such as müllerian inhibiting substance (MIS) and aromatase, which are known to have a role in the developmental biology of the reproductive tract. Preliminary studies suggest that the SRY gene product binds to a DNA regulatory element upstream of the MIS gene and increases the transcription of this gene. An increase in MIS leads to the regression of the müllerian system. SRY also appears to decrease the transcription of aromatase, the critical enzyme in estrogen synthesis. In rare cases the SRY gene can cross over from the Y to the X chromosome in a developing spermatogonia. If a sperm bearing a copy of SRY on an X chromosome fertilizes an oocyte, the resulting 46,XY individual will develop testes rather than ovaries. If the SRY gene is deleted from the Y chromosome, the resulting 46,XX individual will develop ovaries rather than testes.[206]

Differentiation of the indifferent male gonad into a testis begins 6 weeks after conception. Differentiation of the indifferent female gonad into an ovary usually begins approximately 12 weeks after conception. At this time, the cortical or secondary sex cords develop. The cortical cords arise by the invagination of the coelomic epithelium into the ovarian mesenchyme. Entry of primordial germ cells into these cortical cords gives rise to the primordial follicles. These germ cells, now *oogonia*, are incorporated into the cortical sex cords. Mitosis ceases, and the oogonium differentiates into a primary oocyte. The primary oocyte progresses into the prophase of the first meiotic division and then becomes dormant, entering a period of cellular hibernation, which lasts until puberty. The primary oocyte is surrounded by flattened follicular cells derived from the secondary sex cords and is destined to become granulosa

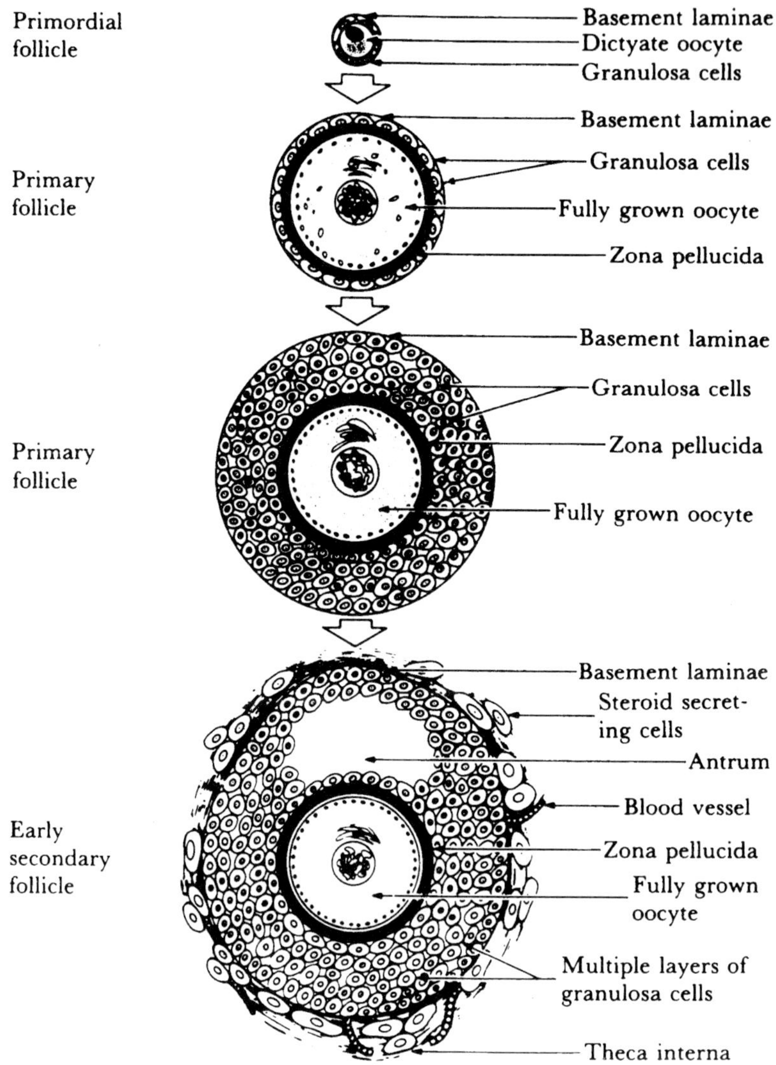

Fig. 9-1. Structure of the ovarian follicle.

cells. The oocyte and the surrounding granulosa cells form a unit called the primordial follicle. During fetal life, the ovary is relatively quiescent. This contrasts with the fetal testis, which makes large amounts of testosterone.

ANATOMY

The ovary has three major anatomic connections. The inferior pole of the ovary is attached to the uterus by a fibromuscular cord, the uteroovarian ligament. The upper pole of the ovary is attached to the distal portion of the oviduct and is supported by the infundibulopelvic ligament. This ligament represents the upper margin of the broad ligament lateral to the tubal ostium and contains the ovarian vessels. The lateral portion of the ovary is attached to the posterior surface of the broad ligament by the mesovarium, a thin fold of tissue by which blood vessels and nerves enter the hilus of the ovary.

The arterial supply of the ovary is provided by the ovarian artery and by the branches of the uterine artery. The ovarian artery arises from the aorta opposite the second and third lumbar vertebrae and crosses the psoas muscle in its descent to the pelvic brim. The ovarian artery enters the infundibulopelvic ligament and divides to give off small branches to the oviduct. The main ovarian artery enters the ovary through the hilus and divides into two medullary branches, which supply the opposite poles of the ovary. The main trunk of the ovarian artery also anastomoses with the ascending division of the uterine artery. The venous drainage of the ovary is similar to the arterial arrangement, except that the right ovarian vein terminates in the inferior vena cava; the left ovarian vein empties into the left renal vein.

The nerve supply of the ovary is derived from branches of the renal and aortic sympathetic plexuses and from the celiac and mesenteric ganglia.

OVARIAN FOLLICLE

The follicle is the functional unit of the ovary. All gametogenic and most endocrine functions of the ovary are controlled by the ovarian follicle. This follicle consists of three key components: (1) the oocyte, (2) granulosa cells, and (3) thecal cells. An understanding of the development and interrelationships of these three components is best obtained by tracing the development of a *primordial follicle* (Fig. 9-1).

The primordial follicle consists of an oocyte arrested in the diplotene stage of meiotic prophase and surrounded by a single layer of flattened granulosa cells. The primordial follicle exists in a state of cellular hibernation until it is recruited to enter a growth phase. The factors that stimulate the primordial follicle to enter a growth phase have not been identified, but it is suspected that this process is independent of gonadotropin secretion. The number of primordial follicles that enter the growth phase each cycle appears to be a fixed proportion of the primordial follicles remaining in the ovary. This is a critical characteristic of the regulation of the ovarian follicular pool. Growth in the primordial follicle is characterized by an increase in the size of the oocyte, a change in shape of the granulosa cells from flattened to cuboidal, and an increase in the number of gap junctions between the granulosa cells and oocyte.

Growth of a primordial follicle into a healthy preantral follicle is dependent on gonadotropin stimulation, especially follicle-stimulating hormone (FSH). The preantral follicle; is characterized by the following: (1) an enlarged oocyte; (2) the development of the zona pellucida, a membrane that surrounds the oocyte; (3) a multilayer proliferation of granulosa cells; and (4) the development of an outer layer of theca cells derived from the ovarian stroma (Fig. 9-1). The key to the growth of the preantral follicle is the stimulation of granulosa cell growth by FSH and estradiol. Multiple "positive" feedback loops help propel the growth of the preantral follicle. For example, estradiol stimulates the production of FSH receptors, thereby increasing granulosa cell sensitivity to FSH. This process results in a magnification of FSH stimulation.[128] High local concentrations of estradiol and FSH stimulate the production of fluid in the interstices of the granulosa cells (Call-Exner bodies). Eventually the fluid coalesces to give rise to the antral follicle. It is likely that the follicle with the greatest blood flow and the highest intrafollicular concentration of FSH and estradiol will be selected to ovulate. Estradiol production in the antral follicle is controlled by both the thecal and granulosa cells. This is the two-cell theory of follicular estrogen production (Fig. 9-2).

The basic components of the two-cell theory of follicular estrogen production are as follows: (1) the theca cells express luteinizing hormone (LH) receptors but not FSH receptors; (2) LH stimulation of the theca results in the production of androstenedione (the theca does not contain high concentrations of the enzyme aromatase and cannot convert the androstenedione to estrogen); (3) the granulosa cells express FSH receptors, and FSH stimulates the production of the enzyme aromatase, which can convert the thecal androstenedione produced by the theca to estrone; and (4) the granulosa cell contains large amounts of an estrogen-specific 17-ketosteroid reductase enzyme, which can convert the estrone to estradiol but does not efficiently convert androstenedione to testosterone.[12] The antral follicle accounts for 95% of the estradiol production during the reproductive life of a woman. The remaining 5% of the estradiol arises from the extraovarian aromatization of androgens in tissues such as fat and muscles.

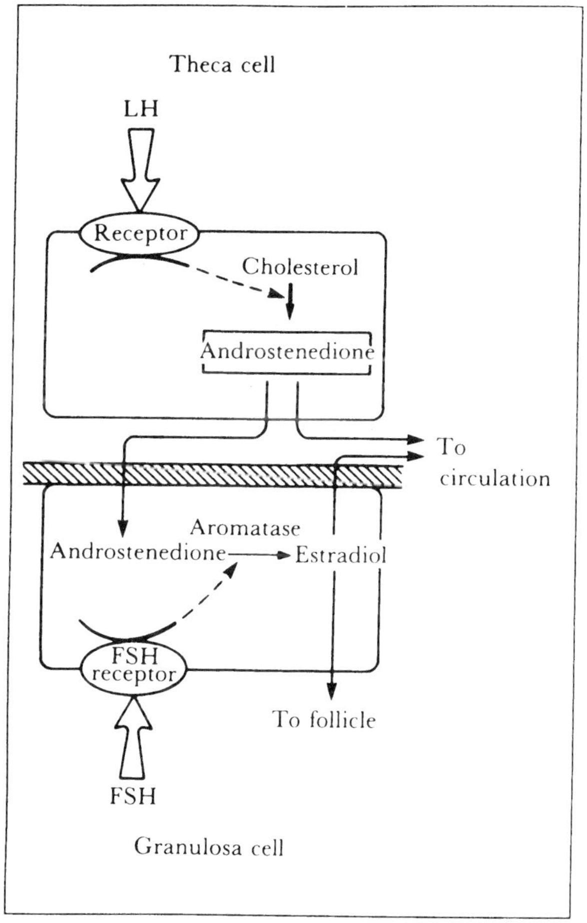

Fig. 9-2. Two-cell, two-gonadotropin theory of follicular estrogen production.

Experiments in nonhuman primates have documented that the large antral follicle controls the timing of ovulation. The ovary, not the hypothalamic-pituitary unit, is the timekeeper (Zeitgeber) of the menstrual cycle. The preovulatory antral follicle contains a large number of granulosa and thecal cells, both of which contribute to estradiol production. When the antral follicle reaches a diameter of 18 to 25 mm, it contains approximately 40 to 60 million granulosa cells. A follicle of this size can secrete approximately 400 μg of estradiol per day, which results in circulating estradiol concentrations of 200 to 300 pg/mL. When circulating estradiol is maintained in the range of 200 to 300 pg/mL for 48 hours, an LH surge is triggered. The LH surge produces a number of changes in the antral follicle: (1) a marked increase in granulosa cell cyclic adenosine monophosphate, which leads to an increase in progesterone production and a decrease in estradiol production; (2) accelerated maturation of the oocyte, which leads to the dissolution of the nuclear membrane (germinal vesicle breakdown) and the completion of meiosis I (extrusion of the first polar body); and (3) an increase in production of follicular prostaglandins, collagenase, and plasmin, which results in the dissolution of the follicle wall and the extrusion of the oocyte. Ovulation occurs approximately 36 to 42 hours after the initiation of the LH surge.

After ovulation, the basement membrane of the follicle dissolves, blood vessels grow into the follicle, luteinization of the theca and granulosa cells is completed, and the follicle is transformed in a corpus luteum (Latin for "yellow body"). The corpus luteum is 20 to 30 mm in diameter. The most important endocrine feature of the luteal phase of the menstrual cycle is the large amount of progesterone (25 mg/day) secreted by the corpus luteum. During the luteal phase of the cycle, progesterone is secreted as pulses in response to LH pulses secreted by the pituitary. The peak steroidogenic activity of the corpus luteum is reached 7 to 8 days after the LH surge, and the functional demise of the corpus luteum begins 2 to 3 days before the onset of menses. The life span of the corpus luteum is 12 to 14 days unless pregnancy occurs, and unless the human chorionic gonadotropin (hCG) secreted by the trophoblast rescues the corpus luteum. The precise mechanisms that govern luteolysis are not known, but an increase in prostaglandin production by the corpus luteum appears to precede luteolysis. With completion of luteolysis, progesterone and estradiol concentrations fall, resulting in the onset of menses.

Recruitment, Selection, and Dominance

At puberty, the ovary contains approximately 200,000 follicles. From this follicular pool, less than 500 follicles will be selected to ovulate. The remaining 199,500 follicles will die without expressing their gametogenic potential. The concepts of recruitment, selection, and dominance help to explain the process by which only 1 of every 400 follicles is chosen for ovulation.[82]

As noted earlier, during each cycle a large number of primordial follicles leave the resting pool of follicles and enter a growth phase. *Selection* is the process by which the initial pool of recruited, growing follicles is winnowed to the species-specific ovulatory quota. The status of the follicular microenvironment is crucial to the process of selection. The inner portion of each follicle is enclosed by a basement membrane of extracellular matrix. No blood vessels cross the basement membrane; therefore, each follicle can create its own unique microenvironment. The small antral follicles that create a microenvironment most conductive to growth continue on a favorable growth trajectory; other follicles undergo atresia. Experimental evidence suggests that the follicles that capture the greatest share of ovarian blood flow and create an intrafollicular microenvironment high in concentrations of FSH and estradiol have the best growth potential.

At the beginning of the follicular phase of the menstrual cycle (day 1 of menses), there are four to six antral follicles 4 mm in diameter in the ovaries. By day 8 of the cycle, one of these follicles has been selected, and the remaining follicles will become atretic. From day 8 of the cycle until the onset of the next menses (day 28 of the cycle), the one selected follicle is dominant and suppresses the growth of all remaining follicles. The dominant follicle prevents the growth of other follicles by secreting sufficient estradiol and inhibin to suppress the production of pituitary FSH, the key hormone governing follicular growth. Surgical removal of the dominant follicle is followed by the growth of a new cohort of small antral follicles that compete to become dominant. The processes of selection and dominance help ensure that, on average, only one egg is ovulated each cycle.

Ovarian Follicular Pool

The peak number of ovarian follicles is approximately 6×10^6 and occurs in fetal life at approximately 20 weeks of gestation.[9, 24] During the late second trimester, and throughout the third trimester of fetal life, a marked loss of germ cells occurs, resulting in approximately 2×10^6 ovarian follicles at birth. By the first menses (median age 12.8 years), the number of remaining follicles is approximately 200,000. By 53 years of age, the majority of women have lost all functional ovarian follicles, and menopause has begun (Fig. 9-3).

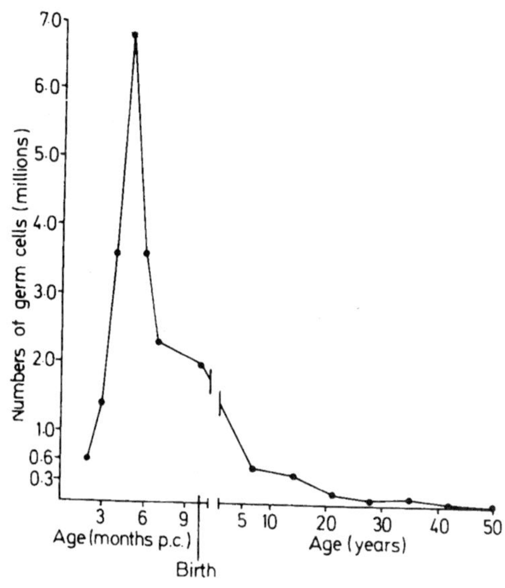

Fig. 9-3. Two-cell, two-gonadotropin theory of follicular estrogen production.

Careful analysis of the rate of loss of follicles in humans and rodents suggests that the loss of ovarian follicles is best described by an exponential function.[60] During each time period *t*, a fixed percentage of the total number of remaining follicles in the ovaries are lost. Over the life of the ovary, fewer follicles are lost during each succeeding time period *t* because fewer follicles are present at the beginning of each succeeding time period *t*.

The fact that follicular loss is governed by an exponential function has important clinical implications. The surgical removal of one ovary or the removal of 50% of each ovary (50% loss of all follicles) does not drastically change the age of menopause because the remaining follicles redistribute their entry into a growth phase. Experimental studies in rodents suggest that much more than 50% of all follicles must be destroyed before a significant impact on the age of menopause is apparent.

Prepubertal and Menopausal Ovary

The prepubertal ovary is a small elongated structure 1 to 2 cm in length. Between birth and age 4 years, the hypothalamic-pituitary unit secretes both LH and FSH, and ovarian follicles grow and secrete small amounts of estradiol. Between 4 and 8 years of age, the hypothalamic-pituitary unit secretes very little LH of FSH, and the ovary is quiescent. Starting at age 8 years, the peripubertal increase in LH and FSH leads to ever increasing levels of follicular activity and to estradiol secretion. The increase in ovarian follicular activity ultimately results in menarche (mean age 12.8 years), and the first ovulation occurs approximately 1 year after menarche. Because the prepubertal ovary is relatively quiescent, persistent cystic or solid structures on the ovary greater than 2 cm in diameter warrant investigation.

At menopause, the ovary becomes devoid of functional follicles, and estradiol production ceases, which results in amenorrhea and hot flushes. In normal women the menopausal ovary, stimulated by high concentrations of LH, secretes testosterone from the stroma. Testosterone secretion from the ovary accounts for at least one half of the total testosterone production in the menopausal woman.[110] This ovarian testosterone may play a role in regulating libido and bone density. Because the menopausal ovary consists of stroma but no follicles, it is small (less than 2 × 2 × 1.5 cm). In a menopausal woman a persistently enlarged ovary is cause for concern and requires clinical evaluation.[11]

FUNCTIONAL DISORDERS OF THE OVARY

Corpus Luteum Defect

In 1949 Jones reported that in a study of 255 menstrual cycles in 98 infertile women, a significant percentage of the cycles were characterized by short luteal-phase length as determined by basal body temperature charts, diminished urinary pregnanediol excretion, and an out-of-phase endometrial biopsy.[109] Subsequent studies confirmed that corpus luteum defect, or luteal-phase deficiency, is a common disorder and occurs in as many as 5% of menstrual cycles in normal fertile women and infertile women. The causes of corpus luteum defect are not completely understood. Most investigators believe that abnormalities in the follicular growth before ovulation are associated with subsequent suboptimal corpus luteum performance. Endocrine abnormalities that can result in corpus luteum defect include hyperprolactinemia and abnormally elevated LH pulse frequency. Corpus luteum defect is most accurately diagnosed by obtaining an endometrial biopsy specimen in the mid-luteal or late-luteal phase and by examining the biopsy specimen for evidence of a delay in endometrial maturation. In infertile women with an endometrial biopsy specimen demonstrating a maturation delay of 4 days or greater, the treatment of the corpus luteum defect often will be associated with subsequent pregnancy.

Luteinized Unruptured Follicle

In 1978 Marik and Hulka and Kninckx et al reported the absence of ovulatory stigmata on the ovaries of a number of infertile women during the periovulatory phase of the menstrual cycle.[140] They postulated that in some infertile women experiencing regular cyclic menses and apparently normal ovulatory cycles, failure of the oocyte to escape the follicle might be the cause of the infertility. Subsequent studies suggest that in fertile women, as many as 5% of all menstrual cycles are associated with a luteinized unruptured follicle (LUF). In infertile women the frequency of cycles with LUF may be greater than 5% but LUF rarely occurs in repetitive cycles in the same women. This suggests that LUF may not be a major cause of infertility. Interestingly, recent studies suggest that the administration of antiprostaglandins such as indomethacin to preovulatory women can cause LUF.[117] This suggests that infertile women should refrain from using high doses of antiprostaglandins during the preovulatory phase of the menstrual cycle.

Ovarian Hyperandrogenism

In as many as 5% of women of reproductive age, the ovary produces excess quantities of the androgens androstenedione and testosterone. Excessive ovarian production of androgens results in hirsutism, oligoovulation or anovulation, and menstrual dysfunction, such as amenorrhea or menometrorrhagia. The causes of functional ovarian hyperandrogenism are incompletely understood but include excess pituitary secretion of LH and elevated production of insulin.

In a subgroup of women with functional ovarian hyperandrogenism, LH pulse frequency and pulse amplitude are markedly elevated. Because the LH pulse frequency is elevated, the gonadotropin-releasing hormone (GnRH) pulse frequency is likely elevated.[212] The mechanisms responsible for this increase in GnRH pulse frequency are unclear. However, increases in hypothalamic norepinephrine levels or decreases in hypothalamic dopamine or opioid levels may account in part for the changes in LH pulse frequency. The elevated LH level stimulates ovarian thecal and stromal tissues to produce excessive quantities of androstenedione and testosterone. In addition, the elevated LH level may produce premature luteinization of granulosa cells in 2- to 8-mm antral follicles, which causes the termination of follicular growth. The accumulation of these antral follicles causes the ovaries to develop a polycystic appearance, hence the descriptive term *polycystic ovary syndrome* (PCOS). The premature termination of follicular growth prevents any follicle from reaching a size necessary to trigger an LH surge and ovulation. Consequently, oligoovulation or anovulation develops.

The elevated ovarian secretion of androstenedione and testosterone produces numerous biochemical changes, which include (1) a decrease in sex hormone-binding globulin production from the liver, leading to an increase in free testosterone levels; and (2) an increase in 5 α-reductase activity in the pilosebaceous unit, resulting in an increase in local dihydrotestosterone production. These changes can result in hirsutism and acne.

A unique opportunity to identify a specific molecular and genetic cause of ovarian hyperandrogenism is provided by the recent observation that abnormalities in the insulin receptor gene are often associated with ovarian hyperandrogenism.[13,14] In Kahn type A diabetes, a gene defect results in the inability to produce adequate numbers of functional insulin receptors. This genetic abnormality decreases glucose utilization in muscle and liver, is associated with an increase in circulating glucose levels, and results in a marked increase in pancreatic insulin production. In normal women, circulating insulin concentrations seldom exceed 150 μU/mL after a carbohydrate challenge. In women with Kahn type A diabetes, insulin concentrations can exceed 1000 μU/mL after a carbohydrate challenge. High concentrations of insulin may be able to bind to insulin-like growth factor 1 (IGF-1) receptors and may stimulate the tyrosine kinase activity of this receptor system. Human ovarian stroma and theca contain IGF-1 receptors, and IGF-1 and LH synergize to stimulate androstenedione and testosterone production. Some authorities believe that in patients with Kahn type A diabetes, the marked hyperinsulinemia may synergize with normal or elevated concentrations of LH to stimulate excessive androgen production from the ovary. The association between hyperinsulinemia and hyperandrogenism may also explain the observation that obesity is commonly associated with hyperandrogenism.

Treatment of functional ovarian hyperandrogenism should be direct at normalizing the LH and insulin concentrations. The production of LH can be normalized by administering combined estrogen-progestogen preparations or GnRH agonists. Insulin concentrations can often be lowered in obese individuals if weight is lost. Spironolactone, an inhibitor of the androgen receptor, can be used as an adjuvant to estrogen-progestogen preparations to help decrease facial hair growth.[125] Ovulation induction with clomiphene citrate of human menopausal gonadotropins is often successful in women with ovarian hyperandrogenism, anovulation, and infertility. Women with hyperandrogenism and anovulation are at risk of developing endometrial hyperplasia and endometrial adenocarcinoma. These women should be treated at regular intervals with a 12- to 14-day course of a progestogen to inhibit the development of endometrial hyperplasia and cancer.

McCune-Albright Syndrome

The McCune-Albright syndrome consists of the triad of cafe-au-lait spots, fibrous cysts of the bones, and precocious puberty resulting from the premature activation of ovarian follicular function. Recent studies suggest that in many cases of the McCune-Albright syndrome, cyclic follicular growth and estradiol production occurs independently of pituitary gonadotropin secretion. The McCune-Albright syndrome appears to be associated with an activating mutation in the gene coding for the α-subunit of the guanine nucleotide-binding regulatory protein (G s α), which couples receptors to adenylyl cyclase.[181] Ketoconazole and testolactone, two drugs that directly inhibit steroidogenic enzymes involved in estrogen production, are often used to treat this disorder.[62]

OVARIAN NEOPLASMS

The diagnosis and management of ovarian neoplasms are a major concern for clinicians. This is largely because invasive ovarian carcinoma is responsible for approximately 12,000 deaths annually in the United States. In spite of tremendous improvement in the survival of young women with germ cell ovarian malignancies, patients with epithelial ovarian cancer have shown only modest improvement in survival over the last 20 years. The most important positive prognostic feature continues to be diagnosis at an early stage. This single fact dictates that significant resources be directed toward evaluating ovarian/adnexal masses.

The technology associated with diagnosing and treating ovarian or adnexal pathology is expanding in an exponential fashion. Radiographic examinations, including ultrasonography (US), computed tomography (CT), and magnetic resonance imaging (MRI) are utilized with increasing frequency. Laparoscopic surgery continues to evolve, and physicians must not only maintain the basic skills involved with the procedure but also stay abreast of new equipment and indications for its usage. It is important that the clinician has a clear understanding of the wide range of disease processes that fall under the category of ovarian neoplasia. Developing and maintaining an understanding of the differential diagnosis of ovarian/adnexal pathology will allow a physician to process information as it becomes available and put it into a useful framework.

Epidemiology

Histologic diversity complicates the establishment of risk factors for both benign and malignant ovarian neoplasms. However, focusing specifically on invasive *epithelial* ovarian carcinoma, the most common ovarian malignancy, several investigators have postulated a causal relationship between certain environmental and genetic factors and this malignancy. Cramer et al found that lactose consumption may be a dietary risk factor, especially when combined with an inherited decrease in the levels of the enzyme galactose-1-phosphate uridyl transferase.[45] Significant consumption of animal fat may also be a risk factor.[44] The same investigators established a relationship between exogenous substances, such as asbestos and talc, and the development of ovarian carcinoma.[40,42]

Sustained elevated levels of gonadotropins have been found, in both animal and human studies, to be associated with an increased risk of ovarian cancer. Pelvic irradiation, viruses (particularly mumps), nulliparity, and the non-use of oral contraceptives (OCs) are associated with an increased risk of ovarian malignancy presumably because of sustained elevations of gonadotropins.[33,41,43,48] Hankinson et al reviewed 20 studies that assessed the association of OC use and ovarian carcinoma.[94] They found a relative risk of 0.64 (95% confidence interval: 0.57 to 0.73) associated with overuse of OCs. Many feel that the protective effect of OCs in reducing the risk of subsequent development of ovarian carcinoma should be considered in a woman's decision to use OCs.

Genetics

Gonadoblastoma and dysgerminoma are most frequently associated with dysgenetic gonads and the presence of a Y chromosome.[139,171,203,208] Granulosa-theca cell tumors have an increased incidence in women with Peutz-Jegher's syndrome of familial polyposis. Ovarian fibromas are associated with multiple nevoid basal cell carcinoma. A majority of epithelial ovarian cancer cases occur sporadically. Schildkraut and Thompson, in a population-based case control study, found that an odds ratio for ovarian cancer in first- and second-degree relatives of patients affected with the disease was 3.6 (95% confidence interval: 1.8 to 7.1) and 2.9 (95% confidence interval: 1.6 to 5.3) respectively, when compared with women who lacked a family history for ovarian cancer.[172] When the daughter of a woman with ovarian carcinoma develops this disease, Piver et al reported that it will more likely occur at an earlier age, irrespective of increased overall risk.[155] Evidence indicates that families that have an autosomal dominant pattern of transmission with a variable degree of penetration are at particularly high risk. Three hereditary syndromes associated with the occurrence of familial ovarian cancer have been described. These include the ovarian cancer syndrome, the hereditary breast-ovarian cancer syndrome, and the Lynch II syndrome that includes a predisposition to ovarian, endometrial, and colon cancer.[132-135]

Classification

The most useful classification system is one based on the cell of origin. Histology is the basis for the organization of this chapter. An abbreviated version of the World Health Organization's classification system for ovarian tumors is presented in Table 9-1. This system assigns ovarian neoplasms to one of five major categories:

I. Epithelial tumors
Serous, mucinous, endometrioid, clear cell, Brenner-transitional cell, mixed mesodermal, and undifferentiated tumors are included in the epithelial tumor category and account for approximately 70% of all ovarian neoplasms.

II. Stromal tumors
Approximately 5% to 10% of all ovarian neoplasms are derived from the ovarian stromal cells. These include granulosa stromal cell tumors, Sertoli stromal cell tumors, sex cord tumor with annular tubules (SCTAT), Leydig cell tumors, lipid cell tumors, and gynandroblastoma.

III. Germ cell tumors
Approximately 15% to 20% of all ovarian neoplasms are of germ cell origin. This includes dysgerminoma, endodermal sinus tumor, embryonal carcinoma, polyembryoma, choriocarcinoma, teratoma, mixed forms, and gonadoblastoma.

IV. Metastatic tumors
Approximately 5% of ovarian malignancies are metastatic from another site, most commonly breast and bowel.

V. Other
A small but significant number of ovarian "neoplasms" result from ovarian soft tissue or nonneoplastic processes.

Symptoms

Irrespective of histology, most ovarian neoplasms cause symptoms by exerting pressure on contiguous structures. Pressure symptoms include urinary frequency, pelvic discomfort, and constipation. As the tumor enlarges, abdominal swelling is the most common complaint. Acute abdominal pain secondary to hemorrhage, rupture with leakage, or torsion can all result from tumor growth. Upper abdominal metastases or ascites cause nausea, heart burn, bloating, weight loss, and anorexia, symptoms usually associated with gastrointestinal processes. Irregular vaginal bleeding can accompany any type of ovarian neoplasm. If ascites and hydrothorax are present, shortness of breath can be the presenting symptom. Smith and Anderson reviewed 83 patients with invasive epithelial ovarian carcinoma and found that the most common symptoms, regardless of stage, were abdominal swelling, fatigue, and abdominal pain (Table 9-2).[184] Contrary to popular belief, the authors found that early stage cancers did produce symptoms. Of the broad range of secondary symptoms, only

Table 9-1. Modified World Health Organization Comprehensive Classification of Ovarian Tumors

I. Common "epithelial" tumors
   A. Serous
   B. Mucinous
   C. Endometrioid
   D. Clear cell
   E. Brenner
   F. Transitional
   G. Small cell
   H. Malignant mixed mesodermal
   I. Unclassified

II. Sex cord stromal tumors
   A. Granulosa stromal cell
      1. Granulosa cell
      2. Thecoma-fibroma
   B. Sertoli stromal cell
      1. Sertoli cell tumors
      2. Sertoli-Leydig cell tumors
         a. Well differentiated
         b. Intermediately differentiated
         c. Poorly differentiated
         d. With heterologous elements
      3. Sex cord tumor with annular tubules (SCTAT)
      4. Leydig (hilus) cell tumors
   C. Lipid (lipoid) cell tumors
   D. Gynandroblastoma

III. Germ cell tumors
   A. Dysgerminoma
   B. Endodermal sinus tumor
   C. Embryonal carcinoma
   D. Polyembryoma
   E. Choriocarcinoma
   F. Teratomas
      1. Immature
      2. Mature (dermoid cyst)
      3. Monodermal (struma ovarii, carcinoid)
   G. Mixed forms
   H. Gonadoblastoma

IV. Metastatic

V. Other

menstrual irregularity was likely to convince these early stage patients to see a physician. Late stage cases were most often accompanied by abdominal pain and swelling, but only pain was likely to convince women to seek a diagnosis.

Biologically active hormones, including estrogen, progesterone, testosterone, corticosteroids, and hCG can be produced by a variety of ovarian neoplasms and cause the predicted symptoms associated with each compound. Teratomas can contain thyroid tissue which can produce a hyperthyroid state. In addition, teratomas can cause autoimmune hemolytic anemia by an unknown mechanism of action.[152]

Table 9-2. Distribution of cancer symptoms in women with ovarian carcinoma

	Symptom noticed		**Symptom convinced patient to seek diagnosis**	
Symptom	**%**	**(N)**	**%**	**(N)**
Abdominal swelling	70.4	(38)	63.9	(23)
Fatigue	55.6	(30)	37.9	(11)
Abdominal pain	48.1	(26)	87.0	(20)
Urination problems	37.0	(20)	52.6	(10)
Indigestion	25.9	(14)	46.2	(6)
Irregular vaginal bleeding	22.2	(12)	66.7	(8)
Shortness of breath	22.2	(12)	45.5	(5)
Metrorrhagia	18.9	(10)	50.0	(5)
Constipation/ diarrhea	18.5	(10)	20.0	(2)
Appetite loss	18.5	(10)	30.0	(3)

From Smith EM and Andersen B: The effects of symptoms and delay in seeking diagnosis on stage of disease at diagnosis, among women with cancers of the ovary, *Cancer* 56(11):2727, 1985.

Although hypercalcemia is a paraneoplastic syndrome associated with many gynecologic malignancies, Holtz found that 16 of 27 gynecologic oncology patients with hypercalcemia had ovarian carcinoma.[100]

Gastrointestinal and nervous system disturbances were the most common manifestations of hypercalcemia. Cerebellar degeneration caused by antibodies to Purkinje's cells rarely is due to ovarian malignancy. The degeneration presents with ataxia, vertigo, dysarthria, diplopia, nystagmus, movement alterations, progressive mental changes, and static tremor.[87]

Physical findings

A complete physical examination is imperative when evaluating a patient with a known or suspected pelvic mass, keeping in mind the differential diagnosis. A careful breast examination in both the sitting and supine positions is important. Abdominal examination, including palpation of all four quadrants, can diagnose ascites or an upper abdominal mass. All lymph node-bearing tissue, including axillary nodes, should be palpated carefully. Pleural effusions, a frequent finding in patients with ovarian cancer, are diagnosed with auscultation of both lungs. Examination of both lower extremities can reveal tenderness and a cord, indicating a deep vein thrombosis that can be the presenting symptom in a patient with a pelvic mass.

The pelvic examination is the most important part of the physical diagnosis of a pelvic mass. Always inspect the vulva, vagina, and cervix first and look for the presence of any other disease process and displacement secondary to a mass. A rectal examination is an obligatory component of a routine pelvic examination. Not only is it necessary to evaluate the posterior uterine surface, uterosacral ligaments, pouch of Douglas, and parametria, but also to screen for colorectal cancer. An occult stool guaiac should always be checked, and if positive, a screening flexible sigmoidoscopy or full colonoscopy is recommended by the American Cancer Society. Defining the size and the location of the uterus is important since an adnexal mass is often an enlarged uterus. Palpation of both adnexae should be carefully undertaken. In premenopausal women the ovaries are approximately 3 × 2 × 2 cm. In postmenopausal women they should be approximately the size of an almond (2 × 1 × 0.5 cm). If no mass is palpated but the patient has symptoms, radiographic evaluation is appropriate (see below).

Differential diagnosis of adnexal mass

Nongynecologic

Diverticular disease. Diverticulitis complicated by a sigmoid colon phlegmon or pericolonic abscess may present as a pelvic mass, most frequently in postmenopausal women. The most common symptoms are left lower quadrant pain and obstipation. In addition to the mass, examination reveals a patient with toxicity, fever, localizing peritonitis, and leukocytosis. In the acute setting, this diagnosis is best confirmed by an abdominal-pelvic CT scan.

Appendiceal abscess. Appendicitis complicated by a appendiceal abscess may present as a right-sided pelvic mass. This is commonly found in women of reproductive age. A recent history of increasing right lower quadrant pain, anorexia, fever, a tender right lower quadrant mass, localizing peritonitis, a fluctuant mass palpated on rectal examination, and leukocytosis all help to make this diagnosis. An abdominal CT scan and barium enema are often useful in confirming this diagnosis.

Crohn's disease. Regional enteritis, or Crohn's disease, may also present as a pelvic or abdominal mass. Because of the early age of onset, pelvic or abdominal masses secondary to Crohn's disease present most commonly in women in the second and third decades of life. Like diverticular disease, a mass secondary to Crohn's disease represents either a phlegmon or perienteric abscess. The most common site of this disease is in the terminal ileum, though any portion of the GI tract may be involved. Patients with a Crohn's-related abscess or phlegmon often present with a history of chronic diarrhea, weight loss, and abdominal pain. They also appear acutely ill with fever, localizing tenderness, and leukocytosis. Full GI tract evaluation with a barium enema, and an upper GI with a small bowel follow-through are essential for evaluating this disease. In addition, an abdominal CT scan may be helpful in the workup of a patient with an abscess or phlegmon secondary to Crohn's disease.

Primary nongynecologic malignancy. Lymphoma, retroperitoneal tumor, small bowel tumors and mesothelial tumors are rare pelvic malignancies that are easily confused with gynecologic neoplasms. Gynecologic neoplasms are almost always accurately diagnosed at laparotomy. Colorectal cancer is the second most commonly diagnosed visceral cancer in the United States and must always be kept in mind when evaluating a pelvic mass, especially in postmenopausal women. The American Cancer Society recommends that patients over the age of 50 years undergo a screening flexible sigmoidoscopy every 3 years. Symptoms depend on tumor size and location and commonly include a change in bowel habits, pain, and hematochezia. On physical examination, rectal lesions and metastases to the ovaries can sometimes be palpated. If fecal occult blood is present, a screening evaluation for colorectal cancer should always be undertaken prior to any other procedure.

Pelvic kidney. The incidence of a pelvic kidney in the general population is 1:20,000. That rate increases to 7% to 15% in women with vaginal agenesis. With this in mind, any patient with a gynecologic malformation should undergo a complete urologic workup including an intravenous pyelogram, and if indicated, cystoscopy and retrograde pyelography.

Gynecologic

Tuboovarian abscess. Pelvic inflammatory disease followed by the development of a tuboovarian abscess most commonly results from a sexually transmitted infectious disease such as gonorrhea or chlamydia. Instrumentation (therapeutic abortion) can also be the initiating event. A review of systems usually reveals a fever, bilateral pelvic pain, and vaginal discharge. On physical examination, cervical motion tenderness, bilateral adnexal tenderness, and cervical discharge are often found. There is often a marked leukocytosis, with significant increase in polymorphonuclear leukocytes. Depending upon the patient's overall condition, broad antibiotic coverage should be initiated, sometimes followed by exploration and removal of the abscess. Sometimes total abdominal hysterectomy/bilateral salpingo-oophorectomy (TAH/BSO) is required, although the maintenance of child-bearing potential is often desirable. Drainage under CT guidance has been shown to be effective in some situations.

Ectopic pregnancy. Ectopic pregnancy continues to be a major cause of maternal death in the United States. Its incidence has been rising over the past decade. The triad of irregular menses, unilateral adnexal pain, and adnexal mass combined with a positive urine or serum hCG level represents an ectopic pregnancy until proven otherwise. The management of this disease process often includes laparoscopy with operative pelviscopy both to confirm the diagnosis and to remove the tubal pregnancy. If the patient is hemodynamically unstable, laparotomy is indicated. In some cases, where the ectopic is not visible at the time of laparoscopy but serum hCG levels show that there is not a normal intrauterine pregnancy, systemic methotrexate can be effective therapy.[30]

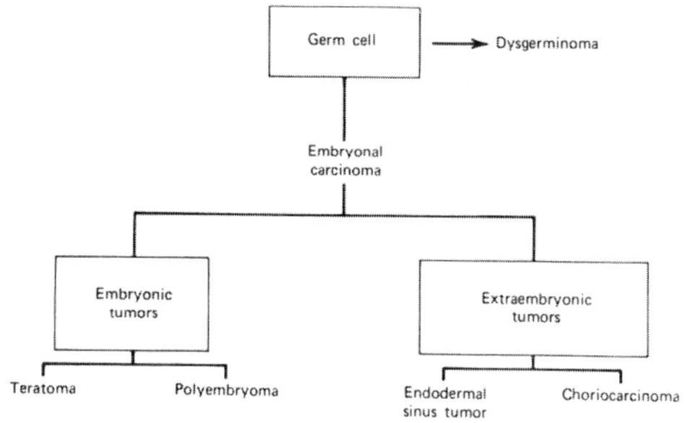

Fig. 9-4. Germ cell tumor derivation. (From Teilum G: *Special tumors of ovary and testis, and related extragonadal lesions: comparative pathology and histologic identification,* ed 2, Philadelphia, 1977, JB Lippincott.)

Leiomyoma. A pedunculated uterine leiomyoma or a primary ovarian leiomyoma can present as an adnexal mass. Most cases are asymptomatic, but torsion can cause abdominal swelling or pain. While the gross appearance is a fleshy, white mass, the microscopic appearance is one of smooth muscle cells with cigar-shaped nuclei. The presence of any mitotic activity raises the suspicion of a sarcoma.

Fallopian tube "neoplasia." Both benign and malignant processes of the fallopian tube present as an adnexal mass and can be confused with an ovarian mass. The differential diagnosis includes pyosalpinx, hydrosalpinx, cystic teratomas, adenomatoid tumor, paratubal cysts, and adenocarcinoma.

Ovarian Neoplasm (see below).
Differential diagnosis of an ovarian mass.

Germ cell tumors. Germ cell tumors are principally diseases of early reproductive women. They are second in frequency (15% to 20%) to epithelial tumors. Because the mean age of occurrence is 19 years, interest in improving survival and maintaining childbearing potential is very keen. The clinical presentation, histology, and biology are quite varied in this group of tumors, with both benign and malignant neoplasms being included. Fig. 9-4 outlines the accepted derivation of germ cell tumors.[202] Gonadoblastoma is the benign tumor of greatest interest because of its frequent association with malignant germ cell tumors. The most common type of malignant germ cell tumor is the dysgerminoma, followed by mixed, endodermal sinus, immature teratoma, embryonal, and choriocarcinoma. Polyembryoma is rare. In general the prognosis for patients with malignant germ cell tumors is much more favorable than those with invasive epithelial tumors. This is a result of early diagnosis and the development of effective chemotherapeutic agents.

Benign germ cell tumors

Gonadoblastoma. Gonadoblastomas are almost always found in patients with gonadal dysgenesis associated with a Y chromosome or Y chromosomal fragment. This tumor, first described by Scully in 1953, is a tumor composed of germ cells mixed with sex cord derivatives.[179] Although this tumor is benign, it is associated with a malignant germ cell tumor in approximately 50% of cases.[95] Karyotyping should be undertaken in any individual with primary or secondary amenorrhea and abnormal sexual development (e.g., lack of secondary sexual characteristics, infantile external and internal genitalia, atrophic vaginal mucosa). If a Y chromosome is present, prompt bilateral gonadectomy is indicated, except in patients with testicular feminization (androgen insensitivity syndrome). In this situation the removal of both gonads can be delayed up to age 30 years because the risk of developing cancer is so low prior to that time.

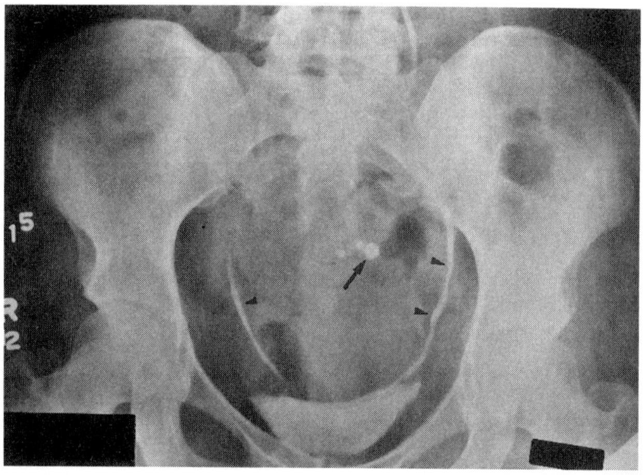

Fig. 9-5. Plain radiograph during intravenous pyelogram demonstrates a calcific density overlying the sacrum (*arrow*) which represents a tooth formed within a dermoid tumor. Also note the ureters *(arrowheads).*

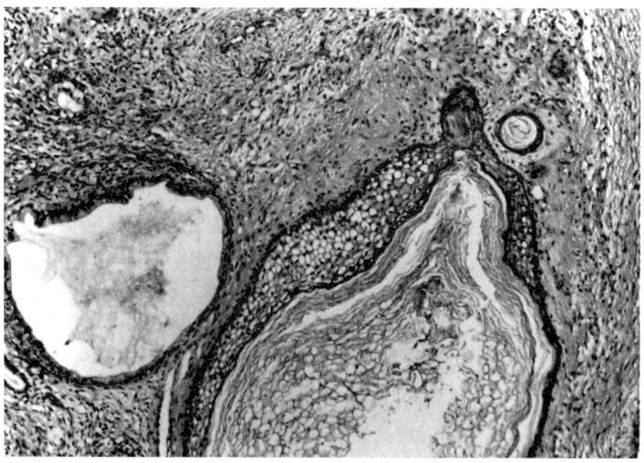

Fig. 9-6. Mature teratoma containing cysts lined by squamous and glandular epithelium of a mature adult type in a benign fibrous stroma.

Teratomas. A single totipotential germ cell gives rise to teratomas. This neoplasm is characterized by the presence of all three germ cell layers: ectoderm, mesoderm, and endoderm. Teratomas can be malignant or benign, as determined by the presence of immature tissue.

The most common benign teratoma is the "cystic teratoma," or "dermoid cyst." This tumor accounts for 25% to 40% of all ovarian neoplasms. While most cases are diagnosed in premenopausal women, 15% of cases occur in postmenopausal women.[85] Most patients will be asymptomatic at the time of diagnosis. Torsion and rupture rarely occur but cause acute peritonitis and necessitate prompt exploratory laparotomy.[191] Physical examination will reveal an adnexal mass that is bilateral in approximately 12% to 15% of cases.[55] Dermoids are often diagnosed by ultasound or plain abdominal radiography (Fig. 9-5). Grossly there is usually a prominent cavity with skin, teeth, bones, hair, and extremities being present. Rokitansky's protuberance represents the part of the dermoid where the greatest variety of tissue is present, grossly appearing as a nodular thickening. Histologically, only mature adult tissue is present (Fig. 9-6).

Autoimmune hemolytic anemia has been found in a small number of patients who have a dermoid present.[152] This is indistinguishable from other causes of the anemia and removal of the tumor resolves the anemia.

The risk of a malignancy arising in a dermoid is small, approximately 1% to 2%, and most commonly occurs in postmenopausal women. Squamous cell carcinoma represents the most common type of malignancy found in a dermoid, followed by carcinoid.

Struma ovarii describes a dermoid where thyroid tissue comprises greater than 50% of the teratomas. This is unusual and accounts for only 2.7% of ovarian teratomas. On gross inspection these tumors are usually unilateral and less than 10 cm. The cut surface is light tan with a glistening appearance. Microscopically, mature thyroid tissue of any type can be found (Fig. 9-7). Rarely is there an associated hyperthyroidism. There have been 45 reported cases of malignant struma ovarii.[81,165]

There have been approximately 200 reported cases of primary ovarian carcinoid.[160,164] It is important to differentiate primary ovarian carcinoid from metastatic carcinoid because of the poorer prognosis associated with carcinoid metastatic to the ovary.[163] Primary carcinoids, almost always associated with other teratoatmous elements, have cells containing nuclei that are round with coarse chromatin (Fig. 9-8). Primary ovarian carcinoids are usually unilateral, in contrast to metastatic carcinoids that are almost always bilateral. Primary carcinoids probably arise from argentaffin cells present in the dermoid. The carcinoid syndrome includes flushing, diarrhea, facial cyanosis, bronchospasm, and evidence of right-sided heart failure. The syndrome is a result of serotonin, bradykinin. and histamine release. Recurrence is rare and approaches only 5% in the Robboy et al series.[160]

Struma carcinoid of the ovary is a teratoma where thyroid tissue develops in association with carcinoid, usually of the trabecular type. Robboy and Scully reported on the largest series to date, which included 50 patients.[162] In this series all tumors were unilateral, none had carcinoid syndrome, and only one patient died of the disease. Twenty-eight percent of the patients in this series were treated with an ovarian conserving procedure, and all of these patients were without evidence of disease at the time of reporting.

Management of Benign Teratomas. Laparoscopy or laparotomy can be used to remove a dermoid and perform a cystectomy in most cases, or oophorectomy when

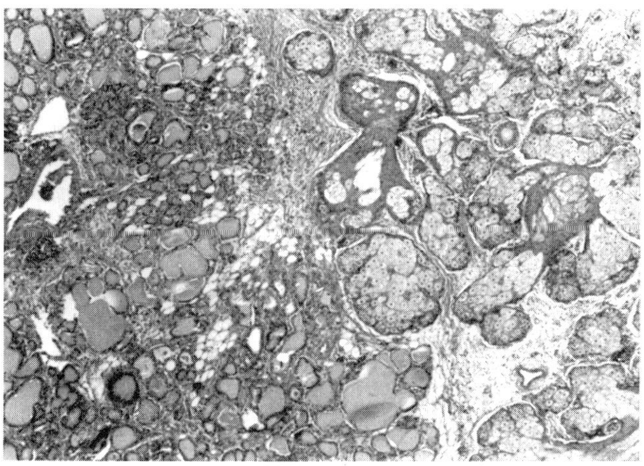

Fig. 9-7. Mature teratoma containing sebaceous epithelium as well as follicles of thyroid-type epithelium (struma ovarii).

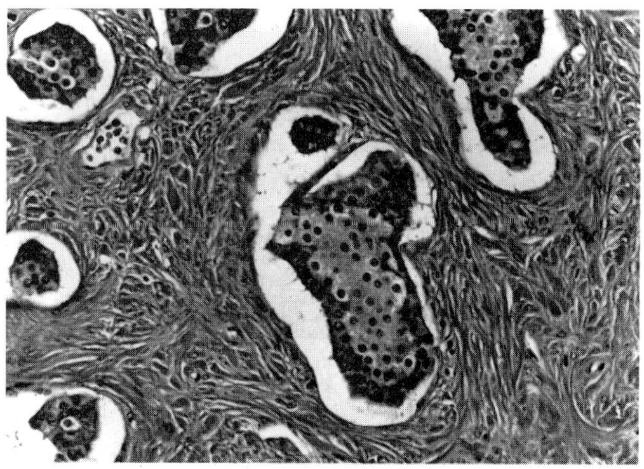

Fig. 9-8. Ovarian carcinoid tumor containing sharply demarcated nests of insular-type carcinoid in a dense desmoplastic stroma. The resultant appearance may be easily confused with that of Brenner tumor.

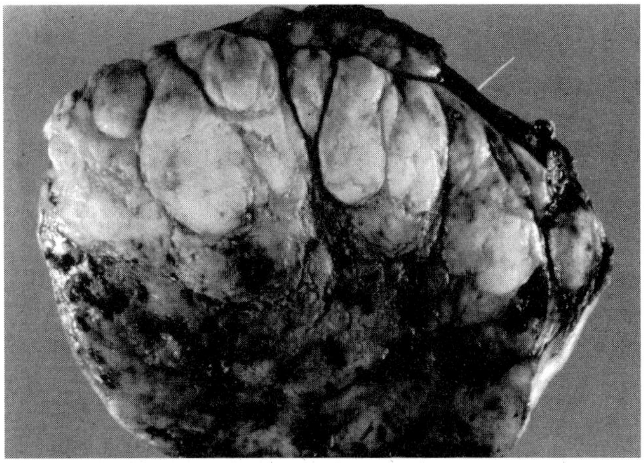

Fig. 9-9. Bisected ovarian dysgerminoma with areas of hemorrhagic infarction as well as lobules of unaltered tumor.

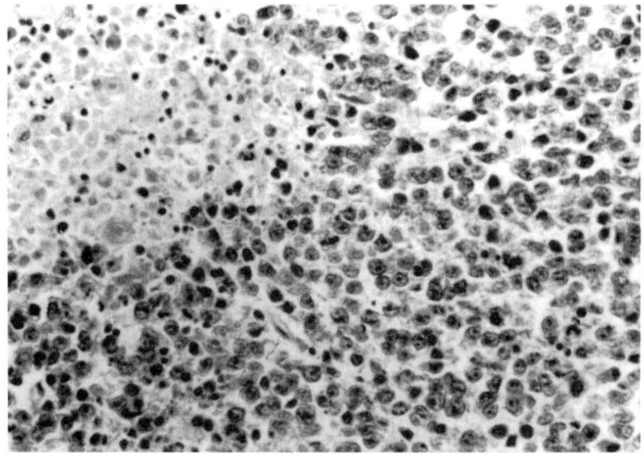

Fig. 9-10. Anaplastic dysgerminoma consisting of sheets of neoplastic cells with numerous mitotic figures, areas of necrosis, but no evidence of differentiation. Lymphocytes are commonly seen with this tumor, but are not obvious here.

necessary. If the dermoid is larger than 6 cm or there is a history of multiple surgical procedures with adhesions, laparotomy is the preferred treatment approach. A frozen section should be obtained in all cases. While careful attention should be given to the other ovary because of the 12% bilaterality rate, routine bivalving of a normal-appearing ovary is not indicated.

Malignant germ cell tumors

Dysgerminoma. This is the most common germ cell malignancy and represents 35% to 45% of all germ cell tumors.[68,84] Grossly this tumor appears lobulated, solid, fleshy, and usually has a smooth external surface; hemorrhage and necrosis are not prominent features (Fig. 9-9). Histologically, aggregates of large hemogeneous polygonal cells are distinguishing features (Fig. 9-10). Lymphocyte infiltration and the presence of delicate fibrous septa are common.[120] Occasionally, multinucleated syncytiotrophoblastic giant cells are present.

It is common for this tumor to be bilateral, either overtly or covertly (10% to 15%).[84] Almost uniquely, dysgerminomas have lymphatic, not hematogenous metastases. The survival rate for patients with early stage disease is greater than 95%.[122,207] Even patients with advanced stage disease enjoy a favorable prognosis of greater than 80%, when appropriate adjuvant therapy is given.

Serum lactic dehydrogenase (LDH) can serve as a useful tumor marker.[130,157,175] Greatly elevated serum LDH levels are the rule in patients with dysgerminoma, in contrast to the minimally elevated levels in a variety of other medical conditions. While the slow fractions of LDH are elevated in most ovarian carcinomas, the fast fractions are increased in patients with dysgerminoma.[67] Serum hCG levels are elevated in a small number of patients as well.

Endodermal sinus tumors. Endodermal sinus tumor (EST), also known as "yolk sac tumor," is an extremely aggressive malignancy, the histology of which previously

A

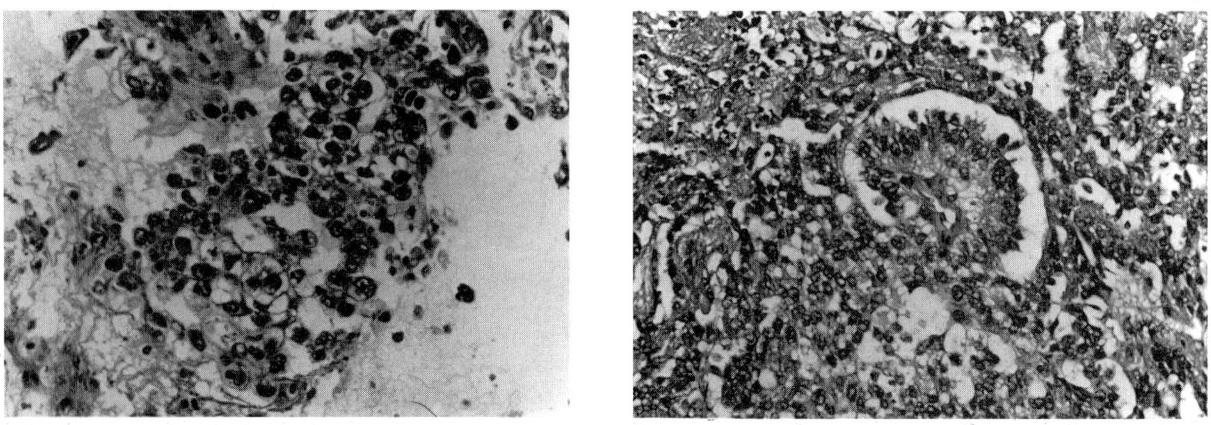

B

Fig. 9-11. A, Yolk sac tumor containing cytoplasmic and extracellular globules of α-fetoprotein. **B,** Yolk sac tumor containing a well-formed Schiller-Duval body with a central papillary tuft surrounded by a glomerulus-like space.

predicted a uniformly poor outcome.[119] Grossly the external surface of this tumor is usually smooth and glistening, with hemorrhage and necrosis being prominent features. Histologically this tumor has several distinctive features including intracellular and extracellular hyaline droplets (periodic acid-Schiff [PAS]–positive), a reticular growth pattern, and the famous Schiller-Duval bodies (a central capillary surrounded by simple papillae) (Fig. 9-11).[201] This tumor is almost never bilateral. Intraperitoneal and hematogenous spread is common; lymph node metastasis is unusual. Commonly these patients present with an acute abdomen, secondary to spontaneous rupture and hemorrhage. While patients with stage I or II have a survival rate in the range of 60% to 100%, patients with stage III or IV have a somewhat lower survival rate of 50% to 75% following appropriate chemotherapy.[73] Platinum-based chemotherapy significantly improves the survival rate of patients with EST.

Most ESTs secrete α-fetoprotein (AFP) and rarely α-1-antitrypsin (AAT).[197] Monitoring serum levels of AFP can be useful when watching a patient's response to therapy and predicting a recurrence.

Immature teratomas. This germ cell tumor represents approximately 20% of all malignant germ cell tumors.[149] While immature tissue from all three germ cell layers is present, the amount of immature glial tissue is the most important from a prognostic point of view (Fig. 9-12). Grade 1 has no more than one focus of immature neuroepithelium per low-power (× 40) field. Grade 2 has immature neuroepithelium present, but not in excess of three low-power fields in any one slide. All grade 3 lesions have immature glial tissue present in four or more low-power fields within individual sections. Spontaneous maturation of extraovarian glial implants is a unique feature of immature teratomas (IT).[161] This entity, termed gliomatosis peritonei, does not confer a negative prognosis.[147] Instead, it has been associated with a favorable outcome. After grade, surgicopathologic stage is the most important prognostic factor. While stage 1, grade 1 lesions enjoy a 100% survival rate, patients with stage 3, grade 1 tumors have a 3-year survival rate of 50%. Fortunately, most patients are diagnosed with early stage disease.

Occasionally, immature teratomas can produce AFP that can be used as a tumor marker, and the same is true for serum LDH and CA-125; hCG is never produced by this tumor.

Embryonal carcinoma. This germ cell tumor is quite rare. Grossly it resembles EST but tends to be larger. Histologically, embryonal glands, gland-like clefts (embryoid bodies), and syntrophoblastic giant cells are present. The tumor is rarely bilateral and tends to spread intraperitoneally. Survival is slightly better than with EST, using the same platinum-based chemotherapy regimens. Both AFP and hCG can serve as tumor markers for this germ cell tumor.

Choriocarcinoma. Nongestational choriocarcinoma of the ovary is extremely rare. It has the same histologic appearance as gestational choriocarcinoma metastatic to the ovaries (Fig. 9-13).[106] Isosexual precocity is present in approximately 50% of prepubertal females diagnosed with this tumor. Serum hCG is produced by this type of germ cell tumor, as it is in gestational choriocarcinoma, and can serve as a useful tumor marker. Although gestational choriocarcinoma is treated successfully in most patients with chemotherapy, remission is less common in patients with nongestational choriocarcinoma. There have been reports of sustained remission in patients with ovarian choriocarcinoma, since the advent of platinum-based chemotherapy.

Mixed. In 10% to 15% of germ cell tumors, more than one histologic type is present, thus the term mixed germ cell tumor.[74] The most frequent combination is dysgerminoma with EST, followed by IT with EST. Embryonal and choriocarcinoma are found much less frequently. The relative amount of the most malignant component and the stage will determine the prognosis. EST has a better

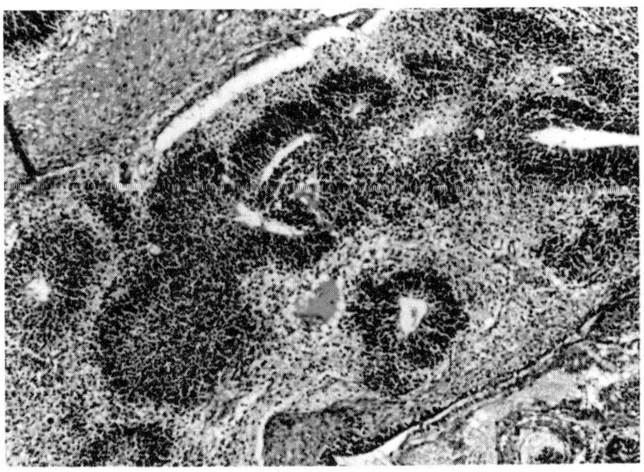

Fig. 9-12. Immature teratoma containing neural-type tissue forming primitive neural tubules.

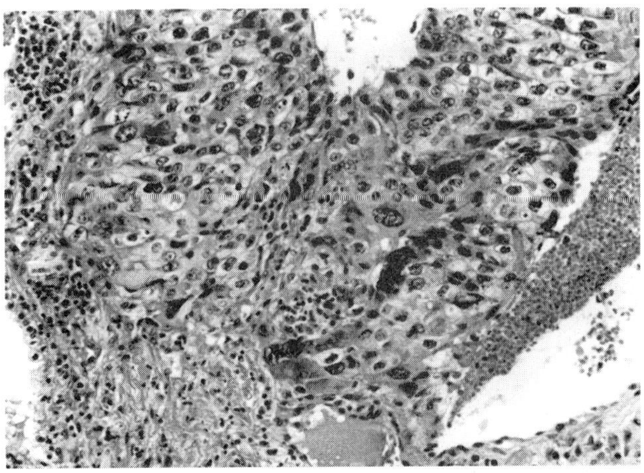

Fig. 9-13. Ovarian choriocarcinoma containing predominantly cytotrophoblastic cells with scattered multinucleated syncytiotrophoblasts.

prognosis when present as a mixed tumor, compared to a pure EST. The tumor marker or markers produced depend on the types of germ cell elements present.

Polyembryoma. This is an extremely rare germ cell tumor, with the histologic appearance of embryoid bodies in different stages of presomite development. Elevated levels of both AFP and hCG have been reported.[195] Chemotherapy has induced remission in only a few reported cases.

Management of malignant germ cell tumors

DYSGERMINOMAS. Fortunately most patients with dysgerminoma have stage I disease. Surgery alone is adequate for cure and consists of unilateral oophorectomy. Careful inspection of the opposite ovary, with biopsy of any suspicious areas, is important because of the risk of overt and covert bilateralism. Formal staging, including an ipsilateral retroperitoneal lymphadenectomy, should always be performed in patients with dysgerminoma because of its tendency for lymph node metastases. All patients with greater than stage I disease should undergo cytoreductive surgery and require additional therapy.[207] While it has been suggested that a patient who has stage I disease with a primary tumor greater than 10 to 15 cm should receive adjuvant therapy, this has not been supported in several large series. Dysgerminomas are exquisitely sensitive to radiation and this has been a mainstay of therapy for patients with metastatic dysgerminoma.[23]

Preservation of ovarian function and fertility is almost always of major importance in these young patients. Because of this and the success of chemotherapy in treating males with seminomas (the male analog to the female dysgerminoma), chemotherapy has replaced radiation therapy as the treatment of choice. Schwartz et al found advanced stage dysgerminomas to be markedly sensitive to vincristine, dactinomycin, and cyclophosphamide (VAC).[174,177] Other authors have found that vinblastine, bleomycin, and cisplatin (VBP) or bleomycin, etoposide, and cisplatin (BEP) have induced a complete response in a greater number of patients.[71,80,174] Etoposide and cisplatin alone have been used as well, with great success.[8] The number of cycles necessary to achieve remission is usually 4 to 6. Serum LDH levels can be helpful in making treatment decisions.

NONDYSGERMINOMATOUS MALIGNANCIES. Unilateral tumors are the rule in patients with nondysgerminomatous germ cell malignancies. Because of this, a unilateral oophorectomy should be performed. This would preserve the contralateral ovary, as long as it appears normal, for hormone production and future child-bearing potential. Staging is important, including a retroperitoneal lymph node dissection, intraperitoneal biopsies, and omentectomy. Although lymph node metastases are unusual, the possibility always exists of dysgerminomatous elements being present (mixed germ cell tumor) but missed on frozen section analysis. Cytoreductive surgery for advanced disease should be undertaken when possible.

As is the case for testicular germ cell tumors, platinum-based combination chemotherapy has had a significant impact on the survival of patients with nondysgerminomatous ovarian germ cell malignancies. The only patients who do not benefit from postoperative chemotherapy are those with immature teratomas, stage IA, grade I. All remaining patients, regardless of histology, receive chemotherapy in either an adjuvant or curative setting. While VAC used to be the combination of choice,[76] platinum-based regimens consisting of either VPB or BEP have shown superior results.[80,200] The Gynecologic Oncology Group found that VAC chemotherapy was not effective in patients with unresectable or incompletely resected nondysgerminomatous or mixed germ cell tumors of the ovary.[183] In another study the effectiveness of VPB in treating the same group of patients was proven.[200]

Maintaining future child-bearing potential is a major issue for many of these young patients, as it is for patients with dysgerminoma. Gershenson et al, and Wu found that the majority of women receiving chemotherapy for ovarian germ cell tumors resumed normal menses after successful chemotherapy.[70,77,217]

The benefit of OCs in preventing ovarian dysfunction in patients receiving chemotherapy has not been established.

Second-look surgery for germ cell tumors is of limited value. Gershenson et al found that 52 of 53 second-look surgeries were negative; only one of the 52 patients recurred and died of disease.[78] With the useful tumor markers and radiographic examinations this surgery is rarely indicated.

Sex cord stromal tumors. The gonadal stroma of the ovary gives rise to approximately 5% of all ovarian neoplasms. The primitive gonadal stroma has the potential to develop in either a male or female direction. Because of this, ovarian stromal tumors can assume histologic and hormonal features consistent with female stroma or can differentiate to assume predominantly male stromal features. While hormone production by stromal tumors is common, including production of estrogen, progesterone, testosterone, other androgenic compounds, and corticosteroids, it is not consistent and cannot be used as a means to classify this group of neoplasms. A majority of these stromal tumors are granulosa-theca cell tumors (female directed). A smaller percentage are Sertoli-Leydig cell tumors (male directed). The gynandroblastoma contains both female- and male-directed cells. Lipid cell tumors are unusual and contain Leydig-like cells, adrenocortical-like cells, or both.

Granulosa stromal tumor

Adult granulosa cell tumors (GCTs). The presence of granulosa cells alone or in combination with theca elements defines GCTs. The term thecoma or theca cell tumor should be used exclusively for tumors consisting only of theca cells. Excess estrogen production is often found in both tumor types, causing isosexual precocious puberty in young women and menometrorrhagia in menstruating or postmenopausal

A 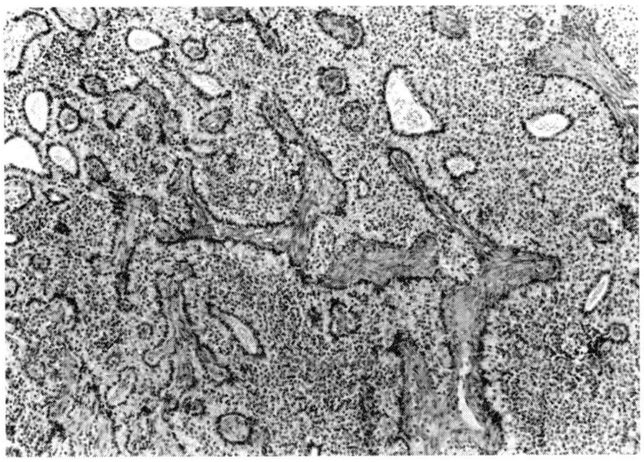 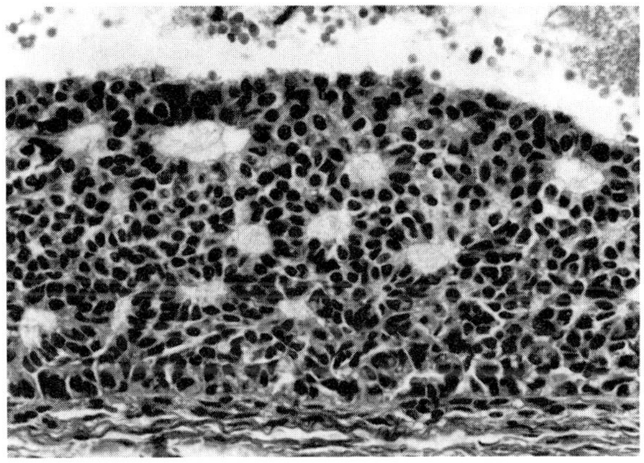 B

Fig. 9-14. A, Ovarian granulosa cell tumor consisting of well-differentiated granulosa cells with prominent cytoplasm. The complex cell nests show peripheral nuclear pallisading. **B,** Granulosa cell tumor containing multiple Call-Exner bodies consisting of extracellular spaces surrounded by neoplastic granulosa cells.

women. Endometrial hyperplasia or carcinoma is as high as 60% in patients with this tumor.[59] More than 50% of GCTs occur in postmenopausal women; fewer than 5% occur in prepubertal girls. Rupture with intraabdominal bleeding is commonly the presenting situation in this group of patients. On gross examination these tumors are solid with cystic areas. Hemorrhage is a common feature. Different microscopic patterns have been described, including microfollicular, macrofollicular, trabecular, insular, and diffuse. Histologic features associated with a poor prognosis included diffuse growth pattern, increased mitotic figures, and cellular atypia. Call-Exner bodies are pathognomonic of this tumor type and are present in the microfollicular pattern (Fig. 9-14).

GCTs are indolent tumors and if clinically confined to the ovary, they infrequently relapse and are rarely lethal.[64,65,150,190] In one report of 118 patients, 10% were stage III, none had stage IV, and only 6.2% with stage IA1 died of the disease.[59] In contrast, 54% of patients with stage III died of the disease. The average time between the initial diagnosis and the first recurrence was 6 years, but one patient recurred 23 years after diagnosis. Seventy-two percent of patients who had a recurrence died of disease. This tumor often produces estradiol, which can serve as a useful tumor marker. Levels greater than 30 picograms in postmenopausal women are abnormal and represent exogenous tumor production.

Juvenile granulosa cell tumors. Juvenile GCTs differ from the adult type with regard to clinical and pathologic features (Table 9-3). As is the case in adult GCTs, bilaterality is rare and the vast majority of patients have stage IA disease. Young et al reviewed 125 cases of juvenile GCTs that show a mortality rate of 1.5% for patients with stage IA disease, but a ten fold increase for the unusual patient with greater than stage IA disease.[222]

Fibromas. Fibromas are almost always unilateral and are most commonly diagnosed in the fifth decade of life. Hormone production is unusual, with estrogen being the most common compound produced. On gross appearance these tumors are usually white and fleshy. Microscopically the appearance is one of intersecting bundles of spindle cells. Two unusual clinical syndromes are associated with fibromas. Fibromas with ascites and hydrothorax represent Meigs' syndrome, which can easily be mistaken for an ovarian malignancy.[143] Gorlin's syndrome, an autosomal dominant disorder, consists of a fibroma associated with multiple basal cell nevus, often including dental cysts and skeletal abnormalities.

Fibromas are benign tumors with less than 1% having increased mitotic activity. If 1 to 3 mitoses per high-power field (HPF) are present, the tumor is considered low grade, and is called a cellular fibroma. If greater than 3 mitoses per HPF are present, it is considered a fibrosarcoma. In both cases the tumor is usually larger than a benign fibroma and carries a worse prognosis.

Table 9-3. Differences between adult GCT and juvenile GCT

Adult GCT	Juvenile GCT
Less than 1% prepubertal	50% prepubertal
Usual after 30 years of age	Rare after 30 years of age
Follicles usually regular, without mucin; Call-Exner bodies common	Follicles often irregular, contain mucin; Call-Exner bodies rare
Nuclei pale, commonly grooved	Nuclei dark, rarely grooved
Luteinization infrequent	Luteinization frequent
Recurrence rarely early, often very late	Recurrence typically early

From Young RH, Dickersin GR, Scully RE: Juvenile granulosa cell tumor of the ovary: a clinicopathological analysis of 125 cases, *Am J Surg Pathol* 8(8):575, 1984.

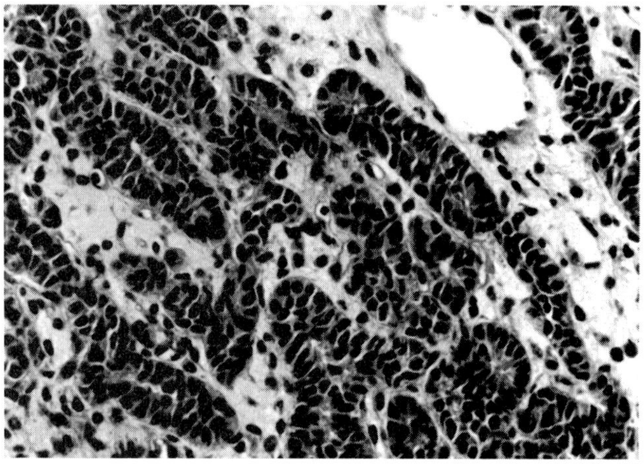

Fig. 9-15. Well-differentiated Sertoli cell tumor consisting of well-developed tubules mimicking testicular seminiferous tubules.

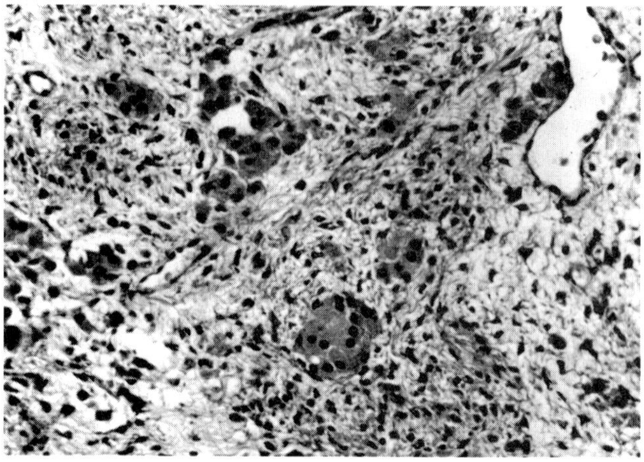

Fig. 9-16. Prominent Leydig cell nests are present in a loose stroma. Elsewhere, this Sertoli-Leydig cell tumor showed clear-cut Sertoli differentiation.

Thecomas. These tumors are very similar to fibromas, and often cannot be distinguished. Clinically the one important difference is that thecomas more commonly produce excess estrogen, which causes postmenopausal bleeding, menorrhagia, amenorrhea, and endometrial hyperplasia or cancer. Grossly they are solid, yellow-orange tumors.

Microscopic examination reveals a significant number of lutein cells and lipid-rich theca cells.

It is unusual for a theca cell tumor to be malignant. The same criteria should be used to define malignant thecoma as are used to define ovarian fibrosarcoma.

Sertoli stromal cell tumors. Arrhenoblastoma or androblastoma are dated terms to describe this group of neoplasms. They represent sex cord stromal tumors that exhibit a testicular or male direction of differentiation. This rare group of tumors represents less than 1% of all ovarian neoplasms. While many of these neoplasms are androgen producing, many are hormonally inert, with estrogen production occurring only occasionally.

Sertoli cell tumors. A pure Sertoli cell tumor of the ovary is composed only of Sertoli cells in a tubular arrangement.[199] Androgens are produced by Leydig cells. This makes the diagnosis of a pure Sertoli cell tumor unlikely in the presence of virilization. Estrogen production can occur. Grossly these tumors are unilateral, solid, and tan on sectioning. Histologically they contain hollow or solid tubules with a fibrous stroma (Fig. 9-15). The average diameter is 9 cm. Rarely is this tumor malignant, but the associated features include large size, infiltration of the stroma with cells, increased mitotic activity, and hemorrhage with necrosis.

Sertoli-Leydig cell tumors. The Sertoli-Leydig cell tumors, also known as arrhenoblastoma, are the most common Sertoli stromal cell tumors. Both Sertoli and Leydig cells are present (Fig. 9-16).

Approximately 40% of patients will show evidence of excess androgen production, or virilization. This includes clitoromegaly, hirsutism, acne, hoarseness, and increased libido. A small percent will show excess estrogen production, while some are hormonally inert. These tumors are almost always unilateral and occur most frequently in the third decade of life. Grossly they are solid, tan, and an average of 13 cm in diameter. Microscopically they have been divided into 4 categories by the World Health Organization (WHO): (1) well differentiated (predominant tubular pattern); (2) intermediate differentiation (sheets of immature Sertoli cells with some stroma present); (3) poorly differentiated (immature Sertoli cells with little or no stroma present); and (4) with heterologous elements. Fifteen percent of patients with heterologous elements will have a retiform pattern, connoting a worse prognosis.[196] Young and Scully, in a review of 207 cases of Sertoli-Leydig cell tumors found that 97.5% of patients had a stage I tumor and only 2.5% had advanced stage disease.[224] The prognosis correlated most meaningfully with the stage and degree of differentiation of the tumor. The high-stage tumors were all clinically malignant. All the well-differentiated tumors were benign, but 11% of those of intermediate differentiation, 59% of poorly differentiated tumors, and 19% of those with heterologous elements behaved in a malignant fashion.

Conservative surgical treatment with preservation of some ovarian tissue is appropriate for most patients with early-stage disease. In those patients with intermediate or poor differentiation, or high-stage tumors, postoperative adjuvant therapy may be indicated.

Sex cord tumor with annular tubules (SCTAT). Histologically this tumor is characterized by simple and complex annular tubules. This tumor is rarely associated with adenoma malignum of the cervix. In 30% of cases it is

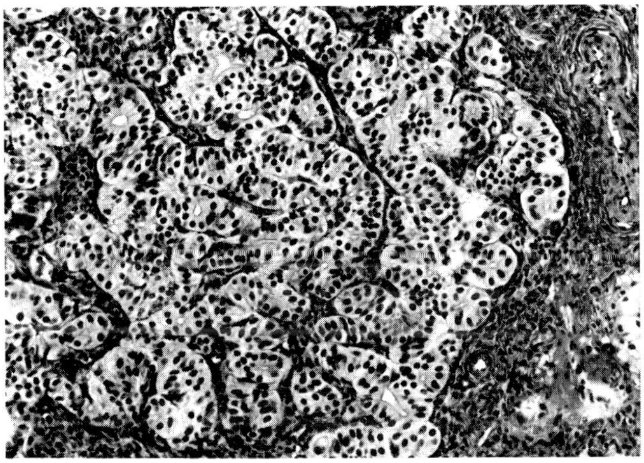

Fig. 9-17. Well-formed tubules indicative of Sertoli cell differentiation are present in this granulosa cell tumor with a secondary Sertoli cell component (Gynandroblastoma).

associated with Peutz-Jeghers syndrome (gastrointestinal polyposis with oral mucocutaneous lesions).[37] When associated with Peutz-Jeghers syndrome, the tumor is usually bilateral, small, and behaves in a benign fashion. When not associated with this syndrome, it is usually unilateral, large, and in one fifth of cases behaves in a clinically malignant fashion. Young et al, in a review of 74 cases of SCTAT, found that 27 patients had Peutz-Jeghers syndrome and small bilateral tumors that behaved in a benign fashion.[225] Signs of increased estrogen production were present in 50% of these patients. All four deaths in this series occurred in patients who did not have an associated Peutz-Jeghers syndrome.

Leydig (hilus) cell tumors. Only Leydig cells are present in this tumor and when these are located exclusively in the hilus, the term hilus cell tumor is applied. This tumor occurs at a mean age of 50 years and almost always behaves in a benign fashion. Testosterone is commonly produced, resulting in mild virilization that develops over a protracted period of time. Grossly these tumors are usually small and reddish brown. Histologically, abundant eosinophilic cytoplasm and little intracellular lipid are seen. The presence of Reinke crystals differentiates this lesion from lipid cell tumors. Testosterone is produced by a majority of these tumors with the associated features of virilization.

Lipid (lipoid) cell tumors. The presence of rounded Leydig-like cells, luteinized stroma, adrenocortical cells, and the absence of Reinke crystals, points to the diagnosis of a lipid cell tumor. These tumors are typically virilizing, with increased levels of serum testosterone and androstenedione. Occasionally other hormones are produced such as estradiol, estrone, and cortisol. Cushing's syndrome is found in approximately 10% of cases, clinically evident as obesity, hypertension, and glucose intolerance.[35,54] In contrast to Leydig cell tumors, 20% of these tumors develop metastases. There is no effective therapy available to treat metastatic disease.

Gynandroblastoma. This diagnosis should be limited to the rare ovarian tumors that contain significant components of both granulosa stromal cell tumors and Sertoli stromal cell tumors (Fig. 9-17).[34] In these cases androgen or estrogen production may be present and the behavior of the tumor is dependent on the individual components.

Evaluation and management of sex cord stromal tumors. The preoperative evaluation of a pelvic mass suspected of being a sex cord stromal tumor is similar to that of any type of ovarian mass. There are two notable exceptions. Firstly, if there is evidence of excess estrogen production, an endometrial biopsy should be obtained prior to laparotomy. In the event that an endometrial carcinoma is found, consideration must be given to performing a TAH. Secondly, if androgen excess is evident, the differential diagnosis includes an adrenal tumor and an ovarian tumor. This is particularly important when there is no ovarian enlargement. Generally, an elevated serum dehydroxyepiandrostenedione (DHEAS) level points to an adrenal source, while an elevated serum testosterone level most likely represents an ovarian process. Radiographic evaluation of the adrenals and the ovaries is appropriate.

The operative management of patients with sex cord stromal tumors is age dependent. For women beyond the reproductive age, TAH/BSO is appropriate. In a younger woman, interested in preserving child bearing potential, a unilateral oophorectomy should be performed. A frozen section analysis should be conducted in either case. If the pathologist is confident of the diagnosis of a sex cord stromal tumor, peritoneal washings, selective biopsies, subtotal omentectomy, exploration for both intraabdominal and retroperitoneal metastases, and careful inspection of the opposite ovary are indicated. In some cases a germ cell tumor cannot be ruled out on frozen section analysis and a retroperitoneal lymphadenectomy should be performed.

The data available on treating patients with advanced or recurrent stromal tumors are limited because of their rarity, multihistologic patterns, and indolent behavior. Even less information is available regarding which patients should receive adjuvant therapy. Gershenson et al reported on the treatment of patients with metastatic stromal tumors using cisplatin, doxorubicin, and cyclophosphamide; there was only a 63% overall response rate.[79] Other combination chemotherapy regimens have been used, with a small number of complete responses in each group.[38] In several small series, pelvic radiation has been found helpful in patients with localized sex cord stromal tumors. Larger prospective studies are needed to fully assess antitumor activity of chemotherapy against this group of tumors.

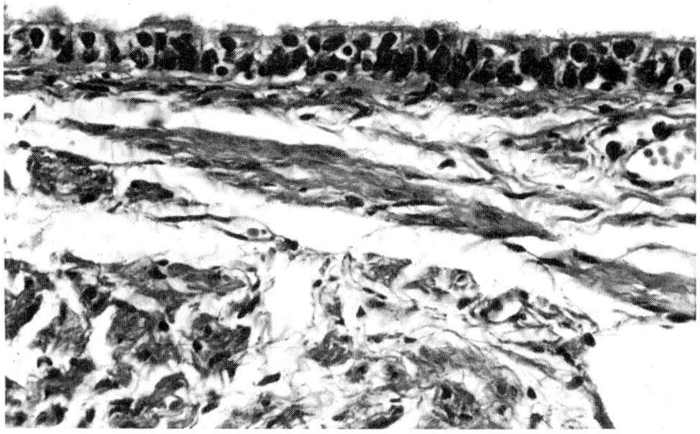

Fig. 9-18. At high magnification, this serous cystadenoma is lined with ciliated, tubal-type epithelium.

While estradiol levels have been a useful tumor marker in many cases of granulosa stromal cell tumors, testosterone levels have been of benefit in some patients with Sertoli stromal cell tumors. In a recent study, inhibin was reported to be a useful tumor marker in patients with granulosa cell tumors.[123]

Epithelial ovarian neoplasia. Almost 85% of all ovarian malignancies are derived from ovarian epithelium, making epithelial malignancies the most commonly encountered ovarian cancer. Each histologic subtype can in most cases be classified as benign, borderline, or malignant.[167] Before discussing the clinical features and management, the histologic subtypes will be detailed.

Issues specific to histologic type

Serous. Benign serous tumors are usually loculated with a single layer of flattened or cuboidal epithelium (Fig. 9-18). Papillations can be present on the external and internal surfaces making it difficult, from a gross perspective, to distinguish this benign tumor from a malignant neoplasm. Mitoses are absent.

Borderline serous tumors account for 10% to 15% of all serous neoplasms. The histologic features that distinguish serous tumors of low malignant potential include a papillary cystic pattern, stratification, tufting, increased mitotic figures, and cytologic atypia (Fig. 9-19). This tumor occurs bilaterally in approximately 15% of cases.

Malignant serous tumors of the ovary are the most common malignant ovarian tumor and account for more than 40% of all invasive epithelial carcinomas. As with borderline tumors, these tumors are commonly bilateral. On gross appearance these are cystic multiloculated tumors with soft friable papillae (Fig. 9-20). On microscopic appearance these tumors are graded as noted above, with significant stromal invasion. Psammoma bodies (calcifications) are present in 32.5% of cases.

Approximately 9% of tumors classified as serous ovarian carcinoma are actually papillary serous carcinoma of the peritoneum. In this situation the ovaries are many times normal-sized or slightly enlarged, with extensive intraabdominal disease. Histologically these tumors resemble malignant serous tumors of the ovary (Fig. 9-21), but only the surface of the ovaries is involved (usually bilateral). Treatment and prognosis are the same as for serous ovarian carcinoma.

Mucinous. Benign mucinous tumors appear with a single layer of tall columnar epithelial cells with clear mucinous-containing cytoplasm (Fig. 9-22). They tend to be larger than serous tumors and are usually smooth-surfaced.

Mucinous tumors of low-malignant potential, or borderline tumors, are distinguished by a complex pattern, 2- to 3-cell layer stratification, cytologic atypia, and the presence of mitotic figures (Fig. 9-23).[96] If there is greater than a 3-cell layer stratification or significant stromal invasion, the diagnosis of carcinoma should be considered. Rice et al studied 80 patients with borderline ovarian tumors; none of the patients had a mucinous borderline tumor greater than stage I disease, and none of the patients in this group recurred.[158]

A

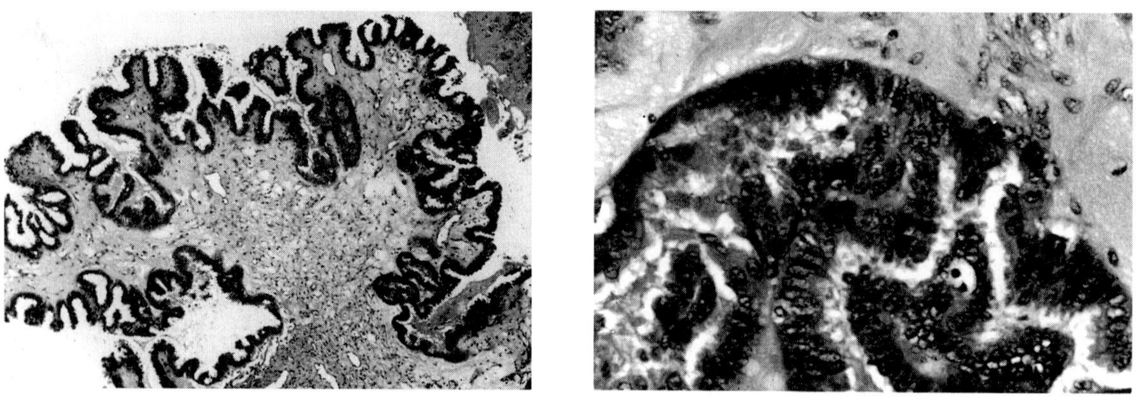

B

Fig. 9-19. A, Serous borderline tumor with papillary fronds lined by mildly atypical serous-type epithelium. There is no stromal invasion. **B,** Borderline serous tumor lined with tubular-type epithelium showing nuclear pseudostratification and moderate nuclear pleomorphism, without invasion of the underlying stroma.

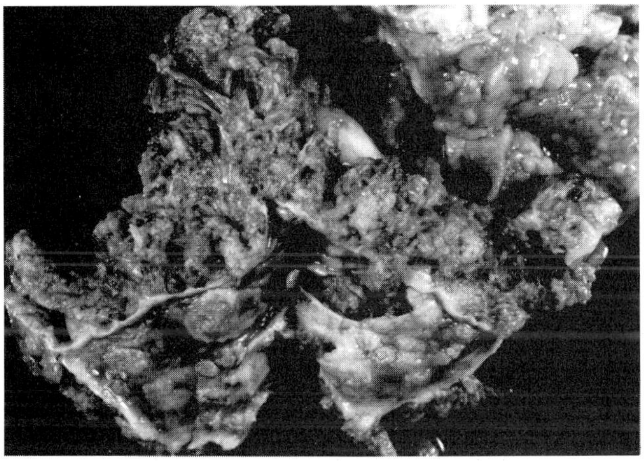

Fig. 9-20. Serous papillary adenocarcinoma produces a cauliflower-like exophytic mass which predominantly involves the surface of the bisected ovary.

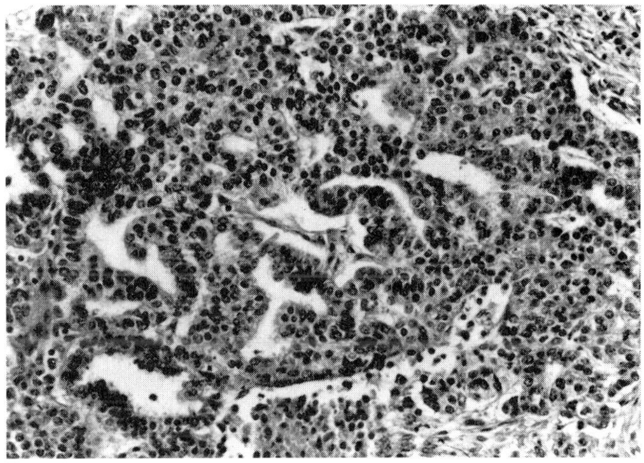

Fig. 9-21. Omental biopsy consisting of moderately differentiated serous papillary carcinoma. The ovaries contained only microscopic foci of similar neoplasia. This patient had serous papillary carcinoma of the peritoneum.

It is reasonable to remove the appendix when a mucinous tumor of the ovary is diagnosed. Several articles have noted an association between appendiceal mucinous neoplasms and mucinous neoplasms of the ovary.[223]

Pseudomyxoma peritonei, defined as the presence of mucinous ascites in association with peritoneal implants (Fig. 9-24), is associated with both appendiceal mucinous neoplasms and mucinous ovarian neoplasms, almost all of which are borderline tumors. The natural history of this clinical syndrome is characterized by repeated recurrences, sometimes necessitating laparotomy or peritoneal lavage for removal of the gelatinous material.[138,154] Casey et al found that positive cytology associated with pseudomyxoma peritonei carried a worse prognosis than negative cytology.[32] Pseudomyxoma peritonei in any clinical setting worsens the prognosis.[126]

Mucinous carcinomas are diagnosed with stage I disease in approximately 50% of cases. This contrasts with serous tumors where the vast majority of patients have advanced stage disease at the time of diagnosis. On gross appearance, mucinous adenocarcinomas are cystic, multiloculated tumors that can reach 50 cm in diameter. The differential diagnosis should always include a gastrointestinal malignancy that has metastasized to the ovary. The histologic features of mucinous ovarian adenocarcinomas are presented in Fig. 9-25. Mucinous tumors of the ovary, compared to other epithelial types, have the greatest heterogeneity in terms of degree of differentiation. Because of this, ample sampling must always be undertaken by the pathologist.

Endometrioid. A benign endometrioid cyst of the ovary is extremely rare. The most common benign endometrial

A

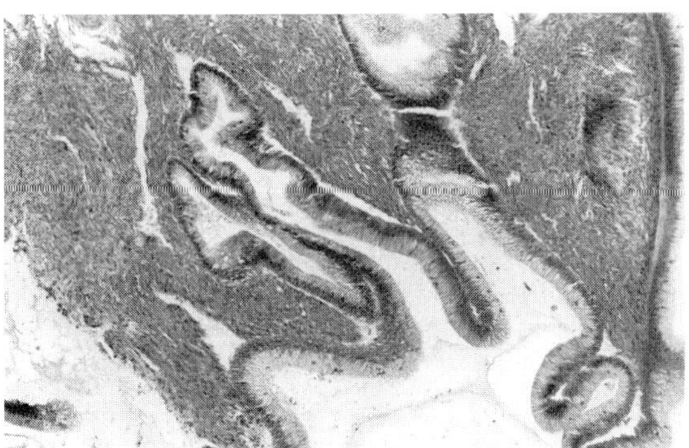

B

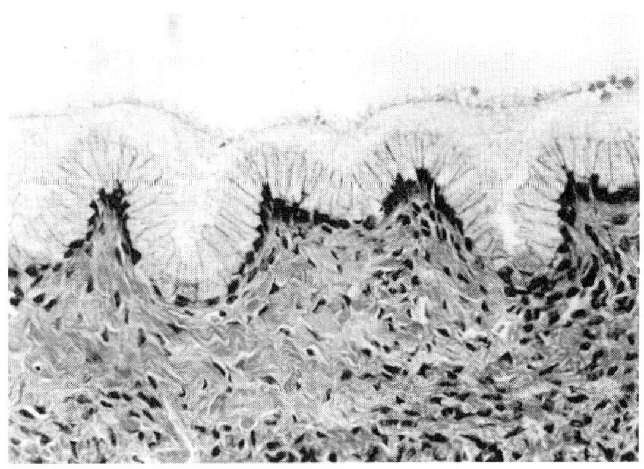

Fig. 9-22. A, Columnar cells with mucin-filled cytoplasm and partially stratified nuclei line this mucinous cystadenoma. **B,** At high magnification, this mucinous cystadenoma is lined with uniform, tall, columnar cells resembling normal endocervical epithelium.

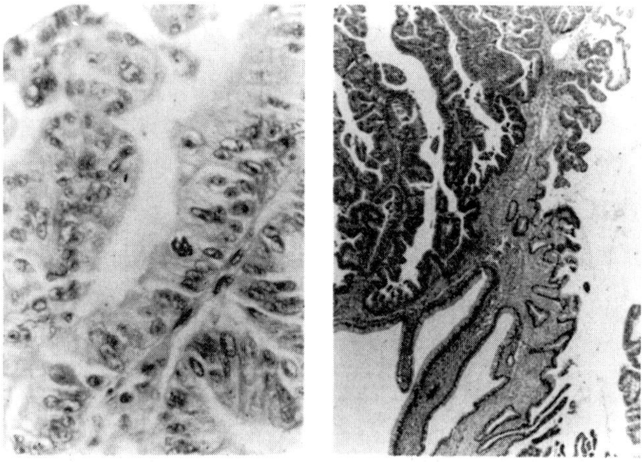

Fig. 9-23. On the left is a low-powered photomicrograph of a borderline mucinous tumor, arising in association with a benign mucinous cystadenoma. A high-powered photomicrography on the right demonstrates stratification, nuclear atypia and mitotic activity.

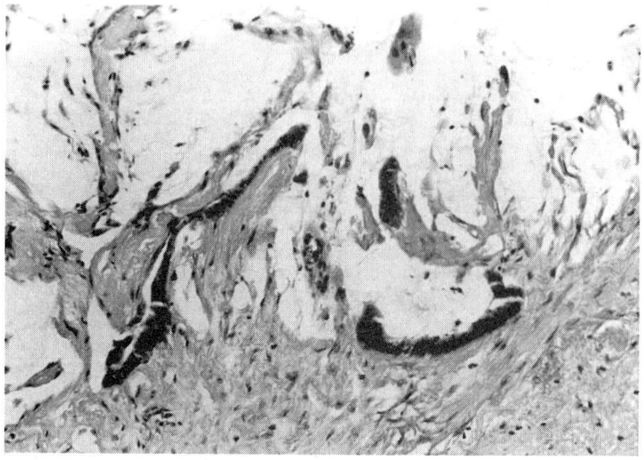

Fig. 9-24. Pseudomyxoma peritonei consisting of a large, acellular mucin pool with rare foci of lining epithelium. The latter manifests minimal nuclear atypia.

tumor of the ovary is the adenofibroma, or cystadenofibroma. This tends to occur in an older age group and can show evidence of epithelial atypia.[111]

Endometrioid borderline tumors of the ovary are rarely reported, but endometrioid carcinoma of the ovary accounts for approximately 10% to 15% of all common epithelial ovarian malignancies.[16,47] In approximately 20% of cases there is a concurrent endometrial carcinoma. Endometriosis is considered a risk factor for this epithelial type.[97] These tumors are usually unilateral and the microscopic appearance is very similar to that of endometrial carcinoma.

Clear cell. Benign or borderline clear cell tumors of the ovary are extremely unusual and are almost always cystadenofibromas. Bell and Scully reviewed 18 patients with adenofibromas; 3 had a benign clear cell adenofibroma component and 12 had clear cell adenofibroma of borderline malignancy.[17] Endometriosis was identified in 7 women in this study. This supported the premise that endometriosis is associated with clear cell tumors of the ovary. The follow-up from this study revealed that the prognosis for patients with this tumor was good and that none of the patients with a benign tumor recurred or died of this disease.

Approximately 5% of ovarian epithelium malignancies are of the clear cell type.[46] As noted above, there is an association with endometriosis which has been reported in more than 25% of cases. Grossly these are large cystic tumors and are bilateral in a small but significant percentage of cases. Microscopically the most common patterns include the tubular glandular, papillary, and cystic types (Fig. 9-26). The so-called hobnail cells are present in a significant number of cases, but not all. Jenison et al reported on 44 patients with clear cell adenocarcinoma of the ovary.[108]

A

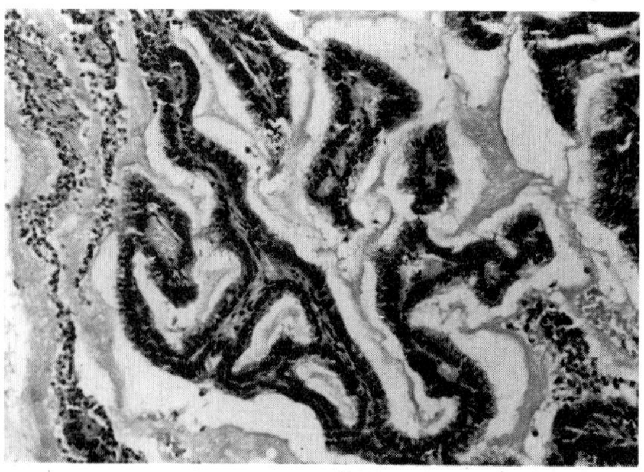

B

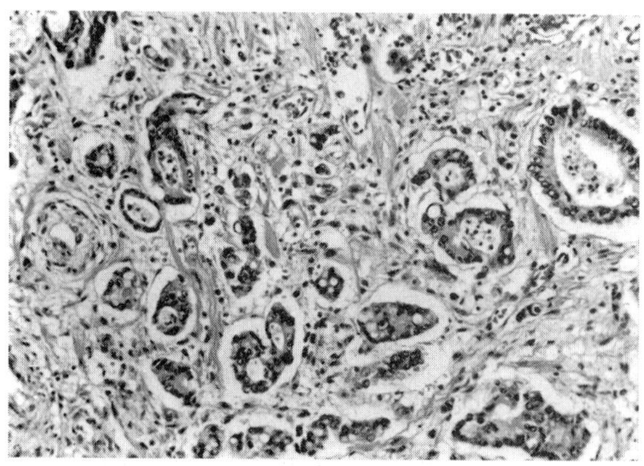

Fig. 9-25. A, Well-differentiated mucinous adenocarcinoma consisting of papillae lined with mucin-secreting cells. **B,** Mucinous adenocarcinoma consisting of well-formed glands resembling those of colonic adenocarcinoma, as well as single malignant cells invading the desmoplastic stroma.

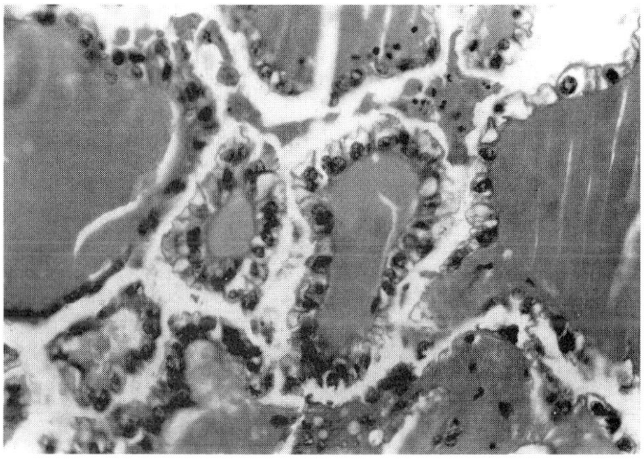

Fig. 9-26. Clear cell carcinoma forms papillae with hyalinized centers, lined with cuboidal cells with prominent clear cytoplasm.

Fifty percent of these patients presented with stage I disease. When compared stage for stage with serous tumors, clear cell tumors were uniformly associated with poorer 5-year survival rates. The authors concluded that ovarian clear cell adenocarcinoma has a distinctly different clinical behavior compared with serous carcinoma and should be regarded as an aggressive epithelial histologic type.

Brenner tumor. Although the cell of origin of Brenner tumors was debated for years, it is now well accepted that these neoplasms are derived from ovarian epithelium that undergoes metaplasia to assume the appearance of urothelial-like epithelium. This rare tumor is bilateral in only a small percentage of cases and tends to occur most commonly in premenopausal women. Grossly it is 2 to 8 cm, solid, and has a white, whirled surface. These tumors are associated with mucinous ovarian tumors in 33% of cases.

Histologically the cells resemble "coffee beans" with a pronounced longitudinal groove in the nucleus (Fig. 9-27, A). The cells form tight nests surrounded by bundles of tightly packed stroma (Fig. 9-27, B). While Brenner tumors were once considered to be benign, studies in the last several decades have established the existence of proliferative and malignant Brenner tumors.[89,168] Woodruff et al reviewed 47 such cases and established their occurrence in an older age group.[216] Other studies have shown that approximately 30% of patients have advanced stage disease at diagnosis and 60% die within 3 years.[6]

Transitional cell carcinoma. The absence of a benign Brenner component separates transitional cell carcinoma (TCC) from a malignant Brenner tumor. They both have a similar-appearing malignant epithelial component that is usually transitional, squamous, or undifferentiated. Malignant Brenner tumors carry a more favorable prognosis than TCC. Silva et al demonstrated an estimated 5-year survival rate of 37% after surgery for patients with a focal or predominant TCC pattern.[182] This survival rate is better than that reported for other epithelial ovarian carcinomas (26% to 29%). Positive prognostic factors included stage, minimal residual tumor, negative second-look laparotomy, a majority of TCC in the carcinoma, and metastases with a predominant TCC component.

Small cell carcinoma. Small cell carcinoma of the ovary is a rare, poorly understood, aggressive tumor of young women and is associated with paraneoplastic hypercalcemia in two thirds of cases. The microscopic appearance is that of small, closely-packed epithelial cells with high mitotic activity.[1] Some authors feel that this tumor is more likely to be of germ cell origin than epithelial, primarily because of the age distribution. The prognosis is poor, with 43 of 49 reported cases dying of the disease.

Malignant mixed mesodermal tumors. Malignant mixed mesodermal tumors (MMMT) of the ovary are rare. They

A

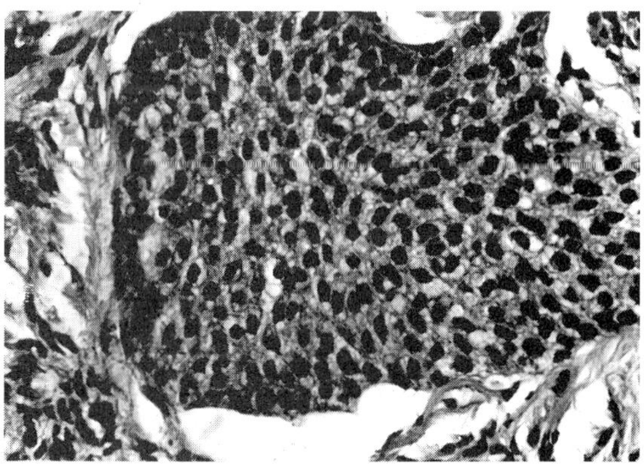

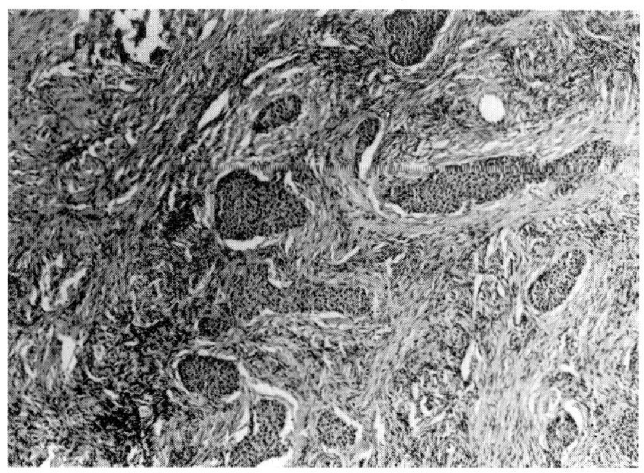

B

Fig. 9-27. A, At high magnification, benign Brenner tumor is composed of sharply demarcated nests of uniform, transitional cell-like epithelium, with a typical "coffee-bean" appearance. **B,** At low magnification, this benign Brenner tumor consists of sharply demarcated epithelial nests in a fibrous stroma.

represent approximately 1% of all ovarian cancers.[53] Grossly these tumors are usually unilateral, cystic, and solid in appearance, with a median diameter of 14 cm. Histologically there are both malignant epithelial and stromal components (Fig. 9-28).

Andersen et al reviewed 10 patients with MMMT of the ovary and confirmed a very poor overall survival, with a median survival of 16 months.[3] A recent study by Barakat et al confirmed the extremely malignant behavior of MMMT and its poor response to chemotherapy.[10] The operative management of this tumor is similar to that for other invasive epithelial ovarian carcinomas. Postoperatively, platinum-based chemotherapy should be given. While patients initially respond to this, a lack of sustained response and a long-term disease-free interval point to the need for investigational studies.

Issues specific to degree of differentiation

Benign epithelial tumors. Benign epithelial ovarian neoplasms are usually uniloculated, smooth lesions that are grossly lobulated. Histologically a single layer of epithelium is present, without stratification, tufting atypia, or invasion of the basement membrane. Conservative surgery with preservation of some ovarian tissue is appropriate in young women. This usually includes an ovarian cystectomy or oophorectomy. In postmenopausal women a TAH/BSO can be considered, to avoid the risk of cancer in the future.

Epithelial ovarian tumors of low malignant potential (borderline tumors). Borderline tumors (BLT) of the ovary were first described in 1929, but it was not until the mid-1970s that they were officially included in the WHO and Federation International of Gynecology and Obstetrics (FIGO) classification systems. Histologically, borderline tumors of the ovary are defined as epithelial tumors where there is stratification and increased atypia but the basement membrane is intact.[5] However, a small subset of patients will have microscopic invasion, defined as small nests of cells just below the basement membrane (Fig. 9-29). Bell and Scully, and Tavassoli, in two separate studies, evaluated this group of patients and established no adverse impact on recurrence or survival when this histologic feature was found.[18,198]

The prognosis for patients with borderline ovarian tumor is much better than for patients with invasive epithelial ovarian carcinoma.[5] This is partly because of the fact that only 20% to 25% of patients with BLT will have extraovarian disease at the time of diagnosis. In addition, patients who have BLT with extraovarian disease have improved survival compared with patients with epithelial ovarian carcinoma. The overall recurrence and death rate is 25%, with recurrence up to 20 years after initial diagnosis. The type of extraovarian implant, whether endosalpingosis, noninvasive, or invasive, is felt by many authors to be important in terms of prognosis. Bell et al found that invasive implants were associated with poorer survival.[19] In contrast, Gershenson and Silva found that survival was unaffected by the type of extraovarian implant.[72]

Borderline tumors of the ovary occur at a mean age of 39 years, compared with 52 years for patients with invasive ovarian carcinoma.[158] Maintenance of future child-bearing potential is an issue. Conservative surgery, with preservation of some ovarian tissue, is appropriate in many cases. In this situation, frozen section analysis is extremely important to rule out the possibility of an invasive carcinoma. If there is any question about the diagnosis, ovarian tissue should be preserved. A second operation might be necessary, if invasive carcinoma is found on final pathology. In women who have completed their child bearing, a TAH/BSO/Omentectomy is appropriate. Surgical staging with retroperitoneal lymphadenectomy and omentectomy should be undertaken, if invasive carcinoma cannot be ruled out on frozen section analysis or in an investigational setting.[219]

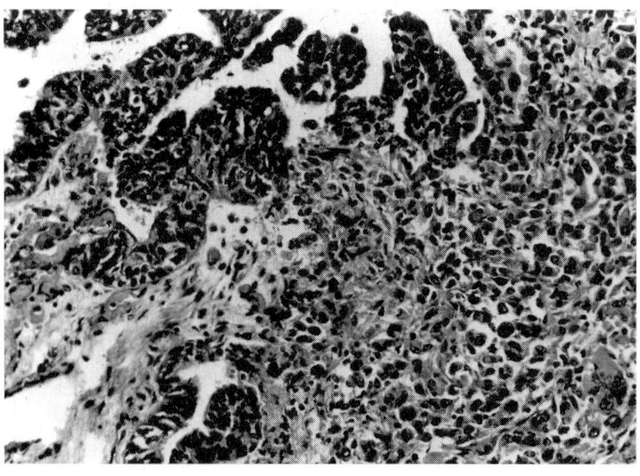

Fig. 9-28. Malignant mixed mesodermal tumor with a malignant papillary epithelial component and an anaplastic stromal component.

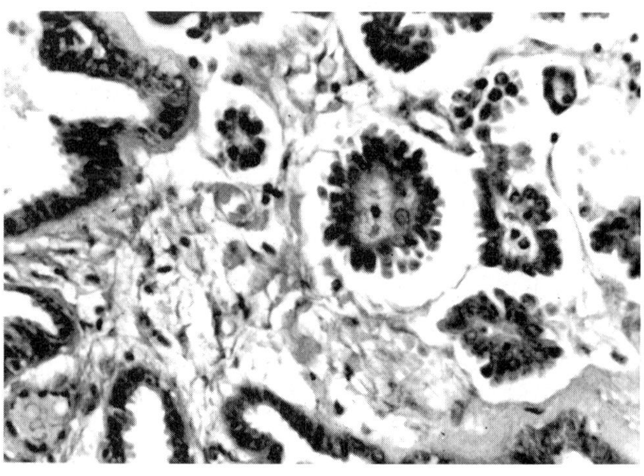

Fig. 9-29. Microscopic stromal invasion is evident here, with nests of cells just below the basement membrane.

CA-125 is a useful tumor marker in patients with serous borderline ovarian tumors of advanced stage. Rice et al found that 75% of patients with stage I serous tumors had a normal preoperative CA-125 level, while 92% of patients with stage II, III, or IV disease had an elevated level ($p < 0.001$).[159]

Postoperative chemotherapy in an adjuvant or curative setting in patients with borderline tumors of the ovary is controversial. There are no prospective controlled studies establishing its efficacy.

Malignant. The gross intraoperative features suggesting an invasive epithelial ovarian carcinoma at the time of laparotomy are presented in Table 9-4. The histologic appearance of a malignant epithelial ovarian carcinoma includes increased mitotic activity, compromise of the basement membrane, and architectural dedifferentiation. These tumors are graded as well differentiated, moderately differentiated, or poorly differentiated, and grade I, II, or III respectively. This grading system is based primarily on the architectural pattern and not on nuclear characteristics. In a large retrospective review of over 500 cases of ovarian carcinoma, Sorbe et al found that histologic grade was the most important prognostic indicator, followed by stage and histologic subtype.[186] Fig. 9-30 shows the influence of histologic grade on survival, in patients with stage IIIB serous carcinoma of the ovary.

STAGE. Invasive epithelial ovarian carcinoma can spread by local extension, lymphatic invasion, intraperitoneal implantation, hematogenous dissemination, and transdiaphragmatic passage, all of which have implications for staging. Ovarian carcinoma has a surgical-pathologic staging system (Table 9-5). Approximately 75% of patients with invasive epithelial ovarian carcinoma will have greater than stage I disease. Stage is a strong predictor of survival (Table 9-6).

Meticulous surgical staging is imperative in patients who have what appears to be an early stage epithelial ovarian carcinoma. Young et al found that 13% of patients referred for treatment of apparent stage I or II ovarian cancer had more advanced disease on further evaluation.[220] In all cases this included a methodical exploration of the entire peritoneal cavity, pelvic and paraaortic lymph node sampling, peritoneal cytology, subtotal omentectomy, and appendectomy, if a mucinous tumor was present.[93,223]

CYTOREDUCTIVE SURGERY. The definition of cytoreductive surgery is the removal of as much of the tumor and its metastases as possible. It includes a TAH, BSO, and complete omentectomy with resection of any metastatic lesions. In some cases a bowel resection and retroperitoneal lymphadenopathy are necessary in order to obtain optimum cytoreduction.[185] Optimum cytoreduction is achieved when the largest residual tumor mass measures less than 1.5 cm. Hacker et al reviewed 47 patients with stage III or IV invasive epithelial ovarian carcinoma who underwent cytoreductive surgery.[88] They found the median survival for the suboptimal group was 6 months, compared with 18 months for patients whose largest residual disease was 0.5 to 1.5 cm and 40 months if residual nodules were less than 0.5 cm ($p < 0.001$). While debulking has been shown to improve survival, Hunter et al raised the question of selection bias.[105] Patients who can be adequately debulked may represent a group that is more sensitive to chemotherapy.

Goodman et al recently reported no survival benefit to patients with stage IV disease who underwent cytoreductive surgery, either initially or on an interval basis, after several courses of chemotherapy.[83]

Table 9-4. Intraoperative findings consistent with an invasive ovarian malignancy

Bilateral
Adherent to adjacent organs
Surface excrescences
Ruptured capsule
Ascites
Peritoneal implants
Hemorrhage and necrosis
Solid areas
Intracystic papillations

Obviously malignant serous carcinoma of the ovary, stage IIIB: 1982-1986. Life table presentation by histologic grade.

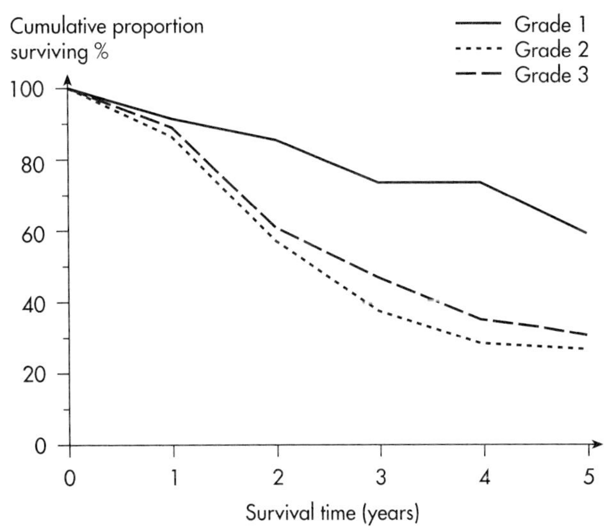

Fig. 9-30. Actuarial survival by year after treatment and by histologic grade for stage IIIB cases. (From Pettersson F, editor: *Annual report of the results of treatment in gynecologic cancer,* vol 36 [suppl], Stockholm, 1990, FIGO.

Table 9-5. Ovarian carcinoma: stage

Stage I	Growth limited to the ovaries
Stage IA	Growth limited to one ovary; no ascites No tumor on the external surface; capsule intact
Stage IB	Growth limited to both ovaries; no ascites No tumor on the external surfaces; capsules intact
Stage IC*	Tumor either stage IA or IB, but with tumor on surface of one or both ovaries; or with capsule ruptured; or with ascites present containing malignant cells; or with positive peritoneal washings
Stage II	Growth involving one or both ovaries with pelvic extension
Stage IIA	Extension and/or metastases to the uterus and/or tubes
Stage IIB	Extension to other pelvis tissues
Stage IIC*	Tumor either IIA or IIB, but with tumor on surface of one or both ovaries; or with capsule(s) ruptured; or with ascites present containing malignant cells; or with positive peritoneal washings
Stage III	Tumor involving one or both ovaries with peritoneal implants outside the pelvis and/or positive retroperitoneal or inguinal nodes; superficial liver metastasis equals stage III; tumor is limited to the true pelvis but with histologically proven malignant extension to small bowel or omentum
Stage IIIA	Tumor grossly limited to the true pelvis with negative nodes but with histologically confirmed microscopic seeding of abdominal peritoneal surfaces
Stage IIIB	Tumor involving one or both ovaries with histologically confined implants of abdominal peritoneal surfaces, none exceeding 2 cm in diameter; nodes are negative
Stage IIIC	Abdominal implants greater than 2 cm in diameter and/or positive retroperitoneal or inguinal nodes
Stage IV	Growth involving one or both ovaries with distant metastases; if pleural effusion is present, there must be positive cytology to allot a case to stage IV

*In order to evaluate the impact prognosis of the different criteria for alloting a case to stage IC or IIC, it would be of value to know (1) if the source of malignant cell detected was (a) peritoneal washings or (b) ascites, or (2) if the rupture of the capsule was (a) spontaneous or (b) caused by the surgeon.

POSTOPERATIVE THERAPY. The postoperative treatment options for patients who have residual disease or are at high risk to recur, include radiation therapy or combination chemotherapy. Young et al identified a small subset of patients who do not benefit from postoperative adjuvant therapy.[221] This group includes patients with stage IA or IB tumors that are either grade 1 or 2. The 5-year disease-free interval is 91% to 98% with or without postoperative therapy. Patients with stage I, grade 3 tumors; all stage IC; and all stage II are at an unacceptable risk of having a recurrence and should receive postoperative adjuvant therapy.

RADIATION THERAPY. The role of radiotherapy in the management of epithelial ovarian cancer is still unclear. In the Princess Margaret Hospital series whole abdomen and pelvic irradiation was as effective as chemotherapy in curing

Table 9-6. Five-year actuarial survival rates for epithelial ovarian cancer (1982 to 1986)*

Stage	
IA	82.3%
IB	74.9%
IC	67.7%
IIA	60.6%
IIB&C	53.8%
III	22.7%
IV	8.0%

From Pettersson F, editor: *Annual report of the results of treatment in gynecologic cancer*, vol 21, Stockholm, 1990, FIGO.
* Based on 10,912 cases

previously untreated patients with minimal residual disease.[49,50] The radiation field extended 1 to 2 cm above the level of the diaphragm and included the entire pelvis. The use of second-line radiotherapy, after initial chemotherapy, has not increased the progression-free interval or cure, and has been shown to have significant increased toxicity.[118]

CHEMOTHERAPY. Platinum-based combination chemotherapy is now the standard postoperative treatment for patients at high risk of having a recurrence (stage I, grade 3; all stage IC; and all stage II) or of having residual disease (stage III or IV).[127,156,204,205] Prior to the development of platinum analogs, oral melphalan was used, which induced a response in approximately 30% of patients with advanced disease. An improved response rate of 60% occurs when platinum-based chemotherapy is used, and the median survival is prolonged by approximately 6 months.[204] While cyclophosphamide, doxorubicin, and cisplatin was the preferred regimen for several years, Omura et al in a randomized study, showed that there was no benefit to the inclusion of doxorubicin.[151] Because of the serious toxicity associated with cisplatin, namely gastrointestinal effects, neurotoxicity, and nephrotoxicity, other platinum analogs have been developed. Carboplatinum is one such analogue, with a very different spectrum of toxicity and an administration protocol that is much less complicated.[213] Swenerton et al showed that carboplatinum-cyclosphosphamide and cisplatin-cyclophosphamide are equally effective; much more toxicity is associated with the latter regimen.[194] Hakes et al showed no survival benefit to administering greater than 6 cycles of chemotherapy after cytoreduction.[91]

Efforts to improve the survival rate in patients with advanced ovarian cancer have been directed at dose intensification of platinum analogs and the development of new chemotherapeutic agents.[90,115,193] Kaye et al found significantly improved survival rates in patients treated with cisplatin 100 mg/m^2, compared with those who received 50 mg/m^2.[113] No other authors have found the same convincing results. Further investigation is needed to establish the effectiveness of dose intensification. Taxol is a new agent, whose mechanism of action involves altering the microtubule apparatus and rendering it dysfunctional.[166] In a recent Gynecologic Oncology Group study, the overall response rate of taxol-cisplatin was significantly higher than cyclophosphamide-cisplatin (79% versus 63%; < 0.01) in patients with advanced stage ovarian cancer.[141] Interestingly the rate of complete pathologic response was no different. Further investigation of this agent will be necessary to establish fully its superiority in treating this group of patients.

INTRAPERITONEAL THERAPY. Intraperitoneal chromic phosphate is presently being investigated by the Gynecologic Oncology Group for treatment of patients with no residual disease but at high risk of recurrence. Intraperitoneal cisplatin has been shown to induce a response rate of 20% to 30% in patients with small-volume residual disease who have previously responded to systemic platinum therapy.[103] Bulky tumor masses cannot be expected to respond to this type of administration because of its lack of penetration to greater than 2 to 3 mm. Patients with significant adhesions will not respond well either, because of the poor distribution. Data collection in a prospective randomized fashion is needed to fully elucidate the role of intraperitoneal therapy in the management of patients with ovarian carcinoma.

SECOND-LOOK PROCEDURE. Second-look surgery is undertaken after the completion of chemotherapy to determine whether the patient has had a complete response and is pathologically free of disease. The most important reason for performing second-look laparotomy after chemotherapy is to identify patients with persistent disease. This provides patients with the opportunity to prolong survival by continuing treatment.[39] There are three important consideration. First, a relapse rate of at least 25% can be expected in patients who have a negative second-look surgery.[75] Second, there are limited salvage therapies available after establishing that residual disease is present.[129] A final important issue is the potential benefit of secondary debulking that resects residual disease present at the time of second-look surgery. There are several small studies available, showing a possible survival advantage to those patients left with microscopic disease. But clearly, gross residual disease connotes poor survival and does not justify a second debulking operation.[22,101] Second-look laparotomy with secondary cytoreduction for the evaluation of experimental adjuvant or salvage therapies may be appropriate in a formal investigation setting.

TUMOR MARKER CA-125. The role of the tumor marker CA-125 in the preoperative evaluation of a woman with a pelvic mass is discussed under the evaluation and management of the adnexal pelvic mass. The CA-125 antigen is elevated in 80% of patients with advanced ovarian carcinoma and in some patients with early stage epithelial ovarian cancer.[15,137] However it is not specific for ovarian cancer. Elevated levels have been found in a variety of benign conditions such as endometriosis, leiomyoma, pregnancy, pelvic inflammatory disease, and several other malignancies.[92,136,153] Lavin et al and Niloff et al demonstrated the utility of serial serum CA-125 assays in the follow-up of patients with confirmed ovarian carcinoma.[124,148] The CA-125 level was elevated before clinical recurrence in 94% of patients, with a median lead time of 3 months.[148]

Metastatic malignancy. Ovarian involvement from extragenital cancer is common.[144,214,215] Approximately 5% of ovarian malignancies are metastases from another site. Yazigi and Sandstad, found the most frequent primary sites to be colon (52%), breast (17%), stomach (10%), and pancreas (10%).[218] The classic Krukenberg tumor is one that metastasizes from the stomach and has the pathognomonic "signet-ring cells" (Fig. 9-31). A careful review of symptoms, a physical examination, and appropriate radiographic studies can assist the clinician in making a diagnosis of the primary tumor, prior to exploring the patient for an ovarian mass. For example, if a patient complains of a change in bowel habits and has an ovarian mass, a barium enema or colonoscopy should be performed prior to laparotomy. Removing the primary colon cancer might be important at the time of exploratory laparotomy. Poor survival in patients with ovarian metastases has proven to be the case in most circumstances.

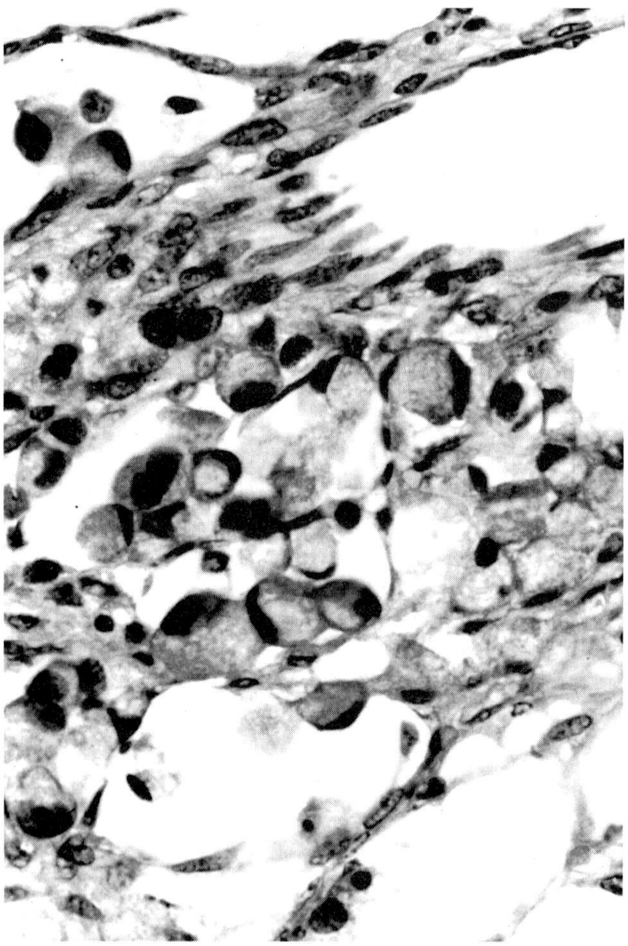

Fig. 9-31. Metastatic mucinous carcinoma (Krukenberg tumor) containing well-formed signet-ring cells with nuclei displaced by cytoplasmic mucin.

Other. This category includes a miscellaneous group of ovarian lesions that comprise less than 5% of the total number of neoplasms.

Nonneoplastic tumorlike conditions

Pregnancy luteoma. This nonneoplastic condition of the ovary must be kept in mind when a solid ovarian tumor develops during pregnancy.[69] Several authors have established that this represents an exaggeration of the luteinization reaction of the ovary. Maternal virilization can occur. Grossly these tumors average 6 cm in diameter and are bilateral in 30% of cases. Microscopically, large luteinized cells in nodules are obvious. Most spontaneously regress postpartum.

Ovarian hyperthecosis. Ovarian hyperthecosis is defined as a nonneoplastic proliferation of ovarian stromal cells that exhibit focal luteinization. Virilization is commonly seen secondary to increased production of ovarian-derived testosterone and androstenedione. Estrogenic manifestations can be present, but much less frequently. Grossly these tumors are white homogenous lesions that are solid on sectioning and usually bilateral. Microscopically there are varying degrees of nodular or diffuse cortical and medullary proliferation of ovarian stromal cells. Normal gonadotropin levels differentiate this lesion from the POCS.

Ovarian edema. Enlargement of the ovary by ovarian edema is rare. The most probable cause is intermittent torsion of the ovarian vessels. The patients are usually young; symptoms include abdominal and/or pelvic pain, menstrual irregularity, and abdominal swelling. In a significant number of patients, virilization will occur. Pelvic examination reveals a palpable unilateral adnexal mass. Abdominal examination will often reveal peritoneal signs, depending upon the degree of torsion. On sectioning, the ovary appears soft and fluctuant with a homogenous gelatinous material present. Histologically, diffuse stromal edema is present. In many cases a unilateral oophorectomy will be necessary because of torsion-induced necrosis of the ovary.

Follicular cyst/corpus luteal cyst. Follicular cysts and corpus luteal cysts represent the two possible etiologies for a solitary functional cyst of the ovary (Fig. 9-32). Follicular cysts (FC) are common during the reproductive years and are probably related to abnormalities in the release of anterior pituitary gonadotropins. Corpus luteal cysts (CLC), which also occur during the reproductive years, result from ovulation. These patients usually present with a palpable adnexal mass, almost always less than 8 cm, with signs of increased estrogen production. Menstrual irregularities are common. On occasion, FC and CLC can present with cyst rupture and intraabdominal hemorrhage. Microscopically, both FC and CLC have a theca and a granulosa cell layer. While most cases of solitary cysts resolve spontaneously, OCs can be used to hasten the process.

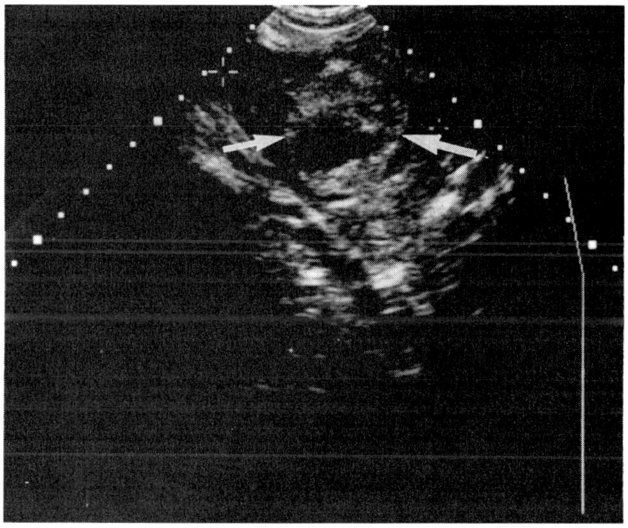

Fig. 9-32. Ultrasound image shows hypoechoic lesion with hypoechoic center *(arrows)* representing a ruptured functional cyst.

Polycystic ovary syndrome. PCOS, also known as Stein-Leventhal syndrome, represents a spectrum of presentations resulting from chronic anovulation and polycystic ovaries. Two major endocrine disturbances associated with PCOS include abnormal gonadotropin release and increased androgen production. PCOS typically presents in the third decade of life with the history of premenarchial obesity and postmenarchial amenorrhea, infertility, and increased androgen production. Hyperestrogenism can occur, but less frequently, and is manifested by menometrorrhagia with or without endometrial hyperplasia or endometrial carcinoma. Grossly the ovaries are typically round and 2 to 4 times larger than normal. There is a thickened white cortex with multiple adjacent cysts. Microscopically the superficial cortex is fibrotic and hypocellular, with an increase in the number of atretic follicles; hyperplasia of the hilus cells is common. Treatment is directed at normalizing cyclic pituitary gonadotropin levels and protecting the endometrium against the unopposed estrogen commonly seen in anovulatory women.

Theca-lutein cyst. Bilateral ovarian enlargement, secondary to numerous luteinized follicle cysts, is commonly seen in theca-lutein cysts. The conditions that most commonly cause this disorder result from increased levels of circulating hCG such as multiple gestations, gestational trophoblastic disease, and RH sensitization with fetal hydrops. Typically the patient presents with pain and a palpable adnexal mass. Virilization, secondary to androgen production, occurs in close to 25% of cases unassociated with trophoblastic disease. Both hemoperitoneum, secondary to rupture, and torsion cause acute abdominal pain, necessitating laparotomy. Ascites are common. Grossly these tumors can reach greater than 20 cm and are usually filled with clear fluid. Histologically there is prominent luteinization of the theca internal layer with marked stromal edema. Regression of these cysts is common when serum hCG levels return to normal.

Endometrioma. Endometriosis commonly occurs in the ovary; when cyclic bleeding occurs, an endometriotic cyst or endometrioma is formed. Accumulation of blood within this cavity results in the classic "chocolate cyst." The pain that is typically produced by endometriosis is similarly produced with endometriomas of the ovary. On physical examination, an adnexal mass will often be felt, as well as the typical findings of endometriosis that include uterosacral nodularity and cul-de-sac tenderness. The preoperative evaluation of a patient with an adnexal mass secondary to an endometrioma is the same as for a patient with any type of adnexal mass. The most important principle is to rule out carcinoma, noting the association between ovarian endometriomas and certain types of ovarian malignancies, particularly clear cell carcinoma and endometrioid carcinoma. Serum CA-125 levels are often elevated in endometriosis and thus would not be helpful in discerning a malignancy.

Germinal inclusion cyst. Germinal inclusion cysts of the ovary result from infolding of the surface epithelium following ovulation. There is no evidence to support an etiologic relationship between these germinal inclusions in the common benign and malignant epithelial neoplasms of the ovary. The theory of incessant ovulation promoting an increased risk of ovarian carcinoma substantiates this concern. These inclusions occur at all ages. Microscopically the epithelium is either flat, cuboidal, or columnar.

Simple cyst. By definition, simple cysts have no identifiable epithelial lining. They are probably derived from follicular cysts, germinal inclusion cysts, or cystadenomas. The most likely cause for the absence or flattening of the epithelium is pressure that results from intracystic fluid.

Mesenchymal tumors

Leiomyoma. Only 30 cases of primary ovarian leiomyoma have been reported in the literature.[61] This process probably originates from the smooth muscle in the wall of a blood vessel. Most patients are postmenopausal and asymptomatic. Grossly, leiomyomas are solid and white. Microscopically the typical appearance is that of uniform smooth muscle cells with cigar-shaped nuclei. Leiomyosarcoma and rhabdomyosarcoma, two other mesenchymal tumors of muscle origin, are extremely rare.

Hemangioma. This tumor of vascular origin is also rare, with the number of well-documented cases reaching 40.[56] Usually this tumor is asymptomatic but occasionally can be quite large. Grossly there are red-purple nodules with a spongy appearance. Histologically it consists of a collection of vascular spaces. Other vascular tumors of the ovary include hemangiosarcoma, lymphangioma, and lymphangiosarcoma.

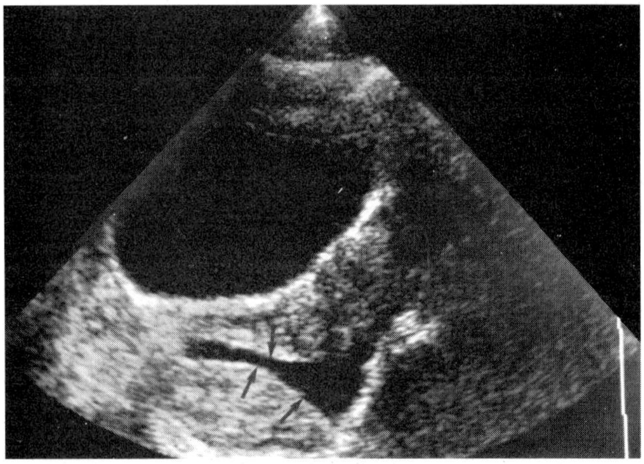

Fig. 9-33. Transverse image shows hypoechoic fluid in Douglas' pouch *(arrowheads).*

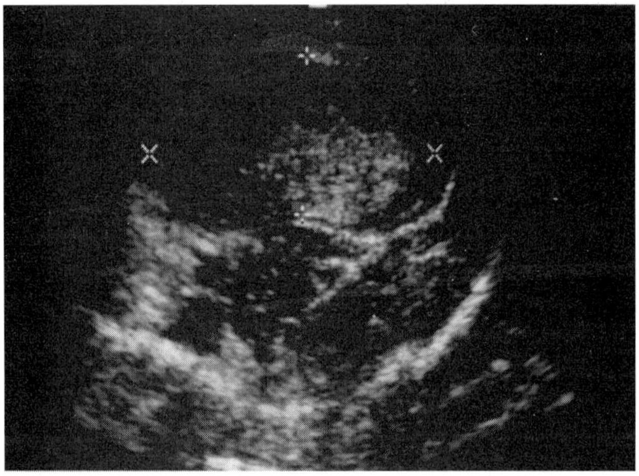

Fig. 9-34. Transverse ultrasound image shows a large mass in the adnexa with mixed echogenicity. These internal echos show that it is definitely not a simple cyst. This was a hemorrhagic functional cyst.

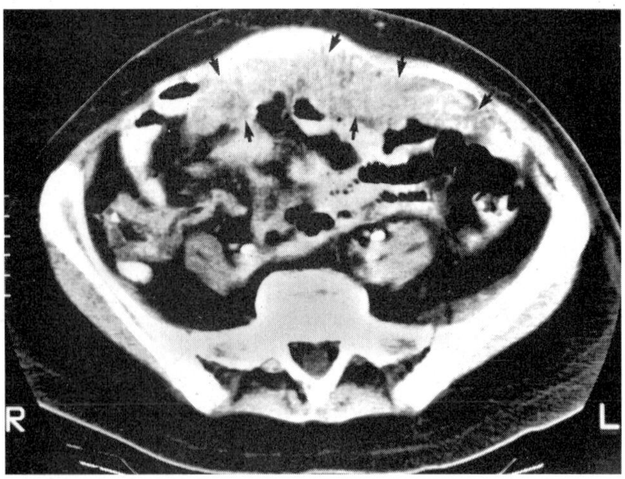

Fig. 9-35. CT scan of the abdomen demonstrates soft tissue density just deep to the abdominal wall. This represents omental cake *(arrows)* from ovarian cancer.

Lymphoma. Primary extranodal malignant lymphoma of the ovary is rare. This diagnosis can only be made if the tumor is confined to the ovary at the time of diagnosis.[36] Lymph node, blood, and bone marrow involvement must be excluded. This is more common in premenopausal women, and the most common complaint is abdominal pain and swelling. Bilaterality is common, with the tumors being lobulated and white. Microscopically a diffuse pattern is most common, usually of the poorly-differentiated type. The patient should be stage properly and treated with radiation or chemotherapy.

Evaluation and management of the pelvic-adnexal mass

Preoperative evaluation. The complete differential diagnosis of a pelvic-adnexal mass must be kept in mind when evaluating a woman of any age with this finding. In a recent study, Killackey and Neuwirth reviewed 540 cases of pelvic-adnexal masses.[116] Of these patients, 291 were operatively evaluated for a pelvic mass of unknown etiology; 249 were operatively evaluated for a suspected leiomyoma; and 44 cancers were diagnosed, 10 of which were nongynecologic malignancies. This report emphasizes the importance of a complete differential diagnosis.

As noted previously, the importance of a complete history and physical examination cannot be emphasized enough.

The radiographic evaluation of a patient with a pelvic-adnexal mass must be tailored to the age of the patient and to the results of the history and physical examination. In a 4-year-old female child, a solid pelvic mass must raise the suspicion of a germ cell malignancy, and ultrasonography would be appropriate. A change in bowel habits in a 50-year-old woman necessitates evaluation for colon cancer, which includes a barium examination and colonoscopy. Hematuria and bladder symptoms would warrant an intravenous pyelogram (IVP) with cystoscopy, urine analysis, and urine cytology.

Ultrasonography has assumed a major role in evaluating pelvic masses.[4,20] Fig. 9-33 shows fluid (ascites) in pouch of Douglas, and Fig. 9-34 shows a complex adnexal mass. Herrmann et al prospectively evaluated 404 women with suspected pelvic masses or a history suggesting ovarian cancer, using abdominal ultrasonography.[98] Three hundred and twelve of these patients were operated on and evaluated within 3 weeks after sonography. The positive predictive value of the sonographic evidence of malignancy was 73% (38 of 52 patients), whereas the negative predictive value was 95.6% (117 of 185 patients). In a similar study, Luxman et al looked at 102 postmenopausal women who underwent abdominal ultrasonography evaluation of adnexal masses prior to surgery.[131] The positive predictive value for abdominal ultrasonography in this group of patients was 39% and the negative predictive value was 94%. If a negative sonogram had been relied upon, 6% of malignant ovarian tumors in postmenopausal women might have been missed.

In recent years, transvaginal ultrasonography has improved the ability of ultrasound to discern an ovarian malignancy. Sassone et al correlated transvaginal sonographic pelvic images of 143 patients with the surgical findings and histopathology.[170] The authors devised a scoring system to delineate benign from malignant lesions, showing a specificity of 83%, a sensitivity of 100%, and positive and negative predictive values of 37% and 100% respectively. Several authors have substantiated the superiority of transvaginal (compared with abdominal) ultrasonography in diagnosing ovarian malignancies.

Color Doppler has been investigated as a means of increasing the specificity of transvaginal ultrasonography. This technique quantifies blood flow in the ovarian vessels. Impedance to blood flow in a malignant ovarian tumor is less than that found in a benign fashion tumor. Further investigation is needed to evaluate this technique fully.

A pelvic CT scan is rarely utilized for primary evaluation of the adnexa. There is controversy regarding its ability to visualize normal ovaries. This radiographic study can be useful in evaluating the extent of metastatic disease in patients with known or strongly suspected ovarian carcinoma (Fig. 9-35).

MRI is another diagnostic modality that has recently been used with greater frequency. There are presently no useful prospective studies evaluating its ability to assess adnexal pathology.

Special consideration must be given to the application of all radiographic techniques in diagnosing and following adnexal masses during pregnancy and childhood, specifically addressing the amount of radiation exposure. Ultrasonography and MRI are superior in that there is no radiation exposure.

The age of the patient is extremely important in determining the appropriate laboratory test. Routine preoperative blood tests in all cases should include SMA-20, CBC, platelets, PT, and PTT. Remembering to order the appropriate tumor marker preoperatively is important (Table 9-7). In patients below the age of 20, with a solid adnexal pelvic mass, a malignant germ cell tumor of the ovary must be considered and serum AFP, serum hCG, and LDH should be ordered as potential tumor markers.

CA-125 is a tumor marker that deserves special attention. While CA-125 has been shown to be elevated in many patients with serous epithelial ovarian carcinoma, it is also elevated (> 35 miu/mL) in a variety of benign and other malignant conditions including adenomyosis, endometriosis, pelvic inflammatory disease, fibroids, pregnancy, liver and renal disease, and colon and breast cancer. In these situations the CA-125 level is usually below 200 miu/mL. Vasilev et al evaluated 182 gynecology patients with pelvic masses and obtained preoperative CA-125 levels in all cases.[211] Fourteen of eighteen malignant masses (77.8%) were identified by a serum level in excess of 35 miu/mL. However, only 14 of 51 patients (27.5%) with elevated

Table 9-7. "Tumor markers" useful with ovarian neoplasms

Substance/marker	Ovarian tumor
AFP	Endodermal sinus tumors; embryonal carcinomas; mixed germ cell tumors (rarely immature teratoma and polyembryoma)
CA-125	All epithelial tumors; especially serous (rarely immature teratoma)
Estradiol	Adult granulosa cell tumors; thecomas
hCG	Choriocarcinoma; embryonal carcinoma; mixed germ cell tumors; polyembryoma
LDH	Dysgerminoma; mixed germ cell tumors
Testosterone	Sertoli cell tumors; Leydig (hilus) cell tumors

CA-125 levels had a malignant tumor. The authors found that increasing the positive cut-off levels to 65 miu/mL did not improve the results. The authors concluded that serum CA-125 levels alone do not sufficiently distinguish benign from malignant masses preoperatively. It is important to recognize that if the preoperative CA-125 level is markedly elevated, an ovarian carcinoma is more likely to be present.

Histologic confirmation is necessary to establish the diagnosis when a pelvic-adnexal mass is present and persistent, either by laparoscopy or laparotomy. However, avoiding surgical intervention for the commonly found functional ovarian cysts is important. These functional cysts do not occur in postmenopausal women, since both CLC and FC are caused by ovulation. For premenopausal women with a simple cyst that measures on transvaginal ultrasound less than 6 cm, a 6-week period of oral contraceptive suppression is appropriate. In a study by Spanos, 81 of 286 premenopausal patients treated with OCs for a cystic adnexal mass required laparotomy for persistence.[187] None of these patients had an FC (Table 9-8).

Taking all the above into consideration, Fig. 9-36 provides a framework for evaluating and treating premenopausal patients with an adnexal mass, and Fig. 9-37 does the same for postmenopausal women.

Operative management. A bowel preparation should always be given to women suspected of having a malignancy or dense pelvic adhesion. This lowers the rate of infectious complications if colorectal surgery is necessary. This will also reduce the need for a colostomy if the colon or rectum is entered. An adequate mechanical bowel preparation is polyethylene glycol electrolyte solution: 4 liters, 8 ounces of which should be given every 10 minutes, the morning before surgery. This should be followed by one gram each

Table 9-8. Operative findings with persistent adnexal masses

Surgical exploration	81
Functional cysts	0
Neoplasm	81
Endometrioma	28
Simple serous cyst	18
Cystadenoma	
Serous	8
Pseudomucinous	6
Dermoid	9
Paraovarian cyst	4
Hydrosalpinx	3
Cystadenocarcinoma	
Serous	3
Pseudomucinous	1
Dysgerminoma	1

From Spanos WJ: Preoperative hormonal therapy of cystic adnexal masses, *Am J Obstet Gynecol* 116(4):551, 1973.

of neomycin and erythromycin given orally at 1:00, 2:00, and 11:00 PM the day before surgery.[146] It is also important that the patient have clear liquids for 24 hours prior to surgery.

Laparoscopy. Laparoscopy is the most commonly performed gynecologic surgical procedure. It continues to be important in confirming the presence and establishing the type of various masses. Its present value is not just in diagnosis but also in treating ovarian masses. With the development of new technology, part or all of an ovarian mass can be removed through the laparoscope. Clinical judgment must be exercised; it is not always easy to distinguish a malignant from a benign ovarian tumor. Laparoscopic removal of an ovarian lesion often results in upstaging, if a malignancy is present. Recently Sainz de la Cuesta et al reported that intraoperative rupture of malignant ovarian neoplasms worsened the prognosis for patients with stage I ovarian cancer.[169] Dembo et al, in a similar study, found results that were not consistent with this finding, but the inclusion criteria in this study were somewhat different.[51] Both of these studies lack sufficient numbers to stratify for grade and treatment. Even in premenopausal women the risk of malignancy should be considered, although clearly that risk is reduced. In a recent study by Mecke et al, 773 patients under the age of 45 underwent pelviscopy.[142] Only two patients (0.26%) had ovarian carcinoma and were operated on by pelviscopy before laparotomy. The authors state that sonography was extremely important in determining whether pelviscopy was appropriate. Patients with multilocular cysts measuring greater than 7 cm in diameter with echodense components should not undergo pelviscopy. This is also the case with a cyst measuring greater than 9 cm, regardless of the ultrasound appearance.

Laparotomy. Laparotomy is the procedure of choice in many situations, as outlined in Figs. 9-36 and 9-37. The surgeon should exercise clinical judgment in determining the type of incision to be used. While a vertical midline incision provides the best exposure, a low transverse incision can be used in premenopausal women not eligible for laparoscopic surgery and with an uncomplicated-appearing ovarian cyst. The patient must clearly understand that if a malignancy is found, a second incision would be necessary for appropriate surgical management. The operation should not be limited by the type of incision. As discussed under laparoscopic surgery, upstaging an ovarian carcinoma with rupture of an ovarian cyst has possible consequence. With that in mind, the surgeon should attempt to remove each ovarian cyst intact.

Conservative surgery with the preservation of reproductive function can be performed but depends on the malignant potential of the ovarian tumor present. Frozen-section pathology can be extremely helpful, but patients must be informed that the final pathology report may differ from the one given at the time of surgery. The ovarian neoplasms, where ovarian conservation is both desired and appropriate, include grade I stage IA epithelial tumors, borderline tumors, germ cell tumors, and stromal cell tumors. Extended surgical staging is imperative in all cases of an even suspected malignancy so that the patient can make an informed decision based on available information. The rate-limiting step should not be histologic information. A detailed discussion of the surgical management of ovarian carcinoma including staging, cytoreductive surgery, and second-look surgery was presented earlier under the epithelial ovarian neoplasm section of this chapter.

Early detection of ovarian cancers

Because ovarian malignancy is such a dreadful illness, both the professional and public communities embrace the concept of "screening." Unfortunately, screening for ovarian cancer is not effective. Programs designed to detect unsuspected ovarian cancer are more accurately described as "earlier detection programs."

Because the incidence of ovarian cancer is relatively low, methods used for detection must have stringent levels of specificity and sensitivity. If the tests do not have a very high specificity, too many women will undergo unnecessary and potentially hazardous operations. If the sensitivity is too low, affected women will pass through the screen undetected. An even more serious barrier to effective screening is the acknowledged lack of a latent or precancerous precursor lesion.[104]

The inability to perform screening in the classical sense does not, however, lessen the need to pursue methods for "early" detection of cancers in stage I. Early detection favorably influences long-term prognosis for the individual and site-specific mortality from ovarian cancer. Proposals of methods for early detection might be especially practical for high-risk women.

Transabdominal ultrasonography. Transabdominal pelvic ultrasonography is effective in measuring the volume and morphologic characteristics of ovaries in postmenopausal women.[26-28,86] In addition, ultrasonography is measurably more accurate than physical examination in detecting adnexal masses.[188] Unfortunately the large prospective screening studies that utilize transabdominal ultrasonography have been hampered by the lack of reliability of ultrasound in distinguishing benign from malignant tissues. This was true even though the units performing the above studies were among the most experienced in the world. Many of the thousands of women screened, were operated upon, but only a very few had ovarian cancer—approximately one case for every one thousand women screened.[29] Moreover, the benefit to the women with ovarian cancer detected by transabdominal US remains to be determined.

Transvaginal ultrasonography. Because the transducer is closer to the area of interest, transvaginal ultrasonography with probes of higher frequency produces images of higher quality and perhaps greater accuracy. Although data regarding ovarian size and morphology are highly reproducible, the use of transvaginal US screening has the same tissue characterization limitations as abdominal ultrasonography.[99] Among the women in these studies who were operated upon as the result of an abnormal transvaginal ultrasound, only a very few had ovarian cancer—approximately 1 per 1000 women screened.[209,210] The additional use of color Doppler as a means of helping to differentiate benign from malignant ovarian lesions has advocates, but there are no data regarding the impact on screening accuracy.[112,173] Currently, transabdominal and transvaginal ultrasound lack adequate specificity to be used alone.

Several authors have developed ultrasonographic morphology scoring systems in an effort to distinguish more reproducibly between benign and malignant lesions.[52] The impact on screening accuracy will require confirmation in randomized prospective trials.

Serum CA-125. The serum marker CA-125 has been evaluated extensively as a screening test for ovarian cancer. It is an antigenic determinant on a high molecular weight glycoprotein which is recognized by the monoclonal antibody OC-125.

The sensitivity of CA-125 prior to the diagnosis of ovarian cancer was determined by the JANUS study.[226] This seminal report involved the retrospective analysis of CA-125 levels in a serum bank of specimens from more than 100,000 individuals between 1973 and 1986. Disappointingly, only 33% of women who developed ovarian cancer had an elevated CA-125 level within 18 months before the diagnosis was established. Only about 20% had an elevated CA-125 level between 18 and 60 months before the diagnosis was established.

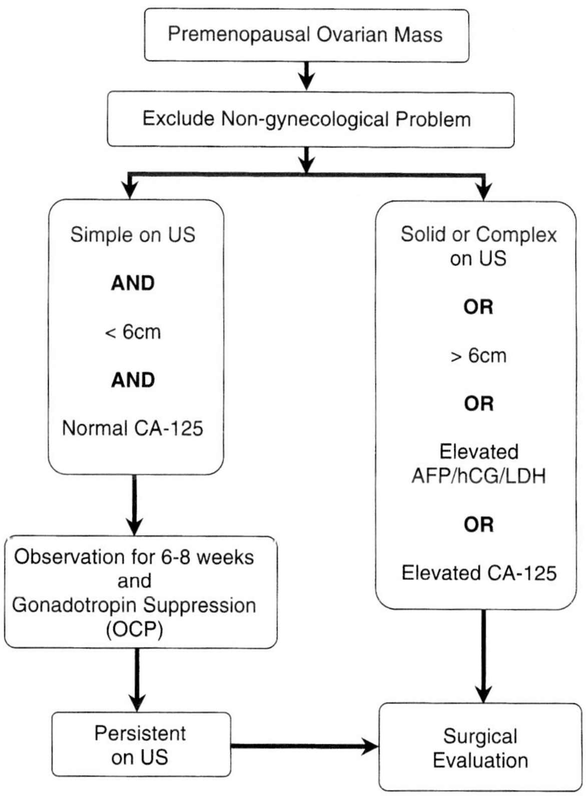

Fig. 9-36. Evaluation and management of a premenopausal ovarian mass.

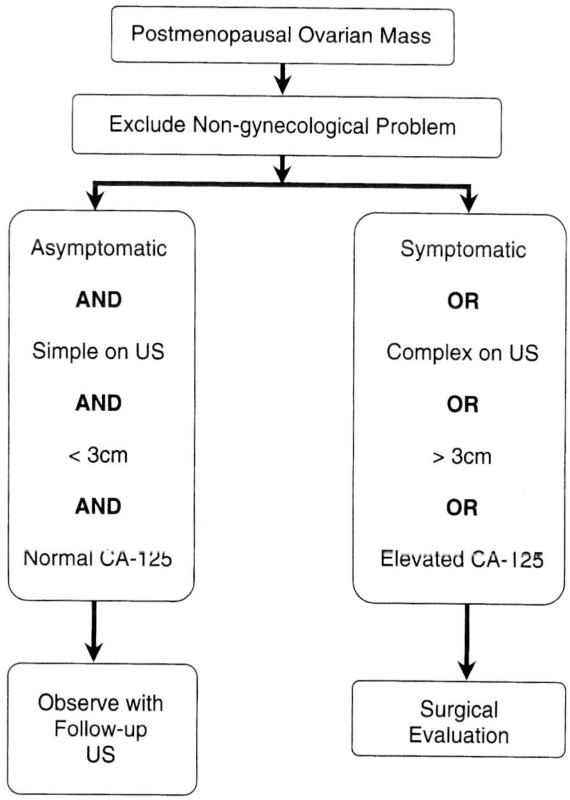

Fig. 9-37. Evaluation and management of a postmenopausal ovarian mass.

Two large prospective studies have confirmed that serum CA-125 lacks satisfactory sensitivity to be used as an independent screening test for ovarian cancer, even when restricted to postmenopausal women.[58,107]

Multimodality screening. A combination of CA-125, US, and physical examination is intellectually appealing.[63] This combination has the potential advantage of improving both the sensitivity and specificity of screening. Jacobs et al used vaginal examination with serum CA-125 as the initial examination (primary screen—higher sensitivity) combined with US for those with abnormalities (secondary screen—higher specificity).[107] They screened 1010 apparently healthy postmenopausal female volunteers. The only case of ovarian cancer that was detected had a 10 cm mass on initial pelvic examination. It is unclear how many women underwent a (potentially unnecessary) surgical procedure because of the screening test and did not have ovarian cancer. Arguably, some of the women may have benefited by detection and removal of nonmalignant processes that would not have been identified, if the women had not participated in the screening program.

Case-finding or screening of high-risk women seems to require the use of multiple modalities to overcome the limitations of the individual procedures. This approach has been applied to self-referred women with a family history of ovarian cancer; the results have been of mixed utility.[57,102,145,176]

Surgical prevention of ovarian cancer. There is no consensus regarding the value of prophylactic oophorectomy as a surgical "routine" when hysterectomy is being performed in women over the age of 40. Boike has suggested that as many as 6% to 8% of women with ovarian cancer have had a previous hysterectomy.[25] He argues that approximately 62 "unnecessary" oophorectomies to prevent each case of ovarian cancer would be acceptable. The operation is justified by the number of cases/deaths from ovarian cancer that might be prevented, if routine oophorectomies were performed at the time of hysterectomy.

Less controversial is the role of prophylactic oophorectomy in patients with familial ovarian cancer syndromes.[31,114,189] Women with one of these syndromes have a lifetime risk of ovarian cancer as high as 50%. Prophylactic oophorectomy in these women will substantially reduce but not eliminate subsequent death from intraabdominal peritoneal carcinomatosis. The unusual ocurrence of disseminated intraabdominal carcinomatosis after prophylactic oophorectomy in women with hereditary ovarian cancer syndromes is well described. Hereditary forms of ovarian cancer are rare (estimated 1% to 3% of ovarian cancer cases). These syndromes (ovarian cancer syndrome; breast-ovarian syndrome; Lynch II colon-ovary-endometrium syndrome) are inherited in an autosomal dominant pattern; many are linked on chromosome 17q.[135] In the absence of a specific genetic marker, women suspected of having a hereditary ovarian cancer syndrome would benefit from formal genetic counseling to determine the presence of an autosomal dominant inheritance pattern.

A history of a family member affected with ovarian cancer is not uncommon. It is very important to distinguish between the women who have family members with ovarian cancer and those with a true hereditary ovarian cancer syndrome, when counseling for possible prophylactic ovariectomy. A 35-year-old without a family history of ovarian cancer has a lifetime risk of about 1.6%. This increases to about 5% if she has one relative and 7% if she has two relatives with ovarian cancer. This risk is in sharp contrast to the 50% risk for the hereditary syndromes.

REFERENCES

1. Aguirre P, Thor AD, Scully RE: Ovarian small cell carcinoma: histogenic considerations based on immunohistochemical and other findings, *Am J Clin Pathol* 92(2):140-149, 1989.
2. Amos CI et al: Age at onset for familial epithelial ovarian cancer, *JAMA* 268(14):1896-1899, 1992.
3. Andersen WA et al: Platinum-based combination chemotherapy for malignant mixed mesodermal tumors of the ovary, *Gynecol Oncol* 32(3):319-322, 1989.
4. Andolf E, Jorgensen C, Astedt B: Ultrasound examination for detection of ovarian carcinoma in risk groups, *Obstet Gynecol* 75(1):106-109, 1990.
5. Aure JC, Hoeg K, Kolstad P: Clinical and histologic studies of ovarian carcinoma: long-term follow-up of 990 cases, *Obstet Gynecol* 37(1):1-9, 1971.
6. Austin RM, Norris HJ: Malignant Brenner tumor and transitional cell carcinoma of the ovary: a comparison, *Int J Gynecol Pathol* 6:29-39, 1987.
7. Awais GM: Dysgerminoma and serum lactic dehydrogenase levels, *Obstet Gynecol* 61(1):99-101, 1983.
8. Bajorin DF et al: Two-drug therapy in patients with metastatic germ cell tumors, *Cancer* 67(1):28-32, 1991.
9. Baker TG: Radiosensitivity of mammalian oocytes with particular reference to the human female, *Am J Obstet Gynecol* 110:746,1971.
10. Barakat RR et al: Mixed mesodermal tumor of the ovary: analysis of prognostic factors in 31 cases, *Obstet Gynecol* 80(4):660-664, 1992.
11. Barber HRK, Graber EA: The PMPO syndrome (postmenopausal palpable ovary syndrome), *Obstet Gynecol* 38:921, 1971.
12. Barbieri RL et al: Rat Leydig cell and granulosa cell 17-ketosteroid reductase activity:subcellular localization and substrate specificity, *Am J Obstet Gynecol* 159:1564, 1988a.
13. Barbieri RL, Ryan KJ: Hyperandrogenism, insulin resistance, and acanthosis nigricans syndrome: a common endocrinopathy with unique pathophysiologic features, *Am J Obstet Gynecol* 147-190, 1993.
14. Barbieri RL, Smith S, Ryan KJ: The role of hyperinsulinemia in the pathogenesis of ovarian hyperinsulinemia, *Fertil Steril* 50:197, 1988b.
15. Bast RC et al: A radioimmunoassay using a monoclonal antibody to monitor the course of epithelial ovarian cancer, *N Engl J Med* 309:883-887, 1983.
16. Bell DA, Scully RE: Atypical and borderline endometrioid adenofibromas of the ovary: a report of 27 cases, *Am J Surg Pathol* 9(3):205-214, 1985.
17. Bell DA, Scully RE: Benign and borderline clear cell adenofibromas of the ovary, *Cancer* 56(12):2922-2931, 1985.
18. Bell DA, Scully RE: Ovarian serous borderline tumors with stromal microinvasion: a report of 21 cases, *Hum Pathol* 21(4):397-403, 1990.
19. Bell DA, Weinstock MA, Scully RE: Peritoneal implants of ovarian serous borderline tumors: histologic features and prognosis, *Cancer* 62(10):2212-2222, 1988.
20. Benacerraf BR et al: Sonographic accuracy in the diagnosis of ovarian masses, *J Repro Med* 35(5):491-495, 1990.

21. Berek JS, Hacker NF: *Practical gynecologic oncology*, Baltimore, 1989, Williams & Wilkins.
22. Berek JS et al: Survival of patients following secondary cytoreductive surgery in ovarian cancer, *Obstet Gynecol* 61(2):189-193, 1983.
23. Bjorkholm E et al: Dysgerminoma: the radiumhemmet series 1927-1984, *Cancer* 65(1):38-44, 1990.
24. Block E: Quantitative morphological investigations of the follicular system in woman, *Acta Anat (Basel)* 14:108, 1952.
25. Boike GM: Surgical prevention of ovarian cancer, *Contemp Obstet Gynecol* 66-78, 1992.
26. Bourne TH et al: Ultrasound screening for familial ovarian cancer, *Gynecol Oncol* 43(2):92-97, 1991.
27. Campbell S et al: Screening for early ovarian cancer, *Lancet* 1:710-711, 1988.
28. Campbell S et al: Transabdominal ultrasound screening for early ovarian cancer, *Br Med J* 299(6712):1363-1367, 1989.
29. Campbell S et al: Novel screening strategies for early ovarian cancer by transabdominal ultrasonography, *Br J Obstet Gynaecol* 97(4):304-311, 1990.
30. Cannon L, Jesionowska H: Methotrexate treatment of tubal pregnancy, *Fertil Steril* 55(6):1033-1038, 1991.
31. Carlson KJ, Nichols D, Schiff I: Indications for hysterectomy, *N Engl J Med* 328(12):856-860, 1993.
32. Casey AC et al: Epithelial ovarian tumors of borderline malignancy: long-term follow-up, *Gynecol Oncol* 50:316-322, 1993.
33. Centers for disease control: Cancer and Steroid Hormone Study: oral contraceptives and the risk of ovarian cancer, *JAMA* 249(12):1596-1599, 1983.
34. Chalvardjian A, Derzko C: Gynandroblastoma: its ultrastructure, *Cancer* 50(4):710-721, 1982.
35. Chetowski RJ et al: Autonomous cortisol secretion by lipoid cell tumor of the ovary, *JAMA* 254(18):2628-2631, 1985.
36. Chorlton I, Norris HJ, King FM: Malignant reticuloendothelial disease involving the ovary as a primary manifestation: a series of 19 lymphomas and one granulocytic sarcoma, *Cancer* 34(2):397-407, 1974.
37. Christian CD: Ovarian tumors: an extension of the Peutz-Jeghers syndrome, *Am J Obstet Gynecol* 111(4):529-534, 1971.
38. Colombo N et al: Cisplatin, vinblastine and bleomycin combination chemotherapy in metastatic granulosa cell tumor of the ovary, *Obstet Gynecol* 67(2):265-268, 1986.
39. Copeland LJ et al: Microscopic disease at second-look laparotomy in advanced ovarian cancer, *Cancer* 55(2):472-478, 1985.
40. Cramer DW, Welch WR: Determinants of ovarian cancer risk. II. Inferences regarding pathogenesis, *J Natl Cancer Inst* 71(4):717-721, 1983.
41. Cramer DW et al: Factors affecting the association of oral contraceptives and ovarian cancer, *N Engl J Med* 307:1047-1051, 1982a.
42. Cramer DW et al: Ovarian cancer and talc: a case control study, *Cancer* 50:372-376, 1982b.
43. Cramer DW et al: Determinants of ovarian cancer risk: reproductive experiences and family history, *J Natl Cancer Inst* 71(4):711-716, 1983.
44. Cramer DW et al: Dietary animal fat in relation to ovarian cancer risk, *Obstet Gynecol* 63(6):833-838, 1984.
45. Cramer DW et al: Galactose consumption and metabolism in relation to the risk of ovarian cancer, *Lancet* 2(8654):66-71, 1989.
46. Czernobilsky B, Silverman BB, Enterline HT: Clear-cell carcinoma of the ovary: a clinicopathologic analysis of pure and mixed forms and comparison with endometrioid carcinoma, *Cancer* 25(4):762-772, 1970.
47. Czernobilsky B, Silverman BB, Mikuta JJ: Endometrioid carcinoma of the ovary: a clinicopathological study of 75 cases, *Cancer* 26(5):1141-1152, 1970.
48. Day NE, Boice JD: Second cancer in relation to radiation treatment for cervical cancer, *International Agency for Research on Cancer,* No. 52, 1983, World Health Organization.
49. Dembo AJ et al: Ovarian carcinoma: improved survival following abdominopelvic irradiation in patients with completed pelvic operation, *Am J Obstet Gynecol* 134(7):793-800, 1979.
50. Dembo AJ et al: The Princess Margaret Hospital study of ovarian cancer: stages I, II, and asymptomatic III presentations, *Cancer Treat Rep* 63(2): 249-254, 1979.
51. Dembo AJ et al: Prognostic factors in patients with stage I epithelial ovarian cancer, *Obstet Gynecol* 75(2):263-273, 1990.
52. DePriest PD et al: A morphology index based on sonographic findings in ovarian cancer, *Gynecol Oncol* 51(1):7-11, 1993.
53. Dinh TV et al: Mixed mesodermal tumors of the ovary: a clinicopathologic study of 14 cases, *Obstet Gynecol* 72(3 pt 1):409-412, 1988.
54. Donovan JT et al: Cushing's syndrome secondary to malignant lipoid cell tumor of the ovary, *Gynecol Oncol* 50(2):249-253, 1993.
55. Doss N Jr et al: Covert bilaterality of mature ovarian teratomas, *Obstet Gynecol* 50(6):651-653, 1977.
56. Ebrahami T, Goldsmith JW, Okagaki T: Hemangioma of the ovary: a case report, *Obstet Gynecol* 38(5):677-679, 1971.
57. Einhorn N: Ovarian cancer: early diagnosis and screening, *Hematol Oncol Clin North Am* 6(4):843-850, 1992.
58. Einhorn N et al: Prospective evaluation of serum CA-125 levels for early detection of ovarian cancer, *Obstet Gynecol* 80(1):14-18, 1992.
59. Evans AT III et al: Clinicopathologic review of 118 granulosa and 82 theca cell tumors, *Obstet Gynecol* 55(2):231-238, 1980.
60. Faddy MJ, Gosden RG, Edwards RG: Ovarian follicle dynamics in mice: a comparative study of three inbred strains and an FI hybrid, *J Endocrinol* 96:23,1983.
61. Fallahzadeh H, Dockerty MB, Lee RA: Leiomyoma of the ovary: report of five cases and review of the literature, *Am J Obstet Gynecol* 113(3):394-398, 1972.
62. Feuillan PP, Jones J, Cutler GB: Long term testolactone therapy for precocious puberty in girls with the McCune-Albright syndrome, *J Clin Endocrinol Metab* 77:647-651, 1993.
63. Finkler NJ et al: Comparison of serum CA-125, clinical impression, and ultrasound in the preoperative evaluation of ovarian masses, *Obstet Gynecol* 72(4):659-664, 1988.
64. Fox H: Sex cord stromal tumors of the ovary, *J Pathol* 145(2):127-148, 1985.
65. Fox H, Agrawal K, Langley FA: A clinicopathologic study of 92 cases of granulosa cell tumor of the ovary with special reference to the factors influencing prognosis, *Cancer* 35(1):231-241, 1975.
66. Fox H, Langley FA: *Tumors of the ovary*, Chicago, 1976, Year Book Medical.
67. Fujii S et al: Analysis of serum lactic dehydrogenase levels and its isoenzymes in ovarian dysgerminoma, *Gynecol Oncol* 22(1):65-72, 1985.
68. Gallion HH et al: Ovarian dysgerminoma: report of seven cases and review of the literature, *Am J Obstet Gynecol* 158(3 pt 1):591-595, 1988.
69. Garcia-Bunuel R, Berek JS, Woodruff JD: Luteomas of pregnancy, *Obstet Gynecol* 45(4):407-414, 1975.
70. Gershenson DM: Menstrual and reproductive function after treatment with combination chemotherapy for malignant ovarian germ cell tumors, *J Clin Oncol* 6(2):270-275, 1988.
71. Gershenson DM: Update on malignant ovarian germ cell tumors, *Cancer* 71(suppl 4):1581-1590, 1993.
72. Gershenson DM, Silva EG: Serous ovarian tumors of malignant potential with peritoneal implants, *Cancer* 65(3):578-585, 1990.
73. Gershenson DM et al: Endodermal sinus tumor of the ovary: the MD Anderson experience, *Obstet Gynecol* 61(2):194-202, 1983.
74. Gershenson DM et al: Mixed germ cell tumors of the ovary, *Obstet Gynecol* 64(2):200-206, 1984.

75. Gershenson DM et al: Prognosis of surgically determined complete responders in advanced ovarian carcinoma, *Cancer* 55(5):1129-1135, 1985.
76. Gershenson DM et al: Treatment of malignant nondysgerminomatous germ cell tumors of the ovary with vincristine, dactinomycin and cyclophosphamide, *Cancer* 56(12):2756-2761, 1985.
77. Gershenson DM et al: Chemotherapeutic complete remission in patients with metastatic ovarian dysgerminoma: potential for cure and preservation of reproductive capacity, *Cancer* 58(12):2594-2599, 1986.
78. Gershenson DM et al: Second-look laparotomy in the management of malignant germ cell tumors of the ovary, *Obstet Gynecol* 67(6):789-793, 1986.
79. Gershenson DM et al: Treatment of metastatic stromal tumors of the ovary with cisplatin, doxorubicin and cyclophosphamide, *Obstet Gynecol* 70(5):765-769, 1987.
80. Gershenson DM et al: Treatment of malignant germ cell tumors of the ovary with bleomycin, etoposide, and cisplatin, *J Clin Oncol* 8(4):715-720, 1990.
81. Gonzalez-Angulo A et al: Adenocarcinoma of thyroid arising in struma ovarii (malignant struma ovarii): report of two cases and review of the literature, *Obstet Gynecol* 21:567-576, 1963.
82. Goodman AL, Hodgen GD: The ovarian triad of the primate menstrual cycle, *Recent Prog Horm Res* 39:1, 1983.
83. Goodman HM et al: The role of cytoreductive surgery in the management of stage IV epithelial ovarian carcinoma, *Gynecol Oncol* 46(3):367-371, 1992.
84. Gordon A, Lipton D, Woodruff JD. Dysgerminoma: a review of 158 cases from the Emil Novak Ovarian Tumor Registry, *Obstet Gynecol* 58(4):497-504, 1981.
85. Gordon A et al: Benign cystic teratomas in postmenopausal women, *Am J Obstet Gynecol* 138(8):1120-1123, 1980.
86. Goswamy RK et al: Ovarian size in postmenopausal women, *Br J Obstet Gynaecol* 95(8):795-801, 1988.
87. Greenlee JE, Brashear HR: Antibodies to cerebellar Purkinje cells in patients with paraneoplastic cerebellar degeneration and ovarian carcinoma, *Ann Neurol* 14(6):609-613, 1983.
88. Hacker NF et al: Primary cytoreductive surgery for epithelial ovarian cancer, *Obstet Gynecol* 61(4):413-420, 1983.
89. Haid M et al: Malignant Brenner tumor of the ovary: electron microscopic study of a case responsive to radiation and chemotherapy, *Cancer* 51(3):498-508, 1983.
90. Hainsworth JD et al: High-dose cisplatin combination chemotherapy in the treatment of advanced epithelial ovarian carcinoma, *J Clin Oncol* 8(3):502-508, 1990.
91. Hakes TB et al: Randomized prospective trial of 5 versus 10 cycles of cyclophosphamide, doxorubicin and cisplatin in advanced ovarian carcinoma, *Gynecol Oncol* 45(3):284-289, 1992.
92. Halila H, Stenman UH, Seppala M: Ovarian cancer antigen CA-125 levels in pelvic inflammatory disease and pregnancy, *Cancer* 57(7):1327-1329, 1986.
93. Hand R et al: Staging procedures, clinical management, and survival outcome for ovarian carcinoma, *JAMA* 269(9):1119-1122, 1993.
94. Hankinson SE et al: A quantitative assessment of oral contraceptive use and risk of ovarian cancer, *Obstet Gynecol* 80(4):708-714, 1992.
95. Hart WR, Burkons DM: Germ cell neoplasms arising in gonadoblastomas, *Cancer* 31(5):1031-1045, 1973.
96. Hart WR, Norris HJ: Borderline and malignant mucinous tumors of the ovary: histologic criteria and clinical behavior, *Cancer* 31(5):1031-1045, 1973.
97. Heaps JM, Nieberg RK, Berek JS: Malignant neoplasms arising in endometriosis, *Obstet Gynecol* 75(6):1023-1028, 1990.
98. Herrmann UJ Jr, Locher GW, Goldhirsch A: Sonographic patterns of ovarian tumors: prediction of malignancy, *Obstet Gynecol* 69(5):777-781, 1987.
99. Higgins RV et al: Interobserver variation in ovarian measurements using transvaginal ultrasound, *Gynecol Oncol* 39(1):69-71, 1990.
100. Holtz G: Paraneoplastic hypercalcemia in gynecologic malignancy, *Obstet Gynecol Surv* 35(3):129-136, 1980.
101. Hoskins WJ et al: Influence of secondary cytoreduction at the time of second-look laparotomy on the survival of patients with epithelial ovarian carcinoma, *Gynecol Oncol* 34:365-371, 1989.
102. Houlston R et al: Use of family history in a screening clinic for familial ovarian cancer, *Gynecol Oncol* 47(2):247-252, 1992.
103. Howell SB et al: Long-term survival of advanced refractory ovarian carcinoma patients with small-volume disease treated with intraperitoneal chemotherapy, *J Clin Oncol* 5(10):1607-1612, 1987.
104. Hulka BS: Cancer screening: degrees of proof and practical application, *Cancer* 62(suppl 8):1776-1780, 1988.
105. Hunter RW, Alexander NDE, Soutter WP: Metaanalysis of surgery in advanced ovarian carcinoma: is maximum cytoreductive surgery an independent determinant of prognosis? *Am J Obstet Gynecol* 166:504-511, 1992.
106. Jacobs AJ, Newland JR, Green RK: Pure choriocarcinoma of the ovary, *Obstet Gynecol Surv* 37(10):603-609, 1982.
107. Jacobs I et al: Multimodal approach to screening for ovarian cancer, *Lancet* 1(8580):268-271, 1988.
108. Jenison EL et al: Clear cell adenocarcinoma of the ovary: clinical analysis and comparison with serous carcinoma, *Gynecol Oncol* 32(1):65-71, 1989.
109. Jones GES: Some newer aspects of the management of infertility, *JAMA* 141:1123, 1949.
110. Judd HL et al: Endocrine function of the postmenopausal ovary: concentrations of androgens and estrogens in ovarian and peripheral vein blood, *J Clin Endocrinol Metab*; 39:1020, 1974.
111. Kao GF, Norris HJ: Cystadenofibromas of the ovary with epithelial atypia, *Am J Surg Pathol* 2(4):357-363, 1978.
112. Kawai M et al: Transvaginal Doppler ultrasound with color-flow imaging in the diagnosis of ovarian cancer, *Obstet Gynecol* 79(2):163-167, 1992.
113. Kaye SB et al: Randomized study of two doses of cisplatin with cyclophosphamide in epithelial ovarian cancer, *Lancet* 340(8815):329-333, 1992.
114. Kerlikowske K, Brown JS, Grady DG: Should women with familial ovarian cancer undergo prophylactic oophorectomy? *Obstet Gynecol* 80(4):700-707, 1992.
115. Khoo SK et al: The prognostic value of clinical, pathologic, and biologic parameters in ovarian cancer, *Cancer* 72(2):531-537, 1993.
116. Killackey MA, Neuwirth RS: Evaluation and management of the pelvic mass: a review of 540 cases, *Obstet Gynecol* 71(3 pt 1):319-322, 1988.
117. Killick S, Elstein M: Pharmacologic production of luteinized unruptured follicles by prostaglandin synthetase inhibitors, *Fertil Steril* 47:773,1987.
118. Kucera PR et al: Whole abdominal radiotherapy for patients with minimal residual epithelial ovarian cancer, *Gynecol Oncol* 36(3):338-342, 1990.
119. Kurman RJ, Norris HJ: Endodermal sinus tumor of the ovary: a clinical and pathological analysis of 71 cases, *Cancer* 38(6):2404-2419, 1976.
120. Kurman RJ, Norris HJ: Malignant germ cell tumors of the ovary, *Hum Pathol* 8(5):551-564, 1977.
121. Kurman RJ: *Blaustein's pathology of the female genital tract*, ed 3, New York, 1987, Springer-Verlag.
122. LaPolla JP et al: Dysgerminoma of the ovary, *Obstet Gynecol* 69(6):859-864, 1987.
123. Lappohn RE et al: Inhibin as a marker for granulosa cell tumors, *N Engl J Med* 321(12):790-793, 1989.
124. Lavin PT et al: CA-125 for the monitoring of ovarian carcinoma during primary therapy, *Obstet Gynecol* 69(2):223-227, 1987.

125. Lobo R: Endocrine therapy of hyperandrogenism. In Barbieri RL, Schiff I, editors: *Reproductive endocrine therapeutics,* New York, 1988, Alan R Liss.
126. Long RT, Spratt JS Jr, Dowling E: Pseudomyxoma peritonei: new concepts in management with a report of seventeen patients, *Am J Surg* 117(2):162-169, 1969.
127. Louie KG et al: Long-term results of a cisplatin-containing combination chemotherapy regimen for the treatment of advanced ovarian carcinoma, *J Clin Oncol* 4(11):1579-1585, 1986.
128. Louvet JP, Vaitukitis JL. Induction of follicle-stimulating hormone (FSH) receptors in rat ovaries by estrogen priming, 99:758, 1976.
129. Luesley D et al: Failure of second-look laparotomy to influence survival in epithelial ovarian cancer, *Lancet* 2(8611):599-603, 1988.
130. Lui TL, Lian IJ, Deppe G: Serum lactic dehydrogenase (SLDH) germ cell malignancies of the ovary, *Gynecol Oncol* 19(3):355-357, 1984.
131. Luxman D et al: The postmenopausal adnexal mass: correlation between ultrasonic and pathological findings, *Obstet Gynecol* 77(5):726-728, 1991.
132. Lynch HT: *Cancer genetics*, Springfield, Ill, 1976, Charles C Thomas.
133. Lynch HT: Genetic risk in ovarian cancer, *Gynecol Oncol* 46(1):1-3, 1992.
134. Lynch HT, Bewtra C, Lynch JF: Familial ovarian carcinoma: clinical nuances, *Am J Med* 81(6):1073-1076, 1986.
135. Lynch HT, Lynch JF: Hereditary ovarian carcinoma, *Hematol Oncol Clin North Am* 6(4):783-811, 1990.
136. Malkasian GD Jr et al: CA-125 in gynecologic practice, *Am J Obstet Gynecol* 155(3):515-518, 1986.
137. Mann WJ et al: Preoperative serum CA-125 levels in patients with surgical stage I invasive ovarian adenocarcinoma, *J Nat Cancer Inst* 80(3):208-209, 1988.
138. Mann WJ Jr et al: The management of pseudomyxoma peritonei, *Cancer* 66(7):1636-1640, 1990.
139. Manuel M, Katayama KP, Jones HW: The age of occurrence of gonadal tumors in intersex patients with a Y chromosome, *Am J Obstet Gynecol* 67:141, 1953.
140. Marik J, Hulka J: Luteinized unruptured follicle syndrome: a subtle cause of infertility, *Fertil Steril* 29:270, 1978.
141. McGuire WP et al: A phase III trial comparing cisplatin/cytoxan and cisplatin/taxol (PT) in advanced ovarian cancer (AOC), *Proc Am Soc Clin Oncol* 12:255, 1993 (abstract).
142. Mecke H et al: Pelviscopic treatment of ovarian cysts in premenopausal women, *Gynecol Obstet Invest* 34(1):36-42, 1992.
143. Meigs JV, Armstrong SH, Hamilton HH: A further contribution to the syndrome of fibroma of the ovary with fluid in the abdomen and chest, Meigs syndrome, *Am J Obstet Gynecol* 42:19-37, 1943.
144. Morrow M, Enker WE: Late ovarian metastases in carcinoma of the colon and rectum, *Arch Surg* 119(12):1385-1388, 1984.
145. Muto M et al: Screening for ovarian cancer: the preliminary experience of a familial ovarian cancer center, *Gynecol Oncol* 51(1):12-20, 1993.
146. Nichols RL et al: Effect of preoperative neomycin-erythromycin intestinal preparation on the incidence of infectious complications following colon surgery, *Ann Surg* 178:453-456, 1973.
147. Nielsen SN, Scheithauer BW, Gaffey TA: Gliomatosis peritonei, *Cancer* 56(10):2499-2503, 1985.
148. Niloff JM et al: The CA-125 assay as a predictor of clinical recurrence in epithelial ovarian cancer, *Am J Obstet Gynecol* 155(1)56-60, 1986.
149. Norris HJ, Zirkin HJ, Benson WL: Immature (malignant) teratoma of the ovary, *Cancer* 37(5):2359-2372, 1976.
150. Ohel G, Kaneti H, Schenker JG: Granulosa cell tumors in Israel: a study of 172 cases, *Gynecol Oncol* 15(2):278-286, 1983.
151. Omura GA et al: Randomized trial cyclophosphamide plus cisplatin with or without doxorubicin on ovarian carcinoma: a Gynecologic Oncology Group study, *J Clin Oncol* 7(4):457-465, 1989.
152. Payne D et al: Autoimmune hemolytic anemia and ovarian dermoid cysts: case report and review of the literature, *Cancer* 48(3):721-724, 1981.
153. Pittaway DE, Fayez JA, Douglas JW: Serum CA-125 in the evaluation of benign adnexal cysts, *Am J Obstet Gynecol* 157(6):1426-1428, 1987.
154. Piver MS, Lele SB, Patsner B: Pseudomyxoma peritonei: possible prevention of mucinous ascites by peritoneal lavage, *Obstet Gynecol* 64 (suppl 3):95S-96S, 1984.
155. Piver MS et al: Epidemiology and etiology of ovarian cancer, *Semin Oncol* 18(3):177-185, 1991.
156. Piver MS et al: Five year survival for stage IC or stage I/grade 3 epithelial ovarian cancer treated with cisplatin-based chemotherapy, *Gynecol Oncol* 46(3):357-360, 1992.
157. Pressley RH et al: Serum lactic dehydrogenase as a tumor marker in dysgerminoma, *Gynecol Oncol* 44(3):281-283, 1992.
158. Rice LW et al: Epithelial ovarian tumors of borderline malignancy, *Gynecol Oncol* 39(2):195-198, 1990.
159. Rice LW et al: Preoperative serum CA-125 levels in borderline tumors of the ovary, *Gynecol Oncol* 46(2):226-229, 1992.
160. Robboy SJ, Norris HJ, Scully RE: Insular carcinoid primary in the ovary: a clinicopathologic analysis of 48 cases, *Cancer* 36(2):404-418, 1975.
161. Robboy SJ, Scully RE: Ovarian teratoma with glial implants on the peritoneum: an analysis of 12 cases, *Hum Pathol* 1(4):643-653, 1970.
162. Robboy SJ, Scully RE: Strumal carcinoid of the ovary: an analysis of 50 cases of a distinctive tumor composed of thyroid tissue and carcinoid, *Cancer* 46(9):2019-2034, 1980.
163. Robboy SJ, Scully RE, Norris HJ: Carcinoid metastatic to the ovary: a clinicopathologic analysis of 35 cases, *Cancer* 33(3):798-811, 1974.
164. Robboy SJ, Scully RE, Norris HJ: Primary trabecular carcinoid of the ovary, *Obstet Gynecol* 49(2):202-207, 1977.
165. Rosenblum NG et al: Malignant struma ovarii, *Gynecol Oncol* 32(2):224-227, 1989.
166. Rowinsky E et al: Phase II study of taxol in advanced ovarian epithelium malignancy, *Proc Annu Soc Clin Oncol* 7:136, 1988.
167. Russell P: The pathologic assessment of ovarian neoplasms: introduction to the common epithelial tumors and analysis of benign epithelial tumors, *Pathology* 11(1):5-26, 1979.
168. Ryback BJ, Ober WB, Bernacki EG Jr: Malignant Brenner tumor of the ovary: report of three cases, *Diagn Gynecol Obstet* 3(1):61-74, 1981.
169. Sainz de la Cuesta R et al: Prognostic Importance of Intraoperative Rupture of Malignant Ovarian Epithelial Neoplasms, *Obstet Gynecol* 84(1):1-7, 1994.
170. Sassone AM et al: Transvaginal sonographic characterization of ovarian disease: evaluation of a new scoring system to predict ovarian malignancy, *Obstet Gynecol* 78(1):70-76, 1991.
171. Schellhas HF et al: Germ cell tumors associated with XY gonadal dysgenesis, *Am J Obstet Gynecol* 109(8):1197-1204, 1971.
172. Schildkraut JM, Thompson WD: Familial ovarian cancer: a population-based case-control study, *Am J Epidemiol* 128:456-466, 1988.
172. Schiller VL, Grant EG: Doppler ultrasonography of the pelvis, *Radiol Clin North Am* 30(4):735-742, 1992.
174. Schwartz PE: Combination chemotherapy in the management of ovarian germ cell malignancies, *Obstet Gynecol* 64(4):564-572, 1984.
175. Schwartz PE, Morris JM: Serum lactic dehydrogenase: a tumor marker for dysgerminoma, *Obstet Gynecol* 72(3 pt 2):511-515, 1988.
176. Schwartz PE et al: Early detection of ovarian malignancy: preliminary results of the Yale Early Detection Program, *Yale J Biol Med* 64(6):573-582, 1991.
177. Schwartz PE et al: Ovarian germ cell malignancies: the Yale University experience, *Gynecol Oncol* 45(1):26-31, 1992.
178. Schwartz SI et al: *Principles of surgery*, ed 4, New York, 1984, McGraw-Hill.

179. Scully RE: Gonadoblastoma: gonadal tumor related to dysgerminoma (seminoma) and capable of sex hormone production, *Cancer* 6:455-463, 1953.
180. Scully RE: Tumors of the ovary and maldeveloped gonads: atlas of tumor pathology, series 2, vascicle 16, Washington, DC, *Armed Forces Institute of Pathology* 117-127, 1979.
181. Shrenrer A et al: Severe endocrine and nonendocrine manifestations of the McCune-Albright syndrome associated with activating mutations of stimulatory G protein GS, *J Pediatr* 123:509, 1993.
182. Silva EG et al: Ovarian carcinomas with transitional cell carcinoma pattern, *Am J Clin Pathol* 93(4):457-465, 1990.
183. Slayton RE et al: Vincristine, dactinomycin and cyclophosphamide in the treatment of malignant germ cell tumors of the ovary: a Gynecologic Oncology Group study, *Cancer* 56(2):243-248, 1985.
184. Smith EM, Anderson B: The effects of symptoms and delay in seeking diagnosis on stage of disease at diagnosis, among women with cancers of the ovary, *Cancer* 56(11):2727-2732, 1985.
185. Soper JT et al: The role of partial sigmoid colectomy for debulking epithelial ovarian carcinoma, *Gynecol Oncol* 41(3):239-244, 1991.
186. Sorbe B, Frankendal B, Veress B: Importance of histologic grading in the prognosis of epithelial ovarian carcinoma, *Obstet Gynecol* 59(5):576-582, 1982.
187. Spanos WJ: Preoperative hormonal therapy of cystic adnexal masses, *Am J Obstet Gynecol* 116(4):551-556, 1973.
188. Sparks JM, Varner RE: Ovarian cancer screening, *Obstet Gynecol* 77(5):787-792, 1991.
189. Speroff T et al: A risk-benefit analysis of elective bilateral oophorectomy: effect of changes in compliance with estrogen therapy on outcome, *Am J Obstet Gynecol* 164(1 pt 1):165-174, 1991.
190. Stenwig JT, Hazekemp JT, Beecham JB: Granulosa cell tumors of the ovary: a clinicopathological study of 118 cases with long-term follow-up, *Gynecol Oncol* 7(2):136-152, 1979.
191. Stern JL et al: Spontaneous rupture of benign cystic teratomas, *Obstet Gynecol* 57(3):363-366, 1981.
192. Su H, Lau YF: Identification of the transcriptional unit, the structural organization and promoter sequence of the human sex determining region Y(SRY) gene, using a reverse genetic approach, *Am J Hum Genet* 52:24, 1993.
193. Sutton GP et al: Phase II trial of ifosfamide and mesna in advanced ovarian carcinoma: a Gynecologic Oncology Group study, *J Clin Oncol* 7(11):1672-1676, 1989.
194. Swenerton K et al: Cisplatin-cyclophosphamide versus carboplatinum-cyclophosphamide in advanced ovarian cancer: a randomized phase III study of the National Cancer Institute of Canada: Clinical Trials Group, *J Clin Oncol* 10(5):718-726, 1992.
195. Takeda A et al: Polyembryoma of ovary producing α-fetoprotein and hCG: imminoperoxidase and electron microscopic study, *Cancer* 49(9):1878-1889, 1982.
196. Talerman A: Ovarian Sertoli-Leydig cell tumor (androblastoma) with retiform pattern: a clinicopathologic study, *Cancer* 60(12):3056-3064, 1987.
197. Talerman A, Haije WG, Baggerman L: Serum α-fetoprotein (AFP) in patients with germ cell tumors of the gonads and extragonadal sites: correlation between endodermal sinus (yolk sac) tumor and raised serum AFP, *Cancer* 46(2):380-385, 1980.
198. Tavassoli FA: Serous tumors of low malignant potential with early stromal invasion (serous LMP with microinvasion), *Mod Pathol* 1(6):407-414, 1988.
199. Tavassoli FA, Norris HJ: Sertoli tumors of the ovary: a clinicopathologic study of 28 cases with ultrastructural observations, *Cancer* 46(10):2281-2297, 1981.
200. Taylor MH, DePetrillo AD, Turner AR: Vinblastine, bleomycin, and cisplatin in malignant germ cell tumors of the ovary, *Cancer* 56(6):1341-1349, 1985.
201. Teilum G: Endometrial sinus tumors of the ovary and testes: comparative morphogenesis of the so-called mesonephroma ovarii (Schiller) and extraembryonic (yolk sac allantoic) structures of the rat placenta, *Cancer* 12:1029, 1959.
202. Teilum G: *Special tumors of ovary and testis, and related extragonadal lesions; comparative pathology and histological identification*, ed 2, Philadelphia, 1971, JB Lippincott.
203. Teter J: Cytogenetics with reference to gonadoblastoma and to gonocytomas. In Lynch HT, editor: *Cancer genetics*, Springfield, Ill, 1976, Charles C Thomas.
204. Thigpen JT et al: Chemotherapy in ovarian carcinoma: present role and future prospects, *Semin Oncol* 16(suppl 4):58-65, 1989.
205. Thigpen T et al: Chemotherapy for advanced or recurrent gynecologic cancer, *Cancer* 60(suppl 8):2104-2116, 1987.
206. Tho SP et al: Absence of the testis determining factor gene SRY in XX true hemaphrodites and presence of this locus in most subjects with gonadal dysgesis caused by U aneuploidy, *Am J Obstet Gynecol* 167:1794, 1992.
207. Thomas GM et al: Current therapy for dysgerminoma of the ovary, *Obstet Gynecol* 70(2):268-275, 1987.
208. Troche V, Hernandez E: Neoplasia arising in dysgenetic gonads, *Obstet Gynecol Sur* 41(2):74-79, 1986.
209. Van Nagell Jr: Ovarian cancer screening, *Cancer* 68(4):679-680, 1991.
210. Van Nagell Jr et al: Transvaginal sonography as a screening method for ovarian cancer: a report of the first 1000 cases screened, *Cancer* 65(3):573-577, 1990.
211. Vasilev SA et al: Serum CA-125 levels in preoperative evaluation of pelvic masses, *Obstet Gynecol* 71(5):751-756, 1988.
212. Waldstreicher J et al: Hyperfunction of the hypothalamic-pituitary axis in women with polycystic ovarian disease: indirect evidence for partial gonadotropin desensitization, *J Clin Endocrinol Metab* 66:165, 1988.
213. Willemse PH et al: Carboplatinum with cyclophosphamide in patients with advanced ovarian cancer: an efficacy and quality-adjusted survival analysis, *Int J Gynecol Cancer* 2:236-243, 1992.
214. Woodruff JD, Novak ER: The Krukenberg tumor: study of 48 cases from the ovarian tumor registry, *Obstet Gynecol* 15:351-360, 1960.
215. Woodruff JD et al: Metastatic ovarian tumors, *Am J Obstet Gynecol* 107(2):202-209, 1970.
216. Woodruff JD et al: Proliferative and malignant Brenner tumors: review of 47 cases, *Am J Obstet Gynecol* 141(2):118-125, 1981.
217. Wu PC et al: Treatment of malignant ovarian germ cell tumors with preservation of fertility: a report of 28 cases, *Gynecol Oncol* 40(1):2-6, 1991.
218. Yazigi R, Sandstad J: Ovarian involvement in extragenital cancer, *Gynecol Oncol* 34(1):84-87, 1989.
219. Yazigi R, Sandstad J, Munoz AK: Primary staging in ovarian tumors of low malignant potential , *Gynecol Oncol* 31(3):402-408, 1988.
220. Young RC et al: Staging laparotomy in early ovarian cancer, *JAMA* 250(22):3072-3076, 1983.
221. Young RC et al: Adjuvant therapy in stage I and stage II epithelial ovarian cancer: results of two prospective randomized trials, *N Engl J Med* 322(15):1021-1027, 1990.
222. Young RH, Dickersin GR, Scully RE: Juvenile granulosa cell tumor of the ovary: a clinicopathological analysis of 125 cases, *Am J Surg Pathol* 8(8):575-596, 1984.
223. Young RH, Gilks CB, Scully RE: Mucinous tumor of the appendix associated with mucinous tumors of the ovary and pseudomyxoma peritonei: a clinicopathological analysis of 22 cases supporting an origin in the appendix, *Am J Surg Pathol* 15(5):415-429, 1991.
224. Young RH, Scully RE: Ovarian Sertoli-Leydig cell tumors: a clinicopathological analysis of 207 cases, *Am J Surg Pathol* 9(8):543-569, 1985.

225. Young RH et al: Ovarian sex cord tumor with annular tubules: review of 74 cases including 27 with Peutz-Jeghers Syndrome and four with adenoma malignum of the cervix, *Cancer* 50(7):1384-1402, 1982.

226. Zurawski VR Jr et al: Elevated serum CA-125 levels prior to diagnosis of ovarian neoplasia: relevance for early detection of ovarian cancer, *Int J Cancer* 42(5):677-680, 1988.

Chapter 10

THE BREAST

Barbara L. Smith

ANATOMY AND DEVELOPMENT

During the fifth week of gestation, a milk streak extending from the axilla to the groin appears and progresses through milk ridge and milk hill stages to form the early breast buds. During this time, mesenchymal cells form the smooth muscle of the nipple and areola while epithelial elements form buds which ultimately give rise to 15 to 25 future ducts and lobules. It is believed that phylogenetically the breast arises as a modified apocrine sweat gland. These early phases of breast development are independent of hormones and occur in fetuses of both sexes. During the third trimester of pregnancy, placental sex hormones cause the previously formed epithelial buds to be converted into hollow ducts. It is these structures which produce the colostrum or "witch's milk" of the newborn that may be observed 4 to 7 days postpartum. These secretions cease over subsequent weeks as the effects of placental hormones wane.

The nipple itself protrudes from the center of the pigmented areola and contains 10 to 15 terminal duct openings. Within the areola are Montgomery's glands, the slightly raised nodules of which are apocrine glands.

As many as 2% to 6% of adult women will have accessory nipples (polythelia) along the milk ridge, most commonly in the axilla or just inferior to the breast. In some instances there will be breast ductal tissue beneath the accessory nipple (polymastia). This breast tissue may enlarge and even lactate as the result of pregnancy. In the axilla this enlargement of axillary breast tissue may need to be distinguished from a breast mass appearing during pregnancy. In general, however, there is no need to remove this accessory nipple or breast tissue, other than for cosmetic purposes or unless palpable abnormalities arise.

Asymmetry of the breasts is quite common and can range from slight asymmetry to dramatic hypoplasia on one side. Complete amastia is quite rare and is often accompanied by chest wall deformities. Poland's syndrome produces absence of the breast with defects of varying severity in the underlying pectoralis major muscle and bony chest wall and is often associated with hand abnormalities.

Abnormalities of breast structure may also have an iatrogenic source. Overly extensive excision of the breast bud underneath the nipple and areola during biopsy of a subareolar lesion in a young child can result in removal of tissue critical for breast development and in gross asymmetry after puberty.

SURGICAL ANATOMY OF THE BREAST

The breast overlies ribs two through six and for surgical purposes extends medial to the sternum, superior to the clavicle, lateral to the latissimus dorsi muscle, and inferior below the inframammary fold for a variable distance down the costal margin. These structures serve as the borders of dissection during mastectomy. The blood supply to the breast comes primarily from perforating branches of the internal mammary artery that supplies the medial and central portions of the breast. The lateral thoracic artery supplies the upper and upper-outer portions of the breast with additional minor contributions from the intercostal, subscapular, and thoracodorsal arteries. Venous drainage is via the veins accompanying these arteries.

The breast lies directly over the pectoralis major muscle, which serves as the deep margin of dissection medially and centrally during a mastectomy. The rectus abdominis muscle lies under the most inferior portion of the breast while the serratus anterior muscle lies beneath the most lateral portion of the breast. The latissimus dorsi muscle, as described above, defines the most lateral extension of breast tissue. The latissimus dorsi muscle may also be used for breast reconstruction after mastectomy; the muscle can be detached posteriorly and swung anteriorly based on the thoracodorsal vessels. The rectus abdominis muscle is also used for breast reconstruction after mastectomy; the muscle can be detached from its inferior insertion and swung upward based on the vessels entering superiorly. In general, the contralateral rectus muscle is preferred for reconstruction, although it is also possible to use the ipsilateral muscle.

Lymph from all parts of the breast drains to the axillary nodes and makes the axillary nodes the most appropriate area of sampling for metastatic disease during breast cancer surgery. Studies with radiolabelled colloid have demonstrated that approximately 97% of lymph from the breast drains to the axillary nodes, while only 3% drains to the internal mammary nodes.[91]

Within the axilla the pectoralis minor muscle and the axillary vein define the three surgical levels of dissection. A level I node dissection includes those lymph nodes below the axillary vein, while a level II dissection includes nodes from the axillary vein extending medially behind the pectoralis minor muscle to its medial border. A level III dissection includes lymph nodes medial to the pectoralis minor muscle. Rotter's nodes are those lying between the pectoralis major and minor muscles.

Fewer than 2% of patients will have "skip metastases" with positive nodes only in level III, although as many as 20% of women will have positive nodes in level II but not in level I.[32,142,149,175] As a result, axillary staging generally includes a level I and II node dissection that can be expected to contain nearly all of the relevant staging information and reduce the risk of subsequent lymphedema (see below).

A number of important structures are present within the axilla and must be preserved during the course of axillary dissection for breast cancer staging. The axillary artery lies superior and deep to the axillary vein. The brachial plexus lies just superior to the axillary vein. Parts of the brachial plexus may pass anterior to the vein as it courses laterally. The long thoracic nerve runs along the serratus anterior muscle serving as its motor nerve. Dividing this nerve results in winging of the scapula. The thoracodorsal bundle with its artery, vein, and nerve enters the latissimus dorsi muscle after coursing diagonally downward through the axilla from medial to lateral. The thoracodorsal vein enters the axillary vein, while the thoracodorsal artery and nerve pass posterior to the axillary vein to their origins from the axillary artery and brachial plexus respectively. Injury to the thoracodorsal nerve will result in weakness of the latissimus dorsi muscle but few clinically evident symptoms. The medial pectoral nerve enters the posterior surface of the lateral portion of the pectoralis major muscle just inferior to the point where the axillary vein crosses the lateral border of the pectoralis major muscle. This confusing nomenclature, with the *medial* pectoral nerve entering the *lateral* portion of the muscle, results from the nerve being named for its origin at the medial cord of the brachial plexus. Dividing this nerve during an axillary dissection will result in partial atrophy of the pectoralis major muscle. The intercostal-brachial nerve runs from anterior to posterior across the axilla more or less parallel to the axillary vein and 1 to 2 cm inferior to it. Division of this nerve during axillary dissection will result in anesthesia of the medial portion of the upper arm.

Any of these structures may be involved by metastatic disease within the axilla, although symptoms arise most commonly from compression of the axillary vein or obstruction of lymphatics, either of which can result in swelling of the affected arm.

Lymphedema may also appear after surgical dissection or radiation of the axilla, presumably from progressive scarring and obstruction of the lymphatics draining the arm. To reduce the possibility of this disabling complication, axillary dissection is generally limited to levels I and II, and axillary irradiation is combined with surgery only when specific clinical circumstances demand both modalities. Lymphedema may appear within the first year following surgery or radiation of the axilla, or may have a delayed onset and appear 5 to10 years after treatment of the axilla.

It has been postulated that lymphedema may also result from progressive scarring from repeated infections or inflammation of the ipsilateral arm. Although this mechanism is not clear, patients are admonished to avoid trauma, including phlebotomy, intravenous lines, and other breaks in the skin of the ipsilateral arm which follow axillary dissection for breast cancer.

RISK FACTORS FOR BREAST CANCER

Clinical observations have identified subgroups of women at increased risk for breast carcinoma relative to the general population.[84] Known risk factors include increasing age; genetic and other factors related to a family history of breast cancer[155,159]; hormonal and reproductive factors including early menarche, late menopause, late first pregnancy or nulliparity, and use of exogenous hormones[29,38,84,115,126,163,164,185]; environmental factors including dietary factors and the lifestyle of developed Western nations[6,92,183]; certain pathologic findings within breast tissue that include prior breast cancer and other premalignant lesions[60,132]; and certain other malignancies, such as ovarian and endometrial carcinomas. Recognition of these risk factors allows for appropriate screening and clinical management of the individual patient.

Taking into account various combinations of risk factors, several mathematical models have been developed to quantify a woman's risk of breast cancer relative to that of the general population.[27,61] These models may be useful in counseling a woman as to her degree of risk and in determining appropriate follow-up. It is important to recognize, however, that many women who develop breast cancer have no known risk factors. The absence of risk factors should not prevent full evaluation or biopsy or a suspicious breast lesion.

Age

The risk of developing breast cancer increases in a nearly linear fashion with increasing age. While a woman's annual risk of developing breast cancer is only 1 in 5900 at age 30, it rises to 1 in 590 by age 50, and 1 in 330 by age 70.[166] Approximately 75% to 80% of breast cancers are diagnosed in women over the age of 50.[130,165]

Genetics and family history

It has long been recognized that breast cancers cluster in some families. Relatives of women diagnosed with breast cancer have a higher incidence of the disease than does the average population. Risk is highest when there are multiple affected relatives, when the relatives are more closely related, such as a mother or sister versus an aunt or grandmother, when the age of onset in relatives is young, and when there are relatives with bilateral breast cancer. Even the presence of a third-degree relative with breast cancer can increase an individual's risk.[159] It has been thought that genetic transmission from relatives on the maternal side contributes more risk than the paternal side, although this has been questioned.

Several genetic syndromes have been identified that are associated with a markedly increased risk for development of breast carcinoma. These include the Li-Fraumeni syndrome in which breast and other malignancies including brain, lung, lymphoma, and sarcomas develop at an early age. It has been recognized that this syndrome is caused by germline mutations of the p53 tumor suppressor gene.[107] Germline p53 mutations are thought to account for only 1% of all breast cancers, although many breast cancers will develop somatic p53 mutations during tumor progression. Deletions of chromosome 17 in the q21-23 region have been identified in families with clustering of breast and ovarian cancers, which suggest the presence of a tumor suppressor gene in this area.[76,124] Tentatively named BRCA-1 for "breast cancer gene 1", this 17q-linked gene is being actively studied in several laboratories. It is hoped that germline mutations in this gene will prove relevant to a large proportion of hereditary and perhaps sporadic breast cancers. It has been postulated that this gene may be mutated in 1 in 200 American women, and that a mutated gene confers an 85% lifetime risk of breast cancer and a 65% lifetime risk of ovarian carcinoma.[59] Cowden's disease, a syndrome which produces multiple pathognomonic cutaneous trichilemmomas, is associated with an increased rate of breast cancer that is frequently bilateral.[18] Cowden's disease appears to be inherited as an autosomal dominant pattern and probably accounts for less than 1% of breast carcinomas.

It is important to recognize that family history may interact with other risk factors, and that individuals in families share both genetics and environment. It has been noted that there is an interaction between family history and other risk factors such as body fat distribution, parity and age at first pregnancy,[155] exogenous hormone use,[164] and histologic risk factors.[132]

Histopathologic factors

Certain histopathologic findings are associated with an increased risk of future development of breast carcinoma. Women who have had breast cancer are at increased risk of developing a new breast cancer. This risk is approximately 1% per year and plateaus with a cumulative lifetime risk in the range of 15%. Women with a diagnosis of lobular carcinoma in situ (LCIS) have a 20% to 25% chance of developing an invasive breast carcinoma, usually of ductal histology, over the next 20 to 30 years.[60,132] This risk is equally distributed over both the biopsied and contralateral breasts. An increase in risk of future breast cancer is also seen in women with biopsies showing either atypical ductal hyperplasia or atypical lobular hyperplasia. This risk is in the range of 15% over the next 15 to 20 years, and like LCIS, the risk is equally distributed over both breasts. A small but measurable increase in breast cancer risk is seen in women with proliferative fibrocystic disease without atypia. Nonproliferative fibrocystic disease and simple cysts do not increase the risk of breast cancer.[132]

Dietary and environmental factors

Differences in breast cancer incidence in different countries has led to the speculation that dietary factors influence breast cancer risk. Although some studies have shown a weak association between higher dietary fat intake and increased risk of breast cancer,[87,88] the majority of studies have failed to show an association between fat intake and breast cancer risk.[67,95,99,119,183] These studies do not rule out the possibility that the timing of fat intake, for example fat intake early in life, may influence risk of breast cancer, or that extremely low fat diets may reduce risk. High dietary fiber intake does not appear to reduce breast cancer risk.[183] Women with diets significantly deficient in vitamin A were found to have an increased risk of breast cancer, although diets rich in vitamin A did not reduce the risk of breast cancer. No association was seen between vitamin E or C intake and breast cancer risk.[92] Higher alcohol intakes have been associated with an increased risk, although the mechanism for this association is not clear.[89,184] Recent reports have raised the issue of an increased risk of breast cancer among women exposed to electromagnetic fields,[109] but the methodology of these studies has been severely criticized.[171]

Hormonal and reproductive factors

It has been observed that hormonal and reproductive factors are related to the risk of breast cancer.[84,115,126] Women whose menarche is at or before age 11 have an increased risk of breast cancer relative to those whose menarche is at age 14 or later. Menopause after age 55 also is associated with an increase in breast cancer risk. A full-term pregnancy before age 30 reduces breast cancer risk, while nullliparity or a first pregnancy after age 30 is associated with an increased risk. The mechanism by which age at first birth influences risk is not known, but there may be differentiation of breast tissue at term that permanently reduces risk. There may be a slight reduction of breast cancer risk with increasing parity, although not all studies support this. Lactation for long periods may decrease risk, although this reduction may apply only to premenopausal breast cancer and possibly has no effect on the risk of postmenopausal breast cancer.[126]

Oral contraceptives and breast cancer

Current data suggest that there is no significantly increased risk of breast cancer among women who have used oral contraceptives. A recent meta-analysis of studies examining the possible influence of oral contraceptive use on breast cancer risk found no increase in risk among all those women who had used oral contraceptives when compared with nonusers.[147] However, this analysis found a higher risk of premenopausal breast cancer in women who had used oral contraceptives for a prolonged period of time before their first pregnancy.[147,185] Some of this increased risk observed with prolonged oral contraceptive use before the first pregnancy may actually reflect a delayed first pregnancy or an early menarche, both of which are accepted risk factors for breast carcinoma.[115] However, in view of this potentially increased risk of breast cancer, it would be prudent to avoid early and prolonged oral contraceptive use in young nulliparous women unless they are sexually active and wish to avoid pregnancy.[84]

Postmenopausal hormone replacement therapy and risk of breast cancer

Hormone replacement therapy provides many benefits to postmenopausal women. Estrogens relieve many of the troubling symptoms of menopause and appear to have a favorable effect on the cardiovascular system and on bone density. However, hormone replacement therapy carries with it an increased risk of other problems that include thromboembolic disease, endometrial carcinoma, and potentially breast carcinoma. The balance between risks and benefits for women as a group and for individual patients has been the source of much recent discussion.

A review of overall mortality among users and nonusers of postmenopausal hormone replacement showed a statistically significant decrease in mortality from all causes (relative risk 0.80, $p < 0.0001$) among users versus nonusers of hormone replacement therapy. This benefit seemed to be derived mainly from a reduction in mortality from acute myocardial infarction (relative risk 0.60, $p < 0.001$), but there was also a trend toward decreased mortality from ischemic heart disease, stroke, and cancer of any type.[83]

When breast cancer risk is analyzed separately from other causes of morbidity and mortality, there is a trend toward increased risk of breast cancer among women using hormone replacement therapy. There has been disagreement among studies as to the degree and magnitude of breast cancer risk associated with hormone replacement therapy and whether individual subgroups of women at higher risk could be identified.

A recent meta-analysis of breast cancer risk and hormone replacement therapy found an approximately 10% overall increase in breast cancer risk among women using hormone replacement therapy relative to nonusers.[38] This value was of questionable statistic significance. This analysis also concluded that there was no increase of breast cancer risk in women using conjugated estrogens at dosages higher than 0.625 mg/day. Another meta-analysis used only studies that met certain criteria and found a relative risk of 1.3 for breast cancer among women using hormone replacement therapy for more than 15 years when compared with nonusers.[164] Breast cancer risk was also found to be significantly higher among hormone users with a family history of breast carcinoma with a relative risk of 3.4, when compared to users without a family history of breast carcinoma. A Swedish cohort study found that risk increased with duration of use and showed an increased risk of breast cancer among users of hormone replacement therapy after 9 years of use.[10] The Nurses' Health study found an increase in breast cancer risk among current users of postmenopausal estrogen replacement therapy after prolonged use.[29] However, there was no increased risk of breast cancer seen among previous users of hormone replacement therapy. This suggested that the effect of estrogen on breast cancer risk may be reversible as risks appeared to return to baseline nonuser levels within 2 to 3 years of cessation of hormone replacement therapy.

The addition of progestins to estrogen replacement therapy, while decreasing the risk of endometrial carcinoma, may in fact increase the risk of breast carcinoma.[10] Analysis of breast cancer risk with postmenopausal estrogen use, when combined with other potential breast cancer risk factors, identified certain subsets of patients with significantly increased risk. In addition to a significantly increased risk among women with a family history of breast cancer (relative risk 3.4), an increased risk was also identified among users of hormone replacement therapy who were nulliparous (relative risk 1.5), those with benign breast disease (relative risk 1.7), and among those whose first pregnancy was after age 30 (relative risk 1.7).[164]

Some series have suggested that although the risk of breast cancer is higher among women using hormone replacement therapy, the cancers that arise are detected at an earlier stage and may have a more favorable prognosis.[62,63,163] With longer follow-up, a survival advantage was seen among hormone users who developed breast cancers over nonusers.[62,63] This early detection and its favorable outcome were attributed at least in part to increased patient and physician awareness of the risk of breast cancer and increased access to medical care among hormone users as compared to non-users. It is also possible that estrogen use may select for a different, more favorable type of breast cancer.

Summary

For most women on postmenopausal hormone replacement therapy there appears to be a significant reduction in mortality from all causes, primarily through a reduction in deaths from cardiovascular disease. There also seems to be reasonable evidence that there is a modest increase in the risk of breast cancer associated with postmenopausal hormone replacement therapy, which amounts to an approximately 10% increase in risk for the average woman. The increase in risk may be substantially higher for women with a family history of breast carcinoma or those with other breast cancer risk factors. In clinical practice, it would seem prudent to weigh the individual woman's cardiovascular and perhaps osteoporosis risks against her preexisting risks for breast carcinoma before making a decision about the use of postmenopausal estrogens.

For postmenopausal women with multiple risk factors for breast carcinoma, or for those who are reluctant to increase their breast cancer risk in any way, it may be prudent to deal with cardiovascular and osteoporosis risks through exercise, diet, and other nonhormonal means rather than through hormone replacement therapy. It has been suggested that tamoxifen, which has been successfully used in the treatment of breast cancer, behaves as both an estrogen agonist and antagonist. Tamoxifen appears to have a favorable effect on the lipid profile, on cardiovascular disease mortality, and on bone density.[48] Review of its use has also suggested a slight decrease in contralateral breast cancers among women using tamoxifen after a first breast cancer.[48] These observations have led to the ongoing NSABP Tamoxifen Trial to determine whether tamoxifen can provide cardiovascular and bone benefits while decreasing breast cancer risk for high risk women.

WORKUP OF THE PATIENT WITH A BREAST PROBLEM

Benign breast disease is an extremely common problem among American women, and its symptoms are the chief complaint of many women presenting to their gynecologists. Many additional breast abnormalities are discovered during the course of routine physical examination and mammography. The management of these benign problems is often difficult, and even more important, it may be difficult to distinguish benign breast lesions from malignant lesions. Mammography fails to detect 10% to 15% of all palpable malignant lesions.

Breast problems seen commonly in clinical practice fall into several categories: discrete palpable masses, vague thickening or nodularity, breast pain, nipple discharge, abnormalities during pregnancy or lactation, mammographic abnormalities, and the persistently worried patient with a negative workup. These will be dealt with in the sections which follow, and the associated pathologic entities will be described. From a risk management perspective and for good medical practice, it is important to document any recommendations for mammography, ultrasonography, biopsy, referral, or follow-up interval in the patient's chart. It is also good practice to discuss these recommendations with the patient herself.

A proper evaluation of any breast problem requires a detailed history of the presenting complaint, a review of prior breast problems, a review of risk factors for breast carcinoma, a thorough physical examination of the breasts, appropriate imaging studies, and an evaluation of the patient's general medical condition.

Pertinent history

A history should be taken that includes documentation of the current breast problem, documentation of risk factors for breast carcinoma, and any history of other breast diseases as listed in Table 10-1. The history should first include a complete description of the patient's chief complaint. The patient is asked to describe when the problem was first identified and whether it was identified by self examination, by a physician on routine examination, or by screening mammography. If there are any physical findings, the patient should be asked if the area in question is tender to palpation. Changes in the size or tenderness of any palpable abnormalities since their initial discovery and any changes in the menstrual cycle should be recorded. The patient should also be asked if she has had similar symptoms at any time in the past. Any prior breast problems or breast surgery should be documented, and pathology reports from any prior breast surgery should be obtained. Any prior evaluation of the problem by another health care professional

Table 10-1. Breast-specific medical history

Current age
Race
Age at menarche
Date of last menstrual period/age of menopause
Parity
Age at first pregnancy
Lactation history
Use of oral contraceptives, years of use before first pregnancy
Use of postmenopausal estrogen replacement
Use of other hormones, fertility regimens, DES
Family history of breast cancer, age at diagnosis
Family history of ovarian cancer, age at diagnosis
Family history of other cancers, age at diagnosis
Dates of prior mammograms
Prior breast biopsies and pathologic findings
Other prior breast surgery
Prior personal cancer history
Prior breast problems

should be described and if possible, documentation of the visits obtained. All imaging studies that have been performed to date should be obtained; the reports and the films themselves should be reviewed.

The next section of the history should detail portions of the medical history pertinent to breast cancer risk and include menstrual history, reproductive factors, and hormone exposures. Age at menarche, and if applicable, menopause is recorded. For menstruating women the date of the last menstrual period is recorded. The number of pregnancies and the age at first term pregnancy is determined. Duration of lactation should be recorded. Any use of exogenous hormones is recorded and should include oral contraceptives and years of use before the first term pregnancy, postmenopausal estrogen replacement therapy, and use of any other sex hormones as part of a fertility program or for other purposes. Any family history of breast cancer should be detailed and include at least first-, second-, and third-degree relatives, and the age at diagnosis of the family members. Ovarian cancer in the family should be recorded with age at diagnosis, as should other cancers, particularly those that affected family members at a young age. Any cancer syndromes affecting the family should be recorded. Any personal history of cancer should be recorded with particular attention to prior breast, ovarian, or endometrial cancers. Prior radiation exposures, especially to the chest wall, should be noted.

An overview of the general medical history should be obtained as for any surgical patient and should include current medications, allergies, tobacco and alcohol use, previous surgery of any type, any medical problems, and a brief social history.

Physical examination

Physical examination of the breasts includes inspection of the skin, palpation of the breasts, examination of the nipples for discharge, and palpation of the axillary and supraclavicular node areas. The breasts should be inspected with the patient sitting with her hands behind her head and her elbows back to look for asymmetry, dimpling of the skin, and any areas of erythema or edema. Taking care to include the subaveolar area, the breast should then be palpated and examined systematically from the clavicle to below the inframammary fold and from the sternum to the posterior axillary line. Examination should be performed first with the fingers flat and together using the region between the DIP and PIP joints of the examining hand to press breast tissue back against the ribs looking for masses, areas of thickening, or tenderness. Any questionable areas are then examined in more detail using the fingertips. Examination of both breasts is performed with the patient both supine and sitting. If an abnormal area is identified, a careful description of its size, contour, texture, tenderness, and position should be recorded. A diagram of the lesion is extremely useful for future reference.

The nipples and areolae are best examined with the patient in the supine position and first inspected for any areas of skin breakdown and then squeezed gently to check for discharge. The number and position of any ducts from which discharge is obtained should be documented. The color of the discharge, whether milky, green, yellow, clear, brown, or bloody and its consistency, whether watery, sticky, or thick should be noted. Of most concern is spontaneous, single duct discharge, or any discharge which is bloody. If a discharge is identified on one side, a careful search for a discharge on the other side is important because unilateral, single duct discharge is much more likely to be pathologic and bilateral multiple duct discharge physiologic. Any discharge identified should be tested for occult blood. Cytology of nipple discharge adds expense and rarely adds to the clinical examination in determining the need for biopsy.

The axillary nodes are examined using the examiner's left hand for the right axilla and right hand for the left axilla. The fingers are pressed inward and upward checking for enlarged nodes. In the supine position the shoulder muscles may be relaxed to facilitate the examination by having the patient rest her elbow at her side, or by the examiner supporting the arm with the patient's hand reaching across her body toward her opposite shoulder. In the sitting position the shoulder muscles may be relaxed by the examiner supporting the patient's elbow with one hand while examining the axillary nodes with the other. Supraclavicular nodes may be examined in the supine or sitting position. Should any enlarged nodes be discovered, their size, mobility, and number should be recorded. Any matting of nodes or fixation of nodes to the chest wall is significant and should be noted. Tenderness of enlarged nodes, which may be more suggestive of a reactive process, should be noted.

Imaging studies

Mammography. Although current recommendations state that a baseline screening mammogram need not be performed until age 40, and there is discussion as to whether this should be delayed until age 50, it is reasonable to perform a mammogram for any woman over 35 years of age with a palpable breast mass or with other specific symptoms. Approximately 4% to 5% of breast cancers occur in women under the age of 40 and 25% in women under the age of 50.[130,165] By age 35 and in the presence of a palpable lesion or other abnormality, there is a reasonable probability of finding additional mammographic abnormalities elsewhere in the symptomatic breast or in the opposite breast that would influence management of the presenting problem. However, it must also be remembered that mammography fails to detect 10% to 15% of all malignant lesions. It is least accurate for lobular carcinoma and in those women who have radiographically dense breast tissue.

It is therefore essential to emphasize that a negative mammogram should not influence the decision to biopsy a clinically palpable lesion. Mammography is performed to look for synchronous lesions or nonpalpable calcifications surrounding the palpable abnormality and not to rule out the need for biopsy of the palpable lesion.

The primary value of diagnostic mammography is early detection of breast cancers when they are not clinically evident and when the incidence of nodal spread is significantly lower. In addition, there are certain mammographic features that are strongly suggestive of benign breast disease. Breast compression is necessary to decrease the depth of tissue that must be penetrated and to reduce the dose necessary to obtain an adequate image. When obtaining mammograms at least two views of both breasts are recommended. These should include a mediolateral view of the breast and a craniocaudal view that should be obtained at approximately right angles to the mediolateral view. For the craniocaudal view, the x-ray beam enters the top of the breast and exits to the detector that is underneath the breast. In women with large breasts or breasts that are difficult to evaluate, additional views may be obtained.

Ultrasonography. The primary value of ultrasonography at the present time is in distinguishing cystic from solid lesions. While this distinction is best made for palpable lesions by direct needle aspiration, which is both diagnostic and therapeutic, for nonpalpable lesions ultrasonography can prove the cystic nature of a lesion and can eliminate the need for additional workup or treatment. Although it was initially hoped that ultrasonography would serve as a useful screening tool, it has been found to be totally inadequate for this purpose. Ultrasound does not detect calcifications and also fails to detect a large number of malignancies. In addition, ultrasound identifies a great deal of normal breast texture as potential nodules and produces false-positive readings.

Ultrasound is also useful for directing fine-needle or core biopsy of lesions that are visualized, as manipulation and positioning of the needle can be performed in real time and directly confirmed.

The use of advanced ultrasound technology, including Doppler imaging, for diagnostic purposes in the breast is currently being explored. It has been suggested that detailed analysis of the contour and internal echo texture of a solid lesion can be used to classify lesions as having a very low or very high probability of malignancy. In addition, the vascular pattern seen with Doppler ultrasound may also be of use in distinguishing benign from malignant lesions; greater vessel density and a more chaotic vessel pattern are seen with malignancies.

MANAGEMENT OF SPECIFIC BREAST PROBLEMS

Discrete palpable masses

Discrete masses, or those that are clearly different from surrounding normal breast tissue, may be either solid or cystic. Distinguishing between these two possibilities is important.[36] Cysts are almost always benign and rarely require more than aspiration. Solid masses, on the other hand, require that a tissue diagnosis be obtained to rule out malignancy. Clinical examination is not accurate in distinguishing a cyst from a solid mass. Rosner and Baird found that physical examination correctly identified only 58% of 66 palpable cysts.[151]

Cysts. A palpable mass suspected of being a cyst should be confirmed as such by aspiration, even if previously shown to be a simple cyst by ultrasound. This aspiration confirms that the palpable mass corresponds to the lesion seen on ultrasound. Removal of the mass by aspiration also permits a more thorough examination of the surrounding breast tissue. Bloody cyst fluid or a persistent mass after aspiration is worrisome for malignancy, and the aspirated fluid should be sent for cytologic analysis.[77] Biopsy is generally indicated in this setting even if the cytologic analysis is negative for malignancy. If the cyst fluid is not bloody and no mass remains after aspiration, there is little chance of malignancy, and the fluid need not be sent for cytology. Ciatto et al found no malignancies among 6747 nonbloody cyst aspirations.[24]

If a cyst is aspirated without prior ultrasonography documentation that it was a simple cyst, the patient should be reexamined in 4 to 8 weeks. Fewer than 20% of simple cysts will recur after a single aspiration, and fewer than 9% will recur after two or three aspirations.[106] When the same cyst recurs rapidly after aspiration, it should be reaspirated and the cyst contents sent for cytologic analysis. A biopsy should be performed if the cytology is suspicious or if the cyst recurs. Appearance of a new cyst in a different area of breast tissue, however, does not require this additional workup and should be evaluated and aspirated as a new problem. Additional cysts may be expected in more than half of the patients.[90]

Solid masses. Discrete masses within the breast that are solid, either by ultrasonography criteria or by failing to yield fluid on aspiration attempts, require a tissue diagnosis to exclude malignancy. Physical examination alone correctly identifies a mass as malignant in only 60% to 85% of cases.[14,103] Experienced examiners often disagree on the need for biopsy of a particular lesion. Boyd et al found that four surgeons uniformly agreed on the need for biopsy of only 73% of 15 palpable masses later shown on biopsy to be malignant.[14]

Before biopsy it is appropriate to order a mammogram in a woman over 35 years of age to look for synchronous lesions.

Vague thickening or nodularity

Normal breast texture is often heterogenous, particularly in premenopausal women. These variations in texture may create areas that feel firmer than the surrounding tissue and may or may not be tender to the touch. These vague thickenings or areas of nodularity are quite common and must be distinguished from a true mass.

In clinical practice, areas of nodularity or thickening first should be compared with the corresponding area of the opposite breast for symmetry. Symmetric areas of thickening are rarely pathologic. Asymmetric areas, particularly those that are tender, often represent fibrocystic disease and will often resolve spontaneously. For premenopausal women, such vague areas should be reexamined after one or two menstrual cycles. If the asymmetry resolves, the finding was most likely a result of a benign process such as a fibrocystic condition. Areas of asymmetry which persist, however, must be viewed with some suspicion. Such patients should be referred to a surgeon for evaluation and potential biopsy. It is appropriate to order a mammogram to rule out synchronous lesions at this point for any woman over 35 years of age who has not had a mammogram in the past 6 months. The value of a negative, fine-needle aspiration biopsy of a vague thickening rather than a discrete mass is unclear. Open biopsy is generally required for adequate sampling.

Breast pain

Breast pain, also termed mastalgia, is one of the most common breast symptoms experienced by women of reproductive age, and brings many women to their physicians.[143,144,186] Often the concern is not about the severity of the pain but rather that the pain indicates a more serious condition such as breast cancer. Physiologic breast tenderness varies with the menstrual cycle; greatest tenderness is felt immediately before the menstrual period. In contrast, noncyclic pain bears no relationship to the menstrual cycle, and its cause is unknown. The pain may be intermittent or continuous and is often described by the patient as "burning". Although breast pain is poorly understood, its cyclic nature and resolution at menopause suggest a hormonal cause. Several studies that have measured estrogen levels in women with breast pain have shown no difference in circulating hormone levels compared with pain-free controls. On the other hand, it has been postulated that progesterone levels may be decreased in women with breast pain. In addition, several studies have demonstrated that the administration of thyrotrophin-releasing factor resulted in a large increase in prolactin release in a large group of women with breast pain compared with asymptomatic controls.[180]

While pain is rarely caused by a breast cancer, evaluation of the patient with breast pain first requires that malignancy be ruled out. A careful physical examination should be performed, and any palpable masses should be evaluated as described above. A mammogram should be performed in any woman over the age of 35 with persistent, noncyclic breast pain. It is also important to rule out causes of pain that do not arise from the breast itself, which include muscle strain, costochondritis, and pain of pleural or mediastinal origin. Once these less common causes of pain are excluded, attempts should be made to differentiate between cyclic and noncyclic breast pain.

For the majority of women presenting with breast pain, reassurance that the workup has shown no evidence of breast cancer or other serious abnormality is the only treatment necessary. The patient may also be reassured that breast pain is usually self-limited, often resolving within a few months. During the periods of more severe breast tenderness, symptomatic relief may be obtained with nonnarcotic analgesics, in particular nonsteroidal antiinflammatory agents. Maneuvers such as the elimination of caffeine, chocolate, or salt from the diet, while harmless, are of no proven benefit. It is often useful to reexamine the patient after one or two menstrual cycles to be sure that no palpable abnormality is evolving and to assess her response to conservative treatment.

For the rare patient whose breast pain is severe and unresponsive to conservative measures, pharmacologic therapy may be instituted. Danazol, a gonadotropin inhibitor, is the only drug approved by the Food and Drug Administration in the United States for the treatment of breast pain.[7,102] It has androgenic effects that many patients find unacceptable. Other pharmacologic agents that have been used to treat breast pain include bromocryptine (a prolactin antagonist) and tamoxifen.[46,113] Evening primrose oil has been reported to produce significant or complete pain relief in half of the women with cyclic mastalgia.[135] The oil is obtained from the evening primrose flower and is extremely high in polyunsaturated oils. The oil is ingested orally and has few side effects. Evening primrose oil is now available in the United States and can be purchased at most health food stores.

Nipple discharge and other nipple and areolar pathology

Nipple discharge. A small amount of nipple discharge may be expressed from the nipples of as many as 60% to 70% of healthy women.[140] This is usually yellow to green in color, observed only with attempts to express it rather than spontaneously, and present bilaterally. This is distinguished from galactorrhea, bilateral, often spontaneous, milky discharge that is almost never caused by a breast malignancy. Galactorrhea may be distinguished from physiologic discharge under the microscope by the presence of fat in the secretions. As many as one third of women with galactorrhea will have pituitary tumors, particularly if there is associated amenorrhea. Hypothyroidism may also cause galactorrhea. Other causes of galactorrhea include chest wall trauma and certain pharmacologic agents. The evaluation of galactorrhea includes measurement of serum prolactin concentration and thyroid function tests. If the prolactin level is elevated, an MRI scan of the head with attention to the sella tursica should be performed to rule out a pituitary adenoma.

Unilateral nipple discharge or nipple discharge that is bloody, watery, or sticky may be an indicator of malignancy and should be evaluated further.[21,35,169] A careful physical examination should be performed to identify any palpable masses present, and a mammogram performed for women over 35 years of age. Cytologic analysis is rarely useful because surgical evaluation is required whether the cytology is positive or negative. Ductograms are generally not useful for the same reason; they rarely provide data that change the need for surgery or the surgical procedure performed. Excision of the discharging duct is performed to rule out malignancy.[136,173]

Other nipple and areolar pathology. Erosion or chronic crusting of the nipple raises the suspicion of Paget's disease of the nipple, a variant of infiltrating or intraductal carcinoma arising in the terminal ducts and involving the surface of the nipple itself. A biopsy is required to distinguish Paget's disease from benign dermatologic conditions such as eczema that may also involve the nipple and areola. Subareolar infections are described in the section which follows.

Breast infections

Infections of the breast fall into three general categories: lactational infections, chronic subareolar infections associated with duct ectasia, and other nonlactational abscesses.

Infections and abscesses may occur during lactation and are often associated with periods of weaning or other times when engorgement occurs. Often there is associated breakdown of the skin of the nipple. It is thought that the nursing infant may be the source of recurrent colonization of the nipple which makes weaning necessary. Early-stage infections are treated with oral antibiotics to cover gram-positive cocci, warm soaks, and active attempts to keep the breast emptied, particularly the affected area of the breast. Weaning is not necessary during treatment of these infections, and the infant is not adversely affected by nursing from the breast with the infection.[9,127] Once an abscess forms, however, surgical drainage and weaning are usually required.

Abscesses of the lactating breast only rarely form fluctuant masses because of the network of fibrous septa within the breast.[9] The diagnosis is established by the clinical picture of fever, leukocytosis, and exquisite point tenderness in the breast. The abscesses that form are multiloculated, and all loculations must be broken up to assure resolution of the infection. Needle aspiration of lactating breast abscesses is therefore not adequate. General anesthetic is almost always required for adequate pain relief during drainage of these abscesses as a result of the tenderness of the affected area and the amount of manipulation required to break up the loculated abscess cavity. The cavity should be packed open as for any abscess and weaning is required.

In women who are not lactating, the subareolar ducts of the breast may develop a chronic relapsing form of infection variously known as periductal mastitis or duct ectasia. The subareolar terminal ducts become thinned and filled with secretions. A series of infections with resulting inflammatory changes and scarring may ensue and result in retraction or inversion of the nipple, masses in the subareolar area, recurrent periareolar abscesses, and occasionally a chronic infectious fistula from the subareolar ducts to the periareolar skin.[136,161] Palpable masses and mammographic changes that mimic carcinoma may result. It is not clear whether a chronic infection causes the observed thinning and dilatation of the subareolar ducts or whether the dilatation and accumulation of secretions is the primary event followed by secondary bacterial infection of the accumulated secretions. The infections that result are most often mixed infections and include anaerobic skin flora.[17,177]

The treatment of infections related to duct ectasia or periductal mastitis in the acute phase is incision and drainage combined with antibiotics against skin flora and anaerobes. Antibiotic treatment is often unsuccessful unless anaerobic coverage is included. Repeated infections are treated by excision of the entire subareolar duct complex after the acute infection has completely resolved and with antibiotic coverage during the perioperative period. The need for drain placement is debated. Even with wide excision of the subareolar duct complex and intravenous antibiotic coverage, some patients will have recurrent infections. Excision of the nipple and areola will often resolve the problem for these patients.[73,173]

The nonlactating breast may occasionally develop abscesses or cellulitis related to breaks in the skin or rarely to a cyst that becomes infected. These infections are usually in the peripheral rather than subareolar breast tissues and are treated with antibiotics, warm soaks, and incision and drainage.

Breast abnormalities in pregnant or lactating women

The physical diagnosis of breast malignancy may be extremely difficult in the setting of pregnancy or lactation. While engorgement or diffuse thickening of the breasts may be expected with pregnancy or lactation, distinct masses, asymmetric tissue, or any area of persistent concern to the patient should be evaluated promptly without waiting for delivery or the elective cessation of lactation. Such patients should be referred promptly to a surgeon for evaluation and possible biopsy.

Mammography is generally not performed during pregnancy because of the density of breast tissue and low mammographic sensitivity and because of concern about radiation for the fetus. Mammographic sensitivity is also poor during lactation and for 3 to 4 months following cessation of breast feeding and generally adds little to the evaluation of a palpable mass. Ultrasonography may distinguish cystic from solid lesions as in nonpregnant women but is not useful for screening.

Biopsy can be performed without difficulty during pregnancy. Fine-needle aspiration biopsy can be performed as a first step in many patients. Open biopsy with local anesthetic is well tolerated, and there are usually no difficulties with healing. Unless the lesion is immediately beneath the areola, subsequent breast feeding is usually possible.

In women who are breast feeding, transient plugging of the ducts must be distinguished from true masses. There is usually no difficulty distinguishing a mass from mastitis or an abscess—tenderness and fever make the diagnosis clear. Any persistent mass or residual mass after drainage of a plugged duct or an episode of mastitis should be evaluated. As with any other persistent breast mass, there should be a low threshold for obtaining a tissue diagnosis, either with fine-needle aspiration or with open biopsy. In approximately half of the lactating women who have open biopsy the incision will heal without having to stop breast feeding. The remaining half, however, will develop a milk fistula at their incision and will have to stop breast feeding before the incision will heal.

The causes of breast masses during pregnancy include all the common breast lesions of premenopausal women and include fibroadenomas, fibrocystic change, fibrosis, and occasionally breast carcinoma. Lactating adenomas are benign lesions that grossly resemble fibroadenomas and may also be seen during pregnancy.

Nonpalpable mammographic abnormalities

The widespread practice of mammographic screening has led to an increase in the number of nonpalpable lesions identified by mammography. The most recent survey by the American College of Surgeons' Commission on Cancer found that 56.1% of breast cancers detected in 1990 had an abnormal screening mammogram as one of the presenting complaints, up from 29.6% in 1983.[130] Two thirds of the cancers detected by mammogram in 1990 had no abnormality on physical examination.

The majority of abnormal mammographic findings, however, will be benign. Mammographers have developed a series of criteria by which they grade their suspicion for a malignancy.[25,75,121,156] There have been recent moves to standardize terminology for mammographic findings. In general, the practicing clinician will rely upon the recommendation of the mammographer for biopsy or follow-up.

Different mammographers set different thresholds for recommending biopsy of a mammographic lesion. On average in the United States, 15% to 30% of mammographic lesions for which biopsy is recommended prove to be malignant.[75] Some authors, however, advocate a lower threshold for biopsy, one in which 10% of the lesions recommended for biopsy would prove to be malignant, in order to minimize the chance of missing an early malignancy.[121,187]

It is clearly desirable to minimize the number of benign biopsies prompted by mammographic screening while detecting as many early stage malignancies as possible. Studies have been conducted to assess the effectiveness and safety of close mammographic follow-up of "probably benign" findings. Biopsy is then reserved for lesions which change and become more suspicious during follow-up. The initial determination that the lesion is probably benign takes into account the patient's breast cancer risk factors including personal history of breast cancer, family history, and current physical examination. Sickles reported prospective follow-up of 3184 consecutive "probably benign" mammographic abnormalities on a protocol obtaining repeat mammograms at 6 months after the initial finding, 6 to 12 months later, then annually for two more examinations.[157] Seventeen (0.5%) of these 3184 probable lesions subsequently proved malignant on biopsy: 15 were detected as a change in the mammographic appearance of the lesion, and two were detached as palpable findings. All malignancies were under 2 cm and two were purely in situ, but two had one positive lymph node each. Two smaller series found 0.6% and 1.1% rates of malignancy in mammographic lesions followed as "probably benign".[82,187] Employing this policy of serial mammographic examination of probably benign findings, authors were able to eliminate a number of benign biopsies; approximately 40% of lesions recommended for biopsy proved to be malignant.[82,157]

These results support the balanced use of mammographic follow-up and biopsy to minimize the morbidity, monetary, and psychologic costs of benign biopsies prompted by mammographic screening. In general, if the mammographer recommends that a lesion identified by mammography be removed, a biopsy should be performed. The decision for follow-up versus biopsy of an equivocal mammographic finding should be made by the mammographer and the patient's clinician and take the patient's overall situation, including breast cancer risk into consideration. It is appropriate to refer such a patient to a surgeon for a second opinion about management.

Nonpalpable cysts detected by mammography and ultrasonography and shown to be *simple* cysts (i.e., without debris or ragged walls) need not be aspirated except for relief of pain.

Management of high risk patients

A woman's risk of breast cancer may be increased as a result of family history, prior personal history of breast cancer, personal history of atypia on biopsy, or for other reasons as described above. At present there are three treatment options for such women: close surveillance, prophylactic mastectomy, or chemoprophylaxis such as the NSABP Tamoxifen Trial.

The option of close surveillance is most often chosen. For women with a prior diagnosis of breast cancer, surveillance protocols are based upon the stage of their initial tumor. For women with lobular carcinoma in situ, atypical hyperplasia, or a family history of breast carcinoma, surveillance should include twice yearly physical examinations by a physician. Mammography should be performed annually after diagnosis of LCIS or atypia. For women with a family history of breast cancer, annual mammography should begin at least 5 years before the age at diagnosis of the youngest affected relative and no later than age 35. For women from families with a cancer syndrome, annual screening should begin 10 years earlier than the age of the youngest affected relative.[111]

The persistently worried patient with a negative workup

There are certain patients who remain concerned about the possibility of having breast cancer despite a negative physical examination and mammogram. It is appropriate to refer such a patient to a surgeon for a second opinion.

BIOPSY TECHNIQUES

There are currently several options for obtaining a tissue diagnosis of a palpable breast mass or a mammographic abnormality: fine-needle aspiration, core-needle biopsy, and open surgical biopsy.

Fine-needle aspiration (FNA)

Fine-needle aspiration (FNA) using a 22- to 25-gauge needle may be performed with minimal patient discomfort at the time that a palpable mass is identified on physical examination. Mammography- or ultrasonography-guided FNA may also be performed for nonpalpable lesions. The false-negative rate of FNA ranges from 1% to 35% for palpable lesions and is as high as 68% for nonpalpable lesions.[37,68,78,103] The false-positive rate is generally in the 1% to 2% range but has been reported to be as high as 18% in some series.[78,103] The false-negative and false-positive rates at a given institution are clearly dependent upon both the technical quality of the aspiration itself and the experience of the cytopathologist interpreting the slides. In view of this false-negative rate, an equivocal diagnosis, nonspecific findings such as normal or fibrocystic breast tissue, or any atypical cytology should be evaluated further, usually with an open surgical biopsy.

Core-needle biopsy

A second, nonsurgical form of breast biopsy is core-needle biopsy. Core-needle biopsy obtains a 14- to18-gauge cylinder of tissue from the mass being sampled and is analyzed by conventional pathology rather than by cytology. As with FNA, the false-positive rate is very low. This technique is more uncomfortable for the patient than FNA because it entails the use of a much larger needle and requires that a small nick be made in the skin.

Recently, the development of stereotactic mammographic biopsy techniques has allowed the use of core-needle biopsy to sample nonpalpable lesions detected by mammography. In studies in which a series of mammographically detected lesions were first biopsied by a stereotactic core-needle technique and then excised with needle localization in the standard fashion, the false-negative rate of the stereotactic core technique ranged from 13% to 59%.[37,133,134] The false-negative rate is lower with 14-gauge biopsy needles than with 18-gauge needles.[133] This technique requires that the patient lie prone with her breast passing through an aperture in the table. Mammograms are taken 30° apart with the breast compressed and the three-dimensional coordinates of the lesion calculated. A nick is made in the skin and a 14-gauge biopsy gun advanced into the breast. Mammograms are again taken 30° apart to confirm the needle placement. The biopsy gun is then fired, and repeat mammogram views are taken to ensure that the needle has passed through the lesion. This process is repeated to obtain 4 to 5 core samples of the lesion. During the 30 to 60 minutes this process generally requires, the patient must lie absolutely still with her breast compressed to keep the lesion in the calculated position. There is clearly a learning curve for operators of this technique.[43]

If a malignancy is diagnosed by core-needle biopsy, a needle localization must still be performed to identify the lesion for definitive excision. Some advocates of this technique feel that this allows the surgeon to approach the lesion with the intention of obtaining wide margins. Opponents state that it is not clear how wide the margins should be after core-needle biopsy; the amount of ductal carcinoma in situ, the major determinant of the size of margin required is not fully assessed by core-needle biopsy. There are also reports of lesions found to be malignant by core-needle biopsy that later cannot be identified by mammography for definitive excision.[133] Because of these concerns, many surgeons are reluctant to apply the stereotactic core-needle biopsy technique to mammographic lesions that are suspicious for malignancy.

As is the case for FNA, any atypical or equivocal diagnosis on core-needle biopsy requires open surgical biopsy. The false- negative rate also raises the issue of whether a diagnosis of fibrocystic disease or normal breast tissue should be accepted, or whether open biopsy is necessary.

The cost of a stereotactic core-needle biopsy of a nonpalpable lesion is less than that of an open surgical biopsy in most institutions. Whether it will prove cost effective in the final analysis will depend on the false-negative biopsy rate as the procedure is used by more practitioners, the number of subsequent open biopsies required for equivocal core diagnoses, and physician and patient willingness to leave a mammographic lesion in place after core diagnosis.[93]

Open biopsy

Open surgical biopsy remains the standard for diagnosis of breast lesions, and unlike FNA or core-needle biopsy, has the advantage of removing the lesion and allowing the pathologist to perform a more complete analysis of the lesion, which includes analysis of margins and extent of intraductal disease if the lesion proves to be malignant. Cost, time, and patient discomfort are highest with this approach. For palpable lesions the surgeon should strive to excise the lesion with a narrow rim of normal-appearing breast tissue.

As the majority of breast masses prove to be benign, unnecessary distortion of the breast is avoided.

Nonpalpable lesions require preoperative wire localization by the mammographers to direct the surgeon to the appropriate area. This procedure requires that mammograms be taken in two projections to determine the three-dimensional location of the lesion. With the woman's breast still compressed in the same position, a needle is advanced through the calculated position of the lesion and repeat mammograms taken. A hooked or curved wire is then passed through the needle, and the needle is removed. A final pair of mammograms is taken to document the position of the lesion relative to the wire. The surgeon then removes a core of tissue around the wire so as to include the lesion with a rim of normal-appearing breast tissue. A specimen radiograph should be obtained before the patient leaves the operating room to be sure that the lesion is contained within the specimen.

Most biopsies, including needle-localized biopsy of nonpalpable lesions, are now performed with local anesthetic or local anesthetic with sedation; general anesthetic is reserved for special circumstances including the need for multiple biopsies. The previously standard approach of biopsy under a general anesthetic with frozen section diagnosis and immediate definitive cancer surgery has largely been abandoned. In addition to the logistic difficulties of this approach for both patient and surgeon, it has been shown that there is no improvement in survival or reduction in recurrence rates by performing definitive surgery on the same day as biopsy. Because there are now multiple treatment options for a woman with breast cancer, a staged approach allowing time for discussion of treatment options and decision-making after a diagnosis of malignancy is preferred.

Choice of biopsy technique

Once a decision has been made to biopsy a breast abnormality, it must be determined whether it should be biopsied by fine-needle aspiration, core-needle biopsy, stereotactic mammographic biopsy, or open surgical biopsy. Little is lost by performing a FNA or core biopsy in the office at the time of discovery of a palpable abnormality. As discussed above, however, the decision to biopsy a nonpalpable mammographic lesion by stereotactic core-needle biopsy versus needle-localized open biopsy is more complex and requires an understanding of the patient's risk of malignancy and a willingness to leave a mammographic lesion in place after sampling. The choice is therefore best made by the gynecologist or surgeon treating the patient, rather than the radiologist who first meets the patient at the time of her mammogram.

Analysis of tissue obtained at biopsy

In addition to routine histologic analysis, a number of additional tests that provide prognostic or therapeutic information are now routinely performed on malignant breast tissue.

Hormone receptor levels. Determination of estrogen and progesterone receptor levels in breast carcinomas is essential as these levels predict response to hormonal therapy. In addition, there has been some suggestion that estrogen receptor-positive tumors have a better prognosis than do receptor-negative tumors. Receptor levels may be determined by the measurement of cytosol receptor levels in fresh frozen tissue using a competitive binding assay, or by an immunohistochemical assay that uses a monoclonal antibody to bind to the receptor in fresh or fixed tissue samples. The immunohistochemical assay is being used with increasing frequency because it is applicable to even the smallest tumors, while the cytosol assay requires 300 to 500 mg of fresh frozen tissue.

DNA ploidy and S-phase fraction. It has been observed that malignant cells frequently contain aberrant amounts of DNA relative to normal cells. Such abnormal DNA levels are termed aneuploid as compared to normal or diploid DNA levels. S-phase refers to the fraction of cells within a population that are synthesizing DNA in preparation for cell division. This value is used to estimate the growth rate of a tumor. It has been suggested that breast cancers with a high S-phase fraction have a poorer prognosis than do tumors with a low S-phase fraction.

Both DNA content and S-phase fraction may be measured by flow cytometry. DNA content at present does not appear to be a good predictor of prognosis.

Molecular markers and other prognostic factors. As molecular biology and immunology have increased our understanding of the properties of tumor cells, a number of molecular markers have been identified that may have implications for the prognosis or treatment of cancers. The true clinical value of these various tumor markers remains to be determined, but a number of them have already been analyzed for their relevance to breast cancer.[42,64]

At present the marker with the greatest clinical relevance is Her–2–neu. Her–2–neu, also called erbB-2, is an oncogene — a gene that when overexpressed contributes to malignant cell behavior. The Her–2–neu protein is a transmembrane protein thought to be involved in the control of cell growth. Studies have suggested that Her–2–neu overexpression was an independent predictor of poor prognosis in breast cancer.[71,158] Recent studies have also suggested, however, that Her–2–neu overexpression is a predictor of a poor response to chemotherapy in node-positive breast cancer.[70,137]

Measurements of density of neovascularization,[180,181] cathepsin D, myc, ras, and p53 have been performed on breast tumor specimens.[42] These studies remain investigational, and their impact on clinical practice remains undetermined. The proposed breast cancer risk gene BRCA-1 on chromosome 17q is being actively investigated in a number of laboratories and may be available for clinical testing some time in the future.[76,124]

Prioritizing the tissue—deciding which tests to perform

Every breast biopsy should be performed as if the tissue obtained is going to be malignant. Therefore, all tissue obtained by open biopsy or by core-needle biopsy should be sent to pathology with a request for processing for estrogen and progesterone receptors. While many institutions are now able to perform these tests on fixed tissue, some institutions prefer or require that these studies be performed on fresh tissue. If this is the case, all breast biopsies should be sent for frozen section analysis so that appropriate studies may be performed if the specimen contains a malignancy. In addition, it is possible to perform receptor studies on fine-needle aspiration samples if the sample is appropriately processed at the time of aspiration.

BREAST CANCER SCREENING

Theory and current modalities

Breast cancer is a common and frightening disease in the Western world. Although recent developments in molecular biology have begun to shed light on the causes of breast cancer, there is still no way to prevent it. Early detection remains the cornerstone of efforts to reduce breast cancer mortality. This goal of early detection has led to the development of screening programs designed to seek out breast cancers at the earliest point in their history, when treatment is thought to have the greatest impact on clinical outcome.

Most breast cancers are believed to pass through a clinically occult phase during which the number of malignant cells is too few to be detected by current imaging studies or by physical examination. As the malignancy progresses, it becomes large enough to be detected by mammographic imaging and usually at a later point by physical examination. Although it is possible for even a very small tumor to metastasize, as a tumor becomes larger there is a progressively greater chance that metastatic clones will emerge. While metastatic disease can sometimes be controlled, very few patients with metastatic disease are ever cured. Screening programs are therefore directed at detecting breast cancers at the smallest size possible, hopefully before metastases have occurred.

Mammography can detect cancers smaller than can be detected by even a skilled examiner, either as calcifications without an associated palpable mass, or as very small or deep masses. Mammography has therefore been a central component of screening programs.

Mammography and physical examination are complementary modalities for screening. As many as 10% to 15% of *palpable* breast malignancies are not visualized by mammography because they do not produce calcifications or a density radiologically distinguishable from surrounding breast tissue. A skilled examiner is able to detect smaller masses and be more precise in identifying suspicious masses against a background of normal breast texture than the average woman performing self-breast examination. For this reason periodic physical examination by a skilled examiner, usually a physician or a specially trained nurse, is the second component of most screening programs.

Self-breast examination (SBE) is the third component of breast cancer screening programs. The individual woman is instructed in systematic monthly self-examination to detect palpable abnormalities appearing during intervals between mammograms and examinations by a health care professional. This program also encourages women to report any abnormal findings to their physician without delay. Self-examination may generate anxiety in some women who become alarmed by the irregular or "lumpy" texture of normal breast tissue. However, as more than 40% of breast cancers are still detected by the woman herself, self-examination remains an important component of any screening program.[130] Patient anxiety is best dealt with by education and reassurance that some nodularity is normal, and that most cancers produce hard, distinct lumps that the patient will be able to distinguish from normal breast tissue.

Physical examination and mammography of the breasts are currently the only accepted modalities for breast cancer screening. Ultrasonography is not a useful modality for screening, because it detects many small irregularities in breast texture that raise concerns but are of no proven clinical significance. Ultrasonography should only be used to determine whether a palpable or mammographic lesion is cystic or solid. The role of MRI, CT, PET, thermography, or other imaging modalities in the diagnosis of breast lesions is not yet determined, and none of these techniques is currently appropriate for screening.

Current issues in breast cancer screening

Although there is general agreement about the importance of detecting breast cancers at the earliest possible stage, there has been a great deal of recent controversy about the ability of current screening modalities to achieve this early detection in a cost-effective manner, particularly for women under the age of 50. Both the scientific and lay press have joined in this discussion, which leaves both women and their physicians unsure of how to proceed with screening, while at the same time more aware of the threat of breast cancer. At present 20% to 25% of breast cancers are diagnosed in women under the age of 50, which makes effective screening of this age group a serious concern.[130,165]

In the early 1990s there was a consensus among the dozen or more organizations issuing breast screening guidelines. It was generally agreed that a first mammogram should be obtained by age 40 followed by mammograms every 1 or 2 years from ages 40 to 50, with annual mammography performed after age 50. Physical examination by a health care professional was to be performed annually by age 35 or 40, and monthly SBE was to be taught and encouraged.

The Canadian National Breast Screening study

The screening controversy emerged in 1992 after the publication of results of the Canadian National Breast Screening study. This trial began in 1980 and recruited volunteers in two age groups, 40 to 49 and 50 to 59 at 15 centers across Canada.[117,118] The 50,430 women aged 40 to 49 were divided into two groups; half had an initial physical examination and instruction in self examination with subsequent follow-up by mail. The remaining half had the same initial physical examination and instruction in self examination and were offered annual mammography and an annual physical examination by a health professional. The 39,405 women aged 50 to 59 were given an initial physical examination and then were randomized to annual mammography and physical examination or annual physical examination alone. Mammography was performed using existing equipment and techniques and interpreted by radiologists at the participating centers.[8]

After 7 years of follow-up, there was no reduction in mortality seen in women ages 40 to 49 who were screened annually with mammography and physical examination; an increase in breast cancer mortality was observed in the screened versus unscreened group.[117] For women aged 50 to 59, mammography added no benefit to screening by physical examination alone.[118] These results prompted a reappraisal of older screening data and a critical appraisal of the design and methodology of the Canadian Screening study.

Criticism of the Canadian screening study

Several aspects of the Canadian study have been criticized.[116] Entry into the study involved randomization to the screened or unscreened group *after* a physical examination. Of the 24 women with advanced breast cancer (four or more positive axillary lymph nodes) at entry into the study, 19 were assigned to the screening group, and deaths among these poor-prognosis women counted as failures of screening. Critics have calculated the probability that this disproportionate assignment of advanced patients was due to chance at 0.0033.[13] Survival among the unscreened control group was also unexpectedly high and better than the overall Canadian breast cancer mortality.[100]

Critics have also stated that the technical quality of the mammograms in the Canadian screening study was poor and reduced its sensitivity as a screening tool. Problems cited included poor patient positioning and the failure to use scatter reduction grids to improve image quality. An outside review found that a significant proportion of films, particularly in the early years of the study, were of unacceptable or poor technical quality and not representative of the sensitivity of current mammography in the United States. Moreover, review by outside radiologists showed that 25% of films initially read as negative by the study radiologists did show a malignancy. These interpretation errors resulted in delays of at least 1 year in diagnosing these screened women.[100,122]

As a result, critics have cautioned against major shifts in screening policy based upon the results of the Canadian Screening study.[13,100] The finding that there is no benefit from mammographic screening for women ages 50 to 59 differs from most other screening studies and has largely been disregarded by groups considering revision of existing screening guidelines. However, the observation that screening by mammography and physical examination has no value in women ages 40 to 49 has become the focus of heated debate and has prompted the review of previously collected data on breast cancer screening in this age group.

Reappraisal of prior screening studies

In response to the emerging screening debate, the National Cancer Institute (NCI) convened the International Workshop on Screening for Breast Cancer in 1993 to review the existing body of data related to breast cancer screening and to make recommendations for further investigation. Eight prospective randomized trials of breast cancer screening among women aged 40 to 74 were reviewed, and a metaanalysis of six of the studies was also performed.[44,56,94] After review of this data, it was concluded that for women aged 50 to 69, all studies showed mortality reductions with screening (approximately 30% fewer deaths from breast cancer in screened versus unscreened populations at the 10- to 12-year follow-up). Data from two of the studies were statistically significant.[56,94]

For women aged 40 to 49, there was no benefit after 5- to 7-years of follow-up. Four of six studies showed no benefit-years of at the 10- to 12-year follow-up point. An analysis of Swedish studies showed a 13% benefit at 12 years that was not statistically significant,[129,168] while HIP data showed a 25% decrease in mortality in women aged 40 to 49 at the 10- to 18-year follow-up point.[23] Additional analysis of the breast cancers identified through screening in Swedish studies predicts that screening will translate into improved survival in women aged 40 to 49.[167] The nonrandomized BCDDP study suggested a benefit in younger women in its 14-year follow-up report.[160] There were too few women over age 70 in the studies to permit adequate analysis of this age group. It was concluded that there was still much to be learned about screening.

Based on this review, the NCI has suggested that breast screening guidelines should be revised.[94] For women over 50 years, it is recommended that mammography be performed every 1 to 2 years with a physical examination performed annually. For women aged 40 to 49, an annual physical examination is recommended as "prudent practice", and it is recommended that "women discuss with a health professional the advisability of breast cancer screening with mammography, which takes into account family history of breast cancer and other risk factors." Women aged 70 and older should be screened with a physical examination and mammography unless otherwise indicated by health status. Monthly breast self-examination is recommended.

There has been considerable resistance to changing current breast cancer screening guidelines in response to the conclusions of the Canadian Breast Screening study and the NCI's screening workshop. The American Cancer Society has not found the current data compelling enough to change its screening guidelines.

The International Union Against Cancer (UICC) has also reviewed the results of existing screening studies and concluded that no previous study, including the Canadian Screening study, was designed with sufficient statistical power in the 40-to 49-year-old subgroup to address adequately the issue of screening in this population.[41] It was felt that further retrospective analysis of these studies would probably not resolve the issue. The UICC has therefore proposed that these questions be answered definitively with a new study that would randomize women of age 40 to 42 to no screening, annual screening, or every other year screening regimens. To achieve sufficient statistical power to settle these issues, it is proposed that 1.5 million women be randomized in the United States and Europe and strong emphasis be placed on the quality of mammography and careful interpretation of films. Enrolled women will be followed for 10 years, and differences in outcome will be determined.

Recommendations for current screening practice

Even with the ongoing debate, there remain certain areas of agreement about screening for breast cancer in current clinical practice. Monthly SBE is encouraged for all women. Annual physical examination by a health professional is recommended after age 40, although some groups would lower this age to 35 or younger. Mammographic screening is recommended every 1 to 2 years after the age of 50 and should continue as long as the woman is in sufficiently good health to tolerate excision of a mass or other abnormality with local anesthetic. For the ages of 40 to 49, current data support any mammography regimen ranging from no screening to annual mammography. Most would agree that it is reasonable to adjust this screening regimen based on the individual patient's risk of breast cancer, with high-risk women having annual mammograms. For high-risk women, screening may also begin at an earlier age than for the general population, as discussed earlier (management of high-risk patients).

CARCINOMA OF THE BREAST

Eleven percent of American women will develop breast cancer at some time in their lives. Treatment options are increasingly being tailored to the specifics of an individual woman's situation, including her own preferences, and to the specific histopathology and other features of her tumor.

Table 10-2. TNM Clinical classification

T–Tumor	
TX	Primary tumor cannot be assessed
T0	No evidence of primary tumor
Tis	Carcinoma in situ: intraductal carcinoma, or lobular carcinoma in situ, or Paget's disease of the nipple with no invasive tumor
T1	Tumor ≤ 2 cm in greatest dimension
	T1a: ≤ 0.5 cm
	T1b: from 0.5 to 1 cm
	T1c: from 1 to 2 cm
T2	Tumor from 2 to 5 cm in greatest dimension
T3	Tumor > 5 cm in greatest dimension
T4	Tumor of any size with direct extension to chest wall or skin
T4a	Extension to chest wall
T4b	Edema (including peau d'orange), or ulceration of the skin of the breast, or satellite skin nodules confined to the same breast.
T4c	Both 4a and 4b
T4d	Inflammatory carcinoma
N–Regional Lymph Nodes	
NX	Regional lymph nodes cannot be assessed (e.g., previously removed)
N0	No regional lymph node metastasis
N1	Metastasis to moveable ipsilateral axillary node(s)
N2	Metastasis to ipsilateral axillary node(s) fixed to one another or other structures
N3	Metastasis to ipsilateral internal mammary lymph node(s)
M–Distant Metastasis	
MX	Presence of distant metastasis cannot be assessed
M0	No distant metastasis
M1	Distant metastasis (includes metastasis to supraclavicular lymph nodes)

From the American Joint Committee on Cancer: *Manual for staging for breast carcinoma,* ed 3, 1989.

STAGING OF BREAST CANCER

Several staging systems have been used for breast cancer. Two staging systems are now commonly used. The first is the tumor node metastases (TNM) staging system which categorizes tumors as to primary tumor size, nodal disease, and distant metastases. The currently used TNM staging categories are shown in Table 10-2.[3] Breast cancer is also characterized as stage I through IV based on specific combinations of tumor size, nodal status, and metastases. This staging system and its relation to the TNM staging system is presented in Table 10-3.[189]

EVOLUTION OF TREATMENT FOR BREAST CANCER

Breast cancer was recognized as a clinical entity in ancient times and was described, including early attempts at treatment, in the records of ancient Egypt and Greece. The ability of physicians to improve the lot of women with breast

Table 10-3. Stage grouping

Stage 0	Tis	N0	M0
Stage I	T1	N0	M0
Stage IIA	T0	N1	M0
	T1	N1	M0
	T2	N0	M0
Stage IIB	T2	N1	M0
	T3	N0	M0
Stage IIIA	T0	N2	M0
	T1	N2	M0
	T2	N2	M0
	T3	N1,N2	M0
Stage IIIB	T4	Any N	M0
	Any T	N3	M0
Stage IV	Any T	Any N	M1

From Yeatman TJ, Bland KI: Staging of breast cancer. In Bland KI, Copeland EM, editors: *The breast: comprehensive mangement of benign and malignant diseases*, Philadelphia, 1991, WB Saunders.

cancer was extremely limited until late in the nineteenth century. Before the1880s, breast cancer was almost always locally advanced at presentation and was generally viewed as a fatal disease. Attempts to perform local excision during these early years were met with local recurrence rates ranging from 50% to 100% and high complication rates.

With improvements in anesthetic and aseptic techniques, larger surgical procedures for breast cancer were explored and included procedures resecting the entire breast and all or part of the pectoralis major muscle. Axillary lymph nodes began to be included in the dissection. Unfortunately, operative mortality was high and few patients demonstrated a survival benefit from these larger procedures. These failures led both patients and physicians to conclude that most women with breast cancer were better off without surgical treatment.

This fatalistic era was ended by the introduction of the Halsted radical mastectomy. The Halsted radical mastectomy, described in 1882, consisted of excision of the entire breast with all overlying skin and a complete, level III axillary node dissection. The pectoralis major muscle and later the pectoralis minor muscles were included in the specimen. The amount of skin removed required a skin graft for closure. Halsted's 1894 series reported a local recurrence rate of only 6%, in contrast to the 50% to 100% local recurrence rates seen with earlier local excision attempts. This success gave physicians the opportunity to study the natural history of breast cancer in the absence of rapid local failure, and the significance of distant metastases was recognized.

The Halsted radical mastectomy became the treatment of choice for breast cancer for more than 70 years. This success of a more extensive surgical procedure, where lesser procedures had failed, changed the way physicians viewed breast cancer. The favored biologic model became one that viewed breast cancer spread as centrifugal and extending outward in a "permeative" fashion from the primary tumor to reach other parts of the body. This led to the design of progressively larger surgical procedures for breast cancer in the hope that a large enough procedure could encompass all spreading tumor cells and eradicate the disease.

This model of breast cancer biology ushered in the surgical era of breast cancer treatment that included trials of the supraradical mastectomy of Wangensteen, a procedure consisting of a radical mastectomy, a supraclavicular lymph node dissection, and a median sternotomy taking bilateral internal mammary lymph node chains. Urban designed the extended radical mastectomy that included a radical mastectomy with resection of the internal mammary nodes and overlying ribs and sternum in continuity.[173] A fascia lata graft was used to close the pleural defect created by this procedure. As might be expected, both of these ultraradical procedures had increased morbidity and mortality and, unfortunately, provided no significant improvement in survival.

The failure of increasingly radical surgical procedures to improve the survival of breast cancer patients led to disillusionment with surgery and required a revision of the existing model of breast cancer progression. It became clear that breast cancer spread was not only centrifugal but also embolic via the blood stream and lymphatics. It also became clear that micrometastases may arise very early in a tumor's course. This led to the hypothesis that metastatic potential was biologically predetermined and unaffected by local control measures. This paradigm led to trials of limited surgery alone or radiation alone in the treatment of breast cancer. During the 1960s and 1970s, these efforts were organized into prospective randomized clinical trials exploring the use of smaller surgical procedures and included modified radical mastectomy, simple mastectomy, local excision alone, or radiation following incisional or excisional biopsy of the primary tumor.

The NSABP B-04 study and other series showed that the modified radical mastectomy had a survival rate equivalent to the Halsted radical mastectomy and led to the abandonment of the radical mastectomy as a treatment option for breast cancer.[52,112,172] This study also showed that simple mastectomy without axillary dissection had a survival rate equivalent to radical or modified radical mastectomy, but resulted in an 18% increase in the rate of development of subsequent palpable axillary disease. Although these axillary failures could be salvaged by a delayed axillary dissection, this failure rate was generally considered unacceptable and left the axillary dissection as an integral part of breast cancer surgery.

Trials of radiation alone for treatment of breast cancer demonstrated its limited ability to control bulky disease but its effectiveness in providing local control in the setting of minimal residual disease.[20] Trials of limited surgery plus radiation as an alternative to mastectomy were undertaken. Prospective randomized trials in both the United States and Europe compared mastectomy with lumpectomy or with lumpectomy plus radiation.[47,54,152,176] One of the most important of these trials was the NSAPB B-06 trial that randomized 1843 women with stage I and II breast cancers and primary tumors up to 4 cm in size to (1) modified radical mastectomy versus (2) segmental mastectomy with axillary dissection and no radiation versus (3) to segmental mastectomy with axillary dissection and 5000 cGy of radiation to the entire breast. Pathologically clean margins were required, with patients undergoing mastectomy if the margins of resection on the partial mastectomy specimen were positive. Survival was found to be equivalent in all three groups. Lumpectomy with radiation gave a local recurrence rate of 10% at 8 years. Without radiation, however, there was a 28% local recurrence rate at 5 years and 39% at 8 years.[47,54]

Similar conclusions were drawn in the Milan Trial from 1973 to 1980 that enrolled 701 patients under 70 years of age with tumors less than 2 cm in size. Patients were randomized to a radical mastectomy or to quadrantectomy with axillary dissection and radiation consisting of 5000 cGy to the whole breast and a 1000 cGy boost to the tumor bed. Overall and disease-free survival was equivalent in the two treatment arms.[174,176]

A randomized trial of modified radical mastectomy versus local excision, axillary dissection, and 6000 cGy of radiation from Villejuif also showed no difference in survival with smaller surgery versus mastectomy.[152] Other studies from the NCI, EORTC, and WHO have also found no difference in survival with mastectomy versus limited surgery plus radiation. However, the Guy's Hospital trial comparing radical mastectomy versus local resection and only 3800 cGy of radiation showed both increased local recurrence rates and lower survival in the limited surgery plus radiation arm, which demonstrated the importance of adequate doses of radiation.[81]

RADIATION THERAPY FOR BREAST CANCER

Current radiation therapy regimens consist of approximately 5000 cGy delivered in fractions of 200 cGy per day to the whole breast, and in most cases a boost of an additional 1000 to 1500 cGy to the tumor bed. Axillary node fields are not treated unless axillary dissection findings suggest a high risk of axillary relapse. Combining surgery and radiation increases the risk of lymphedema of the arm. These modalities are combined therefore only when the risk of axillary relapse justifies the increased risk of complications. Radiation to supraclavicular node fields is also generally restricted to those patients with multiple positive axillary nodes and where the suspicion of occult supraclavicular disease is higher. The internal mammary nodes are not commonly irradiated prophylactically.

Radiation is delivered to the chest wall after mastectomy mainly for T3 or T4 primary tumors, particularly when multiple axillary lymph nodes are positive. It is recognized that large primary tumor size and significant axillary disease are both predictive of higher rates of chest wall recurrence after mastectomy.

Radiation therapy to the breast or chest wall is generally well tolerated with only minor side effects in most women. These include transient erythema or desquamation of the treated skin and mild fatigue. A small amount of lung volume is included in the fields, resulting in what is usually a clinically insignificant but measurable reduction in lung function. The heart will receive some radiation with treatment of the left breast or chest wall with a slightly increased risk of future myocardial infarction. There is also a 1% to 2% risk of a second malignancy induced by the radiation, which include sarcomas, leukemias, or a second breast carcinoma. These radiation-induced malignancies may appear after a long lag time of 7 to 15 or more years following treatment.

ELIGIBILITY FOR LUMPECTOMY AND RADIATION

As previously discussed, clinical trials in the 1970s and 1980s clearly demonstrated that limited surgery consisting of lumpectomy or quadrantectomy, axillary dissection, and radiation gave overall rates of survival equivalent to treatment with radical or modified radical mastectomy for eligible women with stage I and stage II breast carcinoma.[47,54,152,176] Table 10-4 lists categories of patients who are clearly eligible for breast conservation and radiation therapy. For these patients, the long term survival with breast conservation and radiation is equivalent to that of modified radical mastectomy, and local recurrence rates are in the 5% to 10% range or lower. For patients in these categories, the choice of mastectomy versus limited surgery and radiation is made on the basis of patient and physician choice, access to radiation therapy, or other contraindications to radiation. It has been estimated that although approximately

Table 10-4. Patients eligible for breast conservation and radiation therapy

- Primary size up to 5 cm
- Lobular or ductal histology
- Any location of primary within breast, if acceptable cosmetic result following lumpectomy to clean margins (including central lesions)
- Clinically suspicious but mobile axillary nodes
- Any ER or PR status
- Any patient age

two thirds of women with breast cancer fall into these categories and are eligible for breast conservation, many women are still undergoing mastectomy.[45,104,105,125,131]

Contraindications to breast conservation

There are other groups of patients for whom mastectomy is still clearly the preferable treatment. These indications for mastectomy fall into several broad categories, namely, (1) contraindications to radiation therapy, (2) technical and cosmetic limitations of lumpectomy, (3) issues of local recurrence, and (4) issues of prophylaxis for high-risk patients.

Contraindications to radiation therapy

There are certain patients for whom radiation therapy is contraindicated. This would include patients who choose not to undergo radiation therapy, either because of the inconvenience of receiving treatment or because of concerns about potential complications including the induction of second malignancies. Further, there are patients for whom access to radiation therapy is extremely difficult, either as a result of living in a rural area or because of physical difficulties in making daily trips for therapy. There are also patients with psychiatric or other disorders who would find it extremely difficult to comply with the daily treatment schedule over the 6 or more weeks necessary to administer adequate radiation therapy. Additional patients have other medical contraindications to radiation therapy and include women who are pregnant or those who have received prior radiation to the chest wall for other conditions. In general, this category includes women who have had previous treatment with radiation for breast carcinoma that has recurred locally. Although there is some literature supporting the use of repeat local excision without further radiation therapy for local recurrence after radiation, most authors would favor completion mastectomy.[74,101]

Technical and cosmetic issues related to lumpectomy

There are certain patients in whom resection of the primary tumor to clean margins leaves a cosmetically unacceptable appearance of the remaining breast tissue. For these patients, mastectomy with immediate reconstruction may be cosmetically preferable to lumpectomy with radiation. This category would include patients with large primary tumors relative to their breast size and for whom resection of the primary tumor would remove a significant portion of breast tissue. Also included in this category are patients with multiple primary tumors who, in addition to having a higher local recurrence rate (below), would likely require removal of an unacceptable amount of breast tissue to obtain adequate margins around all tumors. Patients with superficial central lesions that would necessitate excision of the nipple and areola for clean margins are, however, eligible for conservative surgery and radiation. It has been shown that with excision to clean margins including the nipple and areola, survival and local recurrence rates are equivalent to other groups of patients undergoing lumpectomy and radiation.[26,55,79] For many women, the cosmetic result after this procedure is preferable to that obtained with an immediate reconstruction, and the option remains for later reconstruction of the nipple and areola for cosmetic purposes. Many surgeons still favor a mastectomy for patients presenting with Paget's disease, although many now consider local excision with radiation an appropriate treatment if pathologically negative margins can be obtained before radiation.

Local recurrence

For most women with breast carcinoma, the appearance of distant metastases heralds incurable and ultimately fatal disease. In contrast, local recurrence after breast conservation appears to have little or no impact on overall survival. In prospective randomized trials, it has been difficult to show a statistically significant reduction in survival among women who have had a local recurrence after limited surgery and radiation. Local recurrences do not therefore seem to be the source of subsequent distant metastases. Biologically the ability of a breast malignancy to recur locally within the breast appears to be different from the ability to grow in a distant, metastatic location. It remains possible that some decrement in survival will eventually be identified in some of those patients who have locally recurring malignancy.[80] However, even without a decrement in survival, there certainly is a cost in patient anxiety; follow-up testing is required, and subsequent treatments must be taken into account when estimating the impact of local recurrence.

It is therefore worthwhile to identify those patients most likely to develop a local recurrence after breast conservation and radiation therapy. Such patients may choose a primary mastectomy to avoid the potential problems of local recurrence. There are several characteristics of primary tumors that have been identified as indicating a higher rate of local recurrence after limited surgery and radiation.

The features of a primary tumor indicating increased risk of local recurrence after breast conservation are as follows:

- Gross residual disease after lumpectomy
- Multiple primary tumors within the breast
- Extensive intraductal component
- Large tumor size
- Lymphatic vessel invasion
- Lobular histology

In practice, obtaining clean margins is probably the most critical factor in reducing the risk of local recurrence. The difficulty of obtaining microscopically clean margins in tumors with an extensive intraductal component and in lobular carcinomas may account for the higher local recurrence rates seen with these tumor types. Histologic analysis of mastectomy specimens from patients with tumors with an extensive intraductal component has shown that these tumors have a high rate of multifocality.[85] It is likely that this residual disease is the cause of a local recurrence.

BREAST RECONSTRUCTION AFTER MASTECTOMY

Breast reconstruction after mastectomy may provide both cosmetic and psychologic benefits. Reconstruction may be performed at any time after mastectomy. Until recently reconstruction was generally delayed for 1 to 2 years following mastectomy. It is now most often performed immediately as part of the same surgical procedure as the mastectomy. This has been shown to have no significant impact on recurrence or survival and no significant delay in the detection of local recurrence or in the administration of adjuvant chemotherapy.[40] Reconstruction options include the placement of subpectoral saline implants either immediately or following tissue expansion, latissimus dorsi, myocutaneous flap reconstruction, or transverse rectus abdominous muscle (TRAM) flap reconstruction. Free flaps may also be employed under special circumstances.

SYSTEMIC THERAPY FOR BREAST CANCER: CHEMOTHERAPY AND HORMONE THERAPY

Despite improvements in surgery and radiation therapy for local control of breast cancer, many patients still developed distant metastases and ultimately died of their disease. The ability of cytotoxic chemotherapeutic drugs or hormones to treat metastatic disease was explored. The superiority of multiple agent "combination" chemotherapy versus single agent chemotherapy was demonstrated in early trials.[12,53] It also became clear that chemotherapy and hormone therapy were limited in their ability to control bulky distant metastases, although occasional patients had dramatic partial responses or even complete responses to therapy.

In an effort to treat micrometastases from breast cancer when they are thought to be most susceptible to treatment, systemic therapy is now administered in an adjuvant setting, when there is no evidence of distant metastases but only sufficient suspicion.[66] Until the late 1980s chemotherapy was given in this "adjuvant" setting primarily to women with axillary nodal metastases but with no other evidence of disease. Studies suggested that premenopausal women benefited most from adjuvant chemotherapy and had less benefit from adjuvant hormone therapy. On the other hand, for node-positive postmenopausal women, hormone therapy gave benefits equivalent to those of chemotherapy with less toxicity.[30]

This philosophy changed in 1988 when a clinical alert was issued by the NCI stating that there was sufficient evidence to recommend adjuvant chemotherapy or hormone therapy for even node-negative breast cancer patients.[28]By this time a number of studies had shown a survival benefit with the use of adjuvant chemotherapy in node-negative breast cancer.[28,48,51,114] A consensus conference of experts in the field suggested that this adjuvant therapy be limited to women with primary tumors greater than 1 cm in size.[128] In 1992 a metaanalysis was published reviewing the treatment of 75,000 women in 133 randomized clinical trials of adjuvant therapy for breast cancer.[39] This study concluded that there was a 20% to 30% improvement in overall survival among node-negative premenopausal women who received chemotherapy compared with those who did not. This benefit also appeared to extend to postmenopausal women who were 50 to 60 years of age. For older node-negative postmenopausal women, tamoxifen conferred a similar 20% to 30% survival advantage over no adjuvant therapy. Hormone therapy did not appear to offer significant benefit to women under the age of 50.

CARCINOMA IN SITU

Ductal carcinoma in situ. With the increasing use of mammography, ductal carcinoma in situ (DCIS) without invasion makes up an increasing proportion of breast cancer cases. DCIS is now found on 6.6% of all needle-localized breast biopsies and makes up 30% of all mammographically detected malignancies.[60] The diagnosis of DCIS is now made in 1.4% of breast biopsies for palpable lesions.[60] It was recognized early that DCIS had a very favorable prognosis compared with other forms of breast cancer; long-term survivals approach 100% after treatment with mastectomy. Axillary lymph nodes are positive in only 1% to 2% of patients, particularly those with large or palpable lesions or comedo histology.

DCIS is believed to be a true anatomic precursor of invasive breast cancer. There are several lines of evidence that support this conclusion. First, review of cases of DCIS treated with biopsy alone (usually because the DCIS was missed at initial biopsy and only found on review of the slides at a later date) show a 25% to 50% rate of development of invasive carcinoma at the site of the initial biopsy. All of these tumors appear within 10 years and are of ductal histology. Secondly, approximately half of patients with local recurrence of DCIS after breast conservation show invasive ductal carcinoma in their recurrence. The true relationship between in situ and invasive ductal carcinoma awaits a better understanding of the molecular biology of breast cancer development.

There have been few clinical trials to date devoted exclusively to the management of DCIS. Preliminary results of the NSABP B-17 study, which tested the role of radiation for DCIS, have been reported.[49] Although details of the size and histologic types of the lesions treated were not included in this initial report, it was suggested that the addition of radiation therapy cuts the recurrence rate approximately in half, from 16.4% with wide excision alone to 7.0% with wide excision and radiation at the 43 month follow-up point. There was also the observation that radiation may result in fewer invasive recurrences than after wide excision only.

Current treatment of DCIS. Surgical treatment options for DCIS are similar to those employed for invasive breast cancer. There is an increased risk of local recurrence after breast conservation for DCIS relative to mastectomy, but a very low probability of metastatic disease with either surgical option. Wide excision to microscopically clean margins followed by radiation therapy has become an accepted alternative to mastectomy. If clean margins cannot be obtained or if the cosmetic result is expected to be poor after excision to clean margins, mastectomy should be performed.

The majority of patients whose DCIS is identified as a mammographic abnormality will have the option of either mastectomy or wide excision with or without radiation, each of which gives very similar and excellent long-term survival rates. Although local recurrence rates are higher after wide excision and radiation, and highest with wide excision alone, most patients can be salvaged by mastectomy at the time of local recurrence. Axillary dissection is not usually performed with lumpectomy for DCIS without invasion as the probability of positive nodes is low. A low axillary dissection is often added to mastectomy for large, particularly comedo DCIS lesions, as the risk of positive axillary nodes is higher and little morbidity is added.

If DCIS is discovered during biopsy of a benign lesion that measures less than 0.5 cm in diameter, has noncomedo histology, and no associated mammographic abnormality, the patient clearly has the option of wide excision rather than mastectomy. On the other hand, there are certain patients with DCIS for whom mastectomy remains the preferred treatment. This category would include patients with lesions measuring more than 5 cm in greatest dimension, patients with large (greater than 2.5 cm) comedo lesions, and those with palpable DCIS. The local recurrence rate after breast conservation, even with radiation therapy, is high enough in these patients that there is concern that survival will be slightly lower than that with mastectomy. These DCIS patients are also at highest risk for positive axillary nodes, and a level I axillary node dissection should be performed with the mastectomy.

Lobular carcinoma in situ. Lobular carcinoma in situ (LCIS), also referred to as lobular neoplasia, does not have the same clinical implications as invasive ductal or invasive lobular carcinoma or DCIS.[72] It is now generally accepted that LCIS is a marker for an increased risk of subsequent breast carcinoma rather than a marker of the site at which the future carcinoma will arise.[50,148] This increased risk is equally distributed over both the biopsied and contralateral breasts. A unilateral mastectomy is therefore an inappropriate treatment as the contralateral breast is at equal risk for future development of carcinoma as the biopsied breast. Appropriate treatment options include careful observation with physical examination two or three times annually with annual mammograms or prophylactic bilateral simple mastectomies with or without reconstruction. The risk contributed by LCIS may be additive with other risk factors such as family history and reproductive and menstrual factors.[60,132] The overall risk for subsequent invasive carcinoma is thought to be 20% to 25% with the majority of those carcinomas showing ductal histology.[60,150] At present most patients are choosing careful follow-up rather than prophylactic mastectomy. There are some patients, however, for whom prophylactic mastectomy is still a good option either because of patient anxiety or other concurrent risk factors.[98] Patients with a diagnosis of LCIS are also candidates for the NSABP Tamoxifen chemoprevention trial and will likely be included in other chemoprevention trials under consideration.

TREATMENT OF EARLY INVASIVE BREAST CANCER

Although there continues to be active investigation of the optimum treatment of breast cancer, there is some consensus as to the currently favored treatment.

Local treatment

For local treatment of stage I and II breast cancer, lumpectomy to microscopically clean margins with axillary dissection and radiation therapy appears to give long-term survival equivalent to that of mastectomy. Patients undergoing lumpectomy and radiation do, however, have a risk of local recurrence in the treated breast and a risk of developing a new primary in remaining breast tissue. These local recurrences can generally be salvaged by mastectomy and make overall survival equivalent to that of women who underwent mastectomy at the time of initial diagnosis. Local recurrence therefore does not generally translate into decreased overall survival, although there may be significant anxiety over recurrence and some morbidity and potentially mortality from a second surgical procedure. There remains the possibility that a small number of women will have decreased survival as the result of their local recurrence.

On the other hand, patients who choose mastectomy as their initial surgical treatment face the psychologic consequences of losing a breast. Although these patients have a lower risk of local recurrence, their overall survival does not seem to be significantly improved over that of patients undergoing lumpectomy, axillary node dissection, and radiation. Each physician and patient must weigh the inconvenience and potential complications of radiation therapy and the risk of local recurrence against the value of breast preservation, while knowing that survival does not appear to be significantly altered by these choices.

Adjuvant therapy

The current consensus is that adjuvant chemotherapy, hormone therapy, or a combination of the two should be considered for all women with tumors greater than 1 cm in diameter. Very small tumors, those less than 1 cm in size, are felt to be already of such a favorable prognosis that any potential benefit of adjuvant therapy is outweighed by its risks. For premenopausal women, adjuvant therapy should consist of combination chemotherapy, with hormone therapy reserved for clinical trials. For women who are postmenopausal, hormone therapy, generally consisting of tamoxifen 10 mg bid is the first line of treatment. There has been a reassessment of the concept of using menopause as the cut off for consideration of chemotherapy. For healthy women of ages 50 to 60, the decision to use hormonal therapy versus chemotherapy plus hormonal therapy is made on an individualized basis and takes into account the woman's overall health and the specifics of her tumor.

For women with node-positive disease, combination chemotherapy is used for premenopausal women and for healthy postmenopausal women up to at least the age of 60. For node-positive postmenopausal women over the age of 60 or those in poor health, hormone therapy is generally the treatment of choice, particularly those with estrogen receptor-positive tumors. Recent data suggest that even estrogen receptor-negative postmenopausal women may benefit from tamoxifen therapy. There is currently a renewed interest in hormonal manipulations such as oophorectomy or chemical castration for premenopausal women at high risk of metastatic disease.[153]

TREATMENT FOR ADVANCED BREAST CANCER

Patients with locally advanced breast cancer, which includes those with primary tumors greater than 5 cm (T3), fixed or matted N2 axillary nodes, and inflammatory breast carcinoma are generally treated with chemotherapy as the first treatment modality. This "neoadjuvant" chemotherapy serves to downstage local disease and in some cases makes inoperable tumors amenable to surgical resection. Patients with locally advanced disease are therefore treated with needle or incisional biopsy to obtain a tissue diagnosis and hormone receptor data. These patients are also carefully staged to identify any distant metastases. Chemotherapy is administered first and is followed by surgery and/or radiation if the tumor responds to chemotherapy. Most patients require all three modalities.

PREGNANCY AND HORMONE REPLACEMENT AFTER BREAST CANCER

Pregnancy after breast cancer

There has been concern that the hormonal milieu of pregnancy would stimulate the growth of occult metastases and would have a negative impact on outcome. Available clinical data do not seem to support this concern and suggest that women who become pregnant after treatment for breast cancer do as well as or better than those who do not become pregnant.[178]

A number of series have reported outcome among breast cancer patients who have had subsequent pregnancies. White found 67% had a 5-year survival rate and 58% had a 10-year survival rate among 12 patients with subsequent pregnancies.[183] Rissanen followed 53 patients and recorded 77% had a 5-year survival rate and 69% had a 10-year survival rate.[146] A series of 52 patients from Holleb and Farrow showed a 5-year survival of 52% .[86] Other series have reported 50% and 29% 5-year survivals in patients with a pregnancy, following treatment for breast cancer.[5,22]

There is likely some degree of selection bias in these figures—women with a better prognosis are more likely to proceed with pregnancy than those with a poor prognosis. There may also be a selection bias in the tracking and reporting of patients who become pregnant after treatment for breast cancer, which favors reporting of those patients who have done well.[141] However, series which have included controls matched for age and clinical stage also showed equivalent or improved survival among those who became pregnant. Peters compared 96 breast cancer patients with subsequent pregnancies to age- and stage-matched controls who did not become pregnant and found the group with pregnancies had better overall and disease-free survival.[138] Similarly Cooper and Butterfield compared 40 breast cancer patients who later became pregnant with 80 controls matched for age and stage and found increased survival among those who became pregnant—the pregnancy group had a 5-year survival of 80%.[31]

Given the limitations of available data on the impact of subsequent pregnancy on outcome after breast cancer treatment, it has been common practice to advise patients to wait several years after treatment for breast cancer before becoming pregnant. This waiting period is thought to allow aggressive, rapidly recurrent disease to declare itself. A frank discussion with the patient about her expected prognosis is also important to allow her to make an educated choice about pregnancy. With increased use of adjuvant chemotherapy for premenopausal women in all but the best prognostic categories, and the premature ovarian failure commonly associated with such chemotherapy, the option of pregnancy subsequent to treatment for breast cancer will likely remain an option open mainly to those women with the best prognosis.

Hormone replacement therapy after breast cancer

Concerns about possible stimulatory effects of exogenous estrogens on occult breast metastases have left many practitioners reluctant to prescribe hormone replacement therapy, (HRT) for women who have been treated for breast cancer. There are little data on this question.

There are clearly certain patients, for example those with DCIS that were treated by mastectomy, for whom the risk of both local recurrence and occult metastases is very low. While these women are at some increased risk of a future contralateral breast cancer, their risk of morbidity and mortality from cardiovascular disease and osteoporosis may outweigh their risk from a future breast cancer. For these women estrogen replacement therapy may reduce overall morbidity and mortality. The situation is not as clear for the majority of women who have been treated for an invasive breast cancer or for those who have had breast conservation after DCIS. These women are at some risk of both local and distant recurrence, and it is not clear whether estrogen replacement therapy would increase these risks, or whether any such increase in risk would be offset by decreased cardiovascular and osteoporosis risks. At present there are no ongoing, large-scale clinical trials to test the risks and benefits of estrogen replacement therapy after treatment for breast cancer. Clarification of this issue therefore awaits better understanding of the biology of breast cancer. It is hoped that tamoxifen or some other estrogen agonist-antagonist will ultimately provide both protection from breast cancer and protection from cardiovascular disease and osteoporosis.

The use of estrogen replacement therapy after treatment for breast cancer is currently determined on an individual basis and takes into account the individual's breast cancer risk and her cardiovascular and osteoporosis risks. In the absence of evidence of its safety, most centers are presently discouraging the use of estrogen replacement therapy and addressing cardiovascular and osteoporosis risks through nonhormonal means including diet and exercise programs.

FUTURE DIRECTIONS IN THE TREATMENT OF BREAST CANCER

Surgery and radiation

There continues to be exploration of the smallest possible treatment that will achieve the optimum control rate of breast cancer. Current trials are underway to explore the need for radiation therapy in favorable small tumors or in tumors consisting of pure ductal carcinoma in situ. Preliminary results of the NSABP B-17 study have been reported.[49] Although details of the size of DCIS and the histologic types were not included in this preliminary report, it was suggested that the addition of radiation therapy cuts the recurrence rate in half and may result in fewer invasive recurrence than wide excision only.

The selection of favorable invasive tumors for management with wide excision without radiation has also been reported in preliminary form. Veronisi et al from Milan reported preliminary results of wide excision only of invasive tumors measuring less than 2.5 cm versus wide excision plus radiation therapy.[174] There was a significantly higher local recurrence without radiation, although this rate was only 3.3% in women over the age of 55 and it was suggested that there may be an age difference in the risk of recurrence without radiation. These patients will be followed to determine the longer term outcomes of these various treatments.

At present it seems that it is not possible to clearly identify either in situ or invasive tumors for which radiation therapy may be safely omitted. All patients undergoing lumpectomy for invasive tumors should receive radiation therapy other than in the setting of a clinical trial. For patients with areas of DCIS measuring less than 1 cm in the greatest dimension, it may be possible to omit radiation in some cases, although this is a complex decision that should be based on the patient's histology and other risk factors.

There are currently trials underway to explore the possibility of wide excision plus tamoxifen as an alternative to wide excision plus radiation for elderly women. Preliminary studies from Great Britain have suggested that the local recurrence rate is higher with wide excision plus tamoxifen than it is with wide excision plus radiation, although other larger trials are underway to test this hypothesis (NSABP B-24).

There has been discussion of omitting axillary dissection in clinically node-negative patients and using features of the primary tumor alone to determine the need for adjuvant therapy. Newer data suggest decreased survival among women who do not undergo axillary dissection, possibly because more accurate staging allows more appropriate use of adjuvant therapies,[19] or because of decreased survival relative to local recurrence.[69,80]

The appropriate follow-up testing regimen after treatment for breast cancer is also under discussion and includes issues of cost effectiveness and the quality of life.[34,65]

Systemic Therapy

Many current chemotherapy trials for breast cancer are focusing on increasing the efficacy of treatment through dose intensification.[188] Trials of high-dose chemotherapy with growth-factor support or autologous bone marrow transplantation are underway with the hope that higher doses of chemotherapy will result in improved response rates and improved duration of response. Early results of bone marrow transplantation have been somewhat disappointing with median survival prolonged only 7 to 10 months over more standard chemotherapy. However, bone marrow transplantation has resulted in a small but significant number of long-term survivors who remain free of disease for more than 5 years after treatment of breast cancer with 10 or more positive lymph nodes.[139] It is hoped that a better understanding of breast cancer on the molecular level will lead to better selection of patients for aggressive chemotherapy and better identification of those patients who are equally well served by treatments with less morbidity.[42,64] It has been suggested that an elevated level of erbB-B2 predicts for a more aggressive form of disease and a poorer response to standard chemotherapy.[1,71,123] It is also hoped that a better understanding of the mechanisms of tumor growth will make it possible to design synergistic combination chemotherapeutic regimens. There is still no definitive evidence that currently available biologic therapies or immune therapies have a significant impact on breast cancer. These areas continue to be actively explored.

CHEMOPREVENTION OF BREAST CANCER

At present efforts to reduce breast cancer mortality are limited to attempts at early detection followed by aggressive treatment of the breast cancers that are discovered. Although continued attempts to achieve earlier detection and to improve therapy are important, it would be highly desirable to have interventions that prevent breast cancer from developing in the first place. This will become increasingly important as the understanding of breast cancer risk factors is refined and as individuals carrying mutations in risk-conferring genes such as BRCA-1 are identified. This concept of chemoprevention that uses a medication or other treatment to prevent the initiation and/or progression of breast cancer is now in the early phases of testing.

The first major national chemoprevention trial, the NSABP Tamoxifen Trial is based on the observation that women receiving tamoxifen for node-positive breast cancer developed fewer contralateral cancers than did the women in the control group not receiving tamoxifen.[48] There was a 50% decrease in the observed rate of contralateral cancers in the NSABP-B-14 study. In addition, there have been suggestions that tamoxifen reduces cardiovascular morbidity and improves lipid profile, while it potentially also increases bone density. The NSABP tamoxifen trial was begun in 1992 and plans to enroll 16,000 high-risk women, half of whom will receive tamoxifen 10 mg bid for 5 years; the other half will receive a placebo. To participate in the trial, a woman must be over 35 years of age and have a risk of developing breast cancer over the next 5 years, a risk equivalent to that of a 60-year-old woman. The risk is assessed using the Gail model that takes into account patient age, first degree relatives with breast cancer, age at menarche, age at first pregnancy, and prior biopsies, particularly those showing atypical hyperplasia.[61] Lobular carcinoma in situ is an automatic entry criterion. Patients are to be monitored for side effects and potential complications of tamoxifen therapy that include endometrial carcinoma and thromboembolic disease.

Other chemoprevention trials are under consideration or under development. Other potential chemoprevention agents include retinoids, protease inhibitors, and dietary modifications.

Silicone breast implants

Silicone gel-filled breast implants have been used for breast augmentation or reconstruction for nearly 3 decades. These implants became the subject of controversy in 1991 when concerns were raised that silicone implants were contributing to or causing autoimmune disorders. These concerns led the Food and Drug Administration (FDA) to institute a voluntary moratorium on the use of silicone breast implants in 1991 and to conclude in 1992 that proof of safety and efficacy had not been adequately established for silicone breast implants.[96] It was recommended that additional controlled clinical trials be conducted to examine the safety of silicone implants for breast reconstruction and augmentation. The form and size of these trials is currently under discussion.[2]

There is currently no clinical evidence that silicone implants increase the incidence of breast carcinoma, from studies that now have more than 10 years of follow-up.[11,33] Upon review of the data suggesting a link between silicone implants and collagen vascular disorders, a consensus review and an FDA advisory panel concluded that there was insufficient evidence to prove an association between silicone implants and any autoimmune disorder.[16,58] For these reasons, it has not been recommended that women with silicone implants have their implants removed empirically.

However, more recent reports are again raising the issue of a relationship between silicone implants and autoimmune disorders,[4,97,162] with some studies identifying circulating autoantibodies as a variety of connective tissue related peptides,[15] or types I and II collagen, or antinuclear antibodies in women with silicone implants.[145] These new findings indicate the need for additional examination of the relationship between silicone and autoimmune disorders before any widespread use of silicone implants resumes.

A recent small study raised the possibility of a scleroderma-like esophageal motility disorder in breast-fed infants of mothers with silicone implants in place.[108] It has been hypothesized that mother-to-child transmission of silicone or maternal antibodies could serve as an initiating insult in this process.[57] Further study of this issue has been recommended.

Although the moratorium on the use of silicone implants has been lifted and replaced with specifically controlled use,[154] nearly all breast reconstructions and augmentations are being performed now with saline-filled implants. It is recommended that women with saline or silicone implants in place have routine breast examination and mammography as appropriate for any woman of their age and risk profile. Some degree of capsule formation will be present with any breast implant, and if severe, may result in a firm to hard breast texture. Capsule formation does not, however, create masses or nodularity, and any palpable masses in women with implants should be evaluated with mammography and biopsy of any persistent masses.

Leak or rupture of an implant may be identified as a change in the size or shape of the augmented or reconstructed breast on physical examination or with variable success by ultrasound, mammography, or MRI. Gross rupture is generally treated with replacement of the implant.

REFERENCES

1. Allred DC et al: HER–2–neu in node-negative breast cancer: prognostic significance of over expression influenced by the presence of in situ carcinoma, *J Clin Oncol* 10:599-605, 1992.
2. AMA Council on Scientific Affairs: Silicone gel breast implants, *JAMA* 270:2602-2606, 1993.
3. American Joint Committee on Cancer: *Manual for staging for breast carcinoma*, ed 3, 1989.
4. Appleton BE, Lee P: The development of systemic sclerosis (scleroderma) following augmentation mammoplasty, *J Rheumatol* 20:1052-1054, 1993.
5. Applewhite RR, Smith LR, DeVicenti F: Carcinoma of the breast associated with pregnancy and lactation, *Am Surg* 39:101-104,1973.

6. Armstrong B, Doll R: Environmental factors and cancer incidence and mortality in different countries, with special reference to dietary practices, *Int J Cancer* 15:617-631, 1975.
7. Baker H, Snedecor P: Clinical trial of danazol for benign breast disease, *Am Surg* 45:727, 1979.
8. Baines CJ: The Canadian National Breast Screening Study: a perspective on criticisms, *Ann Intern Med* 120:326-334, 1994.
9. Benson EA: Management of breast abscesses, *World J Surg* 13:753-756, 1989.
10. Bergvist et al: The risk of breast cancer after estrogen and estrogen-progestin replacement, *N Engl J Med* 321:293-299, 1989.
11. Berkell H, Birdsell DC, Jenkins H: Breast augmentation: a risk factor for breast cancer? *N Engl J Med* 326:1649-1653, 1992.
12. Bonadonna G et al: Current status of Milan adjuvant chemotherapy trials for node-positive and node-negative breast cancer, *NCI Monogr* 1:45-49, 1986.
13. Boyd NF et al: A critical appraisal of the Canadian National Breast Cancer Screening Study, *Radiology* 189:661-663, 1993.
14. Boyd NF et al: Prospective evaluation of physical examination of the breast, *Am J Surg* 142:331-334, 1981.
15. Bridges AJ et al: A clinical and immunological study of women with silicone breast implants and symptoms of rheumatic disease, *Ann Intern Med* 118:929-936, 1993.
16. Brody GS et al: Consensus statement on the relationship of breast implants to connective-tissue disorders, *Plast Reconstr Surg* 90:1102-1104, 1992.
17. Brook I: Microbiology of nonpuerperal breast abscesses, *J Infect Dis* 157:377-379, 1988.
18. Brownstein MH, Wolf M, Bikowski JB: Cowden's disease: a cutaneous marker of breast cancer, *Cancer* 41:2393-2398, 1978.
19. Cabanes et al: Value of axillary dissection in addition to lumpectomy and radiotherapy in early breast cancer: the Breast Carcinoma Collaborative Group of the Institut Curie, *Lancet* 339:1245-1248, 1992.
20. Calle R et al: Conservative management of operable breast cancer: ten years experience at the Foundation Curie, *Cancer* 42:2045-2053, 1978.
21. Chaudary M et al: Nipple discharge: the diagnostic value of testing for occult blood, *Ann Surg* 196:651, 1982.
22. Cheek JH: Cancer of the breast in pregnancy and lactation, *Am J Surg* 126:729-731, 1973.
23. Chu KC, Smart CR, Tarone RE: Analysis of breast cancer mortality and stage distribution by age for the Health Insurance Plan clinical trial, *J Natl Cancer Inst* 80:1125-1132, 1988.
24. Ciatto S, Cariaggi P, Bulgaresi P: The value of routine cytologic examination of breast cyst fluids, *Acta Cytol* 31:301-304, 1987a.
25. Ciatto S, Cataliotti L, Distante V: Nonpalpable lesions detected with mammography: review of 512 consecutive cases, *Radiology* 165:99-102, 1987.
26. Clarke DH et al: Analysis of local regional relapses in patients with early breast cancers treated by excision and radiotherapy: experience of the Institut Gustave Roussy, *Int J Radiat Oncol Phys* 11:137, 1985.
27. Claus EB, Risch N, Thompson WD: Autosomal dominant inheritance of early-onset breast cancer: implications for risk prediction, *Cancer* 73:643-651, 1994.
28. National Cancer Institute, National Institute of Health: Clinical alert from the National Cancer Institute, Department of Human Services, May 16, 1988.
29. Colditz GA, Stampfer MJ, Willett WC: Prospective study of estrogen replacement therapy and risk of breast cancer in postmenopausal women, *JAMA* 264:2641-2653, 1990.
30. Consensus Conferences: Adjuvant chemotherapy for breast cancer, *JAMA* 254:3461-3463, 1985.
31. Cooper DR, Butterfield J: Pregnancy subsequent to mastectomy for cancer of the breast, *Ann Surg* 171:429-433, 1970.
32. Danforth DN et al: Complete axillary lymph node dissection for stage I-II carcinoma of the breast, *J Clin Oncol* 4:655, 1986.
33. Deapen DM, Brody GS: Augmentation mammoplasty and breast cancer: a 5-year update of the Los Angeles study, *Plast Reconstr Surg* 89:660-665, 1992.
34. Del Turco MR et al: intensive diagnostic follow-up after treatment of primary breast cancer: a randomized trial, *JAMA* 271:1593-1597, 1994.
35. Devitt JE: Management of nipple discharge by clinical findings, *Am J Surg* 149:789-792, 1985.
36. Donegan WL: Evaluation of a palpable breast mass, *N Engl J Med* 327:937-942, 1992.
37. Dowlatshahi KD et al: Nonpalpable breast lesions: findings of stereotaxic needle-core biopsy and fine-needle aspiration cytology, *Radiology* 181:745-750, 1991.
38. Dupont WD, Page DL: Menopausal estrogen-replacement therapy, *Arch Intern Med* 151:67-72, 1991.
39. Early Breast Cancer Trialists' Collaborative Group: Systemic treatment of early breast cancer by hormonal, cytotoxic, or immune therapy, *Lancet* 339:71-85, 1992.
40. Eberlein TJ et al: Prospective evaluation of immediate reconstruction following mastectomy, *Ann Surg* 218:29-36, 1993.
41. Eckhardt S, Badellino F, Murphy GP: UICC meeting on breast-cancer screening in premenopausal women in developed countries, *Int J Cancer* 56:1-5, 1994.
42. El-Ashry D, Lippman ME: Molecular biology of breast carcinoma, *World J Surg* 18:12-20, 1994.
43. Elliott RL et al: Stereotaxic needle locationization and biopsy of occult breast lesions: first year's experience, *Am Surg* 58:126-131, 1992.
44. Elwood JM, Cox B, Richardson AK: The effectiveness of breast cancer screening by mammography in younger women, *Online J Curr Clin Trials*, document 32, 1993.
45. Farrow DC, Hunt WC, Samot JM: Geographic variation in the treatment of localized breast cancer, *N Engl J Med* 326:1097-2101, 1992.
46. Fentiman et al: Double-blind controlled trial of tamoxifen therapy for mastalgia, *Lancet* 1:287, 1986.
47. Fisher B et al: Five-year results of a randomized trial comparing total mastectomy and segmental mastectomy with or without radiation in the treatment of breast cancer, *N Engl J Med* 312:665-673, 1985a.
48. Fisher B et al: A randomized trial evaluating tamoxifen in the treatment of node-negative breast cancer women who have estrogen-receptor positive tumors, *N Engl J Med* 320:479-484, 1989b.
49. Fisher B et al: Lumpectomy compared with lumpectomy and radiation therapy for the treatment of intraductal breast cancer, *N Engl J Med* 328:1581-1586, 1993.
50. Fisher B et al: A randomized clinical trial evaluating sequential methotrexate and fluoracil in the treatment of patients with node-negative breast cancer who have estrogen-receptor negative tumors, *N Engl J Med* 320:473-478, 1989a.
51. Fisher B et al: Ten-year results of a randomized clinical trial comparing radical mastectomy and total mastectomy with or without radiation, *N Engl J Med* 312:674-681, 1985b.
52. Fisher B et al: Systemic adjuvant therapy on treatment of previous operable breast cancer: NSABP experience, *NCI Monogr* 1:35-43, 1986.
53. Fisher B et al: Eight-year results of a randomized trial comparing total mastectomy and lumpectomy without irradiation in the treatment of breast cancer, *N Engl J Med* 320:822-828, 1989c.
54. Fisher B, Wolmark N: Limited surgical management for primary breast cancer: a commentary on the NSABP reports, *World J Surg* 9:682, 1985c.
55. Fisher ER, Fisher B: Lobular carcinoma of the breast: an overview, *Ann Surg* 195:377, 1977.
56. Fletcher SW et al: Report of the International Workshop on Screening for Breast Cancer, *J Natl Cancer Inst* 85:1644-1656, 1993.

57. Flick JA: Silicone implants and esophageal dysmotility: are breast-fed infants at risk? *JAMA* 271:240-241, 1994.
58. Food and Drug Administration General and Plastic Surgery Devices Panel Meeting, February 18-20, 1992, Freedom of Information Services Inc documents 100714, 107031, and 107032.
59. Ford D et al: Risks of cancer in BRCA1-mutation carriers, *Lancet* 343:692-695, 1994.
60. Frykberg ER, Kirby IB: Management of in situ and minimally invasive breast carcinoma, *World J Surg* 18:45-57, 1994.
61. Gail MG et al: Projecting individualized probabilities of developing breast cancer for white females who are being examined annually, *J Natl Cancer Inst* 1:1879-1886, 1989.
62. Gambrell RD Jr: Proposal to decrease the risk and improve the prognosis of breast cancer, *Am J Obstet Gynecol* 150:119-128, 1984.
63. Gambrell RD Jr: Breast cancer: improved prognosis in hormone users and decreased incidence in oestrogen-progestogen users. In Mann RD, editor: *Hormone replacement therapy and breast cancer risk,* Park Ridge, New Jersey, 1992, Parthenon Publishing Group.
64. Gasparini G, Pozza F, Harris AL: Evaluating the potential usefulness of new prognostic and predictive indicators in node-negative breast cancer patients, *J Natl Cancer Inst* 85:1206-1219, 1993.
65. GIVIO Investigators: Impact of follow-up testing on survival and health-related quality of life in breast cancer patients, *JAMA* 271:1587-1592, 1994.
66. Goldhirsch A, Gelber RD: Understanding adjuvant chemotherapy for breast cancer, *N Engl J Med* 330:1308-1309, 1994.
67. Goodwin PJ, Boyd NF: Critical appraisal of the evidence that dietary fat intake is related to breast cancer risk in humans, *J Natl Cancer Inst* 79:473-485, 1987.
68. Grant CS et al: Fine-needle aspiration of the breast, *Mayo Clin Proc* 61:377-381, 1986.
69. Graverson HP et al: Breast cancer: risk of axillary recurrence in node-negative patients following partial dissection of the axilla, *Eur J Surg Oncol* 14:407-412, 1988.
70. Gullick WJ et al: C-erbB-2 protein overexpression in breast cancer is a risk factor in patients with involved and uninvolved lymph nodes, *Br J Cancer* 63:434, 1991.
71. Gusterson BA et al: Prognostic importance of c-erbB-2 expression in breast cancer: International (Ludwig) Breast Cancer Study Group, *J Clin Oncol* 10:1049, 1992.
72. Haagensen CD et al: Lobular neoplasia (so-called lobular carcinoma in situ) of the breast, *Cancer* 42:737, 1978.
73. Hadfield J: Excision of the major duct system for benign disease of the breast, *Br J Surg* 47:472-477, 1960.
74. Haffty GB et al: Conservative surgery with radiation therapy in clinical stage I and II breast cancer: results of a 20-year experience, *Arch Surg* 124:1266, 1989.
75. Hall FM et al: Nonpalpable breast lesions: recommendations for biopsy based on suspicion of carcinoma at mammography, *Radiology* 167:353-358, 1988.
76. Hall JM et al: Linkage of early-onset familial breast cancer to chromosome 17q21, *Science* 250:1684-1689, 1990.
77. Hamed H et al: Follow-up of patients with aspirated breast cysts is necessary, *Arch Surg* 124:253-255, 1989.
78. Hammond S et al: Statistical analysis of fine-needle aspiration cytology of the breast: a review of 678 cases plus 4265 cases from the literature, *Acta Cytol* 31:276-280, 1987.
79. Harris JR, Hellman S, Kinne DW: Limited surgery and radiotherapy for early breast cancer, *N Engl J Med* 313:1365, 1985a.
80. Harris JR, Osteen RT: Patients with early breast cancer benefit from effective axillary treatment, *Breast Cancer Res Treat* 5:17-21, 1985b.
81. Hayward J, Caleffi M: The significance of local control in the primary treatment of breast cancer, *Arch Surg* 122:1244-1247, 1987.
82. Helvie MA et al: Mammographic follow-up of low-suspicion lesions: compliance rate and diagnostic yield, *Radiology* 178:155-158, 1991.
83. Henderson BE, Paganin-Hill A, Ross RK: Decreased mortality in users of estrogen replacement therapy, *Arch Intern Med* 151:75-78, 1991.
84. Henderson IC: Risk factors for breast cancer development, *Cancer* 71(suppl):2127-2140, 1993.
85. Holland R et al: The presence of an extensive intraductal component following a limited excision correlates with prominent residual disease in the remainder of the breast, *J Clin Oncol* 8:113-118, 1990.
86. Holleb AI, Farrow JH: The relation of carcinoma of the breast and pregnancy in 283 patients, *Surg Gynecol Obstet* 115:65-71, 1962.
87. Howe GR et al: A cohort study of fat intake and risk of breast cancer, *J Natl Cancer Inst* 83:336-340, 1991.
88. Howe GR et al: Dietary factors and risk of breast cancer: combined analysis of 12 case-control studies, *J Natl Cancer Inst* 82:561-569, 1990.
89. Howe G et al: The association between alcohol and breast cancer risk: evidence from the combined analysis of six dietary case-control studies, *Int J Cancer* 47:707-710, 1991.
90. Hughes LE, Bundred NJ: Breast macrocysts, *World J Surg* 13:711-714, 1989.
91. Hultborn KA, Larsen LG, Raghnult I: The lymph drainage from the breast to the axillary and parasternal lymph nodes: studied with the aid of colloidal Au^{198}, *Acta Radiol* 43:52, 1955.
92. Hunter DJ et al: A prospective study of the intake of vitamins C, E, and A and the risk of breast cancer, *N Engl J Med* 329:234-240, 1993.
93. Jackson VP, Reynolds HE: Stereotaxic needle-core biopsy and fine-needle aspiration cytologic evaluation of nonpalpable breast lesions, *Radiology* 181:633-634, 1991.
94. *J Natl Cancer Inst News,* 1993.
95. Jones DY et al: Dietary fat and breast cancer in the National Health and Nutrition Examination Survey. I. Epidemiologic follow-up study, *J Natl Cancer Inst* 79:465-471, 1987.
96. Kessler DA: The basis of the FDA's decision on breast implants, *N Engl J Med* 326:1713-1715, 1992.
97. Kessler DA, Merkata RB, Schapiro R: A call for higher standards for breast implants, *JAMA* 270:2607-2608, 1993.
98. Kinne D: Clinical management of lobular carcinoma in situ. In Harris JR et al, editors: *Breast diseases*, Philadelphia, 1991, JP Lippencott.
99. Knekt P et al: Dietary fat and risk of breast cancer, *Am J Clin Nutr* 52:903-908, 1990.
100. Kopans DB, Feig SA: The Canadian National Breast Screening Study: a critical review, *AJR* 161:755-760, 1993.
101. Kurtz JM et al: Results of wide excision for local recurrence after breast-conserving therapy, *Cancer* 61:1969, 1989.
102. Lauerson N, Wilson K: The effect of danazol in the treatment of chronic cystic mastitis, *Obstet Gynecol* 48:93, 1976.
103. Layfield LJ, Glasgow BJ, Cramer H: Fine-needle aspiration in the management of breast masses, *Pathol Annu* 24:23-62, 1989.
104. Lazovich D et al: Underutilization of breast conserving surgery and radiation therapy among women with stage I or II breast cancer, *JAMA* 266:3433-3438, 1991.
105. Lee-Feldstein A, Anton-Culver H, Feldstein PJ: Treatment differences and other prognostic factors related to breast cancer survival: delivery systems and medical outcomes, *JAMA* 271:1163-1168, 1994.
106. Leis HP Jr: Gross breast cysts: significance and management, *Contemp Surg* 39(2):13-20, 1991.
107. Levine AJ: The p53 tumor-suppressor gene, *N Engl J Med* 326:1350-1351, 1992.
108. Levine JJ, Ilowite NT: Scleroderma-like esophageal disease in children breast-fed by mothers with silicone breast implants, *JAMA* 271:213-216, 1994.
109. Loomis DP, Savitz DA, Ananth CV: Breast cancer mortality among female electrical workers in the United States, *J Natl Cancer Inst* 86:921-925, 1994.
110. Love RR et al: Effects of tamoxifen on bone mineral density in postmenopausal women with breast cancer, *N Engl J Med* 326:852-856, 1992.

111. Lynch HT, Marcus JN, Watson P: Familial breast cancer, family cancer syndromes, and predisposition to breast neoplasia. In Bland KI, Copeland EM III, editors: *The breast—comprehensive management of benign and malignant diseases,* Philadelphia, 1991, WB Saunders.
112. Maddox VA et al: Does radical mastectomy still have a place in the treatment of primary operable breast cancer? *Arch Surg* 122:1317-1320, 1987.
113. Mansel R, Preece P, Hughes L: A double-blind trial of the prolactin inhibitor bromocriptine in painful benign breast disease, *Br J Surg* 65:724, 1978.
114. Mansur E G et al: Efficacy of adjuvant chemotherapy in high-risk node-negative breast cancer, *N Engl J Med* 320:485-490, 1989.
115. Marchant DJ: Estrogen-replacement therapy after breast cancer, *Cancer* 71(suppl):2169-2176, 1993.
116. Mettlin CJ, Smart CR: The Canadian National Breast Screening Study: an appraisal and implications for early-detection policy, *Cancer* 72(suppl):1461-1465, 1993.
117. Miller AB et al: Canadian National Breast Screening Study 1. Breast cancer detection and death rates among women aged 40-49 years, *Can Med Assoc J* 147:1459-1476, 1992.
118. Miller AB et al: The Canadian National Breast Screening Study. 2. Breast cancer detection and death rates among women aged 50-59 years, *Can Med Assoc J* 147:1477-1488, 1992.
119. Mills PK et al: Dietary habits and breast cancer incidence among Seventh-Day Adventists, *Cancer* 64:582-590, 1989.
120. Morehead JR: Anatomy and embryology of the breast, *Clin Obstet Gynecol* 25:353-357, 1982.
121. Moskowitz M: The predictive value of certain mammographic signs in screening for breast cancer, *Cancer* 51:1007-1011, 1983.
122. Moskowitz M: Guidelines for screening for breast cancer: is a revision in order? *Radiol Clin North Am* 30:221-233, 1992.
123. Muss HB et al: C-erB-2 expression and response to adjuvant therapy in women with node-positive early breast cancer, *N Engl J Med* 330:1260-1266, 1994.
124. Narod SA et al: Familial breast-ovarian cancer locus on chromosome 17q21-q23, *Lancet* 338:82-83, 1991.
125. Nattinger AB et al: Geographic variation in the use of breast-conserving treatment for breast cancer, *N Engl J Med* 326:1102-1107, 1992.
126. Newcomb PA et al: Lactation and a reduced risk of premenopausal breast cancer, *N Engl J Med* 330:81-87, 1994.
127. Niebyl JR, Spence MR, Parmley TH: Sporadic (nonepidemic) puerperal mastitis, *J Reprod Med* 20:97-100, 1978.
128. NIH Consensus Conference: Treatment of early-stage breast cancer, *JAMA*, 265:391-397, 1991.
129. Nystrom L et al: Breast cancer screening with mammography: overview of Swedish randomized trials, *Lancet* 341:973-978, 1993.
130. Osteen RT et al: 1991 national survey of carcinoma of the breast by the Commission on Cancer, *J Am Coll Surg* 178:213-219, 1994.
131. Osteen RT et al: Regional differences in surgical management of breast cancer, *Cancer* 42:39-43, 1992.
132. Page DL, Jensen RA: Evaluation and management of high risk and premalignant lesions of the breast, *World J Surg* 18:32-38, 1994.
133. Parker SH et al: Stereotactic breast biopsy with a biopsy gun, *Radiology* 176:741-747, 1990.
134. Parker SH et al: Nonpalpable breast lesions: stereotactic automated large-core biopsies, *Radiology* 180:403-407, 1991.
135. Pashby NL et al: A clinical trial of evening primrose oil in mastalgia, *Br J Surg* 68:801-805, 1981.
136. Passaro ME et al: Lactiferous fistula, *J Am Coll Surg* 178:29-32, 1994.
137. Perren TJ: C-erbB-2 oncogene as a prognostic marker in breast cancer (editorial), *Br J Cancer* 63:328, 1991.
138. Peters MV: The effect of pregnancy in breast cancer. In Forrest APM, Kunkler PB, editors: *Prognostic factors in breast cancer*, Baltimore, 1968, Williams & Wilkins.
139. Peters WP: High-dose chemotherapy and autologous bone marrow support for breast cancer. In DeVita VT Jr, Hellman S, Rosenberg SA, editors: *Important advances in oncology,* Philadelphia, 1991, JB Lippincott.
140. Petrakis NL: Physiologic, biochemical, and cytologic aspects of nipple aspirate fluid, *Breast Cancer Res Treat* 8:7-19, 1986.
141. Petrek JA: Incidence of pregnancy-associated breast cancer. In Harris JR et al, editors: *Breast diseases,* Philadelphia, 1991, JB Lippincott.
142. Pigott J et al: Metastases to the upper levels of the axillary nodes in carcinoma of the breast and its implications for nodal sampling procedure, *Surg Gynecol Obstet* 158:255, 1984.
143. Preece R, Mansel R, Bolton P: Clinical syndromes of mastalgia, *Lancet* 2:670, 1976.
144. Preece R, Mansel R, Hughes L: Mastalgia: psychoneurosis or organic disease? *Br Med J* 1:29, 1978.
145. Press RI et al: Antinuclear antibodies in women with silicone implants, *Lancet* 340:1304-1307, 1992.
146. Rissanen PM: Carcinoma of the breast during pregnancy and lactation, *Br J Cancer* 22:663-668, 1968.
147. Romieu I, Berlin JA, Colditz GA: Oral contraceptives and breast cancer: review and meta-analysis, *Cancer* 66:2253-2263, 1990.
148. Rosen PP: Lobular carcinoma in situ and intraductal carcinoma of the breast, *Monogr Pathol* 25:59, 1984.
149. Rosen PP et al: Discontinuous or "skip" metastases in breast carcinoma: analysis of 1228 axillary dissections, *Ann Surg* 197:276, 1983.
150. Rosen PP et al: Lobular carcinoma in situ of the breast: detailed analysis of 99 patients with average follow-up of 24 years, *Am J Surg Pathol* 2:225, 1978.
151. Rosner D, Baird D: What ultrasonography can tell in breast masses that mammography and physical examination cannot, *J Surg Oncol* 28:308-313, 1985.
152. Sarrazin D et al: Conservative treatment versus mastectomy in breast cancer tumors with macroscopic diameter of 20 millimeters or less, *Cancer* 53:1209-1213, 1984.
153. Scottish Cancer Trials Breast Group: Adjuvant ovarian ablation versus CMF chemotherapy in premenopausal women with pathological stage II breast carcinoma: the Scottish trial, *Lancet* 341:1293-1298, 1993.
154. Segal M: Silicone breast implants: available under tight controls, *FDA Consumer* June, 1992.
155. Sellers TA et al: Effect of family history, body-fat distribution, and reproductive factors on the risk of postmenopausal breast cancer, *N Engl J Med* 326:1323-1329, 1992.
156. Sickles EA: Mammographic features of 300 consecutive nonpalpable breast cancers, *AJR* 146:661-663, 1986.
157. Sickles EA: Periodic mammographic follow-up of probably benign lesions: results in 3184 consecutive cases, *Radiology* 179:463-468, 1991.
158. Slamon DJ et al: Studies of the HER–2–neu proto-oncogene in human breast and ovarian cancer, *Science* 244:707, 1989.
159. Slattery ML, Kerber RA: A comprehensive evaluation of family history and breast cancer risk, *JAMA* 270:1563-1568, 1993.
160. Smart CR et al: Insights into breast cancer screening of younger women: evidence from the 14-year follow-up of the breast-cancer-detection demonstration project, *Cancer* 72(suppl):1449-1456, 1993.
161. Smith BL: Duct ectasia, periductal mastitis, and breast infections. In Harris JR et al, editors: *Breast diseases*, Philadelphia, 1991, JB Lippincott.
162. Speira H, Kerr LD: Scleroderma following silicone implantation: a cumulative experience of 11 cases, *J Rheumatol* 20:958-961, 1993.
163. Squitieri R et al: Carcinoma of the breast in postmenopausal hormone user and nonuser control groups, *J Am Coll Surg* 178:167-170, 1994.
164. Steinberg KK et al: A meta-analysis of the effect of estrogen replacement therapy, *JAMA* 265:1985-1990, 1991.

165. Public Health Services: Surveillance, epidemiology, and end results: incidence and mortality data, 1973-1977, DHEW (NIH)81-2330, Bethesda, MD, 1981.
166. Public Health Services: Surveillance, epidemiology, and end results, DHEW (NIH) 85-1837, Bethedsa, MD, 1984.
167. Tabar L, Duffy SW, Warren Burhenne L: New Swedish breast cancer detection results for women aged 40-49, *Cancer* 72(suppl) 1437-1448, 1993.
168. Tabar L et al: Update of the Swedish two-county trial of mammographic screening for breast cancer, *Radiol Clin North Am* 30:187-210, 1992.
169. Takeda T et al: Cytologic studies of nipple discharge, *Acta Cytol* 26:35, 1982.
170. Teuber SS et al: Anticollagen autoantibodies are found in women with silicone breast implants, *J Autoimmun* 6:367-377, 1993.
171. Trichopoulos, D: Are electric or magnetic fields affecting mortality from breast cancer in women? *J Natl Cancer Inst* 86:885-886, 1994.
172. Turner L et al: Radical versus modified radical mastectomy for breast cancer, *Ann R Coll Surg Engl* 63:239-243, 1981.
173. Urban J: Excision of the major duct system of the breast, *Cancer* 16:516-520, 1963.
174. Veronesi U et al: Comparison of Halstead mastectomy with quadrantectomy, axillary dissection, and radiotherapy in early breast cancer: long term results, *Eur J Cancer Clin Oncol* 22:1085-1089, 1986.
175. Veronesi U et al: Radiotherapy after breast-preserving surgery in women with localized cancer of the breast, *N Engl J Med* 328:1587-1591, 1993.
176. Veronesi U et al: Distribution of axillary node metastases by level of invasion: an analysis of 539 cases, *Cancer* 59:682, 1987.
177. Veronesi U et al: Comparing radical mastectomy with quadrantectomy, axillary dissection, and radiotherapy in patients with small cancers of the breast, *N Engl J. Med* 312:665-673, 1985.
178. Walker AP et al: A prospective study of the microflora of nonpuerperal breast abscess, *Arch Surg* 123:908-911, 1988.
179. Wallack MK et al: Gestational carcinoma of the female breast, *Curr Probl Cancer* 7:1-58, 1983.
180. Watt-Boolsen S, Eskildsen P, Blaehr H: Release of prolactin, thyrotropin, and growth hormone in women with cyclical mastalgia and fibrocystic disease of the breast, *Cancer* 56:500, 1985.
181. Weidner N et al: Tumor angiogenesis correlates with metastasis in invasive prostate carcinoma, *Am J Path* 143:401-409, 1993.
182. Weidner N et al: Tumor angiogenesis and metastasis - correlation in invasive breast carcinoma, *N Eng J Med* 324:1-7, 1991.
183. White TT: Carcinoma of the breast in the pregnant and the nursing patient, *Am J Obstet Gynecol* 69:1277-1286, 1955.
184. Willett WC et al: Dietary fat and fiber in relation to risk of breast cancer: an 8-year follow-up, *JAMA* 268:2037-2044, 1992.
185. Willett WC et al: Dietary fat and the risk of breast cancer, *N Engl J Med* 316:22-28, 1987.
186. Wingo PA et al: Age-specific differences in the relationship between oral contraceptive use and breast cancer, *Obstet Gynecol* 78:161-170, 1991.
187. Wisbey J, Mansel R, Pye J: Natural history of breast pain, *Lancet* 2:672, 1983.
188. Wolfe JN et al: Xeroradiography of the breast: overview of 21,057 consecutive cases, *Radiology* 165:305-311, 1987.
189. Wood WC et al: Dose and dose intensity of adjuvant chemotherapy for stage II, node-positive breast carcinoma, *N Engl J Med* 330:1253-1259, 1994.
190. Yeatman TJ, Bland KI: Staging of breast cancer. In Bland KI, Copeland EM, editors: *Comprehensive management of benign and malignant diseases,* Philadelphia, 1991, WB Saunders.

Chapter 11

ENDOMETRIOSIS

Mark D. Hornstein
Robert L. Barbieri

Although endometriosis was described in detail more than 100 years ago, it continues to be one of the unsolved, enigmatic diseases affecting women. The first known report was written by Rokitansky in 1860.[92] Following this, only a few scattered reports appeared until about 1900, when Cullen published extensive descriptions of his findings.[24] Yet in 1921, Cattell and Swinton were able to document fewer than 20 reports of endometriosis in the world literature.[17] In the same year, Sampson published the first of his series of reports, and recorded for posterity his theory of retrograde menstruation and implantation as the causative factor in the disease.[94] His articles awakened wide interest, even controversy, and today his theory kindles as much heated debate among physicians as it did following publication of his first reports.

Definitions. Endometriosis may be defined as the presence of functioning endometrial tissue outside the uterus. It is usually confined to the pelvis in the region of the ovaries, uterosacral ligaments, cul-de-sac, and uterovesical peritoneum. The development and extension of endometrial tissue into the myometrium is termed adenomyosis. This disease entity seems unrelated histogenetically and is characterized by a different clinical situation. It should be iterated that the term endometriosis implies proliferating growth and function (usually bleeding) in an extrauterine site. An endometrioma may be defined as an area of endometriosis, usually in the ovary, that has enlarged sufficiently to be classified as a tumor. When an endometrioma is filled with old blood, resembling tarry or chocolate-colored syrupy fluid, it is commonly known as a "chocolate cyst." A corpus luteum hematoma may have an identical gross appearance; therefore, unless confirmed by pathology, chocolate cysts should not be considered to be caused by endometriosis. Even in true endometriomas, the histologic picture may be confusing; endometrial glands and stroma may become compressed by the pressure of the trapped blood, and the pathologist may be unable to make a specific diagnosis. If the endometriosis is not completely burned out, close examination of the wall will usually reveal numerous hemosiderin-laden macrophages, lymphocytes, and patches of condensed endometrial stroma without glands.

ETIOLOGY

The two most popular theories of histogenesis are the transport theory and the coelomic metaplasia theory. The transport theory states that viable fragments of endometrium are carried to intraperitoneal sites by retrograde regurgitation through the oviducts or by transport via lymphatics or vascular channels. The vast majority of endometriosis implants are thought to arise from the regurgitation of small fragments of endometrium via the fallopian tubes. In support of the transport theory are the following observations: (1) during menstruation, retrograde regurgitation of desquamated endometrium has been observed at laparoscopy and laparotomy; (2) some desquamated menstrual endometrium is viable and can seed and grow in intraperitoneal locations; and (3) endometrial tissue can be found in pelvic lymphatic channels. The transport theory also provides a possible explanation for the presence of endometriosis in old laparotomy or laparoscopy sites and for the presence of endometriosis in such distant sites as the lung, pleura, arm, thigh, and pelvic lymph nodes.

The coelomic metaplasia theory states that the ovarian epithelium and pelvic peritoneal mesothelium are capable of differentiating into müllerian elements (e.g., endometrium). The stimuli that cause the transformation of these epithelial elements into endometrium are poorly described. Inflammatory processes, however, such as the irritation of the pelvic peritoneum by regurgitated menstrual blood or by acute infection, may be important stimuli for metaplasia.

The majority of authorities favor the retrograde transport theory over the coelomic metaplasia theory as the most likely explanation for the original source of endometriosis implants. However, a number of findings have yet to be explained by supporters of the retrograde transport theory, most importantly: why is it that not all women with retrograde menstruation develop endometriosis? One possible answer to this question is that there is a dose-response effect; only those women with retrograde menstruation of large amounts of endometrium develop endometriosis. Epidemiologic evidence that supports this concept is presented later.

Another possibility is that immunologic surveillance varies among women; women with local deficiencies in certain immune functions fail to eradicate small implants of endometrium that are regurgitated into the peritoneal cavity. One candidate for an immune mediator in endometriosis is the macrophage. Macrophages are present in high concentrations in peritoneal fluid. There they serve as phagocytic cells and scavengers. In addition, they produce a number of locally active products such as interleukins, cytokines, and prostaglandins, which may serve as local mediators of inflammation. Numerous investigators note an increased concentration of macrophages, particularly well-differentiated, activated macrophages in the peritoneal fluid of women who have endometriosis. This suggests a possible immune mechanism in the etiology of endometriosis.[46]

A key concept in understanding the etiology of endometriosis is that hormonal factors are of central importance in the pathogenesis of this disease. The importance of hormonal factors is highlighted by the following clinical observations: (1) endometriosis is uncommon before the menarche and occurs infrequently after menopause; (2) ovarian ablation usually results in complete and prompt regression of ectopically located endometrial glands and stroma (although scar tissue may persist); (3) endometriosis is rarely observed in amenorrheic women but is common in women who have uninterrupted cyclic menstruation for more than 5 years; (4) endometriosis improves or stabilizes during episodes of physiologically induced (pregnancy) or artificially induced (hormonal) amenorrhea; and (5) frequent pregnancies, if initiated early in reproductive life, appear to prevent the development of endometriosis.

Little experimental evidence concerning the hormonal requirements of endometriosis implants is available, but it is known that normal endometrium and the endometriosis implants contain estrogen, androgen, and progesterone receptors. It is likely that the endometriosis implants retain patterns of hormonal responsiveness similar to those of normal endometrial cells. The following observations are true in normal endometrium: (1) estrogen in physiologic doses stimulates endometrial hyperplasia in a dose-dependent fashion if unopposed by progesterone; (2) androgens produce atrophy of the endometrium; (3) physiologic doses of progesterone support endometrial growth and secretory changes; and (4) pharmacologic doses of progestational agents produce a decidual reaction when adequate estrogen is present and produce atrophy when a hypoestrogenic environment exists (Table 11-1). To test the hypothesis that implants of endometriosis retain hormonal responses similar to those of normal endometrium, DiZerega et al studied the effects of estrogen, progesterone, and a placebo on the growth of peritoneal endometriosis implants in castrated monkeys.[31] Estrogen alone was able to support the growth of the endometriosis tissue in the peritoneal cavity. In a hypoestrogenic, hypoprogestational environment, the endometriosis tissue atrophied. Progesterone alone was also able to support the growth of the endometriosis tissue. These hormonal responses of endometriosis tissue form the physiologic underpinning for effective hormonal therapy.

Table 11-1. The effects of estrogens, androgens, and progestins on endometrial tissue

	Physiologic doses	Pharmacologic doses
Estrogens	Growth	Hyperplasia
Androgens	—	Atrophy
Progestins	Secretory changes	Decidual reaction

The pelvic peritoneum and ovary are the most common anatomic sites of endometriosis, and both the peritoneal fluid and the ovaries contain very high concentrations of estradiol. In normal ovulatory women, the circulating estradiol concentration usually does not exceed 0.4 ng/mL. However, the concentration of estradiol in cul-de-sac fluid is in the range of 1 ng/mL, and the concentration of estradiol in ovarian follicular fluid can be in the range of 1000 ng/mL. The high local concentration of estradiol in peritoneal fluid and in the ovary probably plays an important role in supporting the growth of endometriotic implants.

EPIDEMIOLOGY

The epidemiology of endometriosis is poorly defined; the incidence and risk factors for endometriosis are the subject of much controversy. The main problem hindering a clear exploration of the epidemiology of endometriosis is that this disease can only be definitively diagnosed by a surgical procedure (laparoscopy or laparotomy). Ethical considerations preclude random laparoscopy of large groups of women; until a noninvasive method of diagnosing endometriosis is discovered, investigation of the epidemiology of endometriosis will be hampered by methodologic problems.

Endometriosis can occur in women between the ages of 10 and 60 years. The average age at first diagnosis is 27 years. Most women with endometriosis have had symptoms of the disease for 2 to 5 years before diagnosis.

Endometriosis is an exceedingly common gynecologic problem, but precise incidence and prevalence figures are not available. A study of discharge records from acute care, nonfederal hospitals in 1980 revealed that approximately 8% of all women with gynecologic admissions had endometriosis as a discharge diagnosis.[22] Of all women admitted to the hospital, 0.6% had a discharge diagnosis of endometriosis. Of all women between the ages of 15 and 44 years, 0.9% had a discharge diagnosis of endometriosis. These and similar studies suggest that in the general population of reproductive age women, the prevalence of endometriosis is at least 1%. In certain high-risk populations, the prevalence of endometriosis is much higher. For example, in female partners of infertile couples, the prevalence of endometriosis is approximately 30% to 50%.

Genetic factors may play a role in endometriosis. Familial clustering of endometriosis is a common clinical observation. In families with endometriosis, the disease is often confined to the maternal line and is 7 times more common in first-degree relatives than in the general population. In future studies, evaluation of DNA polymorphism may identify specific genes involved in the development of endometriosis.

Menstrual factors appear to play an important role in the development of endometriosis. Women with the disease more often report menstrual cycles of less than 27 days with greater than 8 days of menstrual flow (Table 11-2).[23] Women with müllerian anomalies, in whom normal menstrual egress is blocked by cervical stenosis or vaginal septa, often develop endometriosis. Of special interest, women with double uteri and only one blocked uterine outflow tract, often develop endometriosis on the pelvic structures ipsilateral to the blocked outflow tract but not on the contralateral pelvic structures. Evidence to support this contention comes from a mathematical model of factors that control the directionality of menstrual flow. At small cervical os diameters, a greater flow was seen through the fallopian tubes. This suggests that women with reduced cervical os diameters may be at greatest risk for the development of endometriosis.[4] These findings support the concept that increasing amounts of retrograde menstruation increase the risk of developing endometriosis.

Other epidemiologic studies suggest that multiple pregnancies and the prolonged use of low-dose oral contraceptives may decrease the risk of developing endometriosis. Both exposures probably decrease the cumulative amount of retrograde menstruation. Of special interest are recent studies that suggest that conditioning exercises may be associated with a decreased risk of developing endometriosis. For example, Cramer et al observed that women who exercise regularly, started exercising before age 15 years, and exercise more than 7 hours/week are at a low risk of developing endometriosis.[23] These findings have important public health implications.

Table 11-2. Menstrual characteristics in relation to relative risk for endometriosis

	Relative risk for endometriosis
Cycle (days)	
≤ 27	2.1
28–34	1.0
≥ 35	0.6
Duration of flow	
≤ 7	1.0
≥ 8	2.4
Menstrual pain	
None	1.0
Mild	1.7
Moderate	3.4
Severe	6.7

(From Cramer DW: Epidemiology of endometriosis. In Wilson EA editor: *Endometriosis*, New York, 1987, Alan R Liss.)

PATHOLOGY

The four basic structures seen microscopically in endometriosis are endometrial epithelium, glands or gland-like structures, stroma, and hemorrhage (Fig. 11-1). Continuing function in areas of endometriosis tends to destroy its microscopic characteristics; as Hertig observed, "the more advanced the lesion clinically, the poorer the histologic detail." Early lesions, particularly those in the cul-de-sac, if totally excised and properly oriented for the pathologist, usually demonstrate classic histology. However, the large endometrial cysts of the ovary, which are obvious to the

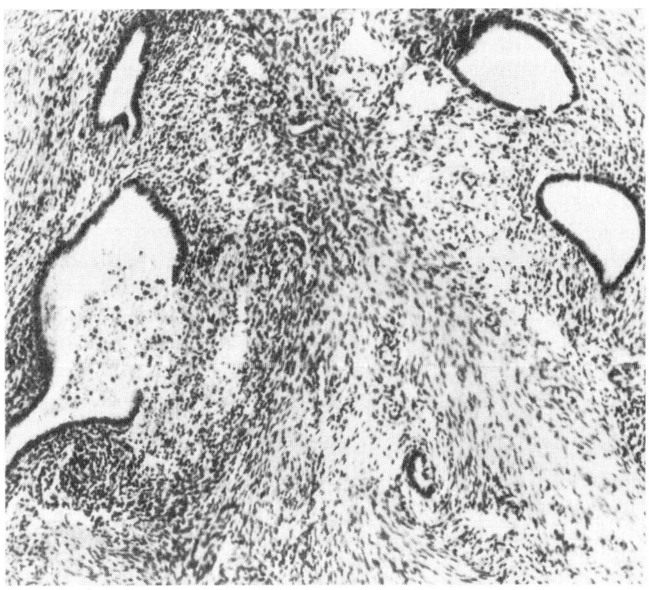

Fig. 11-1. Endometriosis of uterosacral ligament. Typical endometrial glands and stroma are evident in the fibrous connective tissue of the ligament.

gynecologist at the operating table, may show only hemosiderin-laden macrophages with varying amounts of fibrous connective tissue and inflammatory cells. It is important to remember that endometrial stroma, not the glands or epithelium, is responsible for bleeding in endometriosis. In the presence of stroma alone, an experienced gynecologic pathologist can usually make the diagnosis of endometriosis without difficulty. The presence of a decidual reaction or a typical "naked nuclei" cellular pattern surrounded by a delicate reticulum or spiral arterioles with adjacent predecidua, either with or without old or recent hemorrhage, is sufficient to permit the diagnosis to be made without glands.

The most common site of endometriosis is the ovary, and in about 50% of patients both ovaries are involved. Other areas and organs affected (in order of incidence) are the posterior cul-de-sac, anterior uterovesicle peritoneum, posterior broad ligament, uterosacral ligaments, fallopian tube, uterus, rectovaginal septum, sigmoid colon, cervix, vulva, vagina, umbilicus, small intestine, laparotomy or episiotomy scars, ureter and bladder mucosa, arm, leg, pleura, and lung (Fig. 11-2).

Endometriosis has many visual manifestations. The classic visual appearance of endometriosis is the "powder burn" lesion, a small punctate brown or purple discoloration of the peritoneum or ovarian surface. Endometriosis may also appear in other forms. Attention in recent years has focused on the diagnosis of "atypical" endometriosis. Lesions may take on a red, white, or even glandular appearance.[65] Histologic confirmation of the presence of endometriosis in atypical lesions has been reported in over 75% of biopsies of red and white areas with less frequent pathologic confirmation in adhesions.[76] Endometriosis lesions may also be invisible to the human eye. Published reports describe the occurrence of microscopic foci of endometriosis on the pelvic peritoneum that cannot be visually detected by the surgeon. The benign endometrial cyst of the ovary varies from microscopic size to a mass 8 to 10 cm in diameter. The cysts may be multiple in the early stages of the disease but subsequently coalesce into a single large cyst. During the early stage of development, endometriosis cysts are usually mobile and have smooth surfaces. As growth progresses and surface bleeding occurs, the cyst becomes densely adherent to the surrounding structures, particularly to the serosa of the sigmoid colon. The convex border (lateral aspect) of the ovary is more often involved and may adhere to the ileum or lateral pelvic peritoneum. Frequently the ovary shows multiple areas resembling "powder burns", as a result of changes in blood pigments. Minute red or blue cystic areas (raspberry or blueberry spots) with adjacent puckering may be identified on the ovarian surface but are noted more often on the uterosacral ligaments or pelvic peritoneum. The lining of the endometrial cyst varies from red to dark brown, depending on the extent and duration of bleeding. The cyst wall may be thin and smooth or thick and velvety, depending on the preponderance of fibrous tissue or functioning endometrium within it. If discrete papillary or polypoid lesions are found within the cyst cavity, the possibility of malignancy should be considered. The contents of the cyst are usually thick and resemble chocolate syrup or tar.

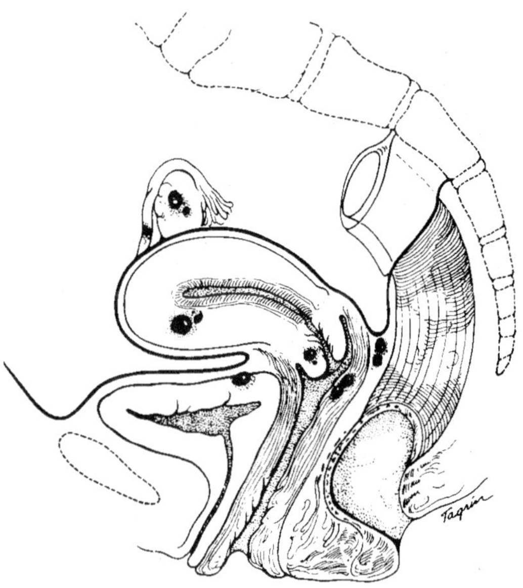

Fig. 11-2. Common sites of pelvic endometriosis.

The uterosacral ligaments or rectovaginal peritoneum may be involved separately, or there may be a fused mass incorporating both structures (Fig. 11-3). The discovery of bluish-red or brown nodules with surrounding areas of puckering on the uterosacral ligaments, adjacent cul-de-sac, peritoneum, or serosa of the sigmoid is a characteristic finding. If these reach adequate size, they may be palpated easily on rectovaginal examination. Eventually an intense fibrous connective tissue reaction occurs, with fusion of the rectosigmoid to the back of the cervix and vagina. Masses of this type may become so firm that malignancy is suspected.

The lower genital tract may occasionally be the site of endometriosis; lesions of the cervix, vagina, and vulva have been reported. Usually there is a history of antecedent trauma such as cervical cauterization or conization, vulvar surgery, or episiotomy. Surface endometriosis of this variety is almost certainly derived from implantation of viable endometrium and generally responds actively to estrogen and progesterone. When endometriosis involves the portio vaginalis of the cervix, the gross examination is usually pathognomonic; blue-black, elevated nodules, either discrete or confluent, will be evident on speculum examination.

The round ligament is occasionally the site of endometriosis. A lesion that exceeds 0.5 cm in diameter can usually be palpated by examination of the inguinal areas. Subjective complaints in the region of the internal inguinal ring, or canal of Nuck, are frequently cyclic and may be correlated with the menses.

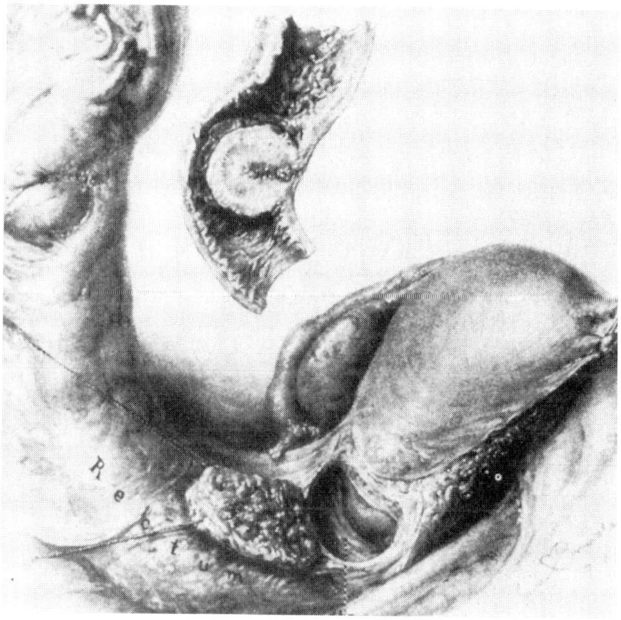

Fig. 11-3. Endometriosis of the sigmoid extending deeply into the bowel lumen. Extensive cul-de-sac endometriosis is shown invading the vagina and rectum. (From Cullen TS: The distribution of adenomyosis containing uterine mucosa, *Arch Surg* 1:215, 1920.)

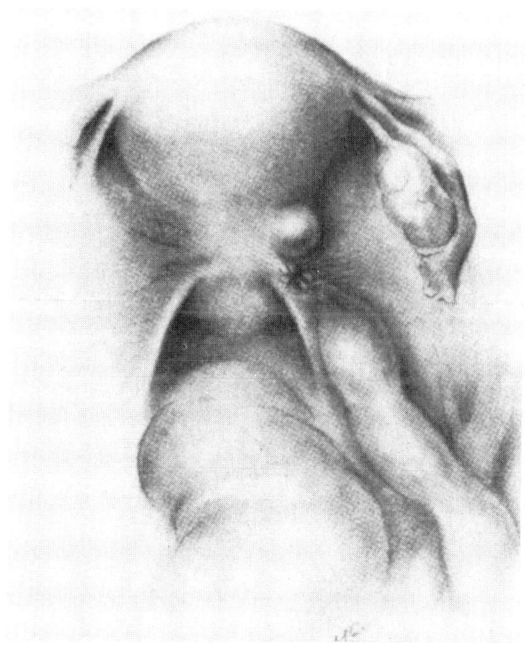

Fig. 11-4. Endometriosis invading the right uterosacral ligament, with fibrosis producing marked hydroureter. (Courtesy Dr. Thomas Leavitt.)

Small bowel involvement is rare (about 0.1% to 0.2%) but may lead to an erroneous preoperative diagnosis. Scar tissue often twists or coils around the lesion and results in symptoms of nausea, diarrhea, and crampy midabdominal or periumbilical pain. When lesions invade the bowel mucosa, patients may present with rectal bleeding. Cyclic monthly hematochezia associated with the menses is highly suggestive of intestinal endometriosis. Grossly the mucosal surface is usually smooth with subjacent fibrosis and scarring. In extensive pelvic endometriosis, several loops of ileum may be involved by contiguity so that resection of the areas is necessary. Similarly the serosa of the appendix is often involved.

Urinary tract endometriosis is not common but probably occurs more often than is reported in the literature. The involvement of the serosal surface of the bladder is seen rather frequently but is usually asymptomatic. By the time the muscularis or mucosa is involved, the patient has usually noted cyclic hematuria and pain. Cystoscopy may show typical bluish "mulberry" lesions, and endoscopic biopsy usually confirms the diagnosis. Ureteral involvement has been reported and probably explains some cases of idiopathic, unilateral hydronephrosis in women (Fig. 11-4). Cyclic flank pain, fever, and pyuria may occur as a result of intermittent ureteral obstruction. The excretory urogram may show beginning ureteral dilation, if obtained at the optimum time in the cycle. A tentative diagnosis may be confirmed by noting cessation of symptoms and improvement in the urogram, following prolonged periods of induced anovulation.

Only limited data are available on the natural course of endometriosis. Thomas and Cooke reported in 1987 that 8 of 17 patients treated with a placebo demonstrated progression of their disease on second-look laparoscopy, after a 6-month interval.[108] Three of the patients developed new adhesions during the observation period. The magnitude of the disease progression, however, was small. A retrospective review of seven patients who had undergone repeated laparoscopic examinations of varying intervals without any treatment estimated that the disease progressed at a rate of 0.3 points per month using the revised American Fertility Society's staging system.[1] Overall, five of the seven women underwent disease progression during the period under observation.[57]

Several cases are now on record of biopsy-proved pleural and pulmonary endometriosis, in which a hematogenous or lymphatic mode of dissemination must be postulated.

In summary, the pathologic process of endometriosis, although microscopically benign, produces havoc in the pelvis as important structures become involved. The process is unique in that it spreads like cancer and produces fibrosis and scarring. The end result may be ovarian destruction, oviduct deformity, bladder dysfunction, large bowel obstruction, and ureteral constriction.

Malignancy in endometriosis is rare. Criteria for the diagnosis of carcinoma arising from endometriosis were outlined by Sampson in 1925, namely: (1) the ovary must be the site of benign endometriosis, (2) there must be a genuine adenocarcinoma, and (3) a transition from benign to malignant areas must be demonstrated.[95] Of interest is the observation that many cases of clear cell carcinoma of the ovary are associated with endometriosis.[97]

Pathologists have noted that approximately 4% of all endometrial lesions demonstrate features of epithelial atypia including cellular crowding, pseudostratification, hyoperchromatic nuclei, and pleomorphcom.[25] Women with endometrial lesions demonstrating epithelial atypia may be at high risk for developing epithelial malignancies of the pelvis, such as clear cell or endometrioid carcinoma.[71] Long-term follow-up of 10 women with endometriosis and epithelial atypia showed that two of the women developed clear cell carcinoma, and one woman developed endometrioid carcinoma.[20]

CLINICAL FEATURES

Symptoms

The characteristic symptoms associated with endometriosis are (1) progressive, acquired, severe pain associated with or occurring just before menstruation; (2) dyspareunia; (3) painful defecation; (4) premenstrual staining and hypermenorrhea; (5) suprapubic pain, dysuria, and hematuria; and (6) infertility (Table 11-3). Some patients do not have "acquired" dysmenorrhea but state that they have always had painful periods. Most, however, will admit to a recent increase in the severity of their pain. In many patients the pain cannot be classified as dysmenorrhea but is actually premenstrual. The pain, which is usually bilateral, varies from mild to severe discomfort in the lower abdomen and is often associated with rectal pressure. A constant soreness in the lower abdomen or pelvis throughout the cycle, which is aggravated just before the menses or during coitus, may be the only complaint. The cause of pain with endometriosis is unknown but is probably related to miniature menstruation and bleeding and to the release of prostaglandins. That the pain is due to intermittent stimulation and withdrawal of hormones is substantiated by the fact that dysmenorrhea is not evident if amenorrhea is induced.

Pain is not always associated with endometriosis even when the disease is extensive. Bilateral, large, ovarian endometriomas are frequently asymptomatic unless rupture occurs. On the other hand, incapacitating pelvic discomfort may be associated with minimal amounts of active endometriosis. Often the surgeon can find only puckering and scarring of the posterior cul-de-sac and an adherent rectosigmoid to account for the multiplicity of symptoms.

Signs

Endometriosis cannot be definitively diagnosed by physical examination; however, many women with endometriosis have physical findings that suggest the presence of the disease (Table 11-3). Women with endometriosis may have tender uterosacral ligaments that are thickened ("banjo strings") and nodular. Rectovaginal examination may demonstrate a thickened rectovaginal septum and an indurated cul-de-sac. In women with endometriomas, fixed adnexal masses may be noted.

DIAGNOSIS AND STAGING

Although the diagnosis of endometriosis may be suggested by the medical history and physical examination, it can be made definitively only by laparoscopy or laparotomy. In patients with mild to moderate endometriosis, laparoscopy reveals the classic "powder burn" lesions. These consist of small (less than 5 mm) purple, blue, or red spots that are visible on the pelvic peritoneum. Scarring and adhesions are commonly seen in association with cases of moderate to severe endometriosis. Evaluation of ovarian masses by laparoscopy is difficult, and the definitive diagnosis of ovarian endometriomas should not be made by laparoscopic evaluation. Aspiration of ovarian masses at the time of laparoscopy may increase the number of endometriomas accurately diagnosed during this procedure. A biopsy of small endometrial lesions, via the laparoscope, can help to confirm the diagnosis. It should be remembered that some endometrial implants may contain only stroma with hemorrhage, thus making the diagnosis difficult for the pathologist.

Currently, intensive efforts are being made to develop noninvasive methods of diagnosing endometriosis. In women with endometriomas, ultrasonography can help confirm the mass and provide a noninvasive method of following the size of the mass. Pelvic ultrasonography, however, is of little value in screening for endometriosis because ultrasonography cannot diagnose peritoneal implants or adhesions. Transvaginal ultrasonography has shown promise in distinguishing endometriomas from other adnexal masses. A recent report demonstrated that this technique can correctly identify endometriomas with a sensitivity of 84% and a specificity of 90%, in the setting of an ovarian mass.[73] Studies also suggest that nuclear magnetic resonance imaging (MRI) may be the noninvasive procedure with the highest sensitivity and specificity for diagnosing endometriosis.[84] Many endometrial implants have unique and intense relaxation signals that identify them. Fat-saturation techniques appear to improve the distinction between blood and fat within ovarian masses. This may aid in the detection and characterization of endometriosis by MRI.[105] Much more research is needed to clarify the role of MRI in the diagnosis of endometriosis. The high cost of MRI studies may preclude the widespread clinical application of this technique.

Table 11-3. Symptoms and signs of endometriosis

Symptoms:	
	Progressive dysmenorrhea
	Dyspareunia
	Infertility
	Premenstrual staining
	Painful defecation
Signs:	
	Cul-de-sac induration
	Uterosacral ligament nodularity
	Fixed ovarian masses

Recently the potential clinical utility of the measurement of serum CA-125 for the diagnosis of endometriosis was described. In the late 1970s, Knapp and Bast produced a panel of monoclonal antibodies to membrane antigens of human ovarian epithelial cancers. They accomplished this goal by immunizing B alb/C mice with tumor cells from a human serous papillary cystadenocarcinoma. Spleen cells from the immunized mice were fused with cells from the P3/NS-1 plasmacytoma cell line. The fused cells were then diluted so that only one cell was present in each culture well. As the cells grew, each culture well contained only one clonal colony of homogeneous daughter cells. Because each daughter cell was derived from the same parental cell, each culture well contained only one type of antibody, a monoclonal antibody. Evaluation of hundreds of clones revealed one antibody that was of particular interest. This monoclonal antibody was designated OC-125.[13] The antigenic determinant defined by OC-125 was designated CA-125. With the use of the monoclonal antibody OC-125 and the biotin-avidin immunoperoxidase technique, various tissues were screened for the antigenic determinant CA-125. In adult human tissues, CA-125 was detected in the endocervix, endometrium, fallopian tube, peritoneum, pleura, and pericardium. In human fetal tissues, CA-125 was detected in the müllerian epithelium, amnion, umbilical epithelium, peritoneum, pleura, and pericardium. The normal adult and fetal ovary were both negative for CA-125. The majority of human epithelial ovarian cancers were positive for CA-125. Endometriomas were also noted to stain with the antibody OC-125 (Fig. 11-5). CA-125 has been partially purified and noted to be a complex membrane glycoprotein with a molecular weight of greater than 200 kilodaltons (kD). On the basis of these observations, it was suggested that CA-125 was an "oncofetal" coelomic epithelial differentiation antigen. The precise function of CA-125 is still unknown.

Bast et al hypothesized that CA-125 might be present in the peripheral circulation because of "shedding" of CA-125 from membrane surfaces.[14] To test this hypothesis, they developed a sensitive immunoradiometric assay to detect CA-125 in the blood. Evaluation of the blood test for CA-125 revealed the following striking findings: (1) greater than 80% of patients with ovarian cancer had elevated blood levels of CA-125, and (2) less than 1% of apparently healthy controls had elevated blood levels of CA-125.[14] Modest elevations in blood CA-125 levels were occasionally also noted in four clinical situations other than ovarian carcinoma: (1) in pregnant women in the first trimester, (2) in women with acute pelvic inflammatory disease, (3) in women following gynecologic surgery, and (4) in some women who had endometriosis.

To investigate further the relationship between elevated blood CA-125 levels and endometriosis, Barbieri et al prospectively measured serum CA-125 preoperatively in 147 consecutive patients undergoing diagnostic laparoscopy or laparotomy.[9] They noted that patients with advanced endometriosis (stages III and IV) had elevated blood CA-125 levels compared to women with normal diagnostic laparoscopies (66.5 units/mL versus 8.2 units/mL, $p > 0.001$) (Fig. 11-6). Patients with stage II endometriosis also had

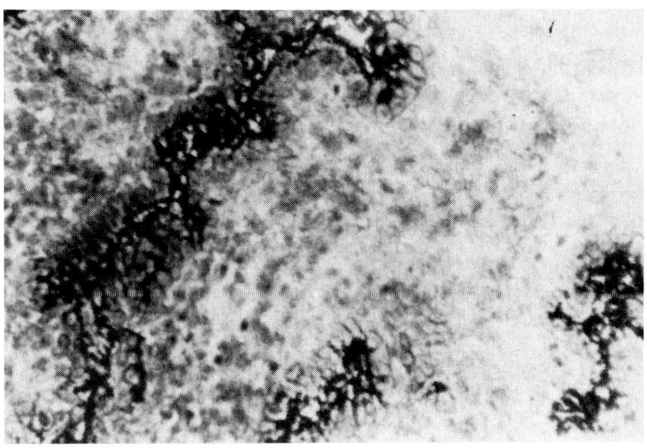

Fig. 11-5. Cryostat section of ovarian endometrioma stained with OC-125 antibody and the avidin-biotin immunoperoxidase technique and counterstained with hematoxylin. Normal ovarian tissue present in the upper right portion of the figure does not stain with OC-125 antibody. The endometrioma tissue stains with the OC-125 antibody. (From Barbieri RL et al: Elevated concentrations of CA-125 in patients with advanced endometriosis, *Fertil Steril* 45:630, 1986.)

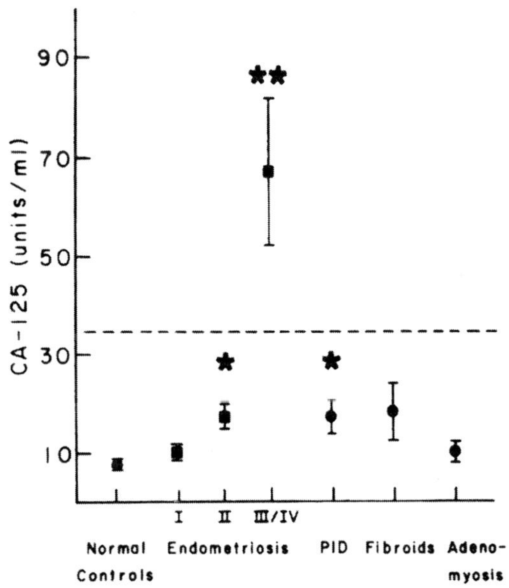

Fig. 11-6. CA-125 concentrations before diagnostic laparoscopy or laparotomy. Mean ± SEM. $*p < 0.05$, $**p < 0.001$ compared with controls. Normal controls were patients with visually normal pelvic organs at the time of diagnostic laparoscopy. (From Barbieri RL et al: Elevated concentrations of CA-125 in patients with advanced endometriosis, *Fertil Steril* 45:630, 1986.)

serum CA-125 levels greater than controls (17.3 units/mL versus 8.2 units/mL, $p > 0.05$), but there was a considerable overlap in the CA-125 levels between these two groups. For the diagnosis of stages III and IV endometriosis, serum CA-125 measurements had a sensitivity of 0.54, a specificity of 0.96, a positive predictive value of 0.58, and a negative predictive value of 0.96 in a population with a 9% prevalence of stage III/IV endometriosis.[9] These results have been confirmed by other investigators (Table 11-4). Menstrual cyclicity of serum CA-125 levels has also been observed in patients with endometriosis. CA-125 levels tend to be higher during menses and lower in the follicular and luteal phases of the menstrual cycle. However, the use of CA-125 values obtained during menses does not improve the diagnostic acuity of the test for endometriosis.[56]

Serum CA-125 measurements may also have value in monitoring disease activity. Investigators have observed that after effective surgical or medical therapy of endometriosis, serum CA-125 levels decrease. Recurrence of disease is often associated with an increase in the serum CA-125 level (Fig. 11-7).[9]

An important unanswered question is why the CA-125 level is elevated in the blood of women with advanced endometriosis. Two mechanisms may be responsible for elevated blood levels of CA-125. First, endometrial lesions appear to have a greater membrane concentration of CA-125 than normal endometrium. This observation suggests that even if endometriosis arises from retrograde transport, it must still undergo a "biochemical coelomic metaplasia" to express more of the CA-125 antigen. Secondly, the inflammation associated with endometriosis may increase the rate at which CA-125 is shed from the membranes of endometrial lesions and increase the rate at which CA-125 enters the circulation (leaky capillary endothelium). This "inflammation mechanism" may also explain why some patients with acute pelvic inflammatory disease also have elevated blood levels of CA-125.[2]

Most patients with endometriosis have stage I or II disease. The major problem with the clinical application of serum CA-125 measurements for diagnosis of endometriosis is that serum CA-125 has a very low sensitivity (0.17) for the diagnosis of stage I and II disease. It may be possible to develop a more sensitive and specific blood test for endometriosis. If endometrial lesions contain membrane antigens that are specific for the disease, it may be possible to develop antibodies to these antigens. Indeed, radiolabeled monoclonal antibodies to CA-125 have been used with immunoscintigraphy. Although severe endometriosis has been detected by this technique, it remains investigational.[67] If these antigens appear frequently in the circulation of patients with endometriosis but not in patients without endometriosis, a useful blood test for endometriosis could be developed. A blood test for endometriosis would represent a significant advance in gynecology.

A critical concept is that endometriosis is a heterogeneous disease that ranges in severity from minimal to severe. Therefore surgical pathologic staging is of utmost importance for planning therapy, determining prognosis, communicating with other physicians, and standardizing research reporting. In the 1970s both Acosta and Kistner proposed descriptive clinical staging systems. These systems have generally been replaced by the revised American Fertility Society's (AFS) staging system (Fig 11-8.).[1]

In the AFS system, points are assigned for severity of endometriosis based on the size and depth of the implant and for the severity of adhesions. The points are summed

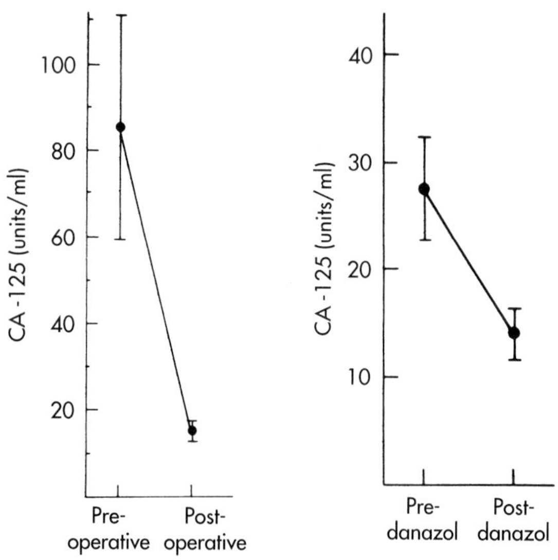

Fig. 11-7. A, Preoperative and postoperative serum CA-125 concentrations in six patients with advanced endometriosis who had total abdominal hysterectomy–bilateral salpingo-oophorectomy (TAH-BSO). Postoperative serum CA-125 concentration was measured 3 months after surgery. **B,** Serum CA-125 concentrations before and after danazol therapy in 10 patients with endometriosis. Patients underwent laparoscopy before and after danazol therapy to monitor disease activity. The American Fertility Society's endometriosis score before therapy was 26 and after therapy was 14.

Table 11-4. Serum CA-125 concentration in women with endometriosis

	Investigator			
	Barbieri et al[9]	Pittaway and Fayez[89]	Malkasian et al[74]	Fedele et al[41]
Disease status	Serum CA-125 (units/mL)			
Normal controls	8	8	—	16
Endometriosis				
Stage I	10	14	30	23
Stage II	17	23	28	24
Stage III/IV	67	33	53	33

Patient's name ______________________________ Date ____________

Stage I (Minimal) - 1-5
Stage II (Mild) - 6-15
Stage III (Moderate) - 16-40
Stage IV (Severe) - >40
Total ____________

Laparoscopy ________ Laparotomy ________ Photography ________
Recommended treatment ______________________________
____
Prognosis ____________________

	ENDOMETRIOSIS		<1 cm	1-3 cm	>3 cm
PERITONEUM		Superficial	1	2	4
		Deep	2	4	6
OVARY	R	Superficial	1	2	4
		Deep	4	16	20
	L	Superficial	1	2	4
		Deep	4	16	20

POSTERIOR CULDESAC OBLITERATION	Partial	Complete
	4	40

	ADHESIONS		<1/3 Enclosure	1/3-2/3 Enclosure	>2/3 Enclosure
OVARY	R	Filmy	1	2	4
		Dense	4	8	16
	L	Filmy	1	2	4
		Dense	4	8	16
TUBE	R	Filmy	1	2	4
		Dense	4*	8*	16
	L	Filmy	1	2	4
		Dense	4*	8*	16

*If the fimbriated end of the fallopian tube is completely enclosed, change the point assignment to 16.

Additional endometriosis: ______________________________
____
____
____

Associated pathology: ______________________________
____
____
____

To be used with normal tubes and ovaries

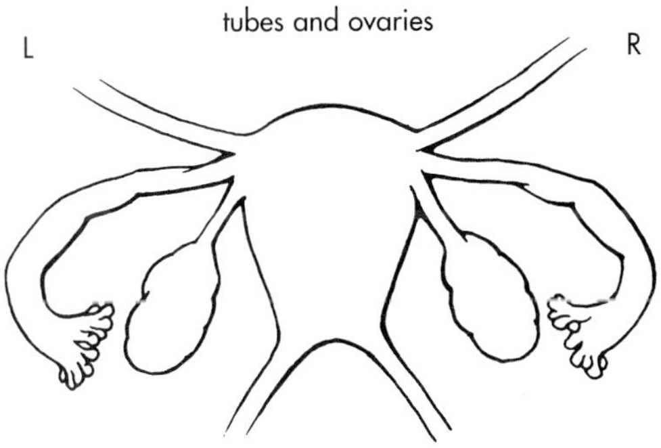

To be used with abnormal tubes and/or ovaries

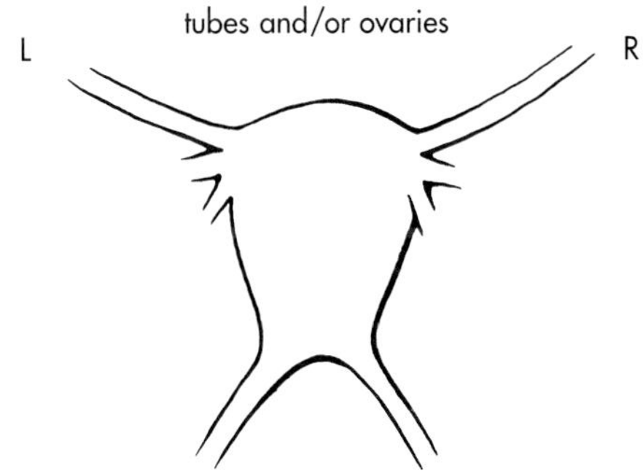

Fig. 11-8. Revised AFS classification for endometriosis. (Courtesy American Fertility Society.)

EXAMPLES & GUIDELINES

STAGE I (Minimal)

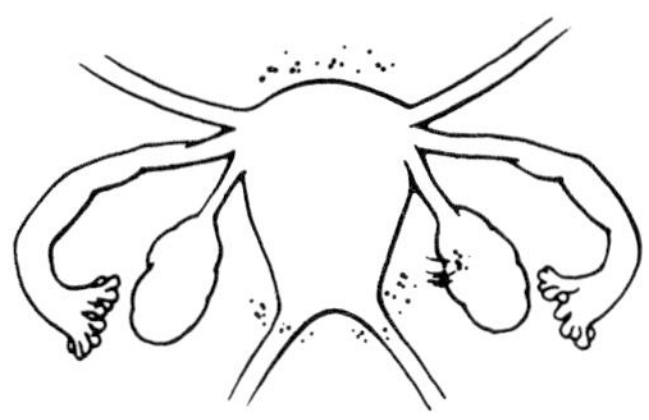

Peritoneum			
Superficial endo	—	1-3 cm	- 2
R. Ovary			
Superficial endo	—	< 1 cm	- 1
Filmy adhesions	—	< 1/3	- 1
Total Points			4

STAGE II (Mild)

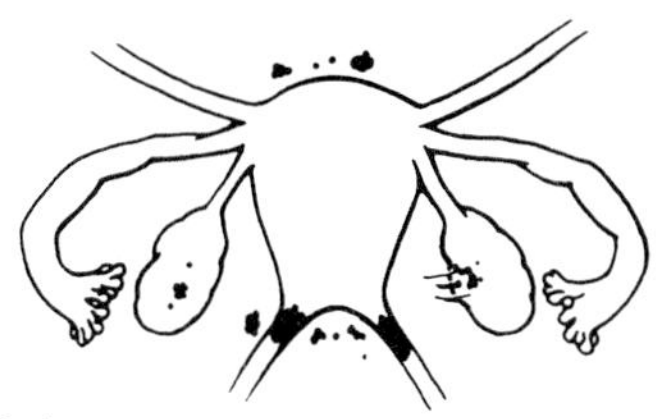

Peritoneum			
Deep endo	—	> 3 cm	- 6
R. Ovary			
Superficial endo	—	< 1 cm	- 1
Filmy adhesions	—	< 1/3	- 1
L. Ovary			
Superficial endo	—	< 1 cm	- 1
Total Points			9

STAGE III (Moderate)

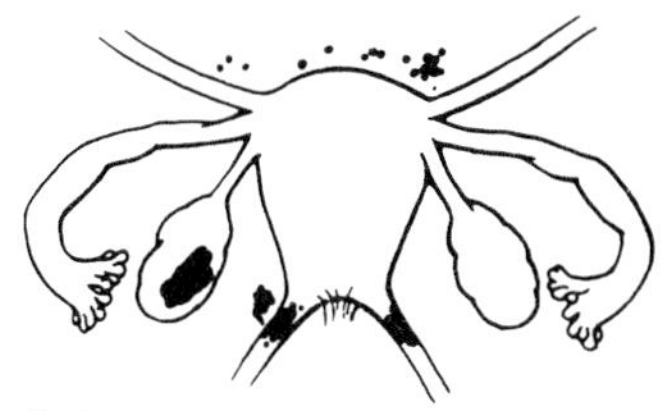

Peritoneum			
Deep endo	—	> 3 cm	- 6
Culdesac			
Partial obliteration			- 4
L. Ovary			
Deep endo	—	1-3 cm	- 16
Total Points			26

STAGE III (Moderate)

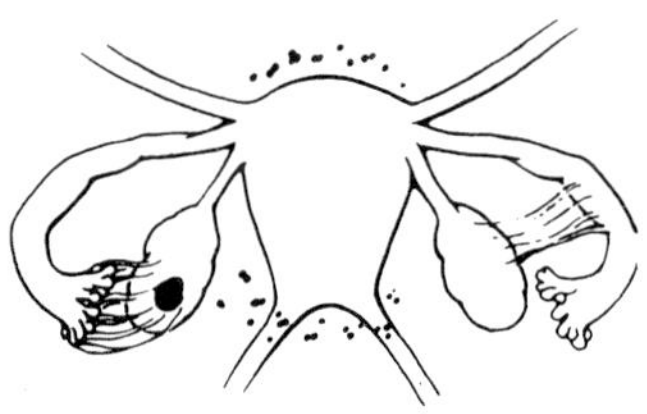

Peritoneum			
Superficial endo	—	> 3 cm	- 4
R. Tube			
Filmy adhesions	—	< 1/3	- 1
R. Ovary			
Filmy adhesions	—	< 1/3	- 1
L. Tube			
Dense adhesions	—	< 1/3	- 16*
L. Ovary			
Deep endo	—	< 1 cm	- 4
Dense adhesions	—	< 1/3	- 4
Total Points			30

STAGE IV (Severe)

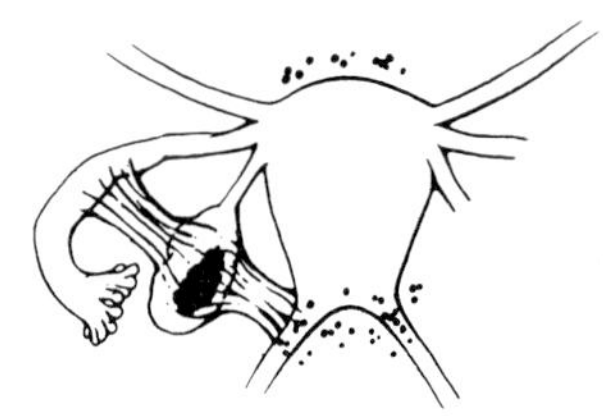

Peritoneum			
Superficial endo	—	> 3 cm	- 4
L. Ovary			
Deep endo	—	1-3 cm	- 32**
Dense adhesions	—	< 1/3	- 8**
L. Tube			
Dense adhesions	—	< 1/3	- 8**
Total Points			52

*Point assignment changed to 16
**Point assignment doubled

STAGE IV (Severe)

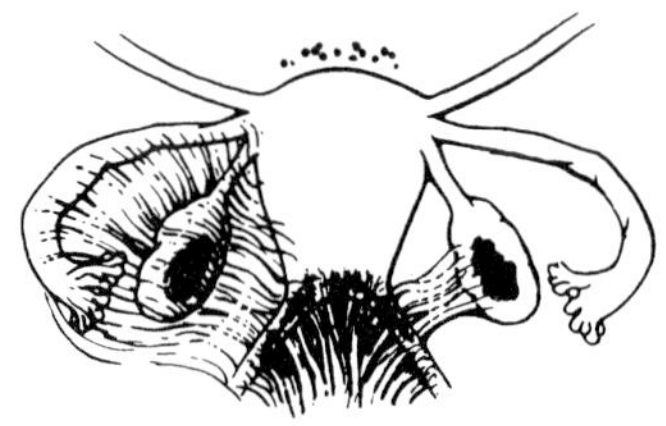

Peritoneum			
Deep endo	—	> 3 cm	- 6
Culdesac			
Complete obliteration			- 40
R. Ovary			
Deep endo	—	1-3 cm	- 16
Dense adhesions	—	< 1/3	- 4
L. Tube			
Dense adhesions	—	> 2/3	- 16
L. Ovary			
Deep endo	—	1-3 cm	- 16
Dense adhesions	—	> 2/3	- 16
Total Points			114

Fig. 11-8, cont'd. Revised AFS classification for endometriosis. (Courtesy American Fertility Society.)

and the patients are assigned to one of four stages: stage I—minimal disease, 1 to 5 points; stage II—mild disease, 6 to 15 points; stage III— moderate disease, 16 to 40 points; and stage IV—severe disease, more than 40 points. The AFS system standardizes the reporting of endometriosis and allows quantification of endometriosis staging in clinical research. Recently, however, the reproducibility of the system has been examined. While observers generally agreed on the assessment of peritoneal endometriosis and pelvic adhesions, quantifying the degree of ovarian endometriosis proved less consistent.[55] The AFS is currently revising the staging system.

CLINICAL PRESENTATION

Most patients with endometriosis present with pelvic pain, infertility, or a pelvic mass. Therapeutic considerations differ for each presentation (Table 11-5).

Pelvic pain

Pelvic pain is one of the most common presentations of women with endometriosis. Women with pelvic pain that is not relieved by antiprostaglandins (e.g., ibuprofen) or that causes significant disability (e.g., absenteeism from work or school) should consider undergoing a diagnostic laparoscopy. If endometriosis is diagnosed, hormonal treatment of the disease will completely or partially relieve the pain in 90% of treated patients. Interestingly the extent of pain does not correlate with the extent of disease. Patients with stage I or II disease often have more pain that those with advanced disease.[39,45] There may be more pain associated with active lesions in the mild disease than with adhesions in severe endometriosis. The latter may represent "burned-out" endometriosis that may, in the absence of fresh active lesions, result in less pain for the patient. In young women

Table 11-5. Management strategies in the treatment of endometriosis based on the presenting complaint

Stages	Pelvic pain* Family not completed	Pelvic pain* Family completed	Infertility
I and II	Hormonal therapy	Hormonal therapy	Expectant management hormonal therapy or laparoscopic surgery
III and IV	Hormonal therapy, surgery, or both	Hormonal therapy, surgery, or both (TAH/BSO considered)	Conservative surgery with preoperative or postoperative (or both) hormonal therapy; IVF

*Fertility not an immediate issue

with endometriosis and severe pelvic pain, long-term hormonal therapy may be required. Surgery to remove endometrial implants and scar tissue may provide temporary relief from pain, but without postoperative hormonal therapy, the endometriosis will usually recur postoperatively. This will result in the return of the pelvic pain. In general, women with severe endometriosis who are more than 40 years old and who have completed their families are probably best treated by a definitive surgical procedure (e.g., hysterectomy and bilateral oophorectomy).

Infertility

Any discussion of infertility in the patient with endometriosis is complicated by the observation that endometriosis does not usually present an absolute barrier to conception. Nonetheless, clinical evidence suggests that moderate and severe endometriosis can cause subfertility and infertility. In normal couples the monthly fecundability, or monthly chance to achieve pregnancy, is about 0.15 to 0.20.[96] In most studies of women with endometriosis and infertility who did not receive treatment, however, the monthly fecundability diminishes to 0.02 to 0.1.[89] This suggests an association between endometriosis and infertility. The mechanisms responsible for this association include mechanical factors and a host of other poorly defined processes. For example, it is clear that if both ovaries are completely covered by adhesions, the egg and sperm will be unable to interact. This will result in infertility. Less clearly defined is the possibility that an ovarian endometrioma will disrupt egg maturation by intraovarian mechanisms.

Despite the large body of clinical data associating high-stage endometriosis with infertility, convincing data that associates minimal and mild endometriosis with infertility are less prevalent. Recently Hull, in an exhaustive review of infertility diagnoses and treatments, concluded that even patients with "minor" endometriosis had lower conception rates than the normal population.[60] Patients with more severe disease who were not treated fared predictably worse. Additional evidence for subfertility in patients with minimal endometriosis came from a study of patients undergoing artificial insemination by donor. Women with minimal endometriosis had a monthly fecundity that was less than one third (0.036) of normal controls (0.12).[64] Similar results were reported in women with stage I or II disease who were undergoing donor inseminations. Patients with endometriosis had a monthly fecundity of 0.06, compared with a monthly fecundity of 0.14 in controls.[109]

In situations where obvious mechanical factors for infertility are absent, the etiology of endometriosis-related subfertility remains less clear. While several hypotheses have been advanced to explain the origins of infertility in these women, none has conclusively accounted for the subfertility of this group.

Some investigators propose that ovulation disorders contribute to infertility in patients with endometriosis. A minority of patients with endometriosis may be oligoovulatory, but the great majority of women with endometriosis have regular ovulation. In fact the incessant endometrial reflux associated with regular menses may play a role in the implantation of ectopic endometrium.

A more subtle ovulation abnormality, the luteal phase defect, may also be associated with endometriosis. However, in 100 consecutive patients with endometriosis, who had an endometrial biopsy in the late luteal phase of the cycle, none had an out-of-phase endometrium. This suggests that luteal phase deficiency is not especially common in women who have endometriosis.[7]

Increasingly the peritoneal environment of women with endometriosis is being evaluated. Pelvic endometriosis is often associated with diffuse pelvic inflammation and an increase in peritoneal fluid volume and the number of activated peritoneal macrophages. These activated peritoneal macrophages are capable of phagocytosis of sperm, impaired sperm motility and transport, impaired oocyte capture, and secretion of esterases, peroxidases, proteolytic enzymes, cytokines, and lymphokines. These secretions may create an environment hostile to egg and sperm function and interaction, impaired fertilization, and ultimately, diminished embryo survival.[47]

In addition, the concentration of lymphocytes and lymphocyte subpopulations is elevated in patients with stage I and II endometriosis.[52] Numerous investigators have tried to correlate higher levels of peritoneal leukocyte products with endometriosis. The studies attempting to correlate peritoneal prostaglandin concentrations with endometriosis have produced contradictory results. It is hoped that further investigation will clarify the role of the immune system and its products in the etiology of endometriosis-associated subfertility.

Sporadic reports have suggested that endometriosis may be associated with an increased incidence of spontaneous abortions and luteal phase defects. Recent studies suggest that the association between endometriosis and an increased risk of spontaneous abortions is spurious and probably was due to selection bias.[53,88]

TREATMENT

Patients with endometriosis typically present with complaints of a pelvic mass, infertility, or pelvic pain. Therapeutic interventions should be designed to resolve the patient's specific problem.

Adnexal mass

For most women with a persistent adnexal mass, surgical removal of the mass is the treatment of choice. Surgical removal of adnexal masses is simultaneously diagnostic and therapeutic. The surgical removal of an endometrioma should be followed by the development of a long-term treatment plan, because the majority of young women who have had an endometrioma surgically removed will have a recurrence within 5 years. The sequential resection of multiple, recurrent endometriomas may often result in the development of premature menopause. For young patients, long-term hormonal therapy may be necessary to prevent the repetitive recurrence of endometriomas. In many instances this can be accomplished after the resection of an endometrioma by instituting a long-term course of combined estrogen-progestogen oral contraceptives used in a noncyclic manner.

Infertility

In reviewing treatment options for patients with endometriosis and infertility, it is useful to distinguish between patients with minimal and mild disease (AFS stages I and II) and those with moderate and severe endometriosis (AFS stages III and IV). In cases of mild disease, the absence of severe anatomic distortion and the uncertain nature of the causal relationship between endometriosis and infertility may allow a more empiric or even expectant management course. In cases of more severe disease with adhesions and often endometriomas and a clearer cause of infertility, a primary surgical approach appears prudent. This may be followed by in vitro fertilization (IVF).

The first step in treatment is visual confirmation of endometriosis. Currently, in almost all women, laparoscopy is the first-choice surgical method. With better instrumentation available, an initial surgical approach via laparoscopy can be made. Analysis of pregnancy data in women treated laparoscopically for endometriosis-associated infertility is hampered by the use of crude pregnancy rates rather than fecundability, variable classification systems, a lack of randomized studies, and most significantly a lack of proper controls. Overall, however, approximately 60% of patients with stage I or II disease may be expected to conceive after laparoscopic electrocoagulation or laser vaporization of endometriosis.[21] In one randomized, controlled study of laparoscopic electrocoagulation of endometriosis, a pregnancy rate of 61% was seen in treated patients versus 19% in control subjects.[86] Thus an initial operative approach seems prudent in these patients. If conception does not occur in a reasonable amount of time, perhaps 6 to 12 months, completion of the infertility workup followed by one of the empiric therapies appears warranted.

An alternative to the surgical approach is medical management of endometriosis-associated infertility. There are no controlled clinical studies demonstrating that the medical treatment of mild or moderate endometriosis improves fertility. The few randomized, prospective studies that have been completed suggest that hormonal treatment using danazol, medroxyprogesterone acetate, or gonadotropin-releasing hormone (GnRH) agonists for women with minimal or mild endometriosis does not improve fecundability, compared with women who have endometriosis and were not treated.[38,59,98] The use of hormonal or surgical therapy for the treatment of infertility associated with mild or moderate endometriosis is a clinical decision to be made jointly by the physician and the patient after all the alternatives have been explored.

An alternative to medical treatment in women with stage I or II endometriosis is ovulation induction, often coupled with intrauterine inseminations (IUI). This approach does not directly treat the endometriosis but may overcome minor abnormalities associated with follicular development or ovulation in these women. IUI may allow a concentrated fraction of motile sperm to have better access to the female reproductive tract. One randomized, controlled study noted improved pregnancy rates in patients with endometriosis who were treated with clomiphene citrate and IUI.[27] Recently several investigators have advocated combining superovulation and human menopausal gonadotropins (hMG) with IUI in the treatment of minimal or mild endometriosis. This achieves cycle fecundity rates of 0.12 to 0.40.[19,33,61,62] The benefit of superovulation in this setting has been confirmed by Fedele et al. They performed a randomized, prospective trial in which patients with stage I or II were randomized to receive superovulation with hMG or expectant management for 3 cycles. Treated patients had significantly higher monthly fecundability (0.15) compared with controls (0.05).[40] One group of investigators failed to find a significantly improved pregnancy rate in patients with minimal endometriosis who were treated with one of several ovulation induction agents, compared with untreated controls.[100]

A final treatment option for women with low-stage endometriosis is one of the assisted reproductive technologies: IVF or gamete intrafallopian transfer (GIFT). In general, clinical pregnancy rates on the order of 20% per cycle initiated may be expected for IVF with this group. Perhaps slightly higher rates may be seen for GIFT.[78] Since virtually all of these patients will have patent fallopian tubes, GIFT may be an especially rewarding treatment in this setting.

As a result of the often severe anatomic distortions seen with advanced endometriosis, the primary therapy for patients with stage III (moderate) or stage IV (severe) disease should be surgical. As equipment and surgical techniques become more sophisticated and gynecologists gain increased laparoscopic skills, an initial operative laparoscopic approach is often warranted. The same principles of good surgical technique apply whether the resection of endometriosis is by laparoscopy or laparotomy and will be reviewed in greater detail later in the chapter. Following surgery, concerted attempts at conception should be made. In general, postoperative medical therapy for couples attempting pregnancy should be discouraged, since most conceptions following surgical corrections for endometriosis occur in the first postoperative year.[7] If conception fails to occur in 6 to 12 months, empiric therapy using superovulation may be considered in the setting of adequate surgical treatment.

Approximately 40% of women with advanced endometriosis and infertility will be unable to conceive, even after surgical and medical therapy. For these women, IVF and embryo transfer (IVF-ET) or GIFT are viable treatment options. In most large series the success of IVF-ET or GIFT for the treatment of endometriosis and tubal factor infertility is similar. In fact the greater efficacy for IVF in patients who have endometriosis is in those who also have bilateral tubal disease.[102] The clinical pregnancy rate for patients with endometriosis is in the range of 20% per oocyte retrieval.[78] One exception to this observation is that women with advanced endometriosis, who have had multiple previous ovarian cystectomies for endometriomas, often respond poorly to ovarian hyperstimulation and develop less than the expected number of mature ovarian follicles. In turn the poor response to ovulation induction decreases the clinical pregnancy rate for this group of women. The mechanism or mechanisms responsible for this observation are unclear. However, multiple ovarian cystectomies for endometriomas may be associated with the resection of a significant proportion of the total oocyte population.[54]

Pelvic pain

Therapy for endometriosis-associated pelvic pain has been shown to be efficacious and will be discussed under four headings: (1) prophylaxis, (2) observation and analgesia, (3) hormonal therapy, and (4) surgical treatment.

Prophylaxis. Manipulations that produce amenorrhea or cause endometrial atrophy are likely to decrease the chance of developing endometriosis. Early and frequent pregnancies appear to effectively decrease the frequency of endometriosis, but this therapeutic strategy is incompatible with the life plans of most women. Exercise-induced amenorrhea may prove to be an effective prophylactic modality but may also be difficult to achieve for many women.

There is suggestive evidence that women who have been taking oral contraceptives for prolonged periods of time, especially those with a potent progestin and a minimal amount of estrogen, may have a diminished chance of developing endometriosis. This is based on the observation that these agents produce endometrial atrophy and lessen menstrual flow, thus preventing tubal reflux of menstrual debris into the peritoneal cavity.

Observation and analgesia. For some women with endometriosis, expectant management is a viable therapeutic option. For instance, some women with pelvic pain and minimal endometriosis may prefer therapy with analgesics over hormonal therapy with danazol or GnRH agonists. For some young women with infertility and minimal or mild endometriosis, the best way to improve their fecundability may be to ensure that there are no other confounding infertility factors, rather than treating the endometriosis.

Hormonal therapy. During the past 40 years, the medical management of endometriosis has become significantly more sophisticated. In the early 1950s the high-dose estrogen regimen of Karnaky was the only available hormonal treatment for endometriosis. In the 1960s and 1970s, Kistner's "pseudopregnancy" and "progestin-only" regimens dominated the medical management of endometriosis.[69] During the 1980s, danazol became the primary hormonal agent used in the treatment of endometriosis. In the 1990s the GnRH agonists have become the most frequently used drugs for the treatment of endometriosis. These advances have significantly expanded the hormonal armamentarium of the gynecologist when treating endometriosis. Proper use of these agents requires a thorough understanding of the hormonal responses of endometrial tissues and an appreciation of the pharmacologic properties of the available agents.

The central dogma that guides the hormonal therapy of endometriosis is the belief that steroid hormones are the major regulators of the growth and function of endometrial tissue. The majority of endometrial implants contain estrogen receptors, progesterone receptors, and androgen receptors. In general, estrogen stimulates the growth of these implants and androgens induce their atrophy. The role of progesterone in the regulation of endometrial tissue is controversial. Progesterone alone may actually support the growth of endometrial tissue. However, the synthetic 19-norprogestogens, which are derivatives of testosterone and have androgenic properties, appear to inhibit the growth of endometrial tissue.

The polarity of response of endometrial tissue to androgens and estrogens is the basis of all current hormonal therapy

Table 11-6. Hormonal strategies for endometriosis treatment

Hormone strategy	Examples	Estradiol concentration (pg/mL)	Unwanted effects
I. Low estrogen, low androgen	GnRH agonists	20	Vasomotor symptoms, bone loss
	Bilateral oophorectomy	20	Irreversible sterility, vasomotor symptoms, bone loss, lipid changes
II. Low estrogen, high androgen	Danazol	40	Weight gain, acne, oily skin, hirsutism, voice changes

of endometriosis. Three observations complicate this simplistic conceptualization. First, a small percentage of endometrial implants (about 5%) do not contain significant concentrations of either estrogen or progesterone receptors. These lesions may be relatively resistant to hormonal therapy. Second, microheterogeneity within endometrial lesions may make the steroid receptor-positive cell populations more susceptible to hormonal manipulations than the steroid receptor-negative cell populations. Third, some endometrial lesions that contain progesterone receptors do not demonstrate typical functional (increased 17b-hydroxysteroid dehydrogenase enzyme activity) or structural (secretory changes) responses to progesterone stimulation. This observation suggests that in some endometrial implants the intranuclear steroid receptors are uncoupled from their site of action (DNA).

The polarity of response of endometrial tissue to androgens and estrogens is the basis for the two hormonal strategies that are most often used to treat endometriosis. One basic strategy is to create an acyclic, low-estrogen hormonal environment. The low estrogen levels cause atrophy of the endometrial tissues. The acyclic environment helps minimize the chance of miniature "menstruation" in the endometrial implants and prevents reseeding of implants from the retrograde transport of normal endometrium during menstruation. An acyclic, low-estrogen environment is best produced by bilateral oophorectomy or with the use of GnRH agonists. The second basic strategy is to produce a hormonal environment high in androgens. Danazol therapy is the best example of this strategy. The high-androgen environment directly produces atrophy of endometrial implants. The high-androgen strategy also results in low, acyclic estrogen levels by interfering with ovarian follicular development. Table 11-6 summarizes these different strategies.

Danazol. Danazol is an isoxazole derivative of the synthetic steroid 17-ethinyltestosterone (Fig. 11-9). The pharmacology of danazol is exceedingly complex and is best discussed in terms of the molecular pharmacology of the drug.[12] Current laboratory findings suggest that danazol interacts with only two major classes of proteins: (1) steroid hormone receptors and (2) enzymes of steroidogenesis. The entire pharmacologic profile of danazol (and danazol's metabolites) can be explained by danazol's interaction with these two classes of proteins

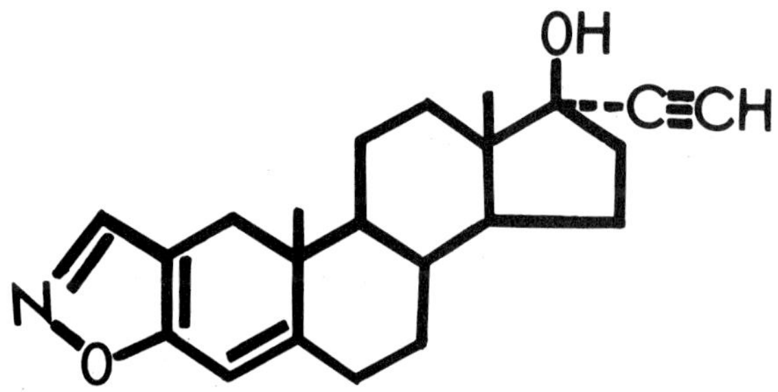

Fig. 11-9. Structure of danazol.

Danazol and Steroid-Binding Proteins. Systematic screening of the interaction of danazol with steroid-binding proteins found that danazol binds to intracellular androgen, progesterone, and glucocorticoid receptors.[8] Numerous investigators have confirmed these original findings (Table 11-7).

The interaction of a steroid with an intracellular steroid receptor system can result in three possible outcomes: (1) the steroid can produce the biologic effects characteristic of that intracellular receptor system (agonist); (2) the steroid can block the biologic effects typically seen after stimulation of the receptor system (antagonist); and (3) the steroid can produce a mixed pattern of agonistic and antagonistic effects. For example, in androgen receptor bioassays (prostatic growth), danazol appears to be a potent androgen agonist. As previously noted, androgens induce atrophy in endometrial implants. The androgenic effect of danazol is one of the main pharmacologic means by which this drug produces atrophy in endometrial tissue.

Danazol has been reported to bind to intranuclear estrogen receptors. However, the affinity of the danazol-estrogen receptor interaction is so weak that this interaction is not believed to have clinical significance. Danazol interacts with glucocorticoid receptors; preliminary evidence suggests that it is a weak glucocorticoid agonist. Danazol also binds to intranuclear progesterone receptors, but its effects in bioassays for progesterone are exceedingly complex. In some bioassays, danazol induces secretory changes in the endometrium which suggests that danazol is a progesterone agonist. In other systems, danazol is able to block the effect of progesterone in the Clauberg assay: a test substance is given to estrogen-primed immature rabbits, and endometrial histologic studies are performed to assess progestational changes. Thus in this circumstance, danazol behaves as an antiprogesterone. Given these diverse bioassay findings, it may be best to classify danazol as a mixed agonist-antagonist with respect to the progesterone receptor system.

In addition to binding to intracellular steroid receptors, danazol also interacts with circulating steroid hormone-binding globulins. Danazol can displace testosterone from sex hormone-binding globulin (SHBG) and cortisol from corticosteroid-binding globulin. Of these two interactions, the danazol-induced increase in the percentage of "bioavailable testosterone" is clinically the more important. In normal women, 40% of testosterone is bioavailable (non-SHBG bound). In women taking danazol, 80% or more of the circulating testosterone is bioavailable (Table 11-8).[83] Therefore part of the androgenic properties of danazol in the human may be due to the dramatic increase in bioavailable androgens caused by danazol. In addition, the observation that danazol can bind to circulating steroid-binding proteins significantly complicates the interpretation of serum total steroid concentrations in patients receiving this drug.

In summary, danazol is an androgen, a glucocorticoid agonist, and a mixed agonist-antagonist with respect to the progesterone receptor system. Part of danazol's androgenic behavior may be due to its ability to displace testosterone from SHBG, which results in an increase in bioavailable testosterone. Danazol's poor ability to bind to estrogen receptors suggests that it has no significant effects in this receptor system. Steroid receptors regulate cell function in a large number of diverse tissues. The effects of danazol on cell function in a variety of steroid receptor-containing tissues will be reviewed briefly.

By acting as an androgen agonist, danazol decreases LH and FSH secretion in castrated animals. One of danazol's main metabolites, ethinyl-testosterone, also suppresses LH and FSH secretion in castrated animals by acting as a progesterone agonist.[29] Although danazol suppresses LH and FSH in castrated animals, the effects of danazol on LH and FSH in animals with intact gonads are complex. The weight of evidence suggests that in women with ovaries, danazol administration does not produce a significant decrease in basal serum LH or FSH levels. This can be explained by the fact that danazol exerts a mild suppressive effect on pituitary secretion of LH and FSH but simultaneously causes a decrease in circulating estradiol levels (by direct actions on the ovary). This in turn stimulates a rise in LH and FSH levels. The overall effect is that danazol does not produce any significant change in basal serum LH or FSH levels in premenopausal women receiving this drug.

Danazol's androgenic properties directly suppress the growth of endometriosis and endometrial tissues. Danazol's lack of estrogenic effects facilitates the androgen-mediated inhibition of growth.

Danazol's androgenic properties probably contribute to the decreased high-density lipoprotein (HDL) cholesterol levels observed in women receiving danazol. The atherogenic risk caused by the decrease in HDL cholesterol levels remains to be fully quantified, but patients with low HDL cholesterol levels may be at increased risk of developing atherosclerosis. Danazol's androgenic and mixed progestational effects probably contribute to the mild increase in insulin resistance that is observed in women receiving this drug.

Danazol's androgenic properties play a major role in altering the production rates of a large number of liver proteins. Danazol increases the production of the following liver proteins: prealbumin, Cl-esterase inhibitor, haptoglobin, transferrin, antithrombin III, prothrombin, and plasminogen. Danazol decreases the production of the following liver

Table 11-7. Interaction of danazol with intracellular androgen, progesterone, and estrogen receptors, and with circulating steroid-binding proteins

	Affinity of danazol for receptor	Biologic consequence
Intracellular receptor system		
Androgen	High affinity	Androgen agonist
Progestin	Moderate affinity	Mixed progestin agonist-antagonist
Estrogen	Low affinity	No estrogenic effects
Circulating steroid-binding proteins		
Sex hormone-binding globulin	Moderate affinity	Causes large increase in free testosterone
Corticosteroid-binding globulin	Moderate affinity	Causes small increase in free cortisol

Table 11-8. Percent of testosterone bound to sex hormone-binding globulin, bound to albumin, and free in women receiving danazol*

	Normal women	Women receiving danazol
SHBG bound	60.1	18
Albumin bound	38.6	79.4
Free testosterone	1.3	2.6

*From Nilsson B et al: Danazol and gestagen displacement of testosterone and influence of sex hormone-binding capacity, *Fertil Steril* 39:505, 1983.

proteins: SHBG, thyroxine-binding globulin, and pregnancy zone protein.

Substantial evidence is accumulating that steroid hormones play a major role in the regulation of the immune system. Glucocorticoid and progestogenic agonists appear to be the most important steroid regulators of the immune system. Danazol, a drug known to interact with both progesterone and glucocorticoid receptors, has been reported to be effective in the treatment of idiopathic thrombocytopenic purpura and systemic lupus erythematosis. Recent in vivo and in vitro studies have demonstrated that danazol can directly suppress leukocyte function.[51]

Danazol and Enzymes of Steroidogenesis. In 1977 it was first reported that danazol inhibits multiple enzymes of steroidogenesis.[5,6] Concentrations of danazol similar to those in the circulation of women who are taking 800 mg/day (2 umol/L) of the drug inhibit multiple enzymes involved in ovarian, testicular, and adrenal steroidogenesis. These enzymes include (1) 3b-hydroxysteroid dehydrogenase isomerase; (2) the 17-hydroxylase, 17-20-lyase complex; (3) 17b-hydroxysteroid dehydrogenase; (4) 11b-hydroxylase; and (5) 21-hydroxylase.[10,11] Steingold et al demonstrated that danazol inhibits steroidogenesis in vivo.[104] They compared the estradiol rise caused by the administration of urinary LH and FSH in five normal women treated with danazol and five normal women not treated with danazol. Danazol treatment resulted in a 50% decrease in serum estradiol. This suggested that danazol inhibited the effects of exogenous gonadotropins by a direct action on the ovary. These investigators also provided evidence that danazol is an inhibitor of the ovarian 17-hydroxylase enzyme in vivo in a second experiment, in which all the experimental subjects were given dexamethasone. The purpose of this manipulation was to ensure that all serum C-21 and C-19 steroids were derived from the ovary. One half of the subjects were then treated with danazol. In the women treated with danazol, a significant increase in serum pregnenolone along with a concomitant decrease in serum 17- hydroxypregnenolone, androstenedione, and dehydroepiandrosterone was observed.[104] These studies suggest that danazol blocks ovarian estrogen production by inhibiting enzymes of steroidogenesis.

An acyclic, high-androgen, low-estrogen environment is extremely hostile to the growth of endometrial tissue. Danazol produces a high-androgen environment because (1) danazol is inherently androgenic and (2) danazol produces high levels of bioavailable testosterone by displacing testosterone from SHBG. A high-androgen environment directly inhibits the growth of endometrial tissue. Danazol produces a low-estrogen environment by (1) inhibiting follicular growth by decreasing LH secretion (and FSH secretion) and (2) inhibiting follicular estrogen secretion via a direct action on follicular steroidogenesis. In addition, the acyclic endocrine environment produced by danazol minimizes the chance of menstruation, which prevents the "reseeding" of the peritoneum with new implants of the retrograde transported endometrium. The acyclic endocrine environment may also decrease pelvic pain by inhibiting bleeding in the endometriotic implants.

Guidelines concerning the use of danazol continue to evolve. The following discussion highlights the areas of consensus and the breadth of disagreement concerning the use of danazol.

Selection of patients for therapy. Most clinicians agree that patients with a suspected diagnosis of endometriosis must have confirmation of the diagnosis by laparoscopy or laparotomy before initiation of therapy.

Initiation of therapy. Danazol should be initiated after the completion of a normal menses. It is important that danazol not be administered to a pregnant woman. Female pseudohermaphroditism is common in female offspring of mothers treated with danazol during the first and second trimesters.[36] Danazol is an effective contraceptive agent (less than 1% incidence of ovulation) at doses of 400 to 800 mg/day. However, patients with poor medication compliance can become pregnant on these doses of danazol because they are taking the drug in an intermittent fashion. Pregnancy testing and careful uterine examinations during danazol therapy will ensure the early detection of an unintended pregnancy. At doses of danazol of less than 400 mg/day, the incidence of ovulation is substantial thus barrier contraceptive should be used. In addition, women taking more than 400 mg/day of danazol should use a barrier contraceptive if their medication compliance is poor.

Dosage. Danazol in doses of 200 mg/day or greater produces pain relief in the majority of patients with endometriosis. However, doses of at least 400 mg of danazol are required to induce amenorrhea reliably (Table 11-9).[15] Given these considerations and a desire to minimize costs, most patients are started on 200 mg of danazol twice daily. For patients with severe endometriosis, consideration can be given to using danazol at a dose of 200 mg four times daily.

Cessation of menses and serum estradiol levels are good clinical and laboratory monitors of danazol therapy. Many experienced clinicians believe that the maximal therapeutic effect of danazol occurs if menses are completely suppressed. The greater the degree of estrogen suppression, the greater the likelihood that amenorrhea will occur. The interval between drug administration appears to play an important role in determining the degree of estrogen suppression. For example, in one study the mean serum estradiol concentration was 40% lower in patients receiving 200 mg of danazol every 6 hours than in patients receiving 400 mg of danazol every 12 hours.[30]

Duration of therapy. Initial trials investigating the efficacy of danazol evaluated a 6-month therapy regimen. This therapy interval need not be followed rigidly. Individualization of care is important when danazol is used to treat endometriosis. For example, in the patient with advanced endometriosis who is scheduled for conservative laparotomy,

Table 11-9. Dose response characteristics of danazol in the treatment of endometriosis after 6 months of treatment

Daily dose of danazol (mg)	Amenorrhea	Percentage of women with symptomatic improvement	Objective improvement
100	29	54	67
200	38	86	79
400	86	74	66
600	88	96	91

(From Biberoglu KO, Behrman SJ: Dosage aspects of danazol therapy in endometriosis: short-term and long-term effectiveness, *Am J Obstet Gynecol* 139:645, 1981.)

a 12-week preoperative course of danazol might be appropriate. For the patient with painful endometriosis who does not desire pregnancy and who is adamantly opposed to surgery, a 52- to 78-week course of danazol is reasonable if side effects and laboratory parameters are carefully monitored.

Side effects. More than 75% of patients receiving danazol will complain of one or more side effects.[7] The major side effects seen with danazol therapy (in decreasing order of frequency) are weight gain, edema, decreased breast size, acne, oily skin, hirsutism, deepening of the voice, headache, hot flashes, changes in libido, and muscle cramps. Significant weight gain (2 to 10 kg) is not uncommon.

Contraindications. In nonpregnant, nonbreast-feeding patients with documented endometriosis, relatively few absolute contraindications to danazol therapy exist. Danazol is metabolized largely via hepatic mechanisms and has been reported to produce mild changes in liver function tests (elevated serum transaminase levels) in some patients. Therefore danazol is contraindicated in patients with hepatic dysfunction. Since danazol can induce marked fluid retention, patients with severe hypertension, congestive heart failure, or borderline renal function may experience deterioration of their medical condition following the initiation of danazol therapy.

Timing of attempts at conception after completion of therapy. Dmowski and Cohen reported a high number of second- and third-trimester intrauterine fetal deaths in patients who conceived within the first three cycles after discontinuation of danazol.[32] They suggested that this degree of fetal wastage may be secondary to implantation in an atrophic endometrium; following a course of danazol, one full menstrual cycle with normal flow and duration should be observed before any attempts to conceive. In contrast to these observations, Daniell and Christianson observed no increase in fetal wastage in patients that conceived within 3 months of completing a course of danazol.[26] Barbieri, Evans, and Kistner confirmed that danazol therapy was not associated with increased fetal wastage.[7] Further information is needed to resolve these discrepancies.

Use of danazol with surgery in the treatment of the infertility of endometriosis. In patients with infertility and advanced stages of endometriosis, surgery is usually necessary to repair anatomic abnormalities and to remove implants of endometriosis. Few experimental data concerning the value of danazol in the preoperative or postoperative management of endometriosis are available. Some experienced clinicians suggest that danazol has little value in the preoperative management of endometriosis. Others believe that danazol may improve the prognosis for infertile women with endometriosis, by decreasing the number and size of endometrial areas and thereby minimize the extent of surgery. In addition, the preoperative use of danazol eliminates the chance of traumatizing a corpus luteum. Use of danazol in the postoperative management of the infertile patient with endometriosis is also controversial. Most conceptions following surgical therapy occur within the first 12 months after surgery. By treating surgical patients with danazol for a prolonged period postoperatively, the time interval with the highest fertility potential may be passed over. Therefore danazol may be used in patients preoperatively, but short courses of postoperative danazol therapy should be reserved for women with residual disease who are not attempting conception.

Use in the treatment of endometriosis in patients not desiring fertility. For the patient who is older than 40 years, has symptomatic endometriosis, and who has completed her family, definitive therapy consisting of total abdominal hysterectomy and bilateral salpingo-oophorectomy (TAH-BSO) is usually recommended. However, some patients may want to postpone or avoid major surgery. For these patients, a trial of danazol may be reasonable. For the young, symptomatic patient with endometriosis who intends to delay pregnancy, danazol therapy is highly effective in relieving symptoms and physical findings.

Treatment of endometriomas. There has been no systematic study assessing the effect of danazol on endometriomas. Clinical experience suggests that danazol can often reduce the size of small endometriomas, but it is unusual for danazol to cause complete regression of an endometrioma. In general, danazol is more effective in causing regression of peritoneal endometrial implants of small diameter than in ablating cysts. Large ovarian masses generally require surgical exploration.

Use in metastatic endometriosis. For the majority of patients with endometriosis that involves organs outside the pelvis, TAH-BSO is necessary. Certain patients will refuse surgery, and others are extremely poor operative risks. In these patients, danazol therapy is a last resort. Danazol has been successful in the treatment of pulmonary endometriosis, bowel obstruction, and ureteral obstruction caused by endometriosis. However, once hormone therapy is discontinued, the disease often recurs.

Recurrence rates after therapy for endometriosis. A major problem in the treatment of endometriosis is that the disease tends to recur unless definitive surgical therapy is performed. Following a course of danazol therapy, the recurrence of symptoms and physical findings is at least 20% per year and is generally higher in patients with endometriomas.[7] A second course of danazol therapy is often successful in inducing a remission of disease symptoms and physical findings.

Danazol versus pseudopregnancy. Few data that directly compare the efficacy of danazol versus a pseudopregnancy regimen in the treatment of endometriosis are available. The results of one small, prospective, randomized trial of danazol versus a combination of mestranol and norethynodrel were reported by Noble and Letchworth.[85] A total of 86% of the patients treated with danazol reported improvement in their symptoms. Only 30% of the pseudopregnancy group reported symptomatic improvement, and improvement in objective findings was demonstrated in 84% of patients treated with danazol, compared with only 18% of patients on the pseudopregnancy regimen. Side effects were a major problem for patients receiving both therapeutic regimens. Only 4% of the danazol group but 41% of the pseudopregnancy group discontinued therapy because of side effects.

Gonadotropin-releasing hormone agonist therapy. GnRH is a hypothalamic decapeptide that controls LH and FSH secretion. In primates, pulses of GnRH in the range of one pulse per hour are associated with a normal pattern of LH and FSH secretion, normal follicular and corpus luteum development, and cyclic menses. Administration of GnRH at a high pulse rate (more than five pulses per hour) or in a continuous fashion produces an initial increase in LH and FSH secretion. This is followed by a drastic decrease in LH and FSH secretion with cessation of ovarian follicular activity, hypoestrogenism, and amenorrhea. This may be due to downregulation or desensitization of pituitary GnRH receptors by continuous infusion of GnRH.[70]

The natural decapeptide GnRH has a short half-life because of its degradation by tissue and circulating peptidases. Therefore it is difficult to produce a constant circulating concentration using native GnRH. By the chemical alteration of amino acid 6 of GnRH, analogs can be synthesized that have two useful properties: (1) high affinity for the pituitary GnRH receptor and (2) a very long half-life because of the resistance to cleavage by endopeptidases. Initially, many investigators believed that these synthetic derivatives of GnRH would be superagonists and potent fertility-enhancing agents, hence the term GnRH agonists. Unexpectedly, GnRH agonists proved to be potent inhibitors of gonadal function. Their administration to men or women causes a transient 1- to 2-week increase in the production of LH and FSH by the pituitary gland and then a dramatic and sustained decrease in pituitary production of bioactive LH and FSH. The ability of the GnRH agonists to downregulate pituitary secretion of gonadotropins has not been fully explained. Numerous GnRH agonists, including nafarelin, leuprolide, buserelin, goserelin, histrelin, and triptorelin are currently available or being evaluated in clinical trials (Table 11-10). No GnRH agonist is effective when given orally. These agents, however, can be administered by monthly intramuscular depot injections or implants, or by daily subcutaneous injections, or nasal sprays (Table 11-11).

Treatment with GnRH agonists results in the reversible suppression of gonadal steroid production in men and women. Consequently many diseases that are modulated by the gonadal steroids testosterone and estradiol can be successfully treated with GnRH agonists.

For example, GnRH agonists have been reported to be successful in the treatment of leiomyomata uteri, polycystic ovarian disease, precocious puberty, and premenstrual syndrome and as an adjuvant for the induction of ovulation in women and in the treatment of prostatic cancer in men. The first report of the use of a GnRH agonist in the treatment of endometriosis came from Meldrum et al.[79] Although used for only a 1 month trial, the study demonstrated the efficacy of this class of compounds in therapy for endometriosis.

Henzl et al reported on the comparative efficacies of danazol and the GnRH agonist nafarelin in the treatment of endometriosis.[49] The study was large, randomized, and double blind, and it included an objective assessment of the response

Table 11-10. Structures of gonadotropin-releasing hormone agonists with documented efficacy in the treatment of endometriosis

Native GnRH	***p* Glu-His-Trp-Spr-Tyr-Gly-Leu-Arg-Pro-Gly-NH2** 6	10
Leuprolide	D-Leu	-NHEt
Buserelin	D-Ser(t-Bu)	-AzA-Gly
Nafarelin	D-NAL(2)	—

Table 11-11. Doses of gonadotropin-releasing hormone agonists used in the treatment of endometriosis

Leuprolide acetate	0.5-1.0 mg subcutaneously daily
Leuprolide acetate-Depo formulation	3.75-7.5 mg intramuscularly monthly
Nafarelin	0.4-0.8 mg intranasally daily

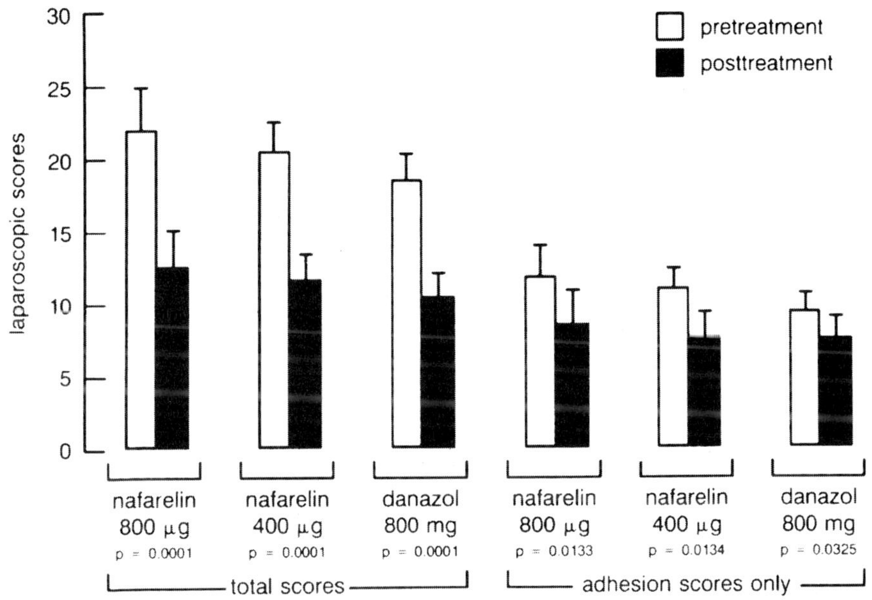

Fig. 11-10. Pretreatment and posttreatment American Fertility Society endometriosis scores in women receiving 6 months of nasal nafarelin or oral danazol therapy. (From Henzl M et al: Administration of nasal nafarelin as compared with oral danazol for endometriosis: a multicenter double-blind comparative clinical trial, *N Engl J Med* 318:485, 1988.)

to therapy by a comparison of laparoscopic examinations performed before and after treatment. The investigators tested two dosages of nasal nafarelin (400 and 800 µg/day) and one dosage of oral danazol (800 mg/day). Drug therapy was continued for 6 months. More than 80% of the patients treated with either nafarelin or danazol had symptomatic and objective improvement in their condition. Nafarelin and danazol were found to be quantitatively similar in efficacy (Fig. 11-10). However, the side effects of the two drugs differed substantially. The women who received danazol reported weight gain, edema, and myalgia. They had increased circulating levels of serum aspartate aminotransferase and alanine aminotransferase and decreased levels of HDL cholesterol. In contrast, the principal side effects reported by women who received nafarelin were hot flashes, decreased libido, and vaginal dryness.

Similar prospective, randomized, comparative trials of other GnRH agonists and danazol report comparable efficacy and side effects. Matta and Shaw utilized buserelin,[77] Wheeler et al used leuprolide depot,[115] the Nafarelin European Endometriosis Trial group studied nafarelin,[81] and Shaw and Rock et al investigated goserelin.[91] In all cases the GnRH agonists proved efficacious and safe.

The major safety concern raised with this class of drugs relates to their hypoestrogenic effects. The initial experience with the GnRH agonists demonstrates that patients using the agonists experience a variety of hypoestrogenic symptoms, including hot flashes and vaginal dryness. In addition, urinary calcium studies suggest an increase in calcium excretion similar to that seen in menopausal women. There is thus a concern that patients taking GnRH agonists are at risk of losing trabecular bone.[103] The spongy trabecular portion of bone that is found in the spine and hip is more sensitive to the loss of estrogen than the cortical bone found in the shaft of the long bones. Numerous investigators have examined the extent of bone loss during short courses of GnRH agonists. Although the sites measured, the method of measurement, and the drug used have differed, most studies demonstrate an approximate 2% to 7% loss in bone density over 6 months of GnRH agonist treatment, with complete or partial recovery over a 6-month, follow-up interval.[42]

Because of the concern about hypoestrogenic effects, most notably on bone, there has been a recent trend to combine hormonal "add-back" with the use of GnRH analogs. One strategy has been to combine progestins with GnRH agonists. The combination of medroxyprogesterone acetate with GnRH agonist treatment diminished hot flashes and protected bone but failed to improve endometrial symptoms.[18] The use of a different progestin, norethindrone, produced symptomatic relief but failed to protect bone density.[106] The same progestin (norethindrone) now used in a higher dose of 5 to 10 mg/day yielded symptomatic relief of endometriosis, with laparoscopically proven efficacy, and had a protective effect on bone.[107] However, this high dose of norethindrone led to adverse effects on serum lipids and cholesterol subfractions.

Another strategy in reducing the hypoestrogenic effects of GnRH analogues has been to "add-back" small doses of estrogens, in addition to progestins, to alleviate the adverse effects of severe hypoestrogenemia while preserving the beneficial effects of GnRH agonist therapy. This treatment regimen is predicated on the hypothesis that estrogen-dependent tissues vary in their responsiveness to estrogen. An "estrogen threshold" may exist for each estrogen-dependent disease; therefore clinical improvement in the underlying disease may occur with only minimal adverse effects of hypoestrogenism.[3,44] Thus an estradiol therapeutic window may exist in which maximum benefit can occur with minimal hypoestrogenic sequelae. Two recent studies suggest that such an estrogen-progestin "add-back" is efficacious and safe. In a small retrospective study, Friedman and Hornstein demonstrated continued reduction in pelvic pain with diminished AFS endometriosis scores in patients who had endometriosis and were followed for 2 years.[43] They were placed on a regimen of 3.75 mg of leuprolide acetate depot every 4 weeks, with 0.625 mg of conjugated equine estrogens and 2.5 mg of medroxyprogesterone acetate daily. No loss of bone density was seen in these women. In addition, Howell et al showed that patients who had endometriosis and were treated for 6 months with goserelin combined with transdermal estradiol and medroxyprogesterone acetate suffered less bone loss than women treated with goserelin alone.[58] Critical evaluation of the efficacy of the steroid add-back approach will await the results of large-scale, definitive, randomized, clinical trials.

The large numbers of recent publications on the use of the GnRH agonists for endometriosis serve to emphasize that the use of these agents continues to evolve. Nonetheless, it is now possible to present some guidelines for the use of these compounds with the caveat that many disagreements among experts still exist. The format below is similar to that used in the discussion of danazol and may allow the reader to contrast the clinical use of these two pharmacologic approaches.

Selection of patients for therapy. As in the case of danazol, because of the side effects and cost of GnRH agonists, patients with suspected endometriosis should have confirmation of the disease by laparoscopy or laparotomy before the therapy.

Initiation of therapy. It is possible to initiate GnRH analogs at two points during the menstrual cycle. Patients may begin the agonists during a normal menses or in the midluteal phase of the cycle. As these agents produce temporary elevations in the gonadotropins, and it generally takes 8 to 15 days for full pituitary downregulation to occur, it is best not to have the agonist effect coincide with the ovulatory midcycle gonadotropin surge. This is best accomplished with an early follicular or midluteal start. Depot preparation should be given at the time of menses. Although malformations associated with GnRH agonist use have not been reported, the safety of its use in early pregnancy has not been established. Thus it is prudent to avoid inadvertent use in early gestation.

Dosage. The recommended dosages of the GnRH agonists currently available in the United States appear in Table 11-11. These doses have been shown to produce estradiol levels in the range of 15 to 30 pg/mL.

Duration of therapy. The Food and Drug Administration has approved nafarelin and leuprolide depot for a 6-month course of therapy for endometriosis. This regimen was based on early studies that used this duration of treatment and took into account the concerns regarding the long-term loss of bone. For patients with no or minimal loss in bone density, or with bone density above the "fracture threshold" after 6 months of therapy, further treatment may be considered with the patient's consent followed by careful monitoring of bone density every 6 months. Alternatively, appropriate hormonal "add-back" regimens may be considered. Repeated cycles of GnRH agonist are possible, with confirmation of healthy bone density before reinitiating therapy.[48]

Side effects. The profound hypoestrogenia seen with these agents leads to predictable side effects of hot flashes (90%), vaginal dryness, and decreased libido. In addition, more than 20% of patients taking GnRH agonists suffer from headaches.[50] Women with a history of migraines seem to be predisposed to a worsening of their headaches. Androgenic side effects such as acne, oily skin, and hirsutism are predictably rare in women treated with GnRH agonists.

Contraindications. As mentioned previously, GnRH agonists are contraindicated in pregnancy. In addition, women who are breastfeeding or who have undiagnosed vaginal bleeding should not take these agents. Hypersensitivity reactions to GnRH agonists have been reported.

Timing of attempts at conception after therapy cessation. Menses generally resume approximately 6 weeks after the completion of a course of GnRH analogs. Unlike danazol, increased fetal wastage has not been reported with these medications.

Use of GnRH agonists with surgery in treatment of endometriosis. There are no large-scale clinical findings to evaluate the efficacy of GnRH analogs, either preoperatively or postoperatively in patients who have endometriosis. As the optimal time to attempt conception is the first 12 months following surgery, and as menses do not immediately return following GnRH agonist therapy, it seems prudent to refrain from postoperative use of these drugs in infertile patients. However, postoperative use of the analogs may be efficacious in patients in whom pelvic pain returns rapidly following surgery or in whom significant residual disease remains.

Treatment of endometriomas. Medical therapy is unlikely to produce complete regression of large endometrial cysts. Patients with such ovarian masses should have surgical exploration. This is possible in many cases by laparoscopy. One study, however, demonstrated a reduction in the size of ovarian cysts, presumed to be endometriomas, in patients who were treated with buserelin.[34] In general, the cysts were small (3 to 4 cm) and only a small (1 to 2 cm) diminution in their size was reported.

Use in metastatic endometriosis. Endometriosis outside the pelvis generally requires TAH-BSO; however, the use of GnRH agonists for extrapelvic endometriosis has been suggested.[75] An interesting case of catamenial pneumothorax, recurrent pneumothorax associated with menstruation treated by leuprolide depot, has recently been reported.[35] In this case, episodes of pneumothorax ceased during the 1 year the patient was treated with GnRH agonist but recurred when she was changed to daily norethindrone.

Recurrence rates after medical therapy. It is difficult to appreciate fully the recurrence rate after medical therapy for endometriosis. Pelvic pain resulting from other causes may lead to overestimates of recurrence rates, while the recurrence of disease not leading to patient complaints may underestimate reactivation of disease. Waller and Shaw recently reviewed the research of patients with laparoscopically proven endometriosis who were treated with GnRH agonists between 1985 and 1987; recurrence rates up to 7 years from the initial treatment were reported.[112] They found that the cumulative recurrence rate for the fifth year of treatment was 53%. However, patients with minimal disease and severe disease had recurrence rates of 37% and 74%, respectively. This long-term study suggests that recurrence of endometriosis following medical therapy is frequent and more likely in patients with more severe disease.

GnRH agonists versus pseudopregnancy. While relief of pain with pseudopregnancy (oral contraceptive [OC] use) does occur, severe cases of endometriosis are better treated with danazol or a GnRH agonist. OCs, especially used in a noncyclic manner, benefit many women with mild degrees of endometriosis. A direct comparison between OCs and GnRH agonists for treatment of endometriosis has recently been published. Vercellini et al prospectively compared goserelin and a low dose OC that contained 0.02 mg ethinyl estradiol and 0.15 mg desogestrel.[111] While significant pain reduction occurred in both groups, women with deep dyspareunia reported better relief with goserelin than with OCs. The reduction in nonmenstrual pain and return of symptoms was similar in both groups. Both drugs were well tolerated and only one patient (in the OC group) withdrew because of side effects. This study again demonstrated the efficacy of OCs in the treatment of endometriosis, but it also demonstrated that in more severe cases the GnRH agonists may provide greater symptomatic relief.

Guidelines for the use of leuprolide or nafarelin for the treatment of endometriosis are similar to those outlined for the use of danazol; for example, (1) document the presence of endometriosis by laparoscopy or laparotomy; (2) ensure that the patient is not pregnant; (3) employ the drug at a dose that will induce amenorrhea; (4) consider a treatment interval of 6 months; and (5) monitor side effects carefully.

Pseudopregnancy regimens. In response to chronic, noncyclic stimulation by both estrogen and progesterone, the endometrium becomes inactive and demonstrates decidualization. Figs. 11-11 and 11-12 illustrate this phenomenon. This observation is the basis for the use of uninterrupted combined estrogen-progestogen agents in the treatment of endometriosis.[68,69] There is no evidence that any one preparation of estrogen-progestogen pill is uniquely effective in the treatment of endometriosis. Therefore any combined estrogen-progestogen preparation may be employed; however, OCs using an androgenic progestin have theoretical appeal. A standard regimen would employ 0.03 mg of ethinyl estradiol with 0.3 mg of norgestrel (Lo/Ovral) daily. The hormones are given every day for 3 to 4 months. The medication is discontinued for 1 week, and light menstrual bleeding may occur at this time. The medication is then reinstituted for another course. If clinically significant breakthrough bleeding occurs, the hormone dosage can be increased to 0.05 mg of ethinyl estradiol with 0.5 mg of norgestrel (Ovral) daily.

A pseudopregnancy regimen is especially useful in the management of dysmenorrhea caused by endometriosis in the young patient. For example, a 17-year-old teenager with mild endometriosis and incapacitating dysmenorrhea, can be given a pseudopregnancy regimen as previously described. For the teenage patient, a pseudopregnancy regimen is less expensive and often better tolerated than danazol.

Progestin-only regimens. Numerous progestins (e.g., medroxyprogesterone acetate, norethindrone acetate, norgestrel acetate, and lynestrenol) are used as single agents for the treatment of endometriosis.[99] In general, these agents produce a hypoestrogenic-acyclic hormonal environment by suppressing ovarian follicular activity via inhibition of LH and FSH secretion. In addition, these agents may have direct effects on endometrial tissue androgen and progesterone receptors. As noted earlier, many synthetic progestins are weak androgen agonists.

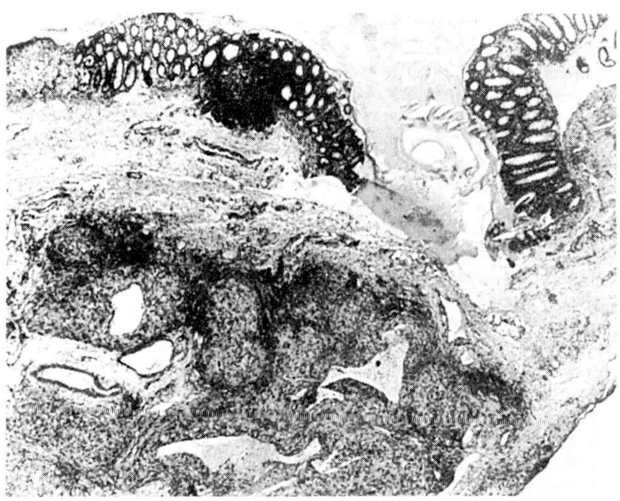

Fig. 11-11. Biopsy of a mass in the rectovaginal septum during the 14th week of pregnancy. Rectal mucosa is seen at the top of the section. Approximately two thirds of the rectal wall has been replaced by endometrial tissue made up of inactive glands and decidua. The endometrial stroma (as decidua) is packed in whorl-like accumulations. (From Kistner RW: The use of steroidal substances in endometriosis, *Clin Pharmacol Ther* 1:525, 1960.)

A major problem with the use of progestins as single agents is that large doses must be given to produce an acyclic-hypoestrogenic environment. These high doses are often associated with side-effects such as bloating, weight gain, depression, and irregular uterine bleeding. Parenteral administration of large doses of medroxyprogesterone acetate in depot form can be effective in the treatment of endometriosis (a dose range of 150 mg every 3 months to 150 mg every month). However, this drug is not recommended as a first-line agent because it can produce prolonged amenorrhea after termination of therapy, and the long-term safety of the agent is still controversial. Oral administration of 30 to 50 mg of medroxyprogesterone acetate daily can be effective in the treatment of endometriosis.[72]

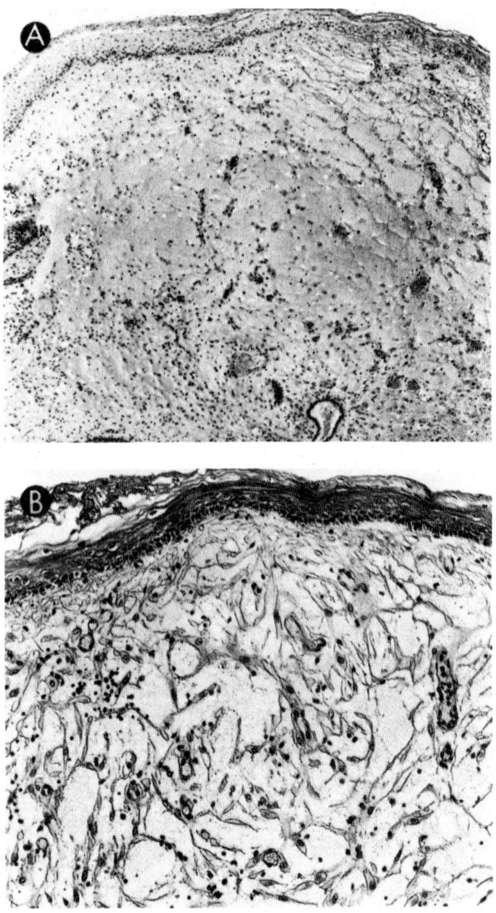

Fig. 11-12. Biopsy of an area of vaginal endometriosis after 12 weeks of continuous norethyndrel with ethinyl estradiol therapy. **A,** There is evidence of marked generalized edema throughout the endometriosis. Under the vaginal epithelium the decidua is well maintained, but most of it is undergoing necrosis. **B,** High-power view of **A.** An unusual pattern of decidual change is present. Most decidual cells remain as naked nuclei or as a cytoplasmic strand in an edematous stroma. A few lymphocytes and macrophages are present and suggest an absorptive process of the necrotic endometriosis. (From Kistner RW: The treatment of endometriosis by inducing pseudopregnancy with ovarian hormones, *Fertil Steril* 10:539, 1959.)

Surgical treatment. In contemplating surgical treatment of endometriosis, one should always bear in mind that functioning ovarian tissue is necessary for the continued activity of the disease. Therefore the successful treatment of endometriosis depends on a knowledge of when it is reasonably safe or desirable to maintain ovarian function and when it is necessary to eliminate it. It is quite obvious that ovarian function should be conserved when treating very early, perhaps symptomless lesions, and eliminated when the pelvic organs are hopelessly invaded by endometriosis or when fertility is no longer a concern. Unfortunately from the standpoint of definite surgical indications, the majority of cases will fall between these two extremes and may present problems in surgical judgment seldom encountered in any other pelvic disease. As knowledge of the life history of endometriosis increases, there is a tendency to become more conservative, particularly in the treatment of early and borderline cases. In general, it is believed that one should err on the side of conservatism. This belief is based on the fact that endometriosis (1) usually progresses slowly over a period of years; (2) only rarely becomes malignant; and (3) regresses at menopause. Current surgical options include laparoscopic surgery, conservative surgery via a laparotomy, and extirpative surgery.

Laparoscopic surgery. The diagnosis of endometriosis requires laparoscopy or laparotomy. At the time of a diagnostic laparoscopy, an attempt should be made to excise all endometrial implants and adhesions. Laparoscopic surgery for advanced endometriosis requires 2 to 3 hours of operative time, advanced technical skills on the part of the surgeon, and specialized equipment. Minimal and mild endometriosis can often be surgically treated at the time of diagnostic laparoscopy without significantly prolonging operative time, and with a minimum of special skills and equipment. Laparoscopic treatment of endometriosis uses a two- or three-puncture technique. Two lower abdominal incisions are often necessary to grasp specific pelvic organs and to allow the use of unipolar or bipolar electrocautery or laser for lysis of adhesions and ablation of implants. Ablation of the uterosacral ligaments at laparoscopy may decrease pain in some patients. There are no studies that directly compare the efficacy of electrocautery and laser in the treatment of endometriosis-associated infertility. Laser surgery has the theoretical advantage, since the depth of tissue injury is often less than that produced by cautery. Advances in laparoscopic surgery are discussed in more detail in Chapter 25.

Conservative surgery technique. If the childbearing function is to be preserved, operative procedures should be as conservative as possible. The approach can usually be through a suprapubic transverse incision. A thorough exploration of the pelvic and abdominal organs should be routinely performed, and a decision should be reached about the performance of either conservative or definitive surgery. Good infertility surgical technique is important. Gentle handling of tissues and meticulous hemostasis are important in minimizing subsequent adhesion formation. The uterus is frequently found to be adherent to the rectosigmoid. These adhesions are separated either by blunt or sharp dissection in the midline, so that the uterus can be brought forward. Traction sutures of 1-0 Mersilene may be placed around the round ligaments to lift the corpus forward and out of the cul-de-sac (Fig. 11-13). With the uterus held forward, further adhesions may then be separated under direct vision. As previously mentioned, the use of hormonal agents for 6 to 12 weeks preoperatively may make the surgery easier to perform. Endometrial implants on the uterosacral ligaments or in the cul-de-sac may be excised, fulgurated by electrocautery, or vaporized by laser. Because some pain-transmitting nerve fibers from the uterus course through the uterosacral ligaments, some gynecologists cut or fulgurate them in the hope of reducing postoperative dysmenorrhea.

Endometrial cysts of the ovary should be excised. These cysts are usually adherent and do not separate as freely as corpus luteum or follicular cysts. After as much of the cyst as possible has been removed, the walls of the ovary are reapproximated with several mattress stitches of fine Vicryl suture and the surface is closed with a running, locked stitch of 4-0 Vicryl. Occasionally all ovarian tissue is destroyed, and oophorectomy is necessary. Nevertheless, an ovarian cyst can be enucleated and a fairly thick capsule of functioning cortical tissue left in situ. Unilateral salpingo-oophorectomy (USO) and resection of 90% of the remaining ovary can result in subsequent ovulation and pregnancy. This is not always the case, however, and some patients have premature menopause following such surgery.

Early implantations on the surface of the peritoneum, wherever they are located, may be excised or destroyed with cautery or the laser. Conservative operations may also be accompanied by correction of uterine displacement, relief of cervical stenosis, and removal of any other concomitant pelvic pathology to aid in the prevention of a recurrence of the condition. Presacral neurectomy, in which the superior hypogastric plexus is divided and ligated, may be performed at the same time to reduce pain associated with endometriosis, in women who wish to preserve childbearing. This procedure works best in women whose pain is primarily in the midline.[16]

The use of intraoperative, intraperitoneal adjuvants to prevent adhesion formation has become widespread in gynecologic surgery, without substantial experimental evidence to support their efficacy. Glucocorticoids, promethazine, high molecular weight dextran, and heparin have all been used in this effort. In addition, some gynecologists have advocated the postoperative use of nonsteroidal antiinflammatory drugs such as ibuprofen to reduce adhesion formation associated with pelvic surgery.

In recent years, Hyskon (a water-soluble glucose polymer of 32% dextran 70 in 10% dextrose) has become popular among gynecologic surgeons. It is widely used as a distending medium for hysteroscopy and is frequently used to prevent adhesions as well.[93] The mechanism of action in minimizing adhesions is unknown but probably occurs because of several of Hyskon's properties. It is hyperosmolar, which induces a temporary ascites and separates serosal layers. It may also inhibit coagulation of fibrin on traumatized serosal surfaces. The solution is easily administered by pouring 50 to 100 mL over the pelvic viscera before closing the peritoneum.

Serious side effects, including anaphylaxis, vulvar edema, and pleural effusions have been reported.[90,110] These complications can be prevented by the prophylactic intravenous use of low molecular-weight dextran (Promit). Promit is a monovalent hapten that prevents the formation of immune complexes of dextran-reactive immunoglobulin (IgG) and thus impedes the occurrence of allergic phenomena. Promit should be given several minutes before Hyskon.

Recent studies have also shown some reduction in postoperative adhesions when antiprostaglandins have been used postoperatively.[66] The use of Hyskon with an antiprostaglandin has provided greater adhesion reduction

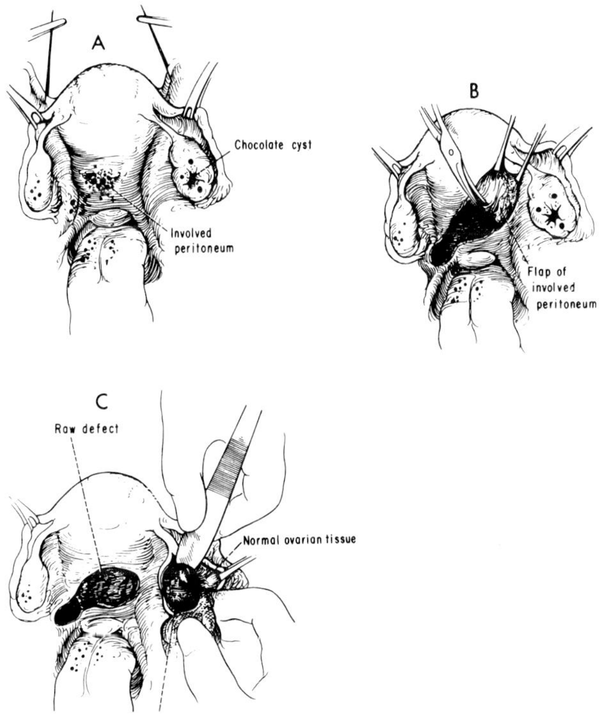

Fig. 11-13. A, The uterus is drawn forward using traction sutures placed around the round ligaments. Areas of endometriosis are shown on the ovaries, posterior aspect of the uterus, and anterior surface of the sigmoid colon. **B,** Serosa of posterior aspect of the uterus involved by endometriosis is excised. Alternatively, endometrial lesions in this area can be fulgurated. **C,** Endometrioma of the right ovary is excised, preserving as much normal ovarian cortex as possible.

than when either agent was used alone.[28] In addition, absorbable barriers have been tested in the attempt to reduce postoperative adhesions. A form of oxidized regenerated cellulose has shown promise in some studies in reducing pelvic adhesions.[63]

Despite a number of studies showing benefits from the use of these adhesion prevention modalities, some investigators have found no benefit. Simple use of Ringer's lactated solution may provide protection against adhesions equal to that achieved by other means and produces fewer side effects.[37]

Hormonal therapy is generally given for approximately 3 months after surgery, if all areas of endometriosis cannot be excised; then concerted efforts are made toward conception. About one half of women so treated will become pregnant, if no other cause for infertility exists.

The incidence of pregnancy following conservative surgery varies widely and is dependent on such factors as extent of the disease, age of the patient, frequency of coitus, previous parity, and the presence of other pelvic pathologic lesions (e.g., leiomyomas, tubal disease, and adhesions) at the time of surgery. It is expected that approximately 40% to 70% of patients who are desirous of childbearing will become pregnant after conservative surgical treatment for endometriosis. Most pregnancies will occur within the first 12 months following conservative surgery.

Extirpative surgery. The treatment of choice for most women with advanced endometriosis who have completed their family is TAH-BSO. From a pathophysiologic viewpoint, it is the bilateral oophorectomy and the concomitant hypoestrogenism that provide relief from the disease process. Many authorities recommend TAH or TAH-USO for the treatment of endometriosis. These authorities argue that leaving one or both ovaries in situ will prevent the sequelae of an early surgical menopause. Although this is true, approximately 50% of women treated with TAH alone will require reoperation because of persistent endometriosis.[80] In a recently reported study, 63% of women who had ovarian preservation at the time of hysterectomy for endometriosis had recurrent symptoms, and nearly half of those women required repeat surgery.[82] A 50% failure rate makes this an unattractive treatment option for advanced endometriosis; however, in cases of mild to moderate endometriosis, TAH-USO may be a reasonable treatment choice.

When definitive surgery for advanced endometriosis is performed, it is important to remove all functioning ovarian tissue. Many women who have advanced endometriosis and who allegedly had TAH-BSO, present with persistent symptoms of disease activity. Uniformly, these women have serum estradiol and FSH concentrations in the premenopausal range. These laboratory studies demonstrate the presence of residual ovarian activity. The high frequency of this scenario prompted the following recommendations: (1) during TAH-BSO for advanced endometriosis, the infundibulopelvic vessels should be ligated high on the pelvic side wall through an incision in the retroperitoneum; (2) every attempt should be made to remove entirely the ovaries along with adherent peritoneal surfaces; and (3) after TAH-BSO, serum FSH and estradiol levels should be monitored monthly, until these hormones enter the menopausal range.

Large, bilateral, ovarian endometrial cysts with extensive peritoneal endometriosis and numerous pelvic adhesions, or with marked invasion of the rectosigmoid and rectovaginal space, constitute the most urgent indications for radical removal of all the pelvic organs, regardless of the age of the patient.

From the operative standpoint, early or moderately advanced endometriosis offers no unusual difficulties, but extensive endometriosis may present many technical problems. Endometriosis, in contrast to pelvic inflammatory disease, produces an extremely dense type of pelvic adhesion with an almost complete absence of planes of cleavage. Therefore much of the dissection must be done with sharp instruments, and the danger of damage to adherent structures is thereby increased. This hazard may be diminished by the use of preoperative danazol or GnRH agonists.

A hysterectomy and BSO can usually be performed on patients with large ovarian endometrial cysts and extensive pelvic adhesions and even on those with marked invasion of the rectovaginal septum. This may be facilitated by incising the posterior peritoneum above the insertion of the uterosacral ligaments. The endopelvic fascia and rectosigmoid may then be reflected, and the danger of fistula formation is minimized. At times it may be necessary to leave a considerable portion of the implants attached to the bowel or other pelvic structures. The fact that these remnants will regress along with other müllerian tissue in the pelvis, following removal of the ovaries, is of great importance in the treatment of this disease. A few cases where this atrophy did not occur have been reported; however, not all ovarian tissue may have been completely removed in some of these cases.

As emphasized, hypoestrogenism "cures" most cases of endometriosis. Paradoxically, most women who have undergone TAH-BSO for advanced endometriosis can use low-dose estrogen replacement therapy without reactivating the endometriosis. If endometriosis is still present approximately 3 months after TAH-BSO, estrogen replacement therapy may be initiated. To reduce hot flashes and to try to reduce residual disease, a course of medroxyprogesterone acetate, 20 mg per day for 3 months, may prove beneficial. At that time, 0.625 mg of conjugated equine estrogens (CEEs) daily or its equivalent is prescribed. With this regimen, fewer than 10% of patients should have reactivation of their disease. If the disease does recur, hormone replacement can be discontinued. Some authorities believe that residual endometriotic implants can undergo malignant transformation when stimulated by continuous unopposed estrogen replacement. These authorities recommend adding a cyclic progestin to the CEE. No well-controlled scientific data to evaluate this practice are available.

REFERENCES

1. American Fertility Society: Revised American Fertility Society Classification of Endometriosis, *Fertil Steril* 43:351, 1985.
2. Barbieri RL: CA-125 in patients with endometriosis, *Fertil Steril* 45:767, 1986.
3. Barbieri RL: Hormone treatment of endometriosis: the estrogen threshold hypothesis, *Am J Obstet Gynecol* 166:740, 1992.
4. Barbieri RL, Callery M, Perez SE: Directionality of menstrual flow: cervical os diameter as a determinant of retrograde menstruation, *Fertil Steril* 57:727, 1992.
5. Barbieri RL et al: Danazol inhibits steroidogenesis, *Fertil Steril* 28:809, 1977a.
6. Barbieri RL, Canick JA, Ryan KJ: Danazol inhibits steroidogenesis in the rat testis in vitro, *Endocrinology* 101:676, 1977b.
7. Barbieri RL, Evans S, Kistner RW: Danazol in the treatment of endometriosis: analysis of 100 cases with a 4-year follow-up, *Fertil Steril* 37:737, 1982.
8. Barbieri RL, Lee H, Ryan KJ: Danazol-binding to rat androgen, glucocorticoid, progesterone, and estrogen receptors: correlation with biological activity, *Fertil Steril* 31:182, 1979.
9. Barbieri RL et al: Elevated serum concentrations of CA-125 in patients with advanced endometriosis, *Fertil Steril* 45:630, 1986.
10. Barbieri RL, Osathanondh R, Ryan KJ: Danazol inhibition of steroidogenesis in the human corpus luteum, *Obstet Gynecol* 57:722, 1981.
11. Barbieri RL et al: Danazol inhibits human adrenal 21- and 11a-hydroxylation, *Steroids* 35:251, 1980.
12. Barbieri RL, Ryan KJ: Danazol: Endocrine pharmacology and therapeutic applications, *Am J Obstet Gynecol* 141:453, 1981.
13. Bast RC et al: Reactivity of a monoclonal antibody with human ovarian carcinoma, *J Clin Invest* 68:1331, 1981.
14. Bast RC et al: A radioimmunoassay using a monoclonal antibody to monitor the course of epithelial ovarian cancer, *N Engl J Med* 309:883, 1983.
15. Biberoglu KO, Behrman SJ: Dosage aspects of danazol therapy in endometriosis: short-term and long-term effectiveness, *Am J Obstet Gynecol* 139:645, 1981.
16. Candiani G et al: Presacral neorectomy for the treatment of pelvic pain associated with endometriosis: a controlled study, *Am J Obstet Gynecol* 167:100, 1992.
17. Cattell RB, Swinton NW: Endometriosis with particular reference to conservative treatment, *N Engl J Med* 241:341, 1936.
18. Cedars M et al: Treatment of endometriosis with a long-acting gonadotropin releasing hormone agonist plus medroxyprogesterone acetate, *Obstet Gynecol* 75:641, 1990.
19. Chaffkin LM et al: A comparative analysis of the cycle fecundity rates associated with combined human menopausal gonadotropin (hMG) and intrauterine insemination (IUI) versus either hMG or IUI alone, *Fertil Steril* 55:252, 1991.
20. Chalas E et al: Nucleolar organizer regions in endometriosis, atypical endometriosis, and clear cell and endometrioid carcinomas, *Gynecol Oncol* 40:260-3, 1991.
21. Cook AS, Rock JA: Surgical management of endometriosis, *Semin Reprod Endocrinol* 9:138, 1991.
22. Cramer DW: Epidemiology of endometriosis. In Wilson EA, editor: *Endometriosis*, New York, 1987, Alan R Liss.
23. Cramer DW et al: The relation of endometriosis to menstrual characteristics, smoking, and exercise, *JAMA* 225:1904, 1985.
24. Cullen TS: Adenomyoma of the round ligament, *Bull Johns Hopkins* 7:112, 1896.
25. Czernobilsky B, Morris WJ: A histologic study of ovarian endometriosis with emphasis on hyperplastic and atypical changes, *Obstet Gynecol* 53:318-323, 1979.
26. Daniell JF, Christianson G: Combined laparoscopic surgery and danazol therapy for pelvic endometriosis, *Fertil Steril* 35:521, 1981.
27. Deaton JL et al: A randomized, controlled trial of clomiphene citrate and intrauterine insemination in couples with unexplained infertility or surgically corrected endometriosis, *Fertil Steril* 54:1083, 1990.
28. DeLeon FD et al: Orally and parenterally administered ibuprofen for postoperative adhesion prevention, *J Reprod Med* 31:1019, 1986.
29. Desaulles PA, Krahenbuhl C: Comparison of the antifertility and sex hormone activities of sex hormones and derivatives, *Acta Endocrinol* 47:444, 1964.
30. Dickey RP, Taylor SN, Curole DN: Serum estradiol and danazol. I. Endometriosis response, side effects, administration interval, concurrent spironolactone, and dexamethasone, *Fertil Steril* 42:709, 1984.
31. DiZerega GS, Barber DL, Hodgen GD: Endometriosis: role of ovarian steroids in initiation, maintenance, and suppression, *Fertil Steril* 33:649, 1980.
32. Dmowski WP, Cohen MR: Antigonadotropin (danazol) in the treatment of endometriosis, *Am J Obstet Gynecol* 130:41, 1978.
33. Dodson WC et al: Superovulation with intrauterine insemination in the treatment of infertility: a possible alternative to gamete intrafallopian transfer and in vitro fertilization, *Fertil Steril* 48:441, 1987.
34. Donnez J et al: Administration of nasal buserelin as compared with subcutaneous buserelin implant for endometriosis, *Fertil Steril* 52:27, 1989.
35. Dotson RL, Peterson M, Doucette RC: Medical therapy for recurring catamenial pneumothorax following pleurodesis, *Obstet Gynecol* 82:656, 1993.
36. Duck SC, Katayama KP: Danazol may cause pseudohermaphroditism, *Fertil Steril* 35:230, 1981.
37. Fayez JA, Schneider PJ: Prevention of adhesion formation by different modalities of treatment, *Am J Obstet Gynecol* 157:1184, 1987.
38. Fedele L et al: Superovulation with human menopausal gonadotropins in the treatment of infertility associated with minimal or mild endometriosis: a controlled randomized study, *Fertil Steril* 58:28, 1992a.
39. Fedele L et al: Stage and localization of pelvic endometriosis and pain, *Fertil Steril* 53:155, 1990.
40. Fedele L et al: Buserelin acetate versus expectant management in the treatment of infertility associated with minimal or mild endometriosis: a randomized clinical trial, *Am J Obstet Gynecol* 166:1345, 1992b.
41. Fedele L et al: CA-125 in serum, peritoneal fluid, active lesions, and endometrium of patients with endometriosis, *Am J Obstet Gynecol* 158:166, 1988.
42. Fogelman I: Gonadotropin-releasing hormone agonists and the skeleton, *Fertil Steril* 57:715, 1992.
43. Friedman AJ, Hornstein MD: Gonadotropin-releasing hormone agonist plus estrogen-progestin "add back" therapy for endometriosis-related pelvic pain, *Fertil Steril* 60:236, 1993.
44. Friedman AJ et al: Efficacy and safety considerations in women with leiomyomata uteri treated with GnRH agonists: the estrogen threshold hypothesis, *Am J Obstet Gynecol* 163:1114, 1990.
45. Fukaya T, Hoshiai H, Yajima A: Is pelvic endometriosis always associated with chronic pain: a retrospective study of 618 cases diagnosed by laparoscopy, *Am J Obstet Gynecol* 169:719, 1993.
46. Halme J et al: Increased activation of pelvic macrophages in infertile women with mild endometriosis, *Am J Obstet Gynecol* 145:333, 1983.
47. Haney AF: Pelvic endometriosis: etiology and pathology, *Semin Reprod Endocrinol* 6:287, 1988.
48. Henzl MR: Gonadotropin-releasing hormone analogs: update on new findings, *Am J Obstet Gynecol* 166:757, 1992.
49. Henzl MR et al: Administration of nasal nafarelin as compared with oral danazol for endometriosis: a multicenter double-blind comparative clinical trial, *N Engl J Med* 318:485, 1988.
50. Henzl MR, Kwei L: Efficacy and safety of nafarelin in the treatment of endometriosis, *Am J Obstet Gynecol* 162:570, 1990.
51. Hill JA, Barbieri RL, Anderson DJ: Immunosuppressive effects of danazol in vitro, *Fertil Steril* 48:414, 1987.

52. Hill JA et al: Characterization of leukocyte subpopulations in the peritoneal fluid of women with endometriosis, *Fertil Steril* 50:216, 1988.
53. Hornstein MD: Endometriosis and spontaneous abortion. In Friedman AJ, editor: *Recurrent pregnancy loss, infertility, and reproductive medicine clinics of North America*, Philadelphia, 1991, WB Saunders.
54. Hornstein MD, Barbieri RL, McShane PM: The effects of previous ovarian surgery on the follicular response to ovulation induction in an in vitro fertilization program, *J Reprod Med* 34:277, 1989.
55. Hornstein MD et al: The reproducibility of the revised American Fertility Society Classification of Endometriosis, *Fertil Steril* 59:1015, 1993.
56. Hornstein MD et al: Menstrual cyclicity of CA-125 in patients with endometriosis, *Fertil Steril* 58:279, 1992.
57. Hoshiai H et al: Laparoscopic evaluation of the onset and progression of endometriosis, *Am J Obstet Gynecol* 169:714, 1993.
58. Howell R et al: A randomized controlled trial of goserelin (zoladex) with add-back hormone replacement therapy (HRT) for endometriosis-effect on bone density. Presented at the 49th Annual American Fertility Society Meeting, Montreal, October 11-14, 1993.
59. Hull ME et al: Comparison of different treatment modalities of endometriosis in infertile women, *Fertil Steril* 47:40, 1987.
60. Hull MGR: Infertility treatment: relative effectiveness of conventional and assisted conception methods, *Human Reproduction* 7:785, 1992.
61. Hurst FS, Bollmann A, Ciangiola C: Treatment of infertility patients with hMG-IUI in a private practice, *Int J Fertil* 38:28, 1993.
62. Hurst BS, Wallach EE: Superovulation with intrauterine insemination: empiric therapy for infertile couples, *Postgrad Obstet Gynecol* 22:1, 1990.
63. Interceed (TC7) Adhesion Barrier Study Group: Prevention of post-surgical adhesions by Interceed (TC7), and absorbable adhesion barrier: a prospective randomized multicenter clinical study, *Fertil Steril* 51:933, 1989.
64. Jansen RPS: Minimal endometriosis and reduced fecundability: prospective evidence from an artificial insemination by donor program, *Fertil Steril* 46:141, 1986.
65. Jansen RPS, Russell P: Nonpigmented endometriosis: clinical, laparoscopic, and pathologic definition, *Am J Obstet Gynecol* 155:1154, 1986.
66. Jarrett JC, Dawood MY: Adhesion formation and uterine tube healing in the rabbit: a controlled study of the effects of ibuprofen, *Am J Obstet Gynecol* 155:1186, 1986.
67. Kennedy SH et al: Immunoscintigraphy of ovarian endometriosis: a preliminary study, *Br J Obstet Gynaecol* 95:693, 1988.
68. Kistner RW: The use of newer progestins in the treatment of endometriosis, *Am J Obstet Gynecol* 75:264, 1958.
69. Kistner RW: The use of steroidal substances in endometriosis, *Clin Pharmacol Ther* 1:525, 1960.
70. Knobil E: The neuroendocrine control of the menstrual cycle, *Recent Prog Horm Res* 36:53, 1980.
71. LaGranade A, Silverberg G: Ovarian tumors associated with atypical endometriosis, *Hum Pathol* 19:1080-1084, 1988.
72. Luciano AA, Turksay RN, Carleo J: Evaluation of oral medroxy-progesterone acetate in the treatment of endometriosis, *Obstet Gynecol* 72:323, 1988.
73. Mais V et al: The efficiency of transvaginal ultrasonography in the diagnosis of endometrioma, *Fertil Steril* 60:776, 1993.
74. Malkasian GD Jr et al: CA-125 in gynecologic practice, *Am J Obstet Gynecol* 155:515, 1986.
75. Markham SM: Extrapelvic endometriosis. In Thomas EJ, Rock JA, editors: *Modern approaches to endometriosis*, Boston, 1991, Kluwer Academic.
76. Martin DC et al: Laparoscopic appearances of peritoneal endometriosis, *Fertil Steril* 51:63, 1989.
77. Matta WH, Shaw RW: A comparative study between buserelin and danazol in the treatment of endometriosis, *Br J Clin Pract* 41 (suppl 48):69, 1986.
78. Medical Research International, Society for Assisted Reproductive Technology, The American Fertility Society: In vitro fertilization–embryo transfer (IVF-ET) in the United States: 1989 results from the IVF-ET Registry, *Fertil Steril* 55:14, 1991.
79. Meldrum DR et al: "Medical oophorectomy" using a long-acting GnRH-agonist: a possible new approach to the treatment of endometriosis, *J Clin Endocrinol Metab* 54:1081, 1982.
80. Montgomery JC, Studd JWW: Oestradiol and testosterone implants after hysterectomy for endometriosis, *Contrib Gynecol Obstet* 16:241, 1987.
81. The Nafarelin European Endometriosis Trial Group (NEET): Nafarelin for endometriosis: a large-scale, danazol-controlled trial of efficacy and safety, with 1-year follow-up, *Fertil Steril* 57:514, 1992.
82. Namnoum AB et al: Incidence of symptom recurrence following hysterectomy for endometriosis. Presented at the 49th Annual American Fertility Society Meeting, Montreal, October 11-14, 1993.
83. Nilsson B et al: Danazol and gestagen displacement of testosterone and influence of sex hormone-binding capacity, *Fertil Steril* 38:48, 1982.
84. Nishimura K et al: Endometrial cysts of the ovary: MR imaging, *Radiology* 162:315, 1987.
85. Noble AD, Letchworth AT: Medical treatment of endometriosis: a comparative trial, *Postgrad Med J* 55(suppl 5):37, 1979.
86. Nowroozi K et al: The importance of laparoscopic coagulation of mild endometriosis in infertile women, *Int J Fertil* 32:442, 1987.
87. Olive DC, Honey AF: Endometriosis associated infertility: a critical review of therapeutic approaches, *Obstet Gynecol* 41:538, 1986.
88. Pittaway DE: Endometriosis and spontaneous abortion, *Semin Reprod Endocrinol* 6:257, 1988.
89. Pittaway DE, Fayez JA: The use of CA-125 in the diagnosis and management of endometriosis, *Fertil Steril* 46:790, 1986.
90. Reisner LS: Anaphylaxis to intraperitoneal dextran, *Anesthesiology* 60:259, 1984.
91. Rock JA et al: Zoladex (goserelin acetate implant) in the treatment of endometriosis: a randomized comparison with danazol, *Obstet Gynecol* 82:198, 1993.
92. Rokitansky C: Uber Uterusdrusen-Neubilding im Uterus und Ovarialsarcomen, *ZKK Gesellch d Arzte zu Wein* 37:577, 1860.
93. Rosenberg SM, Board JA: High molecular weight dextran and human infertility surgery, *Am J Obstet Gynecol* 148:380, 1984.
94. Sampson JA: Perforating hemorrhagic (chocolate) cysts of the ovary, *Arch Surg* 3:245, 1921.
95. Sampson JA: Endometrial carcinoma of the ovary arising in endometrial tissue in that organ, *Arch Surg* 10:1, 1925.
96. Schwartz D, Mayaux MJ: Female fecundity as a function of age: results of artificial insemination in 2193 nulliparous women with ezpospermic husbands, *N Eng J Med* 306:404, 1982.
97. Scully RE, Richardson GS, Barlow JF: The development of malignancy in endometriosis, *Clin Obstet Gynecol* 9:384, 1966.
98. Seibel MM et al: The effectiveness of danazol on subsequent fertility in minimal endometriosis, *Fertil Steril* 38:534, 1982.
99. Semm K, Mettler L: Technical progress in pelvic surgery via operative laparoscopy, *Am J Obstet Gynecol* 138:121, 1980.
100. Serta RT, Ruto S, Seibel MM: Minimal endometriosis and intrauterine insemination: does controlled ovarian hyperstimulation improve pregnancy rates? *Obstet Gynecol* 80:37, 1992.
101. Shaw RW: Zoladex Endometriosis Study Team: an open randomized comparative study of the effect of goserelin depot and danazol in the treatment of endometriosis, *Fertil Steril* 58:265, 1992.
102. Soliman S et al: A randomized trial of in vitro fertilization versus conventional treatment for infertility, *Fertil Steril* 59:1239, 1993.

103. Steingold KA et al: Treatment of endometriosis with a long-acting gonadotropin-releasing hormone agonist, *Obstet Gynecol* 69:403, 1987.
104. Steingold KA et al: Danazol inhibits steroidogenesis by the human ovary in vivo, *Fertil Steril* 45:649, 1986.
105. Sugimura K et al: Pelvic endometriosis: detection and diagnosis with chemical shift MR imaging, *Radiology* 188:435, 1993.
106. Surrey ES et al: The effects of combining norethindrone with a gonadotropin-releasing hormone agonist in the treatment of symptomatic endometriosis, *Fertil Steril* 53:620, 1990.
107. Surrey ES, Judd HL: Reduction of vasomotor symptoms and bone mineral density loss with combined norethindrone and long-acting gonadotropin-releasing hormone agonist therapy of symptomatic endometriosis: a prospective randomized trial, *J Clin Endocrinol Metab* 75:558, 1992.
108. Thomas EJ, Cooke ID: Impact of gestrinone on the course of asymptomatic endometriosis, *Br Med J* 294:272, 1987.
109. Toma SK, Stovall DW, Hammond MG: The effect of laparoscopic ablation or danocrine on pregnancy rates in patients with stage I or II endometriosis undergoing donor insemination, *Obstet Gynecol* 80:253, 1992.
110. Tulandi T: Transient edema after intraperitoneal instillation of 32% dextran 70: a report of five cases, *J Reprod Med* 32:472, 1987.
111. Vercellini P et al: A gonadotropin-releasing hormone agonist versus a low-dose oral contraceptive for pelvic pain associated with endometriosis, *Fertil Steril* 60:75, 1993.
112. Waller KG, Shaw RW: Gonadotropin-releasing hormone analogs for the treatment of endometriosis: long-term follow-up, *Fertil Steril* 59:511, 1993.
113. Wheeler JM, Knittle JD, Miller JD: Depot leuprolide versus danazol in treatment of women with symptomatic endometriosis. I. Efficacy results, *Am J Obstet Gynecol* 167:1367, 1992.

Chapter 12

EVALUATION OF THE INFERTILE COUPLE

Mitchell S. Rein
Isaac Schiff

The definition of infertility is one year of unprotected coitus without conception. The term "primary infertility" is applied to the couple who has never achieved a pregnancy; "secondary infertility" implies that at least one previous conception has taken place. The purpose of the present chapter is to review the investigation of the infertile couple and critically evaluate the predictive value of the traditional diagnostic tests.

Several factors have been identified that contribute to patient satisfaction with the infertility evaluation.[87] The technical skill of the infertility specialist and emotional support from the physician and staff are the most frequent reasons for patient satisfaction. Other important factors include allowing women more control over their evaluation and treatment, explaining procedures, clearly involving men more significantly, and discussing adoption as an alternative. Interestingly, treatment costs and the length of time couples had been trying to conceive are not related to patient satisfaction.

The importance of an efficient and systematic evaluation cannot be overstated. Recently there has been a conscientious effort to simplify the basic infertility evaluation. A thorough evaluation has four important goals:

1. To identify the cause of the infertility
2. To provide a basis for potentially successful treatment options
3. To provide a realistic prognosis, and
4. To offer emotional support

EPIDEMIOLOGY

The epidemiology of infertility is best understood in the context of the probability of fertility. Fecundability is defined as the probability of conceiving during a monthly cycle and provides the basis for estimating fertility over time. The fecundability of "normal" couples using no contraception is estimated at 20% to 25% per cycle.[53] Based on this estimate 50% of couples should conceive after 3 to 4 months and 95% after 12 months. This cumulative fertility is a simple function of fecundability. It provides a basis for the clinical rule that 12 months of unprotected intercourse without conception occurring may define a fertility problem. Using this definition, the National Survey of Family Growth estimates 10% to 15% of couples may be classified as infertile.[159-161] Comparing 1982 and 1988 data, Mosher and Pratt reported that the annual number of women using infertility services increased by 25%.[162] However, the rate of impaired fecundity was unchanged between 1982 and 1988. These authors suggest that the increase in the number of women seeking infertility services was due to delayed childbearing and the entry of baby boom cohorts into the age range of 25 to 44 years.[163]

Unfortunately, a minority of couples with impaired fecundity seek medical assistance. Wilcox and Mosher reported that 43% of all women with infertility obtained some form of infertility service and only 24% obtained specialized infertility treatment.[237] Those most likely to have obtained specialized services were 30 years or older, nulliparous, married, Caucasian women of higher socioeconomic status. Socioeconomic factors are also predictive of successful pregnancy outcomes.[47]

It is important to categorize the nature of the fertility problem based on the pathophysiologic source in the man or woman. The major categories of infertility are male factor, 35%; ovulatory factors, 20%; tubal factor, 20%; cervical factor, 5%; endometriosis, 10%; and unexplained, 10%. It has been estimated that 25% to 35% of all infertility problems are of multiple origin.

Presumptive etiological factors have been identified for some categories of infertility. Iatrogenic factors (conization and cautery), sexually transmitted diseases,[102] and smoking have been associated with the cervical factor.[173] Pelvic inflammatory disease (PID) has been strongly associated with the tubal factor.[233] The increasing incidence of ectopic pregnancy and infertility is largely attributed to the increasing incidence of PID. Other risk factors for the tubal factor include endometriosis, diethylstilbestrol (DES) exposure, intrauterine device (IUD) use, and smoking. Risk factors for endometriosis include menstrual irregularities, dysmenorrhea, and a family history of endometriosis.[55] Exercising and smoking appear to have a protective effect for endometriosis. The etiological factors associated with ovulatory dysfunction include smoking, exercise, body habitus, and genetic factors. Hereditary factors associated with premature ovarian failure (POF) include X chromosome deletions and errors of galactose metabolism. Multiple factors have been associated with male-factor infertility; these will be discussed under the evaluation of the male factor.

The prognosis for infertile couples appears to be strongly affected by their clinical diagnoses, as demonstrated in a group of almost 1300 infertile couples.[49] The cumulative conception rates are shown in Fig. 12-1. Couples with ovulatory disorders seem to have the best prognosis.[50,66] The relatively poor prognosis observed with the tubal and the male factors in the past has improved as a result of in vitro fertilization. The duration of infertility is also a predictor of subsequent pregnancies.[49,231] Couples with less than a 3-year history of infertility are more likely to conceive. A prior pregnancy with the same partner may be the most powerful predictor of a subsequent pregnancy.[49,66]

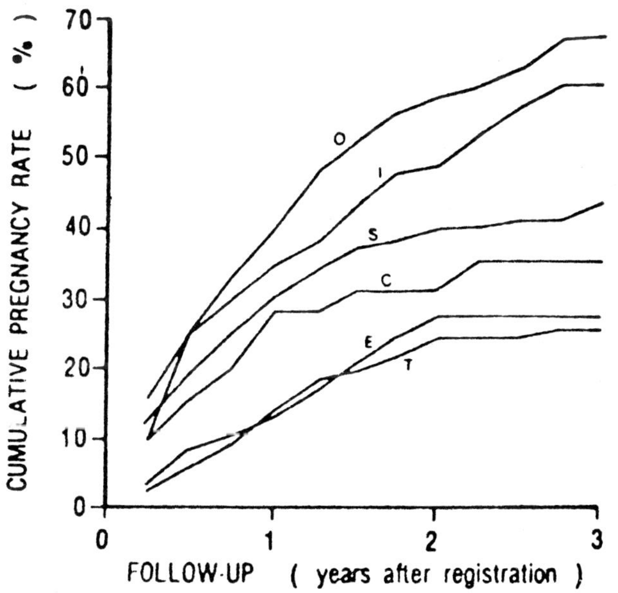

Fig. 12-1. Cumulative pregnancy rates and primary clinical diagnoses among infertile couples. Ovulatory disorders (O); unexplained (I); male factor (S); cervical factor (C); endometriosis (E); tubal factor (T). (From Collins JA: A proportional hazards analysis of the clinical characteristics of infertile couples, *Am J Obstet Gynecol* 148:527, 1984.

In summary, pregnancy rates appear to correlate best with the age of the female, underlying diagnosis, duration of infertility, and pregnancy history. Based on the epidemiological data, couples interested in having children, who have not conceived after 1 to 2 years of unprotected intercourse, are reasonable candidates for an infertility evaluation. Earlier investigation may be recommended on an individual basis, such as younger women with obvious risk factors (i.e., oligomenorrhea, or a history of PID, or women more than 35 years old).

FEMALE REPRODUCTIVE AGING

Data from several sources suggest maternal age may affect fecundability. A multicenter French study evaluated cumulative fertility rates in 2193 multiparous women with azoospermic husbands who underwent artificial donor insemination.[190] The cumulative fertility after 12 cycles of insemination declined after age 30 years. The cumulative fertility after 12 cycles of insemination was 73% for women younger than 25 years, 74.1% for those 26 to 30 years of age, 61.5% for those 31 to 35 years of age, and only 53.6% for women more than 35 years of age. Data extrapolated from the 1976 National Survey of Family Growth similarly suggest a decline in fecundity with increasing maternal age (Table 12-1).[91] A substantial decline in fertility after age 30 years has also been observed among Hutterite women.[220] In summary, fecundity in women is maximal around the age of 25 years, and the incidence of infertility increases after the age of 30 years.

The pathophysiology of female reproductive aging has received relatively little attention. Although there is clear evidence that oocyte quality declines with age, the effect of aging on uterine receptivity remains unclear.[143] Toner et al

Table 12-1. The influence of age on the cumulative pregnancy rate

Age group	Conceiving in 12 months (%)
20-24	86
25-29	78
30-34	63
35-39	52

From Hendershot GE, Mosher WD, Pratt WF: Infertility and age: an unresolved issue, *Fam Plan Perspect* 14:287, 1982.

described the basal, day 3 FSH level as an index of functional ovarian reserve and popularized the phrase "ovarian age".[222] These authors reported that the basal FSH level is a better predictor of in vitro fertilization performance than chronologic age. In contrast, Pearlstone et al concluded that basal FSH levels and chronologic age are equally important predictors of successful pregnancy outcomes.[172] Preliminary data suggests that intercycle variations in basal FSH values do not predict changes in ovarian responsiveness[192]; however, the importance of intercycle variability remains to be determined.

In summary the combined use of age and basal FSH levels may improve the accuracy of the prognosis when counseling patients.

THE INITIAL VISIT

A detailed interview is the critical first step in an infertility evaluation. A major goal during the initial visit is to educate the couple by providing information on reproductive physiology, the causes of infertility, and to provide details of the subsequent infertility evaluation. This will enable the couple to adequately prepare for what is often an emotionally and physically demanding evaluation. During the initial visit both partners should be present and interviewed together. The male partner should be strongly encouraged to attend all visits. On the premise that infertility is often a syndrome of multiple origin, an adequate investigation requires asking about all possible etiologies in both the man and woman. Besides obtaining a complete medical, surgical, and gynecologic history, the physician should elicit information regarding the psychologic, emotional, and sexual behaviors of both partners. This should include questions regarding sexual habits, frequency of intercourse, sexual dysfunction, and stability of the relationship; the couple's motivation to achieve a successful pregnancy should also be questioned. Certain couples may benefit from specific instructions regarding the timing and frequency of intercourse. A frequency of 2 to 3 times per week without the use of lubricants or douches is usually adequate. Coitus every 36 to 48 hours 3 to 4 days before and after the calculated day of ovulation is optimal. The disruption of spontaneous sexuality should be discouraged.

Table 12-2. Important historic points in the male

1. Duration of infertility
2. Prior fertility in other relationships
3. Medical and surgical history (childhood illnesses, venereal diseases, trauma)
4. Medications
5. Alcohol, cigarette, marijuana use
6. Occupational exposures (excessive heat, chemical, radiation)
7. Sexual dysfunction
8. Tight-fitting underwear, hot baths, saunas
9. Previous tests and therapy for infertility

Table 12-3. Important historic points in the female

1. Duration of infertility
2. Detailed menstrual history
3. Prior pregnancies
4. Fertility in other relationships
5. Prior contraceptive use (OCPs, IUD)
6. Frequency of intercourse, sexual dysfunction
7. Gynecologic history (PID, endometriosis, fibroids, cervical dysplasia)
8. DES exposure
9. Medical and surgical history
10. Medications
11. Previous tests and therapy for infertility

The important historic points in the evaluation of the male and female partners are outlined in Tables 12-2 and 12-3. During the physical examination of the woman, particular attention should be given to height, weight, hair distribution, and presence of galactorrhea; the pelvic examination should be thorough. Examination of the man by a urologist is often recommended if there is a persistent abnormality in the semen analysis.

An explanation of the causes of infertility provides an ideal introduction to the nature of the subsequent evaluation. The schedule for the planned investigation should be flexible. The majority of the investigation, however, should be completed within 3 to 6 months. The sequence in which specific infertility tests should be offered will depend on the etiological factors that are suggested by the history and physical examination. These specific tests will be discussed in the context of the multiple causes of infertility.

THE MALE FACTOR

The male factor is frequently cited as the most common cause of infertility. This is somewhat misleading, however, since the present tests available for the evaluation of the man do not easily separate normal fertile men from those with reduced fertility. The evaluation of the man is limited not only by a large overlap in the semen parameters among fertile and subfertile men, but also by the wide fluctuations among sequential semen specimens from the same individual. Since it is relatively rare to identify a male partner with azoospermia (no sperm in the ejaculate), it is often difficult to implicate the male factor as the principal cause for a couple's infertility. Despite its limitations, semen analysis remains the primary screening test for male-factor infertility. If the semen analysis is persistently abnormal, the patient is referred to a urologist for examination and further evaluation. A number of different schemes to categorize the multiple causes of male infertility have been devised. The causes of male infertility are outlined in Table 12-4.

The importance of a thorough physical examination cannot be overstated. Unfortunately, in the majority of cases a specific etiology for male-factor infertility cannot be identified. Varicocele is the most frequently observed correctable cause of male infertility. Over the years the role of varicoceles in male-factor infertility has generated considerable debate. Varicoceles are present in 15% of the normal population and in approximately 40% of men with male-factor infertility. The World Health Organization recently evaluated 9034 infertile couples and concluded varicocele is clearly associated with impairment of testicular function and infertility.[241] Gorelick and Goldstein demonstrated that the incidence of varicocele is much higher in male-factor secondary infertility compared with primary infertility, which suggests varicocele causes progressive impairment in spermatogenesis.[83] Madgar et al reported the first prospective, randomized, controlled clinical trial demonstrating the efficacy of varicocelectomy.[132] In summary, repair of varicocele is recommended when the couple has documented male-factor infertility, the female infertility evaluation is normal, and a varicocele is present on examination.

A karyotype, vasography, and testicular biopsy may be recommended for patients with azoospermia or severe oligozoospermia. Endocrine studies measuring serum testosterone, luteinizing hormone (LH), follicle-stimulating hormone (FSH), thyroid-stimulating hormone (TSH), and prolactin levels should be considered for patients with azoospermia, oligozoospermia, or oligoasthenospermia (poor motility). Immunologic factors may be suggested by sperm agglutination, oligoasthenospermia, or poor cervical mucous penetrability. Immunologic infertility will be further discussed in the section on the cervical factor. Microbiologic studies should be recommended if there is any suggestion of genital tract infections.

The interpretation and clinical value of the various tests available for the evaluation of seminal fluid, sperm cell properties, and sperm cell function will be presented after a brief review of male reproductive physiology.

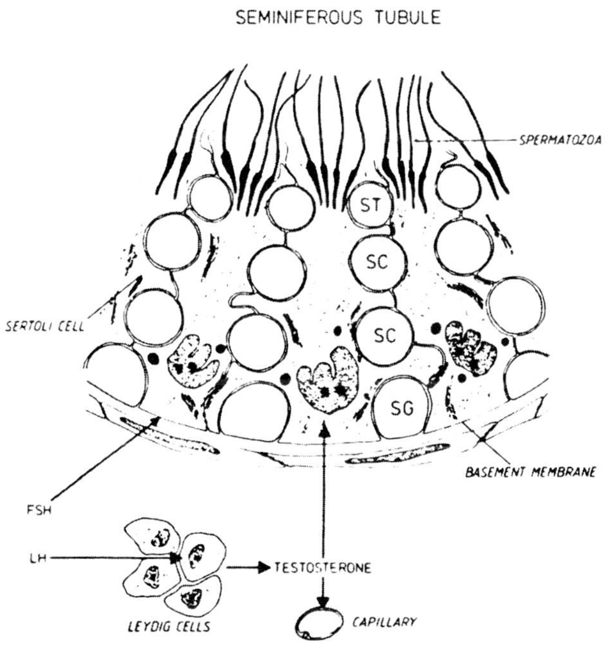

Fig. 12-2. Spermatogenesis. A schematic illustration of the cellular composition and structural relationship between different cell types in the testis. (From Hargreave TB: editor, *Male Infertility,* New York, 1993, Springer-Verlag, p 89.)

Table 12-4. Causes of male infertility

Anatomic Factors
- Varicocele
- Cryptorchidism
- Ductal obstruction (Young's syndrome)
- Congenital anomalies (hypospadias, epispadias, cystic fibrosis, testicular hypoplasia or aplasia, and partial or total absence of the vas deferens)

Endocrine Factors
- Gonadotropin deficiency
- Kallman's syndrome
- Pituitary tumors (Cushing's disease, acromegaly)
- Dwarfism
- Hypothyroidism
- Fertile eunuch syndrome
- Enzymatic defects in testosterone synthesis
- Androgen receptor deficiency
- Congenital adrenal hyperplasia

Genetic Factors
- Klinefelter's syndrome
- Down's syndrome
- 47 XYY
- Autosomal translocations

Inflammatory Factors
- Orchitis
- Epididymitis
- Prostatitis
- Urethritis

Immunologic Factors
- Systemic
- Local

Sexual Dysfunction/Faulty Coital Technique
- Impotence
- Retrograde ejaculation
- Premature ejaculation
- Spermicidal lubricants

Exogenous Factors
- Medication (antihypertensives, antipsychotics, antidepressants, cimetidine, chemotherapy)
- Radiation
- Alcohol
- Marijuana
- Trauma
- Excessive heat (hot tubs)
- Cigarettes

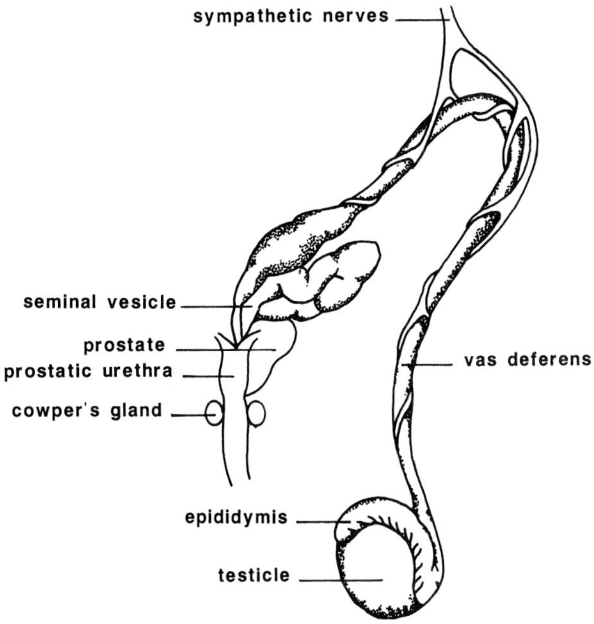

Fig. 12-3. Anatomy of the male reproductive tract.

Male reproductive physiology

The testes contain two cell types (Fig. 12-2). Sertoli cells contain spermatogonia and line the seminiferous tubules. Leydig cells are the androgen-producing cells located in the interstitial tissue. The epididymis is a reservoir for sperm storage and the site of sperm maturation. The vas deferens connects the epididymis with the ejaculatory ducts. The prostate, seminal vesicles, and the bulbourethral (Cowper's) glands secrete the seminal fluid. The anatomy of the male reproductive tract is depicted in Fig. 12-3.

Spermatogenesis is the process of formation and development of the spermatozoon. The transformation of spermatogonia into spermatids involves a series of mitotic and meiotic divisions. The differentiation of spermatids into mature spermatozoa is termed spermiogenesis. In man spermatogenesis is a continuous process; approximately 74 days are required for the conversion of spermatogonia into spermatozoa. When spermatozoa enter the epididymis they are functionally inactive; however, after an average of 12 days of further maturation they are capable of progressive motility.

The endocrinology of spermatogenesis involves pituitary secretion of LH and FSH and the testicular secretion of testosterone and inhibin. Whereas LH stimulates Leydig cell synthesis and secretion of testosterone, FSH stimulates Sertoli cell secretion of inhibin. High levels of intratesticular testosterone are required to support spermatogenesis.

During ejaculation the contents of the distal vas deferens and prostatic fluid are initially released and followed soon after by the release of seminal vesicle secretions. Although semen coagulates during ejaculation to form a gel, liquefaction occurs within 20 to 30 minutes as a result of the proteolytic enzymes in prostatic fluid. Seminal spermatozoa are not capable of fertilization. The process by which sperm acquire the ability to fertilize ova is termed capacitation. Capacitation appears to take place in the cervical mucus. However, a period of time in the female reproductive tract is not required since sperm are capable of fertilization in vitro. This poorly defined series of biochemical and biophysical changes in the sperm surface membrane gives sperm the capacity to undergo the acrosome reaction.

The acrosome reaction involves the breakdown and fusion of the sperm plasma membrane with the outer acrosomal membrane (Fig. 12-4).[22] Several enzymes within the acrosome appear to be important for sperm penetration of the cumulus cell mass, corona radiata, and zona pellucida. Species-specific sperm receptors exist on the zona pellucida. During sperm penetration the oocyte initiates the cortical reaction, the process by which further sperm are prevented from penetrating the oocyte. The cortical reaction involves the breakdown and dispersion of the secretory granules that lie just below the vitelline membrane.[17]

Diagnostic tests for the evaluation of the male

Semen analysis. Since there is no laboratory test to definitively predict the potential for fertility in the male, semen analysis remains the primary diagnostic test for evaluating the male factor. The basic semen analysis measures volume, pH, fructose, liquefaction, round cells, sperm density, motility, and morphology. Prior to obtaining the semen specimen, the patient is instructed to abstain from ejaculation for a minimum of 48 hours and no longer than 7 days. The method of choice for collection is masturbation with avoidance of potential spermicidal lubricants. These specimens should be collected in a clean container and brought to the laboratory within 1 to 2 hours. Several (two or three) samples should be analyzed over a period of 1 to 3 months because of individual fluctuations. The semen analysis may be evaluated by an experienced technician or semiautomated computers.

The optimal period of sexual abstinence has not been determined. There are no scientific data to support the recommendation that having intercourse every other day is more likely to result in conception than having intercourse every day. Recent evidence suggests that the optimal period of abstinence may vary from individual to individual. Ejaculate volume, sperm concentration, and sperm count tend to rise continuously for up to 10 days of abstinence.[28] In contrast, sperm motility does not appear to be affected by ejaculatory frequency.[188] Frequent ejaculation may be associated with decreased semen volume and decreased total motile sperm,[88] whereas infrequent ejaculation has been associated with decreased normal morphology.

Normal semen volumes range from 2 to 6 mL. A very small semen volume may be associated with retrograde ejaculation. The absence of fructose and an acidic pH may

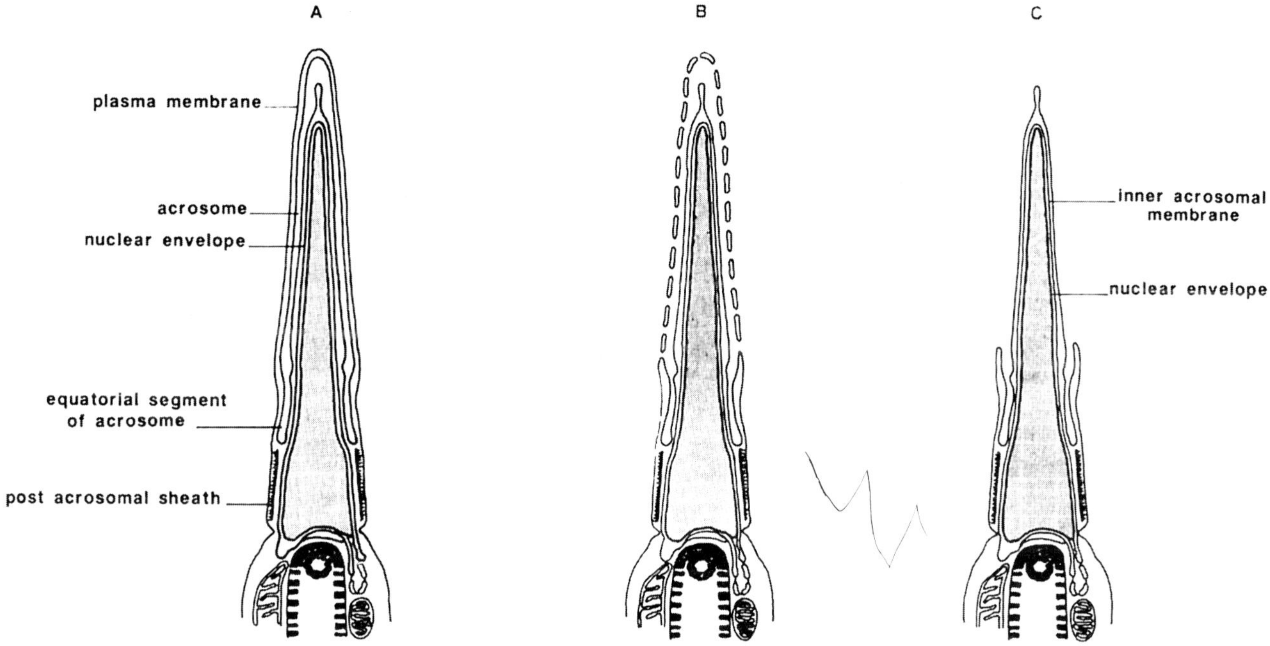

Fig. 12-4. Diagramatic representation of the acrosome reaction. **A,** Intact unreacted spermatozoon; **B,** The acrosome reaction; **C,** Acrosome-reacted spermatozoon. Adapted from Mortimer D: Male factor in infertility. II: Sperm function testing, *Curr Probl Obstet Gynecol*, p 1 8:8, 1985.

suggest seminal vesicle dysfunction or ejaculatory duct obstruction. The absence of liquefaction may result in relatively immobilized spermatozoa. Leukocytospermia and/or an abnormal number of immature germ cells may be suggested by an abnormal number of round cells (greater than 1×10^6/mL). Unfortunately, total round cell counts are poorly predictive of leukocytospermia, and white blood cells (WBCs) are often difficult to distinguish from immature germ cells by conventional microscopy.[176]

An immunoperoxidase staining technique (Endtz test) specific for WBCs is widely used and recommended by the World Health Organization.[240] Studies investigating the role of leukocytospermia in male-factor infertility have yielded conflicting results. Tomlinson et al reported that leukocytes in the semen had no influence on fertilization.[221] In contrast, other investigators have demonstrated a significant inverse relationship between fertilization rates and leukocyte numbers.[44,229] An abnormal number of immature germ cells may be the result of a defect in spermatogenesis and appears to be associated with reduced fertilization.[221]

The interpretation of sperm density, motility, and morphology may be difficult for several reasons. As previously mentioned, there are wide fluctuations in sequential semen analyses from the same individual and significant overlap between fertile and subfertile men. Further difficulty correlating semen parameters with fertility potential occurs because fertility is a function of both partners and not the man alone. An additional drawback is that semen analysis does not measure all of the functional properties of spermatozoa such as capacitation, cervical mucous interaction, penetrating ability, and fertilization. The predictive inadequacy of the seminal parameters is illustrated by the difficulty in determining the lower limits of the fertile range. This is further exemplified by the relatively high pregnancy rates of vasovasostomized men with oligozoospermia and by the normozoospermic men whose sperm fail to penetrate their partner's ova at the time of in vitro fertilization. Nevertheless, among all the tests and parameters available, sperm density, motility, and morphology have been most consistently correlated with fertility status.

Sperm density is a measure of the number of sperm in the ejaculate per milliliter. Based on studies of "fertile" men undergoing vasectomy and follow-up studies of infertile groups,[29,65,164,202] the lower limit of the fertile range appears to be 5 million sperm/mL. Studies comparing sperm density and in vitro fertilization rates seem to suggest a slightly higher cutoff for the "normal" range of 10 to 20 million sperm/mL.[20,98,133] Despite these recent studies the most widely accepted lower limit of the "normal" range continues to be 20 million sperm/mL, based on the landmark studies of MacLeod and Gold.[130] When a higher cutoff is applied there is an increase in sensitivity at the expense of a decrease in specificity. Patients with persistent sperm density less than 20 million/mL are considered to have maleactor infertility and are often referred for further urological evaluation. In contrast, the lower cutoff of 5 million sperm/mL is often used for therapeutic recommendations such as therapeutic donor insemination.

The assessment of sperm motility is as important as the determination of sperm density. Sperm motility should be evaluated within 2 hours after the specimen is produced. Sperm motility is most often expressed as the percentage of progressively motile sperm; however, similar to sperm density, estimating the percentage of progressively motile sperm does not accurately separate fertile men from subfertile men. The recommended lower limits of normal motility is 20% to 60%.[9,30,42,131,177] Data obtained from in vitro fertilization suggest that a cutoff of 50% motility has significant prognostic value.[133] Sperm motility that is persistently less than 50% usually warrants further urologic evaluation.

In an attempt to improve the predictive value of the semen analysis, the analysis of sperm movement has expanded to include the evaluation of linear velocity and the amplitude of lateral head displacement. Mortimer has provided a detailed review of recent developments in the objective analysis of sperm movement characteristics.[158] Various computer technologies have been developed for the evaluation of sperm movement but the clinical usefulness of more complex motility data remains to be determined.

Sperm morphology is another semen parameter that appears to be associated with fertility potential. All semen specimens contain a certain percentage of abnormal spermatozoa. Morphologic abnormalities may involve the sperm head, midpiece, or tail. Abnormalities of the head are most frequently associated with infertility.[31] Based on a number of clinical studies, the recommended cutoffs for normal sperm morphology range from 40% to 60% normal forms.[31,133] Patients with persistently fewer than 40% morphologically normal spermatozoa are considered to have teratozoospermia and are then referred for urologic evaluation. Although abnormal morphology is often associated with reduced sperm density and motility, isolated abnormalities of sperm morphology are not uncommon.[121,182] Using strict criteria, Kruger et al suggested that sperm morphology may be a powerful predictor of successful in vitro fertilization. In vitro fertilization rates were found to be significantly reduced in cases with normal sperm morphology below a critical threshold of 14%. The impairment in fertilization was even more pronounced when the number of normal forms was below 5%. Based on these studies, Kruger's morphology criteria have been adopted in many andrology labs.

Although separate evaluation of each seminal variable is important, there may be advantages in combining semen variables. Mathematical manipulations allow for the expression of the total number of motile sperm and the total number of morphologically "normal" motile sperm per ejaculate. The combination of seminal variables avoids the interpretation of several different "normal" standards. Although a total motile count of less than 20 million has been associated with lower pregnancy rates,[201] the prognostic superiority of combining semen variables remains to be established.

Although the semen analysis remains the primary screening test for male-factor infertility, additional diagnostic tests have been developed in an attempt to define more precisely the reproductive potential of sperm. The majority of these tests assess the functional properties of spermatozoa. The sperm penetration assay (SPA) has been widely applied to clinical practice. Unfortunately, as in the case of the semen analysis, the SPA has significant limitations.

Sperm penetration assay. The SPA, also known as the zona-free hamster egg penetration test, was developed in an attempt to improve the evaluation of male-factor infertility. This assay is believed to assess the ability of sperm to (1) undergo capacitation and the acrosome reaction, (2) fuse with and penetrate the egg membrane, and (3) undergo chromosomal decondensation. Sperm are washed free of seminal plasma and incubated in a protein-enriched medium that promotes capacitation. After incubation, motile sperm are separated and used to inseminate hamster eggs that have previously been enzyme-treated so that the cumulus and zona pellucida have been removed. The SPA does not test the ability of sperm to penetrate the zona pellucida. Sperm from a donor of proved fertility is always tested simultaneously as a positive control. Following several hours of insemination, the hamster eggs are examined for sperm penetration. Penetration rates less than 10% to 15% are considered abnormal. Although the initial studies suggested a high degree of sensitivity and specificity,[113,183] subsequent studies have been unable to substantiate the excellent early results.[138,236] After reviewing the world's literature, Mao and Grimes concluded that the validity, reproducibility, and utility of the SPA have not been established.[134] They recommend that the SPA not be used to evaluate infertile couples.

The utility of the SPA for predicting success during in vitro fertilization remains controversial. Although an abnormal SPA is not always associated with an inability to penetrate human eggs, there does appear to be a correlation between the SPA and in vitro fertilization rates. The SPA appears to be less predictive of fertilization success or failure in patients with abnormal semen parameters than in patients with unexplained or tubal factor infertility.[2,139] The long-term prognostic ability of the SPA is difficult to determine since prospective studies have yielded different results. Aitken and co-workers found that 0% was the only SPA value diagnostic of infertility.[3] It remains uncertain if additional information is gained from the SPA when compared with traditional semen analysis. The SPA is therefore rarely recommended. With these limitations, the SPA may be offered to couples with persistently abnormal semen analyses. Whereas a markedly abnormal SPA may have prognostic and therapeutic implications, a normal test result should not be regarded as reassuring.

Future diagnostic studies. A variety of new methods have been described to evaluate sperm function. The hypoosmotic swelling test measures the functional integrity of sperm membranes by placing specimens in hypoosmotic fluids.[108] This assay has been correlated with successful in vitro fertilization.[228] Sperm nuclear maturation can be determined by staining with acidic aniline blue,[219] acridine orange fluorescence,[217] or sodium dodecyl sulfate decondensation.[23] Several monoclonal antibodies that can be used to detect the acrosome reaction are available.[239] These immunofluorescence assays determine whether a sperm population has the capacity to undergo the acrosome reaction. Other simple techniques for assessing the acrosome include the triple stain[213] and fluorescein isothiocyanate labeled lectins.[56,213] The hemizona test assesses the ability of spermatozoa to bind to the zona pellucida.[34] The human zona pellucida is bisected with one half of the zona incubated with donor sperm, and the other hemizona incubated with the sperm from an infertility patient. Liu et al established a similar sperm-zona pellucida binding test using oocytes that failed to fertilize in vitro.[124] Liu and Baker recently reviewed the development of new tests of human sperm function. They concluded that normal morphology using strict criteria such as linearity, acrosome status, and sperm-zona pellucida binding were the most important characteristics for predicting fertilization in vitro.[123] Although the new sperm function tests appear to provide additional valuable information, their clinical utility remains unclear. Further studies will be required to determine if these tests predict fertility in vivo.

THE CERVICAL FACTOR

The uterine cervix appears to have several important roles in reproduction and is often considered the gateway to the upper reproductive tract. During parturition, massive dilation of the cervix is required for a normal vaginal delivery. In the nonpregnant state, its primary physiologic function is the secretion of cervical mucus which functions as a biologic valve. During midcycle, cervical mucus facilitates the transport of spermatozoa. At other times during the menstrual cycle, cervical mucus functions as a barrier by preventing the passage of foreign material into the upper reproductive tract.

The cervical factor is best defined as the midcycle interaction of spermatozoa and cervical mucus. The postcoital test (PCT) remains the standard for assessing the cervical factor and is often recommended early in the evaluation of most infertile couples. The clinical value of the multiple in vitro studies such as the slide test,[145] the capillary tube test,[119] and the in vitro cervical mucus penetration test remains to be demonstrated.[4] At the present time in vitro tests for the cervical factor are rarely employed in clinical practice. In the following sections the physiology of cervical mucus will be reviewed and the evaluation of the cervical factor will be discussed.

Cervical mucus physiology

Cervical mucus is a heterogeneous secretion produced primarily by the secretory cells of the endocervix. The cervical mucus pool may contain a small amount of endometrial, tubal, and follicular fluid, cellular debris, and leukocytes. Cervical mucus contains 92% to 98% water. The physical properties of cervical mucus are due to its mucinous glycoproteins. Biochemical studies have demonstrated that cervical mucus is a fibrillar system and mucin fibrils originate in the endocervical canal.[78] Other constituents of cervical mucus include carbohydrates, lipids, proteins, proteolytic enzymes, and inorganic salts. During coitus, 200 to 500 million spermatozoa are delivered to the cervix and posterior vaginal fornix, but less than 200 attain close proximity to the egg.[194] Moghissi described several functional properties of the cervix and its secretions that are important for sperm migration[150]: (1) the cervix appears to be the site of sperm capacitation, (2) the fibrillar structure of cervical mucus contributes to sperm transport, (3) the nutrients in cervical mucus provide a supplemental energy source for sperm, (4) cervical mucus protects sperm from the hostile acidic environment of the vagina, (5) cervical mucus has a filtering effect, and (6) the cervical crypts are responsible for the storage and gradual release of spermatozoa to the upper reproductive tract.

The physical properties and certain constituents of cervical mucus display cyclic variations. The secretion of cervical mucus by the endocervical glands is stimulated by estrogen and inhibited by progesterone. The estrogen effect may be assayed by gross inspection or by microscopic examination. Around the time of ovulation, the mucus forms a thin, continuous thread as it is pulled apart—a phenomenon called Spinnbarkeit. This physical characteristic is a function of increasing levels of estrogen and disappears after the appearance of progesterone. Microscopically, when preovulatory mucus is allowed to dry on a slide it reveals a characteristic crystallization pattern called ferning. Preovulatory mucus also becomes more profuse, watery, alkaline, and acellular. Cyclic changes in the physical properties and chemical constituents of cervical mucus may influence sperm migration. Despite individual variation, sperm penetrability begins around the ninth day of the menstrual cycle and is optimal around the time of ovulation.[151,153] Within 1 to 2 days after ovulation, sperm migration is usually inhibited.[147] A scoring system to evaluate the quality of cervical mucus is illustrated in Table 12-5.

The postcoital test

The PCT, also known as the Sims-Huhner test, was first described in 1866 by Marion Sims.[200] However, Huhner is credited for popularizing the test as an index of sperm-cervical mucus interaction. The PCT is often considered an integral part of the routine evaluation of the infertile couple. Even so the clinical value of the PCT in predicting fertility remains controversial. In recent years there has been a gradual trend towards eliminating the PCT from the routine evaluation of the infertile couple. The major problem

Table 12-5. Evaluating the quality of cervical mucus

AMOUNT ______	VISCOSITY ______
0 = 0	0 = thick, highly viscous
1 = 0.1 mL	1 = intermediate viscosity
2 = 0.2 mL	2 = mildly viscous
3 = 0.3 mL or more	3 = normal
FERNING ______	CELLULARITY ______
0 = no crystallization	0 = 11 cells/HPF
1 = atypical pattern	1 = 6-10 cells/HPF
2 = primary and secondary stems	2 = 1-5 cells/HPF
3 = tertiary and quarterly stems	3 = 0 cells/HPF
SPINNBARKEIT ______	TOTAL SCORE ______
0 = ≤ 1cm	>10 = normal
1 = 1-4 cm	5-10 = unfavorable
2 = 5-8 cm	<5 = hostile
3 = ≥ 9cm	

From Belsey et al: *Laboratory manual for examination of human semen and semen-cervical mucus interaction,* Geneva, 1980, World Health Organization.

with the PCT is that it lacks standardization and as a result there is considerable disagreement regarding the timing and interpretation. In addition, the increasing popularity of superovulation and intrauterine insemination has limited the usefulness of the PCT in guiding treatment options.

The PCT should be performed as close to the time of ovulation as possible. The couple is instructed to abstain from intercourse for 2 days prior to having intercourse for the test. Douches or intravaginal medications should not be used during the 48 hours preceding the test. A nonlubricated speculum is inserted into the vagina and a sample of cervical mucus obtained. A number of techniques for collecting cervical mucus have been described. A long, narrow, dressing forceps with a small oval aperture at the tip is often used (Fig. 12-5). Alternatively, if the cervical os is too small to admit a metal instrument, an angiocatheter and a syringe may be used to aspirate a sample of cervical mucus. More recently a flexible suction device, the mucus sampler, has become commercially available (Cheshire Medical Specialties, Cheshire, CT). The cervical mucus should be placed on a glass slide, covered with a cover slip, and examined under the microscope. The number of spermatozoa per high-power field, percent motility, and the quality of forward progression should be noted. Whenever possible, the quality of the cervical mucus should also be described.

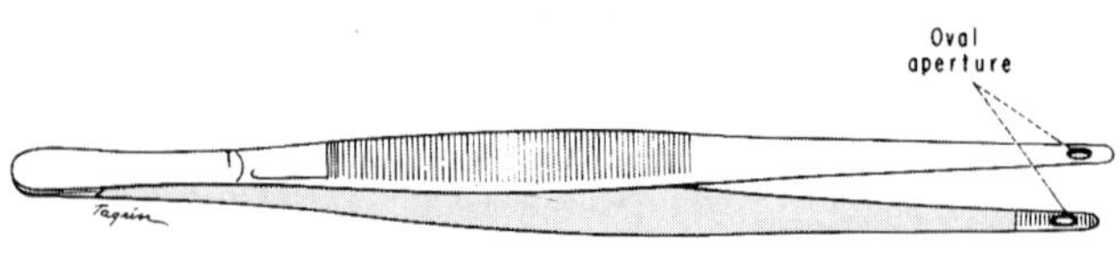

Fig. 12-5. Long dressing forceps adapted for collection of seminal fluid from the endocervical canal.

The controversy regarding the timing of the PCT in relation to coitus has been previously addressed.[216] Several authors have recommended performing the PCT 2 to 3 hours after coitus since this is the time when sperm concentration is highest.[58,224] In contrast, many authors recommend delaying the PCT until at least 6 hours after coitus which emphasizes the role of the cervix as a reservoir for spermatozoa. Moghissi recommends performing the PCT initially at 6 to 8 hours after coitus.[149] Taymor and Overstreet emphasize the importance of sperm longevity and the impracticality of having intercourse several hours before going to the physician's office.[216] They recommend having intercourse "at bedtime" and performing the PCT 10 to 16 hours after coitus. Performing the PCT 10 to 16 hours after coitus allows greater flexibility in the timing of intercourse. If the initial PCT is abnormal earlier timing should be considered.

As previously mentioned the clinical value of the PCT in predicting subsequent fertility is highly controversial. Well-designed prospective studies that demonstrate significant prognostic value for the PCT are balanced by equally well-designed studies that demonstrate no predictive value.[50,86,107] The lack of predictive value is further supported by several laparoscopic studies in which peritoneal fluid was recovered around the time of ovulation and examined for spermatozoa.[11,209] Stone observed numerous motile sperm in the peritoneal fluid in 56% of patients with poor to absent cervical mucus and repetitively poor PCT results (less than five sperm per HPF).[209] In contrast, sperm was recovered from only 53% of control subjects with normal PCT results. Thus several studies highlight the limitations of the PCT in the evaluation of sperm migration and sperm longevity.

Because of conflicting studies there is some debate about what constitutes a normal PCT result. Moghissi's criteria for a normal PCT result is 10 or more sperm with directional motility per HPF.[149] Several other investigators contend that five or more actively motile sperm per HPF may be considered satisfactory.[59,224] Jette and Glass have observed that a PCT result with greater than 20 motile sperm per HPF is associated with an increased likelihood of pregnancy and a normal semen analysis.[107] Although often quoted, these authors have emphasized that no specific number of motile spermatozoa in the PCT result should be judged as "normal."

Interpretation of the PCT result is further complicated by the difficulty in determining the day of ovulation. "Abnormal" cervical mucus is often the result of inaccurate timing with respect to ovulation. If the initial PCT result is abnormal and associated with unfavorable cervical mucus, it should be repeated with consideration of additional testing to determine the day of ovulation (see the discussion of ovulation prediction). If ovulation cannot be determined with a reasonable degree of accuracy, serial PCTs may be considered.

The multiple causes of an abnormal PCT result are listed in Table 12-6. Persistently abnormal PCT results suggest either oligoasthenospermia, abnormal cervical mucus, faulty coital technique, or abnormal cervical mucus-spermatozoa interaction. Male-factor infertility is often suggested when multiple abnormal PCT results are associated with a persistently abnormal semen analysis.

Abnormal cervical mucus may be due to hormonal, anatomic, or infectious etiologies. Any hypoestrogenic state may be associated with unfavorable cervical mucus. Subtle abnormalities in follicular maturation may lead to a relatively low level of preovulatory estradiol and abnormal cervical mucus. Clomiphene citrate has been clearly associated with poor PCT results.[84,141] The mechanism may be related to an antiestrogen effect at the level of the cervix. Anatomical defects that may contribute to abnormal cervical mucus include the hypoplastic cervix and cervical stenosis. Anatomic variations in the position of the cervix are unlikely to contribute to a poor PCT result. Varicosities of the hypoplastic endocervical canal have been associated with extreme friability and scant cervical mucus.[191] Cervical stenosis may be associated with scant cervical mucus and is most commonly the result of a previous cervical conization. Extensive cauterization or cryotherapy of the endocervix, significant cervical prolapse, and acute and chronic cervicitis may also be associated with abnormal cervical mucus. Faulty coital technique may be suspected when the semen analyses and cervical mucus are relatively normal and there are no spermatozoa seen on the PCT. This may be the result of male or female sexual dysfunction such as impotence, premature or retrograde ejaculation, or vaginismus. In addition, the partners of extremely obese women may not be able to fully penetrate the vagina and deposit their semen in the posterior fornix.

Abnormal cervical mucus–sperm interaction is often suggested when the PCT result is poor and the cervical mucus and semen analysis are normal. In the majority of cases no specific cause can be identified. However, an immunologic cause should be suspected when all spermatozoa are immotile, shaking, or displaying poor forward progression.

The immunology of the male and female reproductive tract has been reviewed.[5,94] Both cellular and humoral immunity appear to contribute to reproductive failure. In vitro the soluble products of macrophages and lymphocytes inhibit sperm motility and penetrability.[95,96] Clinically there appears to be a relationship between immunity to sperm and infertility.[33,85,144]

Antisperm antibodies have been isolated from semen, cervical mucus, and male and female serum. These antibodies may be secreted locally within the reproductive tract or they may be associated with circulating serum antibodies.[86,226] The presence of sperm antibodies in semen and cervical mucus is more strongly associated with reproductive impairment when compared to serum. There is also a lack of correlation between the levels of antisperm antibodies in serum and cervical mucus.[207] The precise mechanisms by which antisperm antibodies contribute to infertility remain to be elucidated, but they may interfere with sperm transport, gamete interaction, and macrophage phagocytosis.[32,129]

Bronson et al have emphasized that immunity to sperm is not an all-or-nothing phenomenon.[33] The extent to which antisperm antibodies are present in the reproductive tract appears to influence the degree of fertility impairment. For example, when less than 50% of sperm was antibody bound, the number of motile sperm in the PCT result was no different from that in antibody-negative couples.[33] In addition, spontaneous remission of immunity to sperm has been reported.[33] The etiology of antisperm antibodies appears to be multifactorial. An increased incidence has been

Table 12-6. Causes of an abnormal postcoital test

MALE FACTORS
Oligospermia
Oligoasthenospermia
Sexual dysfunction
ABNORMAL CERVICAL MUCUS
Poor timing
Hypoestrogenism
Cervical stenosis
Cervical varicosities
Cauterization/cryotherapy
Cervicitis
Cervical prolapse
Clomiphene citrate
ABNORMAL SPERM-CERVICAL MUCUS INTERACTION
Idiopathic
Immunologic

associated with vasectomy,[198] genital tract infections,[238] and gastrointestinal exposure to sperm.[33]

A relationship between decreased fertility and antisperm antibodies has been more clearly established in men than in women. In a study of 254 infertile men, Rumke et al demonstrated that the prognosis for future pregnancy was inversely correlated with antibody titers.[187] More recently Ayvaliotis et al[12] have shown that when more than 50% of the spermatozoa in the ejaculate are found to have surface-bound immunoglobulins, the pregnancy rate is 15%, compared with 67% when less than 50% of the sperm are antibody bound. The role of immunologic factors in the cervical mucus and upper reproductive tract remains unclear. Patients with persistent unexplained infertility have a significantly higher incidence of sperm antibodies in their cervical mucus (18.4%) than patients with persistent explained infertility (7.1%).[152]

Several different assays for the detection of antisperm antibodies have been described. The incidence of abnormal test results varies according to the patient population, the individual test, and the titer that is considered abnormal. The Isojima immobilization test result is abnormal in 5% to 10% of women with unexplained infertility.[105] Although no single assay has proved to be superior, the immunobead assay appears to be the most popular. This assay has the advantages of determining the proportion of antibody-bound sperm, immunoglobin subclass specificity, and localization of sperm attachment. A brief description and the relative advantages and disadvantages of several of the tests for antisperm antibodies are outlined in Table 12-7. Flow cytometry has recently been utilized to verify IgG antisperm antibodies.[168]

An antisperm antibody profile is recommended for all couples with poor PCT results. There is a poor correlation, however, between an abnormal PCT result and the presence of antisperm antibodies,[1,45] since approximately one third of female patients with antisperm antibodies have a satisfactory PCT result.[150] The PCT should not be used as the sole screening test for antisperm antibodies. Couples with long-standing unexplained infertility or a history of recurrent or chronic genital tract infections should also have an antisperm antibody profile. The direct and indirect immunobead test is often used to detect antisperm antibodies in cervical mucus, semen, and serum.

Table 12-7. Tests for detecting sperm immunity

Isojima's Immobilization Test (complement-dependent cytotoxity)
- Measures the ratio of motile sperm in control and test serum
- Test for IgG, IgM (IgAs do not fix complement)
- Highly specific; lacks sensitivity (false negatives common)

Kibrick, Friberg-Trey Agglutination Test (sperm agglutination)
- Classical serum tests measures agglutinating antibodies
- False positives result from non specific binding

Enzyme-Linked Immunosorbent Assay (ELISA)
- Antiglobulin binds to human immunoglobulin on sperm surface
- False positives and false negatives result from fixation process and membrane damage, (i.e., membrane extracts may not contain relevant antigens)

Fluorescein-Conjugated Antiglobulins
- False positives common

Radiolabeled Antiglobulin Assay
- High specificity and sensitivity when utilized with living sperm
- Does not determine regional specificity of binding
- Does not determine proportion of antibody-bound sperm

Mixed agglutination reaction
- Utilizes sensitized Rh-positive red blood cells and IgG antiglobulin
- Limitations similar to radiolabeled antiglobulin assay

Immunobead Test
- Detects sperm coating immunoglobulins in seminal plasma and cervical mucus
- Subclass specific (IgM, IgG, IgA)
- Can determine regional specificity
- Can determine proportion of antibody-bound sperm

From Bronson R et al: Sperm antibodies: their role in infertility, *Fertil Steril* 42:171, 1984.

THE OVARIAN FACTOR

Ovulatory disorders include anovulation, oligoovulation, and luteal phase defects. Regular menstrual cycles occurring at intervals of 25 to 35 days, particularly when associated with mittelschmerz, suggest ovulation. In contrast, ovulatory disorders are often associated with irregular menstrual cycles, oligomenorrhea, or amenorrhea. A history of obesity, excessive weight loss, galactorrhea, hirsutism, or acne is often associated with ovulatory disorders. The major clinical entities associated with anovulation and infertility are the polycystic ovary syndrome (PCOS), premature ovarian failure (POF), hyperprolactinemia, and hypothalamic amenorrhea. Certain disorders of the adrenal and thyroid gland may be associated with ovulatory dysfunction. Luteal phase defects appear to be a relatively uncommon cause of infertility. Following a discussion of these major clinical diagnoses, the techniques for documenting ovulation and an adequate luteal phase will be presented.

Polycystic ovarian disease

In 1935 Stein and Leventhal called attention to the syndrome PCOS. It has become increasingly clear that PCOS is a heterogeneous disease. As originally described the hallmark features of this disorder are androgen excess and chronic anovulation. Clinically the most common symptoms associated with PCOS are hirsutism (90%), menstrual irregularities (90%), and infertility (75%). Obesity is found in approximately 50% of cases. In the past the diagnosis was based on the anatomical findings of polycystic or sclerocystic ovaries. The ovaries are large and the surface appears thickened, pale, and smooth. When the ovary is bisected, numerous cystic follicles may be identified beneath the capsule (Fig. 12-6). Microscopically there is fibrosis of the cortical stroma with areas of hyalinization

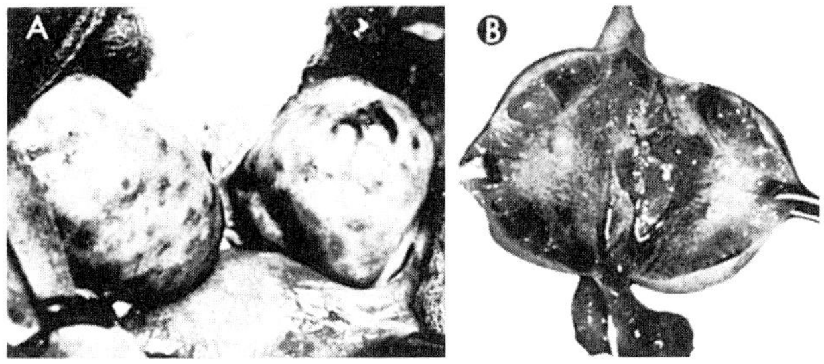

Fig. 12-6. Polycystic ovaries. **A,** Gross appearance. **B,** On bisection.

(Fig. 12 7). Examination of the cystic follicles reveals an unusual activity of the theca interna cells with luteinization. Corpora albicans and corpora lutea are usually absent, but on occasion one or more may be identified. Although at one time this microscopic picture was thought to be pathognomonic of PCOS, present evidence suggests that it is merely representative of prolonged periods of anovulation from various causes. Polycystic ovaries may be observed in women with hyperandrogenism, which includes Cushing's syndrome, congenital adrenal hyperplasia, ovarian and adrenal tumors, hyperprolactinemia, hypothyroidism, and acromegaly. In contrast, one third of women with symptoms and hormonal parameters suggestive of PCOS may have normal-appearing ovaries.

There is no universal agreement regarding the pathophysiology of PCOS. Recent reviews have suggested a multifactorial etiology.[15] At least five major systems may contribute to the development of PCOS: (1) hypothalamus and pituitary, (2) ovary, (3) skin, (4) adrenal, and (5) pancreas. The characteristic biochemical abnormalities include ovarian hyperandrogenism, adrenal hyperandrogenism, inappropriate gonadotropin secretion, peripheral

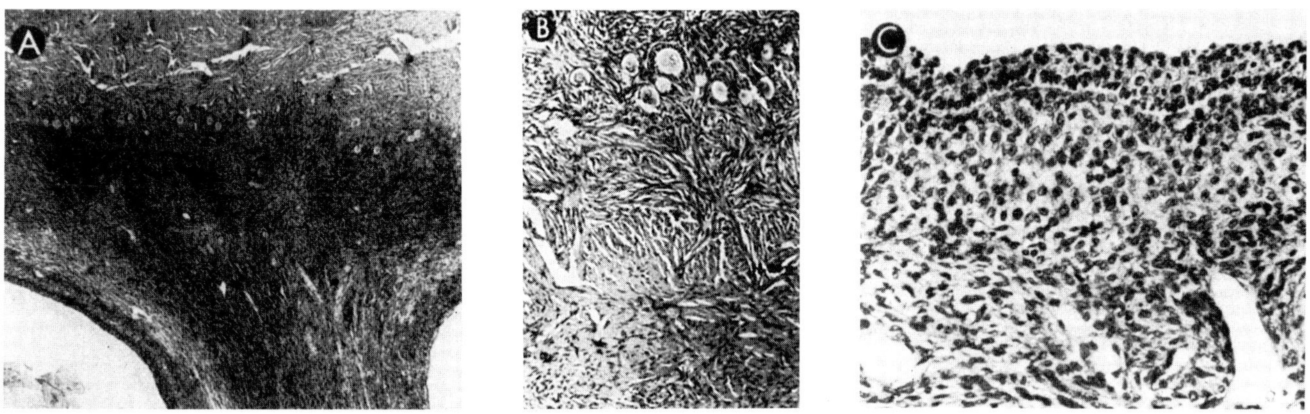

Fig. 12-7. Microscopic appearance of polycystic ovaries. **A,** Low-power view. Note cystic follicles and collagenous character of the cortex. **B,** Higher-power view. Numerous primordial follicles are seen in the zone between the normal cortex and the hyperplastic fibrotic cortex. **C,** High-power view showing the wall of a cystic follicle with a narrow layer of granulosa cells toward the lumen of the cyst and a wide layer of luteinized theca cells.

hyperestrogenism, and hyperinsulinemia. It has been suggested that these hormonal abnormalities represent a vicious cycle of events that perpetuate PCOS.

The inappropriate gonadotropin secretion involves an elevated level of LH and a normal or low level of FSH.[128] The mechanisms that are responsible for the inappropriate gonadotropin secretion remain to be fully elucidated. Centrally, a relative deficiency of dopamine and a relative excess of norepinephrine may contribute to the elevated secretion of LH.[127,242] Peripherally, relatively constant levels of estrogen result from the extraglandular conversion of androstenedione to estrone. Since estrogen may enhance LH secretion, the chronic secretion of estrogen in PCOS may contribute to the persistently elevated levels of LH. The suppression of FSH and the resultant anovulation may be partially due to the chronically elevated levels of estrogen, an increased secretion of inhibin, or both.[214] Several investigators have suggested that the primary defect in the PCOS lies in the hypothalamus. It is possible that an increase in endogenous gonadotropin-releasing hormone (GnRH) may contribute to the increased LH level. Several studies have demonstrated an increased LH pulse frequency and amplitude in PCOS.[116a,178a,243a,243b] In combination the relatively constant levels of estrogen may contribute to the increased sensitivity of the pituitary to GnRH stimulation of LH release and decreased pituitary sensitivity to GnRH stimulation of FSH release.

Several lines of evidence suggest that the adrenal gland may be important in the pathogenesis of PCOS. Approximately 50% of patients with PCOS have elevated levels of dehydroepiandrosterone sulfate (DHEAS).[101,125] The mechanism of excess adrenal androgen production in PCOS is unknown. However, patients with PCOS and elevated levels of DHEAS appear to have adrenals that are extremely sensitive to adrenocorticotropin (ACTH) stimulation.[40]

The association of hyperinsulinemia with PCOS has been manifested clinically by acanthosis nigricans and termed the HAIR–AN syndrome.[14] The severity of the insulin resistance is strongly correlated with the degree of hyperinsulinemia which in turn is highly correlated with the severity of the hyperandrogenism. The hyperinsulinemic state appears to cause the hyperandrogenism and not vice versa. This is supported by the observation that the insulin resistance and acanthosis nigricans are not affected by lowering ovarian androgen production.[15]

Table 12-8. Diagnostic criteria for PCOS

Perimenarcheal onset of menstrual irregularity
Androgen excess
Chronic anovulation
Inappropriate gonadotropin secretion (LH:FSH > 3)
Obesity
Euprolactinemia

From Lobo RA: Polycystic ovary syndrome in infertility, contraception and reproductive endocrinology. In Mishell DR, Davajan V, editors: *Infertility, contraception and reproductive endocrinology*, Oradell, NJ, 1986, Medical Economic Books.

Because PCOS is a heterogeneous syndrome there has been considerable debate regarding the diagnostic criteria. The Lobo's criteria are listed in Table 12-8.[126] Some patients considered to have PCOS may not meet these strict criteria, however. The most consistent finding in PCOS appears to be a mildly elevated serum testosterone level in the range of 70 to 120 ng/dL. In patients with a serum testosterone level greater than 150 ng/dL, the diagnosis of ovarian stromal hyperthecosis is more likely and the possibility of an androgen-secreting tumor should be considered. The presence of mild hyperandrogenism does not differentiate between PCOS, adult onset congenital adrenal hyperplasia (CAH), and Cushing's syndrome. The diagnoses of CAH and Cushing's syndrome may be confirmed with an ACTH stimulation test and dexamethasone suppression test, respectively.

Premature ovarian failure

Premature ovarian failure is defined as a failure of ovarian estrogen production in the setting of hypergonadotropism before the age of 35. The etiology of POF appears to be multifactorial. Most cases are idiopathic. Significant evidence suggests that specific genetic defects may cause POF.[118] POF may be the result of a reduced number of primordial follicles or an increased rate of atresia. Infectious and iatrogenic destruction of primordial follicles may occur as a result of mumps oophoritis, irradiation, or chemotherapy. Documentation of antiovarian antibodies and the association of POF with other immunologic endocrine disorders supports the hypothesis that POF may be an autoimmune disease. An increased incidence of POF has also been associated with abnormal galactose metabolism.[115]

The clinical presentation of POF is quite variable. Patients at varying ages may have symptoms of amenorrhea, infertility, or both. Symptoms suggestive of menopause, including hot flashes, vaginal dryness, sleep disturbances and mood disturbances, may be present. Ovarian failure may be temporary, with spontaneous return of menstrual function. Associated autoimmune disorders include Addison's disease, thyroiditis, hypoparathyroidism, diabetes, pernicious anemia, myasthenia gravis, and vitiligo. Because of the associated polyendocrine autoimmune syndromes, patients should be screened for diabetes, anemia, thyroid, adrenal, and parathyroid insufficiency. The diagnosis is confirmed by elevated gonadotropin levels, particularly FSH levels greater than 40 mIU/mL. All patients less than 30 years of age with POF should have a chromosomal analysis to identify any patients with a Y chromosome who are at risk for the development of a gonadal tumor.

Recently a subgroup of patients with unexplained infertility has been described as having incipient ovarian failure.[222] These patients are characterized by elevated day

3 FSH levels greater than 20 mIU/mL. These patients often have normal, ovulatory menstrual cycles but respond poorly to human menopausal gonadotropins. Similar to patients with POF, these patients have an extremely poor prognosis for future fertility in the absence of in vitro fertilization with donor oocytes.

Hyperprolactinemia

The association of ovulatory dysfunction and hyperprolactinemia is well documented.[106] The primary mechanism appears to be inhibition of pulsatile GnRH secretion and results in a hypoestrogenic state.[155] Elevated prolactin levels may cause direct inhibition of steroidogenesis at the level of the ovary.[142] A number of clinical conditions may cause elevated prolactin levels. These include pituitary tumors, various medications, chest wall trauma, chronic renal insufficiency, hypothyroidism, the empty sella syndrome, pituitary stalk transection, and rarely, nonpituitary tumors. Medications that commonly cause hyperprolactinemia include phenothiazines, tricyclic antidepressants, estrogens, oral contraceptive agents, butyrophenones, metoclopramide, reserpine, amphetamines, and methyldopa. Transient elevated levels of prolactin have also been associated with beer and protein ingestion, *Herpes zoster*, nipple stimulation, stress, sexual intercourse, and hypoglycemia. Although associated galactorrhea is common, not all women with hyperprolactinemia have this symptom. Even though pituitary adenomas tend to be associated with high levels of prolactin they may be associated with any degree of hyperprolactinemia. Therefore evaluation with magnetic resonance imaging is recommended for all patients with persistent hyperprolactinemia, regardless of the absolute level.

Hypothalamic amenorrhea

Hypothalamic amenorrhea is a diagnosis of exclusion. Despite multiple etiologic factors, the primary mechanism appears to be an alteration in GnRH secretion. This results in decreased gonadotropin secretion, a failure in the stimulation of follicular development, and a diminution in gonadal steroidogenesis. Therefore any process resulting in a disturbance of GnRH production may lead to hypothalamic amenorrhea. In contrast to PCOS, hypothalamic amenorrhea is associated with a hypoestrogenic state. Hypothalamic amenorrhea must be distinguished from other forms of hypoestrogenic amenorrhea such as hyperprolactinemia, POF, and Asherman's syndrome (see the discussion of the uterine factor). The diagnosis is confirmed by normal or low gonadotropin levels and a normal progestin challenge. The causes of hypothalamic amenorrhea include exercise, weight loss, and stress. Rare causes include anorexia nervosa, Kallmann's syndrome, and nonfunctional hypothalamic pituitary tumors. In a large percentage of cases there may be no obvious underlying cause. The most common clinical problem associated with hypothalamic amenorrhea is infertility. In contrast to patients with POF, symptoms of estrogen deficiency are relatively rare.

Luteal phase defect

A luteal phase defect (LPD) refers to a relative deficiency in the secretion of progesterone by the corpus luteum. Progesterone is important for the implantation of the embryo and the maintenance of early human pregnancy. The progesterone deficiency may be in the amount or duration (or both) of secretion. The short luteal phase refers to a shortening of the interval between ovulation and the onset of menses to 10 days or less. The short luteal phase may be associated with a normal peak value of progesterone. The inadequate luteal phase refers to a luteal phase of normal length with lower than normal progesterone secretion. The incidence of a luteal phase defect as a pathologic condition is difficult to determine. This is largely due to the lack of uniform diagnostic criteria in the various epidemiologic reports. In addition, there is a limited amount of data to address the incidence of LPD in the "normal" population. Davis et al recently reported that the incidence of LPD in normal fertile women was 6.6%.[60] The incidence of LPD as a cause for infertility is between 3% and 20%.[109,110,232] Because the majority of series estimate the incidence at 3% to 10% LPD may not represent a clinically significant cause of infertility. However, the frequency of luteal phase defects appears to be much higher in certain clinical situations. For example, patients with recurrent miscarriages appear to have an incidence as high as 35%.[174] Luteal phase defects appear to be more common in patients with hyperprolactinemia; other conditions such as strenuous exercise, significant weight loss, and hyperandrogenism may be associated with an increased incidence. Luteal phase defects also appear to be more common at the extremes of reproductive life. The anovulatory patient requiring ovulation induction may demonstrate a residual luteal phase defect which appears to be particularly common among women treated with clomiphene citrate.[77]

The endometrial biopsy appears to be the most practical standard for diagnosing luteal phase defects. The endometrial biopsy not only identifies inadequate progesterone production by the corpus luteum but also identifies abnormal endometrial responsiveness. The usefulness of the endometrial biopsy is highlighted by the studies of Daly et al[57] which demonstrate that the biopsy is predictive of therapeutic outcome. As previously mentioned, the optimal criteria for diagnosing LPD remain controversial. The most widely accepted criterion for diagnosing a luteal phase defect is endometrial dating, which lags behind the time in the cycle by more than 2 days when derived retrospectively in two separate cycles. Attempts have been made to utilize a midluteal serum progesterone level for the diagnosis of luteal phase defect. A midluteal serum progesterone level of greater than 10 ng/mL has been associated with adequate luteal function.[86] The basal body temperature chart is notoriously inaccurate for detecting luteal phase defects. However, evidence of a luteal phase of less than 10 days on basal body temperature charts does appear to correlate with the presence of a short luteal phase.[67] The importance of luteal phase defect as a primary cause of infertility remains to be proved. Therefore the endometrial biopsy should not be recommended as a routine part of the infertility evaluation. Evaluation for luteal phase defect is usually limited to patients with clinical conditions associated with a higher frequency of luteal phase defects.

Thyroid disease

Both hyperthyroidism and hypothyroidism may be associated with menstrual irregularities and ovulatory dysfunction. The underlying mechanism appears to be related to alterations in the metabolism of androgens and estrogens. Thyroid disease may also be associated with abnormalities in gonadotropin secretion. Although many studies suggest a clear association between clinical hypothyroidism and ovulatory disorders, those demonstrating an association between hyperthyroidism and ovulatory disorders are lacking. Hypothyroidism and hyperthyroidism appear to be associated with decreased libido and this may be another mechanism of thyroid-related infertility.

Although few reported cases of pregnancy in patients with hypothyroidism and myxedema exist, myxedematous women appear to be anovulatory.[99,156] Hypothyroidism is associated with alterations in the metabolism of testosterone and estradiol. There is a decrease in sex hormone-binding globulin levels, an increase in the metabolic clearance rate of testosterone, an increase in the conversion of androstenedione to testosterone, and an increase in the conversion of testosterone to estradiol.[82] In hypothyroidism the chronic anovulation appears to be the result of alterations in the metabolism of estradiol and inappropriate estrogen feedback. There is a shift in the normal 2-hydroxylation with an increase in 16-hydroxylation and an increase in the estriol level.[73] Yen has postulated that this increase in the level of the less potent estriol results in inappropriate feedback, abnormal gonadotropin secretion, and chronic anovulation.[243] Hypothyroidism may be associated with hyperprolactinemia and is an additional mechanism for the abnormal gonadotropin secretion associated with hypothyroidism.

Despite its popularity the efficacy of thyroid hormone therapy for euthyroid women remains unsubstantiated. Several well-controlled clinical studies have demonstrated no benefit from the use of thyroid hormone in euthyroid infertile women.[38,243] The role of thyroid hormone therapy for patients with subclinical hypothyroidism (i.e., elevated TSH level and normal thyroxine and triiodothyronine levels) remains unclear and warrants further investigation. In comparison, patients with clinical hypothyroidism may benefit from thyroid hormone replacement with a resumption of normal ovulatory function. In patients with panhypopituitarism, it is imperative that the adrenal insufficiency be corrected before thyroid hormone replacement is initiated since this may result in fatal adrenal insufficiency.

Hyperthyroidism may be associated with menstrual irregularities because of alterations in testosterone and estradiol metabolism. There is an increase in the level of plasma sex hormone-binding globulin, a decrease in the metabolic clearance rate of androgens and estrogens, an increase in the level of plasma testosterone, an increase in the conversion of testosterone to androstenedione, and an increase in the concentration of estrone.[43,82,185] Hyperthyroidism is also associated with an increase in 2-hydroxylation.[74] The menstrual irregularities associated with hyperthyroidism appear to be related to inappropriate feedback with elevated LH secretion and normal FSH secretion.[205] This is similar to the inappropriate gonadotropin secretion associated with PCOS. Despite a clear pathophysiological basis, however, an association between hyperthyroidism and infertility remains to be demonstrated.

Adrenal disease

Certain disorders of the adrenal may be associated with ovulatory disorders. Autoimmune adrenal insufficiency (Addison's disease) may be associated with POF as part of the syndromes of polyglandular failure.[165] Cushing's syndrome, characterized by an overproduction of glucocorticoids, may mimic PCOS by producing obesity, hirsutism, menstrual irregularities, and enlarged polycystic ovaries. Cushing's syndrome may result from an overproduction of ACTH or the autonomous production of glucocorticoids. Cushing's disease is the result of pituitary ACTH hypersecretion and hypercortisolism. The clinical manifestations of Cushing's syndrome are listed in Table 12-9. The mechanisms by which Cushing's syndrome lead to ovulatory dysfunction are not clear. Similar to PCOS, there appears to be an increase in the peripheral production of estrogen that results in inappropriate acyclic feedback. In addition, there appears to be an abnormality in the pulsatile secretion of GnRH.[243] Cushing's syndrome may be

Table 12-9. Clinical manifestations of Cushing's syndrome

Symptom	%
Obesity	95
Moonfaced	95
Hypertension	85
Glucose intolerance	80
Menstrual irregularities	75
Androgen excess	72
Striae	67
Proximal muscle weakness	65
Easy bruisability	55
Osteoporosis	55
Depression	50

distinguished from PCOS with a dexamethasone suppression test and/or 24-hour urine collection for free cortisol. Dexamethasone (1 mg) is given at bedtime and a fasting cortisol level is measured the following morning. If the plasma cortisol level is less than 5 μg/100 mL, the diagnosis of Cushing's syndrome is excluded. Though an abnormal value of greater than 5 μg/100 mL is not diagnostic it does warrant further evaluation.

The adult-onset form of CAH may also mimic PCOS. The subject of CAH has been recently reviewed.[235] Relative deficiencies of 21-hydroxylase and 11-hydroxylase may be associated with hirsutism, menstrual irregularities, and ovulatory dysfunction. Because of these enzymatic defects, the normal biosynthetic pathways are interrupted and an accumulation of adrenal androgens results. Since there appears to be a strong genetic predisposition, a family history of hirsutism, menstrual disorders, and infertility may be suggestive of CAH. A fasting, morning 17-hydroxyprogesterone level is often obtained in the follicular phase as a screening test. In patients with a 17-hydroxyprogesterone concentration of greater than 2 ng/mL, the diagnosis of late-onset CAH should be pursued with an ACTH or cosyntropin stimulation test.[13,166]

TECHNIQUES FOR PREDICTING AND DETECTING OVULATION

Besides pregnancy, recovering an ovum from the female genital tract is the only direct evidence of ovulation. This is obviously impractical for clinical practice. Therefore a variety of diagnostic tests that indirectly predict and detect ovulation are commonly employed. The diagnostic tests commonly used to confirm ovulation include the basal body temperature (BBT) chart, midluteal serum progesterone levels, and the endometrial biopsy. The diagnostic tests that predict the time of ovulation include the BBT chart and the serial assessment of plasma or urinary LH levels.

Basal body temperature chart

All infertility patients should be instructed to take their temperature with a basal thermometer. The BBT chart not only is able to provide indirect evidence of ovulation but may aid in the timing of intercourse, inseminations, and other diagnostic procedures such as the postcoital test. The reading is taken each morning and recorded on a chart, with day 1 corresponding to the first day of menses (Fig. 12-8). Basal body temperature thermometers show a range of only a few degrees and are easier to read. The reading is most accurate when taken immediately on awakening before any activity. During the follicular phase the temperature will usually be 97° F to 98° F. During the luteal phase the temperature is generally greater than 98° F. The mechanism for the elevation in temperature appears to be related to the thermogenic properties of progesterone on the central nervous system. It is often difficult to pinpoint the exact day of ovulation. A significant rise in temperature is not noted until 2 days after the LH peak and coincides with a rise in the serum progesterone level to greater than 4 ng/mL.[153] Ovulation probably occurs on the day prior to the first temperature elevation and may be marked by a dip in the temperature to the lowest level of the cycle. This is supported by the observation that the most likely time for conception based on a single artificial insemination is the day before the temperature rise.[167] The absence of a biphasic temperature pattern is suggestive but not diagnostic of anovulation. In approximately 75% of monophasic cycles hormonal evidence of ovulation has been documented.[21,148] A slow rise in a biphasic chart is not necessarily an indication of an ovulatory disorder. However, a temperature elevation of less than 10 days' duration is suggestive of a short luteal phase. In summary, the BBT chart is very helpful when it is clearly biphasic. When the chart is monophasic or difficult to interpret another diagnostic method should be pursued.

Midluteal serum progesterone

A single, midluteal serum progesterone level greater than 3 ng/mL is indirect evidence of ovulation. Several investigators have suggested that a midluteal progesterone level of greater than 10 ng/mL is associated with adequate corpus luteum function.[92,135,178] Although a single midluteal progesterone determination offers a practical and cost-effective approach to the evaluation of LPD, there are limited data to support these recommendations. In fact other investigators have demonstrated significant overlap among single serum progesterone levels obtained from LPD patients and normal controls. There is also a poor correlation between serum progesterone levels and endometrial biopsy in the evaluation of luteal phase defects.[19,195] The difficulty encountered in the interpretation of a single midluteal serum progesterone level may be due to the pulsatile nature of progesterone secretion.[72,203] Although extremely accurate for confirming ovulation, a single midluteal serum progesterone level is much less reliable for evaluating the adequacy of the luteal phase.

Over the years considerable efforts to improve the diagnostic accuracy of serum progesterone levels in the evaluation of LPD have focused on increasing the frequency of blood sampling. Luteal phase progesterone production is determined by integrating the area under the curve generated by multiple progesterone determinations.[61] Because there is general agreement that the majority of cases of LPD are associated with decreased progesterone secretion, it is not surprising that increasing the frequency of blood sampling increases the diagnostic accuracy. Unfortunately there is no consensus regarding the optimal number and timing of multiple progesterone determinations. Moreover the absolute level of progesterone production that accurately reflects normal luteal function has not been determined. The major disadvantages of multiple blood sampling include the inconvenience and expense.

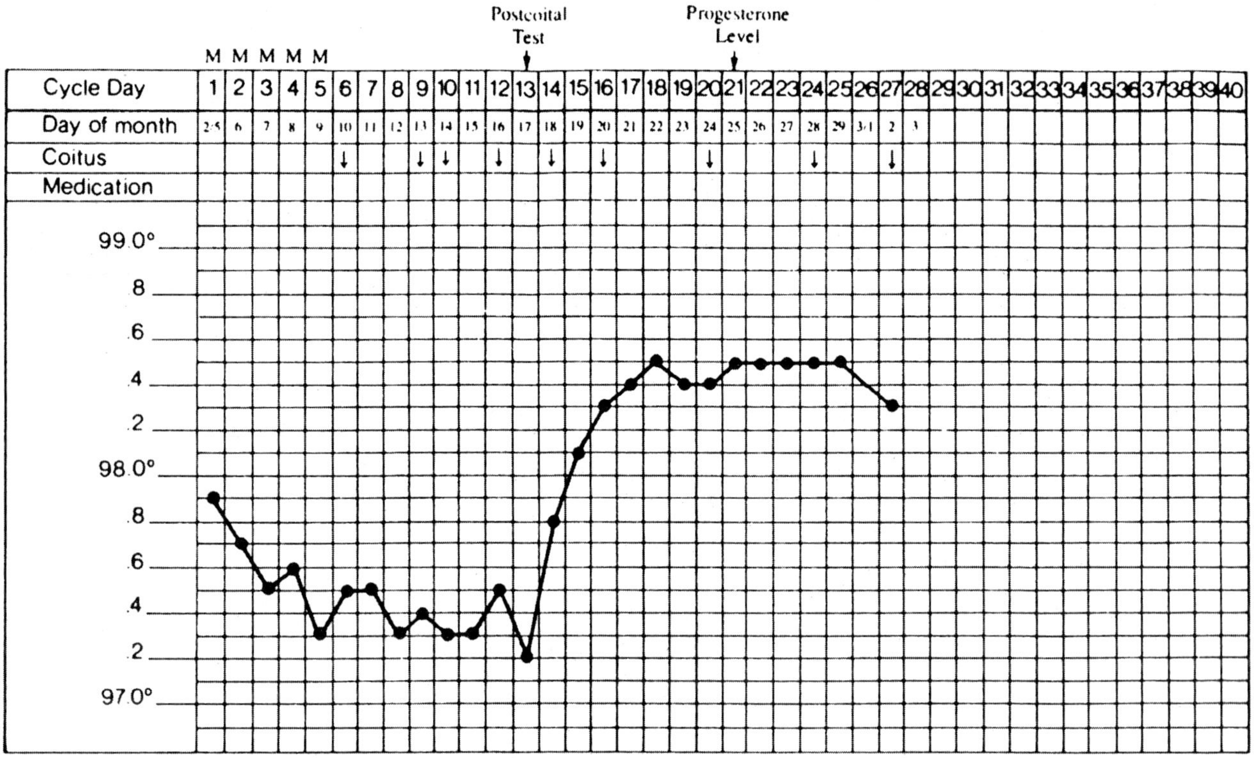

Fig. 12-8. Basal body temperature chart. This example of a BBT chart indicates a biphasic pattern with notations for the days of menstruation (M) and the timing of coitus (arrows).

Endometrial biopsy

The finding of secretory endometrium on an endometrial biopsy is additional indirect evidence of ovulation. Although relatively safe and rarely uncomfortable, the endometrial biopsy should not be performed routinely for confirmation of ovulation because of the availability of accurate noninvasive studies. The role of the endometrial biopsy in the infertility investigation is for the diagnosis of luteal phase defects. Traditionally the biopsy is performed 2 to 3 days prior to the expected menses. If the biopsy is performed prior to the 25th day there is an increased rate of false-negative results. Accurately timing the endometrial biopsy is often difficult in patients with slightly irregular menstrual cycles. Recent studies have focused on improving the timing and interpretation of the endometrial biopsy by determining the "theoretical" cycle day prospectively rather than retrospectively. Shoupe et al correlated endometrial maturation in fertile women with four methods for estimating the day of ovulation.[197] An endometrial biopsy was performed in 13 normally cycling women 8 to 11 days after the predicted day of ovulation. The determination of the day of ovulation with ultrasound, serum-luteinizing hormone measurements, and BBT correlated well with the endometrial histology. In contrast, when the day of ovulation was determined retrospectively as 14 days before the onset of the subsequent menses, the endometrial histology was in error more than 2 days in 35% of the specimens. The authors concluded that an accurate interpretation of the endometrial biopsy should be based on days since ovulation rather than onset of menses. Li et al similarly demonstrated an improved accuracy for dating the endometrial biopsy based on serum-luteinizing hormone determinations when compared with subsequent menses.[122]

A sensitive serum pregnancy test should be offered to the patient in an attempt to prevent the interruption of an early pregnancy. A pelvic examination should precede the biopsy so that the position and size of the uterus can be determined. The cervix is exposed with a speculum and cleansed with an antiseptic reagent. Premedication with a nonsteroidal anti-inflationary agent and a paracervical block using 1% or 2% chloroprocaine may minimize patient discomfort. A tenaculum is attached to the anterior cervix. A Duncan, Novak, or Pipelle curette is placed high in the anterior uterine fundus and the specimen obtained by using a firm stroke extending from the fundus to the cervix. The biopsy tissue is immediately fixed in Bouin's solution.

The interpretation of the endometrial biopsy is based on the dating criteria of Noyes.[169] The accuracy of the endometrial biopsy as a diagnostic test is highly dependent on the experience of the pathologist interpreting the histologic specimen. However, there appears to be significant intra-observer variability.[193] Proliferative endometrium is diagnostic of anovulation. Dated secretory endometrium should be compared with the retrospectively derived cycle day. The first day of bleeding is arbitrarily considered cycle day 28. A single normal endometrial biopsy is often termed "in phase" and is usually considered sufficient to exclude the diagnosis of LPD. An abnormal biopsy is generally required in two separate cycles to make the diagnosis of LPD because an isolated" out-of-phase" biopsy is not uncommon in normally fertile women.[60]

Ultrasound monitoring

Serial ultrasound examinations can demonstrate the growth of a follicle. The disappearance of a dominant follicle combined with the presence of free fluid in the cul-de-sac suggests follicular rupture and is presumptive evidence of ovulation. Ultrasonography may be helpful in assessing corpus luteum formation. Because of the wide range of the preovulatory follicle's diameter (17mm to 26 mm), ultrasound examination appears to be an inaccurate predictor of ovulation. Ultrasound monitoring is rarely used as a primary diagnostic aid for confirming ovulation.

Ultrasound examination may be useful in the diagnosis of the luteinized unruptured follicle syndrome (LUFS). The LUFS is characterized by a normal pattern of gonadotropin secretion, regular menses, and no evidence of follicular rupture.[137] The absence of follicular rupture is associated with entrapment of the oocyte and subsequent luteinization. The LUFS has been associated with unexplained infertility, endometriosis, and pelvic adhesions. Ultrasound criteria include the persistence of an echo-free dominant follicle beyond 36 hours after the LH peak.[181] The absence of stigmata of ovulation at laparoscopy has also been suggestive of LUFS. There is no general agreement regarding the incidence of LUFS among the fertile or infertile patient population. At the present time a causal relationship between LUFS and infertility remains to be established since LUFS does not appear to be recurrent. Therefore routine ultrasound evaluation of infertile couples for LUFS is not recommended.[114] The major usefulness of ultrasound monitoring appears to be limited to the timing of human chorionic gonadotropin (hCG) administration during ovulation induction protocols.

Luteinizing hormone monitoring

The measurement of daily preovulatory serum LH levels appears to be the standard for predicting ovulation which occurs approximately 34 to 36 hours after the onset of the LH surge.[100] A twofold rise above the baseline serum LH level is suggestive of the onset of the LH surge. The accuracy of monitoring the serum LH level must be weighed against the relative inconvenience and significant cost of daily blood testing. In the past decade simple urinary LH ovulation detection kits have become readily available. The accuracy of these kits compared to serum LH and BBT charts for timing intercourse and inseminations remains controversial. Several studies have demonstrated that certain home urinary LH assays are quite accurate.[68,230] Several new techniques are currently being investigated for their accuracy of predicting ovulation. These include salivary detection kits for LH and progesterone and the determination of salivary or vaginal electrical resistance.[71]

TUBAL AND PERITONEAL FACTORS

The etiologic factors for tubal disease, pelvic adhesions, and endometriosis have been previously described. There are no identifiable risk factors in approximately 50% of patients with documented tubal or peritoneal factors.[184] The routine infertility evaluation commonly includes a test for tubal patency. In certain situations, such as the anovulatory patient undergoing ovulation induction with clomiphene citrate or the infertile couple with a moderate to severe male factor, some clinicians recommend postponing an evaluation of tubal patency.

Hysterosalpingography

In the past, uterotubal insufflation (Rubin's test) was used as a screening procedure to determine tubal patency. Hysterosalpingography (HSG) has replaced uterotubal insufflation as the most commonly employed screening test because of the increased accuracy and additional information gained from HSG. In addition to assessing tubal patency, HSG may provide useful information about the uterine cavity (see the discussion of uterine factors). HSG is an outpatient procedure that is usually performed in conjunction with the department of radiology. The procedure is scheduled before ovulation, usually between cycle days 5 and 11, to prevent the possible irradiation of a fertilized ovum. The patient is placed in the dorsolithotomy position and a single-tooth tenaculum is placed on the anterior cervix. A cannula is snugly inserted into the cervical canal and a sterile, radiopaque contrast medium is slowly injected through the cannula. The injection phase of the procedure is best visualized under fluoroscopy. When a fluoroscopy is not available, radiographs should be taken after the sequential injection of 3 to 5 mL of dye. Depending on the size of the uterus, 8 to 10 mL of contrast material may be required.

A radiograph should be taken when the uterine cavity is filled. HSG often provides evidence suggesting proximal tubal obstruction. Several studies have demonstrated that among infertile women with abnormal hysterosalpingograms the site of tubal obstruction appears to be cornual approximately 50% of the time.[76,180] Salpingitis isthmica nodosa (SIN) was first described in 1887 and is a rare cause of proximal tubal obstruction.[41] SIN is characterized by numerous small diverticuli involving the interstitial segment or isthmus (or both) of the fallopian tube. Although the etiology remains unknown SIN is often found in association with chronic inflammation. A second radiograph is taken as the ampullae fill. The presence of mucosal rugae appears to be a favorable prognostic factor for subsequent pregnancy and the absence of rugae suggests damaged tubal epithelium. Young et al demonstrated a 60.7% pregnancy rate in cases with rugal folds compared with a 7.3% pregnancy rate when rugal folds were absent.[244] Distal tubal occlusion is suggested when there is partial filling of the fallopian tube but no peritoneal spillage. This may occur in the isthmic, ampullary, or fimbrial portion of the fallopian tube and is often associated with radiographic evidence of hydrosalpinges. An irregular distribution of loculated contrast medium around the fimbriated end of the tube suggests periadnexal adhesions. Whenever possible a final radiograph demonstrating free intraperitoneal contrast material should be taken to document tubal patency. Fig. 12-9 shows the normal findings obtained by HSG and the findings seen in chronic PID. The accuracy of HSG will be discussed in the following section on laparoscopy.

The optimal contrast medium for HSG remains controversial.[204] A water-soluble contrast medium may be used and excellent quality radiographs obtained; disadvantages are the possible increase in abdominal cramping and a slight loss in image resolution. The use of a water-soluble rather than an oil-based contrast medium avoids the potential complications of lipid granulomas and lipid embolization. Lipid embolization is the result of the injection of contrast medium into the myometrium with subsequent intravasation into the venous or lymphatic system. Siegler has reported nine deaths attributable to the intravasation of dye.[199] Bateman et al have reported 13 cases of contrast medium intravasation in a series of 533 HSGs performed with an oil contrast medium.[18] However, only six of these patients had embolization of dye, and there was no associated morbidity or mortality. These authors state that the use of fluoroscopy allows for early detection of intravasation and minimizes complications. Whenever there is evidence of intravasation injection should be discontinued immediately, regardless of the contrast media employed. The appearance of intravasation includes a network of streak-like opacities adjacent to the uterine cavity that extend toward the pelvic side walls and subsequently migrate in a cephalad direction.

The use of fluoroscopy combined with the use of the less viscous contrast medium ethiodized oil, may minimize the risk of a fatal oil embolus. The popularity of ethiodized oil in certain centers is due to its possible value as a therapeutic agent. Despite numerous anecdotal cases, the therapeutic benefit of HSG remains controversial. Although several studies have demonstrated no increase in the pregnancy rate following HSG[8] several other studies seem to suggest an increased pregnancy rate.[171] Moreover, several studies suggest an increased pregnancy rate with an oil contrast compared with a water-soluble contrast medium.[62,79] DeCherney et al studied 339 patients over a 4-month period and demonstrated a 29% pregnancy rate using an oil medium compared with 13% with a water-soluble medium.[62] The mechanisms by which HSG may enhance fertility include (1) a mechanical lavage of a partially obstructed tube, (2) stimulation of the tubal cilia, and (3) inhibition of hostile peritoneal fluid immune cell function.[81,211]

The absolute contraindications for performing HSG include a possible pregnancy and a history of acute PID. Relative contraindications include a history suggestive of PID, recent uterine instrumentation, and iodine allergy. The risk of PID following HSG has been estimated at 1% to 3%.[180,210] A sedimentation rate may be helpful for screening patients at risk for an acute flare of PID. Although routine antibiotic

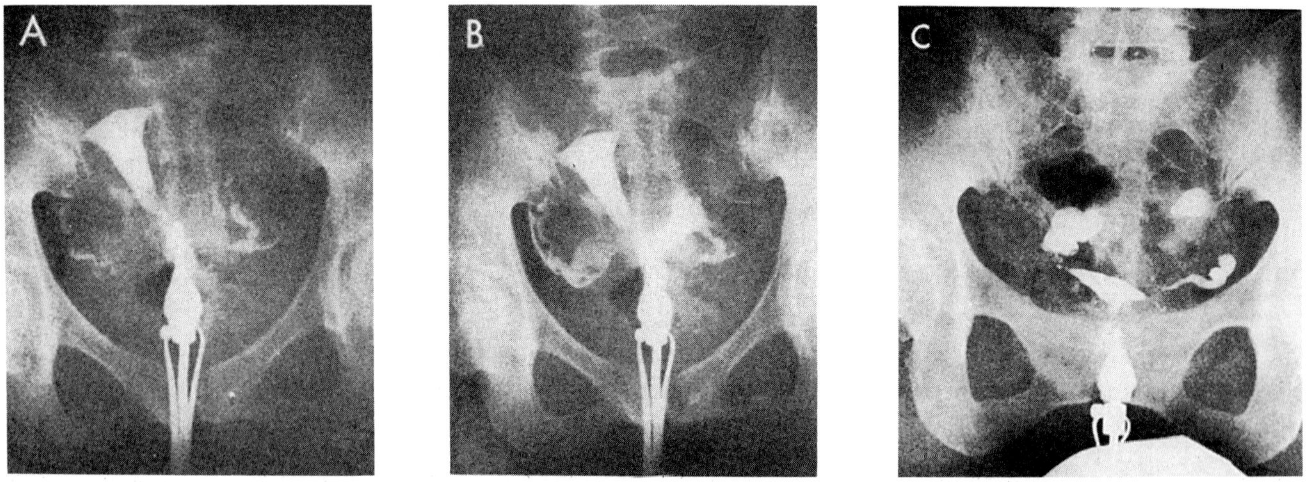

Fig. 12-9. Hysterosalpingograms. **A,** Visualization of uterus and both oviducts in a normal patient. **B,** Second film showing free passage of the dye from the oviduct into the peritoneal cavity. **C,** Patient with chronic PID and bilateral hydrosalpinges.

prophylaxis has not been demonstrated to be efficacious,[210] patients at risk for acute PID may benefit from antibiotic therapy.[175] Generally antibiotic prophylaxis with doxycycline is recommended for 3 days for all patients. For patients at significant risk for an acute flare of PID, laparoscopy with tubal lavage is recommended in lieu of HSG for the evaluation of tubal patency.

Laparoscopy

Laparoscopy with tubal lavage is considered the standard for evaluating tubal patency and other peritoneal factors. Laparoscopy offers the advantage of directly visualizing the pelvic anatomy. During laparoscopy, in addition to assessing tubal patency, the appearance of the fimbria, the anatomical relationship between the fimbria and the ovary, and the presence of periadnexal adhesions and endometriosis can be determined. The technique of laparoscopy is thoroughly reviewed by Wheeless and Katayama.[234] Laparoscopy is usually performed as a day surgical procedure using general anesthetic. However, the procedure may be performed using sedation with local anesthesia or regional anesthesia. The patient is placed in the lithotomy position and a cannula is placed through the cervical canal for the injection of indigo carmine dye. A thin Verres needle is placed through an intraumbilical incision into the peritoneal cavity for the instillation of carbon dioxide. Approximately 2 to 3 L of CO_2 provides an adequate pneumoperitoneum so that the larger trochar may be inserted into the peritoneal cavity. The laparoscope is inserted through this trochar (Fig. 12-10). A second suprapubic puncture may be necessary to adequately expose the pelvic anatomy. Tubal lavage should be performed with indigo carmine dye to assess tubal patency.

The diagnostic accuracy of HSG has been evaluated in many studies that compare HSG and laparoscopy. Although HSG is not a perfect predictor of tubal factor, HSG is in agreement with the laparoscopic findings approximately two thirds of the time. The major inadequacy of HSG is the failure to detect significant periadnexal adhesions. El Minawi et al studied 352 cases of infertility in which both laparoscopy and HSG were performed.[69] There was complete agreement in 56.7% of the cases. Pelvic adhesions were suggested by HSG in 76 cases compared with 151 cases documented by laparoscopy. Moreover, laparoscopy was able to document pelvic adhesions or endometriosis in 57% of patients with previously unexplained infertility.[69] Collins et al estimated the aggregate sensitivity and specificity of HSG to be 76% and 83%, respectively.[46] Therefore laparoscopy will be required among women with a normal HSG to identify a certain percentage of patients with tubal and peritoneal factors. The decision of when to proceed with laparoscopy following a normal HSG should be individualized based on the history, physical examination, and the remainder of the initial infertility evaluation.

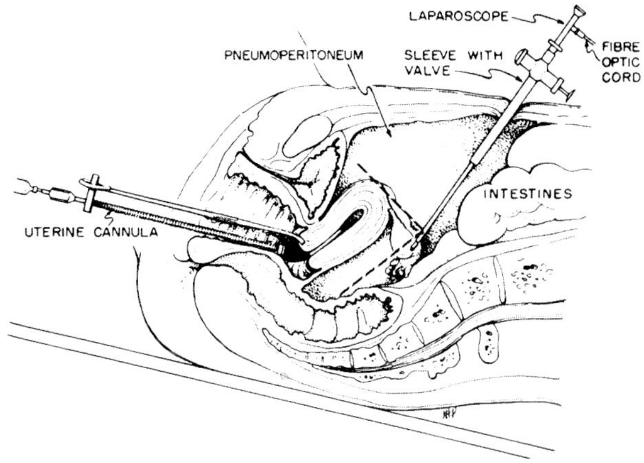

Fig.12-10. Schematic diagram of pelvis at laparoscopy. (From Cohn MR: *Laparoscopy, culdoscopy, and gynecography,* Philadelphia, 1970, WB Saunders.)

In contrast, whenever HSG suggests a tubal factor, laparoscopic confirmation is essential because of the relatively high incidence of false positives. The most common cause of a false-positive HSG is a cornual spasm. In an attempt to eliminate the complication of a cornual spasm, Hutchins studied 62 patients under general anesthesia.[103] This study revealed that 45 of 62 patients (73%) with proximal tubal occlusion on HSG had laparoscopic evidence of normal oviducts with evidence of tubal patency by methylene blue insufflation. Because of the high incidence of false cornual obstruction, two to three separate tubal studies should be considered before the diagnosis of proximal tubal obstruction is confirmed.

Opsahl et al recently reported a practical classification system for HSG based on 756 patients.[170] Hysterosalpingograms were classified as normal, abnormal (bilateral, distal tubal obstruction), or suspicious (all others). Moderate to severe pelvic disease was found at laparoscopy in 16.2% of normals, 53.9% of suspicious, and 81.7% of abnormals. These authors concluded abnormal hysterosalpingograms are highly predictive of severe pelvic disease and do not require diagnostic laparoscopy for counseling of treatment options. Among patients with suspicious hysterosalpingograms, the authors recommend confirmatory laparoscopy by a qualified operative pelviscopist. Although normal HSGs have a high negative predictive value, the authors recommend laparoscopy if nonsurgical treatment is unsuccessful.

The most common laparoscopic finding is post infective tubal disease.[46] This may include pelvic adhesions, phimotic fimbria, hydrosalpinges, or tubal obstruction. Significant pelvic adhesions may also be the result of previous abdominal surgery. Myomectomy, ruptured appendicitis, or any other cause of peritonitis may lead to pelvic adhesion formation. The second most common laparoscopic finding is endometriosis and the prevalence among women undergoing diagnostic laparoscopy for infertility has been reported at 5% to 25%. Laparoscopic visualization, biopsy, or both are required for the diagnosis of endometriosis since there are no specific screening tests. The subject of endometriosis was extensively reviewed in Chapter 11.

The American Fertility Society's classifications of adnexal adhesions, distal tubal occlusion, and endometriosis is based on laparoscopic findings and provides a rational foundation for therapy.[10,37] Recent advances in operative laparoscopy and laser technology have allowed for lysis of adhesions, fulguration of endometriosis, and tubal reconstruction at the time of diagnostic laparoscopy. The techniques of diagnostic and operative laparoscopy are further discussed in Chapter 25.

Future diagnostic procedures

Recent studies suggest a potential role for evaluating tubal patency with ultrasonography.[6] Tufekci et al compared transvaginal sonosalpingography with chromolaparoscopy in 42 patients.[225] Ten to forty mL of isotonic saline was injected into the uterine cavity through a semirigid Foley catheter. These authors demonstrated a 76% concordance rate by accurately revealing patency in 26 patients and bilateral nonpatency in three patients. The addition of pulsed wave and/or color Doppler may improve the predictive value of transvaginal sonosalpingography.[63,206]

Although HSG is an adequate screening procedure for assessing tubal patency, and laparoscopy can accurately confirm tubal patency and detect peritoneal factors, there is no routine procedure to evaluate the functional integrity of the fallopian tube. Although fallopian tube physiology remains poorly understood, the ciliated tubal epithelial cells are thought to be important for ovum and embryo transport. Salpingoscopy (falloposcopy) allows for the endoscopic evaluation of the endosalpinx and may help identify an abnormal mucosal pattern, intratubal adhesions, or both. The technique of salpingoscopy may allow for a better understanding of tubal physiology, which includes the mechanisms of bidirectional tubal motility. Salpingoscopy may be performed at the time of laparoscopy or laparotomy. Kerin et al reported a diagnostic classification system for tubal lumen disease based on falloposcopy.[117] They concluded that falloposcopy may be therapeutic by dislodging intraluminal debris and breaking down filmy adhesions in minimally diseased tubes. Shapiro et al reported 17 patients who underwent salpingoscopy at the time of laparoscopy or laparotomy and found a 23.5% discordance rate between the fimbrial appearance at surgery and the salpingoscopic findings.[196] Marconi et al similarly demonstrated abnormal endosalpingeal salpingoscopic findings in 37% of patients with a normal laparoscopy.[136] In the future, salpingoscopy may aid in the often difficult therapeutic decision between reconstructive tubal surgery and in vitro fertilization.

UTERINE FACTORS

Although uterine abnormalities are often associated with recurrent pregnancy loss, they are not generally considered a cause of infertility. The association between uterine factors and infertility remains unclear since the hormonal and immunologic prerequisites for normal implantation and early embryo development remain poorly understood. A large number of progesterone-dependent endometrial and decidual proteins have been characterized. These proteins may be important for the implantation of the embryo.[24]

The possible association of DES exposure and infertility may be partially the result of uterine factors and impaired implantation.[12] The relationship between DES and infertility remains controversial. Several investigators have reported an increased incidence of infertility in DES-exposed women.[26,27,93,116] In contrast, other investigators have reported no significant difference.[16,52] The conflicting results are likely related to confounding factors and inadequate control groups. Nevertheless, many DES-exposed women have associated abnormalities that are presumed to be the etiology of their infertility. DES exposure is not only associated with abnormal uterine contours but also with an increased incidence of tubal disease, endometriosis, and cervical factor.[54,208]

Uterine leiomyomas or myomas are often implicated as a cause for infertility, even though well-controlled epidemiologic and clinical studies are lacking. A review of the literature suggests that myomas alone are an infrequent cause of infertility.[36] The mechanisms by which myomas may cause infertility include mechanical obstruction of sperm transport and suboptimal implantation. Before myomectomy is considered, the other potential causes of infertility should be evaluated and treated. In patients undergoing myomectomy, the preoperative gestational size and location of the leiomyomas are important prognostic factors with regard to subsequent fertility.[36] In general, anatomic location is more important than myoma size.

Congenital uterine anomalies such as uterine didelphis and uterine septa are also much more commonly associated with midtrimester loss and early fetal wastage when compared with infertility (Fig. 12-11). Asherman's syndrome (intrauterine synechiae) is commonly associated with amenorrhea, menstrual irregularities, habitual abortion, and poor obstetric outcome. It also may be associated with infertility. Patients with severe intrauterine adhesions may have mechanical obstruction of sperm migration and an unfavorable endome trial environment for implantation.[189]

Although the significance of uterine factors may be difficult to determine, women at high risk for intrauterine pathology deserve further evaluation. HSG is considered an excellent screening test for uterine factors since false-negative diagnoses are uncommon. The diagnostic accuracy of HSG for the evaluation of uterine factors has been evaluated in many studies that compare HSG and hysteroscopy.[70,215,227] Although HSG should be considered

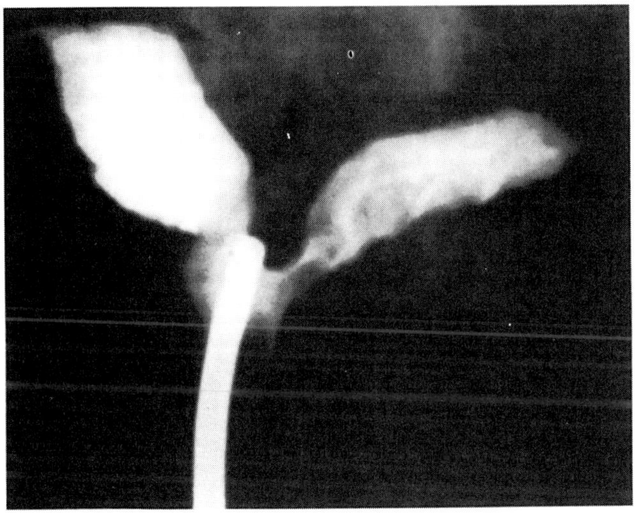

Fig. 12-11. Hysterosalpingogram demonstrating a congenital uterine anomaly. This may represent a bicornuate uterus or a uterine septum. Laparoscopic and hysteroscopic visualization of the external and internal uterine surface are required to distinguish these two entities.

the initial screening test, it often suggests subtle insignificant uterine factors. Hysteroscopy remains the method of evaluating the uterine cavity and is required to confirm any suspected diagnoses or the extent of any pathology. The techniques of diagnostic and operative hysteroscopy are extensively discussed in Chapter 25.

UNEXPLAINED INFERTILITY

Perhaps the most frustrated patients and the most frustrating to take care of are the couples with unexplained infertility. Moghissi and Wallach defined unexplained infertility as "any couple who has failed to establish a pregnancy despite an evaluation that uncovers no obvious reason for infertility or after correction of the factor(s) identified as responsible for the infertility."[154] The incidence of unexplained infertility appears to be decreasing, most likely as a result of improvements in the diagnostic evaluation, and it has been estimated to be approximately 15%.[48,218] Although unexplained infertility may represent the inability of the present diagnostic tests to identify a potential cause, alternatively it may represent a lack of understanding of some aspect of the reproductive process.

Coulam et al suggested that additional testing may reduce the incidence of unexplained infertility.[51] If the initial evaluation of BBT, semen analysis, PCT, HSG, and laparoscopy are all normal, additional testing should be considered. This may include an endometrial biopsy for luteal-phase defect, antisperm antibodies for immunologic infertility, a day-3 FSH level for incipient ovarian failure, and/or a sperm penetration assay to evaluate sperm function. If this additional evaluation fails to identify a particular etiology, empiric therapy should be considered.

MYCOPLASMA AND CHLAMYDIA

Despite a large body of literature, the role of subclinical genital tract infections in infertility remains enigmatic. In particular the role of *Mycoplasma* in infertility remains rather controversial. Although *Chlamydia* appears to be clearly associated with tubal-factor and male-factor infertility, its role in cervical-factor infertility remains unclear.

Isolation rates of *Mycoplasma (Ureaplasma urealyticum, Mycoplasma hominis)* vary depending on a number of socioeconomic factors and on the number of sexual partners. Whether there is a significant difference between fertile and infertile patient populations remains controversial since clinical studies have provided conflicting results.[64,80,140] Several studies suggest that there may be an increased incidence of *Ureaplasma urealyticum* in certain etiologic categories of infertility. For example, couples with the male factor and unexplained infertility appear to have an increased incidence of *Ureaplasma urealyticum*.[39,104] In the male, subclinical genital tract infections including those caused by *Mycoplasma* have been found to be associated with decreased sperm motility[75]; with adequate therapy there appears to be improvement.[212] Unfortunately, well-controlled, prospective studies of the subsequent pregnancy rates have yielded conflicting results.[89,97,223] Several other proposed mechanisms of *Mycoplasma*-related male infertility include the association of antisperm antibodies and abnormal egg penetration.[35,238] In comparison, there is insufficient evidence to support a primary role for *Mycoplasma* in tubal-factor or cervical-factor infertility. Several studies have demonstrated that *Ureaplasma urealyticum* does not alter the physiologic characteristics of cervical mucus or sperm penetration and viability.[104,179] In summary, critical analysis of epidemiologic studies fails to provide significant evidence that *Mycoplasma* is causally related to infertility. There is no role for routine *Mycoplasma* cultures or empiric treatment with doxycycline.

Unlike *Mycoplasma, Chlamydia trachomatis* has clearly been identified as an etiologic agent for infertility. *Chlamydia* has been shown to be a major pathogen in acute salpingitis and therefore has been associated with tubal-factor infertility. Several studies have shown that at least 20% of cases of acute salpingitis have been associated with chlamydial infection. However, whether patients previously exposed to *Chlamydia* are at risk for tubal-factor infertility remains controversial. Several studies suggest that serologic evidence of previous chlamydial infection is associated with an increased risk of asymptomatic tubal disease.[111,157] Minassian and Wu reported chlamydia antibody values by enzyme-linked assay (ELISA) that strongly correlated with salpingitis, tubal occlusion, and pelvic adhesion scores.[146]

Although leukocytospermia and acute chlamydial urethritis are associated with abnormal semen parameters, the importance of subclinical chlamydial infection in male-factor infertility remains controversial.[90] Similarly there is no evidence to suggest that previous or asymptomatic chlamydial infection is associated with cervical-factor infertility. These studies, however, are not readily available since asymptomatic *Chlamydia* cervicitis is rather uncommon in the infertility patient population. It is recommended that only patients with evidence of leukocytospermia, active cervicitis, or acute PID are cultured for *Chlamydia*, and if positive, antibiotic therapy is initiated.

SUMMARY

The investigation of the infertile couple requires a thorough and systematic approach. The initial evaluation should be explained to the couple in the context of the multiple causes of infertility. The basic evaluation should include a semen analysis, documentation of ovulation, assessment of tubal patency, and perhaps a PCT. If the initial evaluation is normal, diagnostic laparoscopy should be considered to exclude the possibility of pelvic adhesions and endometriosis. The results of the diagnostic tests should be reviewed with the couple. Ideally the evaluation should alter the probability of pregnancy and lead to effective therapy. In the majority of cases, the probable cause or causes for the infertility can be determined. If the initial evaluation does not reveal an explanation for the infertility, additional testing should be recommended. The role of the physician is to synthesize the clinical information and provide a choice of reasonable treatment options. Regular review sessions are essential to provide the couple with additional treatment options, emotional support, and a realistic prognosis for future fertility. The treatment of infertility will be discussed in the next chapter.

REFERENCES

1. Ainmelk Y et al: Primary infertility: correlation between sperm migration test and humoral immunity, *Int J Fertil* 27:52, 1982.
2. Aitken RJ: Diagnostic value of the zona-free hamster oocyte penetration test and sperm movement characteristics in oligospermia, *Int J Androl* 8:348, 1985.
3. Aitken RJ et al: A prospective study of the relationship between semen quality and fertility in cases of unexplained infertility, *J Androl* 5:297, 1984.
4. Alexander JA: Evaluation of male infertility with an in vitro cervical mucus penetration test, *Fertil Steril* 36:201, 1981.
5. Alexander NT, Anderson DJ: Immunology of semen, *Fertil Steril* 47:192, 1987.
6. Allahbadia GN: Fallopian tubes and ultrasonography: the Sion experience, *Fertil Steril* 58:901, 1992.
7. Alper MM, Garner PR: Premature ovarian failure: its relationship to autoimmune disease, *Obstet Gynecol* 66:27,1985.
8. Alper MA et al: Pregnancy rates after hysterosalpingography with oil and water-soluble contrast media, *Obstet Gynecol* 68:6, 1986.
9. Amelar RD, Dubin L, Schoenfeld C: Sperm motility, *Fertil Steril* 34:197, 1980.
10. American Fertility Society: The American Fertility Society classifications of adnexal adhesions, distal tubal occlusion, tubal occlusion secondary to tubal ligation, tubal pregnancies, müllerian anomalies, and intrauterine adhesions, *Fertil Steril* 49:944, 1988.
11. Asch RH: Laparoscopic recovery of sperm from peritoneal fluid in patients with negative or poor Sims-Huhner test, *Fertil Steril* 27:1111, 1976.
12. Ayvaliotis B, et al: Conception rates in couples where autoimmunity to sperm is detected, *Fertil Steril* 43:739, 1985.
13. Azziz R, Zacur HA: 21-Hydroxylase deficiency in female hyperandrogenism: screening and diagnosis, *J Clin Endocrinol Metab* 69:577, 1989.
14. Barbieri RL, Ryan KJ: Hyperandrogenism, insulin resistance, acanthosis nigricans: a common endocrinopathy with distinct pathophysiological features, *Am J Obstet Gynecol* 147:90, 1983.
15. Barbieri RL, Smith S, Ryan KJ: The role of hyperinsulinemia in the pathogenesis of ovarian hyperandrogenism, *Fertil Steril* 50:197, 1988.
16. Barnes et al: Fertility and outcome of pregnancy on women exposed in utero to diethylstilbestrol, *New Engl J Med* 302:609, 1980.
17. Barros C, Yanagimachi R: Induction of zona reaction in golden hamster eggs by cortical granule material, *Nature* 233:2368, 1971.
18. Bateman BG, Nunley WC Jr, Kitchin JD: Intravasation during hysterosalpingography using oil-base contrast media, *Fertil Steril* 34:439, 1980.
19. Batista MC et al: Midluteal phase endometrial biopsy does not accurately predict luteal function, *Fertil Steril* 59:294, 1993.
20. Battin DA et al: In vitro fertilization rates of male factor patients, *Fertil Steril* 41:42S, 1984.
21. Bauman JE: Basal body temperature: unreliable method of ovulation detection, *Fertil Steril* 36:729, 1981.
22. Bedford JM: Sperm capacitation and fertilization in mammals, *Biol Reprod* 2(suppl 2):128, 1970.
23. Bedford JM, Best MJ, Calvin H: Variations in the structural character and stability of nuclear chromatin in morphologically normal human spermatozoa, *J Reprod Fertil* 33:19, 1973.
24. Bell SC et al: Protein synthesis and secretion by the human endometrium during the menstrual cycle and the effect of progesterone in vitro, *J Reprod Fertil* 77:221, 1986.
25. Belsey MA et al: *Laboratory manual for examination of human semen and semen-cervical mucus interaction*, Geneva, 1980, World Health Organization.
26. Berger M, Alper M: Intractable primary infertility in women exposed to diethylstilbestrol in utero, *J Reprod Med* 31(4):231, 1986.
27. Bibbo M et al: Follow-up study of male and female offspring of DES-exposed mothers, *Obstet Gynecol* 49:1, 1977.
28. Blackwell JM, Zaneveld LJD: Effect of abstinence on sperm acrosin, hypoosmotic swelling, and other semen variables, *Fertil Steril* 58:798, 1992.
29. Bostofte E, Serup J, Rebbe H: Relation between sperm count and semen volume, and pregnancies obtained during a 20-year follow-up period, *Int J Androl* 5:267, 1982.
30. Bostofte E, Serup J, Rebbe H: Relation between number of immobile spermatozoa in pregnancies obtained during a 20-year follow-up period, *Andrologia* 16:136, 1984.
31. Bostofte E, Serup J, Rebbe H: The clinical value of morphological rating of human spermatozoa, *Int J Fertil* 30:31, 1985.
32. Bronson R, Cooper G, Rosenfeld D: Ability of antibody-bound human sperm to penetrate zona-free hamster ova in vitro, *Fertil Steril* 36:778, 1981.
33. Bronson R, Cooper G, Rosenfeld D: Sperm antibodies: their role in infertility, *Fertil Steril* 42:171, 1984.
34. Burkman LJ et al: The hemizona assay (HZA): development of a diagnostic test for the binding of human spermatozoa to the hemizona pellucida to predict fertilization potential, *Fertil Steril* 49:688, 1988.
35. Busolo F, Zanchetta R: The effect of *Mycoplasma hominis* and *Uureaplasma urealyticum* on hamster egg in vitro penetration by human spermatozoa, *Fertil Steril* 43:110, 1985.
36. Buttram BC, Reiter RC: Uterine leiomyomata: etiology, symptomatology, and management, *Fertil Steril* 36:433, 1981.
37. Buttram VC: Evolution of the revised American Fertility Society's classification of endometriosis, *Fertil Steril* 43:347, 1985.
38. Buxton CL, Herrman WL: Effect of thyroid hormone on menstrual disorders and sterility, *JAMA* 155:1035, 1954.
39. Cassell GH et al: Microbiologic study of infertile women at the time of diagnostic laparoscopy, *N Engl J Med* 308:502, 1983.

40. Chang RJ et al: Circulating levels of plasma adrenocorticotropin in polycystic ovary disease, *J Clin Endocrinol Metab* 54:1265, 1982.
41. Chiari H: zur Pathologischen Anatomie des Eileitercatarrhs, *Z Heilkunde* 8:457, 1887.
42. Chong AP, Walters CA, Weinrieb SA: The neglected laboratory test, *J Androl* 4:280, 1983.
43. Chopra IJ, Tulchinsky D: Status of estrogen-androgen balance in hyperthyroid men with Grave's disease, *J Clin Endocrinol Metab* 38:269, 1974.
44. Cohen J et al: In vitro fertilization: a treatment for male infertility, *Fertil Steril* 43:422, 1985.
45. Collins JA: Diagnostic assessment of the infertile female partner, *Curr Probl Obstet Gynecol Fertil* 2:27, 1988a.
46. Collins JA: Diagnostic assessment of the infertile female partner, *Curr Probl Obstet Gynecol Fertil* 11:27, 1988b.
47. Collins JA, Burrows EA, Willan AR: Occupation and the follow-up of infertile couples, *Fertil Steril* 60:477, 1993.
48. Collins JA, Crosignani PG: Unexplained infertility: a review of diagnosis, prognosis, treatment efficacy, and management, *Int J Gynecol Obstet* 39:267, 1992.
49. Collins JA et al: A proportional hazards analysis of the clinical characteristics of infertile couples, *Am J Obstet Gynecol* 148:527, 1984a.
50. Collins JA et al: The postcoital test as a predictor of pregnancy among 355 infertile couples, *Fertil Steril* 41:703, 1984b.
51. Coulam CB, Moore SB, O'Fallon W: Investigating unexplained infertility, *Am J Obstet Gynecol* 158:1374, 1988.
52. Cousins L et al: Reproductive outcome of women exposed to diethylstilbestrol in utero, *Obstet Gynecol* 56:70, 1980.
53. Cramer DW, Walker AN, Schiff I: Statistical methods in evaluating the outcome of infertility therapy, *Fertil Steril* 32:80, 1979.
54. Cramer DW et al: The relation of endometriosis to menstrual characteristics, smoking, and exercise, *JAMA* 255:1904, 1986.
55. Cramer DW et al: Association of endometriosis with maternal diethylstilbestrol (DES) exposure, *Fertil Steril* 65:185, 1986.
56. Cross NL et al: Two simple methods for detecting acrosome-reacted human sperm, *Gamete Res* 15:213, 1986.
57. Daly DC et al: Endometrial biopsy during treatment of luteal phase defects is predictive of therapeutic outcome, *Fertil Steril* 40:305, 1983.
58. Davajan V: Postcoital testing. In Mishell DR, Davajan V, editors: *Infertility, contraception, and reproductive endocrinology*, Oradell, NJ, 1985, Medical Economics.
59. Davajan V, Kunitake GM: Fractional in vivo and in vitro examination of postcoital cervical mucus in the human, *Fertil Steril* 20:197, 1969.
60. Davis OK et al: The incidence of luteal phase defect in normal fertile women, determined by serial endometrial biopsies, *Fertil Steril* 51:582, 1989.
61. Daya S, Ward S, Burrows E: Progesterone profiles in luteal phase deficient cycles and outcome of progesterone treatment in patients with recurrent spontaneous abortion, *Am J Obstet Gynecol* 158:255, 1988.
62. DeCherney AH et al: Increased pregnancy rate with oil soluble hysterosalpingography dye, *Fertil Steril* 33:407, 1980.
63. Deichert U et al: Transvaginal hysterosalpingo-contrast sonography for the assessment of tubal patency with gray scale imaging and additional use of pulsed wave Doppler, *Fertil Steril* 57:62-67, 1992.
64. DeLouvois J et al: Frequency of mycoplasma in fertile and infertile couples, *Lancet* 1:1073, 1974.
65. Derrick FC, Johnson J: Reexamination of normal sperm count, *Urologie* 3:99, 1974.
66. Dor J, Homburg R, Rabau E: An evaluation of etiologic factors and therapy in 665 infertile couples, *Fertil Steril* 28:718, 1977.
67. Downs KA, Gibson M: Basal body temperature graph and the luteal phase defect, *Fertil Steril* 40:466, 1983.
68. Elkind-Hirsch K et al: Evaluation of the Ovu-Stick urinary luteinizing hormone kit in normal and stimulated menstrual cycles, *Obstet Gynecol* 67:450, 1986.
69. El Minawi MF et al: Comparative evaluation of laparoscopy and hysterosalpingography in infertile patients, *Obstet Gynecol* 51:29, 1978.
70. Fayez JA, Mutie G, Schneider PJ: The diagnostic value of hysterosalpingography and hysteroscopy in infertility investigation, *Am J Obstet Gynecol* 156:558, 1987.
71. Fernando RS, Regas J, Betz G: Prediction of ovulation with the use of oral and vaginal electrical measurements during treatment with clomiphene citrate, *Fertil Steril* 47:409, 1987.
72. Filcori M, Butler JP, Crowley WF: Neuroendocrine regulation of the corpus luteum in the human: evidence for pulsatile progesterone secretion, *J Clin Invest* 73:1638, 1984.
73. Fishman J, Hellman L, Zumoff B: Influence of thyroid hormone on estrogen metabolism in man, *J Clin Endocrinol Metab* 22:389, 1962.
74. Fishman J et al: Effect of thyroid on hydroxylation of estrogen in man, *J Clin Endocrinol Metab* 25:365, 1965.
75. Fowlkes DM, Dooher GB, O'Leary WM: Evidence by scanning electronmicroscopy for an association between spermatozoa and T mycoplasmas in men of infertile marriage, *Fertil Steril* 26:1203, 1975.
76. Gabos P: A comparison of hysterosalpingography and endoscopy: an evaluation of tubal function in infertile women, *Fertil Steril* 27:238, 1976.
77. Garcia J, Jones GS, Wentz AC: The use of clomiphene citrate, *Fertil Steril* 28:707, 1977.
78. Gibbons RA, Mattner P: The chemical and physical characteristics of the cervical secretion and its role in reproductive physiology. In Sherman AI, editor: *Pathways to conception*, Springfield, Ill, 1971, Charles C Thomas.
79. Gillespie HW: The therapeutic aspect of hysterosalpingography, *Br J Radiol* 38:301, 1965.
80. Gnarpe H, Friberg J: *Mycoplasma* in human reproductive failure, *Am J Obstet Gynecol* 114:727, 1972.
81. Goodman SB, Rein MS, Hill JA: Hysterosalpingography contrast media and chromotubation dye inhibit peritoneal lymphocyte and macrophage function in vitro: a potential mechanism for fertility enhancement, *Fertil Steril* 59:1022, 1993.
82. Gordon GG et al: Effect of hyperthyroidism and hypothyroidism on the metabolism of testosterone and androstenedione in man, *J Clin Endocrinol Metab* 29:164, 1969.
83. Gorelick JI, Goldstein M: Loss of fertility in men with varicocele, *Fertil Steril* 59:613-616, 1993.
84. Graff G: Suppression of cervical mucus during clomiphene therapy, *Fertil Steril* 22:209, 1971.
85. Haas GG, Cines DB, Schreiber AD: Immunologic infertility: identification of patients with antisperm antibody, *N Engl J Med* 180:303, 1980.
86. Hall MG, Savage PE, Bromham DR: Prognostic value of the postcoital test: prospective study based on time-specific conception rates, *Br J Obstet Gynaecol* 89:299, 1982.
87. Halman LJ, Abbey A, Andrews FM: Why are couples satisfied with infertility treatment? *Fertil Steril* 59:1046, 1993.
88. Hargreave TB, Nillson S: Seminology. In Hargreave TB, editor: *Male infertility*, New York, 1983, Springer-Verlag.
89. Harrison RF et al: Doxycycline treatment in human infertility, *Lancet* 1:605, 1975.
90. Hellstrom WJG et al: Is there a role for *Chlamydia trachomatis* in genital *Mycoplasma* in male infertility? *Fertil Steril* 48:337, 1987.
91. Hendershot GE, Mosher WD, Pratt WF: Infertility and age: an unresolved issue, *Fam Plan Perspect* 14:287, 1982.
92. Hensleigh PA, Fainstat T: Corpus luteum dysfunction: serum progesterone levels in diagnosis and assessment of therapy for recurrent and threatened abortion, *Fertil Steril* 32:396, 1979.
93. Herbst AL et al: A comparison of pregnancy experience in DES-exposed and DES-unexposed daughters, *J Reprod Med* 24:62, 1980.

94. Hill JA, Anderson DJ: Immunological mechanisms of female infertility. In Johnson PM, editor: *Bailliere's clinical immunology and allergy: immunologic disease in pregnancy*, London, 1988, Bailliere Tindall.
95. Hill JA, Cohen J, Anderson DJ: The effects of lymphokines and monokines on human sperm fertilizing ability in the hamster egg penetration test, *Am J Obstet Gynecol* 160:1154, 1989.
96. Hill JA, Haimovici F, Anderson DJ: Effects of soluble products of activated lymphocytes and macrophages (lymphokines and monokines) on human sperm motion parameters, *Fertil Steril* 47:460, 1987.
97. Hinton RA et al: A double blind crossover study of the effect of doxycycline on *mycoplasma* infection and infertility, *Br J Obstet Gynaecol* 86:379, 1979.
98. Hirsch I et al: In vitro fertilization in couples with male factor infertility, *Fertil Steril* 45:659, 1986.
99. Hodges RE, Hamilton AG, Keetel WC: Pregnancy in myxedema, *Arch Intern Med* 90:863, 1952.
100. Hoff JD, Quigley ME, Yen SS: Hormonal dynamics at midcycle: a reevaluation, *J Clin Endocrinol Metab* 57:792, 1983.
101. Hoffman D, Lobo RA: The prevalence and significance of elevated DHEA-S levels in anovulatory women, *Fertil Steril* 39:404, 1983.
102. Horne HW et al: Subclinical endometrial inflammations and T mycoplasma, *Int J Fertil* 18:226, 1973.
103. Hutchins CJ: Laparoscopy and hysterosalpingography in the assessment of tubal patency, *Obstet Gynecol* 49:325, 1977.
104. Idriss WM, Patton WC, Taymor ML: On the etiologic role of *Ureaplasma urealyticum* (T mycoplasma) infection in infertility, *Fertil Steril* 30:293, 1978.
105. Isojima S, Li T, Ashitaka Y: Immunologic analysis of sperm-immobilizing factor found in sera of women with unexplained sterility, *Am J Obstet Gynecol* 101:677, 1968.
106. Jacobs HS: Prolactin and amenorrhea, *N Engl J Med* 295:954, 1976.
107. Jette NT, Glass RH: Prognostic value of the postcoital test, *Fertil Steril* 23:29, 1972.
108. Jeyendran RS et al: Development of an assay to assess the functional integrity of the human sperm membrane and its relationship to other semen characteristics, *J Reprod Fertil* 70:219, 1984.
109. Jones GES: The luteal phase defect, *Fertil Steril* 27:351, 1976.
110. Jones GES, Pourmand K: An evaluation of etiologic factors and therapy in 555 private patients with primary infertility, *Fertil Steril* 13:389, 1962.
111. Jones RB et al: Correlation between serum antichlamydial antibodies and tubal factor as a cause of infertility, *Fertil Steril* 38:553, 1982.
112. Karande VC et al: Are implantation and pregnancy outcome impaired in diethylstilbestrol-exposed women after in vitro fertilization and embryo transfer? *Fertil Steril* 54:287, 1990.
113. Karp LE et al: Sperm penetration assay: useful test in evaluation of male fertility, *Obstet Gynecol* 57:620, 1981.
114. Katz E: The luteinized unruptured follicle and other ovulatory disorders, *Fertil Steril* 50:839, 1988.
115. Kaufman F et al: Ovarian failure in galactosemia, *Lancet* 2:737, 1979.
116. Kaufman RH et al: Upper genital tract changes and infertility in diethylstilbestrol-exposed women, *Am J Obstet Gynecol* 154:1312, 1986.
116a. Kazer RR, Kessel B, Yen SSC: Circulating luteinizing hormone pulse frequency in women with polycystic ovary syndrome (PCO), *J Clin Endocrinol Metab* 65:233, 1987.
117. Kerin JF et al: Falloposcopic classification and treatment of fallopian tube lumen disease, *Fertil Steril* 57:731, 1992.
118. Krauss CM et al: Familial premature ovarian failure due to an interstitial deletion of the long arm of the X chromosome, *N Engl J Med* 317:125, 1987.
119. Kremer J: A simple sperm penetration test, *Int J Fertil* 10:209, 1965.
120. Kruger TF, Acosta AA, Simmons KF et al: Predictive value of abnormal sperm morphology in in vitro fertilization, *Fertil Steril* 49:112, 1988.
121. Kruger TF et al: Sperm morphologic features as a prognostic factor in in vitro fertilization, *Fertil Steril* 46:1118, 1986.
122. Li T-C et al: A comparison between two methods of chronological dating of human endometrial biopsies during the luteal phase, and their correlation with histologic dating, *Fertil Steril* 48:928, 1987.
123. Liu DY, Baker HWG: Tests of human sperm function and fertilization in vitro, *Fertil Steril* 58:465, 1992.
124. Liu DYet al: A human sperm-zona pellucida binding test using oocytes that failed to fertilize in vitro, *Fertil Steril* 50:782, 1988.
125. Lobo RA: The role of the adrenal in polycystic ovary syndrome, *Semin Reprod Endocrinol* 2:251, 1984.
126. Lobo RA: Polycystic ovary syndrome. In Mishell DR, Davajan V, editors: *Infertility, contraception and reproductive endocrinology*, Oradell, NJ, 1986, Medical Economics Books.
127. Lobo RA et al: Psychological stress and increases in urinary norepinephrine metabolites, platelet serotonin, and adrenal androgens in women with polycystic ovary syndrome, *Am J Obstet Gynecol* 145:496, 1983a.
128. Lobo RA et al: Elevated bioactive luteinizing hormone in women with the polycystic ovary syndrome, *Fertil Steril* 39:674, 1983b.
129. London SN, Haney AF, Weinberg JB: Diverse humoral and cell-mediated effects of antisperm antibodies on reproduction, *Fertil Steril* 41:907, 1984.
130. MacLeod J, Gold RZ: The male factor in fertility and infertility: II. Spermatozoan counts in 1000 men of known fertility and in 1000 cases of infertile marriages, *J Urol* 66:436, 1951a.
131. MacLeod J, Gold RZ: The male factor in fertility and infertility: III. Analysis of motile activity, *Fertil Steril* 2:187, 1951b.
132. Madgar I et al: Controlled trial of high spermatic vein ligation for varicocele in infertile men. 86th Annual meeting of the American Urological Association, Toronto, June 1991.
133. Mahadevan MM, Trounson AO: The influence of seminal characteristics on the success rate of human in vitro fertilization, *Fertil Steril* 42:400, 1984.
134. Mao C, Grimes DA: The sperm penetration assay: can it discriminate between fertile and infertile men? *Am J Obstet Gynecol* 159:279, 1988.
135. March CM: Update: luteal phase defects, *Endocr Fert Forum* 10(4):3, 1987.
136. Marconi G et al: Salpingoscopy: systematic use in diagnostic laparoscopy, *Fertil Steril* 57:742, 1992.
137. Mareck J, Hulka JF: Luteinized unruptured follicle syndrome: a subtle cause of infertility, *Fertil Steril* 29:270, 1978.
138. Margalioth EJ et al: Reduced fertilization ability of zona-free hamster ova by spermatozoa from male partners of normal infertile couples, *Arch Androl* 10:67, 1983.
139. Margalioth EJ et al: Correlation between the zona-free hamster egg sperm penetration assay and human in vitro fertilization, *Fertil Steril* 45:665, 1986.
140. Matthews CD et al: The frequency of genital mycoplasma infection in human fertility, *Fertil Steril* 26:988, 1975.
141. Maxson WS et al: Antiestrogenic effect of clomiphene citrate: correlation with serum estradiol concentrations, *Fertil Steril* 42:356, 1984.
142. McNatty KP, Sawers RS, McNeilly AS: A possible role for prolactin in control of steroid secretion by the human graafian follicle, *Nature* 250:653, 1973.
143. Meldrum DR. Female reproductive aging—ovarian and uterine factors, *Fertil Steril* 59:1-5, 1993.
144. Menge AC et al: The incidence and influence of antisperm antibodies in infertile human couples on sperm-cervical mucus interactions and subsequent fertility, *Fertil Steril* 38:439,1982.
145. Miller EG Jr, Kurzrok R: Biochemical studies of human semen, *Am J Obstet Gynecol* 24:19, 1932.

146. Minassian SS, Wu CH. Chlamydia antibody by enzyme-linked immunosorbent assay and associated severity of tubal factor infertility, *Fertil Steril* 58:1245, 1992.
147. Moghissi KS: Cyclic changes of cervical mucus in normal and progestin-treated women, *Fertil Steril* 17:663, 1966.
148. Moghissi KS: Accuracy of basal body temperature for ovulation detection, *Fertil Steril* 27:1415, 1976a.
149. Moghissi KS: Postcoital test: physiologic basis, technique, and interpretation, *Fertil Steril* 27:117, 1976b.
150. Moghissi KS: The cervix in infertility. In Hammond MG, Talbert LM, editors: *Infertility: A practical guide for the physician*, Oradell, NJ, 1985, Medical Economics.
151. Moghissi KS et al: Mechanism of sperm migration, *Fertil Steril* 15:15, 1964.
152. Moghissi KS, Sacco AJ, Borin K: Immunologic infertility. I. Cervical mucus antibodies and postcoital tests, *Am J Obstet Gynecol* 136:941, 1980.
153. Moghissi KS, Syner FN, Evans TN: A composite picture of the menstrual cycle, *Am J Obstet Gynecol* 114:405, 1972.
154. Moghissi KS, Wallach EE: Unexplained infertility, *Fertil Steril* 39:5, 1983.
155. Monroe SE et al: Prolactin-secreting pituitary adenomas. V. Increased gonadotropin responsivity in hyperprolactinemic women with pituitary adenomas, *J Clin Endocrinol Metab* 52:1171, 1981.
156. Montoro MN et al: Successful outcome of pregnancy in women with hypothyroidism, *Ann Intern Med* 94:31, 1984.
157. Moore DF, Foy HM, Daling JR: Increased frequency of serum antibodies to *Chlamydia trachomatis* in infertility due to distal tubal disease, *Lancet* 2:574, 1982.
158. Mortimer D: Objective analysis of sperm motility and kinematics. In Kell BA, Webster BW, editors: *Handbook of the laboratory:diagnosis and treatment of infertility*, Boca Raton, 1989, CRC Press.
159. Mosher W: Fertility and family planning in the United States: insights from the National Survey of Family Growth, *Fam Plan Perspect* 20:207, 1988.
160. Mosher WD: Infertility trends among U.S. couples: 1965-1976, *Fam Plan Perspect* 14:22, 1982.
161. Mosher WD: Reproductive impairments in the United States: 1965-1982, *Demography* 22:415, 1985.
162. Mosher WD, Pratt WF: Fecundity and infertility in the United States: 1965-1988. DHHS publication no. (PHS)91-1250. Hyattsville, Maryland: National Center for Health Statistics: Advance Data no. 192, 1990.
163. Mosher WD, Pratt WF: Fecundity and infertility in the United States: incidence and trends, *Fertil Steril* 56:192-193, 1991.
164. Nelson CMK, Bunge RG: Semen analysis: evidence for changing parameters of male fertility potential, *Fertil Steril* 25:503, 1974.
165. Neufeld M, MacLaren NK, Blizzard RM: Two types of autoimmune Addison's disease associated with different polyglandular autoimmune (PGA) syndromes, *Medicine* 60:355, 1981.
166. New MI et al: Genotyping steroid 21-hydroxylase deficiency: hormonal reference data, *J Clin Endocrinol Metab* 57:320, 1983.
167. Newill RG, Katz M: The basal body temperature chart in artificial insemination by donor pregnancy cycles, *Fertil Steril* 38:431, 1982.
168. Nikolaeva MA et al: Detection of antisperm antibodies on the surface of living spermatozoa using flow cytometry: preliminary study, *Fertil Steril* 59:639, 1993.
169. Noyes RW, Hertig A, Rock J: Dating the endometrial biopsy, *Fertil Steril* 1:3, 1950.
170. Opsahl MS, Miller B, Klein TA: The predictive value of hysterosalpingography for tubal and peritoneal infertility factors, *Fertil Steril* 60:444, 1993.
171. Palmer A: Ethiodol hysterosalpingography for the treatment of infertility, *Fertil Steril* 11:311, 1960.
172. Pearlstone AC, Fournet N, Gambone JC: Ovulation induction in women age 40 and older: the importance of basal follicle-stimulating hormone level and chronological age, *Fertil Steril* 58:674-679, 1992.
173. Phipps WR et al: The association between smoking and female infertility as influenced by cause of the infertility, *Fertil Steril* 48:377, 1987.
174. Phung TT, Byrd JR, McDonough PG: Etiologies and subsequent reproductive performance of 100 couples with recurrent abortion, *Fertil Steril* 132:389, 1979.
175. Pitaway DE et al: Prevention of acute pelvic inflammatory disease after hysterosalpingography: efficacy of doxycycline prophylaxis, *Am J Obstet Gynecol* 47:623, 1983.
176. Politch JA et al: Comparison of methods to enumerate white blood cells in semen, *Fertil Steril* 60:372, 1993.
177. Pryor JB: Seminal analysis, *Clin Obstet Gynecol* 8:571, 1981.
178. Radwanska E, Hammond J, Smith P: Single midluteal progesterone assay in the management of ovulatory infertility, *J Reprod Med* 26:85, 1981.
178a. Rebar R: Characterization of the inappropriate gonadotropin secretion in polycystic ovary syndrome, *J Clin Invest* 57:1320, 1976.
179. Rehewi MSE et al: *Ureaplasma urealyticum* (T mycoplasma) and seminal plasma in spermatozoa from infertile and fertile volunteers, *Eur J Obstet Gynecol Reprod Biol* 8:247, 1978.
180. Rice JB, London SN, Olive DL: Re-evaluation of hysterosalpingography in infertility investigation, *Obstet Gynecol* 67:718, 1986.
181. Richie WG: Ultrasound in the evaluation of normal and induced ovulation, *Fertil Steril* 43:167, 1985.
182. Rogers BJ et al: Sperm morphology assessment as an indicator of human fertilizing capacity, *J Androl* 4:119, 1983.
183. Rogers BJ et al: Analysis of human spermatozoal fertilizing ability using zona-free ova, *Fertil Steril* 32:664, 1979.
184. Rosenfeld DL, Seidman SM, Bronson RA et al: Unsuspected chronic pelvic inflammatory disease in the infertile female, *Fertil Steril* 39:44, 1983.
185. Ruder H et al: Effects of induced hyperthyroidism on steroid metabolism in man, *J Clin Endocrinol Metab* 33:382, 1971.
186. Rumke P: The origin of immunoglobulins in semen, *Clin Exp Immunol* 12:287, 1974.
187. Rumke P et al: Prognosis of fertility of men with sperm agglutinins in the serum, *Fertil Steril* 25:393, 1974.
188. Sauer MV et al: Effect of abstinence on sperm motility in normal men, *Am J Obstet Gynecol* 158: 604-607, 1988.
189. Schenker JG, Margalioth EJ: Intrauterine adhesions: an updated appraisal, *Fertil Steril* 37:593, 1982.
190. Schwartz D, Mayaux MJ: Female fecundity as a function of age: results of artificial insemination in 2193 nulliparous women with azoospermic husbands. Fed Des Sentres d'Etude et de Conservation du Sperme Humain, *N Engl J Med* 306:404, 1982.
191. Scott JZ et al: The cervical factor in infertility: diagnosis and treatment, *Fertil Steril* 28:1289, 1977.
192. Scott RT et al: Intercycle variability of day 3 follicle-stimulating hormone levels and its effect on stimulation quality in in vitro fertilization, *Fertil Steril* 54:297-302, 1990.
193. Scott RT et al: Evaluation of the impact of intraobserver variability on endometrial dating and the diagnosis of luteal phase defects, *Fertil Steril* 60:652, 1993.
194. Settlage DSF, Motoshima M, Treadway DR: Sperm transport from the external cervical os to the fallopian tubes in women: a time and quantitation study, *Fertil Steril* 24:655, 1973.
195. Shangold M, Berkley A, Gray J: Both midluteal serum progesterone levels and late luteal endometrial histology should be assessed in all infertile women, *Fertil Steril* 40:627, 1983.
196. Shapiro BS, Diamond MP, DeCherney AH: Salpingoscopy: an adjunctive technique for evaluation of the fallopian tube, *Fertil Steril* 49:1076, 1988.

197. Shoupe D et al: Correlation of endometrial maturation with four methods of estimating day of ovulation, *Obstet Gynecol* 73:88, 1989.
198. Shulman S et al: Immunologic consequences of vasectomy, *Contraception* 5:269, 1972.
199. Siegler AM: *Hysterosalpinography*, New York, 1974, Medcon Press.
200. Sims JM: *Uterine Surgery*, New York, 1866, William Woods .
201. Small DRJ et al: The interpretation of semen analysis among infertile couples, *Can Med Assoc J* 136:829, 1987.
202. Smith KD, Rodriguez-Rigau LJ, Steinberger E: Relation between indices of semen analysis and pregnancy rate in infertile couples, *Fertil Steril* 28:1314, 1977.
203. Soules MR et al: The corpus luteum: determinants of progesterone secretion in the normal menstrual cycle, *Obstet Gynecol* 71:659, 1988.
204. Soules MR, Spadoni LR: Oil vs. aqueous media for hysterosalpingography: a continuing debate based on many opinions and few facts, *Fertil Steril* 38:1, 1982.
205. Southern AL et al: The conversion of androgens to estrogens in hyperthyroidism, *J Clin Endoccrinol Metab* 38:207, 1974.
206. Stern J, Peters AJ, Coulam CB: Color Doppler ultrasonography assessment of tubal patency: a comparison study with traditional techniques, *Fertil Steril* 58:897, 1992.
207. Stern JE et al: Antisperm antibodies in women: variability in antibody levels in serum, mucus, and peritoneal fluid, *Fertil Steril* 58:950, 1992b.
208. Stillman RJ, Hershlag A: Pathology of infertility and adverse pregnancy outcome after in utero exposure to diethylsteilbestrol. In Gondos B, Riddick DA, editors: *Pathology of infertility*, New York, 1987, Theime-Stratton.
209. Stone SC: Peritoneal recovery of sperm in patients with infertility associated with inadequate cervical mucus, *Fertil Steril* 40:802, 1983.
210. Stumpf PG, March CM: Febrile morbidity following hysterosalpingography: identification of risk factors and recommendations for prophylaxis, *Fertil Steril* 33:487, 1980.
211. Surrey E, Meldrum DR: Pregnancy rates after hysterosalpingography with oil and water-soluble contrast media, *Obstet Gynecol* 69:830, 1987.
212. Swenson CE, Toth A, O'Leary WM: *Ureaplasma urealyticum* in human infertility: the effect of antibiotic therapy on semen quality, *Fertil Steril* 31:660, 1979.
213. Talbot P, Chacon RS: A triple stain technique for evaluating normal acrosome reaction of human sperm, *J Exp Zool* 215:201, 1981.
214. Tanabe K et al: Levels of inhibin activity and steroids in human follicular fluid from normal women and women with polycystic ovarian disease, *J Clin Endocrinol Metab* 57:24, 1983.
215. Taylor PJ: Correlations in infertility, symptomatology, hysterosalpingography, laparoscopy, and hysteroscopy, *J Reprod Med* 8:339, 1977.
216. Taymor ML, Overstreet JW: Some thoughts on the postcoital test, *Fertil Steril* 50:702, 1988.
217. Tejada RI et al: A test for the practical evaluation of male fertility by acridine orange (AO) fluorescence, *Fertil Steril* 42:87, 1984.
218. Templeton AA, Penny GC: The incidence, characteristics, and prognosis of patients whose infertility is unexplained, *Fertil Steril* 37:175, 1982.
219. Terquem A, Dadoune JP: Aniline blue staining of human spermatozoa chromatin: evaluation of nuclear maturation. In Andre J, editor: *The sperm cell,* London, 1983, Martinus Nijhoff.
220. Tietze C: Reproductive span and rate of reproduction among Hutterite women, *Fertil Steril* 8:89, 1957.
221. Tomlinson MJ et al: Round cells and sperm fertilizing capacity: the presence of immature germ cells but not seminal leukocytes are associated with reduced success of in vitro fertilization, *Fertil Steril* 58:1257, 1992.
222. Toner JP, Philput CB, Jones GS: Basal follicle-stimulating hormone level is a better predictor of in vitro fertilization performance than age, *Fertil Steril* 55:784-91, 1991.
223. Toth A et al: Subsequent pregnancies among 161 couples treated for T mycoplasma genital tract infection, *N Engl J Med* 308:505, 1983.
224. Treadway DT et al: Significance of timing of postcoital evaluation of cervical mucus, *Am J Obstet Gynecol* 121:387, 1975.
225. Tufekci EC et al: Evaluation of tubal patency by transvaginal sonosalpingography, *Fertil Steril* 57:336, 1992.
226. Uehling DT: Secretory IgA in seminal fluid, *Fertil Steril* 22:769, 1971.
227. Valle RF: Hysteroscopy and the evaluation of female infertility, *Am J Obstet Gynecol* 137:425, 1980.
228. Van der Ven HH et al: Correlation between human sperm swelling in hypoosmotic medium (hypoosmotic swelling test) and in vitro fertilization, *J Androl* 7:140, 1986.
229. Van der Ven HH et al:Leucospermia and the fertilizing capacity of spermatozoa, *Eur J Obstet Gynecol Reprod Biol* 4:49, 1987.
230. Vermesh M et al: Monitoring techniques to predict and detect ovulation, *Fertil Steril* 47:259, 1987.
231. Weir W, Cicchinelli AL: Prognosis for the infertile couple, *Fertil Steril* 15:625, 1964.
232. Wentz AC: Endometrial biopsy in the evaluation of infertility, *Fertil Steril* 33:121, 1980.
233. Westrom L: Effect of acute pelvic inflammatory disease on fertility, *Am J Obstet Gynecol* 146:153, 1983.
234. Wheeless CR, Katayama KP: Laparoscopy and tubal sterilization. In Mattingly RF, Thompson JD, editors: *Operative gynecology*, ed 6, Philadelphia, 1985, JB Lippincott.
235. White PC, New MI, Dupont B: Congenital adrenal hyperplasia, *N Engl J Med* 316:1519, 1987.
236. Wickings EJ et al: Heterologous ovum penetration test and seminal parameters in fertile and infertile men, *J Androl* 4:261, 1983.
237. Wilcox LS, Mosher WD: Use of infertility services in the United States, *Obstet Gynecol* 82:122, 1993.
238. Witkin SS, Toth A: Relationship between genital tract infections, sperm antibodies in seminal fluid, and infertility, *Fertil Steril* 40:805, 1983.
239. Wolf D et al: Acrosomal status evaluation in normal ejaculated sperm with monoclonal antibodies, *Biol Reprod* 32:1157, 1985.
240. Wolf H, Anderson DJ: Immunohistologic characterization and quantitation of leukocyte subpopulations in human semen, *Fertil Steril* 49:497, 1988.
241. World Health Organization: The influence of varicocele on parameters of fertility in a large group of men presenting to infertility clinics, *Fertil Steril* 57:1289-1293, 1992.
242. Yen SSC: The polycystic ovary syndrome, *Clin Endocrinol* 12:177, 1980.
243. Yen SSC: Chronic anovulation caused by peripheral endocrine disorders. In Yen SSC, Jaffe RB, editors: *Reproductive endocrinology*, Philadelphia, 1986, WB Saunders .
243a. Waldstreicher et al: Hyperfunction of the hypothalmic-pituitary axis in women with polycystic ovarian disease: indirect evidence for partial gonadotroph desensitization, *J Clin Endocrinol Metab* 66:165, 1988.
243b. Yen SSC, Vela P, Rankin J: Inappropriate secretion of follicle-stimulating hormone and luteinizing hormone in polycystic ovarian disease, *J Clin Endocrinol Metab* 30:435, 1970.
244. Young PE et al: Reconstructive surgery for infertility at the Boston Hospital for Women, *Am J Obstet Gynecol* 108:1092, 1970.

Chapter 13

INFERTILITY TREATMENT

R. Ian Hardy
Janis Fox

Despite the perception that the treatment of infertility is a relative newcomer to the field of gynecology, gamete and embryo investigations have intrigued the basic scientist and practitioner for the past century. The first successful transfer of embryos from one rabbit species to another was described in the nineteenth century.[96] In the ensuing one hundred years, numerous investigators have studied the complexities associated with the conception of life. The clinician today is able to reap the clinical benefits of these studies but is also obliged to consider the ethical questions that accompany these new technologies. This chapter will familiarize the reader with current techniques used in the treatment of infertility. The clinician's approach to infertility treatment must be based on an appropriate evaluation of the infertile couple and an understanding of the indication for and efficacy of specific treatments.

TREATMENT OF MALE-FACTOR INFERTILITY

It is estimated that a male factor contributes to infertility in at least 40% of infertile couples. In many cases the couple with male-factor infertility will initially seek advice from the gynecologist. Although a urology referral is often indicated, it is incumbent upon the gynecologist to have a basic understanding of available treatments for male-factor infertility.

Varicocelectomy

Varicoceles are present in 15% of the normal population and in approximately 40% of men presenting with infertility. Subclinical varicoceles are those that are detectable with Doppler ultrasound examination in patients with an otherwise negative physical examination. Varicocelectomies involve the high ligation of the internal spermatic vein above the internal inguinal ring. There is a long-standing controversy over the value of varicocelectomy in infertile males because the improvement in semen parameters following the procedure has not been shown to consistently improve pregnancy rates. Following varicocelectomy, an increase in testicular volume in addition to an improvement in semen quality has been observed.[33,75] Most studies demonstrate an improvement in both sperm motility and morphology. Steckel et al studied the relationship between varicocele size and response to surgery. Preoperatively, men with large varicoceles had lower sperm counts and motility that improved to a greater degree postoperatively.

Some long-term follow-up studies after varicocelectomy have shown no difference in pregnancy rates. Pregnancies have even been demonstrated to occur earlier in couples with the nonoperated male patient.[189] Others, however, have reported improved conception rates following varicocelectomy.[165] The current recommendations of the American Fertility Society (AFS) are that varicocelectomy is indicated when one of the following conditions is met: (1) the couple has documented infertility; (2) the couple consists of a normal or potentially fertile female partner, but the male has one or more abnormal semen parameters; and (3) a varicocele is present on physical examination. According to the AFS, repair is contraindicated when semen parameters are normal or when a thorough evaluation of the female partner has not been completed.

Clomiphene citrate

The use of clomiphene citrate (CC) has been advocated to improve fertility in oligospermic men.[182] The efficacy of this therapy is questionable. A controlled comparison between CC and placebo over a twelve-month period demonstrated significantly higher levels of serum luteinizing hormone (LH), follicle stimulating hormone (FSH), and testosterone (T) in the CC group. Clomiphene treatment also resulted in increased LH, FSH, and T responses to gonadotropin-releasing hormone (GnRH). However, there were no reported differences between treatment with placebo or CC in sperm penetration assays or semen parameters.[210] Furthermore, Shanis et al have reported a significant deterioration of sperm morphology in patients treated with CC for greater than 4 months.[201] Finally a multicenter, randomized, double-blind study demonstrated no difference in cumulative life-table pregnancy rates between CC and placebo-treated male infertility patients.[238] These studies suggest that CC has no place in the treatment of male infertility.

GnRH pump

Pulsatile GnRH therapy has been utilized in infertile males with hypogonadotrophic hypogonadism. Crowley and Whitcomb reported successful GnRH pump (25 to 600 ng/kg/120 minutes) induction of normal gonadotropin and testosterone secretion in 51 male patients with isolated gonadotropin deficiency. Spermatogenesis was induced successfully in 34 of the 51 men, and eight of nine patients seeking fertility achieved pregnancies following treatment. Seventy-five percent of the pregnancies occurred with sperm counts less than 15 million/mL, which highlighted the fertility potential of this group of patients despite the fact that many demonstrated subnormal semen parameters after GnRH treatment. Case reports of successful pulsatile GnRH therapy (5 mcg/90 minutes) have been described in men with Kallman's syndrome[25] or panhypopituitarism who failed human menopausal gonadotropin therapy.[227] A less clear indication for GnRH therapy is in the male with idiopathic oligozoospermia and a selective elevation of FSH with normal LH and testosterone levels. Men with selective elevation of FSH levels have demonstrated decreased LH pulse frequency.[79] Pulsatile GnRH is effective in decreasing serum FSH levels, but it is unclear whether spermatogenesis and fertility are improved.[15,148]

Treatment of antisperm antibodies

Antisperm antibodies have been found in about 8% of men with infertility and in 60% to 80% of men following vasectomy. Antisperm antibodies can also be found in female serum and cervical mucus. The role of antisperm antibodies in preventing fertilization is controversial. Immunoglobulins directed to antigens on the head of sperm may cause head-to-head agglutination and impaired zona pellucida binding. Antigens on the sperm tail may result in decreased motility and tail-to-tail agglutination. There is no correlation between the titer of antisperm antibodies and their capacity to influence sperm function—it is the nature of the target antigens which is of significance rather than the antibody concentration.[9]

Some clinicians question the value of measuring antisperm antibodies because of the limited efficacy of current treatment.[10] Proposed treatments have included the following: (1) condom use in an attempt to reduce antigenic stimuli[72]; (2) glucocorticoid therapy in both men and women to reduce circulating antibodies[11]; (3) sperm processing in an attempt to dissociate the antibodies with washing[82]; (4) intrauterine insemination[145]; and (5) in vitro fertilization that limits the exposure of sperm to antibodies within human serum. Only the latter option has proved to be effective and then only for female serum antisperm antibodies. Follow-up studies have not demonstrated any benefit after condom use, which was conceptually difficult to prescribe for the couple seeking fertility. Glucocorticoid treatment cannot be recommended given its lack of effectiveness and potential side effects including aseptic hip necrosis. The high affinity of antisperm antibodies for sperm surface antigens makes current sperm washing techniques ineffective. Finally, intrauterine insemination may actually increase the risk of developing systemic antisperm antibodies.[74]

Gamete micromanipulation

Micromanipulation of gametes provides hope for couples who do not qualify for in vitro fertilization due to profoundly abnormal semen parameters, or for couples who have repeatedly failed to achieve fertilization in their IVF attempts. Patients with normal semen but defective sperm-zona pellucida binding and penetration may also benefit from micromanipulation.[16] Several techniques have been described including (1) partial zona dissection (PZD) to facilitate sperm penetration,[42] (2) subzonal sperm injection (SUZI) (also referred to as microinsemination sperm transfer [MIST]),[166] and (3) intracytoplasmic sperm injection (ICSI) that involves the microinjection of a single spermatozoon into the ooplasm of metaphase II oocytes.[175] Nonmotile and perhaps even nonviable spermatozoa may be used with ICSI.[123] Fig. 13-1 summarizes the microinsemination techniques. Despite the numerous pregnancies reported after micromanipulation-assisted fertilization, the overall delivery rates for PZD and SUZI are in the range of 1% to 5%.[69] However, recent reports from one center with experience in ICSI describe a

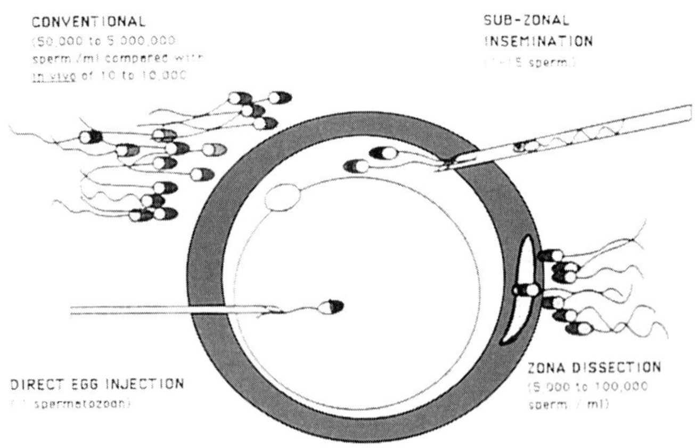

Fig. 13-1. Diagrammatic representation of different micromanipulation insemination techniques. (From Tucker MJ et al: Treatment of male infertility and idiopathic failure to fertilize in vitro with under zona insemination and direct egg injection, *Am J Obstet Gynecol* 169 (13):324, 1993.)

fertilization rate of 61% and a clinical pregnancy rate of 31% per treatment cycle.[228] If these results are successfully duplicated by other centers, ICSI will likely become the preferred form of assisted fertilization for couples with severe, male-factor infertility.

Vasectomy reversal

Approximately 3% of patients undergoing vasectomies request reversal of the procedure. Pregnancy rates after vasectomy reversal vary among different reporting surgeons. In a poll of urologists the average patency and pregnancy rates following vasovasotomy were 73% and 47% respectively; patency and pregnancy rates following vaseopididymostomy were 45% and 18%, respectively.[63] Not all patients have normal semen parameters postoperatively. Under optimal conditions in patients with consistently normal postoperative semen analyses, nearly two thirds can expect to achieve pregnancy.[202] The interval between vasectomy and its reversal correlates inversely with pregnancy rates.

Microsurgical aspirations of sperm from the epididymis is indicated in male patients with failed vasoepididymostomies, congenital absence of the vas, or cystic fibrosis.[146] The low number of sperm aspirated with this technique requires that it be used in conjunction with assisted reproduction technology (ART) procedures.

Artificial insemination

One of the oldest treatments of infertility still in current use is artificial insemination. There is a long history of anecdotal and uncontrolled studies claiming increased success rates with artificial insemination of the husband's semen (AIH). Despite its long history of use, AIH has never been proved to be more effective than intercourse except when significant abnormalities prevent deposition of sperm in close proximity to the uterus and cervix, (e.g., severe hypospadias, retrograde ejaculation, or impotence).[104,243] AIH has not been shown to be effective in couples with poor postcoital tests.[76]

It is important to distinguish AIH from intrauterine insemination (IUI) that involves the direct intrauterine placement of approximately 0.3 cc of processed or washed semen using a designated catheter. Processing of sperm permits capacitation and increases the percentage of motile sperm to be transferred into the uterus. Four commonly used techniques for sperm preparation include the following: (1) simple dilution and washing; (2) sperm migration (swim-up or swim-down), either direct from liquefied semen as a suspension of washed spermatozoa or from a washed sperm pellet; (3) selective washing procedures (Percoll or Nycodenz density gradients); and (4) adherence methods for the elimination of debris and dead spermatozoa (glass wool, glass beads, and Sephadex columns).[157] Direct swim-up from semen remains the simplest way to obtain populations of highly motile spermatozoa. At Brigham and Women's Hospital, Percoll gradients are generally done for both intrauterine inseminations and in vitro fertilization semen preparation.

Experimental semen enhancement procedures are being tried in some centers. Pentoxifylline, a phosphodiesterase inhibitor that maintains high intracellular cAMP, has been used to enhance sperm motility and fertilization.[240] The techniques of flow cytometric DNA analysis and flow sorting have been successfully used to separate X and Y chromosome-bearing sperm populations for couples concerned about transmission of X-linked disease. The DNA content of human X-chromosome sperm is greater than Y-chromosome sperm by 2.8%, permitting selection based on DNA content. Recent reports utilizing DNA flow cytometry were capable of accurate sex selection in 82% of attempts.[115,116]

Proper timing of inseminations is crucial to optimize pregnancy rates. Several methods of ovulation detection are available (and are discussed later in this chapter). Some investigators have proposed that the increased pregnancy rates associated with IUIs on two consecutive days can be explained by the inaccurate timing of single inseminations.[206] A significant decrease in semen volume, sperm concentration, and sperm motility has been demonstrated on the second day of consecutive inseminations.[103] Theoretically, with the more precise and quantitative blood LH measurement, a single IUI should be sufficient. Patients using urine LH detection may benefit from two consecutive-day IUIs.

Fallopian tube sperm perfusion (FSP) has been proposed as an alternative to IUI.[122] FSP is a combination of superovulation with intrauterine and intrafallopian tube insemination that uses a sperm suspension of 4 mL volume. Although one might predict that this large volume of injected sperm would flush the oocytes from the fallopian tubes, initial studies with human menopausal gonadotropins (hMG/FSP) report a pregnancy rate of 29% per cycle and comparative studies show it to be more successful than IUI.[121]

Direct intraperitoneal insemination (DIPI), also known as in vivo transperitoneal fertilization (IVTPF), has been advocated as a first approach to infertility treatment in couples with male subfertility.[131] The technique involves injection of processed spermatozoa through the posterior vaginal fornix into the pouch of Douglas using a 19-gauge butterfly needle. It is of historic interest that the original trials with DIPI were intended as a noninvasive, inexpensive, and in vivo approach to fertilization and embryo transfer. Embryos were collected by repuncturing the pouch of Douglas 48 to 72 hours following DIPI and transferred to the uterus. When a patient conceived following a failed embryo retrieval, it became apparent that DIPI alone, without embryo retrieval and transfer, was a reasonable first approach in patients with male-factor or unexplained infertility. The largest study of the DIPI technique reports a clinical pregnancy rate of 9% per patient and 7% per cycle.[131] Intrafollicular insemination for male-factor infertility has also been reported.[242]

Donor sperm insemination

More than thirty thousand babies are conceived by donor insemination each year in the United States.[26] This is

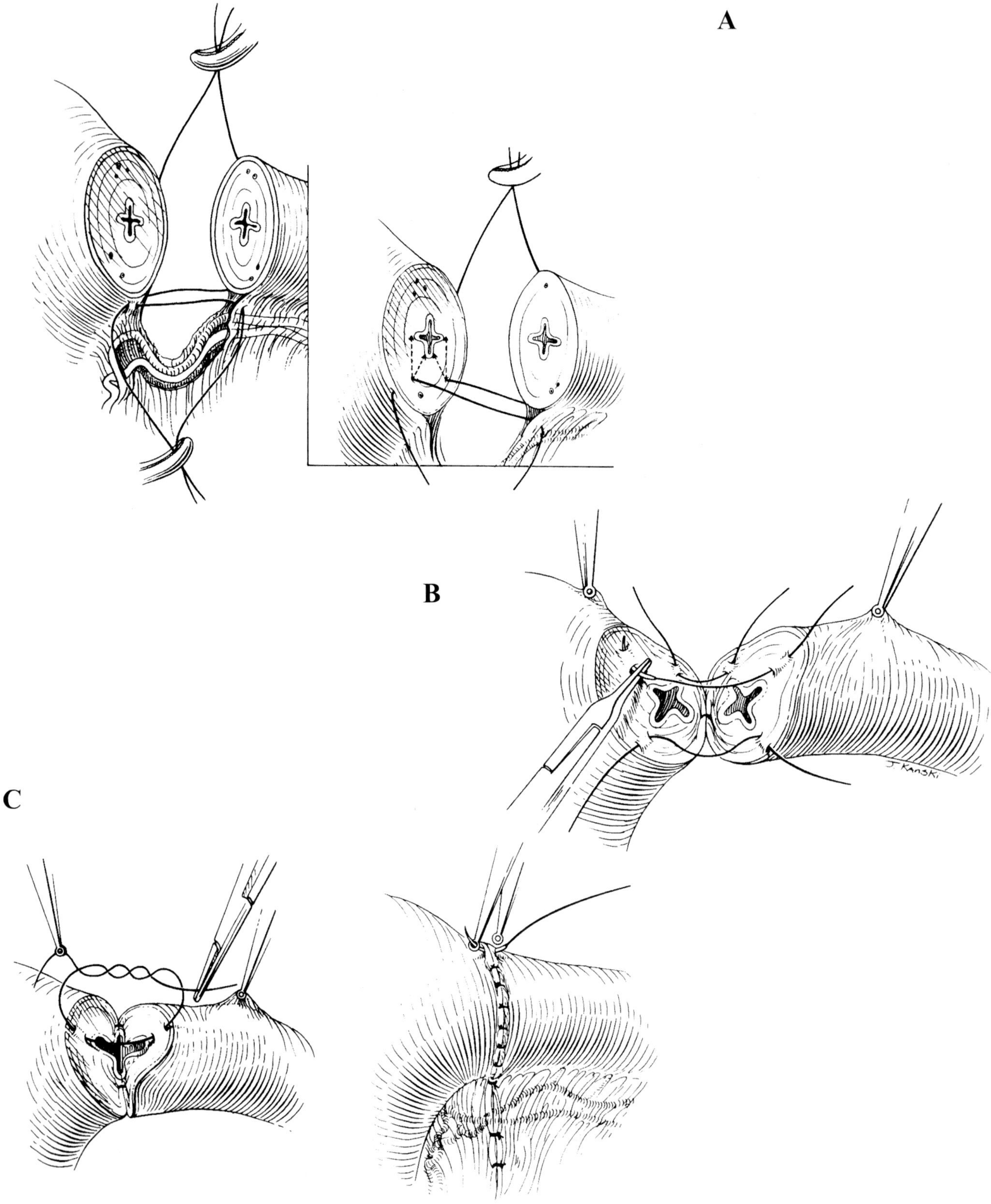

Fig. 13-2. Tubal ligation reversal technique. **A,** After preparing patent proximal and distal tubal segments, stay sutures are placed to align the tubal lumina. **B,** Four 8-0 sutures are placed under microscopic visualization within the tubal muscularis. **C,** The sutures are instrument tied with a surgeon's knot and if distal flow is demonstrated with chromotubation, the serosal layer is reapproximated. (From Hurt RB, editor: *Atlas of female infertility surgery,* ed 2, St. Louis, 1992, Mosby Year Book.)

the only available treatment for azoospermic males with spermatogenic defects and may also be utilized by many couples with severe male-factor infertility who do not wish to pursue IVF with micromanipulation. Prior to initiating donor inseminations, it is important to evaluate the male partner to rule out possible chromosomal or anatomical defects (Chapter 12). Although cycle fecundity is greater with fresh donor sperm,[214] the Food and Drug Administration (FDA), Centers for Disease Control (CDC), and the American Fertility Society (AFS) currently recommend the use of frozen donor sperm in order to prevent human immunodeficiency virus (HIV) transmission. The current method for using frozen semen involves quarantining the specimen from an HIV-negative donor for 60 to 180 days and releasing the specimen only after a follow-up HIV antibody titre is also negative.

Donor insemination raises many complex questions for the couple. The recognition that secrecy raises difficult social, psychologic, and ethical questions despite practical and emotional appeal is a major unresolved issue in the practice of donor insemination.[128,161] The availability of "yes" donor sperm allows for disclosure of the donor's identity at some future date should the couple or offspring so choose.

With isolated male-factor infertility, *donor* inseminations should be continued for at least six cycles before considering assisted reproductive technologies. Intrauterine insemination (IUI) of cryopreserved sperm appears to increase cycle fecundity by 18.3% versus 3.9% when compared to intracervical insemination (ICI).[110] In one study of 2998 treatment cycles with cryopreserved semen, the affects of age, gravidity, and male infertility status on cumulative conception rates after donor insemination were investigated. The cumulative conception rates after 3, 6, and 12 cycles of treatment were 21%, 40%, and 62% respectively for patients < 30 years of age compared with 17%, 26%, and 44% for those aged ≥ 30 years.[204] In vitro fertilization (IVF) has been shown to be useful in patients who have not conceived following six donor insemination cycles.[194]

TREATMENT OF TUBAL/PERITONEAL DISEASE

Tubal ligation reversal

With the advent of ART, surgery is no longer the only option for patients who wish to conceive following tubal ligation. In carefully selected patients, however, surgery may offer a significantly higher success rate than in vitro fertilization–embryo transfer (IVF-ET). In order to properly counsel the patient, the gynecologist should be aware of the pregnancy rates associated with both options. If the predicted success rate of tubal reanastomosis is felt to be lower than that obtainable through ART, the patient may be better served with the latter technology. However, in many cases tubal ligation reversal (Fig. 13-2) can result in excellent pregnancy rates that exceed those obtained through IVF.

Prognosis for success with sterilization reversal depends on several factors, including postoperative tubal length, method of sterilization, site of ligation, fimbrial status, and technique of reanastomosis. In one study, tubal patency rate was 91% after tubal reanastomosis. In this same study, however, overall successful pregnancy rate (PR) was only 35%. Patients with one tube greater than 7 cm in length postoperatively had a delivery rate of 75% compared with 16% for those with shorter tubes. No pregnancy occurred when the final tubal length after anastomosis was less than 4 cm.[29] The most reversible procedure is Falope ring placement (83% PR) and the least reversible is fimbriectomy (29% PR).[97] Following reversal of cautery sterilization, the estimated cumulative probability of pregnancy at 6, 12, 24, and 36 months following surgery was 22.7%, 37.8%, 52.4%, and 57.9%, respectively.[195] Isthmo-isthmic anastomoses have the best prognosis for normal pregnancy, whereas ampullary anastomoses are at a higher risk of ectopic pregnancies. Another study showed that when a distal segment of the anastomosis included part of the isthmic tube, an 80% delivery rate resulted. It was also found that all ectopic pregnancies occurred when the distal segment consisted only of the ampulla. The risk of ectopic pregnancy in this setting was 23%.[108]

Treatment of endometriosis-associated infertility

Endometriosis affects one in 15 women of reproductive age and is present in approximately 25% of infertile women.[120] Endometriosis is discussed at length in Chapter 11. Focusing here on endometriosis and infertility treatment, the gynecologist should be aware that no convincing evidence is present to suggest that stage I or II endometriosis causes infertility, nor have any controlled clinical trials demonstrated that treatment of early stage endometriosis outside the setting of ART improves fertility.[66,170]

No difference in conception rates has been demonstrated when comparing danazol versus surgical therapy in patients with stage III endometriosis. Mechanical factors associated with stage IV endometriosis may contribute to infertility. Retrospective comparisons of expectant management versus surgical therapy in these patients have demonstrated higher conception rates after surgical intervention.[171]

In IVF-ET patients with endometriosis, "ultralong" (at least 60 days) suppression with GnRH agonist prior to ovarian stimulation has been compared with standard midluteal phase suppression. In one study of 33 patients with varying stages of endometriosis, the clinical pregnancy rate per transfer was superior in the ultralong protocol (67% versus 27%).[162] Similar results were reported with the ultralong protocol in stage I or II endometriosis patients undergoing gamete intrafallopian transfer (GIFT).[191]

Although there exists an enormous volume of literature regarding treatment of endometriosis, no prospective, randomized study exists to adequately demonstrate if any of the available treatments significantly improves pregnancy rates. This literature must therefore be interpreted cautiously. The need for well-designed, prospective, randomized, controlled studies is clear.

Adhesions and adhesion prevention

Although pregnancy may occur in infertile women with periadnexal adhesions, treatment with salpingoovariolysis has been associated with higher pregnancy rates.[223] In one study of patients with filmy tubal adhesions and fimbrial phimosis, 63% of patients achieved pregnancy following microsurgical fimbrioplasty. Of those who conceived, the surgery-to-conception interval was 1 year for 62% of patients and 2 years in 35% of patients.[178] If a hydrosalpinx re-forms at any point after reparative surgery, a second surgical procedure is usually less successful. In a Bourn-Hall study of 58 second salpingostomies, four (8%) achieved term deliveries and nine (18%) resulted in ectopic pregnancies.[32] IVF-ET is therefore the preferred treatment in this group of patients.

Numerous surgical adjuvants including hydrocortisone,[216] dexamethasone and promethazine,[101] nonsteroidal anti-inflammatory drugs,[205] heparin,[113] and dextrose 70 (Hyskon),[7] have been proposed to reduce adhesion formation. Barrier materials including Interceed (TC7, Ethicon) and Gore-Tex have also been introduced in an attempt to diminish adhesion formation on raw tissue surfaces.[6,143] Most of these interventions have fallen into disfavor after randomized studies demonstrated their ineffectiveness.[51] A recent randomized study comparing Ringer's lactate, Interceed, and Gore-Tex found Ringer's lactate to be superior to Gore-Tex in reducing postoperative adhesions and Interceed to be ineffective.[174]

Currently, the most effective technique to reduce adhesion formation is adherence to meticulous surgical technique, including careful hemostasis, prevention of tissue desiccation and ischemia, and use of nonreactive suture materials. In addition, pelviscopic procedures are felt to reduce adhesion formation when compared with similar procedures performed by laparotomy.[139]

Corrective procedures for proximal tubal obstruction

In 1849 Smith reported recanalization of proximally obstructed fallopian tubes using a whale bone sound.[192] Improved flexible catheter technology has resulted in the more recent transcervical approach to proximal tubal obstruction. Numerous catheters, guidewires, balloon-tipped catheters, uterine and tubal probes have been recently promoted. Transcervical cannulation may be approached hysteroscopically,[167] fluoroscopically,[187] sonographically,[136] or with falloposcopy.[126] Although the physician's approach is dependent on equipment familiarity and availability, the hysteroscopic/laparoscopic approach provides the distinct advantage of evaluating distal tubal pathology. Only 10% to 20% of patients with tubal-factor infertility have isolated proximal occlusion. At Brigham & Women's Hospital, a cornual cannulation set (Cook Ob/Gyn #KNCS-553555) is used through the operative hysteroscope port.[167] A 0.46-mm, Teflon-coated, stainless steel wire is advanced to the intramural portion of the fallopian tube. The flexibility of the guide wire is enhanced by increasing the length of the wire exiting a 5.0 French catheter tip. Advancement through the uterotubal junction may be facilitated by displacing or straightening the fallopian tube under laparoscopic guidance. A coaxial 3.0 French radiopaque catheter is then positioned over the guide wire. The guide wire is removed and indigo carmine is injected to evaluate patency. Intraoperative fluoroscopy may also be used in conjunction with the hysteroscopic approach.

With proximal tubal cannulation, successful catheterization is achieved in 80% to 90% of patients with pregnancy rates within the first 6 to 12 months ranging between 23% and 39%.[192] Ectopic pregnancies occur in 5% to 13% of patients. Patients are encouraged to attempt pregnancy soon after successful catheterization as patency at 6-month follow-up ranges is between 35% and 82% (Table 13-1). The benefit of unilateral tubal recanalization is unknown.

Microsurgical reconstruction of the proximal oviduct in tubes with limited distal disease is associated with a live birth rate of 53% within 3 years.[180] However, in patients with postinflammatory occlusion of both the proximal and distal oviduct, the conception rate at 2.5 years has been reported to be 12% with no subsequent live births, which strongly supports the use of IVF in these patients.[181]

Table 13-1. Results of selective tubal catheterization, tubal recanalization rates, pregnancy rates (PR), ectopic pregnancy (EP) rates, and 6-month patency rates in patients with proximal tubal occlusion

Authors	No. of patients	Successful unilateral recanalizations	Early uterine PR	EP rate	Estimated 6-month patency
Thurmond and Rosch[219]	100	86	39	6	75
Platia and Krudy[187]	21	76	38	13	75
Confino et al[43]	77	92	35	5	82
Capitanio et al[37]	108	81	23	0	35
Lisse and Syndow[136]	41	84	31	0	57

(From Risquez F, Confino E: Transcervical tubal cannulation, past, present, and future, *Fertil Steril* 60:211, 1993.)

TREATMENT OF ANOVULATORY INFERTILITY

Ovulatory dysfunction is present in approximately 15% to 25% of all couples coming for an infertility evaluation. When there is no other problem, this is one of the most gratifying groups of patients to treat. This section reviews the indications for various ovulation induction agents including CC, hMG, FSH, bromocriptine, and the GnRH pump.

Success with ovulation induction is strongly dependent upon appropriate patient selection.[140] Patients with anovulation presenting for ovulation induction may be classified into one of three groups, based on the World Health Organization (WHO) classification system.

Group I patients are hypogonadotropic and hypoestrogenic. These patients demonstrate evidence of a low estrogen milieu on physical examination (atrophic vaginal mucosa, poor or absent cervical mucus). Serum gonadotropins may be low or low-normal. Progesterone withdrawal does not induce menstrual bleeding, and an endometrial biopsy is atrophic or proliferative. Although some feel a trial of CC is indicated in this group due to its low cost and low risk, the treatment of choice is usually hMG plus human chorionic gonadotropin (hCG).

Group II patients are normogonadotropic and normoestrogenic. This is the largest group of anovulatory (or oligoovulatory) patients. These women have evidence of endogenous estrogen activity. Also, physical examination may reveal evidence of excess androgen production as well. The cervical mucus is profuse. Endometrial biopsy may reveal a benign hyperplasia or maybe even atypical changes. LH may be elevated or normal. FSH is usually normal. There is withdrawal bleeding in response to progesterone. CC initiation of ovulation is the treatment of choice in this group of anovulatory women.

Group III patients are hypergonadotropic and hypoestrogenic. This group of amenorrheic women may or may not give a history of hot flushes or vasomotor complaints. They are distinguished from group I women by their elevated serum gonadotropins. This group suffers from ovarian failure or premature menopause. This diagnosis is generally considered a contraindication to CC therapy and to ovulation induction in general. These women are best treated with ovum donation, which will be discussed in greater detail later in this chapter.

Clomiphene citrate

CC has revolutionized the practice of reproductive endocrinology and has become the mainstay of ovulation induction therapy. CC was first synthesized in 1956 and was introduced for clinical trials in 1960. FDA approval was granted in 1967. The chemical structure of CC is that of an ethylene (C=C) core, which has been substituted with 3 phenyl rings and a chloride anion. One of the phenyl rings has been further modified by the addition of an amino-alkoxy side chain. In the United States it is provided as a racemic mixture of the trans- and cis-isomers. Clomid is made up of 38% zuclomiphene, which is felt by most to be the active form. A zuclomiphene dosage of 10 mg available abroad is roughly equivalent to 50 mg of Clomid.

Clomiphene citrate is a nonsteroid that is chemically related to stilbestrol and tamoxifen. It is orally administered and rapidly absorbed, with a half-life of about 5 days. Metabolites have been detected as long as 6 weeks after initial consumption. It is metabolized primarily by the liver.[4]

Experimental and clinical evidence suggests that CC acts at multiple target sites. Clomiphene has weak estrogenic and strong antiestrogenic effects. It possesses no known progestational, corticotrophic, androgenic, or antiandrogenic properties. Most researchers feel that the ability of CC to initiate ovulation is primarily due to its ability to be recognized by and interact with estrogen receptors at the level of the hypothalamus. Here its effects are mainly antiestrogenic. A central perception of a hypoestrogenic state ensues and results in an increase in GnRH pulse frequency (not amplitude).[125] The pituitary effects of clomiphene appear to be estrogenic and mainly sensitize the gonadotrope to the action of GnRH. Also there may be a direct stimulatory effect on the pituitary. The ovarian effects also appear to be estrogenic. The mechanism is not well documented, but there may be a direct effect on the ovary or a synergistic effect with pituitary gonadotropins. The peripheral effects on the uterus, cervix, and vagina are antiestrogenic.[3] Despite the increase in peripheral estradiol levels, the quantity and quality of cervical mucus decreases in women taking CC. Approximately 15% to 20% of women on CC therapy develop significant dysmucorrhea. CC has also been observed to decrease the percentage of cornification of vaginal epithelial cell smears and to cause endometrial atrophy.

The current FDA approved CC dosage consists of 50 to 150 mg per day for a maximum of 5 days each cycle. Therapy traditionally begins on day 5 of a spontaneous or progesterone-induced bleed, and continues through day 9; however, studies suggest that therapy can be initiated on cycle days 2 through 5 without any significant change in outcome.[239] Over 50% of patients who ovulate will do so at the 50 mg dosage. An additional 24% will ovulate on a CC dose of 100 mg daily. Despite the FDA guidelines, 26% of patients who eventually ovulated on CC did so on ≥ 150 mg/day,[81] whereas 11.8% ovulated on 200 to 250 mg/day. Therefore despite the FDA recommendations, it is probably worthwhile to pursue these high doses prior to initiating hMG therapy.

In general, if ovulation does not occur at the initial dose of CC, the dose should be increased by 50 mg per day per cycle until ovulation occurs, at which point the minimal effective dose should be maintained for 4 to 6 cycles. More than 90% of clomid-related conceptions will occur within this time frame.

In ovulatory CC cycles, ovulation usually occurs 5 to 10 days after the last dose of CC. Patients can be instructed to have intercourse every other day for one week starting 5 days after the last dose. If more precise prediction of ovulation is necessary or desirable, commercially available urinary dipsticks that identify the LH surge, rapid blood LH measurements, or serial pelvic ultrasonography can be utilized. Since there is no benefit in continuing a patient on the same dosage of CC if ovulation is not achieved, every effort should be made to document ovulation on the first cycle and in any subsequent cycle in which the dosage has been changed. A midluteal-phase serum progesterone level can help to confirm ovulation. A late-luteal phase endometrial biopsy may also be performed to rule out a luteal phase defect resulting from clomiphene's direct antiestrogenic effects on the endometrium. A luteal phase defect can be treated by raising the CC dose or supplementing the luteal phase with progesterone or hCG.

Once the minimal dose to achieve ovulation has been determined, a postcoital test should be performed. Approximately 15% to 20% of women will develop dysmucorrhea secondary to the antiestrogenic effects of CC.[232] If a patient falls into this group, timed intrauterine insemination may be considered. Supplemental follicular phase estrogen has also been tried but does not seem to improve pregnancy rates.[188]

In summary, once a treatment plan has been initiated, patients should be monitored by accurately confirming ovulation and carefully assessing the luteal phase. If the patient has failed to ovulate, the dosage should be increased by 50 mg/cycle/day. If the cervical mucus or the luteal phase are deemed inadequate, adjuvant measures need to be employed.

CC failures fall into two categories: (1) conception failures (i.e., the failure to achieve conception despite successful induction of ovulation); and (2) ovulation failures (i.e., the failure to achieve ovulation despite maximal CC therapy). Conception failures are generally felt to be secondary to luteal phase deficiency, dysmucorrhea, luteinized unruptured follicle syndrome, or coexisting infertility factors such as male-factor or tuboperitoneal disease.[83,84,118]

Ovulatory failure may be overcome by several alternate treatment plans. For example, intramuscular administration of exogenous human chorionic gonadotropin (hCG) (5000 to 10,000 IU) can be used to trigger ovulation. Good candidates for this regimen demonstrate an initial ovarian response to CC as indicated by rising serum estradiol values and/or sonographic evidence of follicular development. The timing of hCG administration can be determined empirically (5 to 7 days after the last CC dose) or by the use of ultrasound monitoring when mean follicular diameter exceeds at least 18 to 20 mm.[68,168] It has also been clearly demonstrated that extending the duration of therapy can be effective in producing an ovulatory cycle where a shorter course at the same dose had not been effective.[2,61]

The combination of CC and dexamethasone may be beneficial to women who have elevated levels of dehydroepiandrosterone sulfate (DHEAS) and who have failed to ovulate on the standard clomiphene treatment plan. In this situation it is generally recommended that the standard treatment plan be utilized first and that corticosteroids be tried only in the face of an ovulatory failure. The recommended dexamethasone dosage is 0.5 mg qhs beginning two weeks prior to menses and taken throughout the CC cycle. The addition of dexamethasone has been demonstrated to improve ovulation rates and lower the dose of CC required to achieve ovulation in women with baseline DHEAS levels > 2.0 to 2.5 µg/mL.[138]

Side effects of CC are relatively infrequent and rarely interfere with treatment. The occurrence and severity of these side effects do not tend to correlate well with the dosage. In order of decreasing frequency, the more common side effects are ovarian enlargement (15%), vasomotor flushes (11%), abdominal discomfort (7.4%), breast tenderness (2.1%), nausea and vomiting (2.1%), nervousness/insomnia (1.9%), and visual symptoms (1.6%).[4] Although mild ovarian enlargement and cyst formation are relatively common occurrences, massive enlargement or full-blown hyperstimulation syndrome is rare and generally only seen if supplemental hCG is used.

One notable risk associated with CC therapy is the increased frequency of multiple gestation. Due to the increased GnRH pulse frequency, recruitment of more than one follicle is not uncommon. Ultrasonographic studies show a 35% to 60% incidence of multiple follicular recruitment in clomiphene treated cycles as compared to a 5% to 10% incidence in spontaneous cycles.[193] Most reviewers cite an incidence of 8% to 10% multiple gestations in CC pregnancies, with less than 1% being of a high order (triplets or more). The spontaneous incidence of twinning is about 1%, so CC appears to increase the likelihood of twinning sevenfold. Post-CC conceptions are not at a significantly greater risk for spontaneous abortion (26.5%) than would be expected from the "infertile" population (22.3%), and a 2.4% incidence of post-CC birth defects is not significantly different than commonly quoted rates for the population at large (2.7%).[5,8] Physicians should be fully aware of the following contraindications to CC use: ovarian cysts, pregnancy, liver disease, visual symptoms, and undiagnosed abnormal uterine bleeding.

Bromocriptine

First-line therapy for ovulation induction in the hyperprolactinemic patient is bromocriptine, not CC. In fact these patients are notoriously resistant to ovulation induction with CC. This may be due to specific effects of prolactin (PRL) or increased dopamine levels on the hypothalamic-pituitary axis that reduce GnRH secretion. These patients have a blunted response or no LH response to estradiol, which suggests an abnormal positive feedback mechanism. It has also been proposed that prolactin has an inhibitory effect at the ovarian level. With bromocriptine therapy, restoration of menses occurs in 90% of hyperprolactinemic women within 6 to 8 weeks.

Elevated PRL levels interfere with the normal function of the menstrual cycle by suppressing pulsatile secretion of

GnRH. Bromocriptine is a dopamine agonist that directly inhibits the pituitary secretion of PRL and thus removes the block to FSH and LH release.

Pregnancy rates of 80% are achieved in patients with amenorrhea, galactorrhea, and hyperprolactinemia with no increase in multiple gestation rates, congenital abnormalities or miscarriages, and no risk of hyperstimulation.

In order to minimize side effects (nausea, diarrhea, dizziness, headache, fatigue), bromocriptine dosing should be gradually increased from 1.25 mg qhs for one week to 1.25 mg bid and if tolerated, up to the usual dose of 2.5 mg bid.[211] If side effects are persistent, bromocriptine can be taken intravaginally.[127]

Response is usually rapid. If ovulation is not seen within 2 months of normalizing PRL levels, CC can be added to the regimen in the usual fashion.[98] The use of bromocriptine in anovulatory, normoprolactinemia patients is controversial and its effectiveness has not been established by controlled studies.[55,173,215]

Human menopausal gonadotropin therapy

The most appropriate candidates for hMG therapy are WHO group I patients with pituitary failure. Patients with hypothalamic amenorrhea may also be good candidates but are probably more safely and easily treated with the GnRH pump. hMG is also used for anovulatory infertility patients who fail to ovulate on CC or who fail to conceive after 4 to 6 ovulatory cycles with clomiphene.

Human menopausal gonadotropin contains 75 u of FSH and 75 u of LH. It is inactive orally and must be given by intramuscular injections. It is expensive (approximately $50/amp) and treatment may cost as much as $2000/cycle for the drug alone. Because of its expense and the greater complication rate associated with its use, patients should have an extremely thorough evaluation. Many reproductive endocrinologists recommend performing a laparoscopy prior to initiating hMG therapy. In addition, patients must be given proper instruction regarding the administration of hMG and careful counseling regarding the risks. The financial, emotional, and time commitment on the part of the couple is enormous.

Access to daily estradiol measurements and daily vaginal ultrasound examinations is necessary in order to adequately monitor patients on hMG. A variable dosage method, of administration is the treatment of choice. Using this method the dosage is individually adjusted and clinical decisions are made based on a patient's response to the drug as measured by her serum estradiol levels and the degree of follicular development.[50,142] A commonly employed regimen at Brigham and Women's Hospital is to begin with 2 ampules (150 u) of hMG on cycle days 4 to 7. Estradiol (E2) is measured on the morning of day 8. If < 150 pg/mL, the dose is increased to 3 ampules. If > 150 pg/mL, daily ultrasound examinations are begun and the patient is continued on 2 amps as long as the E2 level rises appropriately each day. Human chorionic gonadotropin (hCG; 5000 u) is given in order to trigger ovulation once a lead follicle is between 15 to 20 mm mean diameter and serum E2 is between 600 to 1200 pg/mL. The patient is advised to have intercourse on the day of the hCG injection and for the next 2 days. Alternatively an IUI is performed 24 and 48 hours following the hCG injection.

To avoid the risks of hyperstimulation and high-order multiple gestation, it is recommended that hCG may be withheld if serum E2 is > 2000 pg/mL, or there are > 4 mature follicles, or if there are > 2 mature and > 5 intermediate (10 to 14 mm) follicles.[28] The average number of cycles required to achieve a pregnancy is three. The ovulation rate is > 90%, and the pregnancy rate/cycle is approximately 25% for patients with hypothalamic amenorrhea. Cumulative pregnancy rates of 70% can be achieved in this group of patients. The spontaneous abortion rate is approximately 25%, and there is no increase in congenital anomalies.

The multiple gestation rate is approximately 20% (15% twins, 5% high-order multiple gestations).[60] Although multifetal pregnancy reduction is available for patients with high-order multiple gestations, this is a very difficult option for an infertile couple to entertain; every effort should be made to avoid this situation through careful monitoring of the cycle.[27]

Uncontrolled ovarian hyperstimulation results in a massive luteinization of follicles. Careful monitoring with ultrasonography and serum E2 can help reduce the incidence of this potentially life-threatening complication by providing the physician the opportunity to withhold hCG in high-risk cases. If hCG is not given, hyperstimulation is unlikely to occur. Hyperstimulation is a purely iatrogenic disease. In mild cases the syndrome includes ovarian enlargement, abdominal distention, and weight gain. In severe cases a critical condition develops with ascites, pleural effusions, electrolyte imbalance, intravascular volume depletion, oliguria, hemoconcentration, and possible venous or arterial thromboses.[77] The relationship between estrogen levels and ovarian hyperstimulation is not a perfect one. Hyperstimulation has been found with relatively low estrogen levels, and high estrogen is not necessarily followed by hyperstimulation. There does appear to be some correlation between the number of intermediate (i.e., 10 to 14 mm) follicles and the development of ovarian hyperstimulation syndrome, although this too is not a perfect relationship.[164] Using multiple discriminant analysis to predict risk factors for ovarian hyperstimulation in IVF-ET patients, Delvigne reported that the best predictors were the slope of log-estradiol increment, hMG dosage, number of oocytes retrieved, and pre-hMG LH/FSH ratios.[53] With carefully monitored cycles, the incidence of significant ovarian hyperstimulation is generally about 1%. hMG therapy is most appropriately managed in the setting of a reproductive endocrinologist's office that is equipped to provide the extensive patient teaching and cycle monitoring that are necessary.

Pulsatile GnRH therapy

Women with hypothalamic amenorrhea (WHO group I) are the classic candidates for pulsatile GnRH therapy. They must have an intact pituitary gland capable of responding to pulsatile GnRH for the therapy to be successful. Diagnostic workup should confirm low gonadotropins, normal values for TSH, PRL, DHEAS, and TEST, and negative values for β–hCG and radiologic studies (CT or MRI) to rule out CNS defect.

By using the GnRH pump in properly selected patients, the patients' endogenous gonadotropins are stimulated, and the risk of multiple pregnancy and hyperstimulation is greatly reduced compared to hMG/hCG treatment, and therefore less monitoring is required. Pumps can be rented and home IV services are now available for line maintenance, which considerably minimize the demands on the physician and office staff.[135]

GnRH may be given subcutaneously, which is simpler but less reliable and incurs a higher total dose and higher total cost, or intravenously, which entails an increased risk of superficial thrombosis and phlebitis. The latter is generally more reliable and requires a shorter, less expensive course of treatment.[114] A 90-minute pulse interval is generally sufficient. Recommended dose per pulse depends upon route of administration (5 to 20 μg for SC, or 2.5 to 5 μg/pulse for IV). Ovulation usually occurs by day 14 of the treatment, but the range extends from 10 to 22 days, so urinary LH monitoring can be helpful. Use of hCG to trigger ovulation is not necessary; patients will have a spontaneous LH surge. Luteal phase support is necessary since patients do not produce endogenous LH without the pump. This can be accomplished by continuing the GnRH pump for 2 weeks postovulation or by administration of hCG (2500 units q3d × 4 doses).

Multiple pregnancy rates approximate those of CC (approximately 7% to 10%, mainly twins). There is no increase in the miscarriage rate or in congenital anomalies.[100] Ovulation rates of 80% to 95% are reported, with pregnancy rates of 30% to 35% and a cumulative pregnancy rate of 90% in hypothalamic amenorrhea.[198] The pump has been tried with less success in polycystic ovary (PCO) patients after suppressing their gonadotropins with long-acting GnRH agonists.

FSH therapy

Purified FSH urofollitropin is derived from hMG that is passed through anti-LH columns. Anti-hCG antibodies cause absorption of LH, eluting out purified FSH extracts (immunochromatography). One ampule of Metrodin contains 75 IU of FSH and > 1 IU of LH.

There are no randomized studies demonstrating superiority of purified FSH over hMG. Purified FSH must be administered in a regimen similar to that of hMG, and the problems and results of therapy are also similar to those of hMG therapy.[40] Utilizing recombinant DNA technology, recombinant human FSH (rFSH, Org 32489) has been successfully used for ovarian stimulation with resulting pregnancies.[56,58]

Fertility drugs and risk of ovarian cancer

The possibility that fertility drugs may increase a woman's risk for ovarian cancer was raised by a recent report of the Collaborative Ovarian Cancer Group (COCG) that investigated reproductive characteristics and exogenous hormone use in relation to ovarian cancer risk.[236] The report concluded that "at most, a small fraction of the excess ovarian cancer risk among nulliparous women is due to infertility, and that any increased risk associated with infertility may be due to the use of fertility drugs." The paper provides no information about reasons for infertility, the specific fertility drugs used, the dosage, or the number of cycles utilized. Only three of the 12 study analyses contained data about the use of fertility drugs and the risk of ovarian cancer. Only 34 women with ovarian cancer were compared to 23 women without the disease; 12 of the 34 women had used fertility drugs while only 1 of the 23 control women had used a fertility drug. The drugs were given before the 1970s, when gonadotropins were not available for infertility treatment in the United States.[17]

In summary, because of the methodologic shortcomings of the study, it is difficult to draw accurate conclusions. Furthermore, even if there is an increased risk, this would need to be balanced against the benefit of achieving a birth (known to reduce one's risk for ovarian cancer).

The American Fertility Society suggests that women receiving ovulation-inducing agents be informed of the known and possible risks of this therapy[236] but feels that the Whittemore study does not support the hypothesis of an increased risk of ovarian cancer in users of fertility drugs.

The need for a properly designed and well-controlled prospective study is clear. No doubt one will be performed in response to the provocative studies that have been published. Hopefully the results will clarify this controversial issue for physicians and patients.

TREATMENT OF UTERINE FACTOR INFERTILITY

Myomectomy

Leiomyomata, commonly known as fibroids, are the most common solid pelvic tumors in women. It is estimated that 20% to 25% of all reproductive-age women have fibroids. It has been suggested that uterine myomas and infertility are related.[231] Myoma-induced interference with embryo implantation has been proposed and results from endometrial thinning and atrophy,[52] inflammation,[109] or vascular alterations.[71] However, the benefit of myomectomy in these patients has not been clearly established.[183] Many infertility patients undergoing myomectomy have multiple problems contributing to their infertility, which make it difficult to evaluate the relative value of myomectomy alone.

In patients with fibroids but otherwise unexplained infertility, Buttram and Reiter suggest that only fibroids 3 cm or larger, those submucus in locale, or those obstructive to the ostia be considered for removal.[35] Tulandi et al evaluated adhesion formation and reproductive outcome in patients undergoing myomectomy and second-look laparoscopy.[224] They concluded that myomectomy incisions on the posterior uterine wall are associated with quantitatively more and qualitatively worse adnexal adhesions than those on the fundus and anterior wall. Removal of fibroids to prevent an anticipated growth of existing tumors during ovulation induction, estrogen replacement therapy, or pregnancy is not warranted. Despite the general impression of fibroid growth during pregnancy, this is true in only a minority of cases.[159] In those patients with fibroid growth during pregnancy, growth occurs more frequently during the first trimester with subsequent decreased growth rate in the second and third trimesters.[132]

Hysteroscopy

Endoscopic visualization of the uterine cavity was described as early as 1869.[176] More recent advances in optics and resecting instruments have permitted the use of hysteroscopy for both diagnosis and for operative treatment (Chapter 25).

In the patient receiving infertility treatment, it is inappropriate to initiate any form of therapy without defining the uterine cavity. Properly performed hysterosalpingography (HSG) is as accurate as hysteroscopy in the diagnosis of normal or abnormal uterine cavities. However, the nature of the intrauterine filling defect is more accurately revealed by hysteroscopy.[65] HSG or hysteroscopy alone cannot accurately differentiate between bicornuate and septate uteri and therefore in the patient with this differential, based on her HSG, hysteroscopy should be used in conjunction with laparoscopy. MRI may also be used to accurately diagnose uterine anomalies.[106,237]

Operative hysteroscopy is the surgical method of choice in the patient with intrauterine adhesions, submucus fibroids, endometrial polyps, or an intrauterine septum. The procedure is usually performed during the follicular phase to optimize visualization. The preoperative use of progestins to induce endometrial atrophy is rarely indicated. If necessary, dilute vasopressin (20 units in 50 mL of saline) can be injected in the cervical stroma to reduce bleeding and medium intravasation. The vasospastic effect usually lasts approximately 20 to 30 minutes.

The reproductive outcome following hysteroscopic adhesiolysis is dependent on the severity of adhesions. Reported live-birth rates following resection of dense adhesions are approximately 25% to 50%.[144,225] The relatively low pregnancy rate may reflect proximal tubal involvement in these patients.

Hysteroscopic resection of submucus fibroids is performed with a resectoscope loop, taking care to make the cutting strokes away from the fundus towards the cervix. The lowest effective cutting/coagulating current should be utilized to avoid charring and potential adhesion formation. Although the procedure is more commonly performed for symptomatic hypermenorrhea than for infertility, it is reasonable to restore the uterine cavity to normalcy before embarking on assisted reproductive techniques. Reported live-birth rates after hysteroscopic resection of submucus fibroids are encouraging and approach 75% of patients treated.[44,54]

Endometrial polyps are often an incidental finding and probably have little effect on fertility. Visible pedunculated polyps can be removed in the office setting. The presence of multiple polyps is best treated by directed curettage with follow-up hysteroscopy to confirm their absence.

Hysteroscopic incision of a uterine septum is primarily indicated in the fertile patient with recurrent pregnancy losses. Successful use of the neodymium-YAG laser has been reported for septum resection.[39] However, using the laser can be tedious and time-consuming. Resecting or incising the midline septum with semirigid hysteroscopic scissors or with loop electrodes is preferred. Initially there is little bleeding associated with resection of the septum. The development of brisk bleeding usually indicates the transition between septum and myometrium and suggests completion of the procedure. Postoperatively, some practitioners empirically employ the use of intrauterine devices or high doses of hormonal supplements to minimize intrauterine adhesion formation. However, in the absence of such therapies, systematic follow-up hysteroscopies at 1, 2, 4, and 8 weeks postoperatively have not demonstrated intrauterine adhesions. Regular proliferative endometrium was present by 8 weeks in the absence of hormonal supplements.[36] Vercellini et al question the value of intrauterine device insertion or estrogen administration following hysteroscopic metroplasty.[230]

Luteal phase insufficiency

The evaluation of a luteal phase defect in the infertile patient has been previously presented (Chapter 12). In the 45 years since the original description of luteal phase insufficiency, there remains enormous ambiguity regarding both its prevalence and its importance as a cause for infertility.[117] Any treatment rendered should be done so with an awareness of this ambiguity.

Although the endometrial biopsy is the clinical standard for defining luteal phase insufficiency, the relevance of an "abnormal" biopsy is questionable. Davis et al found sequentially abnormal biopsies in 27% of proven fertile subjects.[48] Given the pulsatile nature of progesterone secretion in the mid-luteal to late-luteal phase, single serum progesterone determinations have little role in the diagnosis of luteal phase insufficiency. Roughly 5% of ovulatory cycles have an abnormally short luteal phase. Although luteal phase durations of less than 8 days are likely associated with implantation dysfunction, it has not been adequately demonstrated that 8- to 11-day luteal phases are associated with infertility.[169]

CC has been implicated as both a cure and as a cause of luteal phase insufficiency. Patients prescribed CC for anovulation are more likely to have luteal phase insufficiency while receiving CC therapy; these patients may benefit from supplemental progesterone therapy. However, ovulatory patients with luteal phase insufficiency may normalize with CC therapy.[47]

TREATMENT OF UNEXPLAINED INFERTILITY

The percentage of patients being labeled "normal but infertile" continues to decline as the complexities of reproductive biology and its clinical evaluation are more clearly understood. Even with this decline, the reproductive endocrinologist today is likely to encounter unexplained infertility in approximately 10% of infertile couples. These couples may understand that their workup is "normal", but most will feel compelled to initiate some form of therapy. Is empirical treatment with ovulation induction and intrauterine insemination (IUI) an appropriate first step? Given the need to find a correctable cause for their infertility, are these patients better served by in vitro fertilization and embryo transfer (IVF-ET)?

Before making such a decision, an obvious first approach is to ensure that an adequate evaluation has been performed. This may require the use of diagnostic tools not routinely employed: by adding sperm antibody testing, hamster egg penetration assay (HEPA), and ultrasound monitoring of folliculogenesis, Coulam et al reduced the diagnosis of unexplained infertility by 60%.[45] Identifying a cause results in more focused and efficient clinical management. However, care must be taken before removing the label of unexplained infertility. The clinician must be aware of the limitations of diagnostic tests and incorporate refinements to improve their accuracy. For example, nearly 20% of patients who have a negative HEPA may ultimately demonstrate fertilization in an IVF system.[111] Fluorescence staining of nuclear DNA offers an easier and more confident reading of sperm penetration than the traditional HEPA method of acetolacmoid staining and significantly reduces the false-negative rate.[62]

One might argue that the ultimate assurance of an adequate evaluation would be to incorporate the diagnostic properties of IVF-ET in order to determine the cause of previously unexplained infertility. However, IVF-ET may produce many false conclusions. The absence of fertilization does not conclusively pinpoint the problem, nor does it necessarily imply that such couples would not benefit from ovulation induction with IUI. Many couples who lack fertilization in one IVF cycle demonstrate normal fertilization in subsequent cycles. It is important to fully evaluate the possible causes of fertilization failure, which may include defective oocytes,[64] oocyte nuclear immaturity,[80] chromosomal abnormalities,[226] or the male factor.[137] Tarin et al identified the spermatozoa to be responsible for 41% of fertilization failures, whereas oocyte chromosome abnormalities accounted for 19.3%, oocyte immaturity accounted for 11.8%, and unknown etiology accounted for 41%.[218] Thus IVF-ET may not be the ultimate diagnostic test unless a full evaluation of fertilization failure, is pursued. A complete evaluation should incorporate (1) DNA-specific fluorochromes to evaluate oocyte nuclear maturity, (2) cytogenetic analysis to detect chromosomal abnormalities, and (3) sperm-zona pellucida binding tests to evaluate the male factor. These tests are beyond the scope of most centers.

Even in couples who demonstrate fertilization in an IVF-ET cycle, the diagnostic validity may be flawed because there is no standard evaluation of embryo quality. It may not be correct to assume that gametes are normal because the embryo "looks good" because morphologic assessment of the developing embryo may correlate poorly with pregnancy outcome.[94] Until a more objective assessment of embryo quality is available, it is difficult to reach diagnostic conclusions based on embryo quality in couples with unexplained infertility.

Many practitioners use superovulation and IUI in couples with unexplained infertility. Based on comparison trials, Murdoch et al and Iffland et al independently could not support the use of superovulation with IUI for patients with unexplained infertility because of the low conception rates.[112,160] However, others have demonstrated favorable conception rates in patients receiving empirical ovulation induction while waiting for in vitro fertilization. Simon et al have observed that cumulative pregnancy rates (CPR) of 3 superovulation/IUI cycles equaled one IVF-ET cycle in patients with unexplained infertility.[207] In the superovulation/IUI group, the CPR (44.5%) plateaued after 7 cycles, and in the IVF-ET group (45.6%) after 3 cycles.

In summary, couples with unexplained infertility require an aggressive evaluation in hopes of focusing clinical management. In those couples whose infertility remains unexplained, superovulation with intrauterine inseminations may be an appropriate first step. Nearly one half of these patients may conceive within 6 cycles. Pursuing IVF-ET prior to this may achieve pregnancy more rapidly but may not provide reliable diagnostic information.

ASSISTED REPRODUCTIVE TECHNOLOGY

Within the field of obstetrics and gynecology, it is difficult to find a subspecialty that has made such rapid and exciting advances as those in ART. As a result the reproductive endocrinologist today has an armamentarium of procedures for treatment of the infertile couple.

Human IVF without ET was first reported by Rock and Menkin at the Free Hospital for Women in Boston.[196] McLaren and Biggers were the first to report the successful development and birth of mice that were cultivated in vitro as early embryos.[149] Chang was the first to describe a successful pregnancy and delivery after fertilization outside the body by combining rabbit gametes.[38] This work was followed by that of many investigators using both animal and human models. Robert Edwards and Patrick Steptoe began their research in 1968, applying their respective expertise in gamete physiology and gynecologic laparoscopy. After eight years, the first IVF-ET pregnancy was achieved but unfortunately resulted in an ectopic pregnancy. Finally in 1978, after a 10 year effort and 100 unsuccessful cycles, Louise Brown was born marking the world's first successful IVF and ET[213] and the perseverance of two pioneers in ART.

Since the first success in human IVF, there has been an explosion in activity in the field of assisted reproductive technology. The alphabet soup of ART procedures has grown to include IVF-ET, gamete intrafallopian transfer (GIFT), zygote intrafallopian transfer (ZIFT), pronuclear stage tubal transfer (PROST), tubal embryo transfer (TET), natural oocyte retrieval with intravaginal fertilization (NORIF), and the micromanipulation procedures, including partial zona dissection (PZD), subzonal sperm injection (SUZI) (also referred to as microinsemination sperm transfer [MIST]), and intracytoplasmic sperm injection (ICSI). In 1991 the Society for Assisted Reproductive Technologies (SART) reported that a total of 33,001 ART cycles were performed in the United States.

Assisted reproduction is conceptually a simple process. Oocytes are harvested from the female in either natural or stimulated cycles. These are mixed with sperm and transferred to the fallopian tube or incubated until embryos are formed. The embryos are then transferred back into the uterine cavity for purposes of implantation and gestation.

The following section will provide an overview of ART, including patient selection, ovulation induction and oocyte retrieval, in vitro fertilization and embryo culture, assessment of embryo quality, and embryo transfer. Use of donor oocytes, tubal transfer procedures, natural cycle IVF-ET, and embryo micromanipulation will also be addressed. Oocyte micromanipulation is discussed under the treatment of male infertility.

Patient selection

Appropriate selection of patients for ART is important to ensure a balance between the couple's desire for pregnancy and the realistic prognosis of a successful outcome. As the success rates of IVF have increased, the indications for its use have broadened.[119] Initially IVF-ET was used for tubal-factor infertility. Subsequently, male-factor infertility was found to benefit from IVF-ET with or without micromanipulation. As previously discussed, the use of IVF for unexplained infertility and endometriosis has also been employed. Patients suffering from infertility due to immunologic causes may also benefit from ART, since immunologic barriers to fertility are theoretically removed by bringing gametes together outside the body.

The decreased fertility potential and increased spontaneous abortion rate associated with increased maternal age has led many centers, including the Brigham and Women's Hospital, to utilize an age cutoff for acceptance into the ART program. A negative linear correlation has been demonstrated between female age and pregnancy rate in IVF-ET cycles. In a study of 1101 cycles, the ongoing pregnancy rate per ET for patients younger than 30 years of age was 26% compared with 9% for patients aged 37 years. Patients aged 40 years of age or greater had a 50% miscarriage rate, compared to 29% in patients under the age of 40.[172] At the current time the IVF program at the Brigham and Women's Hospital accepts female patients up to 42 years of age. Women accepted into the IVF program in their 40th year must have an FSH level less than or equal to 15 mIU/mL.

Ovulation induction

The main goal of ovulation induction in ART is to obtain oocytes high in quality and in number, while avoiding the risk of uncontrolled ovarian hyperstimulation. Most investigators believe that the risk of uncontrolled ovarian hyperstimulation is reduced in ART as compared to IUI cycles, presumably because of the aspiration of granulosa cells with oocyte retrieval. Gonen et al demonstrated a significant drop in serum estradiol, progesterone, and hCG levels following follicular aspiration.[78]

There is no consensus among different IVF programs as to which ovulation induction agents are superior. A retrospective study compared three ovarian stimulation protocols for IVF-ET that included (1) CC and hMG, (2) hMG alone, and (3) GnRH-agonist (GnRH-a) suppression plus hMG. The investigators concluded that although the use of GnRH-a reduced the cancellation rate and increased the number of retrieved oocytes, it did not result in higher pregnancy rates per cycle than those achieved by stimulation with CC/hMG (31.4% versus 16.9%).[59] A prospective randomized trial comparing CC/hMG versus GnRH-a/hMG in IVF-ET did not demonstrate a clear superiority of one protocol over the other.[67] Lejeune et al observed a significantly higher pregnancy rate with GnRH-a/hMG treatment as compared with CC/hMG cycles. In an attempt to address the different studies, a meta analysis compared treatment outcomes with different GnRH-a protocols.[107] Clinical pregnancy rate per cycle was significantly improved after GnRH-a use for IVF (common odds ratio [OR] 1.80) and gamete intrafallopian transfer (GIFT, common OR 2.37). Cycle cancellation rates were decreased. The spontaneous abortion rate was similar with and without GnRH-a use. Ultimately the selection of one of the GnRH-a protocols should be individualized for each patient based on previous response with gonadotropin stimulation.

Advantages of GnRH-a use include prevention of a premature LH surge, suppression of endogenous basal LH levels, and recruitment of a larger cohort of follicles. GnRH agonists have been used in different protocols including (1) long protocol with suppression started in the mid-luteal phase, (2) short or flare-up protocol starting GnRH-a on day 2 of the cycle, followed by gonadotropins on day 4 of the cycle, (3) ultralong protocol with depot leuprolide acetate 2 to 3 months prior to ovulation induction, and (4) ultrashort protocol using GnRH-a only during cycle days 1 through 3 (Fig. 13-3).

Muasher reports little beneficial effects from the use of the long protocol in low response patients, which he defined as patients with a basal FSH $\geq$ 15 mIU/mL.[158] In low response patients, the use of the short protocol takes advantage of the initial agonistic stimulatory effect of GnRH-a.

Others have recommended starting both GnRH-a and hMG on cycle day 3 when using the short protocol.[23] In patients with an appropriate response to hMG, San Ramon et al reported similar fertilization, biochemical, and clinical pregnancy rates in patients receiving either the short or long protocol. However, the short protocol was associated with premature luteinization, hyperandrogenemia, higher spontaneous abortion rates, and poorer pregnancy outcome when compared with luteal phase administration of GnRH-a. The Hallam Medical Centre reported that the long protocol is superior to the short protocol with significantly greater follicular recruitment, oocyte recovery and fertilization rates, and significantly greater number of embryos available for transfer.[217] Fewer ampules of hMG are generally needed when using the short protocol. The advantages of using an ultrashort protocol include decreased cost and increased convenience to the patient. A comparison of the short and ultrashort protocols showed fertilization and pregnancy rates to be similar, but the ultrashort protocol did not always prevent an LH surge.[1]

Comparisons have been made between different GnRH agonists for use in IVF-ET cycles. In one study, patients receiving nafarelin acetate required significantly less hMG and had significantly more embryos frozen for later transfer than those receiving leuprolide acetate.[185] In a separate study comparing buserelin acetate and leuprolide acetate, the number of follicles punctured, the number of oocytes retrieved, the percentage of mature oocytes, and the number of embryos suitable for replacement and cryopreservation were significantly higher in patients receiving leuprolide acetate.[18] Parinaud et al reported that E2 levels and E2 level per hMG ampule were both significantly lower in IVF-ET cycles with buserelin than with leuprolide acetate and triptorelin.[177] The pregnancy per stimulated cycle rate was not significantly different among the groups.

The standard protocol for ovulation induction in the Brigham and Women's Hospital IVF program is patterned after the work of Meldrum and associates.[152] After luteal phase GnRH-a suppression (estradiol < 50 pg/mL and progesterone < 1 ng/dL), a cycle-day-2 baseline ultrasound is performed to rule out cystic follicles greater than 30 mm in diameter. Hornstein et al reported that baseline cysts less than 30 mm do not negatively impact ovulation induction or pregnancy rates in IVF-ET.[102] hMG is taken on cycle days 2 to 5 at a standard dose of 3 ampules (patient < 150 pounds) qd or 2 ampules bid (patient > 150 pounds). On the morning of day 6, an ultrasound examination and serum estradiol level are obtained. Therapy is thereafter

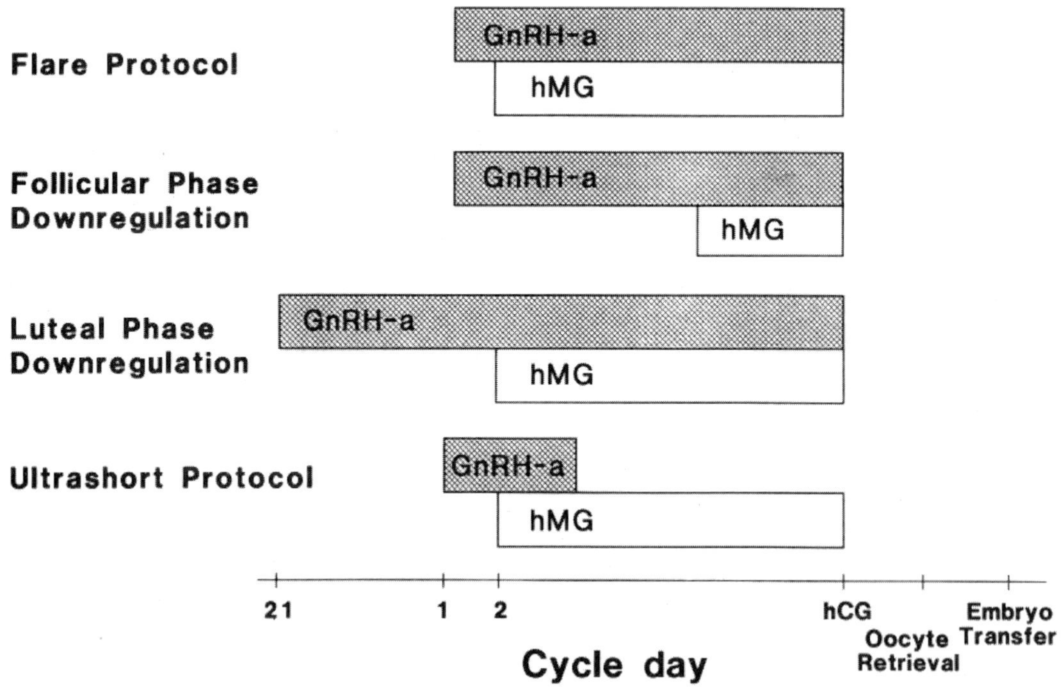

Fig. 13-3. Four different approaches to superovulation using a GnRh-agonist.

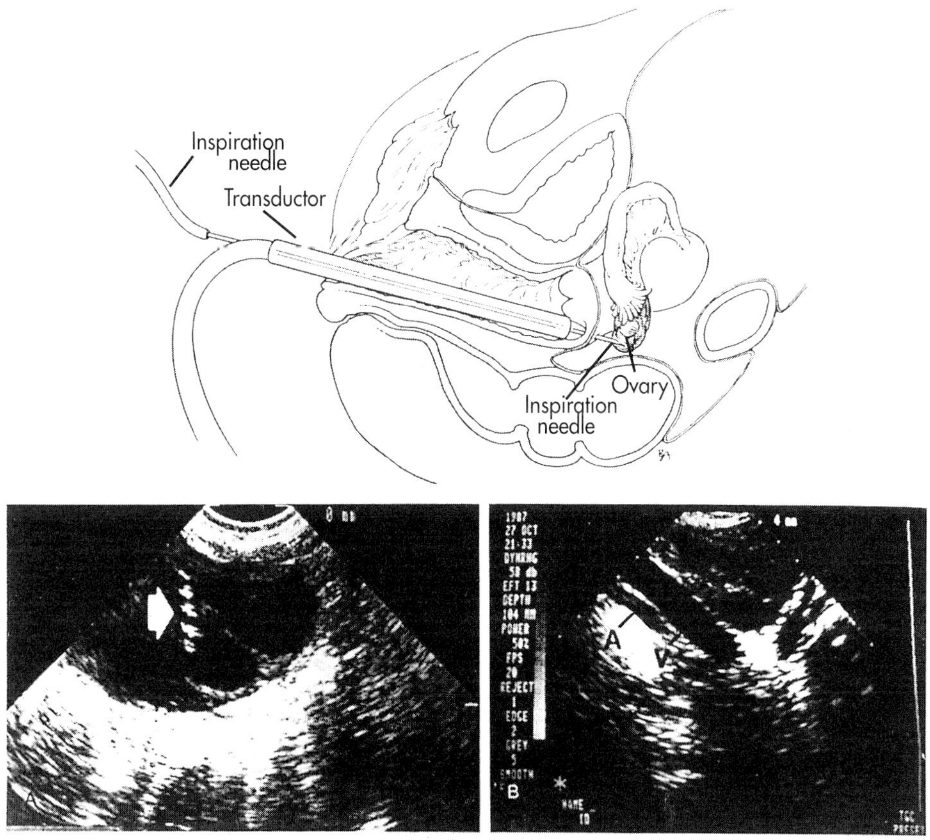

Fig. 13-4. Transvaginal ultrasound-guided oocyte retrieval. With ultrasound, needle (arrow) is easily visualized within the follicle. Care must be taken to avoid the adjacent hypogastric artery (A) and vein (V). (Gershenson DM, DeCherney AH, Curry SL, editors: *Operative gynecology,* 1993, WB Saunders, pp 557-558.)

individualized based on oocyte measurements by ultrasonography and serum estradiol levels. When the estradiol level is greater than 600 pg/mL and at least two follicles with dimensions of 18 x 12 mm are measurable, hCG (10,000 USP units IM) is given.

Oocyte retrieval is scheduled for 36 hours after hCG administration. Oocytes are retrieved transvaginally with ultrasound guidance (Fig 13-4).[200] This technique has replaced the previous use of laparoscopy for oocyte retrieval under direct visualization.[134] The anesthetic for this procedure varies amongst different centers and may involve a paracervical block, conscious sedation, or spinal anesthesia.

Use of donor oocytes

A relatively new application of ART is ovum donation.[141] By using oocytes from suitable donors, women who were previously considered incurably sterile are now able to experience pregnancy and childbirth. It is important for the gynecologist to be aware of this new option. Furthermore, the surgeon should no longer consider bilateral oophorectomy to be an automatic indication for hysterectomy.[163] Women who may benefit from this technique include those with premature ovarian failure, Turner's syndrome, surgically removed ovaries, ovaries that have lost their function because of chemotherapy or radiation therapy, carriers of genetic disorders, women with poor IVF outcomes as a result of low response or oocyte factors, and even perimenopausal or postmenopausal women.[22] This latter group of patients has raised considerable controversy. There is concern about maternal complications arising in pregnant women past their natural reproductive years and concern for their offspring who may become orphans at an early age. Although ovum donation is a very successful and appropriate option for properly selected patients, there remain some serious ethical, legal, and social questions that are still unresolved.

Pregnancy rates per embryo transfer are usually higher in donor oocyte cycles compared to standard IVF-ET. Clinical results from annual national IVF registries demonstrate an average pregnancy rate per transfer of 25% to 30%.[24] Women who have previously conceived following oocyte donation have a high percentage (60%) of conception in repeat trials of in vitro fertilization with same-donor oocytes.[199]

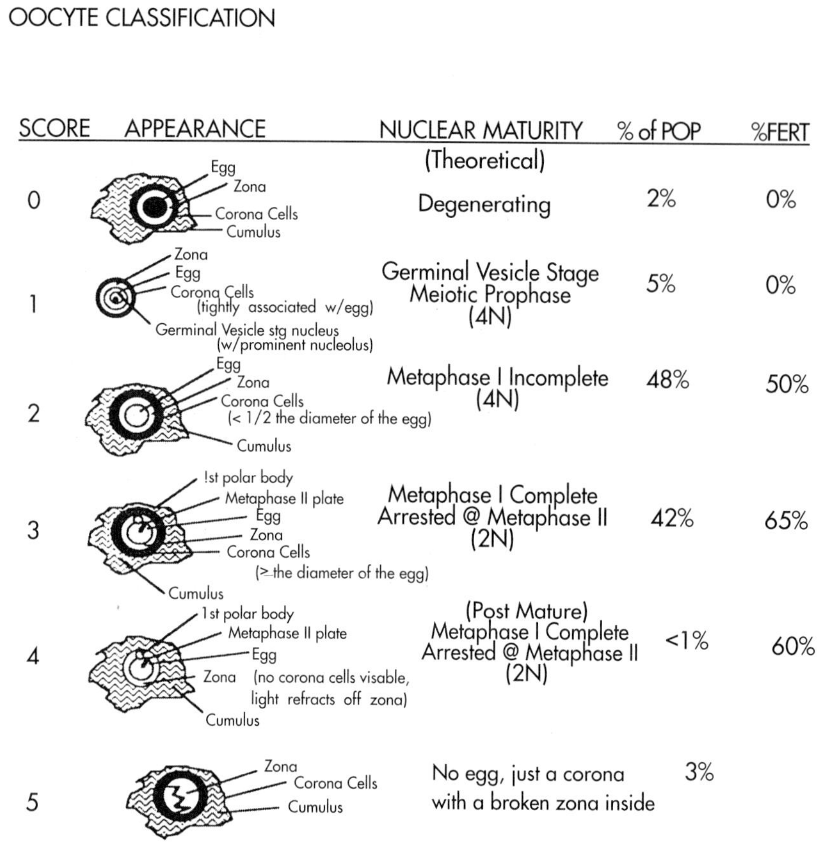

Fig. 13-5. Oocyte classification based on morphologic appearance. (From Brigham & Women's Hospital ART Laboratory Manual, 1993.)

In vitro fertilization and embryo culture

Following oocyte retrieval, the gamete biologist or embryologist assumes the important responsibility of nurturing the reproductive cells until they are returned to the patient's in vivo environment. The retrieved oocytes are initially evaluated for maturity based on the appearance of the cumulus and corona (Fig. 13-5). As fertilization is usually attempted in all oocytes without regard to their maturity, the purpose of oocyte scoring is to permit evaluation of the patient's superovulation regimen for potential future cycles. If a large cohort of oocytes are immature with a resulting low fertilization rate, the next stimulation may be "pushed" to higher estradiol levels. Immature oocytes are occasionally incubated for an additional 12 to 24 hours prior to insemination in hopes of a higher fertilization rate.[147]

The fertilization phase of IVF is entered after the addition of sperm to oocytes. Oocytes are placed in insemination media (0.4% bovine serum albumin (BSA) in Ham's F-10 culture media). No maternal serum (with potential antisperm antibodies) is added to the insemination medium. Insemination normally involves the addition of 150,000 processed sperm per individually cultured oocyte. Approximately 12 to 19 hours after insemination, each oocyte is inspected to document fertilization that is confirmed after the identification of two pronuclei. Polyspermic oocytes (greater than two pronuclei) are discarded. Fertilized oocytes are then placed in "growth" media (7.5% heat-inactivated patient's serum in Ham's F-10 culture media) and returned to the incubator. They are not examined again until just prior to embryo transfer. The expected embryo growth rate is depicted in Fig. 13-6.

In an attempt to mimic in vivo conditions, embryos have been "cocultured" in vitro with human fallopian tube epithelial cell lines.[31] Coculture with fetal bovine uterine fibroblasts,[234] human ovarian follicle and endometrium,[73] and Vero cells has also been described. In comparison, studies with each of these cell lines versus standard culture media, fertilization, blastocyst expansion, and hatching were significantly higher in the coculture groups. In a prospective study of 50 IVF-ET patients, Bongso et al showed improved pregnancy rates after transfer of embryos grown in human fallopian tubal cell coculture.[31] With the increased use of embryo transfer three (as opposed to two) days postoocyte-retrieval, coculture techniques may become increasingly important. Successful pregnancies have been reported after transfer of human embryos cocultured in vitro for 5 days postinsemination.[153] Much further study is needed to define the specific embryotrophic factors produced with coculture technique.

Assessment of embryo quality

One of the primary goals of ART is to acquire many oocytes and subsequent embryos so as to maximize the selection of quality embryos for uterine transfer. In order to select the best embryos for transfer, however, it is necessary to have some objective means to accurately evaluate "good" and "bad" embryos. Unfortunately, no such tool currently exists. Choosing the "right" embryo has been deemed the challenge of the nineties.

Most ART centers continue to assess embryo quality based on morphologic appearance, fully realizing that there is not a perfect correlation between morphologic scoring and rates of embryo implantation.[94] At Brigham and Women's Hospital, embryos are evaluated for number of blastomeres, degree of fragmentation, symmetry, granularity, vacuolation, membrane definition, and number of nuclei per blastomere.

Many investigators have recognized the need for developing better techniques to assess the oocyte and embryo. Proposed methods have included a developmental rating system,[46] fluorescein diacetate fluorescence,[156] immunosuppressive activity in preimplantation culture media,[41] and immunoactive factors in culture media including

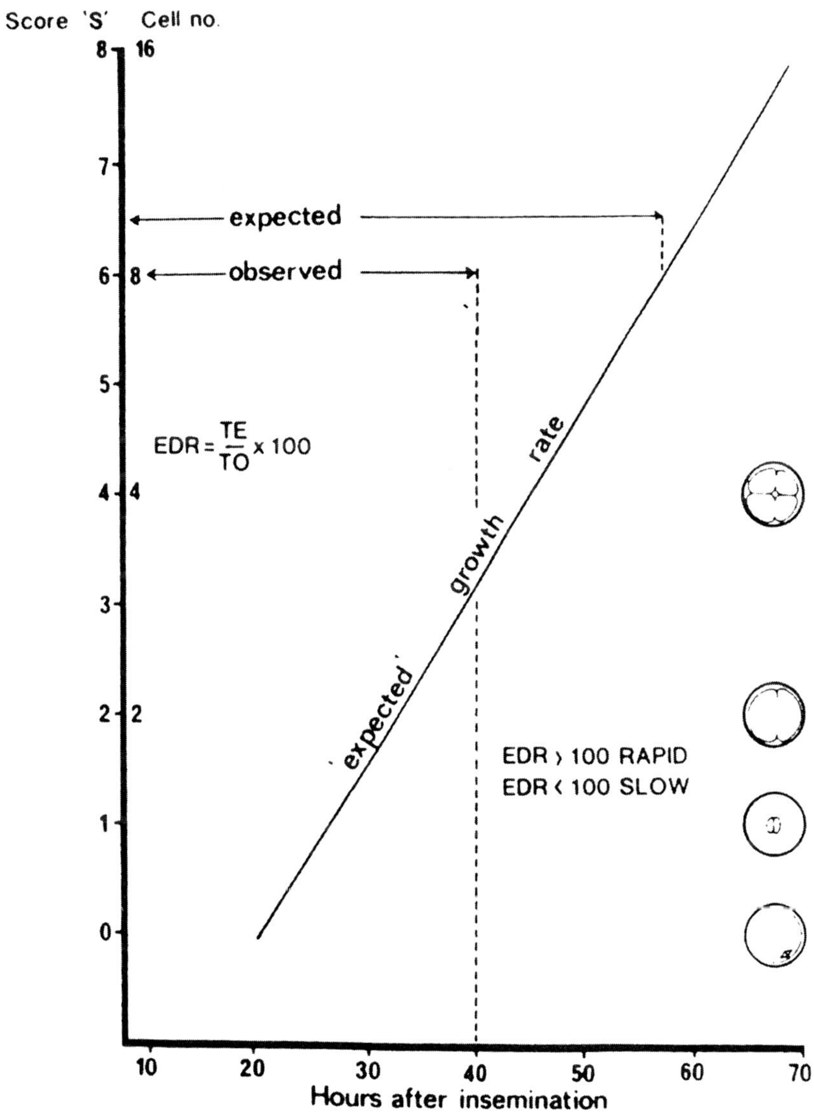

Fig. 13-6. Expected growth of in vitro cultured human embryos. Embryos are compared to an ideal "expected" growth rate, which is a regression of the embryo cell number against time. (From Cummins JM et al: A formula for scoring human embryo growth rates in in vitro fertilization: its value in predicting pregnancy and in comparison with visual estimates of embryo quality, *J In Vitro Fert Embryo Transf* 3(5):284, 1986.)

progesterone,[93] interleukin-1α,[91] and interleukin-1-β.[21] All proposed techniques have limitations, and none are in common use. Preliminary studies on the metabolic assessment of oocyte and embryo quality demonstrate a correlation between NADH laser fluorimetry measurements and mouse embryo development.[92] NADH laser fluorimetry, a well-studied and sensitive indicator of electron transport function in mitochondria, has been shown to be a very efficient method for the nondestructive investigation of cellular metabolism in other systems.

The ability to select embryos for uterine transfer or to evaluate the effects of such interventions as zona drilling, preimplantation embryo biopsy, the use of coculture techniques, and the experimental use of growth factors or cytokines is markedly limited by current assessment techniques. There is a clearly defined need for a technique or assay that could better describe oocyte and embryo quality. This would not only increase IVF-ET pregnancy rates but also further the study of basic reproductive physiology.

Embryo transfer

The technique of ET is relatively simple. Most centers use a side port catheter to prevent clogging of the catheter as it is advanced through the cervix. The embryos are loaded into the catheter in a minimal volume, usually less than 25 μL, and the small catheter is passed into the uterine cavity with or without an introducer. Minimal manipulation of the cervix is employed to decrease the risk of intrauterine irritation and contraction. The ET catheter is placed in the fundal portion of the uterine cavity. The embryos are then injected with minimal pressure and the catheter is held in place for 1 minute. The catheter is removed slowly and gently so as not to disrupt the intrauterine environment. The catheter is then examined microscopically to rule out retention of embryos on the catheter tip. In most ART centers, embryos are transferred approximately 48 hours after oocyte retrieval. In vivo it is believed that gametes spend 3 or more days in the fallopian tube and that the embryo arrives in the endometrial cavity some 3 to 5 days after ovulation.[57] Embryos cultured in vitro develop at a faster rate which may permit their early replacement. ART centers that perform ET 3 days after oocyte retrieval feel that the day 3 transfer is more physiologic. Furthermore the day 3 transfer allows more stringent criteria for embryo selection by avoiding transfer of embryos that have arrested development at the 4-cell stage. The disadvantage of day 3 ET is the prolonged in vitro exposure of the embryo.

The intrauterine transfer of zygotes 1 day after oocyte retrieval has also been reported. Warnes et al found no significant difference in pregnancy rates when comparing intrauterine transfer of embryos 24 or 48 hours after oocyte retrieval.[233] The early intrauterine transfer of embryos again minimizes the duration of in vitro exposure; however, the technique has not become universally adopted because it also reduces the ability to select embryos based on cleavage and development.

The decision on how many embryos to transfer should be individualized for each couple. The goal is to maximize the chance of pregnancy yet minimize the chance of multiple gestations. Factors that should be considered include age of the patient, outcome of patient's prior ART cycles, quality of the available embryos, the couple's acceptance of possible selective reduction, and the center's own statistics on multiple gestation rates. By increasing the number of embryos transferred, the pregnancy rate will accordingly increase—up to a point. Thereafter, the pregnancy rate plateaus and the multiple gestation rate may increase in those patients who would have achieved pregnancy with fewer embryos transferred. The "plateau point" should be independently evaluated for each ART center as this may vary between three to six embryos. This variance is likely dependent on embryo quality. Balen et al report that the incidence of miscarriage increases when fewer embryos are transferred.[19]

After embryo transfer, patients are put on bed rest and observed. In the early days of IVF-ET it was not uncommon to hospitalize a patient overnight after embryo transfer. With improvements in technique and pregnancy rates, the recovery time after embryo transfer has progressively decreased but is still of varied duration among different programs. Decreasing recovery time after embryo transfer to one hour does not adversely affect pregnancy outcome and may result in significant cost savings.[95]

Normal ovarian physiology is most likely disrupted at the time of aspiration of multiple follicles for oocyte retrieval in IVF. Vargyas et al noted a decrease in progesterone level after ovarian aspiration, although the level was higher than in unstimulated patients.[229] In addition, a luteal phase defect may occur with GnRH-a use. Most programs support the luteal phase with progesterone either via an oral, intramuscular (IM), or suppository (vaginal) route. Bioavailability of oral micronized progesterone is approximately 10% of IM administration.[208] Severe thigh myositis can occur following IM progesterone.[186] A prospective randomized comparison of IM progesterone in oil (50 mg/day) and intravaginal micronized progesterone (600 mg/day) in ART cycles showed that despite lower plasma progesterone levels, a lower first trimester abortion rate was found in the intravaginally treated group.[209] At Brigham and Women's Hospital, IM progesterone (50 mg/day) is given on the evening of embryo transfer and continued for 14 days. Thereafter if the patient is pregnant, intravaginal progesterone suppositories (50 mg bid) are continued through the 12th week of pregnancy.

Tubal transfer of gametes and embryos

In 1985 Asch et al introduced the technique of gamete intrafallopian transfer (GIFT).[13] In patients with healthy fallopian tubes, the gametes may theoretically benefit from the tubal microenvironment with its associated proteins and growth factors. Furthermore, the technique reduces the in

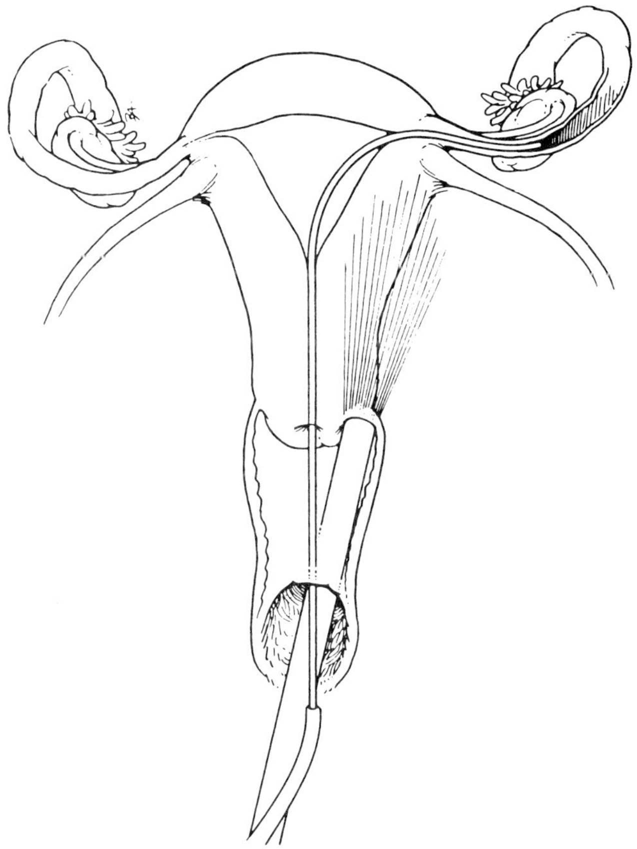

Fig. 13-7. Transcervical approach for intratubal placement of gametes or embryos. (Gershenson DM, DeCherney AH, Curry SL, editors: *Operative gynecology*, 1993, WB Saunders, pp 557-558.)

vitro exposure of gametes. The GIFT procedure involves the same steps as IVF up until oocyte retrieval. Thereafter isolated oocytes and sperm are transferred back into the fallopian tube. The first GIFT procedures utilized laparoscopy for transfer of gametes. Many centers now perform tubal transfer procedures utilizing a transcervical approach guided either by ultrasonography,[34] hysteroscopy,[179] or nonhysteroscopic falloposcopy (Fig. 13-7).[124]

Patients with normal fallopian tubes need not automatically be referred for GIFT as opposed to IVF-ET. The decision to perform GIFT or IVF-ET should be tailored to the experience of the ART program. In programs with experienced gamete biologists as reflected by high IVF-ET pregnancy rates, the patient with normal fallopian tubes may do just as well with IVF-ET and not be exposed to the additional surgical and anesthetic risks associated with laparoscopic gamete transfer. With the increased use of transcervical intrafallopian transfer, this will become less of a consideration. In addition, local anesthetic with conscious sedation has been used successfully for laparoscopic intrafallopian transfer.[155]

ZIFT,[85] also known as PROST,[241] is a two-step procedure involving the tubal transfer of zygotes approximately 24 hours after oocyte retrieval. ZIFT/PROST was developed in an attempt to take advantage of both the tubal microenvironment and reduced in vitro exposure while still being able to confirm fertilization. Prospective randomized studies comparing ZIFT and IVF-ET in couples with male-factor infertility demonstrate no therapeutic advantage of ZIFT over IVF-ET.[220] In couples with nontubal-factor infertility, a prospective randomized trial also failed to demonstrate any therapeutic improvement associated with the increased complexity of ZIFT as compared with standard IVF-ET.[70]

Tubal embryo transfer (TET) is an extension of ZIFT/PROST and involves transfer of cleavage stage embryos within the fallopian tubes as opposed to the uterine cavity. In theory, TET permits the selection of quality embryos that are developmentally competent to undergo cleavage and will potentially benefit from the tubal milieu. Balmaceda et al could not demonstrate any increased pregnancy rates when comparing TET with IVF-ET.[20] The similar pregnancy rates may be explained in part by the possible intrafallopian placement of embryos even with IVF-ET. Placement of a radiopaque contrast medium during "mock" embryo transfers has shown that it is retained in the fallopian tubes in 38% of cases, in the uterine cavity in 68%, in the cervix in 9%, and in the vagina in 12%.[129]

The incidence of multiple pregnancies may be reduced with intrafallopian transfer procedures. In one retrospective study of 1064 cycles in which three embryos or female gametes were transferred, multiple pregnancies at 20 weeks gestation were present in 16% of GIFT pregnancies, 27% of ZIFT pregnancies, and 32% of IVF-ET pregnancies.[30]

Even with the conclusions of prospective comparison studies, the decision to proceed with IVF-ET, GIFT, ZIFT/PROST, or TET should again be tailored to the experience of the ART program. Tubal transfer procedures may be more advantageous in programs with low IVF-ET pregnancy rates. In 1991 the Society for Assisted Reproductive Technology (SART) reported 33,001 cycles of ART treatment, excluding frozen embryo and donor oocyte cycles. Of these, 24,671 cycles were initiated by IVF with 15.2% deliveries per retrieval, 5452 were cycles initiated by GIFT with 26.6% deliveries per retrieval, 2104 were cycles initiated by ZIFT with 19.7% deliveries per retrieval, and 714 were combination cycles of IVF and one of the tubal transfer techniques, which resulted in 19.3% deliveries per retrieval.[14] Care should be taken when comparing pregnancy outcomes between different ART procedures; the associated prognoses of patients within each group should be compared.

Natural cycle IVF-ET

In the first IVF-ET cycles reported by Steptoe and Edwards,[213] superovulation with menotropins was not utilized. Instead, a single oocyte was retrieved during the patient's "natural" cycle. Despite the subsequent evolution of superovulation with its superior pregnancy rates, some programs have renewed interest in the use of natural cycle IVF-ET.[184] Advantages of unstimulated IVF-ET cycles include a reduction in medication costs, multiple pregnancies, and ovarian hyperstimulation. Some argue that because of the increased cancellation rates, decreased success rates, and unavailability of embryos for cryopreservation, the true costs per pregnancy may be similar.[133] Natural cycle IVF-ET is probably best suited for the low response patient who produces only a few follicles despite aggressive menotropine stimulation.

Embryo cryopreservation

Another major development in ART is the cryopreservation of embryos and oocytes.[221] Although cryopreservation of sperm has been available for a long time, only recently have successful pregnancies resulted from cryopreserved embryos. Cryopreservation usually reduces the number of viable embryos because of intracellular ice formation. Embryos that survive the freezing/thawing process and proceed with normal cleavage are not associated with increased chromosomal abnormalities.[203] In 1991 the National IVF Registry reported 4838 frozen embryo procedures. This represents a tenfold increase from the 490 frozen embryo procedures reported in 1987. An average of 11.1% deliveries per frozen embryo procedure was reported in 1991.

Embryo micromanipulation and preimplantation genetic diagnosis

Polymerase chain reaction (PCR) amplification of DNA from a single cell has permitted preimplantation genetic diagnosing at the embryonic stage. The human embryonic genome is activated between the 4- and 8-cell stages and necessitates biopsy of the embryo after this stage to prevent maternal contamination. Embryo biopsy for preimplantation genetic diagnosis is usually performed on day 3 at the 6- to 10-cell stage (i.e., the latest day when embryo transfer is compatible with an acceptable pregnancy rate).[88] Following blastomere biopsy, no adverse effects on in vitro growth of the embryo occur,[86] although nutrient uptake declines in proportion to the reduced cell mass.[90] The ability to amplify DNA sequences a millionfold with PCR may create false-negative or positive results due to implication of contaminating cells. Although less efficient, fluorescent in situ hybridization (FISH) permits numerical and structural analysis of chromosomes of a single cell to be made and is not limited by contamination. Handyside has reported on the successful use of preimplantation genetic diagnosing in pregnancies at risk for cystic fibrosis and X chromosome-linked recessive disease.[87,89] Although these techniques utilize the current scientific technologies, the absence of infertility in many couples seeking preimplantation genetic diagnosis brings into question whether these patients would be equally served by chorionic villus sampling.

ADOPTION

Although there are many treatments available for infertility and our knowledge and understanding is expanding at a rapid rate, some couples are not successful in achieving pregnancy through infertility treatments. Other couples may not choose to pursue a pregnancy through the complex and somewhat invasive technologies currently offered. Adoption is an alternative .

Adoption is not an easy process. Many couples who ultimately turn to adoption in order to start their families are discouraged at the number of "hoops" through which they must jump—applications, evaluations, home visits, lawyers—these can seem overwhelming.

There are many adoption alternatives, such as anonymous adoption, open adoption, or foreign adoption. In general, couples interested in adopting should be referred to a social worker who can discuss the pros and cons of the options, address some of the complex emotional and social issues, and point the couple in the right direction. Consultation with a lawyer familiar with adoption laws is also of tantamount importance as adoption laws may vary from state to state. Several excellent books on adoption are available through RESOLVE, a nonprofit infertility support and education organization.

Physicians should not view adoption as a failure but rather as a success. If the couple are able to start a family, then they have achieved their goal. If the physicians have enabled them to do so by performing a proper workup and reviewing all treatment options, then the physicians can feel good about their role in the process.

Summary

Physicians are more successful in helping couples overcome infertility today than at any other time in history. The development of infertility treatments should be kept in perspective, however. In a dissertation on the history of infertility, DeCherney and Harris outline the development of infertility diagnoses and treatment from Egyptian times to the twentieth century.[49] Although past knowledge of reproduction may seem rudimentary and the treatments crude, previous practitioners in their time had the same conviction in their treatment abilities that physicians have today.

REFERENCES

1. Acharya U et al: Prospective study of short and ultrashort regimens of gonadotropin-releasing hormone agonist in an in vitro fertilization program, *Fertil Steril* 58:1169-1173, 1992.
2. Adams R, Mishell DR Jr, Israel R: Treatment of refractory anovulation with increased dosage and prolonged duration of cyclic clomiphene citrate, *Obstet Gynecol* 39:562, 1972.
3. Adashi EY: Clomiphene citrate mechanism(s) and site(s) of action—a hypothesis revisited, *Fertil Steril* 42:331, 1984.
4. Adashi EY: Clomiphene citrate-initiated ovulation: a clinical update, *Sem Repro Endocrinol* 4:255, 1986.
5. Adashi EY et al: Gestational outcome of clomiphene-related conceptions, *Fertil Steril* 31:620, 1979.
6. Adhesion Study Group: Reduction of postoperative adhesion formation with intraperitoneal 32% dextran 70: a prospective, randomized clinical trial, *Fertil Steril* 40:612, 1983.

7. Adhesion Barrier Study Group: Prevention of postsurgical adhesion by INTERCEED (TC7): a prospective, randomized multicenter clinical study, *Fertil Steril* 51:933, 1989.
8. Ahlgren M, KÑllen B, Rannevik G: Outcome of pregnancy after Clomid therapy, *Acta Obstet Gynecol Scand* 53:371, 1976.
9. Aitken RJ et al: Influence of antisperm antibodies on human sperm function, *Br J Urol* 62:367-373, 1988.
10. Alexander NJ: Treatment for antisperm antibodies: voodoo or victory? *Fertil Steril* 53:602-603, 1990.
11. Alexander NJ, Sampson JH, Fulgham DL: Pregnancy rates in patients treated for antisperm antibodies with prednisone, *Int J Fertil* 28:63-67, 1983.
12. The American Fertility Society: Varicocele and infertility, Guideline for Practice, 1992.
13. Asch RH et al: Gamete intrafallopian transfer (GIFT): a new treatment for infertility, *Int J Fertil* 30:41-45, 1985.
14. Assisted reproductive technology in the United States and Canada: 1991 results from the Society for Assisted Reproductive Technology generated from the American Fertility Society Registry, *Fertil Steril* 59:956-962, 1993.
15. Aulitzky W, Frick J, Hadziselimovic F: Pulsatile LHRH therapy in patients with oligozoospermia and disturbed LH pulsatility, *Int J Androl* 12:265-272, 1989.
16. Baker HWG et al: Diagnosis of sperm defects in selecting patients for assisted fertilization, *Hum Reprod* 8:1779-1780, 1993.
17. Balasch J, Barri PN: Folicular stimulation and ovarian cancer? *Hum Reprod* 8:990-996, 1993.
18. Balasch J et al: The comparison of two gonadotropin-releasing hormone agonists in an in vitro fertilization program, *Fertil Steril* 58:991-994, 1992.
19. Balen AH, MacDougal J, Tan SL: The influence of the number of embryos transferred in 1060 in-vitro fertilization pregnancies on miscarriage rates and pregnancy outcome, *Hum Reprod* 8:1324-1328, 1993.
20. Balmaceda JP et al: Embryo implantation rates in oocyte donation: a prospective comparison of tubal versus uterine transfers, *Fertil Steril* 57:362, 1992.
21. Baranao RI et al: Predictive value of interleukin-1-β in supernatants of human embryo cultures. 48th Annual Meeting of the American Fertility Society, 1992 (abstract).
22. Barri PN et al: Indications for oocyte donation, *Hum Reprod* 7:85-88, 1992.
23. Benadiva CA et al: Comparison of different regimens of a gonadotropin-releasing hormone analog during ovarian stimulation for in vitro fertilization, *Fertil Steril* 53:479-485, 1990.
24. Benshushan A, Schenker JG: Reproductive health care policies around the world; ovum donation—an overview, *J Assist Reprod Genet* 10:105-111, 1993.
25. Berezin M et al: Successful GnRH treatment in a patient with Kallman's syndrome, who previously failed hMG/hCG treatment, *Andrologia* 20:285-288, 1988.
26. Berger GS, Goldstein M, Fuerst M, editors: *The couple's guide to infertility*, 1989, Doubleday.
27. Berkowitz RL et al: Selective reduction of multifetal pregnancies in the first trimester, *N Eng J Med* 318.1043, 1988.
28. Blankstein J et al: Ovarian hyperstimulation syndrome: prediction by number and size of preovulatory follicles, *Fertil Steril* 47:597, 1987.
29. Boeckx W et al: Reversibility after female sterilization, *Br J Obstet Gynaecol* 93:839-842, 1986.
30. Bollen N et al: The incidence of multiple pregnancy after in vitro fertilization and embryo transfer, gamete, or zygote intrafallopian transfer, *Fertil Steril* 55:314-318, 1991.
31. Bongso A et al: Improved pregnancy rate after transfer of embryos grown in human fallopian tubal cell coculture, *Fertil Steril* 52:503-508, 1989.
32. Brinsden PR, Rainsbury PA, editors: *A textbook of in vitro fertilization and assisted reproduction,* Lancs, 1992, Parthenon Publishing Group.
33. Brown JS: Varicocelectomy in the subfertile male: a ten year experience with 295 cases, *Fertil Steril* 27:1046-1053, 1976.
34. Bustillo M, Schulman JD: Transcervical ultrasound-guided intrafallopian replacement of gametes, zygotes, and embryos, *J In Vitro Fert Embryo Transf* 6:321, 1989.
35. Buttram VC, Reiter RC: Uterine leiomyomata: etiology, symptomatology, and management, *Fertil Steril* 36:433-445, 1981.
36. Candiani GB et al: Repair of the uterine cavity after hysteroscopic septal incision, *Fertil Steril* 54:991-994, 1990.
37. Capitanio L et al: Transcervical selective salpingography: a diagnostic and therapeutic approach to cases of proximal tubal injection failure, *Fertil Steril* 55:1045-1050, 1991.
38. Chang MC: Fertilization of rabbit ova in vitro, *Nature* 184:406, 1959.
39. Choe JK, Baggish MS: Hysteroscopic treatment of septate uterus with Neodymium-YAG laser, *Fertil Steril* 57:81-84, 1992.
40. Claman P, Seibel MM: Purified human follicle-stimulating hormone for ovulation induction: a critical review, *Semin Reprod Endocrinol* 4:277, 1986.
41. Clark DA et al: Immunosuppressive activity in human in vitro fertilization (IVF) culture supernatants and prediction of the outcome of embryo transfer: a multicenter trial, *J In Vitro Fert Embryo Transf* 6:51-58, 1989.
42. Cohen J et al: Implantation of embryos after partial opening of oocyte zona pellucida to facilitate sperm penetration, *Lancet* 2:162, 1988.
43. Confino E et al: Transcervical balloon tuboplasty: a multicenter study, *JAMA* 264:2079-2082, 1990.
44. Corson SL, Brooks PG: Resectoscopic myomectomy, *Fertil Steril* 55:1041, 1991.
45. Coulam CB, Moore SB, O'Fallon W: Investigating unexplained infertility, *Am J Obstet Gynecol* 158:1374-1381, 1988.
46. Cummins JM et al: A formula for scoring human embryo growth rates in in vitro fertilization: its value in predicting pregnancy and in comparison with visual estimates of embryo quality, *J In Vitro Fert Embryo Transf* 3(5):284, 1986.
47. Daly DC: Current treatment strategies for luteal phase deficiency, *Clin Obstet Gynecol* 34:222-231, 1991.
48. Davis OK et al: The incidence of luteal phase defect in normal, fertile women, determined by serial endometrial biopsies, *Fertil Steril* 51:582, 1989.
49. DeCherney AH, Harris TC: The barren woman throughout history. In DeCherney AH, editor: *Reproductive failure*, New York, 1986, Churchill Livingstone.
50. DeCherney AH, Laufer N: The monitoring of ovulation induction using ultrasound and estrogen, *Clin Obstet Gynecol* 27:993, 1984.
51. DeLeon FD, Peters AJ: What's new in adhesion prevention? *Contemp Obstet Gynecol* 39:15-32, 1994.
52. Deligdish L, Lowenthal M: Endometrial changes associated with myomata of the uterus, *J Clin Pathol* 23:676-680, 1970.
53. Delvigne A et al: The ovarian hyperstimulation syndrome in invitro fertilization: a Belgian multicentric study. II. Multiple discriminant analysis for risk prediction, *Hum Reprod* 8:1361-1366, 1993.
54. Derman SG, Rehnstrom J, Neuwirth RS: The long-term effectiveness of hysteroscopic treatment of menorrhagia and leiomyomas, *Obstet Gynecol* 77:591, 1991.
55. DeVane GW, Guzick DS: Bromocriptine therapy in normoprolactinemic women with unexplained infertility and galactorrhea, *Fertil Steril* 46:1026, 1986.
56. Devroey P et al: Successful in vitro fertilisation and embryo transfer after treatment with recombinant human FSH, *Lancet* 339:1170, 1992 (letter).
57. Diaz S, Ortez ME, Croxatto HB: Studies on the duration of ovum transport by the human oviduct, *Am J Obstet Gynecol* 137:116, 1980.

58. Donderwinkel PFJ et al: Pregnancy after induction of ovulation with human recombinant FSH in polycystic ovary syndrome, *Lancet* 340:983, 1992 (letter).
59. Dor J et al: The relative success of gonadotropin-releasing hormone analogue, clomiphene citrate, and gonadotropin in 1099 cycles of in vitro fertilization, *Fertil Steril* 58:986-990, 1992.
60. Dor J et al: Cumulative conception rates following gonadotropin therapy, *Am J Obstet Gynecol* 136:102, 1980.
61. Drake TS, Tredway DR, Buchanan GC: Continued clinical experience with an increasing dosage regimen of clomiphene citrate administration, *Fertil Steril* 30:274, 1978.
62. El Danasouri I et al: Fluorescence staining of nuclear DNA facilitates accurate assessment of hamster egg penetration, *Fertil Steril* 57: April 1992 (suppl).
63. Engelmann UH et al: Vasectomy reversal in central Europe: results of questionnaire of urologists in Austria, Germany and Switzerland, *J Urol* 143:64-67, 1990.
64. Ezra Y, Simon A, Laufer N: Defective oocytes: a new subgroup of unexplained infertility, *Fertil Steril* 58:24-27, 1992.
65. Fayez JA, Mutie G, Schneider PJ: The diagnostic value of hysterosalpingography and hysteroscopy in infertility investigation, *Am J Obstet Gynecol* 156:558-560, 1987.
66. Fedele L et al: Buserelin acetate versus expectant management in the treatment of infertility associated with minimal or mild endometriosis: a randomized clinical trial, *Am J Obstet Gynecol* 166:1345-1350, 1992.
67. Ferrier A et al: Evaluation of leuprolide acetate and gonadotropins for in vitro fertilization or gamete intrafallopian transfer, *Fertil Steril* 54:90-95, 1990.
68. Fisch P et al: Unexplained infertility: evaluation of treatment with clomiphene citrate and human chorionic gonadotropin, *Fertil Steril* 51:828, 1989.
69. Fishel S, Symonds M, editors: *Gamete and embryo micromanipulation in human reproduction*, Boston, 1993, Little Brown.
70. Fluker MR, Zouves CG, Bebbington MW: A prospective randomized comparison of zygote intrafallopian transfer and in vitro fertilization-embryo transfer for nontubal factor infertility, *Fertil Steril* 60:515-519, 1993.
71. Forssman L: Distribution of blood flow in myomatous uteri as measured by ocally injected 133 xenon, *Acta Obstet Gynecol Scand* 55:101-104, 1976.
72. Franklin RR, Dukes CD: Antispermatozoal antibody and unexplained infertility, *Am J Obstet Gynecol* 89:6, 1964.
73. Freeman MR et al: Coculture of mouse embryos with cells isolated from the human ovarian follicle, oviduct, and uterine endometrium, *Fertil Steril* 59:138-142, 1993.
74. Friedman AJ, Juneau-Norcross M, Sedensky B: Antisperm antibody production following intrauterine insemination, *Hum Reprod* 6:1125-1128, 1991.
75. Gentile DP, Cockett AT: The effect of varicocelectomy on testicular volume in 89 infertile adult males with varicoceles, *Fertil Steril* 58:209-211, 1992.
76. Glazener CM et al: The value of artificial insemination with husband's semen in infertility due to failure of postcoital sperm-mucus penetration—controlled trial of treatment, *Br J Obstet Gynaecol* 94:774-778, 1987.
77. Golan A et al: Ovarian hyperstimulation syndrome: an update review, *Obstet Gynecol Surv* 44:430, 1989.
78. Gonen Y, Powell WA, Casper RF: Effect of follicular aspiration on hormonal parameters in patients undergoing ovarian stimulation, *Hum Reprod* 6:356-358, 1991.
79. Gross KM et al: Evidence for decreased luteinizing hormone-releasing hormone pulse frequency in men with selective elevations of follicle-stimulating hormone, *J Clin Endocrinol Metab* 60:197-202, 1985.
80. Gwatkin RB et al: Failed fertilization in human in vitro fertilization analyzed with the deoxyribonucleic acid-specific fluorochrome Hoechst 33342, *Am J Obstet Gynecol* 160:31-35, 1989.
81. Gysler M et al: A decade's experience with an individualized clomiphene treatment regimen including its effects on the postcoital test, *Fertil Steril* 37:161, 1982.
82. Haas GG Jr, D'Cruz OJ, Denum B: Effect of repeated washing on sperm-bound immunoglobulin G, *J Androl* 9:190, 1988.
83. Hammond MG: Monitoring techniques for improved pregnancy rates with clomiphene ovulation induction, *Fertil Steril* 42:499, 1984.
84. Hammond MG, Halme JK, Talbert LM: Factors affecting the pregnancy rate in clomiphene citrate induction of ovulation, *Obstet Gynecol* 62:196, 1983.
85. Hamori M et al: Zygote intrafallopian transfer (ZIFT): evaluation of 42 cases, *Fertil Steril* 50:519, 1988.
86. Handyside AH: Biopsy of human cleavage stage embryos and sexing by DNA amplification. In Verlinsky Y, Kuliev A, editors: *Preimplantation genetics*, New York, 1991, Plenum Press.
87. Handyside AH, Delhanty JDA: Cleavage stage biopsy of human embryos and diagnosis of X chromosome-linked recessive disease. In Edwards RG, editor: *Preconception and preimplantation diagnosis of human genetic disease*, Cambridge, 1993, Cambridge University Press.
88. Handyside AH et al: Pregnancy from biopsied human preimplantation embryos sexed by specific DNA amplification, *Nature* 344:768-770, 1990.
89. Handyside AH et al: Birth of a normal girl after in vitro fertilization and preimplantation diagnostic testing for cystic fibrosis, *N Engl J Med* 327:905-909, 1992.
90. Hardy K et al: Noninvasive measurement of glucose and pyruvate uptake by individual human oocytes and preimplantation embryos, *Hum Reprod* 4:188-191, 1989.
91. Hardy RI, Anderson DJ, Hill JA: Assessment of pregnancy outcome by the measurement of interleukin-1-alpha in preimplantation culture media, American Fertility Society Annual Meeting, Montreal 1993 (abstract).
92. Hardy RI, Biggers JD, Golan DE: Use of NADH laser fluorimetry for the metabolic assessment of oocyte and embryo quality. Society of Gynecologic Investigations, Annual Meeting, Chicago, 1994 (abstract).
93. Hardy RI et al: Assessment of oocyte and embryo quality by the measurement of progesterone in preimplantation culture media, Society of Gynecologic Investigations, Toronto 1993 (abstract).
94. Hardy RI et al: Does morphologic assessment of the human embryo predict embryo quality and pregnancy outcome? American Fertility Society Annual Meeting, Montreal 1993 (abstract).
95. Hardy RI et al: Decreased recovery time after embryo transfer does not affect pregnancy outcome, Society of Gynecologic Investigations, Chicago, 1994 (abstract).
96. Heap W: Preliminary note on the transplantation and growth of mammalian ova within a uterine foster mother, *Proc R Soc* 48:457-458, 1891.
97. Henderson SR: The reversibility of female sterilization with the use of microsurgery: a report on 102 patients with more than one year of follow-up, *Am J Obstet Gynecol* 149:57-65, 1984.
98. Hirvonen E, Ranta T, Sepp M: Prolactin stimulates clomiphene responsiveness, *Int J Fertil* 21:255, 1976.
99. Hoffman D, Lobo RA: Serum dehydroepiandrosterone sulfate and the use of clomiphene citrate in anovulatory women, *Fertil Steril* 43:196, 1985.
100. Homberg R et al: One hundred pregnancies after treatment with pulsatile luteinizing hormone-releasing hormone to induce ovulation, *B M J* 298:809, 1989.
101. Horne HW et al: The prevention of postoperative pelvic adhesions following conservative operative treatment for human infertility, *Int J Fertil* 18:109, 1973.

102. Hornstein MD et al: The effects of baseline ovarian cysts on the clinical response to controlled ovarian hyperstimulation in an in vitro fertilization program, *Fertil Steril* 52:437-440, 1989.
103. Hornstein MD et al: The effect of consecutive day inseminations on semen characteristics in an intrauterine insemination program, *Fertil Steril* 58:433-435, 1992.
104. Hovatta OL: Artificial insemination—where do we stand now? *Ann Med* 24:79-80, 1992.
105. Howe RS et al: Pelvic infection after transvaginal ultrasound guided ovum retrieval, *Fertil Steril* 49:726, 1988.
106. Hricak H: Current trends in MR imaging of the female pelvis, *Radiographics* 13:913-919, 1993.
107. Hughes EG et al: The routine use of gonadotropin-releasing hormone agonists prior to in vitro fertilization and gamete intrafallopian transfer: a meta-analysis of randomized controlled trials, *Fertil Steril* 58:888-896, 1992.
108. Hulka JF, Halme J: Sterilization reversal: results of 101 attempts, *Am J Obstet Gynecol* 159:767-774, 1988.
109. Hunt JE, Wallach EE: Uterine factors in infertility: an overview, *Clin Obstet Gynecol* 17:44-64, 1974.
110. Hurd WW et al: Comparison of intracervical, intrauterine, and intratubal techniques for donor insemination, *Fertil Steril* 59:339-342, 1993.
111. Ibrahim ME, Moussa MA, Pedersen H: Efficacy of zona-free hamster egg sperm penetration assay as a predictor of in vitro fertilization, *Arch Androl* 23:267-274, 1989.
112. Iffland CA et al: A within-patient comparison between superovulation with intrauterine artificial insemination using husband's washed spermatozoa and gamete intrafallopian transfer in unexplained infertility, *Eur J Obstet Gynecol Reprod Biol* 39:181-186, 1991.
113. Jansen PPS: Early laparoscopy after pelvic operations to prevent adhesions: safety and efficacy, *Fertil Steril* 49:26, 1988.
114. Jansen PPS et al: Pulsatile intravenous gonadotropin-releasing hormone for ovulation induction. I. Safety and effectiveness with outpatient therapy, *Fertil Steril* 48:33, 1987.
115. Johnson LA, Flook JP, Look MV: Flow cystometry of X and Y chromosome-bearing sperm for DNA using an improved preparation method and staining with Hoechst 33342, *Gamete Res* 17:203-212, 1987.
116. Johnson LA et al: Gender selection in humans? Flow cystometric separation of X and Y sperm for the prevention of X-linked diseases, *Hum Reprod* 8:1733-1739, 1993.
117. Jones GES: Some newer aspects of the management of infertility, *JAMA* 141:1123, 1949.
118. Jones GS et al: Pathophysiology of reproductive failure after clomiphene induced ovulation, *Am J Obstet Gynecol* 108:847, 1970.
119. Jones HW Jr: Indications for in vitro fertilization. In Jones HW et al, editors: *In vitro fertilization*, Baltimore, 1986, Williams & Wilkins.
120. Jones HW Jr, Rock JA: Regulation of female infertility. In Diczfalusy E, editor: *Regulation of human fertility*, WHO Symposium, Scriptor, Moscow, 1977.
121. Kahn JA et al: Fallopian tube sperm perfusion (FSP) versus intrauterine insemination (IUI) in the treatment of unexplained infertility: a prospective randomized study, *Hum Reprod* 8:890-894, 1993.
122. Kahn JA et al: Treatment of unexplained infertility: fallopian tube sperm perfusion (FSP), *Acta Obstet Gynecol Scand* 72:193-199, 1993.
123. Katayose H, Matsuda J, Yanagimachi R: The ability of dehydrated hamster and human sperm nuclei to develop into pronuclei, *Biol Reprod* 47:277-284, 1992.
124. Kerin JF et al: Evidence for a hypothalamic site of action of clomiphene citrate in women, *J Clin Endocinol Metab* 61:265, 1985.
125. Kerin JF et al: Falloposcopic classification and treatment of fallopian tube lumen disease, *Fertil Steril* 57:731-741, 1992a.
126. Kerin JF: Nonhysteroscopic falloposcopy: a proposed method for visual guidance and verification of tubal cannula placement for endotuboplasty, gamete and embryo transfer procedures, *Fertil Steril* 57:1133, 1992b.
127. Kletzky OA, Vermesh M: Effectiveness of vaginal bromocriptine in treating women with hyperprolactinemia, *Fertil Steril* 51:269, 1989.
128. Klock SC, Maier D: Psychological factors related to donor insemination, *Fertil Steril* 56:489-495, 1991.
129. Knutzen V, Stratton CJ, Sher G: Mock embryo transfer in early luteal phase, the cycle before in vitro fertilization and embryo transfer, a descriptive study, *Fertil Steril* 57:156, 1992.
130. Lejeune B et al: Use of buserelin acetate in an in vitro fertilzation program: a comparison with classical clomiphene citrate-human menopausal gonadotropin therapy, *Fertil Steril* 54:475-481, 1990.
131. Lesec G et al: In-vivo transperitoneal fertilization. *Hum Reprod* 4:521-526, 1989.
132. Lev-Toaff HS et al: Leiomyomas in pregnancy: sonographic study, *Radiology* 164:375-380, 1987.
133. Levy MJ, Gindoff MD: Who benefits most from natural cycle IVF? *Contemp Obstet Gynecol* 39(2):11-23,1994.
134. Lewin A et al: Ultrasonically guided oocyte collection under local anesthesia: the first choice method for in vitro fertilization—a comparative study with laparoscopy, *Fertil Steril* 46:257, 1986.
135. Leyendecker G, Wildtu L, Hausmann M: Pregnancies following chronic intermittent (pulsatile) administration of GnRH by means of a portable pump (Zyklomat): a new approach in the treatment of infertility in hypothalamic amenorrhea, *J Clin Endocrinol Metab* 51:1214, 1980.
136. Lisse K, Syndow P: Fallopian tube catheterization recanalization under ultrasonic observation: a simplified technique to evaluate tubal patency and open proximally obstructed tubes, *Fertil Steril* 56:198-201, 1991.
137. Liu DY et al: A human sperm-zona pellucida binding test using oocytes that failed to fertilize in vitro, *Fertil Steril* 50:782-788, 1988.
138. Lobo RA, Paul W, March CM et al: Clomiphene and dexamethasone in women unresponsive to clomiphene alone, *Obstet Gynecol* 60:497, 1982.
139. Luciano AA et al: A comparative study of postoperative adhesions following laser surgery by laparoscopy versus laparotomy in the rabbit model, *Obstet Gynecol* 74:220, 1989.
140. Lunenfeld B, Insler V: Classification of amenorrheic states and their treatment by ovulation induction, *Clin Endocrinol* 3:223, 1974.
141. Lutjen PJ et al: The establishment and maintenance of pregnancy using in vitro fertilization and embryo donation in a patient with primary ovarian failure, *Nature* 307:174, 1984.
142. March CM: Improved pregnancy rate with monitoring of gonadotropin therapy by three modalities, *Am J Obstet Gynecol* 156:1473, 1987.
143. March CM: The surgical membrane study group: prophylaxis of pelvic sidewall adhesions with Gore-Tex surgical membrane: a multicenter clinical investigation. *Fertil Steril* 57:921, 1992.
144. March CM, Israel R, March AD: Hysterosocopic management of intrauterine adhesions, *Am J Obstet Gynecol* 130:653-657, 1978.
145. Margalloth EJ et al: Intrauterine insemination as treatment for antisperm antibodies in the female, *Fertil Steril* 50:441-446, 1988.
146. Marmar JL et al: Microsurgical aspiration of sperm from the epididymis: a mobile program, *J Urol* 149:1368-1373, 1993.
147. Marrs RP, Saito H, Yee B: Effect of variation of in vitro culture techniques upon oocyte fertilization-embryo development in human in vitro procedures, *Fertil Steril* 41:519, 1984.
148. Matsumoto AM et al: The luteinizing hormone-releasing hormone pulse generator in men: abnormalities and clinical management, *Am J Obstet Gynecol* 163:1743-1752, 1990.
149. McLaren A, Biggers JD: Successful development and birth of mice cultivated in vitro as early embryos, *Nature* 182:997-998, 1958.

150. Medical Research International: In vitro fertilization/embryo transfer in the United States: 1985 and 1986 results from the National IVF-ET Registry, *Fertil Steril* 49:212, 1988.
151. Medical Research International: In vitro fertilization/embryo transfer in the Unites States: 1987 results from the National IVF-ET Registry, *Fertil Steril* 51:13, 1989.
152. Meldrum DR et al: Evolution of a highly successful in vitro fertilization-n-embryo transfer program, *Fertil Steril* 48:86, 1987.
153. Menezo Y et al: Coculture of embryos on vero cells and transfer of blastocysts in humans, *Hum Reprod* 7:101-106,1992.
154. Menezo Y, Guerin JF, Czyba JC: Improvement of human early embryo development in vitro by coculture on monolayers of Vero cells, *Biol Reprod* 42:301-306, 1990.
155. Milki AA et al: Local anesthesia with conscious sedation for laparoscopic intrafallopian transfer, *Fertil Steril* 58:1240-1242, 1992.
156. Mohr LR, Trounson AO: The use of fluorescein diacetate to assess embryo viability in the mouse, *J Reprod Fertil* 58:189, 1980.
157. Mortimer D, Mortimer ST: Methods of sperm preparation for assisted reproduction, *Ann Acad Med Singapore* 21:517-524, 1992.
158. Muasher SJ: Use of gonadotrophin-releasing hormone agonists in controlled ovarian hyperstimulation for in vitro fertilization, *Clin Ther* 14 Suppl A:74-86, 1992.
159. Muram D, Gillieson MS, Walters JH: Myomas of the uterus and pregnancy: ultrasonographic follow-up, *Am J Obstet Gynecol* 138:16-19, 1980.
160. Murdoch AP et al: Gamete intrafallopian transfer (GIFT) compared with intrauterine insemination in the treatment of unexplained infertility, *Br J Obstet Gynaecol* 98:1107-1111, 1991.
161. Nachtigall RD: Secrecy: an unresolved issue in the practice of donor insemination, *Am J Obstet Gynecol* 168:1846-1849, 1993.
162. Nakamura K et al: Menotropin stimulation after prolonged gonadotropin releasing hormone agonist pretreatment for in vitro fertilization in patients with endometriosis, *J Assist Reprod Genet* 9:113-117, 1992.
163. Navot D et al: The concept of uterine preservation with ovarian malignancies, *Obstet Gynecol* 78:566-568, 1991.
164. Navot D et al: Risk factors and prognostic variable in the ovarian hyperstimulation syndrome, *Am J Obstet Gynecol* 159:210, 1988.
165. Newton R, Schinfeld JS, Schiff I: The effect of varicocelectomy on sperm count, motility, and conception rate, *Fertil Steril* 34:250-254, 1980.
166. Ng SC, Bongso A, Ratnam SS: Pregnancy after transfer of multiple sperm under the zona, *Lancet* 2:790, 1988.
167. Novy MJ et al: Diagnosis of cornual obstruction by transcervical fallopian tube cannulation, *Fertil Steril* 50:434-440, 1988.
168. O'Herlihy C, Pepperell RJ, Robinson HP: Ultrasound timing of human chorionic gonadotropin administration on clomiphene stimulated cycles, *Obstet Gynecol* 59:40, 1982.
169. Olive DL: The prevalence and epidemiology of luteal-phase deficiency in normal and infertile women, *Clin Obstet Gynecol* 34:156-166, 1991.
170. Olive DL, Haney AF: Endometriosis-associated infertility: a critical review of therapeutic approaches, *Obstet Gynecol Surv* 41:538-555, 1986.
171. Olive DL, Lee KL: Analysis of sequential treatment protocols for endometriosis associated infertility, *Am J Obstet Gynecol* 154:613, 1986.
172. Padilla SL, Garcia JE: Effect of maternal age and number of in vitro fertilization procedures on pregnancy outcome, *Fertil Steril* 52:270-273, 1989.
173. Padilla SL et al: The efficacy of bromocriptine in patients with ovulatory dysfunction and normoprolactinemic glactorrhea, *Fertil Steril* 44:695, 1985.
174. Pagidas K, Tulandi T: Effects of Ringer's lactate, Interceed (TC-7), and Gore-Tex surgical membrane on postsurgical adhesion formation, *Fertil Steril* 57:199, 1992.
175. Palermo G et al: Pregnancies after intracytoplasmic injection of single spermatozoon into an oocyte, *Lancet* 34:17-18, 1992.
176. Pantaleoni D: An endoscopic examination of the cavity of the womb, *Med Press Circ* 8:26, 1869.
177. Parinaud J et al: Randomized trial of three luteinizing hormone-releasing hormone analogues used for ovarian stimulation in an in vitro fertilization program, *Fertil Steril* 57:1265-1268, 1992.
178. Patton GW: Pregnancy outcome following microsurgical fimbrioplasty, *Fertil Steril* 37:150-155, 1982.
179. Patton PE, Hickok LR, Wolf DP: Successful hysteroscopic cannulation and tubal transfer of cryopreserved embryos, *Fertil Steril* 55:640, 1991.
180. Patton PE, Williams TJ, Coulam CB: Microsurgical reconstruction of the proximal oviduct, *Fertil Steril* 47:35-39, 1987a.
181. Patton PE, Williams TJ, Coulam CB: Results of microsurgical reconstruction in patients with combined proximal and distal tubal occlusion: double obstruction, *Fertil Steril* 48:670-674, 1987b.
182. Paulson DF, Wacksman J: Clomiphene citrate in the management of male infertility, *J Urol* 115:73-76, 1976.
183. Paulson RJ: Value of myomectomy in the treatment of infertility, *Fertil Steril* 59:1332, 1993.
184. Paulson RJ et al: In vitro fertilization in unstimualted cycles: a clinical trial using hCG for timing of follicular aspiration, *Obstet Gynecol* 76:788, 1990.
185. Penzias AS et al: Nafarelin versus leuprolide in ovulation induction for in vitro fertilization: a randomized clinical trial, *Obstet Gynecol* 79:739-742, 1992.
186. Phipps WR, Benson CB, McShane PM: Severe thigh myositis following intramuscular progesterone injections in an in vitro fertilization patient, *Fertil Steril* 49:536-537, 1988.
187. Platia MP, Krudy AG: Transvaginal fluoroscopic recanalization of a proximally occluded oviduct, *Fertil Steril* 44:704-706, 1985.
188. Quagliarello J, Weiss G: Addition of estradiol benzoate to Clomid in the management of Clomid failures. *Fertil Steril* 31:224, 1979.
189. Rageth JC et al: Long-term results of varicocelectomy, *Urol Int* 48:327-331, 1992.
190. Rein MS, DiSalvo D, Friedman AJ: Heterotopic pregnancy associated with in vitro fertilization and embryo transfer: a possible role for routine vaginal ultrasound, *Fertil Steril* 51:1057-1058.
191. Remorgida V et al: Comparison of different ovarian stimulation protocols for gamete intrafallopian transfer in patients with minimal and mild endometriosis, *Fertil Steril* 53:1060-1063, 1990.
192. Risquez F, Confino E: Transcervical tubal cannulation, past, present, and future, *Fertil Steril* 60:211-226, 1993.
193. Ritchie WGM: Ultrasound in the evaluation of normal and induced ovulation, *Fertil Steril* 43:167, 1985.
194. Robinson JN et al: A controlled study to assess the use of in vitro fertilization with donor semen after failed therapeutic donor insemination, *Fertil Steril* 59:353-358, 1993.
195. Rock JA et al: Tubal anastomosis: pregnancy success following reversal of Falope ring or monopolar cautery sterilization, *Fertil Steril* 48:13-17, 1987.
196. Rock J, Menkin MF: In vitro fertilization and cleavage of human ovarian eggs, *Science* 100:105, 1944.
197. San Roman GA et al: A prospective randomized comparison of luteal phase versus concurrent follicular phase initiation of gonadotropin-releasing hormone agonist for in vitro fertilization, *Fertil Steril* 58:744-749, 1992.
198. Santoro N et al: Intravenous administration of pulsatile gonadotropin-releasing hormone in hypothalamic amenorrhea: effects of dosage, *J Clin Endocrinol Metab* 62:109, 1986.
199. Sauer MV, Paulson RJ: Repeat trials of oocyte donation to women with previous donor oocyte successes, *Hum Reprod* 8:1851-1853, 1993.
200. Schulman JD et al: Outpatient in vitro fertilization using transvaginal ultrasound guided oocyte retrieval, *Obstet Gynecol* 69:665, 1987.

201. Shanis B et al: Adverse effect of clomiphene citrate on sperm morphology, *Arch Androl* 27:109-111, 1991.
202. Sharlip ID: What is the best pregnancy rate that may be expected from vasectomy reversal? *J Urol* 149:1469-1471, 1993.
203. Shaw JM et al: An association between chromosomal abnormalities in rapidly frozen 2-cell mouse embryos and the ice-forming properties of the cryoprotective solution, *J Reprod Fertil* 91:9, 1991.
204. Shenfield F et al: Effects of age, gravidity and male infertility status on cumulative conception rates following artificial insemination with cryopreserved donor semen: analysis of 2998 cycles of treatment in one centre over 10 years, *Hum Reprod* 8:60-64, 1993.
205. Siegler AM, Kontopoulos V, Wang CF: Prevention of postoperative adhesions in rabbits with ibuprofen, a nonsteroidal antiinflammatory agent, *Fertil Steril* 34:46, 1980.
206. Silverberg KM et al: A prospective, randomized trial comparing two different intrauterine insemination regimens in controlled ovarian hyperstimulation cycles, *Fertil Steril* 57:357-361, 1992.
207. Simon A et al: The value of menotrophin treatment for unexplained infertility prior to an in-vitro fertilization attempt, *Hum Reprod* 6:222-226, 1991.
208. Simon JA et al: The absorption of oral micronized progesterone: the effect of food, dose proportionality, and comparison with intramuscular progesterone, *Fertil Steril* 60:26-33, 1993.
209. Smitz J et al: A prospective randomized comparison of intramuscular or intravaginal natural progesterone as a luteal phase and early pregnancy supplement, *Hum Reprod* 7:168-175, 1992.
210. Sokol RZ et al: A controlled comparison of the efficacy of clomiphene citrate in male infertility, *Fertil Steril* 49:865-870, 1988.
211. Soto-Albers CE et al: Titrating the dose of bromocriptine when treating hyperprolactinemic women, *Fertil Steril* 43:485, 1985.
212. Steckel J, Dicker AP, Goldstein M: Relationship between varicocele size and response to varicocelectomy, *J Urol* 149:769-771, 1993.
213. Steptoe PC, Edwards RG: Birth after reimplantation of a human embryo, *Lancet* 2:366, 1978.
214. Subak LL, Adamson GD, Boltz NL: Therapeutic donor insemination: a prospective randomized trial of fresh versus frozen sperm, *Am J Obstet Gynecol* 166:1597-1604, 1992.
215. Suginami H et al: Ovulation induction with bromocriptine in normoprolactinemic anovulatory women, *J Clin Endocrinol Metab* 62:899, 1986.
216. Swolin K: Die einwirkung von grossen, intraperitonealen dosen glukokorticoid auf die bildung von postoperativen adhasionen, *Acta Obstet Gynecol Scand* 46:204, 1967.
217. Tan SL et al: The long protocol of administration of gonadotropin-releasing hormone agonist is superior to the short protocol for ovarian stimulation for in vitro fertilization, *Fertil Steril* 57:810-814, 1992.
218. Tarin JJ et al: Failed in vitro fertilization of human oocytes: a cytogenetic analysis, *Fertil Steril* 56:290-295, 1991.
219. Thurmond A, Rosch J: Nonsurgical fallopian tube recanalization for treatment of infertility, *Radiology* 174:572-3, 1990.
220. Tournaye H et al: Zygote intrafallopian transfer or in vitro fertilization and embryo transfer for the treatment of male-factor infertility: a prospective randomized trial, *Fertil Steril* 58:344-350, 1992.
221. Trounson A: Preservation of human eggs and embryos, *Fertil Steril* 46:1, 1986.
222. Tucker MJ et al: Treatment of male infertility and idiopathic failure to fertilize in vitro with under zona insemination and direct egg injection, *Am J Obstet Gynecol* 169(13):324-332, 1993.
223. Tulandi T et al: Treatment-dependent and treatment-independent pregnancy among women with periadnexal adhesions, *Am J Obstet Gynecol* 162:354-357, 1990.
224. Tulandi T, Murray C, Guralnick M: Adhesion formation and reproductive outcome after myomectomy and second-look laparoscopy, *Obstet Gynecol* 82:213-215, 1993.
225. Valle RF, Sciarra JJ: Intrauterine adhesions: hysteroscopic diagnosis, classification, treatment and reproductive outcome, *Am J Obstet Gynecol* 158:1459-1470, 1988.
226. Van Blerkom J: The origin and detection of chromosomal abnormalities in meiotically mature human oocytes obtained from stimulated follicles and after failed fertilization in vitro, *Prog Clin Biol Res* 296:299-310, 1989.
227. Van de Berk D, Wijnberg M, Van Dop PA: Initiation of spermatogenesis and successful in vitro fertilization in an infertile male with panhypopituitarism; superiority of pulsatile LH-RH over gonadotropins? a case report, *Eur J Obstet Gynecol Reprod Biol* 40:153-157, 1991.
228. Van Steirteghem AC et al: Intracytoplasmic sperm injection (ICSI). Presented at the annual meeting of the American Fertility Society, Montreal, 1993 (abstract).
229. Vargyas J, Kletzky O, Marrs RP: The effect of laparoscopic follicular aspiration on ovarian steroidogenesis during the early preimplantation period, *Fertil Steril* 45:221, 1986.
230. Vercellini P et al: Value of intrauterine device insertion and estrogen administration after hysteroscopic metroplasty, *J Reprod Med* 34:447, 1989.
231. Verkauf BS: Myomectomy for fertility enhancement and preservation, *Fertil Steril* 58:1-15, 1992.
232. Von Campenhout J, Semard R, Liduc B: The antiestrogenic effect of clomiphene in the human being, *Fertil Steril* 19:700, 1968.
233. Warnes GM et al: The effect of transferring pronuclear embryos on pregnancy outcome after in vitro fertilization, *Ann N Y Acad Sci* 541:465, 1988.
234. Weimer KE et al: Coculture of human zygotes on fetal bovine uterine fibroblasts: embryonic morphology and implantation, *Fertil Steril* 52:503-508, 1989.
235. Whamsby H, Fredga K, Liedholm P: Chromosome analysis of human oocytes recovered from preovulatory follicle and stimulated cycle, *N Engl J Med* 316:121, 1987.
236. Whittemore AS, Harris R, Itnyre J: Collaborative Ovarian Cancer Group: Characteristics relating to ovarian cancer risk: collaborative analysis of twelve U.S. case-control studies. II. Invasive epithelial ovarian cancers in white women, *Am J Epidemiol* 136:1184-1203, 1992.
237. Woodward PJ, Wagner BJ, Farley TE: MR imaging in the evaluation of female infertility, *Radiographics* 13:293-310, 1993.
238. World Health Organization: A double-blind trial of clomiphene citrate for the treatment of idiopathic male infertility, *Int J Androl* 15:299-307, 1992.
239. Wu CH, Winkel CA: The effect of therapy initiation day on clomiphene citrate therapy, *Fertil Steril* 52:564, 1989.
240. Yovich JL: Pentoxifylline: actions and applications in assisted reproduction, *Hum Reprod* 8:1786-1791, 1993.
241. Yovich JL et al: Pregnancies following pronuclear stage tubal transfer, *Fertil Steril* 48:851, 1987.
242. Zbella EA, Tarantino S, Wade R: Intrafollicular insemination for male factor infertility, *Fertil Steril* 58:442-443, 1992.
243. Zikopoulos K et al: Homologous intrauterine insemination has no advantage over timed natural intercourse when used in combination with ovulation induction for the treatment of unexplained infertility, *Hum Reprod* 8:563-567, 1993.

Chapter 14

SPORADIC AND RECURRENT SPONTANEOUS ABORTION

Joseph A. Hill

SPORADIC SPONTANEOUS ABORTION

Spontaneous abortion is the most common complication of pregnancy and causes significant emotional distress to couples who desire to have children. Human pregnancy is an inefficient process since 70% to 80% of pregnancies fail to achieve viability and an estimated 50% of pregnancies are lost before the first missed menses.[452,566] Spontaneous abortion is classically defined as a clinically recognized pregnancy loss (by blood test or ultrasonography) before 20 weeks' gestation and is estimated to occur in 10% to 15% of pregnancies.[9,570] Hertig et al were the first to suggest that the actual incidence of pregnancy loss is much higher than clinically observed.[221] In their classic morphologic study of preimplantation embryos obtained at the time of hysterectomy, only 24 of 34 embryos were observed to be normal.[221] Using sensitive assays for human chorionic gonadotropin (hCG), recent studies indicate that the postimplantation pregnancy loss rate is 30% to 40%.[151,356,573] The majority of these cases are believed to be due to chromosomal or other genetic etiologies. Aneuploidic conceptions were reported in 60% of abortuses that were lost before 8 weeks of gestation.[65] Trisomies are the most common anomaly encountered in karyotyped spontaneous abortions. Trisomy 16 comprises nearly one third of all chromosomal abnormalities encountered in early pregnancy.[522] However, the most common single-chromosome abnormality is monosomy X, 45 X (Table 14-1). Confined placental mosaicism may also result in spontaneous abortion.[286]

Spontaneous abortion can be classified as threatened abortion, inevitable abortion, incomplete abortion, complete abortion, missed abortion, and recurrent abortion. Threatened abortion refers to an intrauterine, viable, clinical pregnancy accompanied by an intrauterine source of vaginal bleeding. A subchorionic hematoma caused by partial placental abruption is often the source of bleeding. A subchorionic hematoma, however, is not necessarily associated with ultimate pregnancy loss.[138] A diagnosis of an inevitable abortion is given in the case of vaginal bleeding through a dilated internal cervical os, especially when accompanied by leaking amniotic fluid caused by ruptured membranes. An incomplete abortion is when some but not all of the fetal/decidual tissue has passed through the cervical os. A missed abortion is an early (before 20 weeks of gestation) intrauterine fetal demise, in the absence of vaginal bleeding. Symptoms of pregnancy such as nausea, breast tenderness, and tiredness may or may not be present at the time of pregnancy loss. Pelvic and ultrasound examination will usually lead to the proper diagnosis. The doubling of β-hCG beta subunit levels every 48 to 72 hours is often but not always a diagnostically useful finding.[308] Significant differences in hormonal (e.g., estriol, β-hCG) profiles of chromosomally normal and abnormal pregnancies were reported to help differentiate between pregnancy success and failure.[508]

A "blighted" ovum is also an example of a missed abortion. The term blighted ovum should be discarded; a more precise term is aembryonic pregnancy. Such a pregnancy is a gestation in which embryo development does not occur with or without evidence of early normal trophoblast growth and function as indicated by adequately rising β-hCG subunit levels. The diagnosis of an aembryonic pregnancy is made when neither fetal heart nor fetal pole can be identified by ultrasonography at 6 weeks' gestation.[519] Many women are erroneously given the diagnosis of aembryonic

Table 14-1. Percentage of specific karyotype abnormalities in chromosomally abnormal abortuses

Karyotype	Aarhus Co.	Geneva	London	New York	Honolulu	Hiroshima
Trisomy (including mosaics)	47.9	58.6	53.0	43.2	44.5	55.3
Monosomy X	27.9	19.5	23.7	15.4	24.0	16.9
Triploid	10.0	9.8	12.9	15.7	15.6	20.3
Tetraploid	8.6	3.3	4.2	4.5	6.8	2.5
Structural Anomalies	2.1	5.1	3.1	2.9	3.9	1.3
Other	3.6	3.7	3.1	8.3	5.2	3.8
Number of Abnormal Karyotypes	140	215	287	312	308	237

From Warburton D et al: Chromosome abnormalities in spontaneous abortion. In Porter IH, Hook EB, editors: *Human embryonic and fetal death*, New York, 1980, Academic Press.

pregnancy, based on ultrasound findings after 6 weeks' gestation. While such a pregnancy may be aembryonic at the time of ultrasound screening, often fetal cardiac activity was present earlier in gestation; however, following its demise the fetal pole was reabsorbed. A true aembryonic pregnancy diagnosed at 6 weeks of gestation is often chromosomally abnormal, with the majority being trisomies; however, monosomy X also occurs.[249] Chromosomal abnormalities are more often found in pregnancies not achieving cardiac activity than in pregnancies with documentation of fetal cardiac activity, although these findings are controversial.[359,460]

RECURRENT SPONTANEOUS ABORTION

Recurrent abortion has been traditionally defined as the occurrence of three or more clinically recognized, spontaneous abortions with or without a prior live-born pregnancy and occurs in approximately 1 in 300 pregnancies.[9,151] This definition, however, should be changed to two consecutive pregnancy losses rather than three, to allow for a search for causation. This is especially important in cases where fetal cardiac activity is identified prior to a subsequent pregnancy loss in women older than 35 years of age, in couples having difficulty conceiving, and in couples anxious to initiate investigation.[35,149,311,529] Data derived from epidemiologic surveys indicate that the risk of subsequent abortion following one spontaneous abortion is 24%; after two, 30%; after three, 35%; and approximately 40% after four consecutive clinical pregnancy losses.[414,441,565] These reoccurrence risk data should be kept in mind when reviewing literature that claims potential success rates with various therapies.

Etiologic factors. Many potential etiologies have been proposed for recurrent pregnancy loss (Table 14-2). Recurrent spontaneous abortions within individuals tend to occur at the same developmental stage in consecutive pregnancies.[414] Chromosomal abnormalities can result in pregnancy loss throughout gestation. Hormonal insufficiency or excess generally results in pregnancy loss before 10 weeks' gestation. Infectious, immunologic, and environmental factors generally mediate first-trimester pregnancy loss but may be involved during any trimester of pregnancy. Anatomic factors are generally associated with second-trimester pregnancy loss, although first-trimester losses may also occur.

Genetic factors. The only uncontested cause of recurrent spontaneous abortion is a structural chromosome aberration in one or both partners of the couple who experience recurrent abortions.[140] A family history alone is not sufficient to rule out a potential chromosomal abnormality. Inborn chromosomal aberrations may be inherited or may arise de novo by spontaneous mutation during early embryonic development. Other genetic factors may involve unknown genes but remain uncharacterized.[504] Chromosomal abnormalities occur in 3% to 6% of couples who experience recurrent pregnancy loss.[208,239,298,531,543] The most common chromosomal abnormality that contributes to recurrent abortion is a balanced translocation which most often occurs in the female partner of the couple who have recurrent abortions.[125] Two thirds of translocations are reciprocal; one third are Robertsonian. A reciprocal, balanced translocation results from a crossover or break and exchange of chromatin between any two nonhomologous chromosomes during meiosis, without loss of genetic material. A Robertsonian translocation occurs from a crossover near the centromere, between specific chromosomes, and with the loss of one centromere and the two short arms of the involved chromosomes. This results in a balanced 45 chromosome state in which the involved chromosome contains the long arms of the two acrocentric chromosomes. Chromosomes 6,7,9,16, and 22 are most often involved in reciprocal translocations; chromosomes 13,14,15,21, and 22 in Robertsonian translocations.[100] In Robertsonian translocations, 58% involve the long arms of chromosomes 13 and 14 (13q 14q). Robertsonian translocations that involve homologous chromosomes always result in aneuploidic conceptions, either trisomies or monosomies. The risk of clinically detectable spontaneous abortion for couples with reciprocal translocations is estimated to be 50%, while that for couples where one of the partners is a carrier for a Robertsonian translocation is estimated to be less than 25%.[81,174,379] The chance of detecting a translocation is higher in couples who have not experienced a live birth, although a history of spontaneous abortions, interspersed with stillbirths and live births with or without congenital anomalies, may also yield parental chromosomal abnormalities upon karyotype analysis. Therefore, it is reasonable to ascertain whether potential chromosome abnormalities may be contributing to pregnancy loss in couples who have experienced two or more spontaneous abortions.

Uncharacterized sperm-selecting factors within the female reproductive tract are believed to account for the lower risk of chromosomal anomalies in the conceptus when there is a paternal karyotypic abnormality rather than when a similar maternal abnormality exists. This is because the risk of trisomy 21 at birth is only 2% to 3% with a paternal 14/21 translocation but 10% if this translocation is maternal in origin.[505] Other parental, structural chromosome anomalies may contribute to recurrent pregnancy loss including mosaicism, single gene defects, and inversion, especially of chromosome 14.[357] Inversion involving chromosome 9 frequently occurs in the general population and is considered to be a normal variant that is not necessarily associated with nor contributes to recurrent abortion.[131,165,284,339,394,400] This concept was challenged in the Japanese population where inversion of chromosome 9 was associated with recurrent abortion.[581] Single-gene disorders may be recognized either through an analysis of detailed family histories or by a particular pattern of anomalies that comprise a syndrome with a known inheritance pattern. Rarely, X-linked disorders may result in recurrent abortion of male but not female conceptions. Uniparental disomy for chromosome 16 may also result in intrauterine fetal demise and other adverse obstetrical outcomes.[287] Future studies using sophisticated molecular cytogenetic techniques may provide new insight into potential parental genetic abnormalities that contribute to recurrent spontaneous abortion.[303] Novel cytogenetic approaches in the investigation of recurrent abortion may also involve the analysis of potential chromosome aberrations in spermatozoa.[468]

Table 14-2. Proposed etiologies for recurrent spontaneous abortion

Etiology	Incidence
A. Genetic Factors	5%
Chromosomal	
Multifactorial	
B. Anatomic Factors	10%
1. Congenital	
a. Incomplete müllerian fusion or septum reabsorption	
b. DES exposure	
c. Uterine artery anomalies	
d. Cervical incompetence	
2. Acquired	
a. Cervical incompetence	
b. Synechiae	
c. Leiomyoma	
d. Endometriosis, adenomyosis	
C. Endocrine Factors	17%
1. Luteal phase insufficiency including LH disorders	
2. Thyroid disorders	
3. Diabetes mellitus	
4. Androgen disorders	
5. Prolactin disorders	
D. Infectious Factors	5%
1. Bacteria	
2. Viruses	
3. Parasites	
4. Zoonotic	
5. Fungal	
E. Immunologic Factors	60%
1. Humoral mechanisms	
a. Antiphospholipid antibodies	
b. Antisperm antibodies	
c. Antitrophoblast antibodies	
d. Blocking antibody deficiency	
2. Cellular mechanisms	
a. TH1 cellular immune response to reproductive antigens (embryo/trophoblast–toxic factors/cytokines)	
b. TH2 cytokine, growth factor and oncogene deficiency	
c. Suppressor cell and factor deficiency	
d. Major histocompatibility antigen expression	
F. Miscellaneous Factors	3%
1. Environmental	
2. Drugs	
3. Placental abnormalities	
a. Circumvallate	
b. Marginate	
4. Medical illnesses	
a. Cardiac	
b. Renal	
c. Hematological	
5. Male factors	
6. Dyssynchronous fertilization	
7. Coitus	
8. Exercise	

Anatomic factors. Anatomic factors are associated with recurrent pregnancy loss and are reported to occur in 10% to 15% of women who experience recurrent spontaneous abortion.[239,274,531,543] It is difficult to give a reliable incidence for any of the associated etiologies for recurrent abortion in the general population since all studies suffer from selection bias; however, the incidence of müllerian anomalies in the general population is reported to be 0.06% to 0.48%.[190] A study addressing hysteroscopic sterilization techniques reported a 6% incidence of uterine septum in those fertile women.[103] Association of any abnormality with recurrent abortion cannot be equated with causation; however, they should not be summarily dismissed as unimportant for there are many ways, both documented and theoretical, that anatomic factors may contribute to pregnancy failure.

Anatomic factors for abortion can be divided into both congenital and acquired lesions. The failure of müllerian duct fusion or incomplete caudal to cranial septum reabsorption results in congenital müllerian anomalies that have been associated with recurrent abortion.[79,191,204,216,274,372,508,584] The American Fertility Society classified these congenital müllerian anomalies into seven categories.[15] Of these seven abnormalities, a septate uterus and the diethylstilbestrol drug-related category are the most firmly associated with recurrent abortion.[15,79,219,220,293,350,366,455,486,528] These anomalies are generally associated with second-trimester pregnancy loss because of the limitation of space and an incompetent cervix.[43,52,78,188,487] An incompetent cervix may also result from previous cervical trauma or surgery.[75,266,312,343,348,493] Müllerian anomalies may be involved in first-trimester pregnancy loss caused by (1) a limitation of the blood supply to the affected areas, such as in the case of a uterine septum or (2) by the dyssynchronous hormonal responsiveness within decidual tissue that overlies a septum or other müllerian defects causing inadequate placentation.[78,295,363,528] Nondrug-related congenital müllerian anomalies may have polygenic or multifactorial inheritance patterns. Familial aggregates were reported and an autosomal recessive pattern has also been implicated.[561]

Anomalies of the uterine artery are proposed as a cause of recurrent abortion. Compromised blood flow to endometrial tissues, which results in dyssynchronous decidualization (inadequate hormonal responsiveness) and compromised placentation, is a potential consequence of uterine vascular anomalies. In a series by Burchell et al, the incidence of recurrent spontaneous abortion was greater in women found to have two ascending uterine arteries on each side than in women with a single ascending branch of the uterine artery.[77]

Acquired anatomic factors that potentially contribute to recurrent abortion include intrauterine synechiae (adhesions), leiomyomas, and endometriosis/adenomyosis. Intrauterine adhesions termed Asherman's syndrome are due to sequelae that follow an intrauterine infection or may be the iatrogenic result of prior uterine surgery or instrumentation.[5,30,417,431,479,489] A history of endometritis/salpingitis is associated with both intrauterine adhesions and spontaneous abortion.[217] Cause versus effect mechanisms are difficult to discern. One potential mechanism that remains speculative is adhesion formation which could interfere with normal decidualization and placentation.[164] In a combined series reported by Schenker and Margalioth, 40% of women with untreated Asherman's syndrome experienced abortion, but following correction the subsequent spontaneous abortion rate in these women decreased to 25%.[479]

A cause of anxiety for many women with recurrent abortion is whether a prior elective pregnancy termination could be a factor in subsequent reproductive difficulties. There is no correlation between induced first-trimester abortions and subsequent spontaneous loss.[95,122,207,300,559] The possibility remains that traumatic cervical dilation resulting in cervical laceration could cause cervical incompetence. Also postabortal endometritis could contribute to adhesion formation and later jeopardize subsequent pregnancy. Induced abortion by suction curettage is associated with placenta previa in subsequent pregnancies, although not all investigators substantiate this association.[44,193,541]

Uterine leiomyomas are associated with recurrent pregnancy loss. Cause versus effect mechanisms are difficult to ascribe as there are many women with leiomyomas who have successful pregnancies. Mechanical factors may contribute to abortion depending on the size, ectogenic structure, position, and location of the leiomyoma relative to the placenta.[155] Potential mechanisms of reproductive loss caused by uterine leiomyomas include a decreased blood supply resulting in congestion and venous dilation, dyssynchronous decidualization, disordered implantation/placentation, and increased uterine irritability causing contractions and expulsion of the uterine contents.[80,132,156,258,261,454] Cystine aminopeptidase, which is responsible for the inactivation of oxytocin, was reported to be decreased in women with leiomyomas and may serve as a mechanism for increased uterine irritability.[60] Leiomyoma degeneration could also increase uterine irritability and culminate in pregnancy loss.[399] Embryo implantation on submucous myomas may lead to pregnancy loss because of compromised placentation.[175] Placental abruption is also more common in women with large uterine leiomyomas.[449] Hormonal alterations induced by leiomyomas were also described and could contribute to reproductive failure.[517]

The association of endometriosis/adenomyosis and recurrent abortion is controversial. Many retrospective studies have claimed an association between endometriosis and spontaneous abortion, with 22% to 51% abortion rates in women before the diagnosis.[163,214,326,355,390,407,409,411,413] A causal relationship between endometriosis and spontaneous abortion should be cautiously appraised, since case-selection ascertainment bias renders interpretation of these data difficult. The abortion rates observed in women with endometriosis may be characteristic of women with subfertility and not necessarily unique to endometriosis.[412] Observations that the severity of endometriosis varies inversely with the risk of spontaneous abortion prompted the suggestion that the two could not be causally related.[572] Laboratory studies indicate that the numbers and concentrations of activated macrophages, T lymphocytes, and natural killer cells that are capable of secreting potentially reproductive toxic cytokines[226] are increased in women with minimal and mild endometriosis compared with women who have moderate or severe disease.[236] These data provide a potential immune mechanism for the observed inverse correlation between recurrent abortion and the stage of endometriosis.[572] Other potential mechanisms for endometriosis-associated abortion include increased prostaglandin production[143,365,558] causing uterine contractions and hormonal alterations of corpus luteum progesterone secretion.[412] Clinical research studies with well-selected control groups seriously challenge a causal relationship between endometriosis and recurrent spontaneous abortion.[177,259,391,459,499] The possibility remains that a subgroup of women with endometriosis may be affected. Whether abortion in these women is due to endometriosis itself or to indirect mechanisms through immune activation will require further study.

Adenomyosis, which is similar to endometriosis, is defined as the presence of endometrial glands and stroma within the myometrium. Adenomyosis may be associated with reproductive loss by the anatomic mechanisms previously discussed. Another potential mechanism for abortion may be the myoma-like distortions of adenomyosis which could impinge on decidualization through blood flow abnormalities and serve as foci for uterine irritability and placental abruption. These potential mechanisms remain speculative because definitive data are not available.

Published series indicate that the risk of spontaneous abortion increases after uterine and fallopian tube surgery.[263,499] Salpingostomy[126] and uterotubal implantation[117] are reported to have a higher incidence of subsequent abortion compared with other procedures. Potential mechanisms for this association are unknown, although the tubal isthmus is proposed to have a "gate keeper" function in sperm selection.[2] Following the adoption of microsurgical techniques, the increased risk of abortion (as seen in earlier studies) has not been observed.[136,264]

Endocrine factors. Endocrine factors areproposed to contribute to recurrent abortion in 10% to 20% of women who experience reproductive loss.[239,531,543] A smaller series of couples with recurrent abortion indicated that the incidence of luteal phase insufficiency may be as high as 50%.[38] In other studies, 17% of women with recurrent abortion were found to have a potential endocrine abnormality; the majority had luteal phase insufficiency.[239] Luteal phase insufficiency is classically defined as abnormal corpus luteum function with insufficient progesterone production.[271] Corpus luteum secretion of progesterone is critical for the survival of the pregnancy, until the luteoplacental shift occurs at 7 to 9 weeks' gestation.[119,120] The precise level of progesterone that is needed to achieve and maintain successful pregnancy is not known.[34] Luteal phase insufficiency has been traditionally characterized into short and inadequate luteal phase and involves hypothalamic-pituitary, ovarian, and endometrial defects.[272,511,513,515]

A short luteal phase is defined as less than 10 days without normal corpus luteum transformation from the ovulated follicle, despite an LH surge and progesterone production.[182,515] Inadequate or asynchronous FSH/LH secretion during the follicular phase with reduced estradiol 17 β production has been demonstrated in women with luteal phase deficiency[8,101] as diagnosed by endometrial histology.[383] Deficiency of low-density lipoprotein synthesis, which occurs in individuals with β lipoproteinemia or in low-density lipoprotein delivery to the corpus luteum, could result in decreased progesterone production and thus luteal phase insufficiency.[84] In rare cases, isolated progesterone-receptor defects in the endometrium may be a cause of luteal phase insufficiency.[295]

Recent evidence suggests that the preimplantation embryo may itself produce a gonadotropic stimulus to enhance ovarian steroid secretion.[526] An embryo's inability to produce such a stimulus or the ovary's inability to respond could be a factor in luteal phase insufficiency and pregnancy loss.

Abnormal maternal thyroid function has been implicated in recurrent abortion, with hypothyroidism being most commonly associated with pregnancy loss.[277,545] However, well-controlled, prospective studies that support this association are lacking. Similarly, there is no clear evidence in support of hyperthyroidism as a cause of abortion.[423,447] The potential mechanisms of abnormal thyroid-induced abortion are not clear. Thyroid-stimulating hormone (TSH) is very important in the normal embryonic development in amphibians,[309] which prompted speculation that dysfunction in TSH regulation during human embryogenesis may also contribute to pregnancy loss. An indirect association between antithyroid antibodies and trisomy 21 has been implicated in young women in their conceptions.[167] Increased antithyroid antibodies were also observed in women with a history of recurrent abortion.[520] The potential mechanisms for fetal loss in these individuals is unknown. Whether or not this associated phenomena is indicative of generalized autoimmunity in these women is also unknown.[186]

Diabetes mellitus has been historically associated with recurrent pregnancy loss.[361,535] This concept is controversial because of methodologic differences between the studies. Recent evidence suggests that when diabetes is well controlled, no increased incidence of abortion occurs.[137,186,288,361,535] Inadequate glucose control before conception and during early pregnancy, as evidenced by elevated glycosylated hemoglobin A1c levels, has been associated with subsequent abortion.[578] End-organ damage resulting from vascular complications of diabetes mellitus may be associated with an increased risk of abortion, especially in cases where compromised uterine blood flow leads to placental insufficiency.

Androgen disorders such as polycystic ovarian syndrome (PCOS) form another endocrine category of potential contributors to recurrent abortion.[1,41,242,269,474] A diagnosis of PCOS based on ultrasonography criteria has been reported in 44% to 82% of individuals with recurrent abortion.[474,553] PCOS is a polymorphic condition characterized by inappropriate LH secretion, either as chronic hypersecretion or as a premature surge.[582] Elevated serum LH concentrations have been associated with an increased risk of recurrent spontaneous abortion.[40,63,243,443,568] The mechanism of action for this effect may be due to the ovulation of a prematurely matured oocyte that is either unfertilizable, which leads to infertility,[63] or that when fertilized is prone to early loss.[40,243,443,568] It is possible that premature ovulating oocytes are more likely to result in chromosomal abnormalities caused by disorders in the resumption of meiosis. Unfortunately, karyotype analyses of abortuses that are presumably lost because of LH hypersecretion have not been reported. Another potential mechanism involved in LH hypersecretion that mediates spontaneous abortion is the oversecretion of androgens resulting in corpus luteum deficiency, endometrial asynchrony, and disordered estrogen secretion.[40] PCOS and hyperandrogenism are accompanied by hyperinsulinemia.[42] Insulin or insulin-like growth factors may contribute to reproductive loss through detrimental effects on the oocyte mediated through intraovarian receptors.[42,404] Disordered prostaglandin synthesis within the endometrium in women with PCOS may be yet another mechanism for abortion.[63] Therefore, abnormal LH secretion may mediate abortion directly on the developing oocyte and endometrium or indirectly through elevations in testosterone and estrogen.[568] Oligomenorrhea associated with isolated luteal-phase estradiol secretion has been reported to be predictive of recurrent abortion.[426] Studies addressing the association of LH hypersecretion in recurrent abortion are problematic because LH secretion is pulsatile. A single blood level that is either high or low may not reflect either the minute-to-minute or day-to-day variations that occur during the menstrual cycle.[162,511,513] More studies are needed in women with recurrent abortion and in women with normal pregnancies to produce definitive data.

The association between prolactin disorders and recurrent abortion is also controversial. Elevated levels of prolactin may interfere with normal gonadotropin secretion[556] and corpus luteum secretion,[4,349] which could result in luteal-phase insufficiency. Hyperprolactinemia and hypoprolactinemia have been associated with luteal-phase insufficiency[133,196] and recurrent pregnancy loss, although the correlation between prolactin disorders and luteal-phase defects has not been substantiated by all of the investigators.[23,538] Prolactin is also produced in human myometrial, endometrial, and decidual tissues.[187,336,450,564] Prolactin production may be mediated by insulin-like growth factors and involved in intrauterine fetal growth.[198,199,215,546] Theoretically if a critical level of endometrial or decidual prolactin is necessary for the maintenance of pregnancy, then perturbations in these levels that are either too high or too low may contribute to pregnancy loss. Uterine leiomyomas have been demonstrated to secrete prolactin.[124,336,564] Whether or not prolactin secretion by leiomyomas can disrupt the homeostatic mechanisms involved in maintaining the integrity of the maternal-fetal interface remains unknown. Recently a rare chromosome mosaicism that involves 6p23 deletion was reported in a women with idiopathic hypoprolactinemia and recurrent spontaneous abortion.[121]

Infectious factors. Infectious disease is a significant problem in maternal health. An estimated 5% of maternal deaths reported to the Centres for Disease Control are associated with recurrent spontaneous abortion.[56] Of these deaths, approximately one half are due to infection. Bacterial, viral, parasitic, fungal, and zoonotic infections are associated with recurrent abortion. The association of infection with recurrent abortion is among the most controversial and poorly explored potential etiologies for reproductive loss. In the largest and most recently published series on the etiology of recurrent abortion, a presumed infectious etiology was found in only 5% of individuals.[239] Before a cause and effect relationship between a particular organism and spontaneous abortion can be unequivocally established, the infectious agent must be documented in mother, placenta, and fetal tissue.[451] Unfortunately, few studies in the literature have achieved these requirements.

Bacteria. *Mycoplasmas* including *Mycoplasma hominis* and *Ureaplasma urealyticum* are the most common organisms associated with spontaneous abortion. *T-mycoplasma (Ureaplasma urealyticum)* was first identified in abortal tissues from women with recurrent abortion.[304] However, *Mycoplasma* is common in the genitourinary tract of sexually active men and women.[342] Ascending infections with these organisms can occur causing endometritis and salpingitis.[331] Cases of chorioamnionitis and stillbirth have been reported.[305] Anecdotal reports and other poorly controlled studies suggest that cervical colonization by *T-mycoplasma* is associated with both sporadic and recurrent spontaneous abortion; however, unequivocal data substantiating causation remain elusive.[430,509,530]

Chlamydia trachomatis is another primarily sexually transmitted bacterial organism whose role in spontaneous abortion is speculative. Chlamydial infections of the cervix have been associated with second-trimester abortions and premature rupture of the membranes.[333,536] A higher prevalence of antibodies to *C. trachomatis* has been reported in the sera of women with recurrent abortion, compared with fertile controls, although the mean titer between the groups was not found to be different.[429,577] The fact that the mean titer of IgM to *Chlamydia* was not different between those groups with or without abortion, together with the finding that the incidence of positive cultures between aborters and controls was not different, indicates that the presence of antibodies to *Chlamydia* is due to prior exposure rather than that an active infection as a causal factor of spontaneous abortion.[84] Two other possibilities could explain the association of antibodies to *Chlamydia* and abortion: (1) reactivation of a latent chlamydial infection could result during pregnancy, thus potentially mediating reproductive loss and (2) antichlamydial antibodies may recognize the epitopes shared by both *Chlamydia* and fetal-placental antigens.[577]

β-Hemolytic streptococcus is associated with the premature rupture of membranes and may infect fetal-placental tissues resulting in pregnancy loss.[246,364,442] An association between bacteriuria and abortion has been proposed but not substantiated.[299,401] The precise role of *β-Hemolytic streptococcus* in recurrent abortion remains theoretical.

Listeria monocytogenes is abortifacient in mice, but its role in human recurrent abortion is not clear.[436] An association between *Listeria* and recurrent abortion in women has been reported but not substantiated.[432,577]

A 29% spontaneous abortion rate has been reported in Ugandan women who were hospitalized with endometritis/salpingitis as a result of infection with gonococcus or other sexually transmitted diseases.[189]

Viruses. *Cytomegalovirus* has been associated with sporadic cases of spontaneous abortion but not with recurrent abortion.[10] The virus may cause neurologic deficits and mental retardation in the offspring of mothers who are infected.

The risk of neonatal infection with the *Herpes* virus is well known. There is also an increased risk of spontaneous abortion as a result of infection with this virus.[375,376] A threefold increase in missed abortions has been reported in women with elevated serum antibody titers to the *Herpes* virus, which prompts the suggestion that the reactivation of a latent infection may culminate in an abortion.[195]

The rubella virus is another well-known teratogenic virus that causes abnormalities in various fetal organs. Fetal developmental retardation, blindness, and deafness are common if maternal rubella infection is acquired during the early weeks of pregnancy. Spontaneous abortion may occur also, but there is no evidence that rubella is involved in recurrent spontaneous abortion.

Other viruses have been associated with spontaneous abortion. *Variola* and *vaccinia* may cause abortion, stillbirth, and maternal mortality. Acute maternal infection with *hepatitis* B virus has been associated with sporadic spontaneous abortion, but not recurrent loss.[90] Spontaneous abortion has been associated with rubeola.[186] Two cases of first-trimester spontaneous abortion have been reportedly associated with infection caused by *Coxsackie A16*, which was isolated from spontaneously aborted placentae.[389] Fetal death has been associated with *Parvovirus B19*, the infection that causes fifth disease.[495] Second-trimester spontaneous abortions are most common with this infection, although cases of first-trimester loss have been reported.[233,234,424,461] There is no evidence, however, of parvovirus being associated with recurrent spontaneous abortion. Similarly, there is no data indicating that women with human immunodeficiency virus (HIV) with or without AIDS are more likely to spontaneous abort than women without this disease. HIV infection has been reported to provoke anticardiolipin antibody production but not to effect pregnancy in HIV-infected individuals.[270]

Parasites. Traditionally, infection with *Treponema palladium*, the spirochaete responsible for syphilis has not been considered a likely cause of abortion due to lack of transplacental transport until 16 weeks' gestation. However, the finding of these organisms in elective first-trimester abortuses indicates that transplacental spirochaete passage is possible early in the pregnancy, which suggests that spontaneous abortion may be possible.[212]

Toxoplasmosa gondi is an obligate intracellular parasite that is also a zoonotic infection since the reproductive cycle of this parasite occurs in the cat and oocytes are excreted in cat feces. An intermediate stage of the life cycle, tachyzoites, can be found in the tissues of other animals. Transmission to humans can occur either by ingesting raw or undercooked meat containing tachyzoites or by ingesting cat feces or feces-contaminated soil or food. Congenital infection can occur any time during the pregnancy. Transplacental passages of tachyzoites is possible, and cases of spontaneous abortion attributed to this parasite have been reported, based on serum antibody titers to the organism.[318,490,516] Placental pathology in infected cases includes focal villitis with stromal hypercellularity.

Zoonotic infections. Other zoonotic infections associated with abortion, in addition to listeriosis and toxoplasmosis, include brucellosis, psittacosis, and campylobacteriosis. Zoonotic infections are rare. However, if they are able to cause abortions in animals, the infections may be capable of mediating abortions in women. *Brucella abortus* causes spontaneous abortion in cows, pigs, dogs, and goats. There has been one case report of intraamniotic infection with *Brucella abortus* causing spontaneous abortion in a human.[419] *Chlamydia psittaci,* which causes psittacosis induced abortion in sheep, may be acquired by humans and has been reported as a gynecologic infection that mediates spontaneous abortion in women.[48] *Campylobacter* causes abortion in both sheep and cattle and enteric diarrhea in humans. The infection in humans originates from animal sources, especially milk. Campylobacteriosis has been associated with spontaneous abortion in humans, and chronic asymptomatic human carriers of this organism may exist.[503]

Fungal. Infection with *Candida albicans* is a relatively minor problem in pregnancy; however, 23 cases of chorioamnionitis associated with *C. albicans* have been reported.

Among these cases were three spontaneous abortions and one stillbirth.[245]

Any organism that is capable of transplacental passage may theoretically mediate spontaneous abortion. In addition to the organisms associated with abortion as discussed above, enteric bacteria, staphylococci, streptococci, pneumococci, salmonellae, borrelia and leptospira organisms, *Vibrio cholera*, and *Mycobacterium tuberculosis* may be transplacentally acquired.[318] A case of transplacental infection with *Hemophilus influenza* has been associated with spontaneous abortion.[388]

Mechanisms of abortion as a result of infectious organisms are largely speculative; however, both direct and indirect effects may be involved. Bacteremia regardless of organism may cause an abortion.[90] Direct fetal-placental infection may mediate abortion through vascular changes and disruption of cell function. Viral infections have been proposed to induce hormonal aberrations during pregnancy; this could result in pregnancy loss.[498] Elevation of core body temperature in response to infection may also result in fetal death. Other indirect effects of infections contributing to spontaneous abortion include immune and inflammatory cell activation that causes the secretion of potentially reproductive-toxic cytokines.[224] Cytokines, secreted in response to immune and inflammatory cell activation caused by infection, may also facilitate prostaglandin production and result in premature labor.[465] Metabolic by-products of infectious organisms such as amines and proteases may predispose the membranes to premature rupture. Chronic subclinical infection within endometrial tissues is another possible way that infections may mediate pregnancy loss. Immunologic memory is another potential contributing factor as are antibodies to organisms that may cross-react with epitopes on fetal-placental tissues.

Little attention has been given to the problem of abortion, with respect to infections; however, new molecular immunologic techniques, which enable the isolation and identification of potentially infectious agents from reproductive tissues and products of conception, may provide insight into potential active and latent infections that contribute to both sporadic and recurrent spontaneous abortion.

Immunologic factors. Multiple immunologic theories have been proposed to explain human reproductive loss.[227] (Table 14-2). The immune system is a complicated and integrated system whose purpose is to defend an organism against nonself tissue. The concept that the conceptus is an immunologically foreign graft that must be maternally tolerated for survival was first introduced by Medawer in 1953.[351] Since both the developing embryo and trophoblast are immunologically foreign to the maternal immune system because of their maternally inherited gene products and tissue-specific differentiation antigens, speculation has arisen that abortion may be due to impaired maternal immune tolerance to the semiallogenic conceptus.[222,231,250,251]

Human reproductive tissues are immunologically dynamic and contain a myriad of antigenic and other immune response cells and their secreted products.[76,232] The immune system may be divided into two components: (1) the humoral immune system which is mediated by antibody-secreting plasma cells derived from activated B lymphocytes; and (2) the cellular immune system which is mediated by T lymphocytes, macrophages, and natural killer cells and their secreted proteins, termed cytokines. More specifically, an immune response is elicited when helper-inducer (CD4) T lymphocytes recognize protein antigens, in association with class II major histocompatibility complex determinants on antigen-presenting cells. CD4 T lymphocytes are divided into subsets, termed TH1 and TH2 which are defined according to their pattern of secreted cytokines.[367,368,463,464] TH1 cell secretion principally of interferon gamma, interleukin 2, and tumor necrosis factor results in heightened cytotoxic immunity, either directly or through enhanced antigen presentation, phagocytosis, Fc receptor expression, or nitric oxide and superoxide production. TH2 cell secretion, principally of interleukin 4, interleukin 5, and interleukin 10 results in heightened antibody production and in a generally more protective immune environment. Therefore, induction of cellular immunity through CD4 T lymphocyte activation and TH2 differentiation will ultimately lead to humoral immunity.

Four humoral immune mechanisms have been proposed for recurrent, spontaneous abortion (Table 14-2). Of these four proposed humoral mechanisms, the antiphospholipid antibodies remain the only scientifically well-substantiated humoral immune cause for pregnancy loss. Antiphospholipid antibodies are IgG and IgM autoantibodies with a specificity for negatively-charged phospholipid. The antiphospholipid antibodies most commonly associated with recurrent pregnancy loss are anticardiolipin and antiphosphotidyl-serine. Antiphospholipid antibodies are also characterized by prolong phospholipid-dependent coagulation tests in vitro (known as lupus anticoagulant tests APTT or Russel viper venom), thrombosis in vivo, thrombocytopenia, and fetal loss. The association of antiphospholipid antibodies with one or more of these characteristic clinical features has been termed the antiphospholipid syndrome.[209] Obstetric complications, in addition to recurrent spontaneous abortion in the first or second trimester include premature labor, premature rupture of membranes, stillbirth, intrauterine growth retardation, and preeclampsia.[68] The presence of antiphospholipid antibodies during pregnancy is a major risk factor for adverse pregnancy outcome.[397] The incidence of antiphospholipid syndrome in women who experience recurrent abortion varies between studies. In a series of 300 couples who were evaluated for recurrent pregnancy loss, the incidence was 3%, which was similar to the 4.8% found in other studies.[29,67,239] A smaller series of women with recurrent abortion reported higher percentages—11% to 48%.[150,251,557] These percentages, like all percentages of potential etiologies for recurrent abortion, vary according to physician-referral patterns. The actual frequency of antiphospholipid antibodies in the general population is unknown. The incidence of fetal loss is significantly higher in women with elevated IgG anticardiolipin antibodies, lupus anticoagulant, or both when accompanied by elevated maternal serum α-fetoprotein levels (62%) as compared to women with only elevated antiphospolipid antibodies (47.6%).[501]

Pathophysiologic mechanisms responsible for adverse fetal outcome in women with antiphospholipid antibodies are poorly defined. Most proposed mechanisms involve inhibition of vascular endothelial prostacycline production leading to vasoconstriction and thrombosis.[86] This mechanism, although pathologically plausible has not been uniformly confirmed.[86,146] Other pathophysiologic mechanisms proposed to explain antiphospholipid antibody-mediated abortion include: (1) interception of signal transduction processes, by antibody binding to phospholipid epitopes on second messenger molecules; (2) platelet damage that results from antiphospholipid antibodies causing platelets to bind to vascular endothelium, which results in platelet aggregation and local thrombosis; and (3) impaired fibrinolytic activity, through antiphospholipid interference with protein C activation.[184,210] Protein C is an endogenous anticoagulant that circulates in an inactive form. Antiphospholipid antibodies have been suggested to interfere with the function of anionic phospholipids within the thrombomodulin system, which culminates in thrombosis.[171] Recent in vitro evidence using the trophoblast-derived choriocarcinoma cell line BeWo, indicated that an antibody against phosphatidylserine, especially the IgM isotype, can inhibit syncytial trophoblast formation.[323] Limited direct pathologic evidence exists for the placental vascular damage that is needed to substantiate the association of antiphospholipid antibodies and abortion since not all women with the antiphospholipid syndrome and recurrent abortion have placental infarctions or maternal surface abruption and hemorrhage.[205] Similarly, while the extent of placental pathology appears insufficient to explain fetal death in many cases of antiphospholipid antibody-positive women, other placentae show these characteristic lesions, yet the mother has no hematologic evidence of antiphospholipid antibodies.[317] Therefore, although substantial clinical evidence exists for the antiphospholipid syndrome being involved in recurrent abortion, the direct pathologic evidence remains equivocal.

Spontaneous abortion was shown to occur in animals that were immunized against sperm to produce antisperm antibodies.[353] Women with antisperm antibodies in their serum were reported to be at increased risk for spontaneous abortion.[198,276,576] However, this work has been challenged.[283] An association between circulating IgG antibodies in women with recurrent spontaneous abortion to the sperm tails of their husbands has been reported.[576] In a much larger study using donor sperm, an association between antisperm antibodies and recurrent abortion could not be substantiated.[98] In a series of 300 couples with recurrent spontaneous abortion, antisperm antibodies was found in the cervical mucous of only two women.[239] Therefore, antisperm antibodies appear unlikely as a major cause of recurrent abortion. Unconfirmed reports in subfertile couples indicated that in women with evidence of sperm immunity, the antibody titers were higher against the sperm from their husbands than the sperm from controls.[338] It is possible that sperm and early embryonic fetal-placental antigens share common epitopes.[231] More work is needed to substantiate the hypothesis that antisperm antibodies are involved in recurrent abortion.

The hypothesis that antitrophoblast antibodies are involved in recurrent abortion was proposed but not unequivacably substantiated. Recent reports that associate antithyroid antibodies in 31% of women with recurrent abortion may represent an epiphenomena in women with abortion or generalized nonspecific autoantibody activation.[183,186,421,520] The hypothesis that antithyroid antibodies may recognize shared epitopes on the trophoblast is currently being tested. If this hypothesis is substantiated then antithyroid antibodies may serve as a marker for cross-reactive antibodies against trophoblast, thereby providing a potential antibody-mediated mechanism for spontaneous abortion in women with antithyroid antibodies.

No other immunologic hypothesis proposed for abortion received as much attention as the theory that maternal blocking antibody deficiency is a cause of recurrent spontaneous abortion. Despite numerous papers on the subject, very little substantive data exist in support of this hypothesis. Therefore, most investigators no longer consider this theory valid; however, many other individuals still believe in the suppositions of this hypothesis, which renders it among the most controversial topics in reproductive immunology.

The theory that maternal blocking antibody deficiency is a cause of recurrent abortion was originally based on three suppositions: (1) there is an antifetal, maternal, cell-mediated, immune response that develops in all pregnancies which must be blocked; (2) blocking antibodies develop in all successful pregnancies that prevent this antifetal maternal, cell-mediated immune response; and (3) in the absence of blocking antibodies, abortion of the fetus always occurs. Unfortunately, none of these suppositions have ever been scientifically validated.[478] There remains no direct pathologic evidence that an antifetal, maternal immune response occurs in all pregnancies either with or without purported blocking antibodies. There is also no direct evidence that blocking antibodies occur in all successful pregnancies to prevent this presumed antifetal immune response. A specific verifiable assay to detect these purported immunoglobulin effectors also does not exist.

Mixed lymphocyte culture (MLC) reactivities between maternal responder and paternal stimulator cells have traditionally been used to determine whether blocking activity in response to uncharacterized serum factors exist. Rocklin et al were the first to associate the absence of a serum-blocking factor with recurrent abortion.[456] This work was later extended by others.[49,346] However, this hypothesis was questioned when women with successful pregnancies were found who did not produce serum factors that were capable of mixed lymphocyte culture inhibition, and when not all of the women with successfully pregnancies were found to make antibodies against paternal human lymphocyte antigens (HLA).[17,457] Further doubt concerning the relevance of MLC reactivities in spontaneous abortion remains, since purported blocking factors may be the consequence rather than the cause of pregnancy success, and other pregnancy-related serum factors such as steroid hormones or cytokines may be responsible for the observed effects. The association of HLA-sharing between men and women who experience recurrent abortion was also challenged.[267]

A novel HLA-linked antigen system that was based on polyclonal rabbit antisera cross-reactive with trophoblast and lymphocytes, termed TLX, was proposed to try and explain pregnancy loss.[347] This hypothesis stated that the sharing of TLX antigens that were perhaps cross-linked with HLA antigens caused the inability to produce maternal blocking antibodies. As previously mentioned, blocking antibodies were never adequately characterized. Recent data indicate that rather than defining a new alloantigen system, TLX is CD46, a complement receptor that is found on a wide variety of cells including trophoblast, lymphocytes and spermatozoa explaining the cross-reactive nature of the antisera that originally defined TLX and contributed to the misconception that this antisera defined a new alloantigen system.[22,425]

Neither human nor animal studies support the concept that an intact, maternal, immune system is necessary for maintaining a normal pregnancy. Agammaglobulinemic mice and women are able to successfully reproduce.[458] Similarly, generations of genetically identical mice are bred successfully. Therefore, the hypothesis that HLA antigen dissimilarity is required for successful reproduction or that the production of blocking antibodies are critical for pregnancy maintenance is not scientifically valid. Although no solid evidence exists that immune mechanisms are necessary for successful pregnancy, the possibility still exists that immune mechanisms may be involved in pregnancy failure.

Four cellular immune-related hypotheses have been proposed to explain pregnancy failure (Table 14-2). An abnormal TH1 cellular immune response that involves the cytokines, interferon-γ, and tumor necrosis factor, which are toxic to embryo and trophoblast growth, is the most recent hypothesis proposed for immunologic reproductive failure.[55,149,230,239] This hypothesis states that the conceptus may be a target of local cell-mediated immune responses, culminating in abortion. In women who are affected, trophoblast, sperm, microbial, or other antigens may activate maternal immune and inflammatory cells (macrophages and lymphocytes) to produce a cellular immune response mediated by the TH1 cytokines, interferon-γ, and the tumor necrosis factor that inhibit in vitro embryo development and trophoblast growth and function.[55,199,234,237,239] Tumor necrosis factor-α may also mediate intravascular thrombus formation.[492] Depending on the individual series, 60% to 90% of women with otherwise unexplained recurrent spontaneous abortion were found to have evidence of an abnormal TH1 cellular immune response to trophoblast antigens, while less than 3% of women with normal reproductive histories have cellular immunity to these same trophoblast antigens.[149,234,239,311,580] In contrast to TH1 immunity to trophoblast in women with unexplained recurrent abortion, recent evidence indicates that a majority of women with normal reproduction make a TH2 immune response, which involves the cytokines interleukin 4 and interleukin 10, to the same trophoblast antigens that women with recurrent abortion respond to with TH1 immunity.[234] These data provide evidence for a new nonmajor histocompatibility-related mechanism for reproductive failure. All reports concerning this hypothesis come from only one laboratory. More studies are needed by other investigators to validate this hypothesis. A study from another laboratory however, has indicated that higher levels of tumor necrosis factor and interleukin 2, another TH1 cytokine, were higher in serum samples from women with unexplained recurrent abortion than from controls.[327]

Other immunologic cytokines, growth factors, and oncogenes are involved in mammalian development.[202,255,502] The suggestion that T lymphocyte cytokines are necessary for normal murine pregnancy has been challenged by studies performed in SCID (immunodeficient) mice, which indicates that T lymphocyte-derived cytokines are not necessary for a successful pregnancy.[118,569] The possibility remains that rather than being secreted by classic immune cells, some of these cytokines may be secreted by endometrial/decidual cells themselves.[537] The absence of the cytokine, colony-stimulating factor 1 (oncogene c-fms) has been theorized to contribute to abortion in mice.[569] However, this same cytokine was shown to cause rather than prevent murine abortion in certain strains.[540] The absence of transforming growth factor-β and epidermal growth factor have been shown to cause abortion in mice.[96,552] The oncogene c-mos which is a kinase, can cause mitotic arrest.[585] The aberrant expression of this oncogene during oocyte or embryo development could theoretically lead to pregnancy failure. Thus far the majority of studies regarding deficiencies in cytokines, growth factors, and oncogenes have been performed in mice and other animals. Many of these same factors, however have been identified in human pregnancy.[173,408,532,579] The absence of these factors has been theorized to lead to spontaneous abortion in women.[96,173,294408,532,552,579,585] Further work is needed in humans to validate these theories and to identify the responsible factors and their possible mechanism of action in causing abortion.

Suppressor cell and factor deficiency is another immune mechanism proposed for recurrent abortion. The concept of suppressor cells and their existence is a controversial topic in immunology.[7] The hypothesis of suppressor cell and factor deficiency as a cause of pregnancy loss was based upon the finding of suppressor immune cell deficiency in abortion-prone CBA/J x DBA/2 mice prior to pregnancy loss.[97] The abortifacient effect in this murine model was later found to be due to *Mycoplasma* infection, as antibiotic treatment with tetracycline abrogated the abortion.[203] Although this mouse model is no longer considered a direct immunologic model for abortion, it is useful in discerning potential infection-mediated mechanisms of abortion through indirect effects on the immune system. Data derived from nonprimate animal models that are extrapolated to humans must be cautiously interpreted because of inherent anatomic, morphologic, endocrinologic, and immunologic differences between species. Therefore, results obtained in animal studies cannot be directly transfered to the human condition.

The decidua in human pregnancy was proposed to constitute a distinct immunologic microenvironment.[147] Support for the theory that deficient suppressor cells/factors are involved in human abortion comes from the observation of decidual suppressor cell deficiency in endometrial biopsies from women with failing chemical pregnancies that followed in vitro fertilization and embryo transfer, and also from three women with missed abortion at 2 to 11 weeks of gestation.[129,381] Although these data suggest support for the theory of suppressor cell/factor deficiency for spontaneous abortion, the fact that 3 of 15 women having elective pregnancy termination were also found to have evidence of suppressor cell/factor deficiency compromises this hypothesis.[129] Evidence in support of a suppressor cell/factor deficiency indicates that decidual macrophage and lymphocyte function, which is normally suppressed during human pregnancy, is enhanced in cases of spontaneous abortion; however, all of these findings do not necessarily indicate causality, since all of the observations in support of suppressor cell/factor deficiency as being a cause of abortion may simply reflect the effects of an abortion. Similarly, the factors and cells involved in this theory were not precisely defined, nor was their specificity determined. Larger, better-controlled studies are needed before this intriguing theory can be substantiated.

Normal human syncytiotrophoblast does not express major histocompatibility complex class I or II antigens except for a truncated form of class I on the cytotrophoblast that is termed HLA G.[59,302] As a result of the absence of classic major histocompatibility complex (MHC) determinants, the trophoblast cannot be a classical immunogen for maternal sensitization or serve as a target for MHC-directed cytotoxic T-cells. Human trophoblast is also resistant to a natural killer cell attack. As previously described, non-MHC–related mechanisms may be involved in reproductive failure such as TH1 mediated immunity, but MHC-related mechanisms cannot. The TH1 cytokine interferon-γ was shown to induce major MHC antigen expression, on placental tissues that were derived from human trophoblast and human trophoblast cell lines in vitro.[19,159] If MHC determinants were expressed in vivo, then cytotoxic T-cell attack could occur and potentially culminate in abortion. This theory, although plausible and supportable by in vitro experiments, nevertheless appears unlikely as a major factor for abortion, since recent studies indicate that there is no difference in MHC expression between placentae from women experiencing recurrent, sporadic, or elective abortion.[19,159,238]

Normal human placentae are also replete with complement regulatory and binding proteins which are thought to protect pregnancy from complement-mediated attack.[241] The suggestion was offered that if the trophoblast does not express these regulatory proteins then abortion might occur through complement-mediated immunologic mechanisms.[256] Experimental evidence does not support this hypothesis because trophoblasts both from elective terminations and from recurrent and sporadic abortions clearly express complement regulatory and binding proteins.[238]

Miscellaneous factors

Environmental. Many other factors and associations have been implicated in sporadic and recurrent abortion (Table 14-2). Environmental factors including chronic exposure to chemicals such as organic solvents (e.g., carbon tetrachloride), and heavy metal toxicity resulting from mercury and lead are known to be abortifacient, as is ionizing radiation.[416] Exposure to electromagnetic fields such as might occur in individuals living near high voltage electric power lines or with prolonged exposure to video display terminals has been associated with spontaneous abortion; however, lack of controls and statistical power for these studies seriously challenges their association with abortion.[481,549] Several large collaborative studies have documented the fact that exposure to video display terminals or microwave ovens does not pose a threat to pregnancy.[54,332] Ionizing radiation and exposure to herbicides (e.g., Agent Orange) and pesticides have been proposed to cause abortion, but no definitive data concerning these possibilities have been published.[73,172]

Drugs. Multiple drugs especially antiprogesterones and folic acid antagonists such as RU486 and amphoterin, which are known abortifacient agents are associated with spontaneous abortion. Antineoplastic drugs such as cyclophosphamide, fluorouracil, and doxolubrican cause abortion in animals. Occupational exposure to these drugs by individuals administering these chemotherapy agents was associated with an increased risk of spontaneous abortion in one study but was not substantiated in other studies.[91,371a,485] Anticonvulsion medications such as trimethadione and phenytoin are associated with congenital malformations but not with spontaneous abortion. Valproic acid is associated with spontaneous abortion while both phenobarbital and primidone (mysoline) are considered safe in pregnancy.[340] Exposure to anesthetic gases during pregnancy has been associated with spontaneous abortion; large case-controlled studies have not supported this association.[539] Warfarin derivatives used to achieve anticoagulation are associated with both malformations and spontaneous abortion, presumably by interfering with vitamin K metabolism.[402] Heparin is relatively safe, if administered during pregnancy since its molecular size does not permit transplacental passage. Isotretinoin, the vitamin A congener used to treat severe cystic acne, if taken during pregnancy may cause congenital malformations and spontaneous abortion.[134] Other agents suspected of having abortifacient properties include ethanol, caffeine, nicotine, and the other metabolic products of cigarette smoking. Several prospective, controlled studies suggested that the incidence of spontaneous abortion in both the first and second trimester of pregnancy is twice that of controls in women with alcohol consumption of greater than 1 to 2 drinks per day during early pregnancy, irrespective of smoking.[25,206] Smoking is also associated with an increased risk of spontaneous abortion and has a dose-response relationship.[160,206] Recently, caffeine consumption has been associated with an increased risk of spontaneous abortion.[154] Doses again appear to be among the most important factors relative to risk. Caffeine consumption of less than 300 mg per day (e.g., less than three cups of coffee per day) during early pregnancy does not appear to increase abortion risk; however, the risk of intrauterine growth retardation may be increased.[141,358] Studies regarding attributable risk of environmental factors and other agents must be cautiously interpreted since confounding variables are very difficult to disassociate. Before definitive conclusions can be reached regarding the environmental factors that cause abortion, the following caveats must be considered: gestational age at time of exposure; the amount reaching the conceptus; the duration of the exposure; the impact of other factors or agents to which the mother or her conceptus are simultaneously exposed; the physiologic status of the mother and her conceptus; genetic differences; and the interrelationship between the frequency of exposure, the frequency of effect, and the recognizability of adverse outcome such as spontaneous abortion.[340]

Placental anomalies. Placental abnormalities are other miscellaneous potential causes of pregnancy loss. These rare abnormalities are most commonly associated with second-trimester and later losses that are caused by circumvallate placenta and placenta marginata.[453,550]

Maternal illness. Maternal medical illnesses have been associated with recurrent abortion. Rheumatologic diseases, especially systemic lupus erythematosus with and without antiphospholipid antibodies, have been associated with an increased risk of spontaneous abortion.[317,360] Spontaneous abortion is a known consequence of severe cardiac and renal disease. Vascular compromise, which causes placental insufficiency, appears to be the common denominator for abortion caused by medical illness. Hematologic disorders are another medical problem predisposing humans to recurrent abortion. Hypercoagulability contributes to spontaneous abortion in such instances because of concomitant medical conditions or inherited abnormalities of coagulation in which a physiologic anticoagulant mechanism is defective such as in antithrombin 3, protein C, and protein S deficiencies, or in abnormalities of the fibrinolytic system and dysfibrinogenesis.[488] Factor 12 (Hageman) deficiency which causes enhanced thrombosis was associated with recurrent abortion.[71,482] Impaired fibrinolytic capacity may also predispose to abortion.[194] Platelet disorders are well known to cause adverse obstetrical outcome.[466] Thrombocytosis and thrombocythemia (i.e., platelet counts of greater than 1 million per cubic millimeter) are associated with recurrent pregnancy loss.[81,472] At the Harvard Center for Recurrent Miscarriage at Brigham and Women's Hospital, of 1600 women thus far evaluated for recurrent abortion, 3 women with thrombocythemia as the only predisposing factor for their prior pregnancy losses have been identified. Hematologic disorders, although rarely found, if diagnosed may be life saving since these disorders often have high maternal morbidity and mortality.[362,488]

Male factors. The potential contribution of male factors to recurrent abortion, other than chromosomal anomalies, is poorly understood. Paternal alcohol abuse, but not moderate drinking, appears to be related to recurrent abortion, even when corrected for maternal ethanol use.[201] The mechanism for this association is unknown but may be related to potential mitogenic effects on the spermatozoa. Teratospermia was anecdotally associated with spontaneous abortion but not with cytogenetic abnormalities.[36,387,469] The spontaneous abortion rate in women who receive donor insemination is higher if their sexual partners have oligospermia compared with women whose sexual partners have azoospermia.[18] The mechanisms for this observation are unknown. Two studies that addressed potential semen abnormalities associated with recurrent abortion were recently completed; however, neither sperm count nor morphology were significantly different between men whose partners experienced recurrent abortion and those having a normal pregnancy.[228,233] There was also no difference in semen parameters between these groups and the control standards that were published by the World Health Organization.[228] Therefore, abnormal sperm morphology does not appear to be a major factor in recurrent abortion. This study did not specifically address whether teratospermia was associated with recurrent abortion, but whether men of couples with recurrent abortion had an increased incidence of teratospermia. Comparable granulocyte and total white blood cell concentrations were found in the semen of men from fertile couples and couples with unexplained recurrent abortion. This suggests that couples with unexplained recurrent abortion do not have an abnormally high incidence of subclinical genital infections for which leukocytospermia would serve as a marker.[233] A higher incidence of elevated CD4 and CD8 T lymphocyte concentrations was observed in semen from men whose partners had evidence of TH1 cellular immunity to sperm antigens.[233] The significance of this association remains to be explored.

Dyssynchronous fertilization. Another potential cause of spontaneous abortion may involve dyssynchronous fertilization that causes an abnormal conceptus. This may be due to preovulatory oocyte aging from unknown causes, which could give rise to DNA degeneration predisposing to aneuploidy.[544] Circumstantial evidence for this potential mechanism comes from the observation that more trisomic than karyotypically normal abortuses were found in cases where ovulation occurred after day 18 of the cycle.[64] Postovulatory aging of the secondary oocyte may also contribute to spontaneous abortion.[197] Chromosomal aberration may occur because of the loss of oocyte integrity, and nondisjunction could lead to chromosomal abnormalities that culminate in spontaneous abortion.[32] Polyspermic fertilization that leads to a triploidic conceptus is also more likely to occur in ovulated aged oocytes as a result of a defective corticogranular reaction in the aged oocyte.[319] Aged sperm in both male and female experimental animals were shown to undergo chromosomal breakdown before losing the capacity to fertilize.[334,335] When sperm were retained in the female reproductive tract of rabbits for up to 30 hours before ovulation, abnormal embryo development caused by cytogenetic anomalies resulted.[334] Delaying the insemination of rats was also found to increase the number of abnormal pregnancies.[33] Additional evidence for dyssynchronous fertilization that predisposes humans to reproductive loss is afforded by the observation of an increased frequency of triploid conceptions, when intercourse occurs remote from ovulation as assessed with basal body temperature graphs.[64] There is no evidence that seasonal variation in conception influences the rate of nondisjunction.[144]

Coitus. Coitus during pregnancy was associated with premature labor and premature rupture of membranes, but not by all investigators.[74,306,373,374,378437,551] Potential mechanisms for this controversial association include prostaglandins in semen, orgasm, and excessive catecholamine release mediating contractions.[392,518,563] There is no evidence that mild to moderate exercise during pregnancy in healthy women is associated with an increased incidence of spontaneous abortion. Guidelines for women who exercise during pregnancy were published by the American College of Obstetricians and Gynecologists.[14] Contraindications to exercise include pregnancy-induced hypertension; rupture of membranes; preterm labor during a prior or current pregnancy; incompetent cervix or cerclage; persistent second- or third trimester bleeding; intrauterine growth retardation; and conditions such as active thyroid, cardiac, vascular, and pulmonary disease.[14]

DIAGNOSIS

There is controversy as to when to begin the evaluation of couples with recurrent spontaneous abortion for potential causative factors. Traditionally evaluation focused on couples who experienced three prior pregnancy losses; however, this number was challenged.[35,149,311,529] Investigation is now suggested after two spontaneous abortions, especially in women whose prior pregnancy losses ended after fetal heart development, in women over 35 years of age, in couples having difficulty conceiving, and in couples anxious to initiate investigation; similar predisposing factors may be common to both sporadic and recurrent abortion.[452,567] A scientifically rational and thorough evaluation should be performed (Table 14-3) because many couples have more than one contributing factor for their losses.[239,535,547] Couples should be advised to avoid conception for at least two menstrual cycles, after experiencing a miscarriage. This has been anecdotally suggested, to allow time for proper resumption of ovulatory cycles.[377] During this interim, preconception diagnostic assessment can be initiated for potential contributing factors for abortion.

Table 14-3. Investigative measures potentially useful in the evaluation of recurrent spontaneous abortion

A. History

B. Physical

C. Laboratory
   1. Parental peripheral blood karyotype
   2. Hysterosalpingography followed by hysteroscopy/ laparoscopy if indicated
   3. Luteal phase endometrial biopsy
   4. Thyroid function tests (TSH, T4)
   5. Antiphospholipid antibodies (cardiolipin, phosphatidylserine)
   6. Lupus anticoagulant (APTT or Russell's viper venom)
   7. Compete blood count with platelets
   8. Antisperm antibodies (cervical mucous, peripheral serum)†
   9. Cervical cultures (*Mycoplasma, Chlamydia, β-streptococcus*)†
   10. TH1 embryotoxic cytokines to reproductive antigens‡
   11. Antithyroid antibodies‡
   12. LH testing/ultrasound assessment for PCOS‡

† Last resort
‡ Experimental

Preconception assessment

History. A thorough history obtained from both partners of the couple with recurrent abortion is fundamental. This should include age and past medical, surgical, psychologic, social, and genetic histories. Questionnaires to elicit genetic information were devised by the American College of Obstetricians and Gynecologists.[12] Current medications and other drugs, smoking, and alcohol use should also be recorded. A descriptive sequence of all prior pregnancies is important. The age of gestation (i.e., fetal size) when pregnancy loss occurred may be informative, since most women loose their pregnancies at approximately the same time in sequential pregnancies. Gestational age when the pregnancy loss occurred as determined by the last menstrual period should also be obtained but may not be informative as there is often a two- to three-week delay between fetal death and expulsion.[356,573] The time required for couples to achieve conception should also be ascertained. In a review of couples who registered at the Harvard Center for Recurrent Miscarriage at Brigham and Women's Hospital, approximately one third of over 1600 couples being evaluated for recurrent abortion attempted to conceive for over one year, before achieving a pregnancy. Difficulty in achieving conception may indicate subclinical (preimplantation) loss. A history of malformed children or fetuses, including neural tube defects may provide insight into possible genetic abnormalities. It is important to ascertain karyotypes of previous abortus material as is fetal sex, if known. The review of all histologic assessments made on previous abortuses may provide clues to possible diagnoses such as infections and potential immunologic aberrations. Questions should be asked concerning prior uterine instrumentation, pelvic infections, and in utero exposure to diethylstilbestrol, drugs, radiation, and other environmental pollutants. Menstrual cycle history is important and may give clues regarding possible oligoovulation caused by PCOS or other endocrine abnormalities and dyssynchronous fertilization caused by delayed ovulation or poor timing of intercourse. Detailed family histories from both partners of the couple with recurrent abortion may also be informative as to a family history of recurrent abortion, stillbirth, infertility, and defects caused by chromosomal abnormalities or multifactorial and Mendelian disorders. Reviews of over 1600 records as mentioned previously have not revealed a high association between recurrent abortion and a family history of recurrent abortion, except in one isolated case of a woman who had a monozygotic twin who also experienced recurrent abortion. Correlation for both spontaneous abortion and stillbirth have been reported to be higher between sisters who are monozygotic rather than dizygotic twins.[111]

Physical examination. Physical examination should include height, weight, and blood pressure, followed by a general assessment for signs of metabolic illness. Body habitus should be defined, and the presence of hirsutism or other signs of hyperandrogenism noted. A breast examination should be performed to look for galactorrhea. Particular attention should be given to the pelvic examination. The cervix should be inspected for signs of diethylstilbestrol exposure, previous trauma, and infection. A bimanual examination to assess the adenxae and the uterine size, shape, and mobility should be performed.

Laboratory investigation

Genetic assessment. The laboratory tests that are potentially useful in the evaluation of the couple with recurrent abortion are shown in Table 14-3. Cytogenetic investigation of peripheral blood leukocytes from both partners should be performed using karyotyping with banding techniques, to identify small rearrangements. Should a genetic abnormality be revealed, appropriate referral to a genetic counselor should then be arranged.

Anatomic assessment. Potential anatomical factors should be initially addressed using hysterosalpingography (HSG) with fluoroscopy and water-soluble contrast media rather than oil-based media, to minimize the chance of potential granuloma formation and pulmonary embolism, should intravascular extravasation occur. Contrast media should be instilled slowly without pressure while simultaneously viewing the intracavitary contour under fluoroscopy. Prophylactic antibiotics such as doxycycline, 100 mg twice a day beginning the day before the procedure for six doses may be given as a prophylaxis against an upper genital tract infection from the cervical-vaginal environment, although this is controversial. Taking an antiprostaglandin medication such as 800 mg of ibuprofen 1 hour before the procedure may be helpful in minimizing discomfort caused by the procedure. The purpose of HSG is to screen for intrauterine filling defects. If the diameter of the internal cervical os exceeds 6 mm, the possibility of an incompetent cervix is increased.[328] Ultrasonography, although useful in determining the size and location of leiomyomas is of limited usefulness in diagnosing potential müllerian anomalies associated with spontaneous abortion.[406] Nuclear magnetic resonance imaging is useful; however, the cost of this procedure limits its use. In cases where a bicornuate configuration is revealed with HSG, ultrasonography may differentiate a unified versus a bicornuate external uterine contour; however, laparoscopy and hysteroscopy are clearly superior for diagnostic evaluation and treatment.[216] Both HSG and hysteroscopy are useful in diagnosing intrauterine synechiae.

Endocrine assessment. A well-timed luteal phase endometrial biopsy remains the standard for evaluating the possibility of a luteal phase defect. Endometrial biopsy should not be performed within two cycles of a previous spontaneous abortion because 22% to 45% of women have endometrial abnormalities during this time.[377] These abnormalities may be due to temporary refractoriness of the pituitary to gonadotrophin releasing hormone (GnRH), the persistence of human chorionic gonadotropin (hCG), persistent decidua, or stress.[179,297,521] Therefore, patients should be advised to avoid conception for two cycles following an abortion. Endometrial biopsies have been traditionally performed 2 days before the next menstrual period; however, a more precise method is to perform the biopsy 10 days after the LH surge.[272,273] Midcycle ultrasonography may also be useful in determining ovulation so that more precise dating can be defined.[515] The diagnosis of luteal phase insufficiency is based on classical histologic criteria of the endometrium that is 3 or more days out of phase.[383] Endometrial asynchrony should be confirmed on a subsequent sequential biopsy because of the 31.4% incidence of out-of-phase biopsies in normal fertile women.[127] Conception should not be attempted during a biopsy cycle so that a proper diagnosis can be ascertained. Concerns regarding interrupted pregnancy during a biopsy cycle, although possible, are rare and can be obviated by obtaining a sensitive pregnancy test the day before the scheduled biopsy.[218,262,289] Some authors have suggested that pregnancy success may even be enhanced in such cycles.[470] This may be related to an enhanced decidual reaction that is known to occur in animal models. A recent report on endometrial dating during conception cycles suggests that implantation occurs only in normally developed endometrium.[24] Earlier studies reported that a successful pregnancy could occur even if the endometrium was out of phase.[534,570] A serum progesterone level of greater than 10 ng/mL in the luteal phase was proposed to be efficacious in predicting luteal phase insufficiency.[254] The usefulness of this test is limited. Normal biopsies occur despite low levels of progesterone in peripheral serum.[313] Isolated values of progesterone may be misleading since progesterone in peripheral blood is pulsatile and considerable overlap exists between the normal and abnormal levels.[34,278,512] Therefore, the ascertainment of progesterone levels is not necessarily helpful in the diagnosis of luteal phase insufficiency. Rarely, progesterone receptor defects within the uterus do occur.[295] Serum progesterone determinations in such cases would obviously be useless. In cases where endometrial asynchrony is found and confirmed on subsequent biopsy, serum prolactin, 17 hydroxyprogesterone, and androgen profiles (testosterone, dehydroepiandrosterone sulfate) may be warranted.

To further assess the possible association of PCOS in recurrent abortion, preconception LH determinations and ultrasonography have been suggested.[1,41,242,269,474] Total secretion of LH in the follicular and particularly in the luteal phase may be more informative than individual determinations.[568] This is not surprising since LH is well known to be secreted in a pulsatile manner; however, an LH value of greater than 20 mIU/mL during the early follicular and late luteal phase is clearly elevated. Ultrasound screening may be an even more sensitive diagnostic tool to discern PCOS in women with recurrent abortion.[474] Physicians, however, should be cognizant of the 18% to 22% incidence of polycystic ovaries that are assessed by ultrasonography in the normal fertile population.[418,474] A history of oligomenorrhea may be of more diagnostic benefit than hormonal profiles in predicting pregnancy failure.[101]

Serum should be assayed for TSH using a sensitive assay. An abnormal result should be repeated, together with a serum thyroxine level. Serum T_3, resin uptake, and thyroid binding capacity are not necessary. At this time an assessment of antithyroid antibodies in light of normal thyroid function both clinically and chemically should only be recommended under a study protocol, until more is known concerning the significance of a positive finding. Elevated antithyroid antibodies may identify women at risk for developing autoimmune thyroiditis. Therefore, periodic thyroid function studies may be indicated in these individuals especially once pregnant.

Infectious assessment. Cervical cultures for *Mycoplasma* and *Ureaplasma* are not often helpful but may be considered especially in cases where no other abnormality has been detected or if there is a history of premature rupture of membranes or premature labor. In such cases, consideration should be given to culturing other organisms such as *Chlamydia* and β-*streptococcus*. *Toxoplasmosis, rubella, cytomegalovirus,* and *Herpes Simplex* titers (TORCH) and detection of other antibodies to infectious organisms are unnecessary, except under specific study protocols or in cases where the history is suggestive of a chronic infectious etiology for pregnancy loss.

Immunologic assessment. Antiphospholipid antibody determinations for cardiolipin and phosphatidyl serine, IgG IgM, together with a test for lupus anticoagulant (APTT, Russell's viper venom) should be part of the evaluation.[11,66] Because of differences in methods, standardization, and units of reporting, practitioners should cautiously interpret the values from different laboratories.[403] Until more information is known, the routine assessment of antiphospholipid antibodies other than to cardiolipin and phosphatidyl serine or other autoantibodies is not currently warranted, except under study protocols where the costs of these tests are born by the investigators and not by the couples seeking evaluation or their insurers.[37,385] Antisperm antibody determinations in the woman's serum and midcycle cervical mucus may be obtained as a last resort, but the incidence of a positive result is very low and its clinical significance controversial.

A complete blood cell count including assessment of platelet count should be obtained. Blood type and Rh factor determinations and rubella immune status should also be part of the routine evaluation.

There is no place in the modern management of recurrent abortion for the ascertainment of antinuclear antibodies (ANA), human leukocyte antigen (HLA) profiles, antipaternal cytotoxic antibodies, or MLC reactivities (Table 14-4).

Antinuclear antibodies (ANA) should not be obtained despite the guidelines published by the American Fertility Society because these antibodies are heterogeneous and

Table 14-4. Investigative measures of no benefit in the evaluation of recurrent spontaneous abortion

A. Antinuclear Antibodies
   1. Association with recurrent pregnancy loss controversial
   2. No difference between women with presumed and unknown etiologies for their abortions
   3. Commonly and nonspecifically occur in the general population
   4. Heterogeneous
   5. May be transitory
   6. Clinical significance in reproduction not established

B. Antipaternal Cytotoxic Antibodies
   1. 32% of 256 women achieving a successful pregnancy as compared to 10% of 50 women whose pregnancy ended in a spontaneous abortion
   2. Rarely demonstrable before 28 weeks gestation
   3. Positive values during pregnancy usually disappear between pregnancies

C. Parental HLA Profiles
   1. Reports suggesting an association with recurrent abortion have been generally of limited size, retrospective, and without population-based controls
   2. Prospective, population-based control studies in Hutterites conclusively demonstrated that HLA heterogeneity is not an essential requirement for successful pregnancy
   3. Animal studies also do not support the concept that MHC heterozygosity is required for successful gestation since inbred animal strains have been maintained for generations.

D. MLC Reactivities
   1. Not all women with presumed immunologic pregnancy loss have evidence of suppressed MLC reactivity with their husbands since spontaneous abortion can occur in the presence of "blocking activity"
   2. Not all women with successful pregnancies produce serum factors capable of inhibiting MLC reactions since viable pregnancies can occur in the absence of "blocking activity"
   3. Causal relationships not addressed as MLC hyporesponsiveness may represent an effect of abortion or differences that result from multiple live births rather than being the cause of recurrent abortion
   4. Interpretation of "blocking activity" in maternal serum depends on the equation used for calculating MLC results

commonly and nonspecifically occur in the general population.[16] Their presence is often transitory, and an association of recurrent abortion with subclinical autoimmunity as reflected by a positive ANA titer is at best controversial and speculative.[112,176] There is also no substantive value in obtaining antipaternal cytotoxic antibodies, since they are rarely demonstrable before 28 weeks' gestation and usually disappear between pregnancies.[440] In a small published series antipaternal cytotoxic antibodies were associated with abortion.[341] However, in a larger series approximately 10% of 50 women whose pregnancies ended in spontaneous abortion were positive, while 32% of 256 women achieving successful pregnancies were also found to have positive values.[439] Therefore, the presence of antipaternal cytotoxic antibodies is not a useful screening test for either the diagnosis or prognosis of recurrent abortion.[104,252,279,439,440]

Parental HLA profiles and their association with recurrent abortion, if parental sharing occurred, received much attention in earlier years. These reports, however, were of limited size, retrospective, and without population-based controls. Prospective population-based control studies in Hutterites conclusively demonstrated that HLA heterogeneity is not an essential requirement for successful pregnancy.[384,386] Therefore, the assessment of parental HLA profiles in the evaluation of recurrent abortion is not clinically justified.[104,115,153,267,279]

An assessment of MLC reactivity between partners with recurrent abortion which looks for purported "blocking antibodies" cannot be clinically justified, as the results of these tests reflect the number and duration of prior pregnancies rather than serve as a marker for recurrent abortion.[104,478] The presence of "blocking antibodies" is not necessarily predictive of pregnancy outcome.[115,116,478,507]

Further work is needed before diagnostic capabilities are clinically available to assess the potential TH1 cellular immunity, suppressor cell/factor and other cytokine growth factors, and oncogene mechanisms of recurrent pregnancy loss. Rapid advances in cellular and molecular immunology and reproductive biology are occurring. New diagnostic tests for TH1 cellular immunity in recurrent abortion are being actively pursued and may be clinically available in the near future.

Postconception evaluation

Once pregnancy is established, close monitoring is advised not only for the psychologic well being of the couple but also to confirm the presence of an intrauterine pregnancy. The incidence of ectopic gestations is reported to be 2.2-fold higher in women with a history of recurrent abortion.[105] At the Harvard Center for Recurrent Miscarriage, at Brigham and Women's Hospital, the incidence of ectopic pregnancy is 2.5 times higher than in the general population. The risk of a molar gestation has been reported to be increased in women with recurrent abortion; however, no differentiation was made in that study between partial molar gestations and complete moles.[109] Six complete molar gestations have been observed in 5 of 1600 women, which represents an unusually high occurrence since the expected incidence in the general United States population is 1 in 1200 pregnancies.[37] Therefore, recurrent spontaneous abortion may be a risk factor not only for ectopic gestation but also for complete molar pregnancy. The suggestion that women with recurrent abortion may be at risk for intrauterine growth retardation, preterm delivery, low birth weight infants, and preeclampsia was also made.[307,446] The Harvard Recurrent Miscarriage Center experience indicates that this association is only valid for women with the antiphospholipid syndrome, since the incidence of intrauterine growth retardation and preeclampsia in the referred patient population with recurrent abortion not having antiphospholipid antibodies is no different from that in the general population.

The endocrinologic events in early pregnancy have been studied; however, methodologic differences between reports obscure any definitive conclusions for most hormonal values. hCG determinations are less controversial. Precisely when the β-sub unit of hCG becomes positive following conception is unknown, but evidence indicates that by the time implantation has occurred (6 days following fertilization), β-hCG is positive in most sophisticated assays. β-hCG levels are expected to double every 2 to 3 days for the first 10 weeks of normal gestation.[72] In aembryonic gestation, β-hCG levels have been reported to not rise appropriately, although not by all of the investigators who suggested that failed embryo development has no immediate effect on trophoblast hormone synthesis.[221,314,480,583] Other pregnancies that were found to have fetal cardiac activity but that ultimately aborted were also shown to have inappropriately rising β-hCG levels.[31,46,47,314,413] The gestational age when fetal death occurs undoubtedly affects hormone values, as many pregnancies that end after 6 weeks of gestation have normal hormonal values earlier in the gestation. Pregnancies with an abnormal karyotype that abort later in the first trimester have been shown to have slowly rising β-hCG levels as early as 6 weeks' gestation.[511]

Serum estradiol and progesterone levels have been reported to be of benefit in predicting pregnancy success and failure.[45,53,282,291,314,477,480] Serial measurements of inappropriately rising estradiol and β-hCG have been suggested to be useful in predicting a pregnancy with an abnormal karyotype.[468] While endocrinologic monitoring prior to 6 weeks' gestation may be beneficial in terms of prognosis, the data for this are not so conclusively precise as to warrant intervention (e.g., D&C) before ultrasound documentation of fetal demise. No single hormone determination will predict a subsequent pregnancy outcome any better than another, if fetal heart activity was ultrasonically detected.[477] Hormonal determinations during pregnancy are generally of little benefit, since levels are often normal until fetal death or abortion occurs.[281,571]

Ultrasonography remains the standard for monitoring early pregnancy. Accordingly, serially monitored β-hCG may be from the point of the missed period until the level is between 1000 and 5000 mIU/mL. At that time a sonogram is performed and further blood sampling is discontinued. Sonography is performed every 2 weeks throughout the first trimester or until the time of gestation that the woman previously lost her pregnancies. No other hormonal tests are obtained unless under a specific clinical study protocol. This frequency of ultrasound scanning is not a necessity; however, it is performed for two fundamental reasons: (1) for the psychologic advantage it affords the couple with the knowledge that their pregnancy is still viable; and (2) should there be an absence of fetal cardiac activity, intervention can be recommended to obtain tissue for karyotype analysis sooner than perhaps may otherwise have occurred.

Early observation of fetal cardiac activity is reported to be a good prognostic indicator for ultimate pregnancy success in the general population, with only 2% to 5% of women experiencing subsequent spontaneous abortion following the documentation of fetal cardiac activity.[88,324,506,575] Similar studies performed in infertile populations reported that the incidence of spontaneous abortion following a demonstration of fetal cardiac activity after the fourth, fifth, and sixth week of gestation was 2% to 3% but was 29.9% if fetal cardiac activity was not present until five weeks after conception.[467] Another study reported a 13.9% incidence of subsequent fetal loss in an infertility population where early fetal cardiac activity was ultrasonically documented but associated with small sac size.[139] Two studies in a population of women with recurrent abortion reported widely disparate rates of 55% and 17% for subsequent pregnancy loss, following documentation of fetal cardiac activity.[524,560] In both of these prior studies, ultrasonography was performed after 6 weeks' gestation and potential etiologies for pregnancy loss were not defined. We recently reported that the rate of subsequent spontaneous abortion after ultrasound documentation of fetal cardiac activity at 5 to 6 weeks from the last menstrual period in women with two or more prior spontaneous abortions of unexplained etiology was 22.7%, which was significantly higher than the 3.3% rate of spontaneous abortion in the control group.[311] Neither maternal age nor number of prior pregnancy losses were associated with the risk of subsequent abortion following the documentation of fetal cardiac activity.[311] These findings may be explained by an increased chance of pregnancy loss of chromosomally abnormal conceptions before fetal cardiac activity is established. The incidence of pregnancy loss is reported to be increased with both increasing number of prior spontaneous abortions and increasing maternal age, presumably because of an increased incidence of aneuploidic conceptions with advancing maternal age.[99,213,441,523,565] Maternal age was reported to be a more valid predictor of a potential chromosomal abnormality than a history of prior live births or spontaneous abortions.[113,247] Ultrasonography is useful in determining whether the products of conception are retained following a spontaneous abortion.[473] The use of duplex Doppler ultrasonography may be helpful in determining the existence of residual trophoblast in women with postabortal vaginal bleeding.[3] Failure to detect a fetal pole and fetal heart activity by 7 weeks' gestation is diagnostic for an aembryonic gestation.[404] A gestational sac of greater than 15 mm or crown-rump length of greater than 5 mm without fetal cardiac activity is also diagnostic for a missed abortion.[3]

Later in the pregnancy, fetal assessment, besides including a sonogram, should also include a maternal serum α-fetoprotein determination at 16 to 18 weeks' gestation with high or low values potentially representing fetal neural tube defects and fetal chromosomal abnormalities, respectively.[13,123,337,354] Women with unexplained elevations of serum α-fetoprotein are at an increased risk for second-trimester fetal loss.[325] Fetal chromosome studies are warranted not only for women over 35 years of age but also for all women who have experienced recurrent spontaneous abortion, since these pregnancies are more likely to be aneuploidic than in age-matched controls, even in couples with recurrent abortion who are without chromosomal abnormalities themselves.[145,248,567] Therefore, a history of recurrent abortion may be a risk factor for subsequent aneuploidy.

The techniques available for an assessment of potential fetal karyotype anomalies include chorionic villus sampling (CVS) and amniocentesis. Ultrasonography has been reported to be useful but cannot replace direct karyotype assessment.[50] Knowledge of the gestational age of prior pregnancy losses is important in determining when to assess fetal chromosomes. Fetal karyotype assessment after the pregnancy has progressed past the time of prior pregnancy losses is recommended. Amniocentesis is currently recommended instead of CVS, because of the potential lower risk.[448] Operator experience and timing of the procedure for CVS and amniocentesis are crucial in maximizing procedure safety.[260] Amniocentesis was traditionally performed at 16 to 17 weeks' gestation; however, recent studies indicated relative safety with the procedure being performed as early as 10 to 12 weeks' gestation.[93] In the future, fetal karyotype assessment may be able to be obtained through DNA isolation from nucleated fetal erythrocytes in maternal venous blood.[58] However, many technical difficulties need to be overcome before this possibility becomes a clinical reality.

While amniocentesis may be a better alternative than CVS in assessing fetal karyotype in viable pregnancy, CVS is quite useful in obtaining material for cytogenetic analysis in cases of a missed abortion before a complete evacuation and facilitates cytogenetic evaluation far better than culture of abortus material obtained following either spontaneous expulsion or induced evacuation.[28,269,510] Material obtained through curettage should be karyotyped following microscopic assessment to ensure that fetal-placental rather than decidual tissues are being processed.

Cytogenetic, phenotypic, and histologic analysis of subsequent abortus material is important both in terms of the potential predictive value it may have for future pregnancies, and for providing the couple with a potential reason for their pregnancy loss. Placentae of women with recurrent abortion do not always have distinctive pathologic features nor do they routinely posses histologic features characteristic of "rejection" as seen in transplanted allografts.[51] Decidual vasculitis noted in some aborted tissue specimens was hypothesized to represent pregnancy loss from an immunologic cause; however, cause-versus-effect phenomena for these observations are difficult to discern.[475] Placental morphology was correlated with normal and abnormal abortal karyotypes.[244] However, morphologic assessment does not obviate the need for karyotype analysis since not all investigators were able to document an association between abnormal placental histology and abnormal karyotype.[250,444] When maternal age and duration of pregnancy before loss have been controlled, neither decidual nor placental lesions have been found to be characteristic of a chromosomally abnormal pregnancy loss.[476] However, an increased prevalence of chronic inflammatory lesions such as intervillositis and decidual vasculitis were noted in chromosomally normal spontaneously aborted samples, as have villous infarcts that are not infrequently found in term placentae but are thought to be rare in normal first-trimester pregnancy.[166,265,476] Cause-versus-effect mechanisms cannot be discerned since abnormal histologic findings may be the result of fetal demise rather than its cause. More work is needed to discern the potential histopathology of the maternal-fetal interface in cases of sporadic and recurrent abortion compared with gestational age-matched elective pregnancy terminations.

Therapy

Chromosomal abnormalities. Unfortunately, when diagnostic efforts reveal a chromosomal abnormality in one or both partners of the couple with recurrent abortion, no corrective measures are currently possible. Genetic counseling prior to attempting another pregnancy is warranted. In cases where a Robertsonian translocation involving homologous chromosomes exists, either donor oocyte or sperm, depending on the affected partner, should be recommended since an abnormality always results in an aneuploidic conception. In other cases, synchronization of ovulation and sperm deposition may be of benefit.

Anatomic factors. Müllerian anomalies were traditionally approached through laparotomy techniques. The Jones reconstructive procedure and the Tompkins metroplasty were the two most commonly used procedures for uterine septum correction.[275,548] Hysteroscopic techniques have replaced the need for laparotomy except in extreme circumstances.[158] Hysteroscopic resection is now the treatment of choice for submucous leiomyomas, intrauterine adhesions, an intrauterine septum, and other intrauterine lesions.[92,152,329,380] Ultrasound-guided transcervical metroplasty has also been reported to be safe and effective.[427]

The use of concomitant prophylactic antibiotics and postoperative hormonal therapy have been challenged for all patients having hysteroscopic resection of intrauterine lesions.[330] Postoperative estrogen supplementation, although controversial, may be of benefit in cases following resection of large surface areas such as in the case of intrauterine adhesions; however, this is probably not necessary following hysteroscopic resection of an intrauterine septum.[82] In cases where hormonal supplementation is used, 2.5 mg of oral conjugated estrogen daily for 30 days is recommended; 10 mg of oral progestin is added during the last 10 days. Pregnancy is attempted during the cycle that follows withdrawal bleeding. In cases where a uterine perforation has occurred or abdominal metroplasty was performed, conception should be delayed for at least three cycles to allow uterine healing. Therapeutic options for women with uterine abnormalities as a result of diethylstilbesterol are few. Cervical cerclage using either the Shirodkar or McDonald techniques should be performed around 14 weeks' gestation to prevent fetal loss caused by an incompetent cervix.[110,344,494] In cases where these techniques previously failed, consideration should be given to intraabdominal cerclage, but because of the high complication rate with this technique, intraabdominal cerclage should only be attempted by physicians with considerable experience in using this method.[110,382]

Endometriosis, if encountered upon diagnostic evaluation, should be pelviscopically resected. Consideration should be given for resection of adenomyosis, if it distorts the normal intrauterine contour in the form of an adenomyoma.

Endocrine abnormalities. Luteal phase insufficiency has been managed by either stimulating folliculogenesis and thereby stimulating luteal function or by luteal phase support. This has been accomplished by either ovulation induction with clomiphene citrate, human menopausal gonadotropin (hMG), or exogenous progesterone supplementation. Clomiphene citrate augments gonadotropin secretion, facilitating folliculogenesis and luteal progesterone production.[62,296] Luteal phase defects, however, may be induced by clomiphene citrate through its antiestrogenic effects caused by estrogen receptor binding within the endometrium.[102] Reports of an increased incidence of pregnancy loss in some women undergoing ovulation induction could be due to induced luteal phase deficiency caused by clomiphene citrate.[178] Therefore, it is important to repeat the endometrial biopsy during a treatment cycle to confirm that luteal phase insufficiency was corrected before conception is attempted. The antiestrogenic activity of clomiphene citrate may adversely affect the quantity and quality of cervical mucous.[102,178] Following confirmation that ovulation induction has corrected luteal phase insufficiency, consideration should be given to performing a postcoital test during a conception cycle using clomiphene therapy.

The effect of therapy on pregnancy rates in women with luteal phase deficiency has not been substantiated; however, in cases of pregnancy loss, ovulation induction is advisable, with the documentation of severe luteal insufficiency (greater than 5 days out of phase).[142,290] Progesterone supplementation is acceptable for milder luteal phase defects (3 to 5 days out of phase).[514] If progesterone supplementation is chosen for luteal phase support, therapy consisting of 50 mg twice a day should be initiated 3 days after ovulation and continued through 8 to 9 weeks of gestation. Although higher peripheral blood levels of progesterone may be obtained using intramuscular injections, higher intrauterine levels have been observed using progesterone vaginal suppositories.[316]

Both gonadotropins and gonadotropin-releasing hormone (GnRH) have been successfully used to treat luteal phase insufficiency.[253,320,491] Other attempts to stimulate luteal phase progesterone production have included the use of hCG injections (1500 to 5000 IU) every 2 to 5 days following the LH surge for the first 8 weeks of gestation but were not definitively shown to be efficacious and may even promote follicular atresia if given too early or attenuate progesterone production if administered too late during the luteal phase.[61,211,395,574]

Ovulation induction may be beneficial in women with hyperandrogen and LH hypersecretion disorders by suppressing GnRH-induced release of pituitary LH.[242,553,574] Pituitary desensitization using GnRH agonist therapy has been reported to reduce pregnancy loss in women with PCOS (Table 14-5). Laparoscopic ovarian diathermy has been reported to reduce the incidence of spontaneous abortion (16% versus the expected 30% to 40%) in women with PCOS.[29] Enthusiasm for GnRH agonist therapy and ovarian diathermy for pregnancy loss in women with PCOS should be tempered until well-designed, prospective, randomized, controlled studies are performed. There is no evidence that either in vitro fertilization or other assisted reproductive technologies (IUI, GIFT, ZIFT, etc.) are beneficial in preventing recurrent pregnancy loss in women who are not having difficulty conceiving. An increased incidence of spontaneous abortion caused by chromosomal anomalies has been reported in women following ovulation induction.[64,433,460] Although couples with infertility are at increased risk for malobstetric outcomes including

Table 14-5. Pregnancy loss rates in women with PCOS following ovulation induction with and without GnRH agonist therapy

Study	Clomiphene citrate and/or hMG (%)	GnRH agonist plus FSH or hMG (%)
Johnson, Pearce[269]	11/20 (55)	2/20 (10)
Abdalla et al[1]	5/14 (36)	3/33 (9)
Balen et al[41]	51/108 (47)	15/74 (20)
Homburg et al[242]	37/97 (38)	17/97 (18)
TOTAL	104/239 (44)	37/224 (17)

spontaneous abortion, the difference in miscarriage rates between natural and induced cycles is not surveillance related.[263,301,435,496] Information tabulated by the Society for Assisted Reproductive Technologies of the American Society for Reproductive Medicine indicates that the spontaneous abortion rate following GIFT is higher than following IVF-ET.[352] Whether or not this is an age-related phonomena remains to be explored.

In women found to have thyroid abnormalities, treatment with synthroid may be helpful in cases of hypothyroidism, especially when associated with menstrual and ovulatory disorders. Titration of thyroid medication until a euthyroid state is achieved is essential. Similarly, bromocriptine should be advised only for women found to have hyperprolactinemia with titration of dosage, until normal prolactin levels are attained. There is no place in the modern medical management of recurrent abortion for either thyroid medication or bromocriptine in women who do not have a thyroid or prolactin disorder.

Infections. Antibiotic trials to test efficacy in preventing abortion have not been consistently randomized, double-blind, or placebo-controlled. In one nonrandomized study, *Mycoplasma* was isolated in 84.5% of couples with a history of 237 pregnancy losses and in only 25.4% of controls.[428] A 28-day course of doxycycline, 100 mg twice a day eliminated *M. hominis* in 100% of couples and *M. urealyticum* in 87.6% of couples. In couples where both organisms were cultured, 61.3% were eliminated with this therapy. The groups that were treated also had a significant reduction in pregnancy loss compared with the women who were not treated.[428]

Empiric antibiotic treatment has been advocated in couples with recurrent abortion but is not rational unless either a high index of suspicion exists for an infectious etiology or the cultures have revealed a specific infection potentially responsible for abortion. If an infection or infectious agent is documented, then susceptible antibiotics should be given to both partners with posttreatment cultures to verify elimination of the infecting organism.

Immunologic factors. The desperate desire for children has compelled couples with recurrent abortion to seek many alternative therapies such as immunotherapy. The immunotherapies proposed for recurrent abortion are given in Table 14-6. Despite the multitude of papers recommending treatment, immunotherapy has not been conclusively demonstrated to be efficacious (Table 14-7), and well-designed, prospective, randomized, double-blind, placebo-controlled trials have not been adequately performed.

The rationale for leukocyte transfusion using unrelated third party and later paternal cells was founded on the belief that by doing so, immunologic fetal rejection could be blocked by mimicking fetal antigen presentation during pregnancy. This was supposed to elicit a maternal immunoglobulin effector thought to be essential for pregnancy

Table 14-6. Immunotherapies proposed for recurrent spontaneous abortion

A. Immunostimulation—not substantiated
   1. Leukocyte transfusions
   2. Trophoblast vesicle fluid transfusions
   3. Seminal plasma suppositories

B. Immunosuppression—not substantiated
   1. Intravenous immunoglobulin-antiidiotype binding of idiotypes on T-cell receptor, Fc receptor blockage, inactivation of complement, inhibit B cell function, increase suppressor T-cell function.
   2. Phasmopheresis—removal of autoantibodies
   3. Corticosteroids—suppresses a myriad of immune/inflammatory responses
   4. Aspirin—suppresses platelet adhesiveness and inflammatory responses
   5. Heparin—suppresses platelet aggregation
   6. Progesterone—suppresses macrophage phagocytosis and lymphocyte proliferation
   7. Pentoxifyline—suppresses macrophage activation
   8. Cyclosporine A—suppresses immune responsiveness
   9. Nifedipine—may affect macrophage function

Table 14-7. Summary of immunotherapies

Treatment	Number of individuals treated	Success (%)
Paternal leukocyte immunization	822	73
Third-party leukocyte immunization	79	75
Trophoblast membrane infusion	79	57
Intravenous immunoglobulin	69	68
Seminal plasma suppositories	44	55
Progesterone controls	225	75
Autologous leukocyte immunization	101	60
Intralipid infusion	20	70
Psychotherapy	135	85
Saline alone	32	67
No treatment	304	58

From Johnson PM, Ramsden GH: Recurrent miscarriage, *Baillieres Clin Immunol Allerg,* 2:607-624, 1992.

maintenance. As previously discussed, the prerequisite for a blocking antibody or any maternal immunoglobulin effector for successful pregnancy is not scientifically valid since pregnancy is not dependent on an intact maternal immune system. Major histocompatibility homogeneity, or HLA sharing between aborting partners, MLC hyporesponsiveness, and maternal absence of antipaternal lymphocytotoxic antibodies were all proposed as a rationale for leukocyte immunization therapy, but as previously discussed, their significance in pregnancy has been disproven. Despite the lack of a scientifically sound rationale for leukocyte immunization therapy, a growing number of individuals have initiated leukocyte immunization clinics to meet the patient demand that some form of therapy be offered. Claims of efficacy based on anecdotal reports of a 70% pregnancy success following leukocyte immunization have become the primary rationale for its use.

The dose, route of administration, timing, and frequency of leukocyte immunization varies between centers offering this therapy, as have patient selection criteria and follow-up rates, rendering data comparison between centers problematic. Effective, prospective, randomized, double-blind, placebo-controlled trials are difficult to perform for leukocyte immunization because of the many centers offering this therapy on a fee-for-service basis. However, there were four such studies published.[89,181,240,369] The initial randomized trial published in 1985 revealed a significantly better outcome in women following immunization using paternal leukocytes, compared with control autologous leukocytes (Table 14-8).[369] The validity of this report has been challenged on the grounds of the low success rate in the placebo group.[223] One reason for the low (37%) pregnancy success in the women receiving autologous leukocytes may be because the women were aware that they were in the placebo and not the treatment group. The failure to report the pregnancy outcome of individuals who were excluded from this study also limited proper data analysis.[223] Two other randomized controlled reports showed no statistically significant benefit of paternal leukocyte immunization for recurrent abortion.[89,240] In these later studies, pregnancy success rates reported for the control group (65% to 76%) corresponded to success rates known from epidemiologic studies in women with two to four prior pregnancy losses, which suggests that in these two studies immunization was given in an appropriately double-blind fashion, unlike the earlier study.[9,369,414,441,565,566] The most recently published study that assessed the treatment of recurrent spontaneous abortion by paternal leukocyte immunization indicated that the live-birth rate among women receiving paternal immunization was 68% (13/19), while that for autologous cells was 47% (9/19), a statistically insignificant difference of $p = 0.1$ by the Fisher exact test.[181] However, none of the studies that address leukocyte immunization therapy have included an irrelevant antigen in the study design to determine if any observed benefit could be due to an immunologic phenomena known as antigenic competition[462] or to a statistical phenomena known as regression of the mean.[192,462] The small numbers of women included in these randomized trials have not enabled a definitive statement concerning efficacy.

Four recent metaanalyses of leukocyte immunization for recurrent abortion have been performed to attempt to address the efficacy of this therapy.[169,420] The first published metaanalysis that addressed previously published trials of immunization therapy for recurrent spontaneous abortion indicated that leukocyte immunization was not efficacious in the treatment of recurrent abortion.[169] The second metaanalysis that was also derived from previously published studies of patients who received leukocyte immunization for recurrent abortion suggested a slight beneficial effect but cautioned that these results may not be biologically relevant. The analysis concluded with the recommendation that immunotherapy should not be used unless under protocol and in a randomized controlled trial where the couple or their insurers were not charged a fee.[420] Another metaanalysis sponsored by the American Society of Immunology of Reproduction (ASIR) was performed and indicated that between 11 and 13 women had to be immunized before one achieved a successful birth.[586] Another metaanalysis, which incorporated the original data included in the ASIR study with additional patients, indicated that the live-birth rate was only 7.6% higher in women receiving paternal leukocytes than in controls, and again clinicians were cautioned that this therapy should not be given unless under protocol in well-designed, placebo-controlled trials at no cost to patients or their insurers.[483]

Leukocyte immunization is not without potential risks to both the woman receiving such therapy and her fetus (Table 14-9). Potentially life-threatening graft-versus-host disease was described in a woman receiving paternal leukocytes; however, not all practitioners using this therapy have reported adverse outcomes.[292] The Harvard Center for Recurrent Miscarriage at Brigham and Women's Hospital documented three cases of isoimmunization to blood group antigens (one to Kell and two to "c" antigens) in women who had previously received leukocyte immunzation at other centers.

Table 14-8. Results of prospective, randomized, double-blind, placebo-controlled trials of leukocyte immunization for recurrent abortion

	Paternal cells live born/total (%)	Autologous cells or saline live born/total (%)
Mowbray et al[369]	17/22 (73)	10/27 (37)
Ho et al[240]	31/22 (79)	32/47 (65)
Cauchi et al[89]	13/21 (62)	19/25 (70)
Gatenby et al[181]	13/19 (68)	9/19 (47)

Table 14-9. Potential risks of leukocyte immunization therapy

Anaphylaxis
Serum sickness
Isoimmunization
HIV
CMV
Hepatitis
Graft-versus-host disease
Intrauterine growth retardation
Thrombocytopenia in the fetus

Alternative immunostimulating therapies have been proposed and abandoned. An intravenous infusion of isolated, sterile, syncytiotrophoblast-microvillus, plasma membrane, vesicle preparations was attempted to mimic the fetal cell contact with maternal blood that normally occurs in pregnancy.[280] This approach, unlike leukocyte immunization, had the advantage of using nonviable cellular material that would not provoke sensitization to HLA, blood group, or platelet antigens. A randomized double-blind placebo-controlled trial and comparative open studies using this therapy in well-defined groups of women with unexplained recurrent abortion found no significant difference in subsequent pregnancy outcome, whether immunotherapy with trophoblast membrane, placebo, or no therapy was used.[280]

Third party seminal plasma suppositories have been used to immunize women with recurrent abortion.[107] The scientific rationale for this therapy was initially based on the idea of an idiotype-antiidiotype control circuit which depended on TLX, anti-TLX, and anti-anti-TLX, and the finding of TLX in semen.[285,533,542] The fact that TLX was later shown to be the complement receptor, CD46, seriously challenged the relevance of this hypothesis and thus the rationale involving TLX, seminal plasma insemination and pregnancy, and seminal plasma suppositories in the treatment of recurrent abortion.[345,425]

Other immunoregulating therapies (Table 14-6) have been advocated, especially in cases where abortion was thought to be due to either antiphospholipid antibodies or cellular immunity. Previous studies reported successful pregnancies in women with the antiphospholipid syndrome.[68,69,114,180,257,321,322,393,396,438,471] Definitive statements concerning which therapeutic option is best for antiphospholipid syndrome are difficult because most of these studies included small numbers of patients and differed in regard to selection criteria and diagnosis. Also, very few of the published studies to date were randomized, and none were placebo-controlled. Nevertheless, data to date suggest that successful pregnancies may be achieved by maternal therapy with prednisone, low-dose aspirin, prednisone and low-dose aspirin, or subcutaneous heparin with or without low-dose aspirin. A combination of prednisone and heparin should be avoided because of the potential of severe osteoporosis, leading to fractures. A combination of low-dose aspirin and heparin has been recommended because of the lower incidence of side effects than afforded with low-dose aspirin and prednisone.[69] A multicenter randomized trial found that a combination of low-dose aspirin and heparin was more efficacious than low-dose aspirin and prednisone in preventing recurrent pregnancy loss.[114] These findings, however, have not been substantiated by all investigators.[69] Although the side effects of heparin are not inconsequential (gastric bleeding, osteopenia), the side effects of prednisone may be worse (aseptic hip necrosis). The use of low-dose aspirin alone is not necessarily benign since an increased risk of abruptior placentae was associated with its use in low-risk women.[497]

Low-dose aspirin daily (80 mg) may be used for women with antiphospholipid syndrome even when they are not pregnant because these women are at risk for spontaneous thrombosis. Once a pregnancy is confirmed, heparin therapy is initiated. Currently, 10,000 IU sodium heparin is given subcutaneously twice daily throughout the gestation. APTT is obtained weekly and the dose adjusted until anticoagulation is confirmed. These pregnancies are closely followed by maternal-fetal medicine specialists because of the propensity for these individual to experience premature labor, intrauterine growth retardation, intrauterine fetal demise, and preeclampsia as previously discussed.

Other unsubstantiated approaches been used to treat patients with antiphospholipid syndrome including plasmapheresis and intravenous immunoglobulin.[57,85,135,161,168,398] Plasmapheresis is no longer considered since the only reports that indicated efficacy were compromised by concommitant administration of prednisone, while plasmapheresis alone was not found to be efficacious.[135,161,168] The use of intravenous immunoglobulin in the treatment of antiphospholipid syndrome was based on reports of efficacy with its use for other autoimmune related conditions.[70,148] Intravenous immunoglobulin has been used to treat unexplained recurrent pregnancy loss; however, these reports were of limited sample size, included patients with two prior losses and limited evaluations, and were nonrandomized or otherwise poorly controlled.[94,106,108,370,371] The specific rationale for the use of intravenous immunoglobulin for recurrent abortion is unclear, although known immunoregulating actions of immunoglobulin include antiidiotype binding to idiotypes on the T-cell receptor, blockage of Fc receptors on antigen-presenting cells, inactivation of complement components, enhanced T suppressor-cell function, and down-regulation of B-cell function.[148] Therefore, intravenous immunoglobulin may theoretically be beneficial in treating reproductive failure caused by TH1 immunity. Studies addressing this issue have yet to be performed. Other immunomodulating therapies theoretically useful in treating recurrent abortion attributable to immune activation include cyclosporine, pentoxifylline, and nifedipine; however, the risk of using these agents during pregnancy limits their use.[157]

Table 14-10. Immunomodulating therapies in development

1. Antigen-specific immunotherapy
2. Tolerance induction therapies
   a. antiimmune cells
   b. growth factors
   c. cytokines
   d. anticytokines

Progesterone was anecdotally and empirically used to treat reproductive failure, based on its endocrinologic properties, for over 40 years with limited success.[128,271] Few physicians are aware of the fact that in high doses (10^{-5} M) progesterone also has immunosuppressive properties capable of inhibiting macrophage phagocytosis, lymphocyte proliferation, and natural killer cell activity and was proposed as nature's immunosuppressant for the maintenance of normal pregnancy.[235,500] There is evidence that 10^{-5} M concentrations of progesterone can inhibit in vitro TH1 immunity in response to trophoblast.[415] The method of clinically incorporating this information awaits testing in a double-blind, randomized, placebo-controlled trial in women with evidence of TH1 immunity to trophoblast.[149]

Rapid advances in molecular immunology and transplantation biology will undoubtedly enable the formulation and availability of new, more effective treatment modalities for couples who experience immunologic reproductive failure (Table 14-10). Therapeutic options may include antigen-specific immunotherapy and tolerance induction brought about by antiimmune cell antibodies, growth factors, cytokines, and anticytokines.[547] Treatment modalities are needed for recurrent spontaneous abortion; however, the rationale for therapy must be scientifically well-founded and more innocuous than the disease.[229] There are 10 criteria needed to test therapeutic efficacy (Table 14-11). A compilation of all of the studies published in English that concern immunotherapy, other than for antiphospholipid syndrome for recurrent abortion, reveals no significant difference between current and past therapies and a placebo (Table 14-7).[292] Very few of these studies, however, were well designed. A moratorium should be placed on the publication of retrospective, nonrandomized, nonplacebo-controlled trials of therapies given to inadequate numbers of patients with fewer than four spontaneous abortions. The strength of placebo effects should not be underestimated in immunotherapeutic studies that concern recurrent spontaneous abortion. "Tender loving care" was reported to be efficacious in 80% to 85% of women experiencing recurrent abortion.[531,555]

A caring, empathetic attitude on the part of the physician toward the couple experiencing pregnancy loss is a prerequisite for healing. Fundamental to the teaching of the healing arts among the ancients was the knowledge of the interdependence between body and mind.[200] The acknowledgement to the couple of the pain and suffering that they experienced on account of their losses, and the resulting stress within themselves and within their relationship with each other, friends, and family may act as a catharsis which may enable them to incorporate their experience of loss into their lives rather than their lives into their experience of loss. Appropriate referrals to support groups, behavioral medicine specialists, psychologists, and psychiatrists with an interest in this problem should be offered. Self-help measures including meditation, yoga, or other exercise programs should also be suggested.

Table 14-11. Criteria needed to test therapeutic efficacy

1. Scientifically sound rationale for using a particular therapy
2. Power calculation to ensure the adequate number of subjects needed to test efficacy
3. Inclusion of patients with more than four spontaneous abortions
4. Prospective
5. Groups stratified by maternal age and number of prev losses
6. Randomized
7. Double-blind
8. Placebo-controlled
9. No other concomitant therapy given
10. Follow-up to ensure maternal-fetal safety

PROGNOSIS

Epidemiologic studies indicate that the probability of completing a successful pregnancy even after four consecutive spontaneous abortions is approximately 60%.[9,414,441,562,565] The majority of these epidemiologic studies neither considered the potential underlying etiologies for spontaneous abortion nor the maternal age. However, the prognosis for a successful pregnancy depends on the etiology of previous

Table 14-12. Prognosis for viable birth

		%
A. Following:	One abortion	76
	Two abortions	70
	Three abortions	65
	Four abortions	60
	Ultrasound-detected fetal cardiac activity at 6 weeks' gestation	77
B. With:	Genetic factors	20-78
	Anatomic factors	60-87
	Endocrine factors	> 90
	Infectious factors	70-90
	Antiphospholipid antibodies	70-90
	TH1 cellular immunity	70-87
	Unknown factors	40-86

spontaneous abortions (Table 14-12). The probability of a successful pregnancy for couples found to have chromosomal abnormality as the only predisposing cause for their spontaneous abortions varies between 20% and 78%, depending on the study.[208,543,562] Women with müllerian anomalies following surgical correction have a successful pregnancy rates between 60% and 87%.[130,208,230,543] Correction of a potential endocrine abnormality in women with recurrent abortion has the best prognosis for a successful pregnancy (more than 90%).[547] Antibiotic therapy for a cervical infection that potentially mediates reproductive loss was associated with a subsequent 70% to 90% live-birth rate.[428] Viable pregnancy rates of 70% to 90% have been reported for women receiving therapy for antiphospholipid syndrome.[69,322] An abnormal resistance index as measured with color Doppler ultrasound in women with antiphospholipid syndrome has been reported to predict pregnancies with poor fetal outcome.[87] Measurement of TH1 immunity in the form of immune cell secretion of embryotoxic cytokines (interferon-γ and tumor necrosis factor) was reported to predict pregnancy outcome with a positive and negative predictive value of 0.76 and 0.86, respectively in women with a history of unexplained recurrent abortion. Of 56 women found to be positive for TH1 immunity in early pregnancy, 40 (71%) miscarried, and 16 (29%) delivered a viable infant. Of 85 women found to be negative for TH1 immunity in early pregnancy, only 11 (13%) had a subsequent spontaneous abortion, whereas 74 (87%) delivered a viable infant.[149] The probability of women achieving successful pregnancies in cases where the etiology of their prior losses is unknown is 40% to 86%.[28,422,531,543,554,562] The live-birth rate after the documentation of fetal cardiac activity 5 to 6 weeks from the last menses in women with two or more unexplained spontaneous abortion is approximately 77%.[311]

CONCLUSION

The couple with a history of recurrent spontaneous abortion presents a clinical challenge. Reproductive failure is a frustrating problem, not only for couples experiencing pregnancy loss but for their physicians as well. This frustration often leads to the recommendation of unsubstantiated therapies with little scientific rationale for their use, which results in significant emotional and financial cost to the couple who experience reproductive failure and unnecessary increases in national health care expenditures. The ethical duty of every physician is to be sure that the tests and procedures that they use are worth the money, inconvenience, and risks involved.[445] Understanding the potential mechanisms involved in recurrent spontaneous abortion, together with a caring empathetic attitude toward the couple experiencing reproductive failure will enable the clinician to ameliorate the emotional distress that these couples face and will facilitate a rational, scientific assessment that will lead to appropriate consultation and ultimate therapy.

REFERENCES

1. Abdalla HI et al: Comparative trail of luteinizing hormone-releasing hormone analogue: HMG and clomiphene citrate/HMG in an assisted conception/program, *Fertil Steril* 53:473-478, 1990.
2. Ablogren M: Sperm transport to and survival in the human fallopian tube, *Gynecol Invest* 6:206-214,1975.
3. Achiron R et al: Transvaginal duplex Doppler ultrasonography in bleeding patients suspected of having residual trophoblastic tissue, *Obstet Gynecol* 81:507-511, 1993.
4. Adashi EY, Resnick CE: Prolactin as an inhibitor of granulosa cell luteinization: implications for hyperprolactenemia-associated luteal phase dysfunction, *Fertil Steril* 48:131, 1987.
5. Adoni A et al: The incidence of intrauterine adhesions following spontaneous abortion, *Int J Fertil* 27:117-118, 1982.
6. Adorini L et al: Tolerance induction in mature T-cells, *Immunologist* 1(6):185-190, 1993.
7. Adorini et al: Selective immunosuppression, *Immunol Today* 285-289, 1993.
8. Aksel S: Sporadic and recurrent luteal phase defects in cyclic women: comparison with normal cycles, *Fertil Steril* 33:372, 1980.
9. Alberman E: The epidemiology of repeated abortion. In *Early pregnancy loss: mechanisms and treatment*, New York, 1988, Springer-Verlag.
10. Altshuler G: Immunologic competence of the immature fetus: morphologic evidence from intrauterine cytomegalovirus infection, *Obstet Gynecol* 43:811-816, 1974.
11. Alving BM et al: The dilute phospholipid APTT: sensitive assay for verification of lupus anticoagulants, *Thromb Haemost* 54:709, 1985.
12. American College of Obstetricians and Gynecologists: *Antenatal diagnosis of genetic disorders,* Washington, DC 1987, ACOG, 1-8 (Technical bulletin no. 108).
13. American College of Obstetricians and Gynecologists: *Ultrasound in pregnancy,* Washington, DC 1988, ACOG, 1-3 (Technical bulletin no. 116).
14. American College of Obstetricians and Gynecologists: *Exercise during pregnancy and the postpartum period,* Washington, DC, 1994, ACOG, (Technical bulletin no.189).
15. American Fertility Society: Classification of müllerian anomalies, *Am Fertil Soc* 1988.
16. American Fertility Society: Guideline for practice: recurrent pregnancy loss, *Am Fertil Soc,* 1993.
17. Amos DB, Kostyn DD: HLA: a central immunological agency of man, *Adv Hum Genet* 10:137-141, 1980.
18. Amuzu BJ, Shapiro SS: Variation in spontaneous abortion rate relates to the indication for therapeutic donor insemination, *Obstet Gynecol* 82:128-131, 1993.
19. Anderson DJ, Berkowitz RS: Gamma interferon enhances expression of class I MHC antigens in the early HLA(+) human choriocarcinoma cell live BeWo but does not induce MHC expression in the HLA(-) choriocarcinoma cell live jar, *J Immunol* 135:2498, 1985.
20. Anderson DJ, Hill JA: Cell-mediated immunity in infertility, *Am J Reprod Immunol Microbiol* 17:22-30, 1988.
21. Anderson DJ et al: Adverse effects of immune cell products in pregnancy. In Grill T, Wegmann T, editors: *Molecular and cellular immunobiology of the maternal-fetal interface,* New York, 1991, Oxford Press.
22. Anderson DJ: Trophoblast/leukocyte common antigen is expressed by human testicular germ cells and appears on the surface of acrosome-reacted sperm, *Biol Reprod* 41:285-293, 1989.
23. Ando N et al: Prolactin disorders in patients with habitual abortion, *Nippon Sanka Fujinda Gakkai Zasshi* 44:650-656, 1992.
24. Andoh K et al: Endometrial dating in the conception cycle, *Fertil Steril* 58:1127-1130, 1992.
25. Anokute CC: Epidemiology of spontaneous abortions: the effects of alcohol consumption and cigarette smoking, *J Nat Med Assoc* 78:771-775, 1986.

26. Ansbacker R: Clinical investigation of listeria monocytogenesis as a possible cause of human fetal wastage, *Am J Obstet Gynecol* 94:386-390, 1966.
27. Aoki K et al: Specific antiphospholipid antibodies as a predictive variable in parents with recurrent pregnancy loss, *Am J Reprod Immunol* 29:82-7, 1993.
28. Appleman Z et al: Chorionic villus sampling for fetal karyotyping in missed abortions, *Prenat Diag* 11:55-57, 1991.
29. Armar NA et al: Laparoscopic ovarian diathermy: an effective treatment for antiestrogen-resistant anovulatory infertility in women with the polycystic ovary syndrome, *Br J Obstet Gynaecol* 100:161-164, 1993.
30. Asherman JG: Traumatic intrauterine adhesions, *J Obstet Gynaecol Br Commw* 57:892-896, 1950.
31. Aspillaga MO et al: Endocrinologic events in early pregnancy failure, *Am J Obstet Gynecol* 147:903-908, 1983.
32. Austin CR: Chromosome deterioration in aging eggs of the rabbit, *Nature* 213:1018-1019, 1967.
33. Austin CR: The egg. In Austin CR, Short RV, editors: *Reproduction in mammals I. Germ cells and fertilization*, Cambridge, 1982, Cambridge University Press.
34. Azuma K et al: Is the luteoplacental shift a myth? Analysis of low progesterone levels in successful ART pregnancies, *J Clin Endocrinol Metab* 77:195-198, 1993.
35. Baaklini N et al: Spontaneous abortion: etiology survey, *Rev Fr Gynecol Obstet* 85:667-672, 1990.
36. Bacz A: The early pregnancy: a role of the male factor, *Eur J Obstet Gynecol Reprod Biol* 24:126-129, 1987.
37. Bagshawe KD: *Choriocarcinoma*, Baltimore, 1969, Williams & Wilkins.
38. Balasch J, Vanrell J: Corpus luteum insufficiency and fertility: a matter of controversy, *Hum Reprod* 2:557-567, 1987.
39. Balen AH, Jacobs HS: Gonadotropin surge attenuating factor: a missing link in the control of LH secretion? *Clin Endocrinol* 35:399-402, 1991.
40. Balen AH, Tan SL, Jacobs HS: Hypersecretion of luteinizing hormones: a significant cause of infertility and miscarriage, *Br J Obstet Gynaecol* 100:1082-1089, 1993.
41. Balen AH et al: Miscarriage rates following in vitro fertilization are increased in women with polycystic ovaries and reduced by pituitary desensitization with Busarelin, *Hum Reprod* 8:959-964, 1993.
42. Barbieri RL, Smith S, Ryan KJ: The role of hyperinsulinemia in the pathogenesis of ovarian hyperandrogenism, *Fertil Steril* 50:197-212, 1988.
43. Barres AB et al: Fertility and outcome of pregnancy in women exposed in utero to diethylstilbestrol, *New Eng J Med* 302:609-613, 1980.
44. Barrett JM, Boehm FH, Killam SP: Induced abortions–a risk factor for placenta previa, *Am J Obstet Gynecol* 141:769-772, 1981.
45. Batzer FR: Hormonal evaluation of early pregnancy, *Fertil Steril* 34:1-20, 1980.
46. Batzer FR et al: Serid β-subunit hCG doubling time as a prognosticator of pregnancy outcome in an infertile population, *Fertil Steril* 35: 307-312, 1981.
47. Batzer FR et al: Landmarks during the first 42 days of gestation demonstrated by the β-subunit of hCG and ultrasound, *Am J Obstet Gynecol* 146: 973-979, 1983.
48. Beer RJS, Bradford WP, Hart RJC: Pregnancy complicated by psittacosis acquired from sheep, *Br Med J* 284: 1156-1157, 1982.
49. Beer AE et al: Major histocompatibility complex antigens, maternal and paternal immune responses, and chronic habitual abortion in humans, *Am J Obstet Gynecol* 141:987-999, 1981.
50. Benacerraf BR: The use of sonography for the antenatal-detecting, *Clin Diagn Aneuploidy Ultrasound* 25: 21-54, 1989.
51. Benirschke K, Kaufmann P: Abortion, placentas of trisomies, and immunological considerations of recurrent reproductive failure. In *Pathology of the human placenta*, New York, 1990, Springer-Verlag.
52. Berger MJ, Goldstein DP: Impaired reproductive performance in DES- exposed women, *Obstet Gynecol* 55:25-27, 1980.
53. Bergquist C, Nillius SJ, Wide L: Human gonadotropin therapy. I. Serum estradiol and progesterone patterns during conception cycles, *Fertil Steril* 39:761-765, 1983.
54. Bergquist UO: Video display terminals and health: a technical and medical appraisal of the state of the art, *Scand J Work Environ Health* 10:1-87, 1984.
55. Berkowitz RS et al: Effects of products of activated leukocytes (lymphokines and monokines) on the growth of malignant trophoblast cells in vitro, *Am J Obstet Gynecol* 158:199-203, 1988.
56. Berman SM et al: Deaths from spontaneous abortion in the United States, *JAMA* 253:3119-3123, 1985.
57. Bernstein RM, Crawford RJ: Intravenous IgG therapy for anticardiolipin syndrome: a case report, *Clin Exp Rheumatol* 6:198, 1988.
58. Bianchi DW et al: Isolation of fetal DNA from nucleated erythrocytes in maternal blood, *Proc Natl Acad Sci U S A* 87: 3279-3283, 1990.
59. Billington WD: Maternal-fetal interactions in normal human pregnancy, *Baillieres Clin Immunol Allerg* 2:527-549, 1988.
60. Blum M: Comparative study of serum CAP activity during pregnancy in malformed and normal uterus, *J Perinat Med* 6:165, 1978.
61. Blumenfeld Z, Ruach M: Early pregnancy wastage: the role of repetitive weeks of gestation, *Fertil Steril* 58:19-23, 1992.
62. Bohnet HG et al: Different hormonal patterns in human menopausal gonadotropin-treated, clomiphene-treated, and untreated conception cycles, *Fertil Steril* 45:469, 1986.
63. Bonney RC, Franks S: The endocrinology of implantation and early pregnancy, *Baillieres Clin Endocrinol Metab* 4:207-301, 1990.
64. Boue J, Boue A: Increased frequency of chromosomal anomalies in abortions after induced ovulation, *Lancet* 7804:679-680, 1973.
65. Boue J, Boue A, Laser P: Retrospective and prospective epidemiologic studies of 1500 karyotyped spontaneous abortions, *Teratology* 11:11-26, 1975.
66. Branch DW et al: Association of lupus anticoagulant with antibody against antiphosphotidyl serine, *Clin Immunol Immunopathol* 42:63, 1987.
67. Branch DW, Scott JR: Clinical implication of antiphospholipid antibodies: the Utah experience. In Harris EN et al, editors: *Phospholipid-binding antibodies*, Boca Raton, FL, 1990, CRC Press.
68. Branch DW et al: Obstetric complications associated with the lupus anticoagulant, *N Eng J Med* 313:1322, 1985.
69. Branch DW et al: Outcome of treated pregnancies in women with antiphospholipid syndrome: an update of the Utah experience, *Obstet Gynecol* 80:614-620, 1992.
70. Brand A, Witvliet M, Claas FHJ: Beneficial effect of intravenous gammaglobuline in a patient with complement-mediated autoimmune thrombocytopenia due to IgM-antiplatelet antibodies, *Br J Haematol* 69:507-511, 1988.
71. Braulke I et al: Factor XII (Hageman) deficiency in women with habitual abortion: new subpopulation of recurrent aborters? *Fertil Steril* 59:98-101, 1993.
72. Braunstein GD et al: First-trimester hCG measurements as an aid in the diagnosis of early pregnancy disorders, *Am J Obstet Gynecol* 131: 25-32, 1978.
73. Brent RL: Radiation teratogenesis: fetal risk and abortion, *Med Phys Mmogr* 5:225-252, 1980.
74. Brustmen LE et al: Changes in the pattern of vaginosis or preterm birth uterine contractility in relationship to coitus during pregnancy at low and high risk for premature labor, *Obstet Gynecol* 73:166-168, 1989.

273. Jones GES: The clinical evaluation of ovulation and the luteal phase, *J Reprod Med* 18:139, 1977.
274. Jones HW: Reproductive impairment and the malformed uterus, *Fertil Steril* 36:137-148, 1981.
275. Jones HW, Seagar-Jones GE: Double uterus as an etiological factor in repeated abortion: indications for surgical repair, *Am J Obstet Gynecol* 65:325, 1953.
276. Jones WR: The use of antibodies developed by infertile women to identify relevant antigens. In Diczfalusy E, editor: *Immunological approaches to fertility control*, Stockholm, 1974, Karolinska Institute.
277. Jones W, Man E: Thyroid function in human pregnancy: premature deliveries and reproductive failure of pregnant women with low butanol extractable iodines, *AM J Obstet Gynecol* 104:999, 1969.
278. Jones GS, Aksel S, Wentz AC: Serum progesterone values in luteal phase defects: effects of chorionic gonadotropin, *Obstet Gynecol* 44:26, 1974.
279. Jonson PM et al: Immunological and immunogenetic investigation of recurrent spontaneous abortions, *Dis Markers* 6:163-171, 1988.
280. Jonson PM, Ramsden GH: Recurrent miscarriage, *Baillieres Clin Immunol Allerg* 2:607-624, 199.
281. Jouppila P, Huhtaniemi I, Tapanainen J : Early pregnancy failure: study by ultrasonic and hormonal methods, *Obstet Gynecol* 55: 42-47, 1980.
282. Jovanovich L et al: Hormonal profile as a prognostic index of early threatened abortion, *Am J Obstet Gynecol* 110:274-278, 1978.
283. Juger S, Kremer J, De Wilde-Janssen IW: Are sperm immobilizing antibodies in cervical mucus an explanation for a poor postcoital test? *Am J Reprod Immunol* 5:56-60, 1984.
284. Kajino T, Ferrier A: cytogenetics of aborters and abortuses, *Am J Obstet Gynecol* 131:33-38, 1978.
285. Kajino T, Torry DS, McIntyre JA: Trophoblast antigens in human seminal plasma, *Am J Reprod Immunol Microbiol* 17:91, 1988.
286. Kalousek DK, Barrett IJ, Gartner AB: Spontaneous abortion and confined chromosomal mosaicism, *Hum Genet* 88:642-646, 1992.
287. Kalousek DK et al: Uniparental disomy for chromosome 16 in human; *Am J Genet* 52:8-16, 1992.
288. Kalter H: Diabetes and spontaneous abortion: historical review, *Am J Obstet Gynecol* 156:1243-1253, 1987.
289. Kaminski PF, Lyon DS: Implications of sampling the implantation site in the endometrial biopsy for infertility, *J Reprod Med.* 35:208-210, 1990.
290. Karamardin LM, Grimes DA: Luteal phase deficiency: effect of treatment on pregnancy rates, *Am J Obstet Gynecol* 167:1391-1398, 1992.
291. Karow WG, Gentry W: Corpus leteum function duy pregnancy previously infertile women, *Obstet Gynecol* 48:603-610, 1976.
292. Katz I et al: Cutaneous graft-versus-hostlike reaction after paternal lymphocyte immunization for prevention of recurrent abortion, *Fertil Steril* 57:927-929, 1992.
293. Kauffman RH et al: Upper genital tract changes and pregnancy outcome in offspring in utero to diethylstilbestrol, *Am J Obstet Gynecol* 137:299-308, 1980.
294. Kauma SW et al: Colony stimulating factor-1 c-fms expression in human endometrial tissues and placenta during the menstrual cycle and early pregnancy, *J Clin Endocrinol metab* 73:746-751, 1991.
295. Keller DW et al: Pseudocorpus luteum insufficiency: a local defect of progesterone action on endometrial stroma, *Fertil Steril* 48:127-132, 1979.
296. Kevin JF et al: Evidence for a hypothalamic site of action of clomiphene citrate in women, *J Clin Endocrinol Metab* 61:265, 1985.
297. Keye WR JR., Jaffe RB: Changing patterns of FSH and LH responses to gonadotropin-releasing hormone in the puerperium, *J Clin Endocrinol Metab* 42:1133, 1976.
298. Khods G: Cytogenetics of habitual abortion: a review, *Am J Obstet Gynecol* 29:299-310, 1974.
299. Kincaid-Smith P, Bullen M: Bacteriuria in pregnancy, *Lancet* 1:395-399, 1965.
300. Kline J et al: Induced abortion and spontaneous abortion: no connection? *Am J Epidemiol* 107:290-298, 1978.
301. Kol S et al: The natural history of multiple pregnancies after assisted reproduction: is spontaneous fetal demise a clinically significant phenomenon? *Fertil Steril* 60:127-130, 1993.
302. Kovats S et al: A class I antigen, HLA-G, expressed in human trophoblasts, *Science* 248:220-223, 1990.
303. Kroisel PM, Rosenkranz W: High resolution banding of an unusual reciprocal translocation in recurrent abortions, *Clin Genet* 37:230-234, 1990.
304. Kundsin RB, Driscoll SC: Strain of *Mycoplasma* associated with human reproductive failure, *Science* 157:1573, 1967.
305. Kundsin RB, Driscoll SC, Pelletier PA: *Ureaplasma urealyticum* incriminated in perinatal morbidity and mortality, *Science* 213:474-476, 1981.
306. Kwki T, Ylikorkala O: Coitus during pregnancy is not related to bacterial vaginosis or preterm birth, *Am J Obstet Gynecol* 169:1130-1134, 1993.
307. Labarrere CA, Althabe OH: Hypothesis: primary chronic abortion, preeclampsia, idiopathic intrauterine growth retardation, hydatiform mole, and choriocarcinoma: a unique concept, *Am J Reprod Immunol* 10:156-157, 1986.
308. Lagrew D, Wilson EA, Jawad J: Determination of gestational age by serum concentration of human chorionic gonadotropin, *Obstet Gynecol* 62:37-40, 1983.
309. Larras-Regard E, Tayuog A, Davis ML: Effects of TSH on the thyroid activity of adult or neonate amphibians, CRS Seances, *Soc Biol* 176:795-803, 1982.
310. Lash AF, Lash SR: Habitual abortion: the incompetent internals of the cervix, *Am J Obstet Gynecol* 59:68-76, 1950.
311. Laufer MR, Ecker JL, Hill JA: Pregnancy outcome following ultrasound-detected fetal cardiac activity in women with history of multiple spontaneous abortion, *J Soc Gynecol Invest* 2 138-142, 1994.
312. Leiman G, Harrison N, Rubin A: Pregnancy following conization of the cervix: complications related to the cone size, *Am J Obstet Gynecol* 136:14-18, 1980.
313. Li TC, Dockery P, Cooke ID: Endometrial development in the luteal phase of women with various types of infertility: comparison with women of normal fertility, *Hum Reprod* 6:325-330, 1991.
314. Lird T, Whittaker PG: The endocrinology of early pregnancy failure. In Huisjes HJ, Lird T, editors: *Early pregnancy failure*, New York, 1990, Churchill Livingston.
315. Lishner M, Amato D, Farine D: Different outcomes of pregnancy in women with essential thrombocytosis, *IS J Med Sci* 29:100-102, 1993.
316. Lobo RA et al: Intrauterine and peripheral blood progesterone levels following intramuscular infections and vaginal suppositories.
317. Lockshin MD et al: Antibody to cardiolipin as a predictor of fetal distress or death in pregnant patients with systemic lupus erythematosus, *N Eng J Med* 313:152, 1985.
318. Lolis D, Tzigounis V, Michalas S, et al: Toxoplasma antibodies and spontaneous abortion, *Int J Gynecol Obstet* 15:299-301, 1978.
319. Lopata A et al: The ultrastructure of the preovulatory human egg fertilized in vitro, *Fertil Steril* 33:12-20, 1980.
320. Loucopoulos A, Ferin M: The treatment of luteal phase defects with pulsatile infusion of gonadotropin-releasing hormone, *Fertil Steril* 48:933, 1987.
321. Lubbe WF et al: Fetal survival after prednisone suppression of maternal lupus anticoagulant, *Lancet* 1:1361-1363,1983.
322. Lubbe WF, Liggins GC: Role of lupus anticoagulant and autoimmunity in recurrent pregnancy loss, *Semin Reprod Endocrinol* 6:161-190, 1988.
323. Lyden TW, NG AK, Rote NJ: Modulation of phosphatidyl-serine epitope expression on BeWo cells during forskolin treatment, *Am J Reprod Immunol* 27:24, 1992.

324. MacKenzie WE, Holmes DS, Newton JR: Spontaneous abortion rate in ultrasonographically visible pregnancy, *Obstet Gynecol* 71:81-83, 1988.
325. Maher JE et al: Unexplained elevation in maternal serum α-fetoprotein and subsequent fetal loss, *Obstet Gynecol* 83:138-141, 1994.
326. Malinak CR, Wheeler JM: Association of endometriosis with spontaneous abortion, prognosis for pregnancy, and risk for recurrence, *Semin Reprod Endorinol* 3:361, 1985.
327. Mallmann P, Mallman R, Krebs D: Determination of tumor necrosis factor α and interleukin 2 in women with idiopathic recurrent miscarriage, *Arch Gynecol Obstet* 249:73-78, 1991.
328. Mann ED, McLain WD, Hayt DB: The physiology and clinical significance of the uterine isthmus, *A J Obstet Gynecol* 81:209, 1961.
329. March CM, Israel R: Gestational outcome following hysteroscopic lysis of adhesions, *Fertil Steril* 36:455, 1981.
330. March CM, Israel R: Hysteroscopic management of recurrent abortion caused by septate uterus: with discussion, *Am J Obstet Gynecol* 156:834-842, 1987.
331. Mardh PA, Estrom L: Tubal and cervical cultures in acute salpingitis with special reference to *Mycoplasma hominis* and T.-strain *Mycoplasmas, Br J Vener Dis* 46;179, 1970.
332. Marriott IA, Stuchly MA: Health aspects of work with visual display terminals, *J Occup Med* 28:835-848, 1986.
333. Martin DH et al: Prematurity and perinatal mortality in pregnancies complicated by maternal *Chlamydia trachomatis* infections, *JAMA* 247:1585-1588, 1982.
334. Martin PA, Shaver EL: Sperm aging in utero and chromosomal anomalies in rabbit blastocysts, *Dev Biol* 28:480-486, 1972.
335. Martin-DeLeon PA, Boice ML: Sperm aging the male and cytogenic anomalies: an animal model, *Human Genet* 62:70-77, 1982.
336. Maslar IA, Riddick DH: Prolactin production by human endometrium during the normal menstrual cycle, *Am J Obstet Gynecol* 135:751-754, 1979.
337. Maternal serum–α-fetoprotein measurement in antenatal screening for anencephaly and spina bifida in early pregnancy: report of the UK collaborative study on α-fetoprotein in relation to neural-tube defects, *Lancet* 1:1323-1332, 1977.
338. Mathur S et al : Sperm immunity in infertile couples: antibody titers are higher against the husbands' sperm than to sperm from controls, *Am J Reprod Immunol* 3:18-22, 1983.
339. Mattei MG et al: Partial inversion of the secondary constriction of chromosome 9: does it exist? *Human Genet* 59:310, 1981.
340. Mattison DR: Minimizing toxic hazards to fetal health, *Contemp OB Gyn* 8:81-100, 1992.
341. McConnachie PR, McIntyre JA: Maternal antipaternal immunity in couples predisposed to repeated pregnancy losses, *Am J Reprod Immunol* 5:145-150, 1984.
342. McCormack WM et al: Sexual activity and vaginal colonization with genital *Mycoplasmas, JAMA* 221:1375, 1972.
343. McDonald IA: Incompetent cervix as a cause of recurrent abortion, *J Obstet Gynaecol Br Commw* 70:105-109, 1963.
344. McDonald IA: Cervical cerclage, *Clin Obstet Gynecol* 7:461-466, 1980.
345. McIntyre JA: In search of trophoblast-lymphocyte cross-reactive (TLX) antigens, *Am J Reprod Immunol Microbiol* 17:100, 1988.
346. McIntyre JA, Faulk WP: Recurrent spontaneous abortion in human pregnancy: results of immunogenetical, cellular, and humoral tests, *Am J Reprod Immunol* 4:165-170, 1983.
347. McIntyre JA et al: Human trophoblast-lymphocyte cross-relative (TLX) antigens define a new alloantigen system, *Science* 222:1135-1137, 1983.
348. McLaren H et al: Pregnancy and cone biopsy of the cervix, *J Obstet Gynecol Br Commw* 81:383-387, 1974.
349. McNatty KP, Sawers RS, McNeilly AS: A possible role for prolactin in control of steroid secretion by the human Graafian follicle, *Nature* 250:653, 1974.
350. McShane P, Reilly RJ, Schiff I: Pregnancy outcomes following Tompkins metroplasty, *Fertil Steril* 40:190-194, 1983.
351. Medawer PB: Some immunological and endocrinological problems raised by the evolution of vivi parity in vertebrates, *Symp Soc Exp Biol* 7:320-338, 1953.
352. Medical Research International: In vitro fertilization–embryo transfer in the United States: 1990 results from the IVF-ET registry, *Fertil Steril* 57:15-24, 1992.
353. Menge AC: Immune reactions and infertility, *J Reprod Fertil* 10:171-187, 1970.
354. Merhatz IR et al: An association between low maternal serum α-protein and fetal chromosome abnormalities, *Am J Obstet Gynecol* 148:886-994, 1984.
355. Metzger DA et al: Association of endometriosis and spontaneous abortion: effects of control group selection, *Fertil Steril* 45:18, 1986.
356. Miller JF et al: Fetal loss after implantation: a prospective study, *Lancet* 2:554-556, 1980.
357. Miller K et al: Pericentric inversion 14, *Ann Genet* 33:225-227, 1990.
358. Mills JL et al : Moderate caffeine use at the risk of spontaneous abortion and intrauterine growth retardation, *JAMA* 269:598-603, 1993.
359. Minelli E et al: Cytogenetic findings on echographically defined blighted ovum abortions, *Ann Genet* 36:107-110, 1993.
360. Mintz G et al: Prospective study of pregnancy in systemic lupus erythematosus: results of a multidisciplinary approach, *J Rheumatol* 13:732, 1986.
361. Miodovnik M et al: Spontaneous abortion among insulin-dependent diabetic women, *Am J Obstet Gynecol* 150:372-376, 1984.
362. Mitus AJ, Shafer AI: Thrombocytosis and thrombocythemia, *Hematol Oncol Clin N Am* 4:157-178, 1990.
363. Mizuno K et al: Significance of Jones-Jones operation on double uterus: vascularity and dating of endometrium in uterine septum, *Jap J Fertil Steril* 29:9, 1978.
364. Moller M et al: Rupture of fetal membranes and premature delivery associated with group B Streptococci in urine of pregnant women, *Lancet* 2:69, 1984.
365. Moon YS et al: Prostaglandin F in human endometriotic tissue, *Am J Obstet Gynecol* 141:344, 1981.
366. Morgan CE et al: Pregnancy outcome in 98 women exposed to diethylstilbestrol in utero: their mothers and unexposed siblings, *Obstet Gynecol* 59:315, 1982.
367. Mossmann TR et al: Two types of murine-helper T-cell clones. I. Definition according to profiles of lymphokine activities and secreted proteins, *J Immunol* 136:2348-2357, 1986.
368. Mosmann TR, Coffman RL: TH1 and TH2 cells: different patterns of lymphokine secretion lead to different functional properties, *Ann Rev Immunol* 7:145-173, 1989.
369. Mowbray JF et al: Controlled trial of treatment of recurrent spontaneous abortion by immunostimulation with paternal cells, *Lancet 1*:941-943, 1985.
370. Mueller-Eckhardt G et al: Prevention of recurrent spontaneous abortion by intravenous immunoglobulin, *Vux Sang* 56:151-154, 1989.
371. Mueller-Eckhart G, Huni O, Poltrin B: IVIG to prevent recurrent sponteous abortion, *Lancet* 1:424-425, 1991.
371a. Mulvihill JJ, Stewart KR: Antineoplastic drugs and spontaneous abortion in nurses, *N Eng J Med* 314:1048-1049, 1986.
372. Musich JR, Behrman SJ: Obstetric outcome before and after metroplasty in women with uterine anomalies, *Obstet Gynecol* 52:63-66, 1978.
373. Naeye RL: Coitus and associated amniotic-fluid infections, *N Eng J Med* 301:1198-2000, 1979.
374. Naeye RL: Factors that predispose to premature rupture of the fetal membranes, *Obstet Gynecol* 60:93-98, 1982.

375. Nahmias AJ et al: Perinatal risk associated with maternal genital *Herpes simplex* virus infection, *Am J Obstet Gynecol* 110:825-837, 1971.
376. Naib ZM et al: Association of maternal genital herpetic infection with spontaneous abortion, *Obstet Gynecol* 35:260-263, 1970.
377. Nakajima ST et al: Endometrial histology after first-trimester spontaneous abortion, *Fertil Steril*, 55:32-35, 1991.
378. Neilson JP, Mutambisa M: Coitus, twin pregnancy, and preterm labor, *Am J Obstet Gynecol* 160:416-418, 1989.
379. Neri G et al: Reproductive risk for translocation carries: cytogenetic study and analysis of pregnancy outcome in 58 families, *Am J Hum Genet* 16:535-561, 1983.
380. Neuwirth RS: A new technique for an additional experience with hysteroscopic resection of submucous fibroids, *Am J Obstet Gynecol* 131:91, 1978.
381. Nobel C: Malimplantation—a cause of failure after IVF and GIFT, *Am J Reprod Immunol* 6:56-57, 1984.
382. Novy MJ: Transabdominal cervicisthmic cerclage for the management of repetitive abortion and premature delivery, *Am J Obstet Gynecol*, 143:44, 1982.
383. Noyes RW, Hertig AT, Rock J: Dating the endometrial biopsy, *Fertil Steril* 1:3, 1950.
384. Ober CL et al: Adverse effects of human leukocyte antigen DR sharing on fertility: a cohort study in a human isolate, *Fertil Steril* 44:227-232, 1985.
385. Ober CL et al: Antibodies and pregnancy history in a healthy population, *Am J Obstet Gynecol* 169:143-147, 1993.
386. Ober CL et al: Shared HLA antigens and reproductive performance among Hutterites, *Am J Hum Genet* 35:994-1004, 1983.
387. Oehninger S et al: Corrective measures and pregnancy outcome in invitro fertilization in patients with severe sperm morphology abnormalities, *Fertil Steril* 50:283-287, 1989.
388. Ogden E, Amstey MS: *Hemophilus influenza* septicemia and midtrimester abortion, *J Reprod Med* 22:106-108, 1979.
389. Ogilvie MM, Teare CF: Spontaneous abortion after Hand/Foot and Mouth disease caused by Coxackie virus A16, *Br Med J* 281:1527-1528, 1980.
390. Olive DL, Franklin RR, Gratkins CV: The association between endometriosis and spontaneous abortion, *J Reprod Med* 27:333, 1982.
391. Olive DL, Haney AF: Endometriosis-associated infertility: a critical review of therapeutic approaches, *Obstet Gynecol Surv* 50:538-555, 1986.
392. Omer H: Possible psychophysiologic mechanism in premature labor, *Psychosomatics* 27:580-584, 1986.
393. Ordi J et al: Fetal loss treatment in patients with antiphospholipid antibodies, *Ann Rheum Dis* 48:798-802, 1989.
394. Osztovics MK, Toth SP, Wessely JA: Cytogenetic investigations in 418 couples with recurrent fetal wastage, *Am J Med Genet* 25:232-236, 1982.
395. Ottobre JS, Soiffer RL: Persistant versus transient stimulation of the macque corpus luteum during prolonged exposure to hCG: a function of age of the menstrual cycle, *Endocrinol* 114:475, 1984.
396. Out HJ et al: A prospective, controlled multicenter study on the obstetric risks of pregnant women with antiphospholipid antibodies, *Am J Obstet Gynecol* 167:26-32, 1992.
397. Out HJ et al: "Lupus" anticoagulant and inhibition of prostacyclin formation in patients with repeated abortion, intrauterine growth retardation, and intrauterine deaths, *Br J Obstet Gynaecol* 167:26-32, 1992.
398. Parke A et al: Intravenous gammaglobulin, antiphospholipid antibodies and pregnancy, *Ann Intern Med* 11:495, 1989.
399. Parks J, Barter RH: The myomatous uterus complicated by pregnancy, *Am J Obstet Gynecol* 63:260, 1952.
400. Partnoi MF et al: Karyotypes of 1142 couples with recurrent abortion, *Am J Obstet Gynecol* 72:31-34, 1988.
401. Patrick MJ: Renal infection in pregnancy: the natural development of bacteria in pregnancy, *J Obstet Gynaecol Br Commonw*, 73:793-796, 1966.
402. Pauli RM: Mechanism of bone and cartilage maldevelopment in the warfarin embryopathy, *Pathol Immunolpathol Res* 7:107, 1980.
403. Peaceman AM et al: Interlaboratory variation in antiphospholipid antibody testing, *Am J Obstet Gynecol* 166:1780-1787, 1992.
404. Pekonen F et al: Decreased 34 K insulin-like growth-factor binding protein in polycystic ovarian disease, *Fertil Steril* 51: 972-975, 1989.
405. Pennell RG et al: Prospective comparison of vaginal and abdominal sonography in normal early pregnancy, *J Ultrasound Med* 10:63-67, 1991.
406. Pennes DR, Bowerman RA, Silver TM: Congenital uterine anomalies and associated pregnancies: findings and pitfalls of sonographic diagnosis, *J Ultrasound Med* 4:531, 1985.
407. Petershan L: Fertility in patients with ovarian endometriosis and after treatment, *Acta Obstet Gynecol Scand* 49:331, 1970.
408. Pfeifer-Ohlsson S et al: Cell type specific pattern of myc protooncogene expression in developing human embryos, *Proc Natl Acad Sci U S A* 82:5050, 1985.
409. Pittaway DE: Endometriosis and spontaneous abortions, *Semin Reprod Endocrinol* 6:257, 1988.
410. Pittaway DE, Ellington CD, Klimek M: Preclinical abortions and endometriosis, *Fertil Steril* 49:221, 1988.
411. Pittaway DE, Vernon C, Fayez JA: Spontaneous abortions in women with endometriosis, *Fertil Steril* 50:711, 1988.
412. Pittaway DE, Wentz AC: Endometriosis and corpus luteum function: is there a relationship? *J Reprod Med* 29:712-716, 1984.
413. Pittaway DE et al: The efficacy of early pregnancy monitoring with serial hCG determinations and real-time sonography in an infertile population, *Fertil Steril* 44:190-194, 1985.
414. Poland BJ et al: Reproductive counseling in patients who had a spontaneous abortion, *Am J Obstet Gynecol* 127:685-691, 1977.
415. Polgar K, Hill JA: Progesterone inhibits in vitro embryotoxic factor production in women with recurrent spontaneous abortion, 41st Annual Meeting of the Society for Gynecologic Investigation, Chicago, IL, 1994.
416. Polifka JE, Friedmann JM: Environmental toxins and recurrent pregnancy loss, *Inf Reprod Med Clinic N Am* 2:195-213, 1991.
417. Polishuck WZ, Anteby SO, Weinstein D: Puerperal endometritis and intrauterine adhesions, *Int Surg* 60:418-421, 1975.
418. Polson DW et al: Polycystic ovaries: a common finding in normal women, *Lancet* 11:870-872, 1980.
419. Poole PA, Whitehouse DB, Gilchrist MM: A case of abortion consequent upon infection with *Brucella* aborts biotype 2, *J Clin Pathol* 25:882-884, 1972.
420. Prandiville WJ, Scott JR: Immunotherapy for recurrent miscarriage. In Enkin MW et al, editors: Pregnancy and childbirth module: cochrane database of systematic reviews, Rev no. 06814, Sept 30, 1993.
421. Pratt D et al: Antithyroid antibodies and the association with nonorgan specific antibodies in recurrent pregnancy loss, *Am J Obstet Gynecol* 168: 837-841, 1993.
422. Prazzini F et al: Short-term reproductive prognosis when no cause can be found for recurrent miscarriage, *Br J Obstet Gynaecol* 95:654-658, 1988.
423. Prout TE: Thyroid disease in pregnancy, *Am J Obstet Gynecol* 122:669-676, 1975.
424. Public Health Laboratory Service Working Party on Fifth Disease: Prospective study of human parvovirus (B19) infection in pregnancy, *Br Med J* 300:1166-1170, 1990.
425. Purcell DFJ et al: The human cell surface glycoproteins Hu Ly-M5, membrane cofactor protein (MCP) of the complement system, and trophoblast-lymphocyte cross-reactive (TLX) antigens are CD46, *Immunol* 70:155-161, 1990.

426. Quenby SM, Farquharson RG: Predicting recurring miscarriage: what is important? *Obstet Gynecol* 82:132-138, 1993.
427. Querlen D, Brasme TL, Parmentier D: Ultrasound-guided transcervical metroplasty, *Fertil Steril* 54:995-998, 1990.
428. Quin PA et al: Efficacy of antibiotic therapy in preventing spontaneous pregnancy loss among couples colonized with genital *Mycoplasmas*, *Am J Obstet Gynecol* 145:239, 1983.
429. Quinn PA et al: Prevalence of antibody to *Chlamydia trachomatis* in spontaneous abortion and infertility, *Am J Obstet Gynecol* 156:291-296, 1987.
430. Quinn PA et al: Efficacy of antibiotic therapy in preventing spontaneous pregnancy loss among couples colonized with genital *Mycoplasmas*, *Am J Obstet Gynecol* 145:239-244, 1983.
431. Rabau E, David A: Intrauterine adhesions: etiology, prevention, and treatment, *Obstet Gynecol* 22:626-629, 1963
432. Rabau E, David A: *Listeria monocytogenes* in abortion, *J Obstet Gynecol* 70:481, 1963.
433. Racowsky C, Kaufman ML: Nuclear degeneration and meiotic aberrations observed in human oocytes in vitro: analysis by light microscopy, *Fertil Steril* 58:750-755, 1992.
434. Radwanska E, Frankenberg J, Allen E: Plasma progesterone levels in normal and abnormal early human pregnancy, *Fertil Steril* 30:398-402, 1978.
435. Ransom MX et al: The difference in miscarriage rates between menotropin-induced and natural cycle pregnancies is not surveillance related, *Fertil Steril* 59:567-570, 1993.
436. Rappaport F, Rabinovitz M: Genital *listeriosis* as a cause of repeated abortion, *Lancet* 1:1273, 1960.
437. Reamy K, White S: Sexuality in pregnancy and puerperium: a review, *Obstet Gynecol Surv* 40:1-13, 1985.
438. Reece EA et al: Recurrent adverse pregnancy outcome and antiphospholipid antibodies, *Am J Obstet Gynecol* 163:162-169, 1990.
439. Regan L, Braude PR: Is antipaternal cytotoxic antibody a valid marker in the management of recurrent abortion? *Lancet* 11:1280-1282, 1987.
440. Regan L, Braude PR, Hill DP: A prospective study of the incidence, time of, appearance of, significance of antipaternal lymphocytotoxic antibodies in human pregnancy, *Hum Reprod* 6:294-298, 1981.
441. Regan L, Braude PR, Trembath PL: Influence of postreproductive performance on risk of spontaneous abortion, *Br Med J* 299:541-545, 1989.
442. Regan L, Chao S, James LS: Premature rupture of membranes, preterm delivery and group B *Streptococcal* colonization of mothers, *Am J Obstet Gynecol* 141:184, 1981.
443. Regan L, Owen EJ, Jacobs HS: Hypersecretion of luteinizing hormone, infertility, and miscarriage, *Lancet* 336:1141-1144, 1990.
444. Rehder H et al: Is there a correlation between morphological and cytogenetic findings in placental tissue from early missed abortions? *Hum Genet* 82:377-385, 1989.
445. Relman AS: On controversy in medicine, *Pharos* 18-22, 1978.
446. Repke JT, Hardy JB, McCarthy J: Is a history of prior abortion a risk factor for preterm delivery and now birth weight? 41st Meeting of the Society for Gynecologic Investigation, 1994 (abstract 445).
447. Reynolds WA: Thyroid function in mother, fetus, and neonate, *Obstet Gynecol Ann* 7:67-90, 1978.
448. Rhodes GG et al:The safety and efficacy of chronic villus sampling for early prenatal diagnosis of cytogenetic abnormalities, *N Eng J Med* 320:609-617, 1989.
449. Rice JP, Kay HH, Mahony BS: The clinical significance of uterine leiomyomas in pregnancy, *Am J Obstet Gynecol* 160:1212, 1989.
450. Riddick DH et al: De nova synthesis of prolactin by human decidua, *Life Sci* 23:1913-1922, 1978.
451. Riley LA, Tuomala RE: Infectious diseases and recurrent pregnancy loss, *Inf Reprod Med Clin N Am* 2:165-174, 1991.
452. Roberts CJ, Lowe CR: Where have all the conceptions gone? *Lancet* 1: 498-499, 1975.
453. Robertson WB: Defective haemochorial placentation as a cause of miscarriage: a preliminary study, *Br J Obstet Gynaecol* 94:649-655, 1987.
454. Rock JA, Murphy AA: Anatomic abnormalities, *Clin Obstet Gynecol* 29:886-891, 1986.
455. Rock JA, Jones HA: The clinical management of the double uterus, *Fertil Steril* 28:793-806, 1977.
456. Rocklin RE et al: Maternal-fetal relation: absence of an immunologic blocking factor from serum of women with chronic abortions, *N Eng J Med* 295:1209, 1976
457. Rocklin RE, Kitzmiller JL, Garvey MR: Maternal-fetal relation: further characterization of an immunologic blocking factor that develops during pregnancy, *Clin Immunol Immunopathol* 22:305-315, 1982.
458. Rodger C: Lack of a requirement for a maternal humoral immune response to establish and maintain successful allogenic pregnancy, *Transplant* 40:372-375, 1985.
459. Rodriquez-Escudero FJ et al: Does mild endometriosis reduce fecundity? *Fertil Steril* 522-524, 1988.
460. Roesler M, Wise L, Katayama KP: Karyotype analysis of blighted ova in pregnancies achieved by in vitro fertilization, *Fertil Steril* 51:1065-1066, 1989.
461. Rogers BB et al: Detection of human parvovirus B19 in early spontaneous abortuses using serology, histology, electron microscopy, in situ hybridization, and the polymerase chain reaction, *Obstet Gynecol* 81:402-408, 1993.
462. Roitt IM: *Essential immunology*, Boston, 1980, Blackwell Scientific.
463. Romagnani SI: Human TH1 and TH2 subsets: doubt no more, *Immunol Today* 8:256-257, 1991.
464. Romagnani SI: Human TH1 and TH2 subsets: regulation of differentiation and role in protection and immunopathology, *Int Arch Allergy Appl Immunol* 4:279:85, 1992.
465. Romero R et al: Infection and labor. III. Interleukin 1: a signal for the onset of parturition, *Am J Obstet Gynecol* 160:1117-1123, 1989.
466. Romero R, Duffy TP: Platelet dividers in pregnancy, *Clin Perinatol* 7:327-448, 1980.
467. Rosen GF et al: Predicting pregnancy outcome by the observation of a gestational sac or of early fetal cardiac motion with transvaginal ultrasonography, *Fertil Steril* 54:260-264, 1990.
468. Rosenbuseh B, Sterzik K, Lauritzen C: Cytogenetic analysis of sperm chromosomes in couples with habitual abortion, *Geburtshilfe Frauenheilkal* 51:369-372, 1991.
469. Rosenbusch B, Strehler E, Sterzik K: Cytogenetics of human spermatozoa: correlation with sperm morphology and age of fertile men, *Fertil Steril* 58:1071-1072, 1992.
470. Rosenfeld DL, Garcia CR: Endometrial biopsy in the cycle of conception, *Fertil Steril* 26:1088-1093, 1975.
471. Roseover MH et al: Heparin therapy for pregnant women with lupus anticoagulant or anticoagulant antibodies, *Obstet Gynecol* 75:630-634, 1990.
472. Rosner F, Grunwald HW: Thrombocytosis and spontaneous abortion, *Am J Hematol* 27:233, 1988.
473. Rubin MC, Bornstein SG, Campbell JD: The reliability of ultrasonography in the management of spontaneous abortion, clinically thought to be complete: a prospective study, *Am J Obstet Gynecol* 168:12-15, 1993.
474. Sagle M et al: Recurrent early miscarriage and polycystic ovaries, *Br Med J* 297:1027-1028, 1988.
475. Salafia CM, Burns JP: The correlation of placental and decidual histology with karyotope and fetal viability, *Teratology* 39:478, 1989.
476. Salafia C et al: Placental and decidual histology in spontaneous abortion in detailed description and correlations with chromosome number, *Obstet Gynecol* 82:295-302, 1993.
477. Salem HT et al: Prognostic value of biochemical tests in the assessement of fetal outcome in threatened abortion, *Br J Obstet Gynaecol* 91:382-385, 1984.

478. Sargent IL, Wilkins T, Redman CWG: Maternal immune responses to the fetus in early pregnancy and recurrent miscarriage, *Lancet* 11:1099-1104, 1994.
479. Schenker JG, Margalioth EJ: Intrauterine adhesions: an update appraisal, *Fertil Steril* 37:593-610, 1982.
480. Schneditsch MO et al: Hormonal considerations in early normal pregnancy or blighted ovum syndrome, *Fertil Steril* 31:252-257, 1979.
481. Schnorr TM et al: Video display terminals and the risk of spontaneous abortions, *N Eng J Med* 324:727, 1991.
482. Schved J et al: Factor XII congenital deficiency and early spontaneous abortion, *Fertil Steril* 52:335-336, 1989.
483. Scott J: Controversies in ob/gyn: leukocyte immunization for recurrent spontaneous abortion 41st Annual Meeting of the Society for Gynecologic Investigation, Chicago, IL , 1994.
484. Scott JR et al: Intravenous globulin treatment of pregnant patients with recurrent pregnancy loss due to antiphospholipid antibodies and Rh immunization, *Am J Obstet Gynecol* 159:1055-1056, 1988.
485. Selevan SG et al: A study of occupational exposure to antineoplastic drugs and fetal loss in nurses, *N Eng J Med* 313:1173-1178, 1985.
486. Semmens JP: Congenital anomalies of the female genital tract, *Obstet Gynecol* 19:328-350, 1962.
487. Semmens JP: Congenital defects of the reproductive tract: clinical implications, *Contemp Obstet Gynecol* 5:95, 1975.
488. Shafer AI: The hypercoagulable states, *Am Intern Med* 102:814-828, 1985.
489. Shaffer W: Role of uterine adhesions in the cause of multiple pregnancy losses, *Clin Obstet Gynecol* 29:912-924, 1986.
490. Sharf M, Eibschitz I, Eylan E: Latent toxoplasmosis and pregnancy, *Obstet Gynecol* 42:349, 1973.
491. Shapiro AG: New treatment for the inadequate luteal phase, *Obstet Gynecol* 40:826, 1972.
492. Shiomura K et al: Recombinant human tumor necrosis factor-α: thrombus formation as a cause of antitumor activity, *Int J Cancer* 41:243, 1988.
493. Shirodkar VN: A new method of operative treatment for habitual abortions in the second trimester, *Antiseptic* 52:299-330, 1955.
494. Shirodkar VN: *Surgical treatment of habitual abortion. Tendances actuelles en gynecologie et obstertrique, Geneva*, 1955, Georg O. Cie.
495. Shmoys S, Kaplan C: Parvovirus and pregnancy, *Clin Obstet Gynecol* 33:268-275, 1990.
496. Shoham Z, Zosmer A, Insler V: Early miscarriage and fetal malformations after induction of ovulation (by clomiphene citrate and/or human menotropins), in vitro fertilization, and gamete intrafallopian transfer, *Fertil Steril* 55:1-11, 1991.
497. Sibai BM et al: Prevention of preeclampsia with low-dose aspirin in healthy nulliparous pregnant women, *N Eng J Med* 329:1213-1218, 1993.
498. Siegel M: Congenital malformations following chickenpox, measles, mumps, and hepatitis: results of a cohort study, *JAMA* 226:1521-1524, 1973.
499. Siegler AM, Hellman LM: Tubalplastic surgery: report of a survey, *Fertil Steril* 7:170-177, 1950.
500. Siiteri PK et al: Progesterone and maintenance of pregnancy: is progesterone nature's immunosuppressant? *Ann NY Acad Sci* 286:384-397, 1977.
501. Silver RM et al: Unexplained elevations of maternal serum α-fetoprotein in women with antiphospholipid antibodies: a harbinger of fetal death, *Obstet Gynecol* 83:150-155, 1994.
502. Simmen FA, Simmen RCM: Peptide growth factors and protooncogenes in mammalian conceptus development, *Biol Reprod* 44:1-5, 1991.
503. Simon AE et al: Abortion and perinatal sepsis associated with *Campylobacter* infection, *Rev Infec Dis* 8:397-402, 1986.
504. Simpson JL: Genes, chromosomes, and reproductive failure, *Fertil Steril* 33:107, 1980.
505. Simpson JL, Martin AO: Parental diagnosis of cytogenetic disorders, *Clin Obstet Gynecol* 19:841-853, 1976.
506. Simpson JL et al: Low fetal loss rates after ultrasound-proved visibility in early pregnancy, *JAMA* 258:2555-2557, 1987.
507. Smith JB, Cowchock FS: Immunological studies in recurrent spontaneous abortion: effects of immunization of women with paternal mononuclear cells in lymphocytotoxic and mixed lymphocyte reaction-blocking antibodies and correlation with sharing of HLA antigens and pregnancy outcome, *J Reprod Immunol* 14:99, 1988.
508. Soltes B et al: Hormonal profiles of early gestation with abnormal karyotype, *Fertil Steril* 59:810-814, 1993.
509. Sompolinsky D, Soloman F et al: Infections with *Mycoplasma* and bacteria in induced midtrimester and fetal loss, *Am J Obstet Gynecol* 121:610, 1975.
510. Sorokin Y et al: Postmasterm chorionic villus sampling in correlation of cytogenetic and ultrasound findings, *Am J Med Genet* 39: 314-316, 1991.
511. Soules MR et al: Luteal phase deficiency: abnormal gonadotropins and progesterone secretion patterns, *J Clin Endocrinol Metab* 69:813-820, 1989.
512. Soules MR et al: The corpus luteum: determinants of progesterone secretion in the normal menstrual cycle, *Obstet Gynecol* 71:659, 1988.
513. Soules MR et al: Luteal phase deficiency: characteristics of reproductive hormones over the menstrual cycle, *J Clin Endocrinol Metab* 69:804-812, 1989.
514. Soules MR et al: The diagnosis and therapy of luteal phase deficiency, *Fertil Steril* 28:1033, 1977.
515. Soupe D, Mishell DR Jr, LaCavra M: Correlation of endometrial maturation with 4 methods of estimating day of ovulation, *Obstet Gynecol* 73:88, 1989.
516. Southern PM: Habitual abortion and toxoplasmosis: is there a relationship? *Obstet Gyencol* 39:45, 1972.
517. Spellacy WN et al: Plasma growth hormone and estradiol levels in women with uterine myomas, *Obstet Gynecol* 40:829, 1972.
518. Speroff L, Ramwell PW: Prostaglandins in reproductive physiology, *Am J Obstet Gynecol* 107:111-113a, 1970.
519. Stabile I, Campbell S, Grudzinskas GJ: Ultrasound assessment in complications of first-trimester pregnancy, *Lancet* 2:1237-1239, 1987.
520. Stagnaro-Green A et al: Detection of at-risk pregnancy by means of highly sensitive assays for thyroid autoantibodies, *JAMA* 1422-1425, 1990.
521. Steier JA, Bergsijo P, Myking OL: Human chorionic gonadotropin in maternal plasma after induced abortion, spontaneous abortion, and removed ectopic pregnancy, *Obstet Gynecol* 64:391, 1984.
522. Stein ZA: Early fetal loss: birth defects 17:95-111, 1981.
523. Stein ZA:A woman's age: childbearing and childrearing, *Am J Epidemiol* 121:327-340, 1985.
524. Stern JJ, Coulam CB: Mechanism of recurrent spontaneous abortion. I. Ultrasonographic findings, *Am J Obstet Gynecol* 166:1844-1852, 1992.
525. Stevenson CS: Myomectomy for improvement of fertility, *Fertil Steril* 15:367, 1964.
526. Stewart DR et al: Enhanced ovarian steroid secretion before implantation in early human pregnancy, *J Clin Endocrinol Metab* 76:1470-1476, 1993.
527. Stillman RJ: In utero exposure to diethylstilbestrol: adverse effects on the reproductive tract and reproductive performance in male and female offspring, *Am J Obstet Gynecol* 142:1905, 1982.
528. Stillman RJ, Hershlag A: Pathology of infertility and adverse pregnancy outcome after in utero exposure to diethylstilbestrol. In Gondos B, Riddick DH, editors: *Pathology of infertility: clinical correlations in the male and female,* New York, 1987, Theime Med.
529. Stirrat GM: Recurrent miscarriage: its definition and epidemiology, *Lancet* 336:73-75, 1990.
430. Stray-Pedersen B. Lorentzen-Stry A: Uterine *T. mycoplasma* infections and repeated abortions, *Am J Obstet Gynecol* 128:716, 1977.

531. Stray-Pederson B, Stray-Pederson S: Etiologic and subsequent reproductive performance in 195 couples with a prior history of habitual abortion, *Am J Obstet Gynecol* 148:140-146, 1984.
532. Sui BC et al: Temporal and constitutive expression of homebox-2 gene (Hu-2), human heart-shock gene (hsp-70), and oncogenes C-sis and N-myc in early human trophoblast, *Am J Obstet Gynecol* 150:1195, 1988.
533. Suic-Foca N, Reemisma K, King DW:The significance of the idiotypic antiidiotypic network in humans, *Transplant Proc* 18:230, 1986.
534. Sulewski JM, Ward SP, McGaffic W: Endometrial biopsy during a cycle of conception, *Fertil Steril* 34:548-551, 1980.
535. Sutherland HW, Pritchard CW: Increased incidence of spontaneous abortion in pregnancies complicated by diabetes mellitus, *Am J Obstet Gynecol* 155:135-138, 1986.
536. Sweet RL et al: *Chlamydia trachomatis* infection and pregnancy outcome, *Am J Obstet Gynecol* 156:824-833, 1987.
537. Tabibzadeh S: Human endometrium: an active site of cytokine production and action, *Endo Rev* 12:272-290, 1991.
538. Tambascia M et al: Sustained hyperprolactinemia in a normally menstruating woman with apparently normal ovarian function, *Fertil Steril* 34:282, 1980.
539. Tannebaum TW, Goldberg RJ: Exposure to anesthetic gases and reproductive outcome: a review of the epidemiologic literature, *J Occup Med* 27:659-668, 1985.
540. Tartakovsky B: CSF-1 induced resorption of embryos in mice, *Immunol Letters* 23:65-70, 1989.
541. Taylor VM et al: Placenta previa in relation to induced and spontaneous abortion: a population-based study, *Obstet Gynecol* 82:88-91,1993.
542. Thaler CJ: Immunlogic role for seminal plasma in insemination and pregnancy, *Am J Reprod Immunol Microbiol* 21:147, 1989.
543. Tho PT, Byrd JR, McDonough PG: Etiologic and subsequent reproductive performance of 100 couples with a prior history of habitual abortion, *Fertil Steril* 32:389-395, 1979.
544. Tho SPT, McDonough PG: Genetics of fetal wastage, sporadic and recurrent abortion, *Inf Reprod Med Clin N Am* 5:157-176, 1994.
545. Thomas R, Reid RL: Thyroid disease and reproductive dysfunction: a review, *Obstet Gynecol* 70:789, 1987.
546. Thrailkill KM et al: Insulin-like growth factor I stimulates the synthesis and release of prolactin from human decidual cells, *Endocrinol* 123:2930-2934, 1988.
547. Tisch R, McDevitt HO: Antigen-specific immunotherapy: is it a real possibility to combat T-cell–mediated autoimmunity? *Proc Natl Acad Sci U S A* 91:437-438, 1994.
548. Tompkins P: Comments on the bicornuate uterus and twinning, *Surg Clin North Am.* 42:1049,1962.
549. Tompkins P : Hazards of electromagnetic fields to human reproduction, *Fertil Steril* 53:185, 1990.
550. Torpin R: Placenta circumvallata and placenta marginata, *Obstet Gynecol* 6:277-284, 1955.
551. Toth M et al: The role of infection in the etiology of preterm birth, *Obstet Gynecol* 71:723-726, 1988.
552. Tsutsum I, Oka T: Epidermal growth factor deficiency during pregnancy causes abortion in mice, *Am J Obstet Gyencol* 156:241-244, 1987.
553. Tulppala M et al: Polycystic ovaries and levels of gonadotropins and androgens in recurrent spontaneous abortion: prospective study in 50 women, *Br J Obstet Gynaecol.*
554. Tulppala M et al: A prospective study of 63 couples with a history or recurrent spontaneous abortion: contributing factors and outcome of subsequent pregnancies, *Hum Reprod* 8:764-770,1993.
555. Tupper C, Weil RJ: The problem of spontaneous abortion, *Am J Obstet Gynecol* 83:423, 1962.
556. Tyson JE et al: Inhibition of cyclic gonadotropin secretion by endogenous human prolactin, *Am J Obstet Gynecol* 121:375, 1975.
557. Unander AM et al: Anticardiolipin antibodies and complement in 99 women with habitual abortion, *Am J Obstet Gynecol* 156: 114, 1985.
558. Van Voorhis BJ et al: Prostaglandin synthesis localization in the human uterus and in endometriosis, *Am J Obstet Gynecol* 163:57, 1990.
559. Van Der Slikke JW, Treffers PE: Influence of induced abortion on gestational duration in subsequent pregnancies, *Br Med J* 1: 270-272, 1978.
560. VanLeeuman I, Brarch DW, Scott JR: First-trimester ultrasonography findings in women with history of recurrent pregnancy loss, *Am J Obstet Gynecol* 168:111-114, 1993.
561. Verp MS et al: Heritable aspects of uterine anomalies. I. Three familial aggregates with müllerian fusion anomalies, *Fertil Steril* 40:80-90, 1983.
562. Vlaadneren W, Treffers PE: Prognosis of subsequent pregnancies after recurrent spontaneous abortion in first trimester, *Br Med J* 295: 92-93, 1987.
563. Wagner N, Butler J, Sanders J: Prematurity and orgasmic coitus during pregnancy: data on a small sample, *Fertil Steril* 27:911-915, 1976.
564. Walters C et al: Human myometrium: a new potential source of prolactin, *Am J Obstet Gynecol* 147:639-644, 1983.
565. Warburton D, Fraser FC: On the probability that a woman who has had a spontaneous abortion will abort in subsequent pregnancies, *Br J Obstet Gynaecol* 68:784-787, 1961.
566. Warburton D, Fraser FC: Spontaneous abortion rate in man: data from reproductive histories collected in a medical genetic unit, *J Hum Genet* 10:1, 1963.
567. Warburton D et al: Does the karyotype of a spontaneous abortion predict the karyotype of a subsequent abortion? *Am J Hum Genet* 41:465-483, 1987.
568. Watson H et al: Hypersecretion of luteinizing hormone and ovarian steroids in women with recurrent early miscarriages, *Hum Reprod* 8:829-833, 1993.
569. Wegmann TG: Maternal T-cells promote placental trophoblast growth and prevent spontaneous abortion, *Immunol Letters* 17:297-302, 1988.
570. Wentz AC et al: Cycle of conception endometrial biopsy, *Fertil Steril* 46:196-199, 1986.
571. Westergoard JG et al:Does ultrasound examination render biochemical tests obsolete in the predicting of early pregnancy failure? *Br J Obstet Gynaecol* 92:77-83, 1985.
572. Wheeler JM, Johnston BM, Malinak LR: The relationship of endometriosis to spontaneous abortion, *Fertil Steril* 39:656-660, 1983.
573. Wilcox AJ et al: Incidence of early loss of pregnancy, *New Eng J Med* 319:159-194, 1988.
574. Williams RF, Hodgen GD: Disparate effects of human chorionic gonadotropin during the late follicular phase in monkeys: normal ovulation, follicular atresia, ovarian cyclicity, and hypersecretion of follicle phase in monkeys: Normal ovulation, follicular atresia, ovarian acyclicity, and hypersecretion of follicle-stimulating hormone, *Fertil Steril* 33:64, 1980.
575. Wilson RD et al:Spontaneous abortion and pregnancy outcome after normal first-trimester ultrasound examination, *Obstet Gynecol* 67: 352-355, 1986.
576. Witkin SS, Chaudry A: Association between recurrent spontaneous abortions and circulating IgG antibodies to sperm tails in women, *J Reprod Immunol* 15: 151-158, 1989.
577. Witkin SS, Ledger WJ: Antibodies to *Chlamydia trachomatis* in sera of women with recurrent spontaneous abortions, *Am J Obstet Gynecol* 167:135-139, 1992.
578. Wright AD et al: Spontaneous abortion and diabetes mellitus, *Postgrad Med J* 59:295-298, 1983.
579. Wu M, Yunis AA: Common pattern of two distinct types of colony-stimulating factors in human tissue and cultured cells, *J Clin Invest* 66:772-775, 1980.
580. Yamada H, Polgar K, Hill JA: Evidence of cell-mediated immunity to trophoblast antigens in women with recurrent spontaneous abortion, *Am J Obstet Gynecol*, 170:1339-1344, 1994 (in press).

581. Yamada K: Population studies of INV (9) chromosomes in 4300 Japanese: incidence, sex difference, and clinical significance, *Jap J Hum Genet* 37:293-301, 1992.
582. Yen SSC: The polycystic ovary syndrome, *Clin Endocrinol* 12:177-208, 1980.
583. Yovich JL et al:The prognostic value of hCG, PAPP-A, Oestrodiol-17 bater of progesterone in early human pregnancy, *Aust N Z J Obstet Gynecol* 26:59-64, 1986.
584. Zabriskie JR: Pregnancy and the malformed uterus: report of 92 cases, *West J Obstet Gynecol* 70:293, 1962.
585. Zhao X, Singh B, Batten BE: The role of c-mos protooncogene in mammalian meiotic maturation, *Oncogene* 6:43-49, 1991.
586. The Recurrent Miscarriage Immunotherapy Trialist Group: Worldwide collaborative observational study and metaanalysis of allogenic leukocyte immunotherapy for recurrent spontaneous abortion, *Am J Reprod Immunol* 32:55-72, 1994.

Chapter 15

PRINCIPLES OF BIOSTATISTICS AND EPIDEMIOLOGY FOR GYNECOLOGISTS

Daniel W. Cramer

Readers may begin this chapter with different concepts about "statistics." To some, statistics conveys the notion of assembling and summarizing data. To others, statistics is the end result of description in the community (e.g., birth rates and death rates—vital statistics). To still others, statistics means statistical inference—determining whether observations differ from that expected by chance. Each of these interpretations is considered in the first part of this chapter. Clinical data are generally collected within the context of studies designed to determine the causes of a disease or its treatment. It is necessary for clinicians to have an appreciation of study designs in order to understand the strengths and limitations of published reports. Clinicians must also be knowledgeable about the uses of diagnostic screening tests and the definitions pertaining to them. Study designs and screening tests are the subject of the final part of this chapter.

This broad overview is provided to help clinicians become more critical in their reading of the medical literature. This chapter provides a framework for clinicians who wish to collect and analyze data; reference to statistical texts or packages for personal computers will be necessary for detailed computational formulas. Many basic and advanced statistics texts are available.[1,5,7,16,20] A list of popular statistics software packages for the personal computer and some of their features is shown in Table15-1.

DESCRIPTIVE STATISTICS

Scales of measurement

The description of data collected in medical research depends upon its scale of measurement. Data collected on a *nominal scale* are also referred to as qualitative, attribute, or categorical data. Frequently, nominal data take a simple yes or no form: individuals have or do not have a particular disease; they did or did not have a particular exposure prior to the disease; they survived or they died after therapy. Nominal data may also have more than two categories (e.g., blood groups, histologic types of cancer). When there exists some predetermined order to the various categories, the data are measured on an *ordinal scale* (e.g., cancer stage, disease severity). Data collected on a *numerical scale* are more precise and called quantitative data. *Numeric discrete* data are collected as integers (e.g., number of cigarettes that were smoked), while *numeric continuous* data fall along a continuum (e.g., height/weight ratios).

Data collected on a more precise scale can always be reduced to data on a less precise scale. Continuous data can be reduced to discrete data or further reduced to ordinal data. Commonly, numeric data are *rank ordered* (i.e., from low to high) and the ranks rather than the actual observations are examined in statistics tests. These *nonparametric tests* are used when the distribution pattern for the discrete data deviates widely from a normal distribution.

Numeric data can be further reduced to a dichotomy; for example, when a cutoff value for clinical action is desired. Data collected on a less precise scale cannot be upgraded. Data collection forms are often prepared with numeric data (e.g., age or weight) precoded into ordinal categories. Whenever possible the actual numeric data should be recorded because important information may be lost by collecting data on a less precise scale, thus precluding the use of more powerful statistics tests.

Displaying data

Data for a nominal or ordinal scale variable are displayed by a frequency table. One column shows the count

Table 15-1. Statistics software packages for the personal computer and their features

Software (Version)	Source	Features
SAS/STAT (V6.07)	SAS Institute Inc. Software Sales Department SAS Campus Drive Cary, NC 27513 (919) 677-8000	IBM-PC, Network Wide range of statistical capabilities Imports files from ASCII
SPPS (V4.0)	SPSS Inc. Suite 3000 444 North Michigan Ave. Chicago, IL 60611	Similar to SAS
BMDP/ Dynamic (V7.0)	BMDP Statistical Software, Inc. 1440 Sepulveda Blvd., Suite 316 Los Angeles, CA 90025 (310) 479-7799	IBM-PC, Network Wide range of statistical capabilities Imports files from ASCII, Lotus, Excel, and dBASE Menu-driven module
STATA (V3.1)	STATA Corporation 702 University Drive East College Station, TX 77840 (800) 782-8277	IBM-PC, MAC, Network Wide range of statistical capabilities Imports files from ASCII
StatXact (V2.0)	Cytel Software Corporation 675 Massachusetts Avenue Cambridge, MA 02139 (617) 661-2011	IBM-PC Exact nonparametric statistical inference Imports files from ASCII
EGRET (V3.0)	SERC 909 Northeast 43rd Street Seattle, WA 98105 (206) 632-3014	IBM-PC, Network Logistic regression and survival analysis Imports files from ASCII Menu-driven module
Statistix (V4.0)	NH Analytical Software 1958 Eldride Avenue Roseville, MN 55113 (612) 631-2852	IBM-PC, Network Wide range of statistical capabilities Imports files from ASCII and Lotus Menu-driven module

(frequency) of observations in each category. Another column shows the proportion or percentage of the total, represented by the categories shown in the rows. Bar graphs and pie charts can be used to illustrate the data. A *contingency table* illustrates the count (frequency) for two or more nominal or ordinal variables, usually to determine whether there is a statistical association between the row variables and the column variables. A two-by-two (2×2) contingency table in which the frequencies of two dichotomous variables are displayed is particularly common, since clinical data often take this form (e.g., women with and without endometrial cancer were classified by whether or not they had used unopposed menopausal hormones prior to their cancer; Table 15-2).[3]

Table 15-2. Two-by-two contingency table illustrating prior exposure to unopposed menopausal hormones in women with and without endometrial cancer

	Use of conjugated estrogen	
	yes	no
Endometrial cancer case	73 (39%)	115 (61%)
Control without cancer	86 (20%)	342 (80%)

A table similar to a 2×2 contingency table but conceptually and analytically different, is one that shows how matched pairs differ with respect to a dichotomous variable. For example, Table 15-3 shows the appropriate display of data in which women with a complete molar pregnancy were matched with women who had not had a molar pregnancy. The pair members were examined to determine whether their consumption of the vitamin A precursor, carotene, was above or below the control median.[2] In this type of design only the pairs who were discordant (i.e., one had a value above and one had a value below the median) contribute to the analysis.

Numeric scale data generally have a wide range of values; counts for each number would be cumbersome. A *frequency distribution* consists of a series of ordinal categories together with tallies of the number of observations that fall into ranges that are defined by each category. To set up a frequency distribution, first examine the values observed from low to high, obtain a range by subtracting the low from the high value, select the number of categories desired, and divide the range by the number of categories to obtain the width of each interval. The number of categories desired is arbitrary but should be sufficient to demonstrate the shape of the distribution (5 to 20 categories). The width of each category should be equal and must not overlap. Investigators should first review relevant literature to determine if standard or clinically useful categories have already been accepted; for example, age intervals are commonly stated in 5-year age groups (20 to 24, 25 to 29, 30 to 34, etc.). This process results in a frequency distribution (Table 15-4) which may be graphically illustrated by a *histogram* (Fig. 15-1).

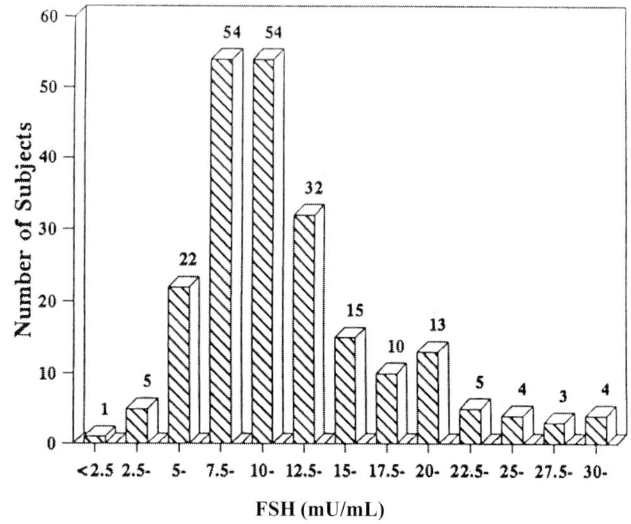

Fig. 15-1. Histogram illustrating the frequency distribution of follicle-stimulating hormone levels in Table 15-4.

Summarizing quantitative data

Nominal data can be summarized by proportions or ratios (e.g., the proportion of treated subjects who survived, the ratio of those who died to those who survived). Quantitative data are more complex and require that at least two characteristics be considered; the central tendency of the distribution and its spread. Frequency distributions generally display a clustering of the middle values. This tendency towards a central value may be summarized by the mean, median, or mode values. The *mean* ($\bar{x}$) is the sum (Σ) of all values (x) divided by the number of observations (n).

$$\bar{x} = \frac{\Sigma x}{n}$$

The *median,* apparent after rank ordering the data, is the middle value for an odd number of observations, or the average of the middle two values for an even number of observations. The *mode* is the value of the observation that occurs most frequently. Distributions may display two or more modes; a bimodal distribution often suggests that the population studied is heterogeneous. In a *symmetric* distribution, the mean, median, and mode values will be identical. Nonsymmetric distributions are referred to as skewed. In distributions with the long tail to the left (negatively skewed), the mean is the smallest number, followed by the median, then the mode. In distributions with the long tail to the right (positively skewed) the order of mean, median, and mode are reversed.

Measures of the spread of data include range and variance. *Range* is the difference between the largest and smallest observations. It unsatisfactorily measures the spread because it depends on only the two extreme values. *Variance* is a measure of spread that is calculated by summing the squares of the differences between each observation and the mean, divided by the number of observations minus one.

Table 15-3. Matched study design examining discordancy in diets above the median for carotene consumption for women with complete molar pregnancy paired to women without molar pregnancy

	Carotene consumption for case pair member	
	Equal or above median	Below median
equal or above median	17	11
below median	28	34

Table 15-4. The distribution of FSH levels during the early follicular phase of the menstrual cycle in women age 26 to 50 at the time of the study (unpublished data by the author)

FSH mU/mL	Number	Percent
< 2.5	1	0.45
2.5	5	2.25
5.0	22	9.91
7.5	54	24.32
10.0	54	24.32
12.5	32	14.41
15.0	15	6.76
17.5	10	4.50
20.0	13	5.86
22.5	5	2.25
25.0	4	1.80
27.5	3	1.35
>30.0	4	1.80
Total	**222**	**100.00**

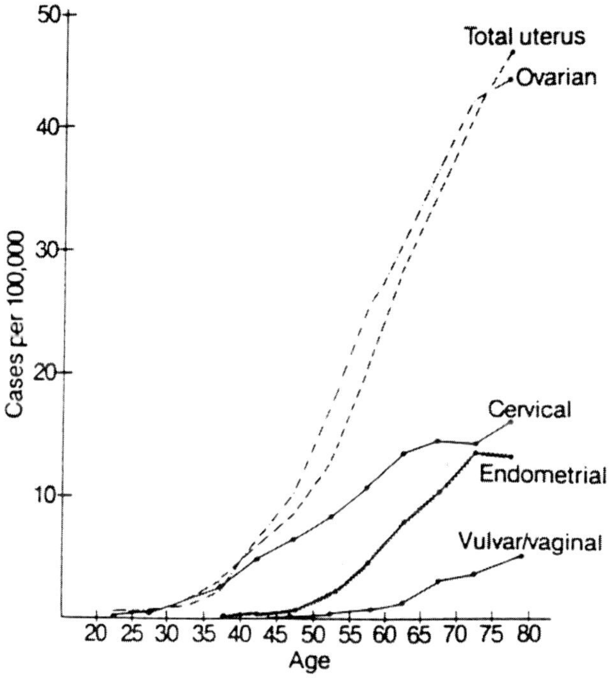

Fig. 15-2. Age-specific mortality rates for the gynecologic cancers. (From Cramer DW: Epidemiologic aspects of gynecologic oncology. In Knapp RC, Berkowitz (editors): *Gynecologic Oncology*, ed 2, New York, 1993, McGraw-Hill.)

$$\text{variance} = \frac{\Sigma(x-\bar{x})^2}{n-1}$$

Justification for this formula, as well as computational formulas for variance, can be found in basic statistics texts. *Standard deviation* (SD) is the square root of the variance and is useful for summarizing the distribution of the observations. In a symmetric, unimodal distribution, 67% of the observations lie between x - 1 SD and x + 1 SD, 95% of the observations lie between x - 2 SD, and x + 2 SD, and 99.7% of the observations lie between x - 3 SD and x + 3 SD.

Standard error or *standard error of the mean* (SE) is the standard deviation divided by the square root of the number of observations.

$$SE = \frac{SD}{\sqrt{n}}$$

The standard error approximates the standard deviation of the means of various samples that might be obtained if the study was repeated numerous times. Features of this "sampling distribution" are important in statistical inference.

The *coefficient of variation* (CV) is the standard deviation divided by the mean and is stated as a percent.

$$CV \ \frac{SD}{\bar{x}}(100)$$

This measure of variation may be used when evaluating the characteristics of a laboratory test or when the same variable is measured in different units (e.g., height in inches or meters).

VITAL STATISTICS

Vital statistics refers to rates of birth, illness, or death and is used in the public health evaluation of a population. A *rate* differs from a proportion in that the element of time is involved. Birth rates, morbidity rates, and mortality rates are all examples of *incidence rates* in which births, new cases of illness, or deaths are counted over a specified period of time and then divided by the time interval of data collection and by the population size. The rate is then multiplied by a base (e.g., 1000, 10,000, or 100,000) to yield numbers that are more easily tabulated and compared. Estimates of the events in the numerator may come from birth or death certificate data or specialized registries. Estimates of the population for the denominator may come from census data. An excellent compendium of public health data sources has been prepared by Gable.[10]

If the incidence rate is not specified with regard to age, it is described as "crude". *Age-specific incidence rates* refer to the number of new events per population time that occur in specific age groups (usually 5- or 10-year groupings). Age-specific mortality rates for the gynecologic cancers illustrate sharp increases during the perimenopausal years (Fig. 15-2).[6]

Because of the marked differences by age for most diseases, age-specific incidence rates are the best way to describe the occurrence of events in a population. An overall rate is useful for comparing disease occurrence in several populations; however, crude incidence may differ between two populations that have identical age-specific incidence rates and a different age structure. The *age-adjusted rate* corrects for differences in age structure in populations. It is derived by multiplying the incidence rate for each age stratum (IR_i) by the proportion of individuals in that age stratum from a "standard" population (W_i) and summing the entire age range.[17]

$$\text{Age-adjusted Rate} = \Sigma(IR_i)(W_i)$$

If the age structure of the standard population is nearly identical to that of the study population, the adjusted rate will match the crude rate.

While incidence focuses on new events over a specified time interval, *prevalence* is the number of individuals with some condition at a particular point in time divided by the population at that point in time. Because prevalence measures disease status in a population rather than events occurring over time, prevalence is a proportion rather than a rate. Examples of prevalence include the proportion of individuals in a population who report that they are smokers; the proportion of women of a particular age who report that they are menopausal; and the proportion of cadavers at the time of autopsy who are found to have occult cancer. Frequently there is confusion in the literature about the use of the terms incidence and prevalence. Incidence is a rate involving time; prevalence is a proportion indicating existing conditions.

STATISTICAL INFERENCE

Statistical inference is the objective process of drawing conclusions from data. It includes the components of hypothesis testing and interval estimation.

Hypothesis testing

The process of hypothesis testing involves the following steps:

1. Observations are made and summarized by some parameter: mean(s), variance(s), proportion(s), rate(s), ratio(s), etc.
2. A research question is stated in terms of a *null hypothesis* that claims there is no difference between the observed parameter(s) and some theoretical value. For example, if one wishes to test whether means from two populations differ, the null hypothesis claims that the difference between the means is zero. An *alternate hypothesis* disagrees with the null hypothesis and need not be explicitly stated for significance testing but is necessary for determining power (see step 7 below).
3. A significance level, or *alpha value,* is chosen. The alpha value reflects the probability of incorrectly rejecting the null hypothesis based upon the data that the investigator is willing to accept, when in reality the null hypothesis is true. This is called a *type I error* and traditionally a value of 5% is chosen. In significance testing, a *p value* indicates the degree of conflict between the observe parameter(s) and that assumed under the null hypothesis.
4. A statistics test is chosen based upon the nature of the parameter being studied (e.g., t test for mean, F-test for variance, chi-square for proportion) and a test statistic is calculated.
5. Appropriate statistics tables are consulted to determine the p value associated with the test result. If the investigator is interested only in deviations from the null value in one direction (e.g., the mean of population A is lower than the mean of population B), a one-tailed p value associated with the test statistic is read. It is more conservative to select a two-tailed value that examines deviations from the null value in either direction.
6. If a p value of less than or equal to the traditional alpha of 5% is observed, the investigator then has sufficient evidence to "reject the null hypothesis."
7. If a p value of greater than 5% is observed, the null hypothesis cannot be rejected; but the investigator may have committed a *type II* or *beta error* by failing to reject the null hypothesis when in reality it is false. *Power* is the probability of not committing a beta error (1-beta). To calculate power, a specific alternate hypothesis must be stated. This is commonly done to determine the sample size necessary to meet certain study objectives. After choosing a specific alternate hypothesis, the sample size may be calculated with the assumption that an alpha of at least 5% and a beta error no greater than 20% (or power of 80%) is desired.

Interval estimation

The process of interval estimation involves the concept of sampling distributions; that is, the distribution of the means or another statistical parameter which might be obtained if the study could be repeated numerous times. Instead of providing a single point estimate for the parameter calculated, the investigator presents a range of values in which it can be stated, with some degree of confidence, that the true value for the parameter is likely to occur. In a study involving at least 50 observations that are distributed normally, the "true" mean for that population has about a 95% probability of residing in the interval as noted below:

$$x \pm 2.0 \frac{SD}{\sqrt{N}}$$

Common errors in statistical inference

1. Errors may be made in choosing and calculating the appropriate test statistic. A chi-square test may be inappropriate for a contingency table with small frequency counts (0 to 5) in some cells of the table (the Fisher-exact test is better). T tests should not be used when distributions deviate widely from the normal; a nonparametric test, such as the Mann-Whitney test, is more appropriate.
2. When the data set involves means from more than two populations, it is appropriate to use analysis of variance (ANOVA) rather than multiple t tests to determine if the subgroups all come from a population having the same mean. If a significant ANOVA is observed, a *multiple comparisons* test (e.g., Tukey's) may be used.
3. Investigators are frequently accused of applying significance testing to a large number of data items and publishing the ones with p values below 5% (data dredging). This potential criticism should not dissuade investigators from making full use of their data. However, they must allow for chance as an explanation in discussions of their study findings.
4. Small studies that find no difference between the treatment modalities are frequently cited as evidence that the therapy had no effect; possibly the size was only sufficient to rule out major differences in efficacy.[9] However, a beta error is only pertinent to studies which have failed to reject the null hypothesis. A small study that has produced a significant p value cannot be accused of having a lack of power for the particular null hypothesis that was tested.

Table 15-5. Classification of study designs

A. Observational, descriptive studies
  1. case series
  2. cross sectional

B. Observational, etiologic studies
  1. cohort
    a. retrospective
    b. prospective
  2. case control

C. Experimental studies
  1. clinical trials—randomized and nonrandomized
  2. field trials—randomized and nonrandomized
  3. community intervention trials

STUDY DESIGN AND EPIDEMIOLOGY

Designs of studies applied to humans may be classified as to whether or not they involve observation, intervention, or experiment. A distinction is further made between observational studies that are purely descriptive and those that have a more rigorous design that permits more formal statements about disease etiology (Table 15-5).

Descriptive studies

Case series. Case reports or series describe the characteristics of patients with a particular condition. They are probably the most frequently seen study design in the medical literature. A case series may be used to identify interesting features or to generate hypotheses about the causes or treatment of a disease that might be pursued further by etiologic or experimental studies. Occasionally, observations from a case series are so persuasive that they alone form the basis for public health decision-making. Silverberg and Makowski reported on 11 cases involving young women who developed endometrial cancer and who were using sequential oral contraceptives.[19] This observation occurred about the same time as the recognition of a link between unopposed menopausal hormones and endometrial cancer. Estrogen-dominant sequential oral contraceptives were withdrawn from the market without a formal etiologic study having been performed.

Cross-sectional studies. Cross-sectional studies collect observations in a broader population and demonstrate relationships in the population at the time of the survey. Cross-sectional surveys generally provide more persuasive data about disease associations than do case-series surveys, but uncertainty about the precise sequence between possible exposures and illness may require a more formal etiologic study.

Correlation analysis. A frequent type of statistical analysis used in both case-series and cross-sectional studies is a correlation analysis. A correlation analysis determines whether a linear relationship exists between two numerical scale variables (symbolized by x and y) and is often illustrated by a scatterplot (Fig. 15-3).[21] The *correlation coefficient(r),* or Pearson product moment correlation may be calculated according to the following formula:

$$r = \frac{\Sigma(x-\bar{x})(y-\bar{y})}{\sqrt{\Sigma(x-\bar{x})^2}\sqrt{\Sigma(y-\bar{y})^2}}$$

The null value for r is zero, indicating that there is no association. Generally, correlations of less than 0.25 show little evidence of a relationship; 0.25 to 0.5 indicate a fair degree of relationship; 0.5 to 0.75 indicate a good relationship; and greater than 0.75 indicate an excellent relationship. The square of r is called the *coefficient of determination* and indicates the degree of variability in one of the measures that is explained by the other measure (e.g., a correlation of 0.5 between a woman's weight and her bone density would indicate that 0.5 x 0.5, or 25% of the variability of bone density is determined by the woman's weight).

Linear regression is an analysis that is related to correlation but is more specific; it states which variable is dependent upon the other. Linear regression is defined by the following equation:

$$y = a + b\,x$$

y is the dependent variable shown on the vertical axis; x is the independent variable shown on the horizontal axis; a is the point where the line intercepts the y, or vertical axis; and b is the slope of the line (Fig. 15-3).

Correlations do not imply causation but only the presence of a linear association; the absence of a correlation implies only the absence of a linear relationship. More complicated associations might exist. Trivial correlations are created whenever one variable is correlated with a function of that same variable (e.g., weight at year x will be correlated with percent weight gain by year x + y). Observations that come from heterogeneous populations may

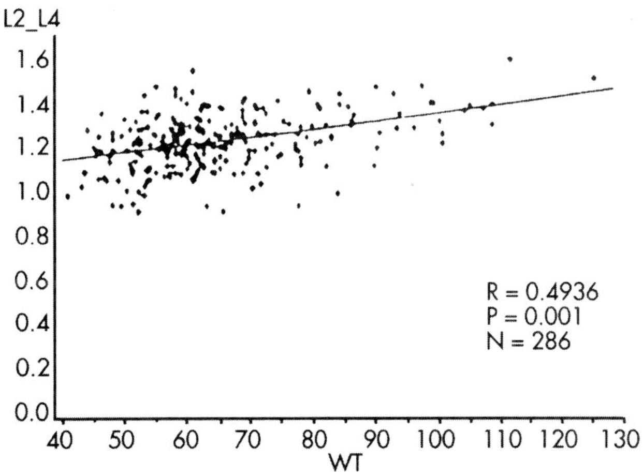

Fig. 15-3. The relationship between weight (kg) and bone density (gm/cm^2) at L2-L4 vertebra on premenopausal women age 35-50. (From Steinberg KK et al: Sex steroids and bone density in premenopausal and perimenopausal women, *JCEM* 69:533, 1989.)

Table 15-6. Comparison of cohort and case-control studies

		Cohort			Case control	
		Exposed	Unexposed		Exposed	Unexposed
Design	Diseased cases	a	b	Cases	a	b
	Person-time	N_1	N_0	Controls	c	d
	Rate difference (attributable risk)	$\frac{a}{N_1} - \frac{b}{N_0}$			Not obtainable directly	
Yield	Relative risk (RR)	$\frac{a/N_1}{b/N_0}$		Exposure odds ratio (RR)	$\frac{a/b}{c/d} = \frac{ad}{bc}$	
Cost/feasibility		Generally costly; more feasible for well-defined exposure and common outcomes. Not efficient for rare outcomes			Generally lower in cost; more efficient for rare disease but not for rare exposure.	
Biases		Selection bias less common, but subject to misclassification and confounding			Subject to selection, recall bias, and confounding	

(From Cramer DW: Epidemiologic aspects of gynecologic oncology. In Knapp RC, Berkowitz RS, editors: *Gynecologic Oncology*, ed 2, New York, 1993, McGraw-Hill).

display an artificial correlation as a result of a mixture of two nonsignificant correlations. Thus while correlations are useful statistical tools, there is the potential for misuse or misinterpretation.[3]

Etiologic studies

While much can be learned about disease associations from case-series and cross-sectional studies, more precise information is often gained from etiologic studies known as cohort and case-control studies (Table 15-6).

The cohort study. In a cohort study, the groups to be studied (the cohorts) are defined by whether or not an exposure has occurred. Each cohort member is examined at a particular time interval after the exposure to determine whether or not death, disease, or some other outcome of interest has occurred. In a retrospective cohort study, the exposures and outcomes occurred before the study began. For example, studies of radiation and subsequent cancer may be based on records of women irradiated for cervical cancer 10 to 30 years previously.

Medical records and death certificates are used to determine those who developed a particular disease after the exposure. In a prospective cohort study, the relevant exposure may have occurred when the study began but the outcome has not yet occurred. After the cohort is selected, the investigator must wait for the outcome to appear in the cohort members.

Cohort studies generally allow the association between an exposure and an illness to be summarized by either of two measures: an attributable risk or a relative risk. An *attributable risk* is the difference in the rates of outcomes between cohorts who were exposed and those who were unexposed. The null value is zero; a positive number may indicate how much disease is caused by the exposure, and a negative number may indicate how much disease is prevented by the exposure. The *relative risk* divides the rate of outcome in those who were exposed by the rate of outcome in those who were unexposed. The null value for the relative risk is one; a value greater than one may indicate that the exposure causes disease, and a value less than one may indicate that exposure prevents disease.

Cohort studies are less susceptible to certain biases and generally allow calculation of both attributable and relative risks. However, they may be costly and take a long time to complete. Cohort studies are most useful for examining the occurrence of common disease(s) after a rare exposure (e.g., the follow-up of atom bomb survivors to determine how many developed cancer). For rare exposures, an investigator may use the general population as the unexposed group. In this case, the observed number of cases in the exposed cohort is divided by the number of cases expected if general population rates had prevailed in the exposed cohort. This comparison is called the *standardized morbidity, or mortality, ratio* (SMR) and is equivalent to the relative risk.

The case-control study. In a case-control study, subjects are selected depending upon whether or not they have disease rather than whether or not they have exposure as in the cohort study. Exposures of potential interest are determined retrospectively from records or interviews. The odds of exposure among cases (i.e., the ratio of exposed cases to unexposed cases) is compared with the odds of exposure among controls. The resulting term is the *exposure odds ratio*. If an entire population could be characterized by its exposure and disease status, the exposure odds ratio would be identical to the relative risk obtained in a cohort study. While it is not feasible to survey the entire population, the exposure odds ratio will approximate the relative risk as long as the sampling of the cases (or controls) from the population was not influenced by their exposure status. Attributable risk is not directly obtainable in a case-control study.

Case-control studies are often referred to as retrospective because the investigator looks backward from the outcome to a past exposure. The cohort study is referred to as prospective because the investigator looks forward from an exposure to an outcome. However, many cohort studies are also retrospective in that the exposure and outcome had already occurred when the study began. Case-control studies are generally lower in cost, easier to conduct, and are most feasible for examining the association between a relatively common exposure and a relatively rare disease. However, they include a greater potential for selection and recall bias.

Interpreting etiologic studies

Both cohort and case-control studies have the potential to define relationships between exposures and outcomes but also the potential for misinterpretation. The features of the association between exposure and outcome that are used to judge scientific merit are considered below.

Validity. Validity means freedom from bias. Bias refers to a systematic error in the design, conduct, or analysis of a study which results in a mistaken conclusion. *Information bias* means that subjects have been classified incorrectly with respect to exposure or disease. This may occur because of incomplete records, or the criteria for exposure or outcome are poorly defined (which leads to *misclassification),* or the cases remember more detail about their past exposures (*recall bias*). Adequate criteria, complete records, and "blindness" of observation may reduce information bias, if researchers can be kept unaware of the status of the subjects or the purpose of the study. *Selection bias* may occur when correlates of the exposure or outcome influence sampling from the larger population of potentially eligible subjects. Using incident cases from a defined geographic area, obtaining high participation rates, and attempting to describe nonparticipants are several means of reducing or estimating selection bias. Confounding is a third source of potential bias in epidemiologic studies. A *confounder* is an extraneous variable that accounts for the apparent effect of the study variable or masks the true association. When cases and controls or exposed and nonexposed individuals differ from each other in the frequency of the confounding factor, then a distortion of the true association between the exposure and disease may be produced. Age, race, and socioeconomic status are likely confounders for an association and are "adjusted for" by statistics techniques that include matching, stratification, and multivariate analysis.[17]

Statistical significance. A variety of statistical tests can determine whether the relative risk or exposure odds ratio differs from the null value of one.[17] Besides statistical significance, the larger the value of the relative risk (its strength) the less likely that the association may be spurious. However, the precision of the estimate and the validity should also be kept in mind. A "weak" association (e.g., a relative risk of less than 2.0) with a narrow confidence interval from a large study that is carefully controlled for biases is more suggestive of a causal association than is a "strong" relative risk with wide confidence intervals from a small study that is poorly controlled for biases.

Dose response. Dose response means that an increase in risk for the disease is observed with an increase in the amount of exposure. Trend tests are used to determine whether a dose response exists.[17]

Consistency and credibility. Agreement among different studies provides reassuring evidence for an association and can be formally tested by the process of meta-analysis. Biologic credibility means that an association is plausible and takes into consideration all that is known about the natural history or demographics of the disease, or all that has been observed in relevant animal studies.

Experimental studies

Because an investigator must assign exposures according to a strict protocol, human experimental studies are limited to the study of measures that will prevent disease or the consequences of the disease. *Clinical trials* evaluate the treatment of disease in humans. The process of randomization is the cornerstone of a good clinical trial. It minimizes the bias that can result from confounding or the preferential assignment of a treatment that is based upon patient characteristics. Randomization involves the process of assigning treatments to subjects by using random numbers. A valid clinical trial will provide a table that shows that the experimental treatment group was similar to the placebo or traditional treatment group, with respect to key factors that might influence outcome. A properly designed clinical trial will enroll a sufficient number of subjects so that a negative study has sufficient power to rule out a treatment effect of clinical interest. A more complete discussion of the design aspects of clinical trials is provided by Mienert.[15]

Field trials generally evaluate the measures that may prevent disease in healthy people. Large numbers of subjects are needed and the disease must have serious consequences to warrant the expense of such studies. Examples of such a design include studies on mammography and breast cancer.[18] When the intervention is assigned on a community-wide basis, the experimental study is called a *community intervention trial*. Early studies involving cervical cytology were conducted as community intervention trials.[13]

Meta-analysis

Meta-analysis is the process of combining results from several independent studies that employed similar designs to examine the same exposure (or treatment) in relation to the same outcome. A more powerful test of the null hypothesis may then be conducted. A meta-analysis is conducted by assembling measures of association, (e.g., relative risks) from each of the various studies, weighting them by the variance observed, and taking an overall average. The weighting is such that studies with the largest sample size will contribute the greatest information. Besides a complete selection of all of the studies on a particular topic, some comment on the overall quality of the studies is desirable. Meta-analysis on the topic of postmenopausal hormone use and breast cancer not only provides a good model for the application of this technique but also the reassurance that the effect of such agents on breast cancer risk is modest.[8]

SCREENING TESTS IN GYNECOLOGY

Definitions of validity measures

The Pap test for cervical cancer, mammography for breast cancer, and ultrasound for ovarian cancer are a few examples of existing or proposed screening tests that are commonly used by gynecologists. It is desirable to have an understanding of the uses and limitations of screening tests. On the simplest level, where a screening test may be designated as positive or negative, and where the population is able to be classified as to whether or not they have the disease, a 2x2 table provides the basis for definitions of the various parameters that are related to screening (Table 15-7).

Cell "a" in Table 15-7 describes true positives, cell "b" describes false positives, cell "c" describes false negatives, and cell "d" describes true negatives. The key measures for the validity of a screening procedure are the following: *sensitivity* which is defined as true positives out of all subjects with the disease [a/(a+c)]; *specificity* which is defined as true negatives out of all subjects without the disease [d/(b+d)]; and the *predictive value of a positive test* which is defined as true positives out of all positive test results [a/(a+b)].

Complexities of screening

Complexities that may arise in the practical application of a screening test include (1) the effect of the prevalence of the disease on validity measures, (2) defining a "positive" and "negative" test result, (3) estimating sensitivity and specificity when the disease status of the entire population is unknown, and (4) the cost issues.

Disease prevalence. The sensitivity and specificity of a screening test are inherent properties of the screening test and do not vary by the prevalence of the disease in the population. This is not true for the predictive value of a positive test. Arithmetically, the predictive value of a positive test can be rewritten to show that it is a function of sensitivity (SN), specificity (SP), and the overall prevalence (P) of the disease in the population screened.

Table 15-7. Definitions of measures of validity for a screening test in a population classified by screening test result and presence or absence of disease.

		True disease state	
		Present	Absent
Screening Test Result	Positive	a (true positives)	b (false positives)
	Negative	c (false negatives)	d (true negatives)

Validity Measure	Definition
Sensitivity	a/(a + c), true positives out of all subjects with the disease
Specificity	d/(b + d), true negatives out of all subjects without the disease
False-negative rate	c/(a + c), false negatives out of all subjects with the disease
False-positive rate	b/(b + d), false positives out of all subjects without the disease
Positive predictive value	a/(a + b), true positive out of all test positives
Negative predictive value	d/(c + d), true negatives out of all test negatives
Overall accuracy	(a + d)/(a + b + c + d), true positives and true negatives out of all tests

(From Goldman L: Quantitative aspects of clinical reasoning. In Braunwald E et al, editors: *Harrison's principles of internal medicine,* New York, 1987, McGraw-Hill.)

$$\text{Positive predictive value} = \frac{\text{SNxP}}{\text{SNxP} + (1 - \text{SP}) \times (1 - \text{P})}$$

The implication of this function is that a positive screening test is more likely to be a true positive in a population at high risk for the disease than it is in a low-risk population. This "prior probability of disease" is frequently taken into consideration in formal treatments of clinical decision-making known as Bayesian analysis. Goldman provides a good discussion of this in Harrison's *Principles of Internal Medicine.*[11]

Definitions of positive and negative screening tests. For screening tests that are read on a numeric scale, a particular value must be chosen as a cutoff point for a positive or negative test result. Since the distribution of screening test results for a population with the disease usually overlaps the distribution of the normal population, the choice of a cutoff point will involve a trade-off between false-positive test results for the normal population and false-negative results for the population with the disease. This is illustrated in Fig. 15-4, which shows the distribution of spine bone mineral density in women with and without a vertebral fracture.[14] In general, the test result that provides the best balance between false-positive and false-negative results will occur at the intersection of the two distribution curves.

For a screening test that is read on a nominal scale there will be a feature that allows the test to be declared positive or negative. The reliability of one observer when replicating a reading on the same specimen (intrarater reliability) and the reliability of two or more observers when reading the same test (interrater reliability) are important measures of the reproducibility of the test. The *kappa* test measures the degree of nonrandom agreement between measurements of the same variable by the same or different observers.

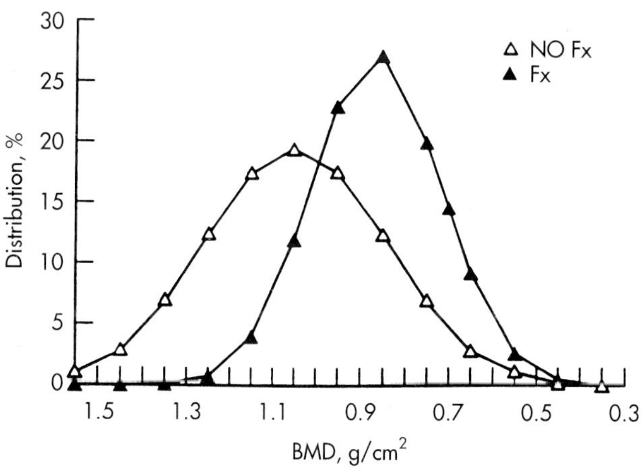

Fig. 15-4. Spine bone mineral density in postmenopausal women with and without vertebral fractures. (From Melton LJ et al: Epidemiology of vertebral fractures in women, *Am J of Epidemiol* 129:1000, 1989.)

$$\text{kappa} = \frac{P_o - P_e}{1 - P_e}$$

In the above formula, P_o is the proportion of times that the measurements agree and P_e is the proportion of times that they can be expected to agree by chance alone. Complete concordance between raters would yield a kappa of 1; if there is no more than chance concordance, kappa would be 0; and if measurements disagree more often than could be accounted for by chance, kappa would be negative.

Estimating sensitivity and specificity. Many clinical studies are constructed so that both a definitive diagnostic test and a screening test are employed and a 2x2 table (Table 15-6) can be reliably constructed. In some circumstances it is not possible to employ a definitive diagnostic test on the entire population (e.g., a cancer screening test in a broad population). However, a definitive diagnostic procedure could be performed on a random subset of individuals whose screening tests were negative. Alternatively the number of false-negative subjects could be estimated by determining how many individuals had negative screening tests but then developed the disease over a "short" period of follow-up. Similarly since the number of nondiseased persons may not be known with certainty, specificity can be approximated from the number of false positives out of the entire population.[4]

$$\text{specificity} \simeq 1 - b/(a + b + c + d)$$

Cost. Issues other than the distribution of screening test values in populations that do and do not have the disease may enter into the choice of the cutoff value that would define a positive or negative test result. What is the "cost" of a false-negative test and the "cost" of a false-positive test in terms of the clinical consequences of missing the diagnosis or in terms of the discomfort and the expense that individuals who do not have the disease will have to bear if they have a false-positive test result. The costs will depend upon whether we wish to maximize sensitivity or specificity. Investigators occasionally construct *receiver-operating characteristic* (ROC) plots that are based upon various cutoff values of the test and illustrate the relationship between sensitivity and specificity.[12,22]

Another "cost" factor that must be considered in the clinical use of screening tests (particularly cancer screening) is whether or not disease prognosis will be improved. Is survival better for a patient whose disease was diagnosed by a screening test because the test reflects the "lead time" between preclinical disease and the onset of clinical disease? The issue of what constitutes a good screening test and whether it is cost effective to employ such a test clinically is very complicated. Definitive answers about cost-effective screening will usually require large collaborative studies and the participation of clinicians, statisticians, and health economists.

CONCLUSION

This chapter provides a broad overview of the statistics and epidemiologic issues that gynecologists may encounter in the performance of clinical research or in its interpretation in the literature. The importance of understanding the scales of measurement of clinical data and how to summarize such data is considered; the principles in the application of hypothesis testing are reviewed; and the distinction between type I and type II errors are emphasized. Knowledge of study designs will enable the clinician to understand the strengths and limitations of various types of clinical research and how to interpret individual studies. Finally, it is important to understand the factors affecting the validity of screening tests that are used in clinical diagnosis and the cost issues pertaining to their application.

REFERENCES

1. Armitage P: *Statistical methods in medical research,* ed 4, New York, 1977, John Wiley and Sons.
2. Berkowitz RS et al: Risk factors for complete molar pregnancy from a case-control study, *Am J Obstet Gynecol* 152:1016-1020, 1985.
3. Buring JE et al: Conjugated estrogen use and risk of endometrial cancer, *Am J Epidemiol* 124:434-441, 1986.
4. Cole P, Morrison AS: Basic issues in population screening for cancer, *JNCI* 64:1263-1272, 1980.
5. Colton T: *Statistics in medicine,* Boston, 1974, Little, Brown and Company.
6. Cramer DW: Epidemiologic aspects of gynecologic oncology. In Knapp RC, Berkowitz RS, editors: *Gynecologic oncology,* ed 2, New York, 1993, McGraw-Hill.
7. Dawson-Saunders B, Trapp RG: *Basic and clinical biostatistics,* Norwalk, 1990, Appleton & Lange.
8. Dupont WD, Page DL: Menopausal estrogen replacement therapy and breast cancer, *Arch Intern Med* 151:67-72, 1991.
9. Freiman JA et al: The importance of beta, the type II error, and sample size in the design and interpretation of the randomized control trial: survey of 71 "negative" trials, *N Engl J Med* 299:690-694, 1978.
10. Gable CB: A compendium of public health data sources, *Am J of Epidemiol* 131:381-394, 1990.
11. Goldman L: Quantitative aspects of clinical reasoning. In Braunwald E et al, editors: *Harrison, principles of internal medicine,* New York, 1987, McGraw-Hill.
12. Hanley JA: Receiving operating characteristic (ROC) methodology: the state of the art, *Crit Rev Diagn Imaging* 29:307-335, 1989.
13. Kaiser RJ et al: Initial effect of community wide cytologic screening on clinical stage of cervical cancer conducted in an entire community. Results of Memphis-Shelby County Tennessee study, *JNCI* 69:349-355, 1982.
14. Melton LJ et al: Epidemiology of vertebral fractures in women, *Am J of Epidemiol* 129:1000-1011, 1989.
15. Meinert CL: *Clinical trials: design conduct and analysis,* New York, 1986, Oxford University Press.
16. Rosner B: *Fundamentals of biostatistics*, ed 3, Boston, 1982, Duxbury Press.
17. Rothman KJ: *Modern epidemiology,* Boston, 1986, Little, Brown and Company.
18. Shapiro S et al: Ten to fourteen year effect of screening on breast cancer mortality, *JNCI* 69:349-355, 1982.
19. Silverberg SG, Makowski EL: Endometrial carcinoma in young women taking oral contraceptive agents, *Obstet Gynecol* 46:503:506, 1975.
20. Snedecor GW, Cochran WG: *Statistical methods*, ed 8, Ames, 1989, The Iowa State University Press.
21. Steinberg KK et al: Sex steroids and bone density in premenopausal and perimenopausal women, *JCEM* 69:533-539, 1989.
22. Zweig MH, Campbell G: Receiver-operating characteristic (ROC) plots: a fundamental evaluation tool in clinical medicine, *Clin Chem* 39:561-577, 1993.

Chapter 16

GESTATIONAL TROPHOBLASTIC DISEASES

Ross S. Berkowitz
Donald P. Goldstein

MANAGEMENT OF MOLAR PREGNANCY AND GESTATIONAL TROPHOBLASTIC TUMORS

Gestational trophoblastic diseases (GTDs) include a group of interrelated diseases including complete and partial molar pregnancy, invasive mole, placental site trophoblastic tumor, and choriocarcinoma that have varying propensities for invasion and spread. Gestational trophoblastic tumor (GTT) is one of the rare human malignancies that are highly curable even with widespread metastases.[4,25] While GTTs most commonly follow a molar pregnancy, they may ensue after any gestation period. Important advances have been made in the diagnosis, treatment, and follow-up of patients with molar pregnancy and GTTs. This chapter will review these advances and discuss basic principles in management based upon the clinical experience accumulated at the New England Trophoblastic Disease Center (NETDC).

Epidemiology

The reported incidence of GTD varies dramatically in different regions of the world. The frequency of molar pregnancy in Asian countries is 7 to 10 times greater than the reported incidence in North America or Europe.[16] While hydatidiform mole occurs in Taiwan in 1 in 125 pregnancies, the incidence of molar gestation in the United States is about 1 per 1500 live births. Variations in the incidence rates of molar pregnancy result partly from differences between hospital-based versus population-based data.

The high incidence of molar pregnancy in some populations has been attributed to socioeconomic and nutritional factors. It was observed in a case-control study that the risk for complete molar pregnancy progressively increases with decreasing levels of consumption of dietary carotene (vitamin A precursor) and animal fat.[6] Parazzini et al also reported from Italy that low carotene consumption was associated with GTD.[41] Global regions with a high incidence of vitamin A deficiency correspond to areas with a high frequency of molar pregnancy. Dietary factors such as carotene may therefore partly explain the regional variations in the incidence of molar pregnancy.

The risk of having a molar pregnancy also increases with advanced maternal age.[16] Women older than age 40 have a fivefold to tenfold greater risk of having a molar gestation. Ova from older women may be more susceptible to abnormal fertilizations. Similarly Buckley et al proposed that low estrogen levels may be associated with abnormal ovulation and may predispose to choriocarcinoma.[17]

MOLAR PREGNANCY

Complete versus partial molar pregnancy

Pathologic and chromosomal features. Hydatidiform mole may be categorized as either complete or partial based upon gross morphology, histopathology, and karyotype (Table 16-1).

Complete hydatidiform moles have no identifiable embryonic or fetal tissues. The chorionic villi have generalized swelling and diffuse trophoblastic hyperplasia (Fig. 16-1). Complete moles usually have a 46, XX karyotype, and the molar chromosomes are derived entirely from paternal origin.[28] Most complete moles appear to arise from an anuclear empty ovum that has been fertilized by a haploid sperm, which then duplicates its own

Table 16-1. Complete versus partial molar pregnancy: histopathologic and chromosomal features

	Complete mole	Partial mole
Fetal or embryonic tissue	absent	present
Hydatidiform swelling of chorionic villi	diffuse	focal
Trophoblastic hyperplasia	diffuse	focal
Scalloping of chorionic villi	absent	present
Trophoblastic stromal inclusions	absent	present
Karyotype	46, XX (mainly) 46, XY	triploid (mainly) diploid

chromosomes.[61] While most complete moles have a 46, XX chromosomal pattern, about 10 % of complete moles have a 46, XY karyotype.[42] The 46, XY complete mole arises from fertilization of an anuclear empty ovum by two sperm. While chromosomes in the complete mole are entirely of paternal origin, the mitochondrial DNA is of maternal origin.[3]

Partial hydatidiform moles are characterized by the following pathologic features: (1) varying sizes of chronic villi with focal swelling and focal trophoblastic hyperplasia, (2) marked villous scalloping and prominent stromal trophoblastic inclusions, and (3) identifiable fetal or embryonic tissues (Fig. 16-2).[51] Partial moles generally have a triploid karyotype that results from the fertilization of an apparently normal ovum by two sperm.[52] Lage et al and Lawler et al reported that 90% and 93%, respectively, of partial moles were triploid.[33,34] When fetuses are identifiable with partial moles, they generally have the stigmata of triploidy including growth retardation and multiple congenital anomalies.

Complete molar pregnancy

Presenting signs and symptoms

Vaginal bleeding. Vaginal bleeding is the most common symptom in patients with a complete mole and occurs in 97% of the authors' patients.[12] The endometrial cavity may be expanded by large volumes of retained blood. When the intrauterine clots undergo oxidation and liquefaction, "prune juice"-like fluid may leak into the vagina.

Excessive uterine size. The uterus is larger than expected for gestational age in about half of the patients with a complete mole.[12] The endometrial cavity may be expanded both by chorionic tissue and by retained clots. Excessive uterine size is generally associated with markedly elevated hCG levels because the uterus is expanded by chorionic tissues with hyperplastic trophoblasts. While excessive uterine size is one of the classic signs of a complete molar pregnancy, half of the patients with a complete mole lack this clinical finding. Because ultrasound is now commonly performed early in pregnancy, even in asymptomatic women, a complete mole may now be diagnosed before these classical signs develop.

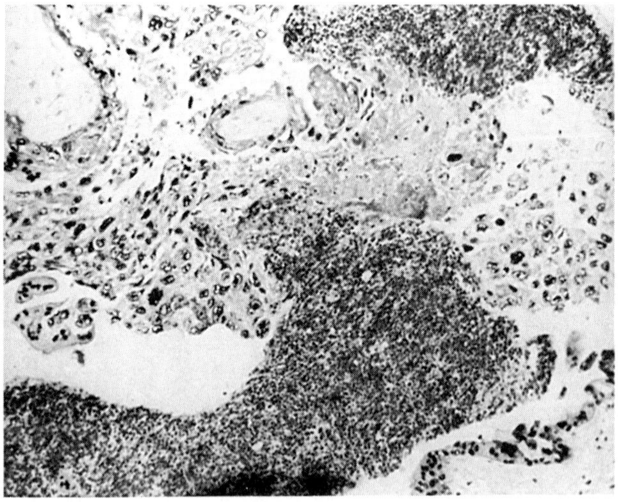

Fig.16-1. Complete hydatidiform mole with marked trophoblastic hyperplasia and atypia. Note syncytial border of villus at lower right and marked trophoblastic hyperplasia in center.

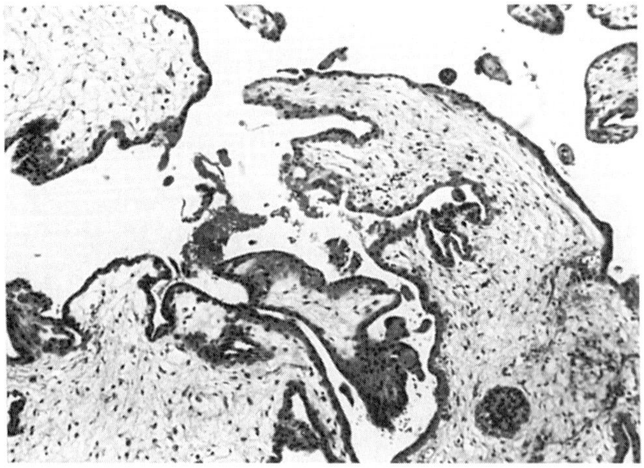

Fig. 16-2. Photomicrograph of partial mode demonstrating varying-sized chorionic villi with focal trophoblastic hyperplasia and villous scalloping and stromal trophoblastic inclusions.

Preeclampsia. Preeclamptic toxemia was diagnosed in 27% of the authors' patients with a complete mole. Although preeclampsia is often associated with hypertension and hyperreflexia, eclamptic convulsions rarely occur. Toxemia develops almost exclusively in patients with markedly elevated hCG values and excessive uterine enlargement. Curry et al[18] also reported that 81% of their patients with molar pregnancy and toxemia had excessive uterine size. The diagnosis of hydatidiform mole should be considered in any patient who develops toxemia early in pregnancy.

Hyperemesis gravidarum. Hyperemesis requiring antiemetic and/or intravenous therapy occurred in 26% of patients with a complete mole. Infrequently, patients may develop severe electrolyte disturbances and require parenteral fluids. Hyperemesis develops primarily in patients with excessive uterine size and markedly elevated hCG levels.

Hyperthyroidism. Hyperthyroidism was diagnosed in 7% of our patients with complete mole. These patients may have symptoms of tachycardia, warm skin, and tremor. The diagnosis of hyperthyroidism is confirmed by detecting elevated serum levels of free thyroxine (T_4) and triiodothyronine (T_3). If hyperthyroidism is suspected, β-adrenergic blockers should be administered before uterine evacuation, since anesthetic or surgery may precipitate a thyroid storm. A thyroid storm may be manifested by hyperthermia, convulsion, atrial fibrillation, or cardiovascular collapse. β-adrenergic blockers may prevent or rapidly reverse many of the metabolic and cardiovascular complications of a thyroid storm.

Some investigators have suggested that hCG is the thyroid stimulator in patients with molar pregnancy.[38] Positive correlations between serum hCG and serum total T_4 or total T_3 concentrations have been observed in some but not all studies. However, when 47 patients with a complete mole were tested for thyroid function, no significant correlation was observed between serum hCG levels and free T_4 or T_3 index values.[1] The identity of the thyrotropic factor in molar pregnancy has therefore not been clearly delineated.

Trophoblastic embolization. Two percent of patients with a complete mole develop acute respiratory distress partly because of trophoblastic embolization to the pulmonary vasculature.[30] Patients may experience tachypnea and tachycardia in the recovery room after molar evacuation. Auscultation of the chest usually reveals diffuse rales, and a chest roentgenogram may demonstrate bilateral pulmonary infiltrates (Fig. 16-3). The signs and symptoms of respiratory distress generally resolve within 72 hours with cardiovascular and respiratory support. However, patients may temporarily require intubation with mechanical ventilation.

Respiratory distress usually develops in patients with markedly enlarged uteri. Twiggs et al reported that 12 (27%) of 44 patients with a molar pregnancy of at least 16 weeks size developed pulmonary complications.[55]

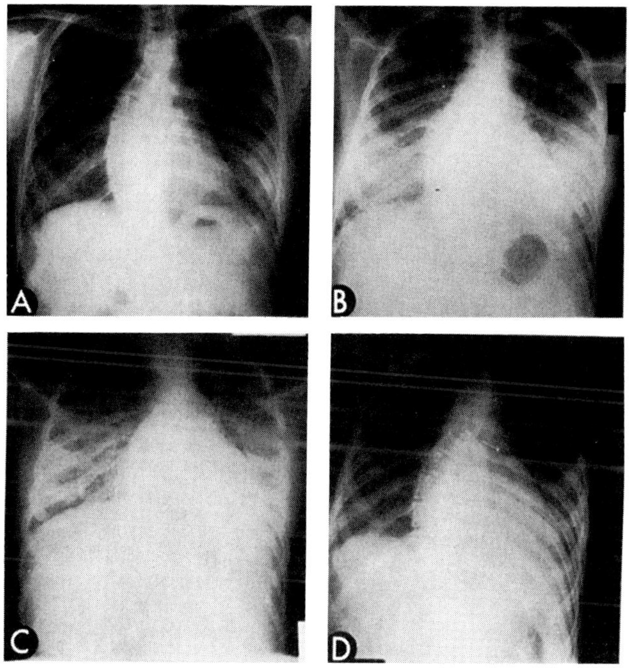

Fig. 16-3. A-D, Chest roentgenograms of patient in whom trophoblastic embolization developed immediately following suction evacuation of molar pregnancy. The condition generally runs its course in 72 to 96 hours, as shown by complete clearing of both lung fields (D).

Hankins et al detected only minimal trophoblastic cells in the pulmonary arterial blood of six women undergoing evacuation of large molar pregnancies.[27] None of these women developed significant pulmonary compromise or hemodynamic instability. These investigators speculated that pulmonary compromise in patients with a mole may be due in part to the cardiopulmonary changes induced by preeclampsia, anemia, hyperthyroidism, and vigorous transfusion therapy.

Theca lutein ovarian cysts. Prominent theca lutein ovarian cysts (> 6 cm in diameter) develop in about half of the patients with a complete mole.[12] The cysts contain amber-colored or serosanguineous fluid and are usually bilateral and multilocular. Ovarian enlargement occurs almost exclusively in patients with markedly elevated hCG levels. The formation of theca lutein cysts may also be related to increased serum levels of prolactin.[40] While theca lutein cysts are usually noted at presentation, they may also develop shortly after uterine evacuation. The mean time for spontaneous regression of theca lutein cysts is 8 weeks.[35] Montz et al reported that only 3 of 99 patients with theca lutein cysts developed acute surgical complications (torsion or rupture).[35] If patients have marked symptoms of pelvic pressure, theca lutein cysts may be safely aspirated percutaneously under ultrasound control or during laparoscopy.

Partial molar pregnancy

Presenting signs and symptoms. Patients with a partial molar pregnancy usually do not present with the classic clinical features that are characteristic of a complete mole. These patients generally present with the signs and symptoms of missed or incomplete abortion. Eighty-one patients were followed with partial mole at the NETDC between January 1979 and August 1984.[6] Excessive uterine size was noted in only three patients, and preeclampsia was noted in only two patients. Szulman and Surti also reported that only nine (11%) of 81 patients with a partial mole had excessive uterine enlargement.[53] None of the patients had prominent theca lutein ovarian cysts, hyperthyroidism, or hyperemesis. Preevacuation hCG values were measured in 30 patients and exceeded 100,000 mIU/mL in only two patients (7%). The diagnosis of partial mole is usually made after histologic review of curettage specimens.

Ultrasonography and diagnosis of hydatidiform mole

Ultrasonography is a sensitive and reliable technique for detecting complete molar pregnancy. Because of marked swelling of the chorionic villi, a complete mole produces a characteristic vesicular sonographic pattern. However, it may be difficult to distinguish an early mole from degenerating chorionic tissues, since molar chorionic villi in the first trimester may be too small to visualize with ultrasound. hCG measurement at the time of sonography may help in differentiating a complete mole from a missed abortion.

Ultrasonography may also contribute to the diagnosis of partial molar pregnancy. Two sonographic findings are significantly associated with the diagnosis of partial mole; cystic changes in the placenta and a ratio of the transverse to anteroposterior dimension of the gestational sac greater than 1.5.[22] When both findings were present, the positive predictive value for a partial mole was 87%. On rare occasions the sonogram shows the presence of a fetus with multiple congenital anomalies and a focally hydropic placenta.

Natural history of molar pregnancy and prognostic factors

Complete hydatidiform moles are recognized to have a potential for developing uterine invasion or distant spread. Following molar evacuation, uterine invasion occurs in 15% of patients and metastasis occurs 4 % of patients.[7]

Eight hundred and fifty-eight patients with a complete mole were reviewed to identify factors that predispose to postmolar tumor. At the time of presentation, 41% of the patients had the following signs of marked trophoblastic proliferation: hCG level greater than 100,000 mIU/mL, uterine size greater than gestational age, and theca lutein cysts greater than 6 cm in diameter. After evacuation, 31% of these patients developed uterine invasion and 8.8% developed metastases. The risk for persistent tumors is considerably less for patients who do not have marked trophoblastic growth. Following molar evacuation, only 3.4% of these patients developed invasion and 0.6% developed metastases. Therefore patients with complete moles, markedly elevated hCG levels, and excessive uterine size are at an increased risk of developing postmolar tumors, and are categorized as high risk.

An increased risk of postmolar GTT has also been observed in women older than age 40 years. Tow reported that 37% of women older than age 40 years with molar pregnancy developed persistent tumors.[54] Complete moles in older women are more frequently aneuploid, and this may be related to their increased potential for local invasion and metastasis. The risk for persistent GTT, however, does not appear to be related to whether a complete mole is homozygous or heterozygous.[37]

The prognostic value of histologic grading of complete moles has been controversial. However, Genest et al performed a thorough clinicopathologic study of 153 cases of complete mole between 1980 and 1990 and determined that histologic grade did not correlate significantly with clinical outcome.[24]

Sixteen (6.6%) of 240 patients who were followed for partial mole at the NETDC developed nonmetastatic persistent GTT.[43] Only one of these patients presented with the classical signs and symptoms of molar disease, including excessive uterine enlargement, theca lutein ovarian cysts, and high hCG levels. Fifteen (94%) patients were thought to have a missed abortion before evacuation. Patients with a partial mole who developed persistent disease did not have the clinical features that distinguished them from patients with a partial mole. Flow cytometric studies of partial moles that developed persistent tumors showed a triploid pattern in 11 (85%) of 13 cases with interpretable histograms.[32] The remaining two cases had a diploid pattern.

The risk of developing persistent GTT after a partial mole has been reported from 0% to 11% (Table 16-2). Summarizing nine published series, 39 (3.5%) of 1125 patients

Table 16-2. Persistent tumor after partial molar pregnancy

Series	Patients	Persistent tumor	Metastases
Stone and Bagshawe[48]	194	5	2
Vassilakos et al[56]	56	0	0
Czernobilsky et al[20]	25	1	0
Szulman and Surti[53]	49	2	0
Wong and Ma[60]	35	4	2
Ohama et al[39]	56	0	0
Lawler et al[34]	51	0	0
Lage et al[32]	310	17	0
Goto et al[26]	349	10	3
TOTAL	1125	39 (3.5%)	7 (0.6%)

(From Goldstein DP, Berkowitz RS: Current management of complete and partial molar pregnancy, *J Reprod Med* 39:139-146, 1994.)

with a partial mole developed persistent GTT and only seven (18%) of these patients had metastases.

Surgical evacuation

After diagnosing a molar pregnancy, the patient should be carefully evaluated to identify the presence of medical complications including preeclampsia, electrolyte imbalance, hyperthyroidism, and anemia that might complicate surgical evacuation. The patient is first stabilized, and then a decision is made concerning the most appropriate method of evacuation.

If the patient no longer desires to preserve fertility, hysterectomy may be performed and prominent theca lutein ovarian cysts may be aspirated at the time of surgery. Although hysterectomy eliminates the risks of local invasion, it does not prevent metastases.

Suction curettage is the preferred method of evacuation, regardless of uterine size, in patients who desire to preserve fertility.[13] As the cervix is being dilated, the surgeon may encounter brisk uterine bleeding because of the passage of retained blood. Shortly after commencing suction evacuation, uterine bleeding is generally controlled and the uterus rapidly regresses in size. If the uterus is larger than 14 weeks gestation size, one hand should be placed on top of the fundus and the uterus should be massaged to stimulate uterine contraction. When suction evacuation is thought to be complete, a sharp curettage should be performed to remove any residual molar tissue. The curettings from suction and sharp curettage are submitted separately for pathologic review. Patients who are Rh negative should receive Rh immune globulin at the time of the evacuation because Rh D factor is expressed on the trophoblast.

The role of prophylactic chemotherapy

The use of prophylactic chemotherapy at the time of molar evacuation remains controversial. However, several investigators have reported that chemoprophylaxis reduces the risk of postmolar tumor.

Kim et al performed an important randomized, prospective trial of chemoprophylaxis in patients with complete mole.[29] Chemoprophylaxis significantly reduced the incidence of postmolar tumor from 47% to 14% in patients with high-risk mole. However, chemoprophylaxis did not significantly influence the occurrence of persistent tumor in patients with low-risk mole.

Prophylactic dactinomycin also reduces the risk of persistent GTT in patients with high-risk complete mole.[13] Only 10 (11%) of 93 patients with high-risk complete mole developed postmolar tumor after prophylactic dactinomycin. Chemoprophylaxis failure more commonly occurred in patients with markedly elevated hCG values. Prophylactic chemotherapy may be of benefit in patients with high-risk complete moles, particularly when hormonal follow-up is unavailable or unreliable.

Hormonal follow-up

After molar evacuation, all patients must be followed with hCG measurements to assure remission. Patients are followed with weekly hCG values until they are normal for 3 weeks and then monthly until normal for 6 months.

Patients are encouraged to use effective contraception during the entire interval of follow-up. Intrauterine devices should not be inserted until the patient achieves normal hCG levels because of the risk of uterine perforation and infection if residual tumors are present. If the patient does not want surgical sterilization, she has the choice of using either hormonal contraceptives or barrier methods.

The incidence of postmolar tumor has been reported to be increased in patients who use oral contraceptives.[49] However, data from the NETDC and the Gynecologic Oncology Group indicate that oral contraceptives do not increase the risk of postmolar trophoblastic disease.[14, 19] The contraceptive method also did not influence the mean hCG regression time. The authors believe that oral contraceptives may be safely prescribed after molar evacuation.

GESTATIONAL TROPHOBLASTIC TUMORS

Pathologic considerations

After a molar pregnancy, persistent GTT may have the histologic pattern of either molar tissue or choriocarcinoma. However, following a nonmolar gestation, persistent GTT may only have the histologic features of choriocarcinoma. Gestational choriocarcinoma does not contain chorionic villous structures but is composed of sheets of both anaplastic cytotrophoblast and syncytiotrophoblast (Fig. 16-4).

Placental site trophoblastic tumor (PSTT) is an uncommon variant of choriocarcinoma.[23] PSTT is composed almost entirely of mononuclear intermediate trophoblast and does not contain chorionic villi. PSTTs secrete very limited amounts of hCG, and therefore a large tumor burden may be present before hCG levels are detectable.

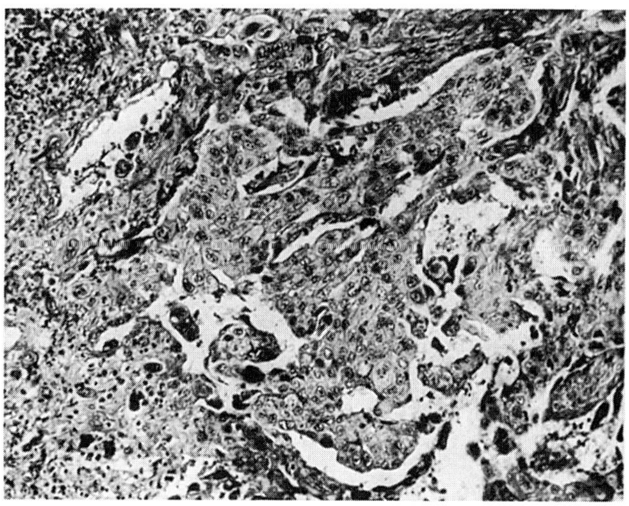

Fig. 16-4. Typical plexiform arrangement of trophoblastic cells in choriocarcinoma.

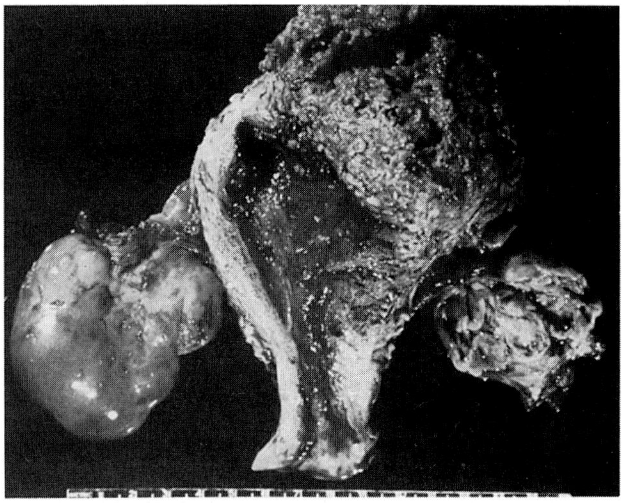

Fig. 16-5. Uterine choriocarcinoma with massive destruction of uterine wall.

Natural history

Nonmetastatic disease. Locally invasive GTT develops in 15% of patients following evacuation of a complete mole and infrequently after other gestations.[13] Trophoblastic tumors may perforate through the myometrium, producing intraperitoneal bleeding, or may erode into uterine vessels, causing vaginal hemorrhage. A bulky necrotic tumor may serve as a nidus for a uterine infection (Fig. 16-5).

Metastatic disease. Metastatic GTT occurs in 4% of patients after the evacuation of a complete mole and infrequently following other pregnancies. Metastatic GTT is often associated with choriocarcinoma. Choriocarcinoma has a propensity for early vascular invasion with widespread dissemination. The most common metastatic sites are the lung (80%), vagina (30%), brain (10%), and liver (10%). Because trophoblastic tumors are perfused by a myriad of fragile vessels, metastases are often hemorrhagic. Patients may present with signs and symptoms of bleeding from metastases such as hemoptysis or acute neurologic deficits. Cerebral and hepatic metastases are uncommon unless there is concurrent involvement of the lungs and/or vagina.

Staging system

The International Federation of Gynecology and Obstetrics has begun to report data on GTT using an anatomic staging system (Table 16-3). Stage I includes all patients with persistently elevated hCG levels and tumors confined to the uterine corpus. Stage II comprises all patients with tumors outside of the uterus but localized to the vagina and/or pelvis. Stage III includes all patients with pulmonary metastases with or without uterine, vaginal, or pelvic involvement. Stage IV patients have far-advanced disease with involvement of the brain, liver, kidneys, or gastrointestinal tract. Patients with stage IV disease are in the highest risk category because they are most likely to be resistant to

Table 16-3. Staging of gestational trophoblastic tumors

Stage	
Stage I	Disease confined to uterus
Stage IA	Disease confined to uterus with no risk factors
Stage IB	Disease confined to uterus with one risk factor
Stage IC	Disease confined to uterus with two risk factors
Stage II	Gestational trophoblastic tumor extending outside uterus but limited to genital structures (adnexa, vagina, broad ligament)
Stage IIA	Gestational trophoblastic tumor involving genital structures with no risk factors
Stage IIB	Gestational trophoblastic tumor extending outside uterus but limited to genital structures with one risk factor.
Stage IIC	Gestational trophoblastic tumor extending outside uterus but limited to genital structures with two risk factors.
Stage III	Gestational trophoblastic tumor extending to lungs with or without known genital tract involvement
Stage IIIA	Gestational trophoblastic tumor extending to lungs with or without genital tract involvement and with no risk factors
Stage IIIB	Gestational trophoblastic tumor extending to lungs with or without genital tract involvement and with one risk factor
Stage IIIC	Gestational trophoblastic tumor extending to lungs with or without genital tract involvement and with two risk factors
Stage IV	All other metastatic sites
Stage IVA	All other metastatic sites with no risk factors
Stage IVB	All other metastatic sites with one risk factor
Stage IVC	All other metastatic sites with two risk factors

Risk factors affecting staging include the following: (1) hCG > 100,000 mIU/mL and (2) duration of disease > 6 months from termination of antecedent pregnancy.

The following factors should be considered and noted in reporting: (1) prior chemotherapy has been given for known GTT; (2) placental site tumors should be reported separately; (3) histologic verification of disease is not required.

Table 16-4. Scoring system based on prognostic factors

Prognostic factors	Score[b] 0	1	2	4
Age (years)	≤ 39	> 39		
Antecedent pregnancy	HM	abortion	term	
Interval[a]	4	4-6	7-12	12
hCG (IU/litre)	10^3	10^3-10^4	10^4-10^5	10^5
ABO groups (female x male)		O x A A x O	B AB	
Largest tumor, including uterine tumor		3-5 cm	5 cm	
Site of metastases		spleen kidney	GI tract liver	brain
No. of metastases identified		1-4	4-8	8
Prior chemotherapy			single drug	2 or more drugs

[a] Interval: time (months) between end of antecedent pregnancy and start of chemotherapy.

[b] The total score for a patient is obtained by adding the individual scores for each prognostic factor. Total score:
≤ 4: low risk
5-7: middle risk
≥ 8: high risk

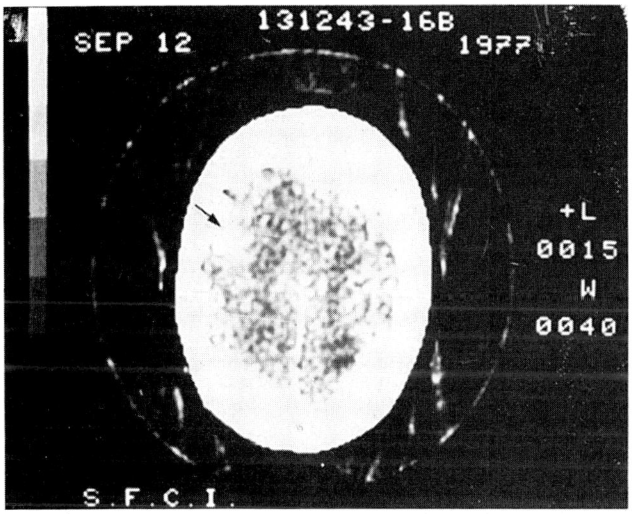

Fig. 16-6. Computed tomographic scan of large intracranial metastasis of choriocarcinoma showing filling defect.

chemotherapy. Stage IV tumors generally have the histologic pattern of choriocarcinoma and commonly follow a nonmolar pregnancy.

It is also helpful to employ prognostic variables to predict the likelihood of drug resistance and to assist selecting appropriate chemotherapy. The World Health Organization published a prognostic scoring system that reliably predicts the potential for chemotherapy resistance (Table 16-4). When the prognostic score is eight or greater, the patient is considered high risk and requires intensive combination chemotherapy to achieve remission. In general, patients with stage I disease have a low-risk score and patients with stage IV disease have a high-risk score. Therefore the distinction between low and high risk primarily applies to stages II and III GTTs.

Diagnostic evaluation

The optimal management of GTTs requires evaluation of the extent of the disease before treatment. All patients with persistent tumors should undergo a thorough assessment including a complete history and physical examination, hCG levels, and hepatic, thyroid, and renal function tests. The metastatic workup should include a chest roentgenogram or computed tomography, ultrasonography of the abdomen and pelvis, head computed tomography or magnetic resonance imaging scans, and in some cases selective angiography of abdominal and pelvic structures. Head computed tomography scans have facilitated the early detection of asymptomatic cerebral lesions (Fig. 16-6).[2]

Management of stage I GTT

Tables 16-5 and 16-6 review the NETDC protocol for the management of stage I disease and the results of therapy. The selection of treatment is based mainly on the patient's desire to preserve fertility.

If the patient no longer wishes to retain fertility, hysterectomy with adjuvant single-agent chemotherapy may be performed as primary treatment. Adjuvant chemotherapy is administered for three reasons: (1) to reduce the likelihood of disseminating viable tumor cells at surgery, (2) to maintain a cytotoxic level of chemotherapy in the bloodstream and tissues in case viable tumor cells are disseminated at surgery, and (3) to treat any occult metastases that may be already present at the time of surgery. Occult pulmonary metastases may be detected by computed tomography scan in about 40% of patients with presumed nonmetastatic disease.[36] Chemotherapy may be safely administered at the time

Table 16-5. Treatment protocol for stage I GTT (New England Trophoblastic Disease Center)

Initial:	Single-agent chemotherapy or hysterectomy with adjunctive chemotherapy
Resistant:	Combination chemotherapy Hysterectomy with adjunctive chemotherapy Local resection Pelvic infusion
Follow-up:	hCG:weekly until normal x 3; Monthly until normal x 12; Contraception: 12 consecutive months of normal hCG levels

Table 16-6. New England Trophoblastic Disease Center
July 1965 - December 1992
Stage I. Confined to uterine corpus

Remission therapy	Number of patients (%)	Number of remissions (%)
Initial:	408 (94)	
Sequential MTX/Act-D		373 (91.4)
Hysterectomy		29 (7.0)
MAC		3 (0.8)
EMA		3 (0.8)
Resistant:	26 (6)	
MAC		10 (38.4)
EMA		11 (42.3)
Hysterectomy		2 (7.7)
Local uterine resection		2 (7.7)
Pelvic infusion		1 (3.9)
TOTAL	434 (100)	434 (100)

MTX = methotrexate
Act-D = dactinomycin
MAC = methotrexate, dactinomycin, cyclophosphamide
EMA = etoposide, methotrexate, dactinomycin

Table 16-8. New England Trophoblastic Disease Center
July 1965 - December 1992
Stage II. Metastases to pelvis & vagina

Remission therapy		Number of patients (%)	Number of remissions (%)
Low Risk		18 (69.2)	
Initial:	Sequential MTX/Act-D		16 (88.9)
Resistant:	MAC		2 (11.1)
High Risk		8 (30.8)	
Initial:	Sequential MTX/Act-D		2 (25.0)
	MAC		4 (50.0)
Resistant:	MAC		1 (12.5)
	CHAMOCA		1 (12.5)
TOTAL		26 (100)	26 (100)

MTX = methotrexate
Act-D = dactinomycin
MAC = methotrexate, dactinomycin, cyclophosphamide
CHAMOCA = Bagshawe multiagent regimen

of hysterectomy without increasing operative complications. Twenty-eight patients were treated by primary hysterectomy and adjuvant chemotherapy at the NETDC, and all achieved complete remission with no additional therapy.

Nonmetastatic PSTTs should be treated with hysterectomy because of their poor response to chemotherapy. Because a PSTT is generally resistant to chemotherapy, there are few long-term survivors with metastases despite intensive multimodal therapy.

Single-agent chemotherapy is the preferred treatment in patients with stage I disease who desire to retain fertility. Primary single-agent chemotherapy induced complete remission in 373 (93.5%) of 399 patients with stage I GTT.

Table 16-7. Treatment protocol for stage II and III GTT (New England Trophoblastic Disease Center)

Low Risk*	
Initial:	Single-agent chemotherapy
Resistant:	Combination chemotherapy
High Risk*	
Initial:	Combination chemotherapy
Resistant:	Second-line combination chemotherapy
Follow-up	
hCG:	Weekly until normal x 3 Monthly until normal x 12
Contraception:	12 consecutive months of normal hCG levels

*Local resection optional

Table 16-9. New England Trophoblastic Disease Center
July 1965 - December 1992
Stage III. Metastases to lung

Remission therapy		Number of patients (%)	Number of remissions (%)
Low Risk		85 (65.4)	
Initial:	Sequential MTX/Act-D		71 (83.5)
Resistant:	MAC		12 (14.1)
	EMA		2 (2.4)
High Risk		45 (34.6)	
Initial:	Sequential MTX/Act-D		13 (28.9)
	MAC		12 (26.6)
	EMA		12 (26.6)
Resistant:	MAC		2 (4.4)
	CHAMOCA		1 (2.2)
	5-FU-Adria		1 (2.2)
	VPB		2 (4.4)
	EMA		1 (2.2)
TOTAL		130 (100)	129 (99.2)

MTX = methotrexate
Act-D = dactinomycin
MAC = methotrexate, dactinomycin, cyclophosphamide
CHAMOCA = Bagshawe multiagent regimen
5-FU-Adria = 5-fluorouracil, adriamycin
VPB = vinblastine, cisplatin, bleomycin
EMA = etoposide, methotrexate, dactinomycin

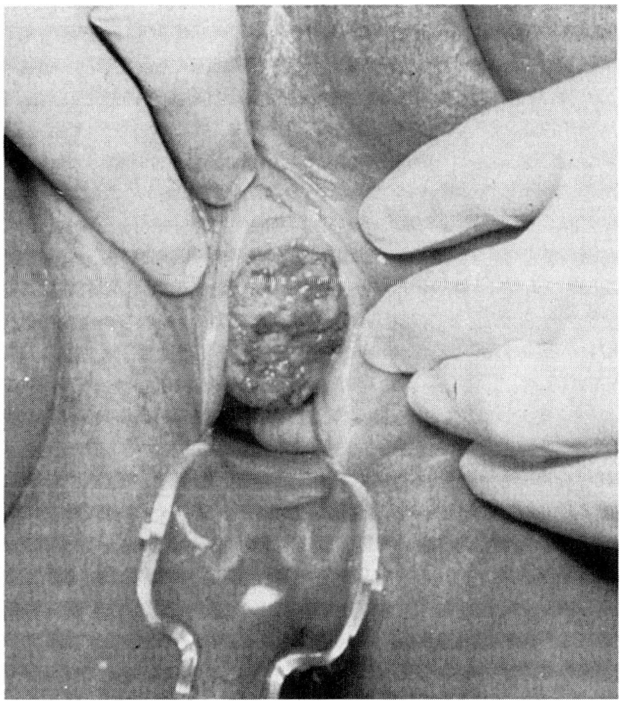

Fig. 16-7. Fungating suburethral metastasis of choriocarcinoma with necrosis and infection.

The remaining 26 resistant patients subsequently attained remission with either combination chemotherapy or surgical intervention. If the patient is resistant to chemotherapy and wants to preserve fertility, local uterine resection may be considered. When local resection is planned, ultrasound, magnetic resonance imaging, and/or arteriogram may identify the site of resistant tumor.

Management of stage II and III GTT

The NETDC protocol for the management of stage II and III disease and the results of treatment are outlined in Tables 16-7 to 16-9. While low-risk patients are treated with primary single-agent chemotherapy, high-risk patients are managed with primary combination chemotherapy.

Between July 1965 and December 1992, 26 patients with stage II disease were treated at the NETDC and all achieved remission. Single-agent chemotherapy induced complete remission in 16 (88.9%) of 18 low-risk patients. In contrast, only two of eight high-risk patients achieved remission with single-agent treatment.

Vaginal metastases may bleed profusely because they may be highly vascular and friable (Fig. 16-7). Bleeding may be controlled by packing the hemorrhagic lesion or by performing wide local excision. The administration of one or two courses of chemotherapy may result in avascular planes around the vaginal tumor. Infrequently angiographic embolization of the hypogastric arteries may be required to control hemorrhage from vaginal metastases.

Between July 1965 and December 1992, 130 patients with stage III tumors were managed at the NETDC and 129 (99.2%) attained complete remission. Single-agent chemotherapy induced complete remission in 71 (83.5%) of 85 patients with low-risk disease and in 13 (28.9%) of 45 patients with high-risk disease. All patients resistant to single-agent treatment later achieved remission with combination chemotherapy.

Thoracotomy has a limited role in the management of stage III GTT. Thoracotomy should be performed if the diagnosis is seriously in question. Furthermore, if a patient has a persistent viable pulmonary nodule despite intensive chemotherapy, pulmonary resection may be performed. However, an extensive metastatic survey should be obtained to exclude other sites of persistent tumor. It is important to emphasize that fibrotic nodules may persist indefinitely on chest roentgenogram after complete gonadotropin remission is achieved.

Hysterectomy may be required with metastatic GTT to control uterine hemorrhage or sepsis. In patients with a bulky uterine tumor, hysterectomy can also reduce the tumor burden and thereby limit the need for chemotherapy.

Management of stage IV GTT

Tables 16-10 and 16-11 outline the NETDC protocol for the management of stage IV disease and the results of treatment. These patients are at high risk for developing rapidly progressive disease despite intensive therapy.

All patients with stage IV disease should be treated with intensive combination chemotherapy and the selective use of radiation therapy and surgery.[50] Before 1975 only 6 (30%) of 20 patients with stage IV disease attained complete remission. However, after 1975, 14 (77.8%) of 18 patients with stage IV tumors achieved remission. This dramatic improvement in survival resulted from the introduction of intensive multimodal therapy early in the course of treatment.

Table 16-10. Treatment protocol for stage IV GTT (New England Trophoblastic Disease Center)

Initial:	
	Combination chemotherapy
	Brain: whole head irradiation (3000 rad)
	Craniotomy to manage complications
	Liver: resection to manage complications
Resistant:	Second-line chemotherapy*
Follow-up:	hCG: weekly until normal x 3
	Monthly until normal x 24
	Contraception: 24 consecutive months of normal hCG levels

* Local resection optional

The management of hepatic metastases is particularly difficult and challenging. If a patient is resistant to systemic chemotherapy, hepatic arterial infusion of chemotherapy may induce complete remission in selected cases. Hepatic resection may also be required to control bleeding or to excise resistant tumors (Fig. 16-8).

Table 16-11. New England Trophoblastic Disease Center July 1965 - December 1992
Stage IV. Distant metastases

Remission therapy*	Number of remissions (%)	Remissions/Patients (%)
Prior to 1975		
Initial: Sequential MTX/ Act-D	5	
Resistant:MAC	1	6/20 (30)
After 1975		
Initial: Sequential MTX/ Act-D	2	
MAC	2	
Resistant: HD**MTX/ Act-D	4	14/18 (77.8)
MAC	1	
CHAMOCA	1	
VPB	1	
EMA	3	

* = Radiotherapy and surgery used when indicated
** = High dose
MTX = methotrexate
Act-D = dactinomycin
MAC = methotrexate, dactinomycin, cyclophosphamide
CHAMOCA = Bagshawe multiagent regimen
VPB = vinblastine, cisplatin, bleomycin
EMA = etoposide, methotrexate, dactinomycin

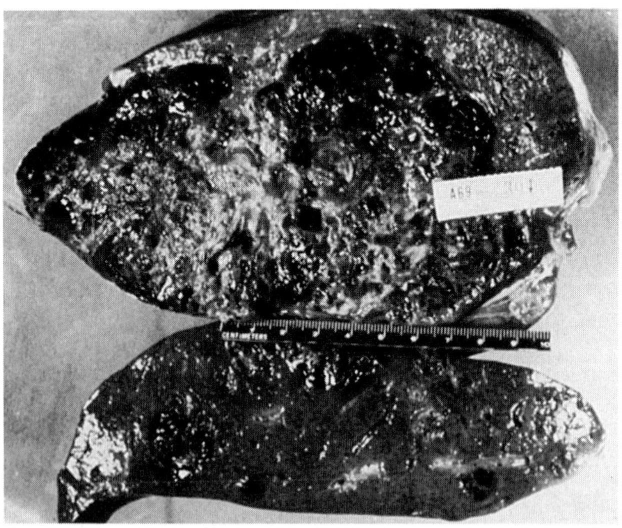

Fig. 16-8. Liver showing diffuse involvement with choriocarcinoma.

If cerebral metastases are detected, whole brain irradiation should be promptly instituted. The risk of spontaneous cerebral hemorrhage may be reduced by the concurrent use of chemotherapy and brain irradiation.[58] Brain irradiation may be both hemostatic and tumoricidal. Yordan Jr et al reported that deaths attributed to central nervous system involvement occurred in 11 (44%) of 25 patients treated with chemotherapy alone, but in none of 18 patients treated with brain irradiation and chemotherapy.[62]

However, Rustin et al have reported excellent remission rates in patients with cerebral metastases who were treated with chemotherapy alone.[45] Thirteen of 15 (86%) patients with cerebral lesions achieved sustained remission with intensive combination chemotherapy, including high-dose intravenous and intrathecal methotrexate. Excellent cure rates can therefore be attained in patients with cerebral metastases with intensive chemotherapy alone.

Craniotomy should be performed to manage life-threatening complications and thereby provide the opportunity for chemotherapy to induce complete remission. Craniotomy may be necessary to provide acute decompression or to control bleeding (Fig. 16-9). Infrequently, cerebral metastases that are resistant to chemotherapy may be amenable to resection. Most patients with cerebral metastases who achieve remission generally have no residual neurologic deficits.

Follow-up

In all patients with stages I, II, and III GTTs, weekly hCG values are followed until normal for 3 weeks, and then monthly hCG values are followed until normal for 12 months. Patients are encouraged to use contraception during the entire interval of follow-up.

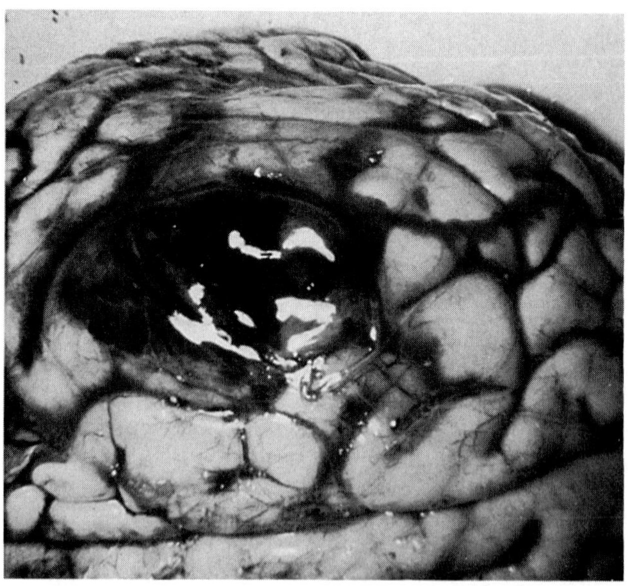

Fig. 16-9. Cerebral metastasis of choriocarcinoma with recent hemorrhage.

Patients with stage IV disease are followed for weekly hCG values until normal for 3 weeks and then are followed monthly for hCG values until normal for 24 months. These patients require prolonged follow-up because they have an increased risk of late recurrence.

CHEMOTHERAPY

Single-agent chemotherapy

Selection of single-agent chemotherapy. Single-agent chemotherapy with either dactinomycin (Act-D) or methotrexate (MTX) has induced comparable and excellent remission rates in both nonmetastatic and metastatic GTTs. [31] An optional regimen should maximize the cure rate while minimizing toxicity.

Methotrexate and folinic acid (MTX-FA) has been the preferred single-agent regimen in the treatment of GTT at the NETDC since 1974.[10] Between September 1974 and September 1984, 185 patients with GTT were treated with primary MTX-FA at the NETDC. Complete remission was induced with MTX-FA in 162 (87.6%) patients, and 132 (81.5%) of these patients required only one course of MTX-FA to achieve remission. MTX-FA induced remission in 147 (90.2%) of 163 patients with stage I GTT and in 15 (68.2%) of 22 patients with low-risk stages II and III GTT. Resistance to MTX-FA was more common in patients with choriocarcinoma, metastases, and pretreatment hCG levels greater than 50,000 mIU/mL. Following MTX-FA treatment, thrombocytopenia, granulocytopenia, and hepatoxicity occurred in only 11 (5.9%), 3 (1.6%), and 26 (14.1%) of patients respectively. No patient required platelet transfusions or developed sepsis from myelosuppression. MTX-FA not only induces an excellent remission rate with minimal toxicity, but also effectively limits chemotherapy exposure.

Administration of single-agent chemotherapy. The hCG level is measured weekly after each course of chemotherapy, and the hCG regression curve serves as the primary basis for determining the need for further treatment. After the first treatment, further chemotherapy is withheld as long as the hCG level is falling progressively. Additional single-agent chemotherapy is not administered at any predetermined or fixed time interval. A second course of chemotherapy is administered under the following conditions: (1) the hCG level plateaus for more than 3 consecutive weeks of reelevates, and (2) the hCG level does not decline by one log within 18 days after completing the first treatment.

If a second course of MTX-FA is required, the dosage of MTX is unchanged if the patient's response to the first treatment was adequate. An adequate response is defined as a fall in the hCG level by one log, following a course of chemotherapy. When the response to the first treatment is inadequate, the dosage of MTX is increased by 2 mg/kg in four divided doses. If the response to two courses of MTX-FA is inadequate, the patient is considered to be resistant to MTX and dactinomycin is promptly substituted.

Combination chemotherapy

A modified triple therapy with MTX-FA, dactinomycin, and cyclophosphamide had been the preferred combination drug regimen at the NETDC.[8] Ten (71.4%) of 14 patients with high-risk metastatic GTT achieved complete remission with this modified triple therapy. However, the triple therapy is inadequate as an initial treatment in metastatic patients with a high-risk score.[7,21] Triple therapy induced remission in only 5 (45%) of 11 patients with a high-risk score.

Etoposide (VB16) has been demonstrated to be a new effective antitumor agent in GTT. Primary oral etoposide induced complete sustained remission in 56 (93.3%) of 60 patients with nonmetastatic or low-risk metastatic GTT. [59] Bagshawe reported an 83% remission rate in patients with a high-risk score using a new combination regimen that includes etoposide.[5] This new regimen includes etoposide, MTX, dactinomycin, cyclophosphamide, and vincristine (EMA-CO) and may currently be the preferred treatment for patients with a high-risk score. Bolis et al and Schink et al have similarly reported that EMA-CO induced complete remission in 13 (76.4%) of 17 patients and in 5 (100%) of 5 patients respectively, with metastatic GTT and a high-risk score.[15,46] The optimal combination drug regimen will most likely include MTX, dactinomycin, and etoposide and perhaps other agents administered in the most dose-intensive manner.[50]

Table 16-12. Subsequent pregnancies in patients with complete mole
(New England Trophoblastic Disease Center
June 1, 1965 - December 31, 1992)

Outcome	Number of pregnancies (%)	Cases/ deliveries (%)
Term delivery	826 (68.5)	
Stillbirth	7 (0.5)	
Premature delivery	90 (7.5)	
Spontaneous abortion		
1st trimester	198 (16.4)	
2nd trimester	18 (1.5)	
Therapeutic abortion	38 (3.2)	
Ectopic	11 (0.9)	
Repeat mole	17 (1.5)	
TOTAL	1205 (100)	
Congenital malformations (major and minor)		38/923 (4.1)
Primary cesarean section		56/318 (17.6)*

* January 1979 to December 1992

From: Berkowitz RS et al: Subsequent pregnancy experience in patients with gestational trophoblastic disease, New England Trophoblastic Disease Center, 1965-1992, *J Reprod Med* 39:228-232, 1994.

Table 16-13. Subsequent pregnancies in patients with partial mole
(New England Trophoblastic Disease Center)
June 1, 1965 - December 31, 1992

Outcome	Number of pregnancies (%)	Cases/deliveries (%)
Term delivery	109 (73.2)	
Stillbirth	1 (0.7)	
Premature delivery	4 (2.7)	
Spontaneous abortion		
1st trimester	22 (14.8)	
2nd trimester	1 (0.7)	
Therapeutic abortion	9 (5.9)	
Ectopic pregnancy	1 (0.7)	
Repeat molar pregnancy	2 (1.3)	
TOTAL	149 (100)	
Congenital malformations (major and minor)		3/114 (2.6)
Primary cesarean section		19/113 (16.8)*

* January 1979-December 1992
From: Berkowitz RS et al: Subsequent pregnancy experience in patients with gestational trophoblastic disease, New England Trophoblastic Disease Center, 1965-1992, *J Reprod Med* 39:228-232, 1994.

Table 16-14. Subsequent pegnancies in patients with gestational trophoblastic tumors
(New England Trophoblastic Disease Center)
June 1, 1965 - December 31, 1992

Outcome	Number of pregnancies (%)	Cases/deliveries (%)
Term delivery	295 (70.2)	
Stillbirth	7 (1.6)	
Premature delivery	18 (4.3)	
Spontaneous abortion		
1st trimester	65 (15.5)	
2nd trimester	7 (1.6)	
Therapeutic abortion	22 (5.2)	
Ectopic pregnancy	4 (1.0)	
Repeat molar pregnancy	2 (0.6)	
TOTAL	420 (100)	
Congenital malformations (major and minor)		7/320 (2.2)
Primary cesarean section		32/214 (15.0)*

* January 1979-December 1992
From: Berkowitz RS et al: Subsequent pregnancy experience in patients with gestational trophoblastic disease, New England Trophoblastic Disease Center, 1965-1992, *J Reprod Med* 39:228-232, 1994.

Patients that require combination chemotherapy must be treated intensively to attain remission. Combination chemotherapy is administered as frequently as toxicity permits until the patient attains three consecutive normal hCG values. After the patient achieves normal hCG levels, additional chemotherapy is administered to reduce the risk of relapse.

SUBSEQUENT PREGNANCIES

Pregnancies after hydatidiform mole

Patients with complete molar pregnancies can anticipate normal reproduction in the future.[11] Patients with complete moles that were treated at the NETDC had 1205 later pregnancies between June 1965 and December 1992. These pregnancies resulted in 826 (68.5%) full-term live births, 90 (7.5%) premature deliveries, 11 (0.9%) ectopic pregnancies and seven (0.5%) stillbirths (Table 16-12). First-trimester spontaneous abortion occurred in 198 (16.4%) pregnancies, and major and minor congenital malformations were detected in only 38 (4.1%) infants. Primary cesarean section was performed in only 56 (17.6%) of 318 subsequent full-term and premature births between January 1979 and December 1992.

Limited information is available regarding the later pregnancy experience in patients with a partial mole (Table 16-13). Between June 1965 and December 1992, patients with partial mole at the NETDC had 149 subsequent gestations that resulted in 109 (73.2%) term live births, 1 (0.7%) stillbirth, 1 (0.7%) ectopic pregnancy, and four (2.7%) premature deliveries. First-trimester spontaneous abortion occurred in 22 (14.8%) pregnancies, and major or minor congenital anomalies were detected in only three (2.6%) infants. The preliminary data concerning subsequent conceptions after a partial mole is therefore reassuring.

When a patient has had a molar pregnancy, she is at increased risk of developing molar disease in later conceptions.[44] Twenty four (1:150) patients have had at least two molar gestations between June 1965 and July 1993. Patients may have an initial complete or partial mole and then in a later pregnancy develop the other type of molar disease. Following two episodes of molar pregnancy, 24 patients had 20 later conceptions resulting in 13 (65%) full-term deliveries, 4 (20%) complete moles, 2 (10%) spontaneous abortions, and one (5%) ectopic pregnancy.

It therefore seems prudent to obtain an ultrasound in the first trimester of any subsequent pregnancy to confirm normal gestational development. Furthermore, the placenta of products of conception from later pregnancies should undergo pathologic review. An hCG measurement should also be obtained 6 weeks after the completion of any future pregnancy to exclude occult trophoblastic mischief.

Pregnancies after GTT

Patients with GTT successfully treated with chemotherapy can also expect normal reproduction in the future.[11,57]

For example, patients treated with chemotherapy at the NETDC had 420 pregnancies between June 1965 and December 1992. These later pregnancies resulted in 295 (70.2%) full-term live births, 18 (4.3%) premature deliveries, four (1.0%) ectopic pregnancies, and 7 (1.6%) stillbirths (Table 16-14). First-trimester spontaneous abortion occurred in 65 (15.5%) pregnancies, and major and minor congenital anomalies were detected in only 7 (2.2%) infants. It was particularly reassuring that the frequency of congenital malformations was not increased because chemotherapy can be taratogenic and mutagenic. Primary cesarean section was performed in only 32 (15.0%) of 214 subsequent full-term and premature deliveries between January 1979 and December 1992. Later pregnancies showed no increased risk for obstetric complications either prenatally or intrapartum.

Song et al performed cytogenic studies on the peripheral lymphocytes of 94 children from subsequent pregnancies and reported no increase in chromosomal aberrations.[47] The growth and development of these children were also evaluated and proved to be normal.

REFERENCES

1. Amir SM et al: Human chorionic gonadotropin and thyroid function in patients with hydatidiform mole, *Am J Obstet Gynecol* 150:723-728, 1984.
2. Athanassiou A et al: Central nervous system metastasis of choriocarcinoma: 23 years' experience at the Charing Cross Hospital, *Cancer* 52:1728-1735, 1983.
3. Azuma C et al: Application of gene amplification by polymerase chain reaction to genetic analysis of molar mitochondrial DNA: the detection of anuclear empty ovum as the cause of complete mole, *Gynecol Oncol* 40:29-33, 1991.
4. Bagshawe KD: Risks and prognostic factors in trophoblastic neoplasia, *Cancer* 38:1373-1385, 1976.
5. Bagshawe KD: Treatment of high-risk choriocarcinoma, *J Reprod Med* 29:813-820, 1984.
6. Berkowitz RS et al: Risk factors for complete molar pregnancy from a case-control study, *Am J Obstet Gynecol* 152:1016-1020, 1985.
7. Berkowitz RS, Goldstein DP: Management of molar pregnancy and gestational trophoblastic tumors. In Knapp RC, Berkowitz RS, editors: *Gynecology Oncology*, New York, 1993, McGraw-Hill.
8. Berkowitz RS, Goldstein DP, Bernstein MR: Modified triple chemotherapy in the management of high-risk metastatic gestational trophoblastic tumors, *Gynecol Oncol* 19:173-181, 1984.
9. Berkowitz RS, Goldstein DP, Bernstein MR: Natural history of partial molar pregnancy, *Obstet Gynecol* 66:677-681, 1986a.
10. Berkowitz RS, Goldstein DP, Bernstein MR: Ten years' experience with methotrexate and folinic acid as primary therapy for gestational trophoblastic disease, *Gynecol Oncol* 23:111-118, 1986b.
11. Berkowitz RS, Goldstein DP, Bernstein MR: Reproductive experience after complete and partial molar pregnancy and gestational trophoblastic tumors, *J Reprod Med* 36:3-8, 1991a.
12. Berkowitz RS, Goldstein DP, Bernstein MR: Evolving concepts of molar pregnancy, *J Reprod Med* 36:40-44, 1991.
13. Berkowitz RS, Goldstein DP, Bernstein MR: Updated approach to complete molar pregnancy, *Contemp Ob/Gyn* 38:78-84, 1993.
14. Berkowitz RS et al:Oral contraceptives and postmolar trophoblastic disease, *Obstet Gynecol* 58:474-478, 1981.
15. Bolis G et al: EMA-CO regimen in high-risk gestational trophoblastic tumor (GTT), *Gynecol Oncol* 31:439-444, 1988.
16. Bracken MB: Incidence and etiology of hydatidiform mole: and epidemiologic review, *Br J Obstet Gynaecol* 94:1123-1135, 1987.
17. Buckley JD et al: Case-control study of gestational choriocarcinoma, *Cancer Res* 48:1004-1010, 1988.
18. Curry SL et al: Hydatidiform mole: diagnosis, management, and long-term follow-up of 347 patients, *Am J Obstet Gynecol* 45:1-8, 1975.
19. Curry SL et al: Hormonal contraception and trophoblastic sequelae after hydatidiform mole: a Gynecologic Oncology Group study, *Am J Obstet Gynecol* 160:805-811, 1989.
20. Czernobilsky B, Barash A, Lancet M: Partial mole: a clinicopathologic study of 25 cases, *Obstet Gynecol* 59:75-77, 1982.
21. DuBeshter B et al: Metastatic gestational trophoblastic disease: experience at the New England Trophoblastic Disease Center, 1965-1985, *Obstet Gynecol* 69:390-395, 1987.
22. Fine C et al: Sonographic diagnosis of partial hydatidiform mole, *Obstet Gynecol* 73:414-418, 1989.
23. Finkler NJ et al: Clinical experience with placental site trophoblastic tumors at the New England Trophoblastic Disease Center, *Obstet Gynecol* 71:854-857, 1988.
24. Genest D et al: A clinicopathologic study of 153 cases of complete hydatidiform mole (1980-1990): histologic grade lacks prognostic significance, *Obstet Gynecol* 78:402-409, 1991.
25. Goldstein DP, Berkowitz RS: *Gestational trophoblastic neoplasms: clinical principles of diagnosis and management*, Philadelphia, 1982, WB Saunders.
26. Goto S et al: Development of postmolar trophoblastic disease after partial molar pregnancy, *Gynecol Oncol* 48:165-170, 1993.
27. Hankins G et al: Trophoblastic embolization during molar evacuation—central hemodynamic observations, *Obstet Gynecol* 69:368-372, 1987.
28. Kajii T, Ohama K: Androgenetic origin of hydatidiform mole, *Nature* 268:633-634, 1977.
29. Kim DS et al: Effects of prophylactic chemotherapy for persistent trophoblastic disease in patients with complete hydatidiform mole, *Obstet Gynecol* 67:690-694, 1986.
30. Kohorn EI: Clinical management and the nepotistic sequelae of trophoblastic embolization associated with hydatidiform mole, *Obstet Gynecol Surv* 42:484-488, 1987.
31. Kohorn EI: Single-agent chemotherapy for nonmetastatic gestational trophoblastic neoplasia: perspective for the 21st century after 3 decades of use, *J Reprod Med* 36:49-56, 1991.
32. Lage JM et al: Flow cytometric analysis of DNA content in partial hydatidiform moles with persistent gestational trophoblastic tumors, *Obstet Gynecol* 77:111-115, 1991.
33. Lage JM et al: A flow cytometric study of 137 fresh hydropic placentas: correlations between types of hydatidiform moles and nuclear DNA ploidy, *Obstet Gynecol* 79:403-410, 1992.
34. Lawler SD, Fisher RA, Dent J: A prospective genetic study of complete and partial hydatidiform moles, *Am J Obstet Gynecol* 164:1270-1277, 1991.
35. Montz FJ, Schlaeth JB, Morrow CP: Natural history of theca lutein cysts, *Gynecol Oncol* 26:414, 1987.
36. Mutch DG et al: Role of computed axial tomography of the chest in staging patients with nonmetastatic gestational trophoblastic disease, *Obstet Gynecol* 68:348-352, 1986.
37. Mutter G et al: Sex chromosome composition of complete hydatidiform mole: relationship to metastasis, *Am J Obstet Gynecol* 168:1547-1551, 1993.
38. Nisula BC, Taliadouros GS: Thyroid function in gestational trophoblastic neoplasia: evidence that the thyrotropic activity of chorionic gonadotropin mediates the thyrotoxicosis of choriocarcinoma, *Am J Obstet Gynecol* 138:77-85, 1980.
39. Ohama K et al: Cytogenetic and clinicopathologic studies of partial moles, *Obstet Gynecol* 68:259-262, 1986.

40. Osathanondh R et al: Hormonal measurements in patients with theca lutein cysts and gestational trophoblastic disease, *J Reprod Med* 31:179-182, 1986.
41. Parazzini F et al: Dietary factors and risks of trophoblastic disease, *Am J Obstet Gynecol* 158:93-100, 1988.
42. Pattillo RA et al: Genesis of 46, XY hydatidiform mole, *Am J Obstet Gynecol* 141:104-105, 1981.
43. Rice LW et al: Persistent gestational trophoblastic tumor after partial hydatidiform mole, *Gynecol Oncol* 36:358-362, 1990.
44. Rice LW et al: Repetitive complete and partial hydatidiform mole, *Obstet Gynecol* 74:217-221, 1989.
45. Rustin GJS et al: Weekly alternating etoposide, methotrexate, actinomycin D/vincristine and cyclophospharide chemotherapy for treatment of CNS metastases of choriocarcinoma, *J Clin Oncol* 7(7):900-903, 1989.
46. Schink JC et al: Etoposide, methotrexate, actinomycin D, cyclophosphamide, and vincristine for the treatment of metastatic, high-risk gestational trophoblastic disease, *Obstet Gynecol* 80:817-820, 1992.
47. Song H-Z et al: Pregnancy outcomes after successful chemotherapy for choriocarcinoma and invasive mole: long-term follow-up, *Am J Obstet Gynecol* 158:538-545, 1988.
48. Stone M, Bagshawe KD: Hydatidiform mole: two entities, *Lancet* 1:535, 1976.
49. Stone M et al: Relationship or oral contraception to development of trophoblastic tumor after evacuation of a hydatidiform mole, *Br J Obstet Gynaecol* 83:913-916, 1976.
50. Surwit EA, Childers JM: High-risk metastatic gestational trophoblastic disease: a new dose-intensive multiagent chemotherapeutic regimen, *J Reprod Med* 36:45-48, 1991.
51. Szulman AE, Surti U: The syndromes of hydatidiform mole. I. Cytogenetic and morphologic correlations, *Am J Obstet Gynecol* 131:665-771, 1978a.
52. Szulman AE, Surti U: The syndromes of hydatidiform mole. II. Morphologic evolution of the complete and partial mole, *Am J Obstet Gynecol* 132:20-27, 1978b.
53. Szulman AE, Surti U: The clinicopathologic profile of the partial hydatidiform mole, *Obstet Gynecol* 59:597-602, 1982.
54. Tow WSH: The influence of the primary treatment of hydatidiform mole on its subsequent course, *J Obstet Gynaecol Br Commonw* 73:545-552, 1966.
55. Twiggs LB, Morrow CP, Schlaerth JB: Acute pulmonary complications of molar pregnancy, *Am J Obstet Gynecol* 135:189-194, 1979.
56. Vassilakos O, Riotton G, Kajii T: Hydatidiform mole: two entities, *Am J Obstet Gynecol* 127:167-170, 1977.
57. Walden PAM, Bagshawe KD: Reproductive performances of women successfully treated for gestation trophoblastic tumors, *Am J Obstet Gynecol* 125:1108-1114, 1976.
58. Weed JC Jr, Hammond CB: Cerebral metastatic choriocarcinoma: intensive therapy and prognosis, *Obstet Gynecol* 55:89-94, 1980.
59. Wong LC, Choo YC, Ma HK: Primary oral etoposide therapy in gestational trophoblastic disease: an update, *Cancer* 58:14-17, 1986.
60. Wong LC, Ma HK: The syndrome of partial mole, *Arch Gynecol* 234:161-166, 1984.
61. Yamashita et al: Human lymphocyte antigen expression in hydatidiform mole: androgenesis following fertilization by a haploid sperm, *Am J Obstet Gynecol* 135:597-600, 1979.
62. Yordan EL Jr. et al: Radiation therapy in the management of gestational choriocarcinoma metastatic to the central nervous system, *Obstet Gynecol* 69:627-630, 1987.

Chapter 17

PSYCHOSOMATIC ISSUES IN OBSTETRICS AND GYNECOLOGY

Susan Caruso Klock

The obstetrician or gynecologist is often a woman's primary care provider and is the first person she consults for medical and psychosomatic problems related to her reproductive functioning. Therefore the obstetrician-gynecologist is in a unique role to identify, assess, and treat psychosomatic disorders among women. Also, as Mathis noted, the obstetrician-gynecologist deals with emotionally laden topics.

> Sex, reproduction, and the reproductive system are almost synonymous with emotional reactions in our culture...The woman who seeks medical attention for her reproductive system deserves a physician who understands the total significance of femininity as well as they know the anatomy and physiology of the female. The physician who assumes this responsibility automatically becomes involved in emotional processes unequaled in any other branch of medicine.[92]

Unfortunately, many obstetricians and gynecologists feel ill-prepared to address psychologic issues with their patients. Also, physicians in busy practices often have little time to spend with their patients or to keep up to date on continually evolving diagnostic and treatment issues in psychosomatic obstetrics and gynecology.

In addition to their pivotal role in women's health care, the obstetrician-gynecologist should be well versed in psychosomatic issues because women are becoming more active and educated consumers of health care. They expect their health care providers to attend to both the physical and the psychologic aspects of their health.[12] The woman's role as a patient has shifted from that of a passive recipient to an active consumer. This shift has been brought about by social change, which includes questions about the traditional patriarchal medical model, increased awareness of women's health issues, and increased dissemination of health information to the public. These changes have increased the need for clinics that specialize in disorders such as premenstrual syndrome and menopausal problems and the use of nontraditional forms of healing and multidisciplinary case management.

There has been a long history of interaction between psychiatry and obstetrics and gynecology, although psychiatric consultation is often underutilized.[19,156] The interaction began as advances in the management of obstetrics were developed. In the late nineteenth century the advent of forceps for delivery, medication for sepsis, and anesthetic for pain control all marked the medicalization of childbirth. During this time, psychiatrists Breuer and Freud considered the role of the female reproductive cycle and sexual functioning to be a critical part of theories of personality and development.[19] Case reports by obstetricians and surgeons reported that hysterectomies could cure hysteria and other maladies. During the 1950s and 1960s, obstetricians began to use psychologic methods to increase women's preparation and control over childbirth; they promoted relaxation and breathing techniques and provided psychosocial support during labor and delivery. During this time, psychiatry began to investigate disorders such as postpartum depression and premenstrual syndrome. Currently there appears to be a convergence of the two disciplines in the subspecialty of psychosomatic obstetrics and gynecology.

This chapter provides a broad overview of several psychosomatic issues related to the reproductive function in women. These issues include premenstrual syndrome, chronic pelvic pain, postpartum depression, the psychologic sequelae of infertility, and menopause. The purpose of this chapter is to provide the physician with a general overview of the research and clinical findings relating to these five topics.

PREMENSTRUAL SYNDROME

Although it may seem to be a recent phenomenon, premenstrual syndrome (PMS) was described over fifty years ago.[40] Frank is credited with coining the phrase *premenstrual tension* when he reported an indescribable tension and increased seizure activity in the late luteal phase among a group of women with seizure disorder. He reported that the tension increased during the late luteal phase and remitted with the onset of menses. Since the publication of Frank's article, there have been thousands of studies investigating various aspects of PMS.

The definition and diagnostic criteria of the disorder have evolved significantly in the past twenty years. The first issue in the diagnosis of PMS is the differentiation of normal premenstrual somatic and psychologic changes from problematic premenstrual symptoms.[13] Blechman emphasized the importance of clearly defined terms for diagnostic accuracy and clarity.[11] She defined *premenstrual changes* as any physical or behavioral experience that is discriminably different during the premenstruum compared to other times in the menstrual cycle. Premenstrual changes can be either positive or negative. It is estimated that 80% of women experience some type of premenstrual change.[89] *Premenstrual symptoms* are those changes that are perceived by the woman to be negative, severe, or limit functioning. Over one hundred symptoms have been identified as part of the PMS profile.[58] These symptoms have been classified by Rubinow and Roy-Byrne and are presented in Table 17-1.[135] Common symptoms include feelings of depression or irritability, decreased concentration, increased food and alcohol consumption, breast pain, edema, headaches, and fatigue. Although some researchers have argued that there are several subtypes of PMS, most patients present with a unique combination of symptoms that vary in degree of intensity and duration.[2,57]

After the symptoms have been identified, a diagnosis of PMS can be considered. The definition of PMS is the "cyclic recurrence in the luteal phase of the menstrual cycle of a combination of distressing physical, psychologic, and/or behavioral changes of sufficient severity that result in deterioration of interpersonal relationships and/or in interference with normal activities."[126] PMS is diagnosed only if the symptoms (1) are reliably related to the luteal phase of the menstrual cycle, (2) remit shortly after the onset of menses, (3) are separate from a preexisting psychiatric disorder, and (4) significantly impair the patient's functioning.[152] It is estimated that 10% to 30% of women have some form of PMS, although rates vary depending on the stringency of the diagnostic criteria and the accuracy of assessment.[150]

In an attempt to refine the diagnosis of PMS, in 1987 the American Psychiatric Association developed diagnostic criteria for late luteal phase dysphoric disorder (LLPDD). This diagnosis obtained provisional acceptance in the *Diagnostic and Statistical Manual of Mental Disorders*.[4] The inclusion of this diagnostic category in the DSM-III-R was controversial but provided a much needed revision of previously confusing and nonspecific diagnostic criteria.[151] The diagnostic criteria for LLPDD are presented in Table 17-2.

These criteria specify that a woman must have at least one prominent mood symptom, four other somatic or behavioral symptoms, and the symptoms must be prospectively confirmed via daily symptom ratings for at least two cycles. These criteria clarify some of the diagnostic inaccuracies that existed before 1987. Since the development of the LLPDD criteria, PMS refers to a general syndrome with numerous symptoms that are related to the premenstruum, and LLPDD refers to a specific psychiatric disorder with a defined set of symptoms of significant severity, duration, and functional impairment. LLPDD is considered to be a more severe disorder with well-defined, predictable symptoms.

Table 17-1. Common symptoms of premenstrual syndrome

Affective	*CNS*
Sadness	Clumsiness
Anxiety	Seizures
Anger	Dizziness
Irritability	Vertigo
Labile mood	Paresthesia
	Tremors
Cognitive	*Fluid/Electrolyte*
Decreased concentration	Bloating
Indecision	Weight gain
Paranoia	Oliguria
"Rejection sensitive"	Edema
Suicidal ideation	
Pain	*Dermatologic*
Headache	Acne
Breast tenderness	Greasy hair
Joint and muscle pain	Dry hair
Neurovegetative	*Behavioral*
Insomnia	Decreased motivation
Hypersomnia	Poor impulse control
Anorexia	Decreased efficiency
Craving for certain foods	Social isolation
Fatigue	
Lethargy	
Agitation	
Libido change	
Autonomic	
Nausea	
Diarrhea	
Palpitations	
Sweating	

From Rubinow D, Roy-Byrne P: Premenstrual syndromes: overview from a methodologic perspective, *Am J Psychiatr* 141:163, 1984.

Table 17-2. Diagnostic criteria for late luteal phase dysphoric disorder (LLPDD)

A. In most menstrual cycles during the past year, symptoms in B occurred during the last week of the luteal phase and remitted within a few days after onset of the follicular phase. In menstruating females, these phases correspond to the week before and a few days after the onset of menses. (In nonmenstruating females who have had a hysterectomy, the time of luteal and follicular phases may require measurement of circulating reproductive hormones.)

B. At least five of the following symptoms have been present for most of the time during each symptomatic late luteal phase, with at least one of the symptoms being either (1), (2), (3), or (4):

(1) marked affective lability (e.g., feeling suddenly sad, tearful, irritable, or angry)
(2) persistent and marked anger or irritability
(3) marked anxiety, tension, feeling of being "keyed up," or "on edge"
(4) markedly depressed mood, feeling of hopelessness, or self-deprecating thoughts
(5) decreased interest in usual activities (e.g., work, friends, hobbies)
(6) easy fatigability or marked lack of energy
(7) subjective sense of difficulty in concentrating
(8) marked change in appetite, overeating, or specific food cravings
(9) hypersomnia or insomnia
(10) other physical symptoms such as breast tenderness or swelling, headaches, joint or muscle pain, a sensation of "bloating," and weight gain

C. The disturbance seriously interferes with work or with usual social activities or relationships with others.

D. The disturbance is not merely an exacerbation of the symptoms of another disorder such as major depression, panic disorder, dysthymia, or a personality disorder (although it may be superimposed on any of these disorders).

E. Criteria A, B, C, and D are confirmed by prospective daily self-ratings during at least two symptomatic cycles. (The decision may be made provisionally before this confirmation.)

From American Psychiatric Association: *Diagnostic and statistical manual of mental disorders*, ed 3 revised, Washington, DC, 1987, American Psychiatric Association.

It is estimated that 5% of women in the general population and 24% of women from a psychiatric population meet the diagnostic criteria for LLPDD.[34,131] In a recent multicenter study the prevalence of LLPDD was estimated from a sample of 670 women seeking evaluation for PMS.[68] The typical patient in this study was 34-years-old, Caucasian, employed, and college educated with two children and had an 8-year history of premenstrual difficulties. Using three different scoring methods for daily symptoms the rates of LLPDD varied from 14% to 38%. Of note, 27% of the sample had a current coexisting psychiatric disorder and 50% had a history of other psychiatric disorders. Others have noted the high prevalence of personality and other psychiatric disorders among patients presenting for a PMS evaluation.[34,56] Therefore it is important to differentiate LLPDD from other psychiatric disorders.

Given the previous confusion surrounding the definitions of PMS and LLPDD, it is not surprising that the assessment of PMS and LLPDD has changed significantly in the past three decades. In the 1950s Dalton simply asked patients if they had symptoms that varied with their cycles to confirm a diagnosis of PMS.[24] Unfortunately, as recent research has demonstrated, retrospective reports of premenstrual symptomatology are often inaccurate.[136] Other studies compared the relationship between prospective and retrospective ratings of symptoms and found that they are not highly correlated.[165] Therefore it is recommended that the assessment of PMS and LLPDD includes the following: (1) a complete gynecologic exam to rule out a somatic cause(s) for the symptoms, (2) a daily symptom rating for three consecutive cycles, and (3) a psychologic evaluation.[72]

An example of a daily symptom rating sheet is given in Fig. 17-1.[127] This form is easy both for the patient to use and the clinician to interpret. Other measures such as the Premenstrual Assessment Form and Daily Rating Form, the Moos Menstrual Distress Questionnaire, and visual analog scales are available.[58,99,15] Other psychometric tests such as the Minnesota Multiphasic Personality Inventory (MMPI) can determine the presence of coexisting psychopathology.[17]

Table 17-3. Theories of the etiology of premenstrual syndrome

Excess estrogen
Progesterone deficiency
Fluid retention
Hyperprolactinemia
Vitamin B_6 deficiency
Hypoglycemia
Prostaglandin deficiency
Prostaglandin excess
Endogenous hormone allergy
Endogenous opiates
Psychogenic
Thyroid abnormality
Serotonin deficiency

From Smith S, Schiff I: The premenstrual syndrome—diagnosis and management, *Fertil Steril* 52:527, 1989.

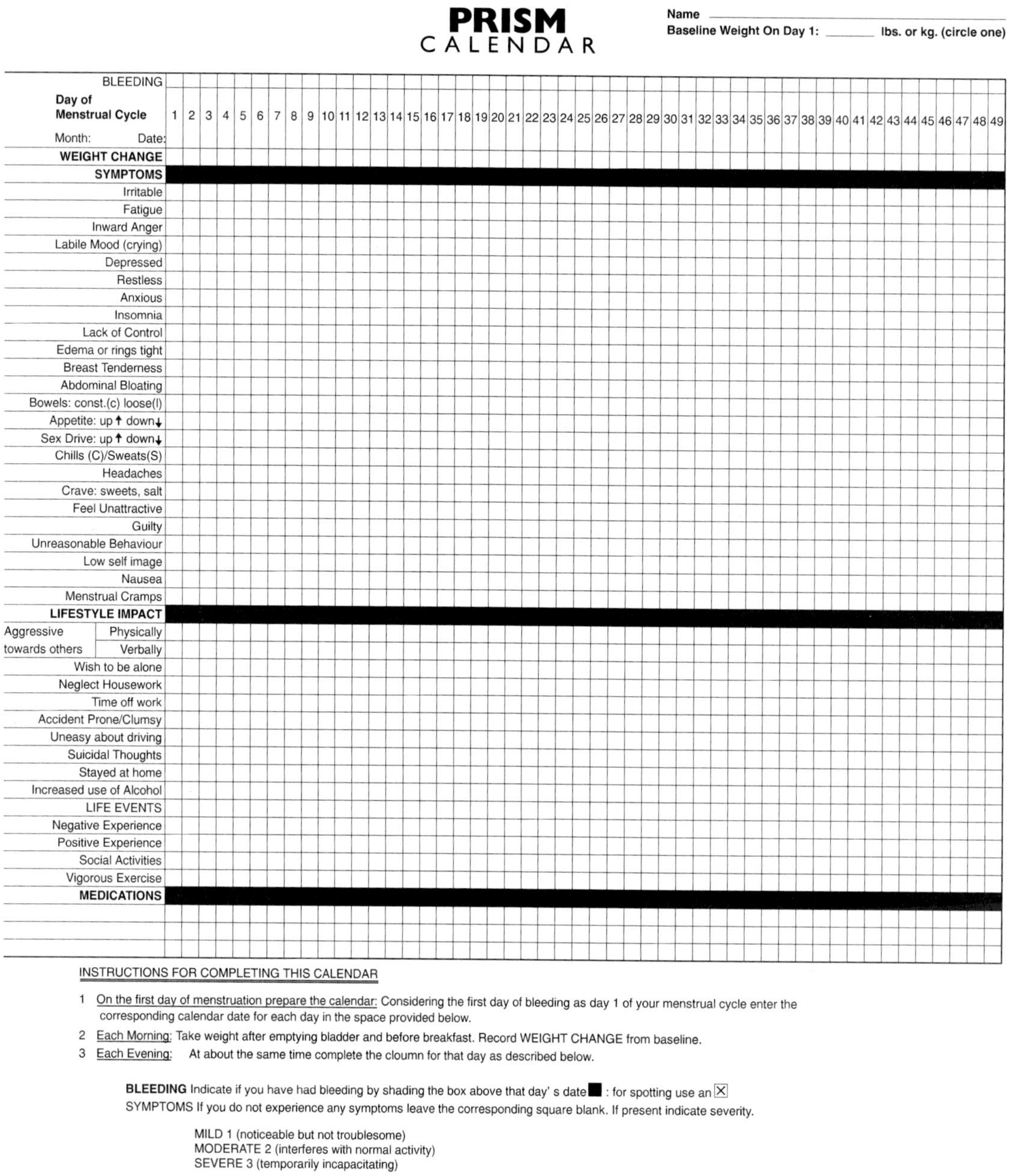

Fig. 17-1. The prospective record of the impact and severity of menstrual symptomatology (PRISM). (From Reid R: Premenstrual syndrome, *Endocrinol Metab* 5:1, 1987.)

Despite the widespread recognition of PMS and LLPDD and its inclusion in the psychiatric nomenclature, the etiology and treatment of the disorder remain unclear. Several thorough reviews of the etiology of PMS and LLPDD are available.[128,135,150] Table 17-3 includes a summary of the most common theories of the etiology of PMS and LLPDD.

The three most commonly proposed etiologies explaining LLPDD are the ovarian hormones, beta endorphin, and psychosocial theories. The ovarian hormone theory refers to the hypothesis that PMS and LLPDD are due to an imbalance in the ratio of estrogen to progesterone, with a relative deficiency in progesterone. This theory was first popularized by Dalton who believed that PMS is caused by a deficiency of progesterone and consequently treated patients with progesterone suppositories.[26] Recent studies investigating the levels of progesterone in women with PMS have been inconclusive because of methodologic difficulties. These difficulties include inconsistent diagnostic criteria, lack of matched controls groups, lack of daily ratings of premenstrual symptoms, and inconsistent assessment of the duration and severity of symptoms.[93,100]

Another hypothesis about the etiology of PMS and LLPDD is the beta endorphin theory.[128] It has been hypothesized that during the late follicular and early to midluteal phases, a woman with PMS or LLPDD becomes "addicted" to her own beta endorphin. When the level of beta endorphin drops precipitously in the late luteal phase she experiences symptoms of opioid withdrawal such as depression, irritability, increased appetite, etc. Alterations in peripheral endogenous opioids may account for the changes in electrolyte balance and its related symptoms. Choung et al tested this hypothesis in a study during which naltrexone was given to the patient in the follicular phase to block the initial beta endorphin dependence.[18] In an open clinical trial they reported general improvement of PMS symptoms but significant side effects were noted.

A final group of hypotheses regarding the etiology of PMS are the psychosocial theories.[3] Early psychoanalytic theorists believed that PMS was a conscious manifestation of a woman's unconscious conflicts about femininity and motherhood.[133] Psychoanalytic thinkers proposed that the premenstrual physical changes reminded the woman that she was not pregnant and therefore not fulfilling her traditional feminine role. Although this hypothesis was compelling to many psychoanalytically oriented clinicians, it was impossible to substantiate via scientific methods.

Cognitive and social learning theory models have also been proposed.[11,124] These models suggest that the onset of menses is an aversive psychologic event for the woman susceptible to PMS or LLPDD. The woman dreads the onset of menses and as a result develops an increased psychologic arousal and a vigilance for cues that it is about to begin. Over time these cues combine with the aversive event (menses) and normal premenstrual changes become premenstrual symptoms. In addition, these women may also have negative cognitive expectations which reinforce the aversiveness of the premenstrual symptoms. The reporting of symptoms becomes reinforced by reliably predicting the aversive event (menses). The woman then develops maladaptive coping strategies such as mood changes, social withdrawal, missed work, and increased eating to reduce the immediate stress. The immediate reduction of stress in the short term reinforces these behaviors and over time they occur regularly during the premenstruum.

From a sociocultural perspective, some writers have noted that PMS and LLPDD are manifestations of the negative attitudes and beliefs about menstruation pervasive in our culture.[173] Others note that PMS and LLPDD are cultural expressions of women's anger and discontent not only over traditional female roles in American society but also over the constant role strain many experience.[52] The role of a productive worker conflicts with that of a traditional woman for whom childrearing activities are central.[70] Some feminist thinkers argue that PMS and LLPDD are psychiatric "disorders" created by the medical establishment to medicalize a normal biologic process and to prevent women from engaging in activities with responsibility and power within society.[39] Because only women can be diagnosed with LLPDD, it is cited as discriminatory. Blechman objected to the creation of a new diagnostic category for a premenstrual disorder.[11] This objection is based on the belief that many women experience premenstrual symptomatology at other times during the menstrual cycle and therefore a diagnosis implying a premenstrual causal factor is inappropriate. They feel that a new psychiatric diagnosis is unnecessary because the symptoms experienced by this small group of women can be subsumed under preexisting psychiatric diagnoses.

There is a wide range of treatments for PMS and LLPDD including lifestyle changes, psychotherapy, and medications.[73] Lifestyle changes include the following: (1) dietary modifications with avoidance of simple carbohydrates, frequent small meals and reduction or elimination of salt, caffeine, sugar, and alcohol; (2) decreased tobacco use; (3) increased aerobic exercise (20 to 30 minutes three times per week)[119,153]; and (4) a decreased stress level managed by techniques such as assertiveness training, time management, progressive muscle relaxation, and guided imagery.[48]

Several studies have investigated the use of progesterone in treating premenstrual symptoms. Although some studies reported positive results, these studies were marred by methodologic problems, which included nonrandom assignment of treatment groups, small sample sizes, and lack of a placebo control group.[5,26,54,87,93,137] Recently Freeman et al demonstrated in a double-blind, placebo-controlled study that progesterone suppositories are an ineffective treatment for PMS.[42] Other hormonal preparations such as the oral contraceptive pill and GnRH agonists have been used to alter ovarian hormone function. Results of oral contraceptive use are inconclusive, since some patients report improvement in symptoms and others report the opposite.[53,117] The use of GnRH agonists is reported to relieve symptoms,[59,104] but the long term use of these agents is questionable because of the long term side effects of maintaining a hypoestrogenic state. Many psychotropic medications such as fluoxetine, nortryptyline, and alprazolam have been used to treat PMS and LLPDD.[62,63,95,157,176] These medications are given in a variety of regimens targeted to specific symptoms. Referral to a psychiatrist is recommended for the management of these psychiatric medications.

In summary, many women report premenstrual changes but only 5% to 10% meet criteria for LLPDD. Prominent symptoms of LLPDD are emotional lability, depression or irritability and complaints of numerous physical and behavioral changes that occur the week before the beginning of menses. Careful documentation of symptoms is necessary to establish the relationship between symptom onset and its remission relative to the menstrual cycle. Symptoms must be present for two to three consecutive cycles. Although the cause of LLPDD is nebulous, several treatments have been developed. Progesterone and other hormone preparations have had mixed effectiveness in treating LLPDD. Lifestyle changes and psychotherapy also have had mixed results, although psychoactive medications may be used to treat specific symptoms. A careful diagnosis that includes the exclusion of a preexisting psychologic disorder is critical.

POSTPARTUM DEPRESSION

Pregnancy and childbirth are significant developmental milestones for most women. Physical, intrapersonal, and relational adaptations are needed to successfully adjust to pregnancy and delivery. The stresses that a new mother experiences are numerous and include disruption in routine, sleep deprivation, decreased independence, social isolation, and changes in status at the workplace. The well-adjusted woman is able to anticipate these changes and prepare for them accordingly. Unfortunately, a minority of women may experience postpartum depression, a serious psychiatric disorder that afflicts the new mother. The pregnancy, delivery, and postpartum care of a woman are medical events controlled or overseen by the obstetrician. Therefore it is important for obstetricians to be well versed in the course and the treatment of postpartum depression.

Postpartum depression should be taken seriously for several reasons. It can cause significant suffering for the afflicted woman, has a relatively high prevalence, can be of long duration, and can have deleterious consequences for the newborn.[116] The adverse impact of postpartum depression on infants has been noted and is receiving increased attention in the literature.[21,103,132]

Postpartum depression is characterized by depressed affect, loss of interest in activities, change in appetite, fatigue, sleep difficulties, difficulty caring for the baby, guilt, low self-esteem, difficulty concentrating, psychomotor retardation or agitation, and suicidal ideation. It is much more serious and persistent than the "maternity blues," which is a transient emotional reaction that women experience shortly after birth that subsides without intervention.[67] Hayworth et al noted that postpartum depression can begin 2 to 8 weeks after delivery and can persist from 2 weeks to several months.[64] Estimates of the prevalence of postpartum depression vary depending on the method of assessment. Based on self-report data, Dalton reported that 7% of women were depressed in the postpartum period.[25] Cutrona reported that 3.5% of a sample of pregnant women were depressed during their pregnancy and the postpartum, based on DSM-III depression criteria.[23] O'Hara et al found a 9% rate of depression during pregnancy and 12% in the postpartum, using research diagnostic criteria.[112] Dennerstein et al reported a 14% rate of postpartum depression among women in a multicenter study.[31] Gotlib et al in a prospective study found that 10% of women were depressed during pregnancy and 7% were depressed in the postpartum, using research diagnostic criteria.[50] The percentages rose to 22% during pregnancy and 26% during the postpartum, using the Beck Depression Inventory, a self-report measure of depression. In general, the base rate of postpartum depression is approximately 10%.[111]

Several factors have been investigated as possible causes of postpartum depression. Biologic variables, including hormones and neurotransmitters, have been investigated for their hypothesized relationship to postpartum depression. Dalton proposed that progesterone played a significant role in the etiology of postpartum depression, although no data supporting the hypothesis was reported.[25] Nott et al measured levels of LH, FSH, estrogen, progesterone, and prolactin in a prospective study and correlated them with depressive symptoms.[108] They found a moderate correlation between irritable mood and estrogen levels and an inverse correlation between progesterone levels and depression. Unfortunately none of their subjects met criteria for a clinically significant depression. Gordon et al found that estriol levels were inversely correlated to a moderate degree with crying spells in the postpartum.[49] In a prospective study O'Hara et al looked at plasma estradiol, progesterone, prolactin, and cortisol.[110,115,116] Only estradiol showed a relationship to postpartum depression; its levels in the postpartum depressed subjects were significantly lower than those of the nondepressed subjects.

Others have investigated the relationship between postpartum depression and tryptophan, the precursor to and the rate-limiting agent in the production of serotonin.[60,61,155] A decrease in serotonin has been associated with depressive symptoms in psychiatric patients.[22,130] Stein et al found that women with severe postpartum depression had tryptophan levels similar to those of depressed psychiatric inpatients.[155] Plasma tryptophan levels and depressive scores had a correlation coefficient of -0.60, suggesting a moderate relationship. Handley et al found that plasma tryptophan levels rose over the second to fifth postpartum days, although none of their patients was classified as having postpartum depression.[61] In a second study Handley et al found that tryptophan levels were low before delivery, then rose rapidly on postpartum days 1 and 2. The absence of a tryptophan peak after delivery correlated significantly with the "maternity blues" and subsequent depression in the following six months.[60] Treadway et al found no significant correlations in plasma catecholamines and postpartum mood.[164]

The relationship between postpartum depression and psychosocial variables has also been studied. Hopkins et al provided a thorough review of the literature on postpartum depression and on predisposing psychosocial variables.[67] They concluded that there are no significant relationships between postpartum depression and demographic factors such as age or parity. However, there does appear to be a relationship between postpartum depression and the quality of the marital relationship. Several studies have found that poor marital relationships precede postpartum depression.[79,109,169] Also, lack of support from the male partner has been associated with increased severity of the depression.[109,113] Cutrona reported that a lack of perceived social support during pregnancy was associated with the degree of postpartum depression.[23]

Another significant predictor of postpartum depression is depression during pregnancy.[23,112,114] Watson et al reported that depressive symptoms during pregnancy predicted a later diagnosis of postpartum depression.[169] In a recent study Gotlib et al followed a group of 360 pregnant women during and after pregnancy to determine the predictors of depression.[50]

They found that 10% of women met criteria for depression during pregnancy and 7% were depressed during the puerperium. Only half of the cases of postpartum depression were new onset; the remainder of the women, who were depressed during the puerperium, were also depressed during pregnancy. Also, these investigators found that variables that predicted depression during pregnancy differed from those that predicted depression during the postpartum. Factors that predicted depression during pregnancy were young age, less education, multiparity, and lack of outside employment. These variables were not significant predictors of postpartum depression.

Hopkins et al investigated the relationship between infant-related stressors and postpartum depression.[66] In a cross-sectional study they compared life-event stress, neonatal risk status, infant temperament, and social support in groups of depressed and nondepressed women 6 to 8 weeks postpartum. They found that infant-related stressors such as medical complications and maternal perceptions of infant temperament related significantly to postpartum depression. In this study, life-event stress and social support did not relate to postpartum depression.

Another study looked at predictors of postpartum depression in a sample of 115 primiparous women.[171] This study investigated marital adjustment, cognitive attributional style, life stress, maternal expectations and perception of infant behaviors, and depressive symptoms. In this sample 6% of the women had major depression at 8 weeks postpartum. Many variables related to postpartum depressive *symptoms* but only poor marital adjustment and the presence of depressive symptoms during the pregnancy related to the *diagnosis* of postpartum depression.

In another study of postpartum depression, Gotlib et al followed a group of 730 women during pregnancy and through 4 weeks postpartum.[51] In this study 10% of the subjects were diagnosed with depression during pregnancy. An additional 5% of women became depressed during the puerperium. Those women who were depressed during the postpartum reported higher depressive symptom scores during pregnancy, higher perceived stress during pregnancy, lower levels of marital satisfaction, and escapism as a coping strategy. During the puerperium, these two groups also differed on current perceived stress and marital satisfaction.

In the only study using a matched control group, O'Hara et al compared a group of pregnant women with a group of nonpregnant controls to determine if pregnancy and the postpartum were times of increased stress and depression.[116] Women were assessed during the second trimester of pregnancy and again at 9 weeks postpartum. Eight percent of the pregnant subjects met criteria for depression during the second trimester, and 6% of the controls were depressed during the same time period. Ten percent of the pregnant women were depressed at 9 weeks postpartum compared with 8% of the control subjects. The rates, time of onset, and duration of the depression were not significantly different between the two groups. During the postpartum assessment, 26% of the pregnant women had the "maternity blues," and 8% of the controls had the "blues." The authors concluded that the prevalence of a clinical depression may not significantly increase after childbirth but depressive symptoms, or the "maternity blues," are much more likely to occur.

O'Hara et al proposed a diatheses-stress model of postpartum depression that also has been used to describe the causes of other types of depression.[115] In this model, diatheses (vulnerability factors) such as a familial predisposition for depression, history of depressive episodes, or dysfunctional cognitive attributional style may predispose a woman to depression which then emerges as the woman has to cope with stressors related to pregnancy and motherhood. Common stressors during the pregnancy and postpartum are presented in Table 17-4.[6] The preexisting vulnerability to depression in combination with acute stressors may lead to the development of depression. O'Hara et al tested this model of postpartum depression in a study of childbearing women with postpartum depression.[115] The study assessed demographic, psychiatric, social, and cognitive vulnerability variables. Additionally they measured stress, from current life events, peripartum stress, and childcare stress. Hormonal assays were conducted on prolactin, estradiol, progesterone, and cortisol at 34, 36, and 38 weeks of gestation and several days postpartum. The results indicate that depressive history, depression during pregnancy, childcare-related stressors, and peripartum stressors account for 40% of the variance in the diagnosis of postpartum depression. None of the hormonal variables differ significantly for the depressed versus the nondepressed women.

A final study investigating the impact of psychosocial variables on postpartum depression was conducted by Powell and Drotar.[118] In this study women were asked about their mood, stressors, social support, and "daily hassles." Results indicated that prepartum depression, social support, and "daily hassles" are the strongest predictors of postpartum depression. This provides additional evidence for the diatheses-stress model and suggests that both predisposing vulnerability factors and current stressors need to be considered when screening women for postpartum depression.

In summary, the base rate for postpartum depression is approximately 10%. It is unclear whether or not the postpartum period is a time of increased clinical depression among women, although an increase in reporting depressive symptoms is common. For those women who do have postpartum depression the common variables associated with the disorder include the following: (1) a previous history of depression (including depression during pregnancy), (2) a poor marital relationship, (3) difficulties with childcare, (4) inadequate social support, and (5) numerous daily stressors. Women with one or more of these factors may need increased attention during pregnancy and in the postpartum period. The diagnosis of depression is made when the symptoms of depressed mood, emotional lability, decreased interest in

Table 17-4. Postpartum stressors

Category	Examples of items reported	
Physical symptoms (PS)	Fatigue	Eating disturbances
	Nausea/vomiting	GI disturbances
	Bodily pain/discomfort	Bowel/bladder
	Rest/sleep disturbances	
	Physical restrictions	
Changes in living patterns (CLP)	Housing (space, rearrange house)	
	Activities (diet, exercise, smoking)	
	Time schedules (responsibilities)	
	Relocation to new residence	
Body image (BI)	Weight gain	
	Feelings (fat, unattractive, distorted size)	
	Wardrobe not fitting	
	Getting back into shape	
	Physical marks on body	
Monetary stressors (MS)	Money to buy things	
	Bills	
	Concern over insurance coverage	
	Loss of regular income	
Family stressors (FS)	Parents (reactions, pressures, getting along)	
	Support (lack of, far away, too helpful)	
	In-laws	
	General worries	
Emotional stressors (EM)	Changes (moody, irritable, sensitive, lack of patience)	
	Fears/worries/concerns (baby, coping, control)	
	Anger, frustration/ambivalence	
	Depression, loneliness	
	Guilt	
Pregnancy concerns (PG)	Fear of miscarriage	Baby's due date
	Complications—risks	Birth control (spacing)
	Preterm labor	Misc. (technology)
	High blood pressure	
	Insufficient weight gain	
Labor-delivery (LD)	Fears	Outcomes
	Pain/discomfort	
	Complications	
	Waiting	
	Cesarean	
Social stressors (SS)	Decrease in social opportunities	
	Friends' reactions, advice	
	Others (communications of strangers)	
	Single parenting (reactions)	
Job/career/school (JC)	Work (fatigue, limitations, relationships)	
	Change in career plans	
	School (decisions to finish, quit, examinations)	
Mate/spouse issues (MSI)	Time constraints (impact on relationship)	
	Reactions/comments (emotional needs)	
	Arguments/marital problems	
	Sex life (attractiveness, discomfort, decreased frequency)	
	Misc. (husband's responsibility with household, working too much)	
Parenting concerns (PC)	Mothering role and responsibilities	
	Breastfeeding concerns	
	Child-care concerns	
	Newborn care	
	Nightfeedings	
	Misc. (pediatric care, driving with baby, baby classes)	
Newborn behaviors (NB)	Baby crying	
	Identify infant distress signals	
	Colic behaviors	

Table 17-4. Postpartum stressors—cont'd

Category	Examples of items reported
Baby welfare (BW)	Health (baby ok?) Normality (abnormal baby, birth defects) Effects on baby (nutrition, diseases) Anticipation/expectations Sick baby (prematurity, NICU care)
Other children (OC)	Care/responsibilities Sibling rivalry (children fighting) Reactions to new baby

From Arrizmendi T, Affonso D: Stressful events related to pregnancy and postpartum, *J Psychosom Res* 31:743, 1987.

activities, poor concentration, sleep or appetite changes, and difficulty caring for the newborn are present at moderate to severe intensity for at least 2 weeks. It is particularly important to determine if the woman is still able to care for herself and the newborn. Obstetricians can help detect cases of depression at postpartum follow-up appointments. Following completion of the physical examination, a few questions such as, "Have you had any problems with depression since the baby has been born?" or "Do you feel that you have adjusted well to becoming a mother?" can open the door to assessing depressive symptoms. If the woman responds in the affirmative to a general question regarding mood difficulties, obstetricians can conduct further assessment for depression or they can refer the patient to a psychiatrist or psychologist.

There are a variety of treatments available for postpartum depression.[37] Individual psychotherapy can provide the patient with increased social support, emotional expression, stress management skills, and improved cognitive and behavioral coping strategies, which can increase feelings of efficacy and control. Within the context of psychotherapy, antidepressant medications can be used. Sichel recommended early psychopharmacologic stabilization with tricyclic antidepressants.[148] Medication use is often limited among breastfeeding mothers because of concerns about the effects of psychoactive medications ingested by the nursing infant. Some women with severe depression need medication to benefit from other types of interventions. In addition to individual psychotherapy, psychoeducational groups can provide valuable information about parenting and childcare. Support groups allow the patient share her feelings with others and help her to realize that she is not alone in her adjustment to parenthood. Couples counseling also can be used when relationship issues play a significant role in the depression. A common clinical scenario is the postpartum woman who remains at home with the baby while her husband works full time. By the end of the day she needs a break from her responsibilities but her husband feels a need to unwind after work. As a result, neither partner feels able to meet the demands of caring for the baby; traditional role behaviors and lack of assertive communication may trap the couple in a pattern of behavior such that the woman continues to provide the majority of care for the baby. She may be unable to communicate her needs to her husband and may become angry with him for being unresponsive to her needs. Consequently, the husband may sense her anger and withdraw, thus increasing the woman's anger and frustration. Therapy can teach the couple to communicate clearly and to share in household and childcare activities in a mutually agreeable arrangement. Finally, in cases where outpatient management is not possible because severe depression prevents the woman from taking care of herself and/or the baby, hospitalization may be necessary. It also may be indicated when the woman is suicidal, homicidal, or has developed psychotic delusions.

To summarize, numerous variables have been investigated as predisposing factors for postpartum depression. There is no unequivocal evidence for a hormonal cause of postpartum depression, although depression during pregnancy, a history of depression, the quality of the marital relationship, perceived social support, and daily stressors appear to be related factors. Early identification and treatment for postpartum depression is critical for the welfare of the mother and the baby.

CHRONIC PELVIC PAIN

It is estimated that chronic pelvic pain is the presenting complaint in 10% to 30% of all gynecologic visits.[168] Data from several studies have indicated that 12% to 19% of all hysterectomies are performed because of unresolved chronic pelvic pain.[33,43] Hysterectomies are one of the most common surgical procedures in the United States, with a rate of 650,000 per year; approximately 78,000 hysterectomies are performed annually because of chronic pelvic pain.

Though there may be no such thing as "typical" chronic pelvic pain patients, generally they report chronic, debilitating pelvic pain and numerous unsuccessful attempts at relief. Associated symptoms include depressed mood, sleep disturbance, fatigue, impaired work functioning, deteriorating marital or other relationships, decreased sexual interest and activity, and drug use or dependence. There are three main dimensions that define chronic pelvic pain[154] as follows: (1) duration—any type of pelvic pain lasting six months or longer; (2) anatomic—pelvic pain defined by physical findings at laparoscopy; and (3) affective/behavioral—pain accompanied by significantly altered physical activity such as work, recreation, and sex, and changes in mood related to the chronic pain. Clinicians and researchers have used these to classify different types of chronic pelvic pain. Relying on positive physical findings at laparoscopy to diagnose chronic pelvic pain is insufficient because 10% to 80% of women with chronic pelvic pain either do not have any physical cause for their pain or their pain is out of proportion to the extent of disease.[78,83] However, relying only on the behavioral or affective components of pain may prompt the clinician to overlook important somatic causes. It is important for the physician to be knowledgeable about both the physical and psychologic correlates of chronic pelvic pain.

Investigators have studied the occurrence of pelvic pathology and psychologic disturbance among chronic pelvic pain sufferers. Many studies have looked at the incidence of positive physical findings among chronic pelvic pain patients.[78,120,134] Kresch et al conducted a prospective study of physical and psychologic variables among a group of 100 women with chronic pelvic pain and a control group having a laparoscopy for sterilization.[78] They found that 83% of the chronic pelvic pain group had pelvic pathology compared with only 29% of the control group. The most common types of pathology in the pain patients were pelvic adhesions, endometriosis, and bowel and liver adhesions. In another prospective study Rosenthal et al found that 75% of his sample of 100 chronic pelvic pain patients had pelvic pathology at laparoscopy.[134] These abnormalities included adhesions, endometriosis, and ovarian cysts. The results of similar studies are summarized in Table 17-5. Steege et al summarized the findings of several other studies that indicate that of 2624 women studied 16% had endometriosis, 20% had adhesions, and 36% had negative findings at laparoscopy.[154] Therefore although many women with chronic pelvic pain had an identifiable physical problem that could account for some or all of the pain, over one third of the

Table 17-5. Summary of studies of laparoscopy findings among chronic pelvic pain patients

Author/Date	No. of patients	Endometriosis No.	Endometriosis %	Adhesions No.	Adhesions %	Negative No.	Negative %	R/P†	Controls
Pent, 1972	38	7	18	13	34	18	47	R	None
Lundberg et al, 1973	95	13	14	29	31	40	42	R	None
Semchyhyn et al, 1976	198	22	11	24	12	131	66	R	None
Beard et al, 1977	35	3	17	6	33	17	49	P	Nine asymptomatic women (no laparoscopy)
Goldstein et al, 1980*	140	66	47	28	20	19	14	R	None
Cunanan et al, 1983	1194	43	4	229	19	355	30	R	None (included acute and chronic pain)
Rosenthal et al, 1984	60	10	17	33	55	15	25	P	None
Magni et al, 1984	29	6	20	3	10	11	38	P	n = 11 women with perianal pain
Kresch et al, 1984	100	32	32	38	38	17	17	p	n = 50 laparoscopic sterilization: Endometriosis: 15% Adhesions: 39%
Levitan et al, 1984	186	4	2	14	8	168	92	R	None
Magni et al, 1986	30	2	7	61	20	14	47	P	n = 30 no laparoscopies on controls
Rapkin, 1986	100	37	37	216	26	36	36	R	n = 88 infertility patients Endometriosis: 33% Adhesions: 39%
Goldstein, 1989*, **	282	126	45	37	13	71	25	R	None
Vercellini et al, 1989*	47	18	38	3	6	19	40	R	None
Stout et al, 1991***	90	46	51	35	39	19	21	P	n = 12 laparoscopic sterilization: Endometriosis: 25% Adhesions: 25%
Total	2624	435	16.5	524	20	950	36.2		

*Adolescent population; **Pain duration 3 months; ***35% of laparoscopies done to investigate infertility
†R = retrospective; P = prospective
From Steege J, Stout A, Somkuti S: Chronic pelvic pain: toward an integrative model, *J Psychosom Obstet Gynecol* 12(suppl):3, 1991.

women who were studied had no positive finding. Also, there are numerous nongynecologic causes of chronic pelvic pain including gastrointestinal problems such as idiopathic constipation and irritable bowel syndrome. Urologic problems such as urethral syndrome, interstitial cystitis, and bladder spasms are also possible causes of chronic pelvic pain.[162] Musculoskeletal problems can be a predisposing factor; King et al found faulty posture to be common among a group of chronic pelvic pain patients.[74] In their study women reported significant relief upon correction of posture with physical therapy.

The investigation of the relationship between psychosocial problems and chronic pelvic pain has a long history. Early reports from the 1960s focused on the clinical speculation that women with chronic pelvic pain had deep-seated emotional conflicts about their feminine identities and roles.[16,46] Recently investigators have studied psychiatric comorbidity among women with chronic pelvic pain. Walker et al studied two groups of women; a chronic pelvic pain group and a group of women who were having a tubal ligation or an infertility-related diagnostic laparoscopy.[168] Each group had a laparoscopy with classification of adhesions, a structured psychiatric interview that explored a possible history of sexual abuse, a family psychiatric history interview, and a self-report measure of psychiatric symptoms. The groups were then divided into subgroups based on whether or not any physical pathology was found at the laparoscopy. This resulted in the following groups: (1) chronic pelvic pain with physical pathology; (2) chronic pelvic pain without physical pathology; (3) control group with physical pathology; and (4) control group without physical pathology. The psychologic data were then compared within groups, but analyses indicated no significant differences in the psychologic variables between groups 1 and 2 or between groups 3 and 4. That is, the psychologic variables did not correlate with physical findings at laparoscopy. The data from groups 1 and 2 (chronic pelvic pain) and groups 3 and 4 (controls) were compared based on the various psychiatric variables. The authors found that the rates of current and past psychiatric disorders were significantly higher for the chronic pelvic pain patients than for the control group. For example, 28% of the chronic pelvic pain group had a current depressive disorder compared with 17% of the control group and 32% of the chronic pelvic pain group had a current phobia compared with 10% of the control group. Significantly, 64% of the chronic pelvic pain group had a history of sexual abuse compared with only 23% of the control group. Finally, the chronic pelvic pain group had significantly more sexual dysfunction than the control group, both in terms of inhibited desire and inhibited orgasmic function. Walker et al discussed their findings in the context of the correlation of depression to chronic pain syndromes in general. They noted that depression is related to higher utilization of medical services, numerous somatic complaints, and other types of pain syndromes such as chronic back, pelvic, and head pain. In the case of pelvic pain Walker et al speculated that the history of sexual abuse may play a role in determining the localization of the pain. They hypothesized that chronic pelvic pain occurred in women who come from multiproblem families in which the girl was not adequately protected from a sexual abuser. As a result the girl is sexually abused and develops sexual dysfunction in adulthood. The woman develops chronic pelvic pain as a way to avoid sexual interactions. Reiter and Gambone also found higher levels of sexual abuse histories in women with chronic pelvic pain.[129] They found that 48% of patients with chronic pelvic pain had a history of sexual abuse compared with only 6% of a control group. They noted that women with chronic pelvic pain used three times the amount of prescription medications and that they had a history of significantly more surgical procedures than the controls. In contrast to these studies Rapkin et al compared the sexual abuse histories of chronic pelvic pain patients, other pain patients, and a group of controls[122]; the rates of sexual abuse were not significantly

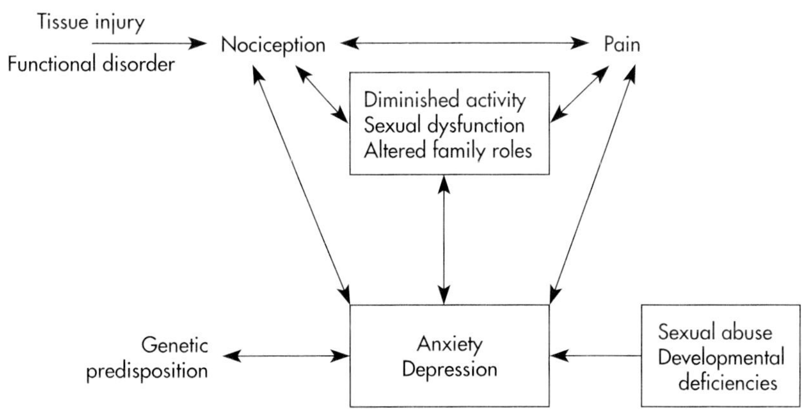

Fig. 17-2. An interactive model of chronic pelvic pain. (From Steege J, Stout A, Somkuti S: Chronic pelvic pain: toward an integrative model, *J Psychosom Obstet Gynecol* 12(suppl):3, 1991.

higher among the chronic pelvic pain patients compared with the other two groups (19% for chronic pelvic pain, 16% for other pain patients, and 12% for controls).

Other studies have looked at chronic pelvic pain and psychopathology. Stout and Steege found that 50% of their patients who presented with chronic pelvic pain had clinically significant depression.[158] Rosenthal et al found that 80% of patients with chronic pelvic pain had significant psychopathology indicated by their profiles on the MMPI.[134] There were no significant differences in MMPI profiles among women with and without documented pelvic pathology. A schematic representation of the interaction of physical and psychologic factors in the development of chronic pelvic pain is provided by Steege et al and is presented in Fig. 17-2.[154]

The clinical picture in chronic pelvic pain is complicated by physical and psychologic factors. There is a significant number of chronic pelvic pain patients who have a history of psychosexual trauma and psychologic disorders. Therefore a multidisciplinary assessment and treatment approach is recommended.[121,123,154,175] Rapkin and Kames have described a series of behavioral signs that in their experience indicate that a patient may be unresponsive to the traditional medical treatment of chronic pelvic pain.[121] A list of their signs is presented in Table 17-6.

Rapkin and Reading provided a thorough overview of a multidisciplinary treatment plan.[123] During the first visit, a thorough history is taken and includes the nature, location, intensity, and variability of the pain. In addition, questions about the impact of the pain on areas of functioning (such as work, home, and relationships) are asked. A thorough medical, obstetric, gynecologic, and psychologic history should be taken, followed by a complete physical examination and laboratory studies. The patient is then instructed to note the intensity, frequency, location, and duration of the pain in a diary. Other factors such as medication use, activity level, and stressors that affect the pain should also be noted in the diary.

Table 7-6. Indications for multidisciplinary treatment of chronic pain

1. Pain/disability greatly disproportionate to the pathology
2. Excessive pain behavior, such as nonverbal cues (e.g., moaning, splinting movement)
3. Poor response to appropriate treatment
4. Immediate relief followed by worsening or moving pain
5. Unusual reaction to specific treatment modalities
6. Withdrawal from normal life activities (e.g., work, school, sexual activity)
7. Significant time spent lying down
8. Severe depression
9. Severe anxiety
10. Physician shopping
11. Unwillingness to admit to any stress or upset whatsoever
12. Blaming all problems on the pain (i.e., "If the pain were gone my life would be perfect.")
13. Extreme unassertiveness
14. Noncompliance with a treatment regime
15. Excessive medication use or drug dependence
16. Significant family, marital or sexual problems
17. History of incest or onset of pain associated with trauma (e.g., rape, abortion)

Adapted from Rapkin A, Kames L: The pain management approach to chronic pelvic pain, *J Reprod Med* 32:323,1987.

During the second visit, all laboratory results and information in the pain diary are reviewed with the patient. Also, an examination of the abdominal, lumbrosacral, and vaginal pain trigger points can be conducted. Review of the pain diary helps to identify psychosocial or behavioral precipitants of the pain, narcotic or other substance use, or abuser dependence. The patient can also have a psychologic consultation with a psychologist or psychiatrist wellversed in chronic pelvic pain. This evaluation may include a complete psychologic interview, a history, and a mental status examination. Extensive evaluation of the psychosocial precursors, the covariates, and the consequences of the pain can be conducted, and the presence of a concurrent psychiatric disorder can be determined. As Rapkin and Kames noted, chronic pelvic pain patients can experience significant amounts of depression, anxiety, and personality dysfunction.[121] Objective psychologic tests can provide standardized information regarding psychologic functioning.

During the third visit, the pain diary can be reviewed again, and a laparoscopy may be scheduled to identify and treat any pelvic pathology. If a laparoscopy indicates the absence of pelvic pathology, treatment can focus on medication and on psychologic treatment of the pain. When prescribed, medications are given at regular intervals instead of on an "as needed" basis to minimize psychologic conditioning that associates severe pain with medication-taking behavior and subsequent pain reduction. Pain-management programs or psychologic intervention can identify the patterns of pain and develop strategies to reduce it and/or its impact on the patient's life. Also, alternative coping skills help to manage the pain. Specific psychologic interventions include relaxation training, stress management, cognitive-behavioral therapy, and sexual or marital counseling.

INFERTILITY

Fertility is highly valued in most cultures and the wish for a child is one of the most basic of all human motivations. For women, pregnancy and motherhood are developmental milestones highly emphasized by our culture.[32,167,173] When an attempt to have a child fails it can be an emotionally devastating experience.[71,90,96]

Infertility is defined as 12 months of appropriately timed intercourse that does not result in conception. Approximately 16% of couples in the United States have difficulty conceiving a child.[105] This appears in part because of the trend for some women to delay childbirth until their mid thirties to late thirties and the associated decrease in fertility after the age of 35. Although there is the perception that infertility is on the rise it is actually an artifact of the large number of women currently in the childbearing years because of the baby boom of the 1950s. The base rate of infertility among women has remained the same, but the absolute number of women in the reproductive years has increased.[102]

Approximately 40% of infertile couples have female factor infertility, 40% have male factor, and 20% have a combination of both or infertility of unknown cause. For decades clinicians have believed that infertility, particularly that of unknown cause, could be caused by psychologic distress.[9,91,138] Investigators tried to identify "unconscious" or other psychologic variables that caused infertility.[35,98,144] In the mid 1980s clinicians and researchers began to question the hypothesis that psychologic distress *caused* infertility. As a result they began to investigate the psychologic distress that was a *consequence* of infertility. Mental health clinicians became increasingly involved in the provision of care to infertile patients.[55,76] This led to increased research on the myriad psychologic aspects of infertility.

In the mid 1980s psychologic researchers began to investigate the emotional impact of infertility. Based on clinical observations of infertile couples, Mahlstedt described a series of losses experienced by the infertile couple; the loss of self-esteem, relationships, health, and financial security.[90] The infertile person experiences a loss of self-esteem by failing to achieve a desired goal (having a baby) despite numerous attempts. The inability to have a child challenges and erodes a person's self-esteem. The problem may worsen significantly if the individual has been highly successful in other areas of life and has not developed the coping skills to deal with failure and loss.

The second loss is the real or feared loss of important relationships. This includes not only the marital relationship but also relationships with family and friends. The marital relationship may be strained or lost because of fears that the fertile partner will leave the infertile partner. The inability to discuss feelings about infertility, the act of blaming one another, and sexual difficulties related to the treatment of infertility can strain the infertile couple's relationship. Several writers have noted that infertile couples have sexual difficulties.[27,38,71,125] Sex may remind the couple of their failure to have a child. In addition to marital difficulties, the infertile couple may experience strain in relationships with family and friends. For example, an infertile women may avoid contact with her mother and sister if they constantly ask her if she is pregnant. Friends who are pregnant serve as a reminder that others can become pregnant with ease. The infertile

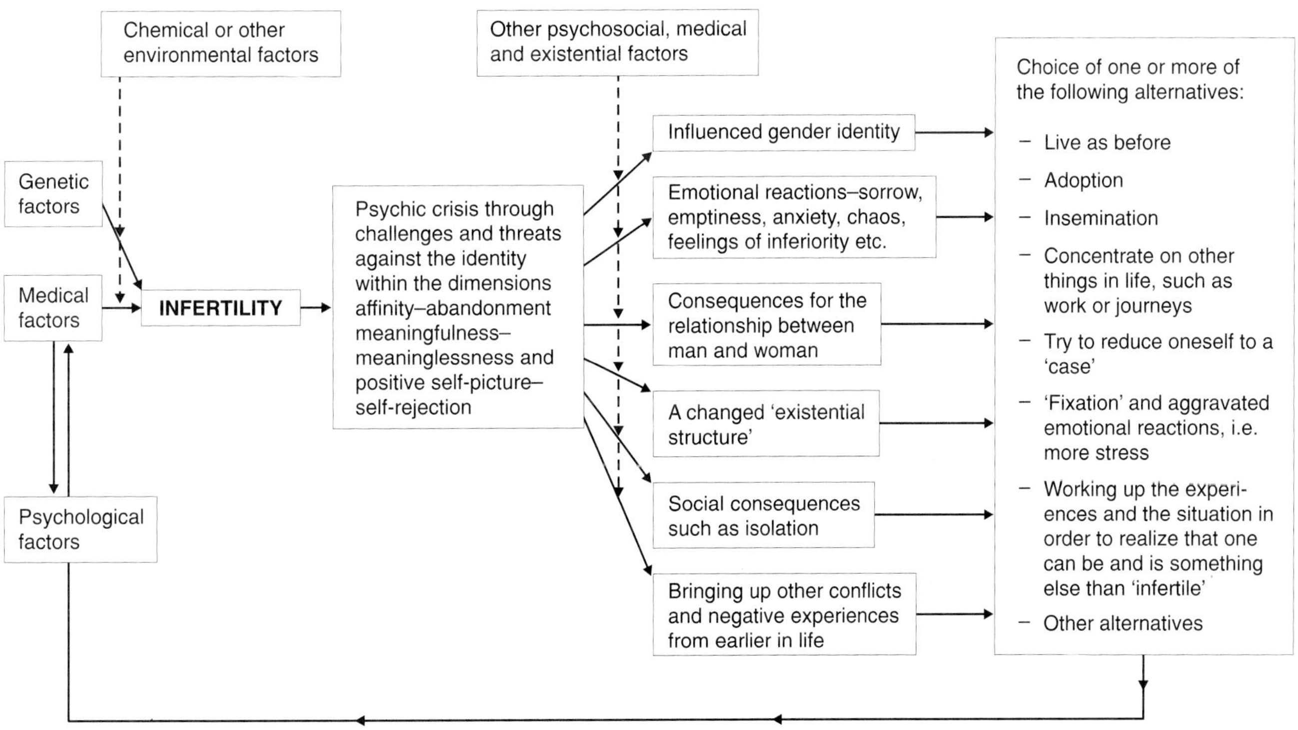

Fig. 17-3. Schema of infertility precursors and consequences. (From Moller A, Fallstrom K: Psychological factors in the etiology of infertility: a longitudinal study, *J Psychosom Obstet Gynecol* 12:13, 1991.)

woman's loss of relationships can deprive her of social support and compound feelings of isolation and depression.

The third loss related to infertility is that of health. The female patient may spend a great deal of time in the infertility clinic for tests and treatments. Although she is not really "sick," she may begin to identify with the "sick" role and feel that her physical health is compromised. Women may report feeling ill also because of the side effects of some of the hormonal medications prescribed to enhance fertility.

The fourth loss is that of financial security. Infertility treatments can be extremely expensive,[44] with one cycle of (IVF) costing approximately ten thousand dollars. A corollary to the financial problems are concerns about job security for women. Because women are frequently the primary focus of the evaluation or treatment, they often have to miss a considerable number of work hours thus placing their jobs in jeopardy. In addition, women often fear telling their employers the reason for their absences. They feel vulnerable to layoffs or firings because employers may assume the treatment will be successful and the woman will be leaving her job to have a child.

The losses related to infertility and other psychologic sequelae can adversely impact on the infertile woman. Moller and Fallstrom provide a useful schema for understanding the interactive effects of the biologic and psychosocial precursors and consequences of infertility.[98] Their model is presented in Fig. 17-3.

Much of the empirical research on the psychologic impact of infertility has focused on IVF patients. In their sample Freeman et al found that approximately half of the women rated infertility as the most stressful experience of their life.[41] In addition, they found that 18% of men and 16% of women had significant psychologic distress that included high levels of depression and somatization. Leiblum et al found that women reported more depression before and after infertility treatment than men and that 34% of the women in the study rated IVF as being "very stressful."[84] A third study of the psychologic impact of infertility and IVF, conducted by Baram et al, surveyed couples after they had completed one cycle of IVF.[8] As an indirect measure of how stressful the procedure was, couples were asked if they would undergo IVF again. The survey reported that 38% of the couples would not undergo IVF again because it was too expensive, the success rate was too low, and the emotional pain of the procedure was too intense. In addition, 18% of the couples reported that infertility negatively impacted on their marriage, 66% of women reported that they became depressed after the procedure, and 13% of the women reported that they had suicidal ideation after an unsuccessful procedure.

The results of these three studies underscored the psychologic component of infertility treatment. Infertility treatment can lead to depression or other adverse psychologic reactions because it is time consuming, emotionally draining, expensive, and has a relatively low (15% to 20%) chance for success. These factors put the infertile woman at risk for psychologic distress.

After documenting that infertility and IVF were psychologically stressful, the next phase of research began to look at variables that would predict the development of psychologic distress among infertile patients. Newton et al investigated pre-IVF psychologic factors that were related to post-IVF adjustment.[107] They found that 14% of women had clinically significant levels of anxiety and 24% had clinically significant levels of depression. They also found that both post-IVF anxiety and depression were best predicted by pre-IVF trait anxiety, depression, and childlessness. Men did not report clinically significant anxiety or depression.

Two recent studies investigated the stress of infertility using a stress and coping model.[82] According to this model, a situation is stressful if it is perceived as a threat to the person and if the person does not feel they have the coping skills to adapt to it. In this model infertility is stressful because it threatens the plan to have a child—an event that is highly valued. The extent to which infertility is stressful is further impacted by the coping skills the person uses. With this model one could identify *a priori* those individuals for whom infertility would be psychologically stressful. A study by Litt et al assessed several variables to determine their contribution to post-IVF distress.[85] These variables included demographic and reproductive history, general appraisal (optimism), situational appraisal (chances for success), and coping skills. Following an unsuccessful IVF cycle, 25% of the woman were clinically depressed. Results indicated that general optimism and perceived low responsibility for the cause of the infertility are protective against post-IVF distress. Feelings of loss of control, perceived contribution to the IVF failure, and the use of escapism as a coping strategy related to increased post-IVF distress. In this study optimism seemed to protect the woman from the threat of infertility. Only one coping strategy, escapism, related to post-IVF outcome indicating that women who used it experienced greater distress.

In a cross-sectional study of infertile patients investigators found that for women the most important factors related to psychologic distress were perceived personal control, optimism that they will eventually have a child, and intensity of motivation to have a child.[1] High levels of perceived personal control and optimism were related to lower distress levels, and high levels of motivation to have a child were associated with increased distress. According to this study, the more important it was to the woman to have a child the more distress she reported related to the experience of infertility.

Several recent papers have tried to demonstrate a relationship between psychologic status and outcome (pregnancy versus no pregnancy).[35,97,159] These studies have found no significant relationship between pretreatment psychologic variables and subsequent pregnancy. Although some investigators have tried to make a strong case for the psychologic cause of infertility, [9,36,91] there is little empirical support for this position.

Many of the studies of infertility have focused on women because they are the primary recipients of infertility treatment. Male factor infertility is also stressful and has been studied in the context of donor insemination.[10,77] Studies have indicated that male infertility can have a detrimental effect on a man's self-esteem and sexual functioning.[75]

In addition to donor insemination, donor oocyte, gestational carrier, and surrogacy procedures have psychologic risks and rewards. As reproductive technologies have expanded, so too has the number of ways in which a couple can have a child.[81] These options have created additional layers of psychologic, social, ethical, and legal entanglements that have not previously encumbered traditional reproduction. Society has not yet caught up with the advances in technology, and therefore the psychologic risk of these treatments is increased as patients are used in test cases to expand the boundaries of parenthood. Further research and discussion is needed to determine the consequences of these treatments and to develop language to describe the relationships between parent and child since the term "parent" now can mean gamete donor, gestational carrier, and/or psychosocial parent. The psychologist or psychiatrist can help screen, educate, and prepare patients for treatment and can treat any psychologic disorders that develop during the course of treatment.

The obstetrician-gynecologist should remember that infertility is a stressful event for both men and women. Women are more likely than men to report psychologic distress in the form of depression and anxiety in relation to infertility. Approximately 20% of women develop an acute clinical depression after a failed IVF attempt. Marital and sexual adjustment can be compromised by infertility. Because infertility is a problem that affects both partners, it is recommended that the couple be seen together in the evaluation and in treatment and that the emphasis is placed on infertility as the *couple's* problem. Perceived control is protective against psychologic distress in infertility treatment. Therefore providing the patient with opportunities to control treatment-related events is of help. Takefman et al have demonstrated that providing patients with basic information about the procedures both increases knowledge about infertility and decreases negative feelings about the experience.[163] Optimistic patients often are less distressed than those who are pessimistic. However the more important it is for the person to have a child, the more stressful the infertility experience will be. It is as important to talk about when to end treatment as it is to talk about the treatment itself.[14] Physicians can provide information in broad terms about the average number of cycles for various types of treatment. In addition, they can encourage the couple to discuss how much time, money, and emotional energy they are willing to devote to infertility treatment. Couples should be encouraged to take breaks from treatment as time permits to allow for physical rest and renewal of psychologic resilience.

In terms of psychologic services for infertility patients, a mandatory psychologic consultation is recommended for all

Table 17-7. Guidelines for infertility counseling

The following guidelines for referral indicate which issues are typically the most stressful or are most likely to cause significant emotional distress and disruption of infertility treatment. They are intended to provide the medical professional with a guide to those issues that are most likely to warrant referral to a qualified infertility counselor.

1. Patients entering treatment with assisted reproductive technologies
   The assisted reproductive technologies include treatment with IVF, gamete intrafallopian transfer (GIFT); other affiliated programs such as treatment with donor gametes (sperm and ovum), surrogacy, and gestational carrier programs; and any other medically assisted means of noncoital reproduction. Considerable research has shown that treatment with assisted reproductive technology is often psychologically as well as physically demanding. Furthermore, the treatment may be perceived by the couple and their caregivers as a last chance at parenthood and considered only after several years of infertility and a myriad of medical treatments. Not all couples *need* supportive and educational counseling. Any couple requesting counseling, showing overt distress, or meeting the description in the following guidelines would likely profit from referral to a qualified infertility counselor.
2. Psychiatric illness (past and present)
   A. A history of psychiatric illness with clear vulnerability to the current stressor
   B. Current significant psychiatric symptoms or illness
3. History of pregnancy complications or loss
   A. A history of traumatic perinatal or fetal loss
   C. A history of unresolved bereavement associated with abortion or perinatal death
   D. A current multiple pregnancy in which the patient is considering fetal reduction
   E. A patient undergoing IVF/genetic screening
4. Significant physical illness (past and present)
   A. Significant illness making pregnancy dangerous
   B. Request for donor gametes because of significant illness or genetic disorder
5. Sexual abuse (past and present)
   A. A history of unresolved rape, incest, or sexual abuse
   B. Current sexual abuse
6. Conflicted gender identity, homosexuality, or bisexuality
   A. Homosexuality or bisexuality interfering with marital stability and infertility treatment
   B. Atypical sexual behavior compromising fertility or infertility treatment
7. Chemical abuse or dependency
   A. Repeated failed attempts at treatment and continued or current abuse
   B. Inability to meet demands of medical treatment owing to abuse or dependence
   C. Even occasional use of drugs that are teratogenic
   D. A pattern of unstable behavior owing to chemical dependency
   E. Drug-seeking behavior
8. Pregnancy after 40 years of age
9. Chaotic social or familial functioning
10. Single women

From Burns L: An overview of the psychology of infertility, *Infertil Reprod Med Clin N Am* 4:433, 1993.

cases of third-party reproduction.[14,76] In addition, a psychologic consultation may be indicated when the patient has had the following: (1) a difficult reproductive history, (e.g., numerous pregnancy losses); (2) significant psychiatric problems (e.g., substance abuse, sexual assault, or psychiatric illness); and/or (3) current significant marital instability. Table 17-7 provides a useful summary of guidelines for referrals to a mental health professional.

MENOPAUSE

For women significant biologic and psychologic changes occur in midlife.[69] Menopause is the time when a woman's menstrual cycle ends because of an estrogen deficiency. This deficiency also produces vaginal atrophy and vasomotor instability (hot flushes). With these biologic changes, significant psychosocial events may occur such as changes in her relationship with her children, loss or illness of her parents, and marital instability or widowhood. Menopause has been described as a psychologically difficult time during which women are subject to moodiness, irritability, and depression.[161] In the late nineteenth century psychiatrists Maudsley and Kraeplin both described a clinical syndrome of depression or melancholia that occurred during the climacteric.[142] Kraeplin is credited with coining the phrase "involutional melancholia," which was used to refer to patients who had depression during menopause. These patients were described as having rigid and obsessive personalities and symptoms of agitated depression with hypochondriacal or nihilistic delusions. Involutional melancholia gained validity as a distinct psychiatric entity by its inclusion in the first and second editions of the *Diagnostic and Statistical Manual of Mental Disorders* (DSM).[4] From the gynecologic perspective Kupperman et al included psychiatric symptoms in the description of menopause.[80] Gynecology textbooks included psychologic symptoms in the descriptions of menopause. Although it was a common belief in gynecology and psychiatry that menopause was a time of increased risk for depression, very few empirical studies had investigated this belief. However, in the past 15 years there has been an increase in the study of the biologic and the psychologic aspects of menopause.

From a psychiatric perspective investigators tried to determine if there was a unique menopausal mood disorder. Weissman studied a group of over 400 psychiatric outpatients.[170] The sample was divided into two groups (those under 45 years of age and those 45 years or older) and assessed them for depressive history and current depressive symptoms. There was no difference in the rates of depression between the two groups. Although Weissman used these findings to call into question the existence of involutional melancholia, the classification of subjects into premenopausal (under the age of 45) and menopausal (45 or older) categories based on age alone was a major flaw in this study. Therefore it is unclear whether the two groups were significantly different in terms of their menopausal status. Winokur studied a group of women admitted to a psychiatric hospital and found that there was no greater risk for an episode of depression during the menopause than at other times during a woman's life.[174]

In a study using nonclinical subjects of all ages Neugarten and Kraines found that menopausal and adolescent women had the highest scores on a symptom checklist that assessed psychologic symptoms associated with the menopause.[106] Although women who were menopausal had high symptom scores, women who were postmenopausal had low symptom scores indicating that the symptom increase at the time of the menopause is not longlasting. These studies provided evidence that menopausal women are at no greater risk for depression during menopause than at other times of life. Despite these findings, gynecologists and psychiatrists often see menopausal women who are depressed.

Many attempts have been made to establish a link between menopause and depression. Researchers have hypothesized that depression during the menopause is caused by declining levels of gonadal hormones or is secondary to fatigue and loss of sleep from nocturnal hot flushes.[69,142] Others believe that depressive symptoms during the menopause are a result of stressful life events and of the transitions of aging.[101] To determine if gonadal hormones play a role in menopausal depression, many studies have investigated the impact of hormone replacement therapy on mood among menopausal women. George et al administered conjugated estrogen in a double-blind, crossover trial to thirteen women who had undergone a hysterectomy with bilateral oophorectomy. The estrogen had no effect on the degree of depressive symptoms reported.[45] Strickler et al found similar results in a group of 20 women who were perimenopausal.[160] There were no differences in reported depressive symptoms between women receiving estrogen and a placebo in this double-blind, crossover study. Unfortunately, these two studies did not control for prior level of depression among the subjects or use a standardized depression measure with adequate psychometric reliability and validity.

Schneider et al investigated the effects of four weeks of treatment with conjugated estrogens on depressive symptoms in a group of twenty menopausal women.[143] In their study pretreatment depression levels were assessed by self-report questionnaires and by a clinical interview. Ten subjects were classified as depressed and ten were not depressed. All were treated for 4 weeks with estrogen, then retested. Nine of the ten nondepressed women had a reduction in depression symptom scores. There were no changes in the reported depressive symptomatology for the group of ten depressed women. Coope also investigated the effect of estrogen on menopausal depressive symptoms.[20] In a placebo-controlled study women were randomly assigned to treatment with either estrogen or placebo. The only symptom that estrogen significantly improved was hot flushes. The results of this study are confounded by the use of antidepressants by one quarter of the sample.

Two rigorous studies on the effects of exogenous hormone treatment on menopausal mood symptoms were conducted by Sherwin et al.[146,147] In one study 42 women who had total hysterectomies were divided into four groups and treated with estrogen, androgen, estrogen + androgen, or placebo.[147] In addition, a group of 10 women with intact ovaries served as controls. Treatments were administered for 3 months. During the fourth month, all patients received a placebo and then were crossed over to a different treatment. Plasma levels of estrone, estradiol, and testosterone, and mood symptoms were assessed four times during the study. Results indicated that estrone and estradiol levels were equivalent across treatment groups and as expected the control group had significantly higher levels of estrogen. Also the estrogen + androgen and the androgen alone treatment groups had significantly higher levels of testosterone than the other groups. In terms of the depressive symptomatology, all the subjects were within the normal range of mood symptoms, although posthoc tests indicated that the placebo group had significantly higher depression scores as compared with the other groups. The placebo group's higher depression scores correlated with lower levels of estradiol, estrone, and testosterone. The authors concluded that exogenous estrogen may help maintain higher central levels of serotonin thereby attenuating depression.

Sherwin investigated the use of estrogen + androgen, estrogen alone, or no treatment in a group of 44 women who had complete hysterectomies.[146] Treatment was provided and hormone levels and psychologic symptoms were assessed at monthly intervals. Results indicated a significant correlation between estrogen levels and composure, elation, and clear-headedness for the treatment groups. Women in these treatment groups also reported feeling more elated, energetic, composed, and confident than those receiving placebo.

Studies have investigated the effect of estrogen and progesterone on naturally menopausal women. Siddle et al examined the use of estrogen and progesterone treatment on naturally menopausal women.[149] Each woman received estrogen continuously for the first month then half of the subjects received 20 mg dydrogesterone for the first 12 days of the cycle, for 3 months. The other half of the subjects had 10 mg of dydrogesterone for the first 12 days of the cycle for 3 months. Results indicated no significant differences between the two levels of progesterone treatment on psychologic symptoms. After collapsing the data across the two progesterone groups, no differences were found in psychologic symptoms levels between the estrogen alone and the estrogen and progesterone groups.

A study by Sherwin looked at the effects of combined estrogen and progesterone treatment on menopausal symptoms.[145] Naturally menopausal women were assigned to four treatment groups of conjugated estrogens and medroxyprogesterone or placebo. Hormonal assays and assessment of psychologic symptoms were conducted at regular intervals throughout the study. Women who received estrogen and the higher dose (5 mg) of medroxyprogesterone reported being significantly more dysphoric than women taking estrogen alone. The study also found that regardless of treatment group, women experienced greater sexual desire during weeks 1 and 2 of the treatment month compared to week 4 when no hormones were taken. Mood scores of the women who received both low (0.625 mg) and high (1.25 mg) doses of estrogen did not differ significantly, whereas the mood scores of the women who received low estrogen (0.625 mg) and high progesterone (5 mg) were significantly more dysphoric than those of women receiving a high dose of estrogen (1.25 mg) alone. The author concluded that progesterone has a mood-dampening effect among menopausal women. It was also noted that the changes in mood were not due to changes in the frequency of hot flushes, since all groups reported similar reduction in hot flushes. Other studies investigating the effect of combined estrogen and progesterone treatment of menopausal women indicate that women receiving estrogen and progesterone have more dysphoric moods compared to women taking estrogen alone.[30,65,88]

In addition to hormonal changes, psychologic changes take place during menopause. Dennerstein and Burrows noted nervousness, irritability, depression, and decreased social adaptation among menopausal women.[29] Another factor that may influence the occurrence of psychologic changes associated with menopause is the negative expectations about menopause that are prevalent in our culture. Women dread the changes that they have heard about from others and this may make them more susceptible to those changes. Interestingly, cross-cultural studies have shown that women in other, non-Western cultures do not have significant menopausal difficulty. In fact in some cultures where women's status rises after menopause there is no noted psychologic change in functioning.[28,166,172]

Others have speculated that the loss of the traditional role of mother and childrearer is particularly difficult during the menopause.[32] The "empty nest" problem of loss of role and identity is a popular clinical myth since there is little scientific support for this view. In fact some studies have found that women reported relief and satisfaction after their children had left home.[47,86]

Changes in sexual desire and arousal may impact the menopausal woman's mental health.[7,94,139-141] Sarrel noted that approximately 20% of referrals to a general sexual dysfunction clinic were for sexual functioning problems related to the menopause.[141] Bachmann et al found that 20% of the menopausal sample reported a decrease in sexual desire.[7] McCoy and Davidson found that among 16 women experiencing a natural menopause, both sexual desire and frequency decreased over the menopause and beyond.[94] Overall, four changes have been noted to take place during the menopause. These changes are diminished sexual responsiveness, dyspareunia, decreased sexual frequency and decreased sexual desire.[141] The hormonal, psychologic, and social changes that take place during the menopausal phase of life influence these changes. In terms of physical changes, decreased genital engorgement, delayed reaction time of the clitoris, and decreased vaginal secretions are attributed to the lowered levels of estrogen and its effect on peripheral blood flow.

The clinical management of menopausal women can focus on both physical and psychologic difficulties. First, the specific symptoms and their severity should be documented. An evaluation of the relative risk to relative benefit of hormone replacement therapy is then considered. If the relative benefit outweighs the risk, the initial trial of hormone replacement therapy may help to alleviate the somatic symptoms and in turn may improve psychologic adjustment. Mood symptoms may be directly or indirectly affected by the hormone replacement therapy. If problematic mood symptoms continue after successful initiation of a hormonal therapy regime, psychologic consultation may be considered. Also, assessment of contributory psychosocial problems may be addressed. If indicated, antidepressant therapy may be initiated after hormonal treatment has been established.

SUMMARY

The interface of obstetrics, gynecology and psychiatry presents many challenges to the physician and mental health professional. This chapter has reviewed the research and clinical literature in five areas commonly seen by the obstetrician or gynecologist. The subspeciality of psychosomatic obstetrics and gynecology continues to grow and thereby increases our knowledge of the special health and psychologic needs of women.[156] As a primary care provider, the obstetrician-gynecologist plays an important role in identifying and treating psychosomatic disorders across the reproductive lifespan. Because of the important role in women's health care, obstetrician-gynecologists should be particularly knowledgeable of and sensitive to the emotional needs of their patients. In addition, a good consultative relationship with a psychologist or psychiatrist often provides multidisciplinary treatment of psychosomatic disorders.

Establishing a collaborative relationship between the obstetrician-gynecologist and the psychiatrist or psychologist poses some difficulty especially during the course of a busy day. When a patient is having an acute psychologic crisis, the pressing concern at that time is patient care. There may be no time to discuss philosophy of treatment, training experience, and role boundaries. These, however, are the factors that promote effective collaboration. Instead of trying to develop a consultative relationship in the midst of a patient crisis, ideally an obstetrician-gynecologist can proactively establish one with a colleague in psychology or psychiatry before such an incident occurs. First, a call to the psychology or psychiatry department in the hospital will determine if any of the practitioners specialize in women's mental health care. If there are such providers at the hospital, arrangements may be made to meet with one to discuss both a mutual interest in psychosomatic obstetrics and gynecology and the clinical needs. Treatment issues such as theoretical orientation, training background, specific areas of specialization, treatment modalities, and referral procedures may also be discussed. In general, psychologists or psychiatrists with doctoral (PhD or MD) levels of training have the most extensive background and experience. Psychologists specialize in many modalities of psychotherapy including psychoanalytic, cognitive, behavioral, couple's, and group. They also administer psychologic tests that assess personality and psychologic functioning. A referral to a psychiatrist is necessary if medications are to be used in the psychologic treatment. The most important part of the psychiatric consultative relationship is the ability of the psychologist or psychiatrist to work well with both the patient and the referring physician. In addition to providing therapy, the mental health professional can also be a resource for programs in the community that may be beneficial to the patient, such as psychoeducational groups or support groups for specific disorders. Finally, a discussion of the roles of each provider will clarify that the primary relationship exists between the obstetrician or gynecologist and the patient; and that the mental health professional's role is consultative. In this context the patient should be informed that the providers will be working together and sharing information with one another on an ongoing basis. This reassures the patient that her care is monitored and that all her providers are well informed. The development of a collaborative relationship between the obstetrician-gynecologist and the mental health professional can insure high quality patient care. Since both demands on the physician's time and energy and attention to consumer satisfaction with medical care is increasing, the mental health consultant can be an important addition in the care of the woman patient.

REFERENCES

1. Abbey A, Halman L, Andrews F: Psychosocial, treatment and demographic predictors of the stress associated with infertility, *Fertil Steril* 57:122, 1992.
2. Abraham G: Nutritional factors in the etiology of premenstrual syndromes, *J Reprod Med* 28:446, 1983.
3. Abraham S, Mira M: Psychosocial forces in premenstrual syndrome. In Demers L et al, editors: *Premenstrual, postpartum and menopausal mood disorders*, Baltimore, 1989, Urban & Schwarzenberg.
4. American Psychiatric Association: *Diagnostic and statistical manual of mental disorders*, ed III-R, Washington, DC, 1952, 1968, 1987, American Psychiatric Association.
5. Andersch B, Hahn L: Progesterone treatment of premenstrual tension, *J Psychosom Res* 29:489, 1985.
6. Arrizmendi T, Affonso D: Stressful events related to pregnancy and postpartum, *J Psychosom Res* 31:743, 1987.
7. Bachmann G et al: Correlates of sexual desire in postmenopausal women, *Maturitas* 7:211, 1985.
8. Baram D et al: Psychosocial adjustment following unsuccessful in vitro fertilization, *J Psychosom Obstet Gynecol* 9:181, 1988.
9. Benedek T: Infertility as a psychosomatic defense, *Fertil Steril* 3:527, 1952.
10. Berger D: Psychiatric and psychological aspects of male infertility, *Prog Reprod Biol* 3:157, 1978.
11. Blechman E: Premenstrual syndrome. In Blechman E, Brownell K, editors: *Handbook of behavioral medicine for women*, New York, 1988, Pergamon.

12. Boston Women's Health Book Collective: *The new our bodies, ourselves*, New York, 1992, Touchstone.
13. Brooks-Gunn J: Differentiating premenstrual symptoms and syndromes, *Psychosom Med* 48:385, 1986.
14. Burns L: An overview of the psychology of infertility, *Infertil Reprod Med Clin N Am* 4:433, 1993.
15. Casper R, Powell AM: Premenstrual syndrome: documentation by linear analog scale compared with two descriptive scales, *Am J Obstet Gynecol* 155:862, 1986.
16. Castelnuevo-Tedesco P, Krout B: Psychosomatic aspects of chronic pelvic pain, *Intl J Psychiatr Med* 1:109, 1970.
17. Choung C et al: The MMPI as an aid in evaluating patients with premenstrual syndrome, *Psychosomatics* 29:197, 1988.
18. Choung C et al: Clinical trial of naltrexone in premenstrual syndrome, *Obstet Gynecol* 72:332, 1988.
19. Cohen R: A brief history of the relationship between obstetrics and the mental health professions. In Cohen R, editor: *Psychiatric consultation in childbirth settings*, New York, 1988, Plenum.
20. Coope J: Is oestrogen therapy effective in the treatment of menopausal depression? *J Roy Col Gen Pract* 31:134, 1981.
21. Cooper P et al: Nonpsychotic psychiatric disorders after childbirth: a prospective study of prevalence, incidence, course and nature, *Br J Psychiatr* 152:799, 1988.
22. Coppen A, Eccleston E, Peet M: Total and free tryptophan in unipolar illness, *Lancet* 2:1249, 1976.
23. Cutrona C: Causal attributions and perinatal depression, *J Abnormal Psychol* 92:161, 1983.
24. Dalton K: *The Premenstrual Syndrome*, Springfield, 1964, Charles Thomas.
25. Dalton K: Prospective study into puerperal depression, *Br J Psychiatr* 118:689, 1971.
26. Dalton K: The premenstrual syndrome and progesterone therapy. In *Progesterone therapy*, ed 2, London, 1984, William Heinemann.
27. Daniluk J: Infertility: intrapersonal and interpersonal impact, *Fertil Steril* 49:982, 1988.
28. Davis D: Women's status and experience of the menopause in a Newfoundland fishing village, *Maturitas* 4:207, 1982.
29. Dennerstein L, Burrows G: A review of studies of the psychological symptoms found at menopause, *Maturitas* 1:55, 1978.
30. Dennerstein L et al: Hormone therapy and affect, *Maturitas* 1:247, 1979.
31. Dennerstein L, Lehert P, Riphagen F: Postpartum depression risk factors. *J Psychosom Obstet Gynecol* 10(Suppl):53, 1989.
32. Deutsch H: *The psychology of women*, vol 2, New York, 1945, Grune & Stratton.
33. Dicker R et al: Complications of abdominal and vaginal hysterectomy among women of reproductive age in the United States: the collaborative review of sterilization, *Am J Obstet Gynecol* 144:841, 1982.
34. Eckerd M, Hurt S, Severino S: Late luteal phase dysphoric disorder: relationship to personality disorder, *J Personality Disorders* 3:338, 1989.
35. Edelmann R et al: Psychogenic infertility: some findings, *J Psychosom Obstet Gynecol* 12:163, 1991.
36. Eisner B: Some psychological differences between fertile and infertile women, *J Clin Psychol* 14:391, 1963.
37. Elliot S: Postnatal depression: consequences and intervention. In Demers L et al, editors: *Premenstrual, postpartum and menopausal mood disorders*, Baltimore, 1989, Urban & Schwarzenberg.
38. Fagan P et al: Sexual functioning and psychological evaluation of in vitro fertilization couples, *Fertil Steril* 46:668, 1986.
39. Faludi S: *Backlash: an undeclared war against American women*, New York, 1991, Crown.
40. Frank R: The hormonal cause of premenstrual tension, *Arch Neurol Psychiat* 26:1053, 1931.
41. Freeman E et al: Psychological evaluation and support in a program of in vitro fertilization and embryo transfer, *Fertil Steril* 43:48, 1985.
42. Freeman E et al: Ineffectiveness of progesterone suppository treatment for premenstrual syndrome, *JAMA* 264:349, 1990.
43. Gambone J et al: Validation of hysterectomy indications and the quality assurance process, *Obstet Gynecol* 73:1045, 1989.
44. Gennaro S, Klein A, Miranda L: Health policy dilemmas related to high technology infertility services, *Image: J Nursing Scholarship* 24:191, 1992.
45. George G, Beumont P, Beardwood C: Effect of exogenous oestrogens on minor psychiatric symptoms in postmenopausal women, *S Afr Med J* 47:2387, 1973.
46. Gidro-Frank L et al: Pelvic pain and female identity, *Am J Obstet Gynecol* 79.1184, 1960.
47. Glen N: Psychological well being in the postparental stage, *J Marr Fam* 37:105, 1975.
48. Goodale I, Domar A, Benson H: Alleviation of premenstrual syndrome symptoms with the relaxation response, *Obstet Gynecol* 75:1649, 1990.
49. Gordon R et al: Predicting postnatal emotional adjustment with psychosical and hormonal measures in early pregnancy, *Am J Obstet Gynecol* 155:80, 1986.
50. Gotlib I et al: Prevalence rates and demographic characteristics associated with depression in pregnancy and the postpartum, *J Consult Clin Psychol* 57:269, 1989.
51. Gotlib I, Whiffen V, Wallace P: Prospective investigation of postpartum depression: factors involved in onset and recovery, *J Abnorm Psychol* 100:122, 1991.
52. Gottlieb A: American premenstrual syndrome: a mute voice, *Anthropol Today* 4:10, 1988.
53. Graham C, Sherwin B: A prospective treatment study of premenstrual symptoms using a triphasic oral contraceptive, *J Psychosom Res* 36:257, 1992.
54. Greene R, Dalton K: Premenstrual syndrome, *Br Med J* 1:1007, 1953.
55. Greenfeld D et al: The role of the social worker in the in vitro fertilization program, *Soc Work Health Care* 10:71, 1984.
56. Hair C et al: Premenstrual syndrome in a psychiatric setting. In New Research Abstracts, 143rd Annual Meeting of the American Psychiatric Association, Washington, DC, 1990, APA.
57. Halbriech U, Endicott J: Classification of premenstrual syndromes. In Friedman R, editor, *Behavior and the Menstrual Cycle*, New York, 1982, Marcel Dekker.
58. Halbriech U et al: The diversity of premenstrual changes as reflected in the Premenstrual Assessment Form, *Acta Psychiatr Scand* 65:46, 1982.
59. Hammarback S, Backstrom T: Induced anovulation as treatment of premenstrual tension syndrome: a double-blind, crossover study of LRH agonist versus placebo. Presented at the Second International Symposium on Premenstrual, Postpartum and Menopausal Mood Disorders. Kiawah Island, SC, Sept 9, 1987 (abstract).
60. Handley S et al: Tryptophan, cortisol, and puerperal mood, *Br J Psychiatr* 136:498, 1980.
61. Handley S et al: Mood changes in puerperium and plasma tryptophan and cortisol concentrations, *Br Med J* 2:18, 1977.
62. Harrison W, Endicott J, Nee J: Treatment of premenstrual depression with nortriptyline: a pilot study, *J Clin Psychiatry* 5:136, 1989.
63. Harrison W, Endicott J, Nee J: Treatment of premenstrual dysphoria with alprazolam, *Arch Gen Psychiatry* 47:270, 1990.
64. Hayworth J et al: A predictive study of postpartum depression: some predisposing characteristics, *Br J Med Psychol* 53:161, 1980.
65. Holst J et al: Progestogen addition during oestrogen replacement therapy—effects on vasomotor symptoms and mood, *Maturitas* 11:13, 1989.
66. Hopkins J, Campbell S, Marcus M: Role of infant related stressors in postpartum depression, *J Abnorm Psychol* 96:237, 1987.

67. Hopkins J, Marcus M, Campbell S: Postpartum depression: a critical overview, *Psych Bull* 95:498, 1984.
68. Hurt S et al: Late luteal phase dysphoric disorder in 670 women evaluated for premenstrual complaints, *Am J Psychiat* 149:525, 1992.
69. Hutchinson K: Psychological aspects of menopause, *Infertil Reprod Med Clin N Am* 4:503, 1993.
70. Johnson T: Premenstrual syndrome as a Western culture-specific disorder, *Culture, Med, Psychiatr* 11:337, 1987.
71. Keye W: Psychosocial response to infertility, *Clin Obstet Gynecol* 27:760, 1984.
72. Keye W: General evaluation of premenstrual symptoms, *Clin Obstet Gynecol* 30:396, 1987.
73. Keye W: Management of premenstrual syndrome. In Demers L et al, editors: *Premenstrual, postpartum and menopausal mood disorders*, Baltimore, 1989, Urban & Schwarzenberg.
74. King P et al: Musculoskeletal factors in chronic pelvic pain, *J Psychosom Obstet Gynecol* 12(Suppl):87, 1991.
75. Klock S: Psychological aspects of donor insemination, *Inf Reprod Clin N Am* 4:455, 1993.
76. Klock S, Maier D: Guidelines for the provision of psychological services for infertility patients at the University of Connecticut Health Center, *Fertil Steril* 56:680, 1991.
77. Klock S, Maier D: Psychological aspects of donor insemination, *Fertil Steril* 56:489, 1991.
78. Kresch A et al: Laparoscopy in 100 women with chronic pelvic pain, *Obstet Gynecol* 64:672, 1984 .
79. Kumar R, Robson K: A prospective study of emotional disorders in childbearing women, *Br J Psychiatr* 144:35, 1984.
80. Kupperman H, Wetchler B, Blatt M: Contemporary therapy of the menopausal syndrome, *JAMA* 171:1627, 1959.
81. Lantos J: Second generation ethical issues in the new reproductive technologies. In Stotland N, editor: *Psychiatric aspects of reproductive technology*, Washington, DC, 1990, American Psychiatric Association.
82. Lazarus R, Folkman S: *Stress, appraisal and coping,* New York, 1984, Springer pg 8.
83. Levitan Z et al: The value of laparoscopy in women with chronic pelvic pain and a normal pelvis, *Intl J Gynecol Obstet* 23:71, 1985.
84. Leiblum S, Kemmann E, Lane M: The psychological concomitants of in vitro fertilization, *J Psychosom Obstet Gynecol* 6:165, 1987.
85. Litt M et al: Coping and cognitive factors in adaptation to in vitro fertilization failure, *J Behav Med* 15:171, 1992.
86. Lowenthal M, Thurnher M, Chiriboga D: *Four stages of life,* San Francisco, 1975, Jossey-Bass.
87. Maddocks S et al: A double-blind-placebo controlled trial of progesterone suppositories in the treatment of premenstrual syndrome, *Am J Obstet Gynecol* 154:573, 1986.
88. Magos A et al: The effects of norethisterone in postmenopausal women on estrogen replacement therapy: a model for the premenstrual syndrome, *Br J Obstet Gynecol* 93:1290, 1986.
89. Magos A, Brincat M, Studd J: Trend analysis of the symptoms of 150 women with a history of premenstrual syndrome, *Am J Obstet Gynecol* 155:277, 1986.
90. Mahlstedt P: The psychological component of infertility, *Fertil Steril* 43:335, 1985.
91. Mai F, Munday R, Rump E: Psychosomatic and behavioural mechanisms in psychogenic infertility, *Br J Psychiatr* 120:199, 1972.
92. Mathis J: Psychiatry and the obstetrician-gynecologist, *Med Clin N Amer* 51:1375, 1967.
93. Maxson W: The use of progesterone in the treatment of premenstrual syndrome, *Clin Obstet Gynecol* 30:465, 1987.
94. McCoy N, Davidson J: A longitudinal study of the effects of menopause on sexuality, *Maturitas* 7:203, 1985.
95. Menkes D et al: Fluoxetine treatment of severe premenstrual syndrome, *Br Med J* 305:346, 1992.
96. Menning B: Psychosocial impact of infertility, *Nurs Clin NAm* 17:155, 1982.
97. Moller A, Fallstrom K: Psychological consequences of infertility: a longitudinal study, *J Psychosom Obstet Gynecol* 12:27, 1991.
98. Moller A, Fallstrom K: Psychological factors in the etiology of infertility: a longitudinal study, *J Psychosom Obstet Gynecol* 12:13, 1991.
99. Moos R: The development of a menstrual distress questionnaire, *Psychosom Med* 30:853, 1968.
100. Morse C: A critical review of methodological issues and approaches to managing premenstrual syndrome, *J Psychsom Obstet Gynecol* 12:133, 1991.
101. Morse C, Dennerstein L: Psychosocial aspects of the climacteric. In Demers L et al, editors: *Premenstrual, postpartum and menopausal mood disorders*, Baltimore, 1989, Urban & Schwarzenberg.
102. Mosher W, Pratt W: Fecundity and infertility in the United States, 1965-1988, *Advance Data* 192:1, 1990.
103. Murray L: Effects of postnatal depression on infant development. In Kumar R, Brockington I, editors: *Motherhood and mental illness,* vol 2, London, 1988, John Wright.
104. Muse K et al: The premenstrual syndrome: effects of medical ovariectomy, *N Engl J Med* 311:345, 1984
105. National Center for Health Statistics: Reproductive impairments among married couples: United States Vital and Health Statistics, Public Health Service, Washington, DC, 1982, US Government Printing Office.
106. Neugarten B, Kraines F: Menopausal symptoms in women of various ages, *Psychosom Med* 27:266, 1965.
107. Newton C, Hearn M, Yuzpe A: Psychological assessment and follow-up after in vitro fertilization: assessing the impact of failure, *Fertil Steril* 54:879, 1990.
108. Nott P et al: Hormonal changes and mood in the puerperium, *Br J Psychiatr* 128:379, 1976.
109. O'Hara M: Social support, life events, and depression during pregnancy and the puerperium, *Arch Gen Psychiatr* 43:569, 1986.
110. O'Hara M: Psychologic and biologic factors in postpartum depression. In Demers L et al, editors: *Premenstrual, postpartum and menopausal mood disorders*, Baltimore, 1989, Urban Schwarzenberg.
111. O'Hara M: Postpartum mood disorders: an overview. Paper presented at the Psychiatric Disorders Associated with Female Reproductive Function Course, Massachusetts General Hospital/Harvard Medical School, June 12, 1993, Boston, MA.
112. O'Hara M, Neunaber D, Zekoski E: Prospective study of postpartum depression: prevalence, course and predictive factors, *J Abnormal Psychol* 93:158, 1984.
113. O'Hara M, Rehm L, Campbell S: Postpartum depression: a role for social network and life stress variables, *J Nerv Ment Dis* 171:336, 1983.
114. O'Hara M, Rehm L, Campbell S: Predicting depressive symptomatology: cognitive behavioral models and postpartum depression, *J Abnorm Psychol* 91:457, 1983.
115. O'Hara M et al: Controlled prospective study of postpartum mood disorders: psychological, environmental, and hormonal variables, *J Abnorm Psychol* 100:63, 1991.
116. O'Hara M et al: Controlled prospective study of postpartum mood disorders: comparisons of childbearing and nonchildbearing women, *J Abnorm Psychol* 99:3, 1990.
117. Paige K: The effects of oral contraceptives on affective fluctuations associated with the menstrual cycle, *Psychosom Med* 33:515, 1971.
118. Powell S, Drotar D: Postpartum depressed mood: the impact of daily hassles, *J Psychosom Obstet Gynecol* 13:255, 1992.
119. Prior J et al: Conditioning exercise decreases premenstrual symptoms: a prospective, controlled 6 month trial, *Fertil Steril* 47:402, 1987.
120. Rapkin A: Adhesions and pelvic pain: a retrospective study, *Obstet Gynecol* 68:13, 1986.
121. Rapkin A, Kames L: The pain management approach to chronic pelvic pain, *J Reprod Med* 32:323, 1987.

122. Rapkin A et al: History of physical and sexual abuse in women with chronic pelvic pain, *Obstet Gynecol* 76:92, 1990.
123. Rapkin A, Reading A: Chronic pelvic pain, *Curr Probl Obstet Gynecol Fertil,* July/August 4:101, 1991.
124. Reading A: Cognitive model of premenstrual syndrome, *Clin Obstet Gynecol* 35:693, 1992.
125. Reading A: Sexual aspects of infertility and its treatment, *Inf Reprod Med Clin N Am* 4:559, 1993.
126. Reid R: Premenstrual syndrome, *Current Prob Obstet Gynecol* 8:1, 1985.
127. Reid R: Premenstrual syndrome, *Endocrinol Metab* 5:1, 1987.
128. Reid R, Yen S: Premenstrual syndrome, *Am J Obstet Gynecol* 139:85, 1981.
129. Reiter R, Gambone J: Demographic and historic variables in women with idiopathic chronic pelvic pain, *Obstet Gynecol* 75:428, 1990.
130. Riley G, Shaw D: Total and nonbound tryptophan in unipolar illness, *Lancet* 2:1249, 1976.
131. Rivera-Tovar A, Frank E: Late luteal phase dysphoric disorder in young women, *Am J Psychiat* 147:1634, 1990.
132. Robson K, Kumar R: Delayed onset of maternal affection after childbirth, *Br J Psychiatr* 136:347, 1980.
133. Rodin M: The social construction of premenstrual syndrome, *Soc Sci Med* 35:693, 1992.
134. Rosenthal R et al: Chronic pelvic pain: psychological features and laparoscopic findings, *Psychosom* 25:833, 1984.
135. Rubinow D, Roy-Byrne P: Premenstrual syndromes: overview from a methodologic perspective, *Am J Psychiatr* 141:163, 1984.
136. Ruble D: Premenstrual symptoms: a reinterpretation, *Science* 197:291, 1977.
137. Sampson G: Premenstrual syndrome: a double-blind controlled trial of progesterone and placebo, *Br J Psychiatry* 135:209, 1979.
138. Sandler S: Emotional stress and infertility, *J Psychosom Res* 12:51, 1968.
139. Sarrel P: Sex problems after menopause: a study of fifty married couples treated in a sex counseling programme, *Maturitas* 4:231, 1982.
140. Sarrel P, Whitehead M: Sex and menopause: defining the issues, *Maturitas* 7:217, 1985.
141. Sarrel P: Sexuality and menopause, *Obstet Gynecol* 75(Suppl):26, 1990.
142. Schmidt P, Rubinow D: Menopausal mood disorders. In Demers L et al, editors: *Premenstrual, postpartum and menopausal mood disorders*, Baltimore, 1989, Urban & Schwarzenberg.
143. Schneider M, Brotherton P, Hailes J: The effects of exogenous oestrogens on depression in menopausal women, *Med J Austral* 2:162, 1977.
144. Shatford L et al: Psychological correlates of dysfunctional infertility diagnosis in an in vitro fertilization program, *Am J Obstet Gynecol* 158, 1099, 1988.
145. Sherwin B: The impact of different doses of estrogen and progestin on mood and sexual behavior in postmenopausal women, *J Clin Endocrin Metab* 72:336, 1991.
146. Sherwin B: Affective changes with estrogen and androgen replacement therapy in surgically menopausal women, *J Affect Dis* 14:177, 1988.
147. Sherwin B, Gelfand M: Sex steroids and affect in the surgical menopause: a double-blind, cross-over study, *Psychoneuroendocrinol* 10:325, 1984.
148. Sichel D: Psychiatric issues of the postpartum period, *Currents in Affect Illness* 11: 5: 1992.
149. Siddle N et al: Endometrial, physical, and psychological effects of postmenopausal oestrogen therapy with added dydrogesterone, *Br J Obstet Gynecol* 97:1101, 1990.
150. Smith S, Schiff I: The premenstrual syndrome—diagnosis and management, *Fertil Steril* 52:527, 1989.
151. Spitzer R et al: Late luteal phase dysphoric disorder and DSM III-R, *Am J Psychiat* 146:892, 1989.
152. Steege J: Symptom measurement in premenstrual syndrome. In Demers L et al, editors: *Premenstrual, postpartum and menopausal mood disorders*, Baltimore, 1989, Urban & Schwarzenberg.
153. Steege J, Blumenthal J: The effects of aerobic exercise on premenstrual symptoms in middle aged women, *J Psychosom Res* 37:127, 1993.
154. Steege J, Stout A, Somkuti S: Chronic pelvic pain: toward an integrative model, *J Psychosom Obstet Gynecol* 12 (Suppl):3, 1991.
155. Stein G et al: Relationship between mood disturbances and free and total plasma tryptophan, cortisol, and puerperal mood, *Br Med J* 2:457, 1976.
156. Stewart D, Stotland N: The interface between psychiatry and obstetrics-gynecology: an introduction. In Stewart D, Stotland N, editors: *Psychological aspects of women's health care*. Washington, DC, 1993, American Psychiatric Association Press.
157. Stone A, Pearlstein T, Brown W: Fluoxetine in the treatment of late luteal phasedysphoric disorder, *J Clin Psychiatr* 52:290, 1991.
158. Stout A, Steege J: Psychosocial and behavioral self reports of chronic pelvic pain patient. Paper presented at the meeting of the American Society of Psychosomatic Obstetrics and Gynecology, Houston, TX, March, 1991.
159. Strauss B, Appelt H, Ulrich D: Relationship between psychological characteristics and treatment outcome in female patients from an infertility clinic, *J Psychosom Obstet Gynecol* 13:121, 1992.
160. Strickland B: Menopause. In Blechman E, Brownell K, editors: *Handbook of behavioral medicine for women*, New York, 1988, Pergamon.
161. Strickler R et al: The role of oestrogen replacement in the climacteric syndrome, *Psychol Med* 7:631, 1977.
162. Summitt R, Ling F: Urethral syndrome presenting as chronic pelvic pain, *J Psychosom Obstet Gynecol* 12(Suppl):77, 1991.
163. Takefman J et al: Sexual and emotional adjustment of couples undergoing infertility investigation and the effectiveness of preparatory information, *J Psychosom Obstet Gynecol* 11:275, 1990.
164. Treadway R et al: A psychoendocrine study of pregnancy and puerperium, *Am J Psychiatr* 125:86, 1969.
165. Valda J, Youdale M, Freeman R: Premenstrual assessment form typological categories: classification of self-defined premenstrually symptomatic and asymptomatic women, *J Consult Clin Psychol* 55:418, 1987.
166. Van Keep P, Kellerhals J: The impact of socio-cultural factors on symptom formation, *Psychother Psychosom* 23:251, 1974.
167. Veevers J: *Childless by Choice*, Toronto, 1980, Butterworth.
168. Walker E et al: Relationship of chronic pelvic pain to psychiatric diagnoses and childhood sexual abuse, *Am J Psychiatr* 145:75, 1988.
169. Watson J et al: Psychiatric disorders in pregnancy and the first postnatal year, *Br J Psychiatr* 144:453, 1984.
170. Weissman M: The myth of involutional melancholia, *JAMA* 242:742, 1979.
171. Whiffen V: Vulnerability to postpartum depression: a prospective multivariate study, *J Abnormal Psychol* 97:467, 1988.
172. Wilbush J: Climacteric expression and social context, *Maturitas* 4:195, 1982.
173. Williams J: *Psychology of Women,* ed 2, New York, 1983, WW Norton.
174. Winokur G: Depression in the menopause, *Am J Psychiatr* 130:92, 1973.
175. Wood D, Wiesner M, Reiter R: Psychogenic chronic pelvic pain: diagnosis and management, *Clin Obstet Gynecol* 33:179, 1990.
176. Wood S et al: Treatment of premenstrual syndrome with fluoxetine: a double-blind, placebo-controlled, crossover study, *Obstet Gynecol* 80:339, 1992.

Chapter 18

UROGYNECOLOGY

Joan M. Bengtson
Eboo Versi

Urogynecology covers all aspects of lower urinary tract functions that fall reasonably within the domain of gynecology. As many patients with lower urinary tract dysfunction also have a concomitant gynecological problem, this subject is of concern for the gynecologist. Obviously there are going to be situations where the interface between urology and gynecology becomes blurred. In such cases surgeons from both specialties need to collaborate. Though urogynecology also includes the management of prolapse, this has been covered in Chapter 5 and will not be discussed here.

EMBRYOLOGY

Kidneys and ureters

The kidneys and ureters are formed through a three-stage process that recapitulates development of the excretory system in primitive vertebrates. During the third week of embryonic life, the mesoderm forming the nephrogenic cord along the dorsal body wall gives rise to several pairs of tubules, the pronephros. This system is transient and nonfunctioning in the human.[15] Formation and degeneration of the pronephros proceeds in a cranial to caudal sequence and is complete by the end of the fourth week. The only persistent component of this system is the pronephric duct. Initially it comprises the union of the pronephric tubules, but as they degenerate the duct continues to grow caudally to join the cloaca during the fifth week. Subsequently, it is retained as the mesonephric duct.

The second primitive kidney, the mesonephros, develops within the nephrogenic cord caudal to the pronephros, beginning in the fourth week. The tubules begin as blind vesicles that grow to join the mesonephric duct laterally. Medially each tubule forms a Bowman's capsule and associates with a vascular glomerulus. The mesonephros probably functions to produce urine in the human fetus during the third and fourth months.[18] In the female the entire system degenerates, leaving only vestigial remnants. The persistent tubules may be identified in the mesovarium of the adult as the epoophoron and paroophoron, while the mesonephric duct becomes Gartner's duct within the broad ligament and lateral paravaginal tissues. In the male the mesonephros also degenerates but the duct persists and, under the influence of androgens, develops into the male genital duct system.

The third and permanent kidney, the metanephros, arises from the metanephric mesenchyme, the most caudal portion of the mesodermal nephrogenic cord. Its collecting system, the ureter, develops as an outbudding of the mesonephric duct. The ureteric bud arises from the caudal end of the mesonephric duct (Fig. 18-1). It grows cranially, pushing into the metanephric mesenchyme and induces this tissue to differentiate into permanent nephrons.[32] Factors originating in the metanephric mesenchyme then induce a series of dichotomous subdivisions in the cranial portion of the ureter that ultimately form the calyceal collecting system. The distal portion elongates to form the permanent ureter. Apparent ascent and medial rotation of the metanephros to its permanent position occur as a result of rapid growth of the caudal structures of the embryo over the ensuing weeks. The metanephros produces urine by the fourth month of fetal life. Fetal urine is a major component of amniotic fluid.

Bladder and urethra

The bladder and urethra are mainly derived from endodermal tissue. The expanded distal portion of the hindgut, the cloaca, is divided by the urorectal fold into the anterior urogenital sinus and the posterior rectum during the fourth week.[82] The urogenital sinus is further divided into the vesicourethral canal that forms the bladder and upper urethra, and the definitive urogenital sinus that forms most of

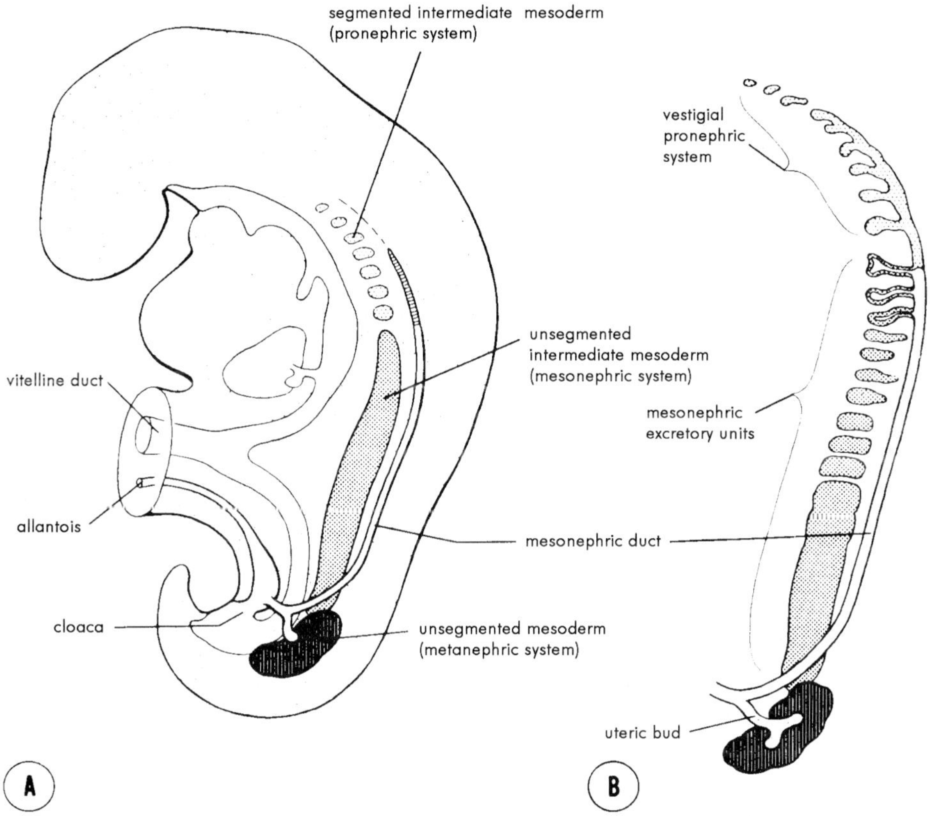

Fig. 18-1. A, Schematic diagram showing the relation of the intermediate mesoderm of the pronephric, mesonephric and metanephric systems. In the cervical and upper thoracic regions, the intermediate mesoderm is segmented, in the lower thoracic, lumbar, and sacral regions, it forms a solid, unsegmented mass of tissue, the nephrogenic cord. Note the longitudinal collecting duct, initially formed by the pronephros but later taken over by the mesonephros. **B**, Schematic representation of the excretory tubules of the pronephric and mesonephric systems in a 5-week-old embryo. The ureteric bud penetrates the metanephric tissue. Note the remnant of the pronephric excretory tubules and longitudinal collecting duct.

the urethra, the paraurethral glands, and the vestibule. Within the base of the bladder is a specialized structure, the trigone, which derives partly from mesoderm. The urorectal fold becomes the perineal body that separates the vestibule and the rectum.[16]

The vesicourethral canal receives the allantois cranially. By the fourth month of fetal life, attenuation and elongation of the allantois results in formation of a ligamentous structure, the urachus. It runs from the bladder dome to the umbilicus. The urachus persists in adult life as the median umbilical ligament of the anterior abdominal wall.

Bilaterally the vesicourethral canal receives the orifices of the mesonephric ducts. The metanephric duct (the ureter) arises as an outgrowth of the mesonephric duct just cranial to this junction. However, differential growth of the ducts results in the establishment of an independent orifice between the metanephric duct and the developing bladder (Fig. 18-2). The mesonephric duct orifice becomes displaced distally and opens into the upper urethra. In the female most of the mesonephric duct undergoes degeneration. The terminal portion ultimately becomes incorporated into the bladder wall and gives rise to a part of the trigone and posterior upper urethra.[77] Thus this segment of the bladder is of mesodermal origin.

Distally the vesicourethral canal elongates and contributes to the formation of the upper anterior urethra. Most of the urethra, however, derives from the urogenital sinus. Paraurethral glands (Skene's glands) arise as outgrowths of the urethral mucosa and are probably homologues of the male prostate gland.[38] The posterior segment of the urogenital sinus further differentiates into the vestibule and the distal vagina.

ANATOMY

Ureters

The ureters are bilateral tubes that function as conduits to convey urine from the kidneys to the urinary bladder. Each ureter is 30 to 34 cm long and 6 to 10 mm in diameter and retroperitoneal throughout its course from the renal pelvis to the bladder. Each ureter has an abdominal portion and a pelvic

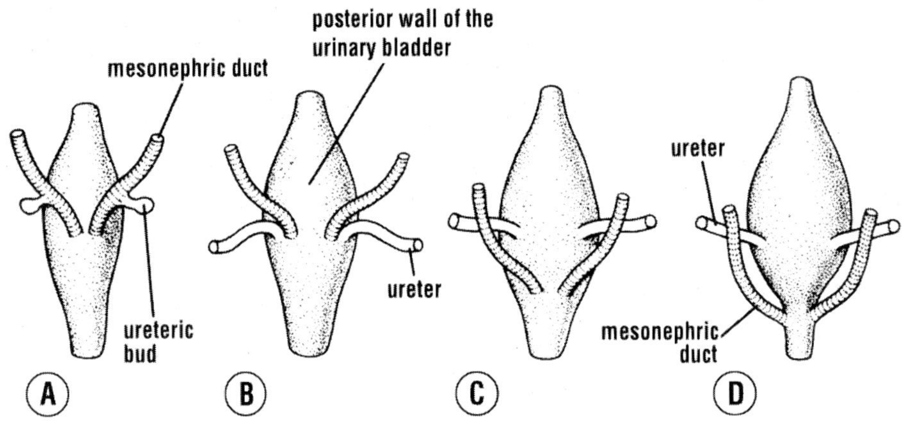

Fig. 18-2. Schematic drawings to show the relationship of the ureters and mesonephric ducts during development. Initially the ureter is formed by an outgrowth of the mesonephric duct, but with time it obtains a separate entrance into the urinary bladder. (From Sadler TW: *Langman's medical embryology*, ed 5, Baltimore, 1985, Williams & Wilkins.)

portion. The abdominal portion comprises the superior 15 cm and runs caudally anterior to the psoas muscle, crossing the genitofemoral nerve. The right ureter is crossed by the duodenum, the right colic and ileocolic vessels, and the terminal ileum. The left is crossed by the left colic vessels and the sigmoid mesentery and vessels.

The pelvic ureter begins near the sacroiliac articulation at the linea terminalis of the iliac bone. As it descends into the true pelvis along the lateral wall, it is crossed by the ovarian vessels coursing within the infundibulopelvic ligament. It crosses the common iliac artery near its bifurcation to lie medial to the visceral branches of the anterior division of the internal iliac artery. As the ureter continues its course into the pelvis, it travels along the superior surface of the levator ani muscle in the cardinal ligament, the most inferior portion of the broad ligament. In this location it is surrounded by the extensive venous plexus of the uterus and crossed superiorly by the uterine artery at approximately the level of the internal cervical os, 1 to 1.5 cm lateral to the cervix.[36] Each ureter then turns medially, coursing closely to the anterior vaginal fornix to enter the base of the bladder. The interstitial portion of the ureter is approximately 1 cm in length and traverses an oblique course anteromedial to open via a slit like orifice at the bladder trigone.[97]

Bladder

The bladder is a highly distensible, hollow organ that changes shape and its superior relations as it fills with urine. The superior segment or dome of the bladder consists of the detrusor muscle. Its surface is covered with visceral peritoneum that reflects onto the bladder from the anterior abdominal wall and off the bladder into the vesicouterine pouch. The inferior surfaces are not covered by peritoneum. Anteriorly the bladder is separated from the pubic bone by a potential retroperitoneal space called the space of Retzius. Posteriorly it is related to the anterior surface of the uterine cervix and anterior fornix of the vagina.

The trigone is a specialized area at the base of the bladder that represents the continuation of the muscular layer of the ureters as they are incorporated into the bladder wall.[97] It is a triangular area delineated by the ureteral orifices, the interureteric ridge forming the base, and the internal urethral meatus at the apex (Fig. 18-3). The ureteral orifices are about 3 cm apart. The trigone forms a relatively fixed, unyielding segment of the bladder and is important in supporting the outlet during storage of urine and in coordinating the funneling effect necessary for efficient emptying of the bladder.[77]

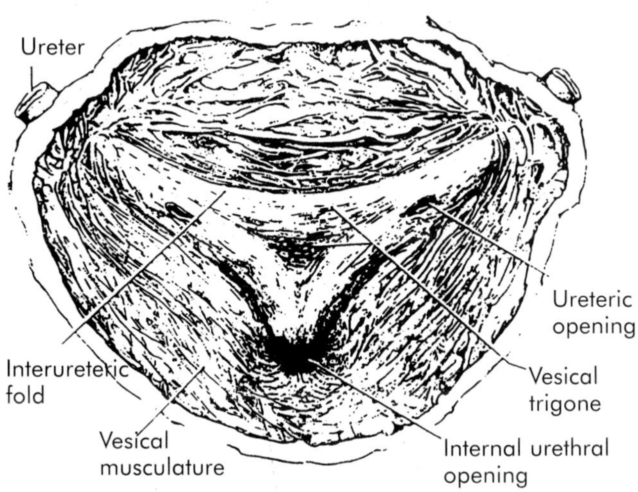

Fig. 18-3. View of the bladder trigone showing ureteral orifices and internal urethral meatus. (From Woodburne RT, *J Urol* 100:478, 1968 ©American Urological Association, Inc.)

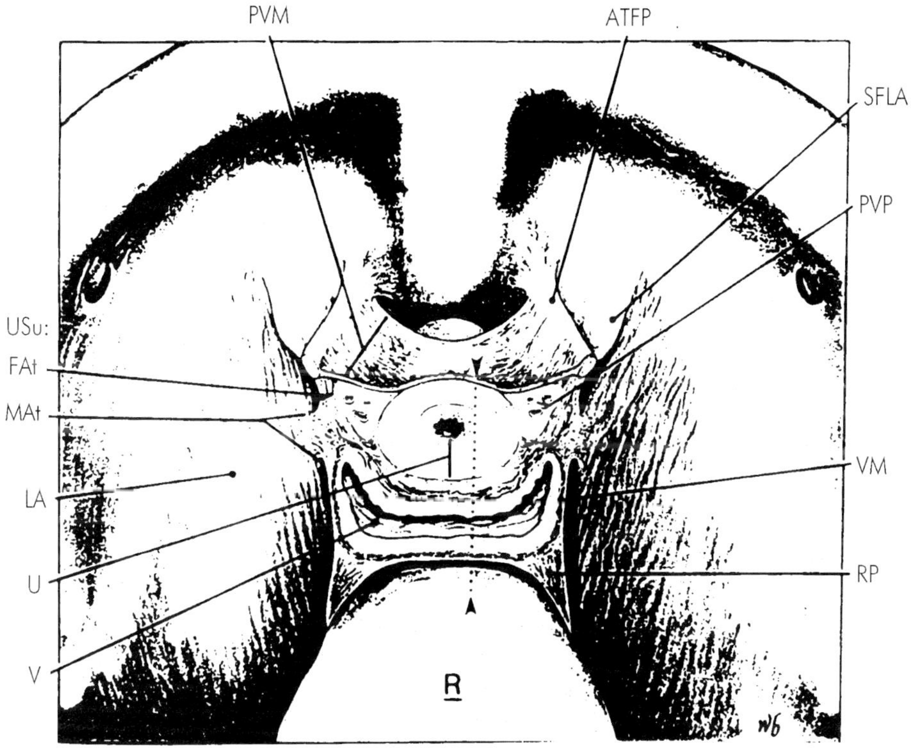

Fig. 18-4. Cross-section of the urethra (U), vagina (V), arcus tendineus fasciae pelvis (ATFP), and superior fascia of levator ani (SFLA) just below the vesical neck (drawn from cadaver dissection). The pubovesical muscles (PVM) lie anterior to the urethra, and anterior and superior to the paraurethral vascular plexus (PVP). The urethral supports (USu) (the pubo-urethral ligaments) attach the vagina and vaginal surface of the urethra to the levator ani muscles (MAt, muscular attachment) and to the superior fascia of the levator ani (FAt, fascial attachment). R, rectum; RP, rectal pillar; VM, vaginal wall muscularis; LA, levator ani. (Dotted line indicated plane of section not shown in this Chapter). (From DeLancey JOL, *Clin Obstet Gynecol*, 33:300, 1990.)

Urethra

The female urethra is approximately 4 cm long. It runs from the bladder base to the vestibule and is positioned behind the pubic symphysis anterior to the vagina. The external urethral meatus forms a slit like orifice in the vestibule about 2 cm posterior to the clitoris. The paraurethral glands of Skene are inconstant, but usually open into the posterior urethra just within the meatus.

The urethral supports are important features of the continence mechanism. The urethra is connected laterally to the fixed bony structure of the pelvis by fascial fibers inserting into the periurethral tissues. They arise from both the levator ani muscle (muscular attachments) and its superior fascia (fascial attachments) (Fig. 18-4). The pubovesical muscle and ligament connect the anterior aspect of the urethra to the posterior aspect of the pubic bone. This muscle may assist in voiding by actively opening the bladder neck at the initiation of micturition.

HISTOLOGY

The histologic structure of the urinary tract from the renal calyces to the urethra is consistent and varies only by an increase in thickness. It is well suited to the functions of storage and propulsion of urine. Three component layers are identified—mucosa, muscularis, and adventitia.[39]

The mucosal lining is transitional epithelium, three to five cells thick in the ureters and up to eight cells thick in the bladder. In the contracted state the epithelium is compact and the cells are round. As the viscus distends to accommodate stored urine, the epithelium becomes thin and the individual cells flatten parallel to the surface. There is no discernible basement membrane. The lamina propria is composed of collagenous and elastic fibers. The distal urethra is lined by nonkeratinizing stratified squamous epithelium. Like vaginal mucosa, it is estrogen sensitive, which is consistent with their common embryologic derivation from the urogenital sinus.[19]

The muscularis is comprised of an inner longitudinal and an outer circular layer with an additional outer longitudinal layer beginning in the distal ureter and continuing in the bladder. The layered arrangement is less discrete in the urinary tract compared with the gastrointestinal tract. This results in a more interlaced, anastomosing pattern in the bladder. The inner longitudinal layer of each ureter flattens out as it enters the bladder to form the sheet like trigone. This layer continues downward into the proximal urethra as well.

The muscularis is surrounded by a fibroelastic adventitia. At the bladder dome this layer provides loose attachments to accommodate the mobility necessary in physiologic filling and emptying. In the periurethral area an extensive vascular plexus courses in the adventitia. When the vessels are engorged they may contribute to urethral closure pressure by creating forces of extrinsic compression.[69]

The bladder outlet lacks a discrete circumferential sphincter, yet several elements participate in this function. In the bladder neck, elastin fibers comprise a passive mechanism that maintains closure at rest.[31,92] In the urethra four components contribute to the sphincter mechanism—smooth muscle, striated muscle, the epithelium, and connective tissue. The outer circular layer of the detrusor muscle is continuous with the urethra and may contribute to the smooth muscle sphincter. However, this layer is poorly developed in females and its contribution to urethral closure is doubted since the detrusor and sphincter muscles function reciprocally.[19] Smooth muscle extending from the trigone into the urethra probably constitutes an intramural sphincter. The urethra also contains the striated urogenital sphincter located from approximately 20% to 80% of total urethral length (Fig. 18-5). It is composed primarily of slow twitch muscle fibers capable of maintaining prolonged basal tone.[30] Additional voluntary sphincter function is provided by decussating striated muscle fibers of the compressor urethrae and the urethrovaginal sphincter muscle of the urogenital diaphragm.[63] The epithelium forms the ultimate watertight closure of the urethral valve. It must be supple and moist to achieve a hermetic seal. Finally abundant collagen and elastin fibers intrinsic to the urethral wall add an additional passive mechanism contributing to closure.

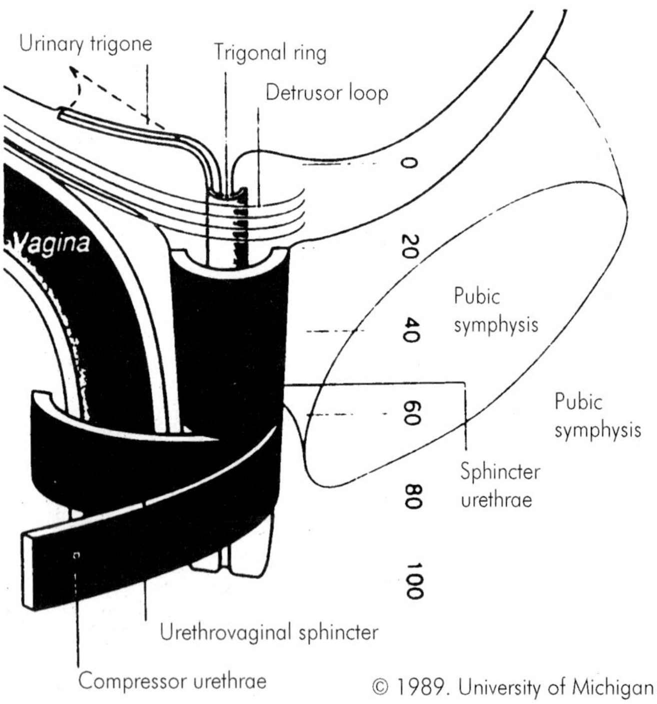

Fig. 18-5. Diagrammatic representation of the components of the internal and external urethral sphincters. (From DeLancey JOL: *Clin Obstet Gynecol*, 33:302, 1990.)

PHYSIOLOGY AND PHARMACOLOGY

Physiology of micturition

The lower urinary tract stores urine until conditions are appropriate to completely expel bladder contents. Its functions are controlled by a complex neurologic system involving both central and peripheral components. In infancy micturition occurs as a reflex and is involuntary. However, with maturation of the cerebral descending pathways, it is brought under voluntary control.

The two components of the lower urinary tract must function reciprocally to accomplish the opposing functions of storing and emptying urine. During storage the detrusor muscle remains relaxed to accommodate increasing urine volumes while the sphincter is contracted to maintain continence. During emptying, the pelvic floor and urethral sphincter relax to provide a low resistance conduit through which the urine passes as the detrusor contracts to expel the bladder contents.

The bladder wall is innervated by sensory fibers that carry sensations of pain, temperature, and proprioception (stretch) to the spinal cord.[8] They synapse in the sacral spinal cord micturition center with efferent motor nerves that return to the bladder to complete a reflex arc. The motor neurons supplying the detrusor muscle originate in the sacral spinal segments S2 to S4. In addition the afferent nerves synapse with other neurons that transmit information about bladder sensation up the cord to the brain stem and cerebral cortex, where other centers coordinating micturition activity are located.

The activity of the efferent neurons controlling detrusor function is modulated by input from bladder afferent nerves as well as from signals originating in the brain stem and the frontal lobe. The basic micturition reflex consists of a detrusor contraction in response to the stretch of bladder filling. Input from higher centers on this reflex is primarily suppressive. Toilet training is a learned response that allows the inhibition of detrusor activity until a socially appropriate time for emptying occurs. Thus the micturition reflex is brought under a degree of voluntary control.

After appropriately integrating the information from the bladder with that from higher centers, the sacral micturition center sends signals to both the detrusor and the urethral sphincter to initiate a coordinated micturition event. Three characteristics of the event are notable. First, the actions of the detrusor and the sphincter must be coordinated so that the bladder empties through an open outlet. This avoids the need to generate excessive intravesical pressures that might create ureteral reflux. Second, the detrusor contraction must be sustained until the entire contents are expelled to avoid residual urine retention in the bladder. Finally, when the bladder is empty, the bladder and sphincter must return to the basal states that promote urine storage.

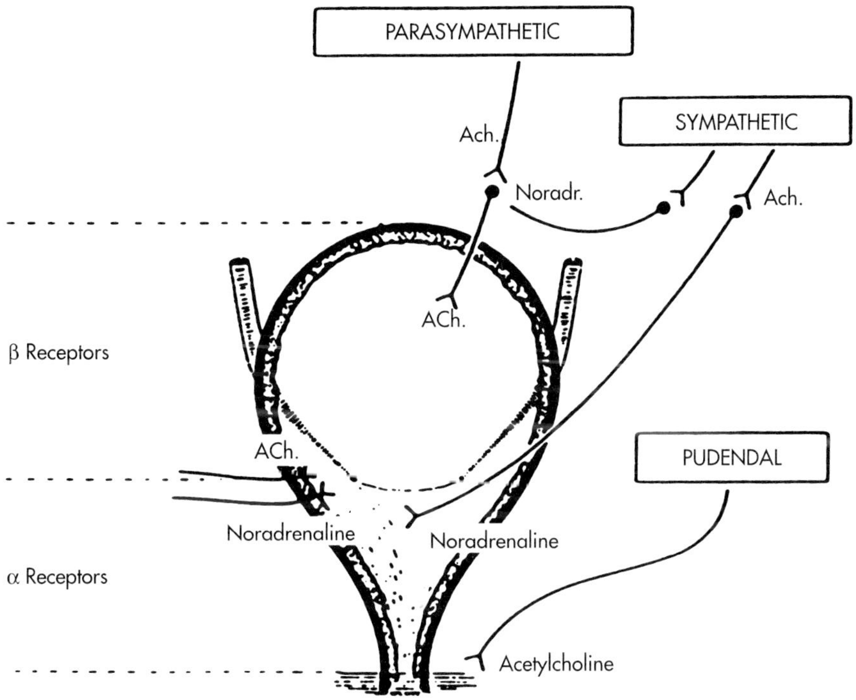

Fig. 18-6. Autonomic innervation of the detrusor muscle and urethral sphincter. (From vanGeelen H, *Internatl Urogynecol J* 1:20, 1990.)

The detrusor motor neurons reach the bladder via the pelvic nerve. They are parasympathetic and thus form ganglionic synapses within the wall of the bladder. Postganglionic neurons then carry information to the smooth muscle cells of the detrusor. Release of the neurotransmitter acetylcholine stimulates a detrusor contraction. The role of the sympathetic nervous system in the control of bladder function is less well established for humans.[31] Preganglionic fibers from the thoracolumbar spinal segments synapse in chain ganglia with postganglionic fibers that travel in the hypogastric nerve to the bladder and sphincter. Sympathetic effects are mediated through alpha and beta receptors. Beta receptors are predominant in the detrusor and stimulation of these is thought to cause inhibition of detrusor contractility. Alpha receptors are abundant in the sphincter region and stimulation causes contraction of these muscle fibers. Thus a picture emerges of autonomic influence on bladder function such that parasympathetic activation initiates bladder emptying while sympathetic activation relaxes the detrusor and stimulates the sphincter to promote the storage function of the bladder (Fig. 18-6).

Despite intense investigative efforts, the mechanism of continence remains incompletely understood. From a simplified point of view, continence is maintained during the bladder storage phase because intraurethral pressure exceeds intravesical pressure at all times. Intravesical pressure remains low during filling due to the relaxed state and high compliance of the detrusor muscle. This allows the bladder to accommodate increasing volumes of urine with only a minimal increase in intravesical pressure. Intraurethral pressure remains high because of a combination of intrinsic and extrinsic factors that contribute to a sphincter-like effect.[39] The intrinsic features of the urethra that determine intraurethral pressure include the following: (1) sympathetically mediated contraction of the smooth muscles of the internal sphincter, (2) contraction of the striated muscles of the external sphincter, (3) tissue turgor resulting from blood flow in the paraurethral vascular bed, and (4) the mucosal seal resulting from the elastic properties of the urethral wall.

Extrinsic structures that support the urethra and bladder comprise an extremely important aspect of the continence mechanism. This is especially true during episodes of increased ambient intraabdominal pressure such as sudden valsalva, coughing, and sneezing. An increase in intraabdominal pressure is transmitted across the wall of the bladder and increases intravesical pressure. As long as the proximal urethra is properly supported and stabilized between the pubic bone and the anterior vaginal wall, the pressure increase is likewise transmitted across its wall and compresses the lumen closed and raises intraurethral pressure to a comparable degree. The pressure relationship between the bladder and urethra is unchanged and continence is maintained. If the supports are damaged and the urethra is allowed excessive downward mobility during stress, adequate compression of the urethra will not occur, and if intravesical pressure increases sufficiently, leakage will result.

Pharmacology of the lower urinary tract

An understanding of the neurophysiology of the lower urinary tract has allowed the application of various pharmacologic agents to the treatment of urinary tract disorders.[20] Drugs that facilitate urine storage are helpful in treating incontinence. They may work either by promoting detrusor relaxation or sphincter contraction. Detrusor relaxation may be induced with anticholinergic agents, direct smooth muscle relaxers, calcium channel blockers, beta receptor agonists, prostaglandin inhibitors, and tricyclic antidepressants. Clinically the most effective are oxybutynin, propantheline, and imipramine.[81] Drugs that promote sphincter closure include alpha agonists, beta antagonists, and possibly estrogen. The mechanism of the beneficial effect of estrogen is thought to be increased blood flow to the paravaginal tissues, increased pliability of the mucosal lining, and increased responsiveness of the smooth muscle to adrenergic stimulation.

Pharmacologic treatment of the disorders of bladder emptying employs drugs with opposite actions on the bladder and sphincter. Drugs that enhance detrusor contractility include parasympathomimetics, choline esterase inhibitors, and beta antagonists. Agents that decrease sphincter closure include alpha-antagonists, beta-agonists, and skeletal muscle relaxants.

MALFORMATIONS

The genital and urinary tracts develop in close association. In the female, normal development of the mesonephric system precedes and is partly responsible for inducing normal development of the müllerian ducts. Following fusion of the caudal ends of the müllerian ducts, the downward growth of the müllerian tubercle separates the urogenital sinus into its urinary and vaginal components. A consequence of this interdependence is that abnormalities in one system are commonly associated with abnormalities in the other.

Some important lower urinary tract malformations become manifest during infancy or childhood and thus are diagnosed by the pediatrician. Others may remain silent into adulthood and are only detected coincidentally as a result of an unrelated imaging study or surgical procedure. Urinary tract malformations of special importance to the gynecologist include the following: (1) unilateral renal agenesis, (2) ureteral duplication, (3) ectopic ureteral orifice, and (4) ureterocele.

Unilateral renal agenesis occurs with an incidence of approximately 1 per 1000.[53] Associated genital tract anomalies, usually partial or complete uterine duplication, occur in 35% to 45% of affected women. Several mechanisms have been proposed including failed differentiation of the nephrogenic ridge, failed differentiation of the mesonephric duct and ureteral bud, and failed development of the metanephric blastema. The earlier in embryonic development the urinary tract aberration occurs, the more severe are the associated abnormalities in the genital tract. The diagnosis of unilateral renal agenesis is usually made while evaluating the patient for symptomatic renal disease or at surgery. When it is identified, a structural evaluation of the genital tract should be done. There is no renal functional derangement unless there is compromise of the single kidney.

Duplication of the ureter may be partial or total and occurs in approximately 1% of the population.[82] The Y-shaped partial duplication results when the ureteral bud branches before establishing contact with the metanephric blastema. Two complete ureters result from growth of a duplicated ureteral bud that arises from the mesonephric duct. The ureters usually cross each other within a common vascular sheath so that the ureter draining the upper renal pole enters the bladder more medial and distal to its mate (the Meyer-Weigert rule). It may occur so inferior that it is considered an ectopic ureter. The interstitial segment of the distal ureter tends to be shorter and thus is prone to vesicoureteral reflux and resulting upper urinary tract infection. In addition to possible reflux, it is important to recognize this condition clinically so that the duplicated ureter may be avoided during surgery.

An ectopic ureteral orifice may open into the urethra, vestibule, vagina, or uterus.[98] Usually it occurs in a duplicated ureter with the ectopic ureter draining the superior renal pole as expected by its more distal position. If the ectopic ureter opens distal to the urethral sphincter or into the genital tract, incontinence results. The usual clinical presentation is constant dribbling of urine with a concurrent normal voiding pattern. In children it may be misinterpreted as enuresis. If the ureter opens to the uterus or vagina, signs and symptoms of vaginitis may be most prominent. Symptomatic ectopia is treated surgically usually by ipsilateral ureteroureterostomy or reimplantation into the bladder.

A ureterocele is a cystic dilatation of the distal ureter.[82] It may be congenital or acquired and usually involves the interstitial ureter. It is probably the result of an incomplete perforation of the bladder by the ureter that results in a localized increase in hydrostatic pressure. The usual clinical presentation is recurrent urinary tract infections due to obstruction. Treatment requires surgical resection of the involved segment with reimplantation into the bladder.

URINARY INCONTINENCE

Urinary incontinence is defined by the International Continence Society as the involuntary loss of urine that is a social and hygienic problem and is objectively demonstrable.[1] Occasional episodes of incontinence are common in women and therefore should not be regarded as abnormal. However, incontinence becomes a medical problem when it interferes with the woman's social life or hygiene. Objective demonstration is important as incontinence can often be confused with vaginal discharge or leakage of amniotic fluid in pregnant women.

Classification

Classification can be based on symptoms, but as these do not correlate specifically to underlying pathology, such a subdivision is less helpful than a classification based on diagnostic pathology. The breakdown of this is shown in Fig. 18-7 where broadly speaking, incontinence can be transurethral or extraurethral. The most common cause is genuine stress incontinence or urethral sphincter incompetence. Detrusor instability can have a neurological basis, but in the vast majority of gynecology patients no concomitant neurological abnormality is detected. Loss of urethral pressure prior to detrusor contraction is a common finding with detrusor instability; however, when seen in the absence of detrusor instability the loss of pressure is termed urethral instability, but this is quite rare. Urinary retention with overflow, more common in the elderly, can also occur in the young. On the other hand congenital abnormalities of the urethra usually present in infancy. There are some incontinent women in whom no underlying causes can be detected. If there is an associated mental disorder, these patients could be classified as having functional incontinence. It is important that the term functional incontinence should not be used as a "trash can" diagnosis. The extraurethral causes of incontinence are either congenital or acquired. The congenital ones are usually diagnosed in childhood; occasionally they may present in the reproductive age group (see section on malformations). Fistulas can either be iatrogenic following surgery or radiotherapy, or result from malignancy. In the developing world they can also result from obstetric trauma.

Prevalence. Most published data on urinary incontinence address prevalence rates in defined groups. While useful these

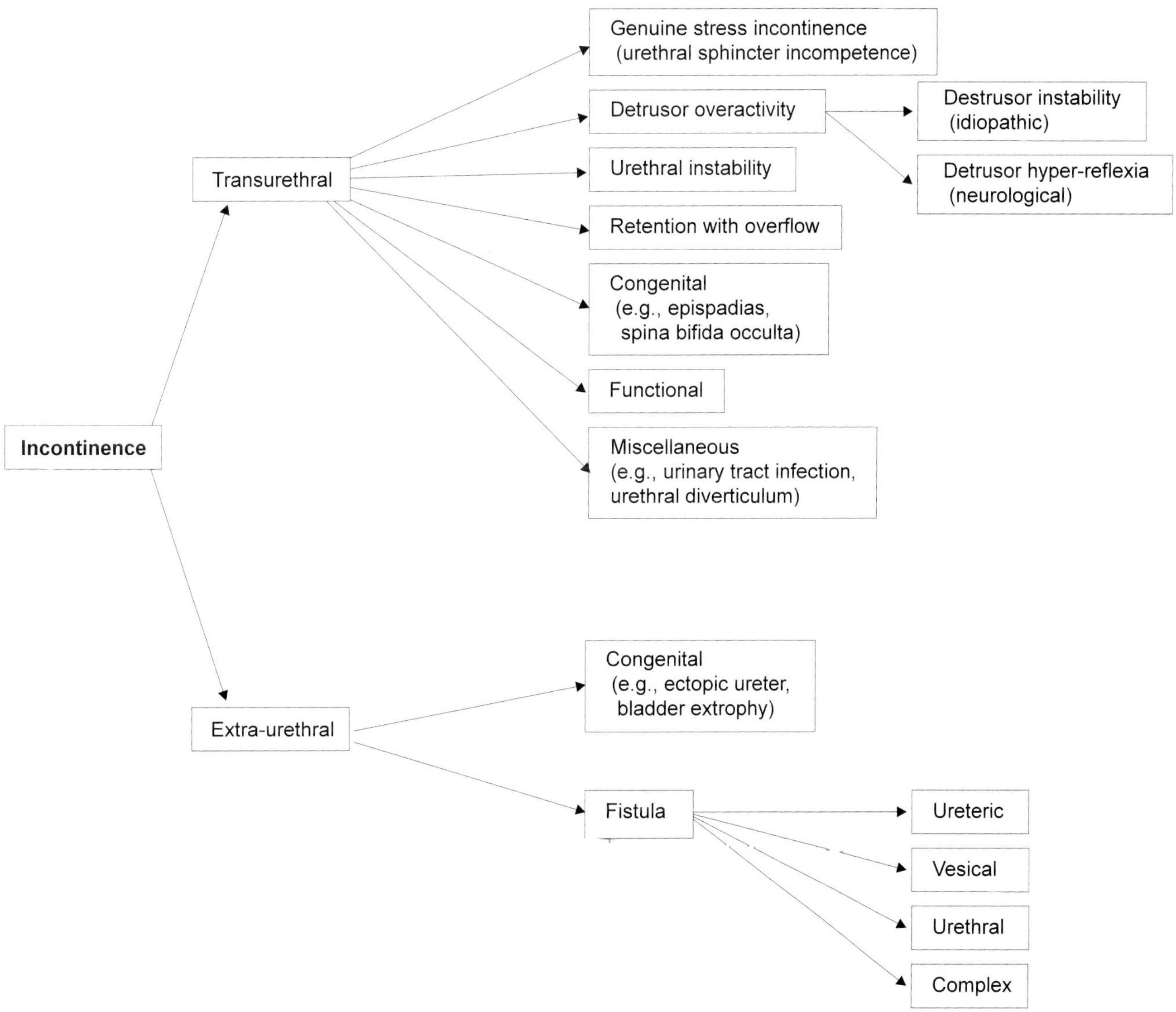

Fig. 18-7. The causes of female urinary incontinence. (Modified from Stanton SL: Classification of incontinence. In Stanton SL editor: *Clinical gynecologic urology*, St Louis, 1984, CV Mosby.)

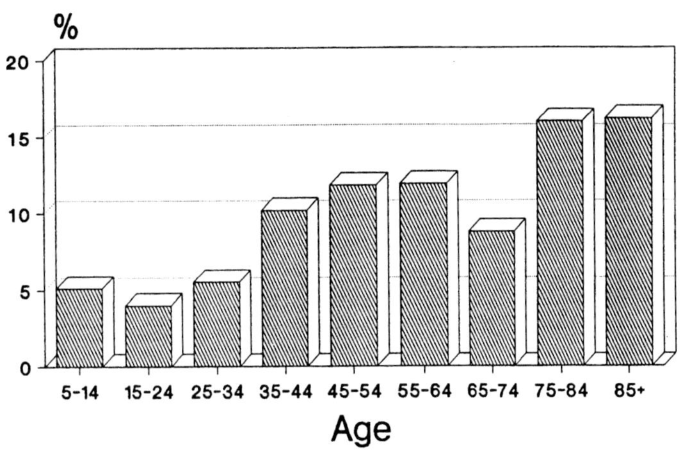

Fig. 18-8. The prevalence of female urinary incontinence at different ages. (Modified from Thomas TM et al: *Br Med J* 28:1243, 1980.)

studies do not yield reliable information on the global problem of female urinary dysfunction. It is generally understood that incontinence is under reported, but inaccuracies can also arise in the data collected from postal questionnaires where reliance is placed on the patient's assessment of urine leakage as opposed to objective demonstration.

Between 5 and 14 years of age 6.9% of males and 5.1% of females complain of regular incontinence whereas for occasional incontinence these figures increase to 10.9% and 11.2% respectively.[79] From 15 years onward the prevalence of female urinary incontinence increases with age and is higher in females than males.[9] However, stress incontinence is more common than urge incontinence although the prevalence of the latter does tend to rise in the elderly.[48]

Menopause has often been proposed as a cause of incontinence, but there is no good epidemiologic evidence to suggest that menopause per se, (i.e., estrogen deficiency), results in incontinence.[87] The reason for this association is that the prevalence of stress incontinence reaches a peak in the 5th and 6th decade and so is coincident with the menopause. However, rates decline thereafter,[41] which is contrary to what would be expected if this was an estrogen deficiency symptom. Analysis of studies using hormone replacement therapy in postmenopausal women for the treatment of genuine stress incontinence does not show a consistent beneficial effect.[13] The prevalence of urge incontinence and detrusor instability appears to rise after the menopause, but this may be an age-related rather than a hormonally-related phenomenon.

Etiology. As incontinence is due to many different causes, a discussion of the etiology of the condition without reference to the type of incontinence is inappropriate. To document the types of incontinence, a urodynamic classification is required. Unfortunately, gross generalizations have been made in the literature leading to difficulty in interpretating the reported studies. For the purposes of this chapter, the etiologies of the different types of incontinence will be covered in the relevant subsection.

Psychosocial. The psychosocial impact of incontinence is considerable with 34% of patients complaining that it interfers significantly with household chores.[56] The psychologic reaction to incontinence appears to be akin to reactive depression. Psychologic symptoms associated with urinary incontinence are phenomena of psychologic tension and sleep disorders. This is confirmed in a report where the psychoneurotic-related incontinence appears to result from the decreased quality of life rather than from underlying personality traits.[46] With regard to quality of life, middle-aged women suffer more than older women, and it is the fact of incontinence rather than the frequency or severity that causes this negative impact.

Costs. It is difficult to estimate the costs of urinary incontinence as good data are lacking. However, in 1987 a figure of $10.3 billion was attributed by Hu,[37] and in 1983 the cost of palliative care in France appeared to be $35 million with an anticipated growth of 30% per annum.[55] Overall in the western world significant incontinence probably afflicts between 4% and 8% of the population, and it is sad that only 5% of these cases have a precise medical diagnosis.[83] Thus the problem of incontinence is widespread and expensive.

Clinical evaluation of the lower urinary tract

History. Lower urinary tract dysfunction will present with one or more of the following symptoms: (1) incontinence, (2) irritative symptoms (urgency, frequency, painful micturition), and/or (3) voiding difficulties.

For diagnostic purposes, symptoms can be misleading. However, a careful history is essential because it clarifies the patient's complaint as opposed to any other co-existing conditions, and allows the diagnostician to put the investigative findings into context. The reason that most women present with mixed symptoms is that the primary pathology induces a behavior modification that itself results in symptoms. For example, a woman with incontinence will learn to reduce her incontinence by keeping her ambient bladder volume at a minimum. This necessitates voiding frequently, and she then also has the complaint of frequency and this often results in urgency. A woman with retention may complain of stress incontinence because when her bladder is full, she may leak urine on coughing. Similarly a full bladder may be an invitation to colonization by bacteria; she may present with recurrent urinary tract infections or symptoms that are primarily irritative.

Stress incontinence is a term used to describe incontinence that occurs involuntarily during physical activity. This activity causes increased intraabdominal pressure, resulting in incontinence. Urge incontinence on the other hand is a strong and sudden desire to void that results in an involuntary loss of urine. Dribbling incontinence is another symptom that may have a variety of underlying causes ranging from retention with overflow to a fistula or an ectopic ureter. Postmicturition dribble is less common in women, but can occur in the presence of a marked urethrocele or urethral diverticulum. Nocturnal enuresis is a term that is applied to bed wetting; however, the patient is awakened by having wet the bed rather than by the desire to void and then have become incontinent. Giggle incontinence is found in younger adolescent girls and is often associated with detrusor instability. Incontinence occurring during coitus is usually associated with genuine stress incontinence, but when it occurs with orgasm, it is thought to be due to detrusor instability.

Frequency of micturition varies considerably amongst normal women, and some may void only twice a day (cameloid bladder). When voiding occurs more than 7 times per day it is thought to be abnormal. Nocturia is a condition of waking up with a strong desire to void. Habitual voiding because the patient wakes up for some other reason is not nocturia. Once per night is normal, and nocturia only becomes significant when it occurs more often. Urgency is the strong and sudden desire to void that can be debilitating as the patient thinks of little else. There are many causes of frequency and urgency and some of them are shown in Table 18-1. When confronted with a patient with incontinence, it is important to consider the potential for other coexisting pathology.

Voiding difficulties in women may present with symptoms of hesitancy, poor stream, straining to void, incomplete bladder emptying, or a combination of these. Again the causes of voiding dysfunction are numerous and are listed in Table 18-2. Dysuria is a confusing term best avoided because it can refer to painful micturition or difficulty with micturition; instead the actual symptoms should be described. Frequency, urgency, and painful micturition have been termed the urethral syndrome. However, this is not a useful term as the causes of this so-called syndrome are various. Treatment is also diverse and ranges from antibiotics for a urinary tract infection to hormone replacement therapy for tissue atrophy. Hematuria can be due to a variety of causes ranging from malignancy to infection. This should always be promptly investigated. Finally backache is a fairly common nonspecific problem associated with incontinence. The cause in many women is a musculoskeletal dysfunction, but it can also be secondary to the presence of uterine prolapse. It is sometimes difficult to differentiate between the two, but in general backache from the former is worse in the morning while backache from the latter gets progressively worse through the day. This back pain should be distinguished from flank pain, which when associated with painful micturition may be due to early pyelonephritis.

Physical examination. As for any surgical or medical condition, a full examination is required. However, for the purposes of lower urinary tract dysfunction, the physician should concentrate on the gynecologic, urologic and neurologic examination. Testing of the sacral nerve roots S_2 to S_4 is important as incontinence may have a neurologic origin. Assessment of the patient's mental state is also

Table 18-1. Causes of frequency and urgency

Structural	Urethral caruncle or diverticulum Bladder mucosal lesion (e.g., papilloma) Small capacity bladder Pelvic mass (e.g., fibroids) Radiation cystitis or fibrosis
Infective/Inflammatory	Urinary tract infection Urethritis or cystitis Chronic retention of urine Bladder calculus Genital warts
Endocrine	Diabetes insipidus or mellitus Hypothyroidism Pregnancy
Life Style	Habit Large fluid intake
Miscellaneous	Idiopathic detrusor instability Upper motor neuron lesion Diuretic therapy or impaired renal function Previous pelvic surgery

Table 18-2. Causes of voiding dysfunction

Neurological	Upper or lower motor neuron lesions
Inflammation	Urethritis, vulvitis, or vaginitis
Drugs	Tricyclic antidepressants Anticholinergic agents Alpha-adrenergic stimulators Ganglion blockers Epidural anesthesia
Obstruction	Urethral stenosis or stricture Edema following surgery or parturition Fibrosis due to repeated dilatations or irradiation Pelvic mass, e.g., fibroids, retroverted gravid uterus, ovarian cyst, faeces etc. Urethral distortion due to a large cystocele
Medical	Diabetic neuropathy Hypothyroidism Psychosis
Atonic detrusor	Secondary to over distention
Functional	Anxiety, apprehension

useful. The physician needs to ascertain if the individual is suitable for behavior modification or conservative therapy that would require comprehension and motivation. When contemplating surgery, the integrity of pelvic floor tissues and the degree of atrophy are important prognostic features. The gynecologic examination should also try to elicit the presence of uterine prolapse. This can be done with the patient standing; however, it is easier when the patient is lying in the "Sims" position on her left side. Anterior, vault, or posterior prolapse should be systematically determined. The normal gynecologic vaginal examination should take place to determine concomitant pathology and also to detect presence of a palpable bladder and localized tenderness. The urethra should be observed while the patient coughs to detect stress incontinence, and it should also be inspected for the presence of a caruncle or urethral mucosal prolapse. It should be palpated throughout its entire length for the presence of a diverticulum. The course of the ureter should be palpated for localized tenderness, and the kidneys examined for enlargement or tenderness.

The Q-tip test assesses the integrity of the ligamentous support of the proximal urethra and determines the presence of urethral hypermobility.[42] A sterile, lubricated cotton swab is placed into the bladder neck. At rest in the lithotomy position, the urethra (and thus the swab) assumes a 0° angle to the horizontal plane. The patient is then asked to perform a Valsalva maneuver. If the proximal urethra is normally supported, straining displaces the distal end of the swab only slightly. However, with loss of support, straining causes the proximal end of the urethra to descend and the distal end of the swab to move upward to an angle that usually exceeds 30° and often approaches 90°.

Frequency volume charts. While a history is essential for obtaining the patient's perception of her problems, this is often at variance with actual events; a frequency volume chart or voiding diary is an important adjunct to the clinical evaluation. There are many different voiding diaries available commercially, but essentially they all elicit similar information (Fig. 18-9). The volumes voided give an indication of whether voiding is premature or whether there is a true diuresis; this can be ascertained by the amount and the type of fluid that is drunk. Also documentation of the changes through the day is useful as simple measures can resolve many of the difficulties. For example, if the patient is prone to drinking large amounts of fluid, especially tea or coffee last thing at night, then nocturia is a likely consequence.

BLADDER RECORD CHART

WEEK COMMENCING ______ NAME ______ ADDRESS ______

ENTER A TICK IN APPROPRIATE SQUARE EACH TIME YOU PASS URINE NORMALLY

		8am	9am	10am	11am	12 noon	1pm	2pm	3pm	4pm	5pm	6pm	7pm	8pm	9pm	10pm	11pm	12mn	1am	2am	3am	4am	5am	6am	7am
NORMAL	MON.																								
	TUES.																								
	WED.																								
	THUR.																								
	FRI.																								
	SAT.																								
	SUN.																								
		MORNING					AFTERNOON					EVENING					NIGHT								

ENTER A TICK IN APPROPRIATE SQUARE EACH TIME YOU ARE WET OR DAMP

		8am	9am	10am	11am	12 noon	1pm	2pm	3pm	4pm	5pm	6pm	7pm	8pm	9pm	10pm	11pm	12mn	1am	2am	3am	4am	5am	6am	7am
INCONTINENT	MON.																								
	TUES.																								
	WED.																								
	THUR.																								
	FRI.																								
	SAT.																								
	SUN.																								

SPECIAL INSTRUCTIONS:

KV 307 12/81

Fig. 18-9. An example of a frequency volume chart or voiding diary (from Kabi Pharmacia).

Basic urodynamic investigations. No matter how careful the physician is in obtaining the history, diagnosis based on the clinical picture alone will commonly be inaccurate.[40,70,72] Even when a computerized questionnaire was used to limit clinician bias, the results (though more predictive than in the previously published studies) displayed an 80% correct classification that is still not acceptable for clinical practice.[90]

Cystometry. In patients suffering from incontinence due to detrusor instability, operations designed to elevate the bladder neck are contraindicated. This is because of the following: (1) anatomical repositioning of the bladder neck is not required, and (2) surgery at the level of the bladder neck often results in a worsening of detrusor instability.

The primary objective of any investigation is to exclude detrusor instability, and the mainstay of basic urodynamic investigations is cystometry. As this requires catheterization, it is important that no patient with a urinary tract infection should undergo this procedure.

As the term implies, cystometry is the measurement of bladder pressure, and it is a dynamic investigation in that the intravesical pressure is measured not only during filling, but also at capacity and during voiding. As the bladder is an intraabdominal organ, any changes that occur in the intraabdominal pressure will also be reflected in the intravesical pressure. Thus to account for this, the intraabdominal pressures are often measured separately. This can be done by measuring the pressure inside the rectum or in the upper third of the vagina. The equation: detrusor pressure = intravesical pressure minus intraabdominal pressure describes three-channel cystometry; the two pressures on the right side of the equation can be measured and the detrusor pressure on the left side of the equation can be calculated.

The standard test for the diagnosis of detrusor instability is three-channel, fluid-filled provocative cystometry. Saline or contrast medium is used because this best approximates urine and during filling measures are taken to provoke abnormal detrusor contractions. The bladder is filled at a rate faster than the physiological rate, the fluid used tends to be at room temperature, and while the bladder is filling, the patient is asked to cough intermittently. Any of these measures may elicit a detrusor contraction. During the filling phase the patient is asked to indicate when she experiences the urge to void. The volume in the bladder at this point is noted and should be between 100 and 300 mL in the average gynecologic patient. Some investigators differentiate between a first desire and a strong desire to void. When the patient is unable to tolerate any further filling, the physiologic capacity is reached, which should be between 400 and 600 mL. If patients have a low-volume first sensation and bladder capacity, then they are deemed to have sensory urgency if no detrusor instability has been noted. If they have a high-volume first sensation and bladder capacity then the diagnosis is a hyposensitive bladder. With a full bladder the patient is asked to change posture from supine to erect and this in itself may induce a detrusor contraction. Should none of these measures result in a wave-like (systolic or phasic) detrusor contraction and if the pressure increase both on filling and on standing is less than 15 cm of water, then the patient is deemed to have a stable detrusor as defined by the International Continence Society Standardization Committee.[1] When the patient has a full bladder in the erect or sitting position, she is asked to cough and the presence of stress incontinence is noted. Should this occur in the absence of any detrusor contraction then the diagnosis is genuine stress incontinence. Following evaluation of the urethral sphincter, the patient is asked to void and during this phase the detrusor (activity) pressure changes are monitored. Voiding pressure per se is not very helpful as it is highly dependent on urethral resistance. Therefore if the pelvic floor and urethra are fully relaxed, then a woman may void with very little increase in her own detrusor pressure. To determine the strength of detrusor activity, the stop test can be applied. The patient is ordered to stop voiding midstream. This results in an instantaneous contraction of the urethral sphincter, but the detrusor muscle does not relax so quickly. Thus an isometric detrusor contraction is noted; the pressure generated by this manoeuver is of more interest for the evaluation of detrusor contractility.

Three-channel cystometry requires a urodynamic system that is either computer based or one that utilizes amplifiers. Both systems require the use of pressure transducers and a printer or chart recorder. In a bid to simplify and reduce the cost of this test, many investigators have tried to use single channel (intravesical) cystometry, but because of the confounding problem of intraabdominal pressure, this technique results in an over diagnosis of detrusor instability. In an attempt to avoid messy fluid-filled systems, CO_2 gas cystometry has been used. Unfortunately carbon dioxide dissolves to form carbonic acid, which is an irritant, and it is thought that this technique also exaggerates the incidence of detrusor instability.

Uroflowmetry. This technique measures rate of urine flow, and the most important diagnostic variable is the peak flow rate. The peak flow rate declines with age, but as a rough guide, peak flows in excess of 15 mL per second are accepted as normal. However, prior to voiding the bladder must contain more than 200 mL otherwise the detrusor muscle is not able to develop an adequate contraction. Following voiding, the residual should be less than 50 mL; if it is greater than 100 mL, it is regarded as abnormal.

Clearly uroflowmetry is an essential investigation in a patient with voiding difficulties, but it is also used for preoperative evaluation of a woman about to undergo bladder neck surgery for genuine stress incontinence. A poor preoperative flow rate is a poor prognostic feature for postoperative voiding, irrespective of the cause. As some women void by abdominal contractions, such a manoeuvre after surgery for stress incontinence will result in closure of the urethra and hence postoperative voiding difficulties.

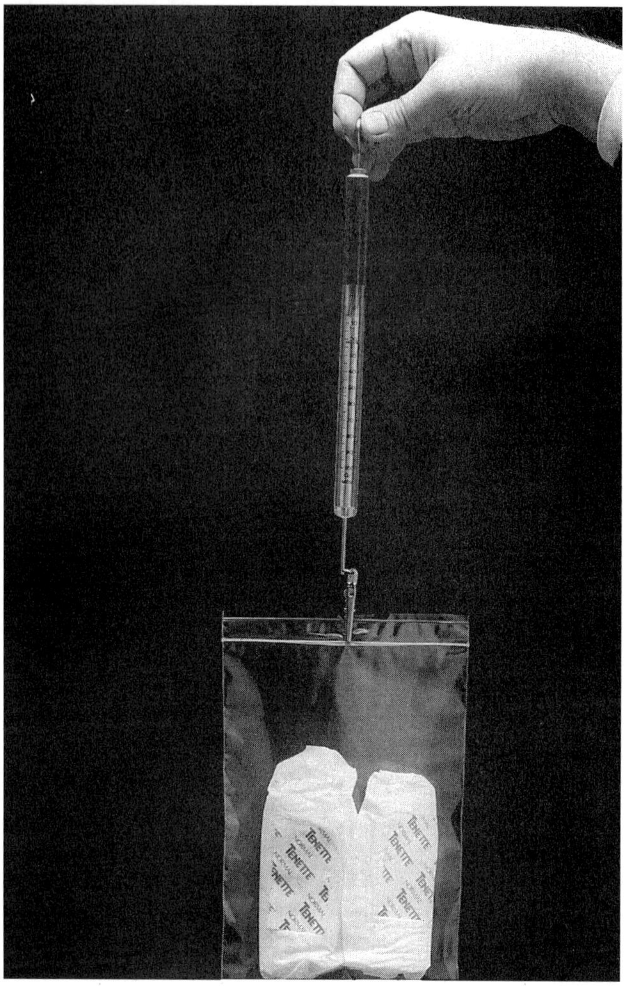

Fig. 18-10. The perineal pad is placed in a self-sealing plastic bag and weighed before and after the test period. The increase in weight is quantification of the degree of incontinence.

Pad testing. Pad tests are important not only for objective verification of urinary incontinence, but also for quantification and hence definition of the magnitude of the problem. However, the degree of incontinence does not always relate to the psychosocial impact as this tends to depend on an individual's background and reaction to the disability.

These tests essentially involve the use of a perineal pad that is weighed before and after the patient has worn it. The difference in weight is interpreted as the weight (volume) of urine that is lost. There are two types of pad tests, those that are done in a hospital setting, and those that are carried out in the home.[52] While the former may be monitored under more controlled conditions, the latter gives a better description of the complaint as it is not set in an artificial environment. Cheap and noninvasive, pad tests can be used not only for diagnosis but also to monitor the progress of treatment. Various commercial kits are available, and when these tests are performed in conjunction with a voiding diary, this simple test can yield much useful information about the patient's disability (Fig. 18-10).

Special urodynamic investigations

Cystourethroscopy. This technique is useful in the older patient where symptoms of frequency and urgency may well be associated with bladder pathology. However, in the absence of hematuria in the young, its use in the investigation of lower urinary tract dysfunction is not so valuable. If routine urodynamic investigations reveal the possibility of a stricture or stenosis, then such an investigation may well be an appropriate next step. The investigation can be carried out with a flexible cystoscope and general anaesthesia is often not required.

Urethral pressure profilometry. This is a technique whereby pressure in the urethra can be measured at different points along the urethra simultaneously with bladder pressure.[22] It is primarily used for diagnosing urethral sphincter incompetence, but can also be used to diagnose urethral instability and urethral strictures and diverticula.

The first person to attempt to measure urethral pressures was Victor Bonney,[7] and he used a technique of retrograde sphincterometry. Subsequently perfusion systems were developed. While perfusion techniques are simple, their reproducibility has been drawn into question. Modern day techniques utilize solid state transducers that are mounted on a catheter.[5] The most commonly used catheter employs two transducers mounted approximately 6 cm apart. The catheter is inserted into the bladder via the urethra until both sensors are inside the bladder. While the catheter is being withdrawn steadily the proximal sensor passes through the urethra and obtains a urethral pressure profile at rest (Fig. 18-11). Many measurements can be taken from the resting profile, but specifically they relate to measures of urethral length or maximum urethral closure pressure. The technique can also be carried out while the patient is coughing to obtain a stress profile. Clearly the latter is more important for investigating the integrity of the urethral sphincter. While the reproducibility of the resting profile is well accepted, the same cannot be said for the stress profile. For this reason urethral pressure profilometry cannot be used accurately for the diagnosis of genuine stress incontinence.[85,91]

Urethral instability can be detected by placing the catheter so that the urethral sensor is at the maximum urethral pressure point. At this point various fluctuations are seen in urethral pressure; there is a small urethral pulse that is in time with the vascular pulse. There is also a fluctuation in the maximum urethral pressure that usually does not vary by more than a third of the resting value.[88] However, in some patients there is a sudden and complete loss of urethral pressure that may be associated with incontinence. This often occurs in patients with detrusor instability prior to an unstable contraction that mimicks the situation during normal micturition. However, in a few patients this loss of urethral pressure occurs in the presence of a stable detrusor and therefore is diagnosed as urethral instability.

A consistent dip in the urethral pressure profile may indicate a urethral diverticulum, and an aberrant point of

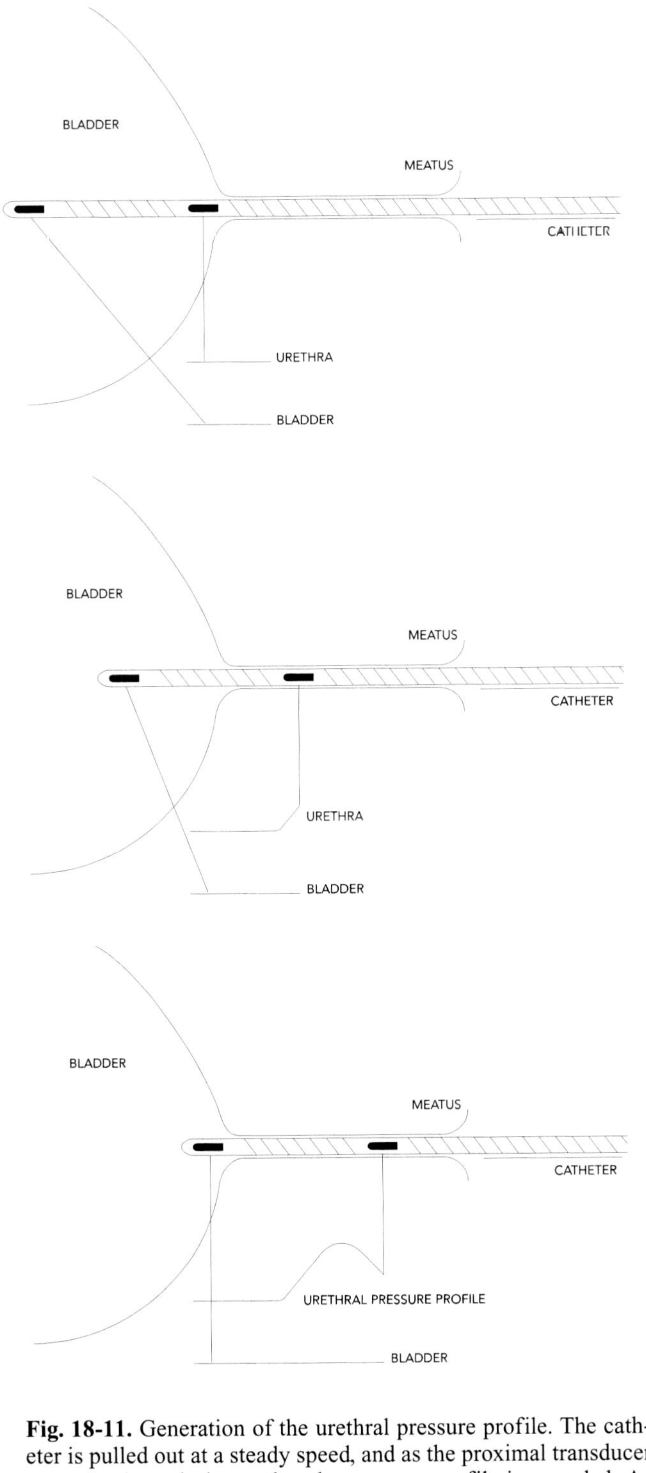

Fig. 18-11. Generation of the urethral pressure profile. The catheter is pulled out at a steady speed, and as the proximal transducer traverses through the urethra the pressure profile is recorded. As the bladder sensor is intravesical throughout no pressure change is registered by this sensor. (From Versi E, Cardozo LD: Urodynamics. In Studd JWW, editor: *Progress in Obstetrics and Gynaecology*, vol 8, London, 1990, Churchill Livingstone.)

abnormally high pressure may be construed as a urethral stricture. These urethral abnormalities are more easily diagnosed by cystourethroscopy or fluoroscopy.

While urethral pressure profilometry is widely used in urodynamic investigations, diagnostic criteria for genuine stress incontinence have been poorly formulated which limits the clinical value of this technique.

Electrophysiological studies. The value of routine electromyography (EMG) as a part of the urodynamic workup for a neurologically intact, incontinent patient is also limited. Although this technique is more useful in research, it has a clinical role in the investigation of voiding disorders and in patients with other concomitant neurological abnormalities.

Patients with voiding difficulties may have detrusor sphincter dyssynergia. In this condition the detrusor muscle contracts, but at the same time the urethral sphincter also contracts, instead of relaxing. Another type of voiding dysfunction observed in neurologically intact young women is caused by pelvic floor contraction at the time of attempted micturition. Both of these abnormalities can be detected by EMG studies.

Imaging studies

Video-urodynamics. Video-urodynamics is the most useful test that can be carried out for evaluation of the lower urinary tract. Essentially the investigation involves cystometry using an X-ray contrast medium and fluoroscopy so that the bladder and urethra can be imaged while the pressure recordings are being made. This "form and function" test can be recorded on video tape and reviewed at a later date for analysis and also for teaching purposes.

This technique is considered the best urodynamic test as it yields a comprehensive array of information about the lower urinary tract. It could be argued that this test is unnecessary for the evaluation of uncomplicated incontinence in a neurologically intact patient. However, the technique will yield more information than simple cystometry. This test is most useful for investigating patients who have undergone previous failed surgery and for those with a voiding dysfunction and/or a neurologic abnormality.

Ultrasonography. With improving resolution of ultrasound imaging and the use of vaginal, rectal, and perineal probes, the definition of lower urinary tract imaging is improving. The main difficulty with these techniques is that the presence of the probe may alter the anatomical configuration of the structures being viewed and so in itself influence the findings.

This modality is most useful in the diagnosis of urinary retention. Urethral catheterization to determine a urinary residual has been replaced by simple transabdominal ultrasonography. The bladder is imaged so that its three dimensions can be measured. The product of these dimensions is multiplied by 0.7 to give a bladder volume that is accurate to an error of less than 20%. The ultrasound equipment automatically measures and calculates the above indices.

Vaginal probes are able to delineate clearly the bladder neck, and on coughing, bladder neck incompetence can be diagnosed.[66] Bladder neck incompetence is of little diagnostic value as many continent women have an open bladder neck at rest and on coughing.[86,92] For the diagnosis of genuine stress incontinence, it is important to be able to see the urethra open throughout its entire length, and this is not always possible using ultrasound because of movement during a cough. Also in patients who have cough-induced detrusor instability, ultrasonic imaging will possibly misdiagnose the condition as urethral sphincter incompetence. There may, however, be a place for ultrasonic imaging in combination with conventional urodynamic pressure studies, but this remains to be evaluated.

Magnetic resonance imaging. This is an exciting new means of viewing the lower urinary tract. In the future, evaluation of pelvic floor muscle bulk may provide useful prognostic information for patients contemplating pelvic floor retraining as a conservative treatment of genuine stress incontinence. However, its clinical application is limited at present as scans are taken with the patient supine and imaging times are in excess of 1 minute. Rapid scans in the erect position would be more useful for assessing lower urinary tract function.

Plain radiology. Micturating cystography is largely outmoded because it is not a dynamic test and so provides little information compared to video-urodynamics. Intravenous urography, while an essential test for investigation of the upper urinary tract, has limited value in the investigation of incontinence. This test should be deferred in favor of the more dynamic tests previously mentioned.

Genuine stress incontinence

Etiology. Genuine stress incontinence is defined as urethral sphincter incompetence. As a result there is an involuntary loss of urine when intravesical pressure exceeds the maximum urethral closure pressure in the absence of a detrusor contraction.[1] Prior to detrusor contraction there is often urethral relaxation. If stress incontinence occurs during urethral relaxation, it is not due to urethral sphincter incompetence and hence the rider about excluding detrusor instability is important.

There may be many causes for genuine stress incontinence and some of these are listed in Table 18-3. Childbirth has definitely been implicated but is not the only cause. Many young nulliparous girls are also incontinent. Thomas et al found that multiparity was a predisposing factor,[79] whereas Jolleys noted the association with obstetric trauma.[41] Recent studies on collagen synthesis suggest that deficiencies in the repair process may contribute to the etiology of prolapse but perhaps not genuine stress incontinence.[62] Electrophysiologic studies have shown that vaginal delivery rather than pregnancy itself can damage the pudendal nerve,[3] but this does not explain why women experience stress incontinence during pregnancy. It may be that during pregnancy women suffer from transient detrusor instability, whereas after delivery any damage that is caused may be more permanent.

Radical pelvic surgery can cause genuine stress incontinence and voiding dysfunction,[25] possibly because of embarrassment of the nerve supply. On the other hand radiotherapy is more likely to result in detrusor instability and a small capacity bladder. There are a few studies to suggest that benign gynecological surgery, in particular hysterectomy, is associated with the development of incontinence.[55] Unfortunately the data are so flawed with confounding variables that a definitive statement is impossible without further studies and subgroup analyses.[84]

Diagnosis. The diagnosis of genuine stress incontinence can be made with cystometry when stress incontinence is noted in the absence of a detrusor contraction. Stress incontinence can be demonstrated by observing the external urethral meatus or by fluoroscopy. Many units throughout the world use urethral pressure profilometry as a means of diagnosing the condition. While this may be adequate in many cases, there are a large number of patients tested with ambiguous results.

Treatment

Conservative management. Nonsurgical management of genuine stress incontinence has been reviewed elsewhere[67]; the types of treatments are listed in Table 18-4. Pelvic floor exercise is the mainstay of treatment,[45] but electrical therapy can be useful as a trophic stimulus to the muscles but more significantly as a biofeedback technique. Contraction of the specific pelvic floor muscles allows the patient to become aware of these muscle groups which aids pelvic floor retraining.[54]

Perineometry works in a similar fashion. A vaginal dilator-shaped device is inserted into the vagina and the patient is asked to contract her pelvic floor. The device measures the strength of the contraction, and the patient receives the biofeedback of pelvic floor activity, thus reinforcing the education process.

Vaginal cones are an interesting innovation (Fig. 8-12). A set of 5 cones identical in size but of different weights are used by the patient. A single cone of the lowest weight is

Table 18-3. Genuine stress incontinence associated features

Pelvic floor damage or denervation	Parturition Pelvic surgery
Urethral damage	Vaginal (urethral) surgery Surgery for incontinence Urethral dilatation or urethrotomy Recurrent urinary tract infections Radiotherapy
Increased intraabdominal pressures	Pregnancy Chronic cough (bronchitis) Abdominal/pelvic mass Fecal impaction Ascites Obesity

Table 18-4. Conservative treatment for genuine stress incontinence

Pelvic floor exercises
Inferential therapy
Faradism
Vaginal cones
Perineometry
Tampons
Mechanical devices
Alpha-adrenergic agonists +/- estrogen replacement therapy

inserted into the vagina by the patient; she is then instructed to hold it in place while walking around. The cones are designed to teach the patient to contract her pelvic floor muscles without contracting her abdominal musculature, otherwise the cone is pushed out of the vagina. When the patient is able to hold a certain weight, she then moves on to the next weight; effectively weight training for the pelvic floor! Patients find the cones acceptable[65] and easy to use.

The cure rate for these physical treatments is limited, but about 70% of patients have significant improvement. The key to successful use of this therapy is patient selection. Women who are highly motivated, young, thin, and fit, and have not undergone incontinence surgery, are the ones most likely to benefit. Other good prognostic features are absence of long standing incontinence, concomitant prolapse, or chronic cough.[54]

Tampons and mechanical devices are useful as they provide temporary occlusion of the urethra. These are inserted into the vagina to prevent leakage in patients who experience stress incontinence only during exercise. They are not useful for the long term because of the problems of a foreign body inside the vagina.

In postmenopausal women, alpha-adrenergic agonists in association with estrogen replacement therapy are effective in the conservative management of genuine stress incontinence.[2] However, given the side effects of these drugs, it is unlikely that many patients will accept this treatment in the long term.

Surgical management. Over 100 operations have been described for the treatment of genuine stress incontinence. Although a full discussion of these operations is beyond the scope of this chapter, they are described elsewhere.[75] The operations can be classified into six groups which are discussed in the next sections.

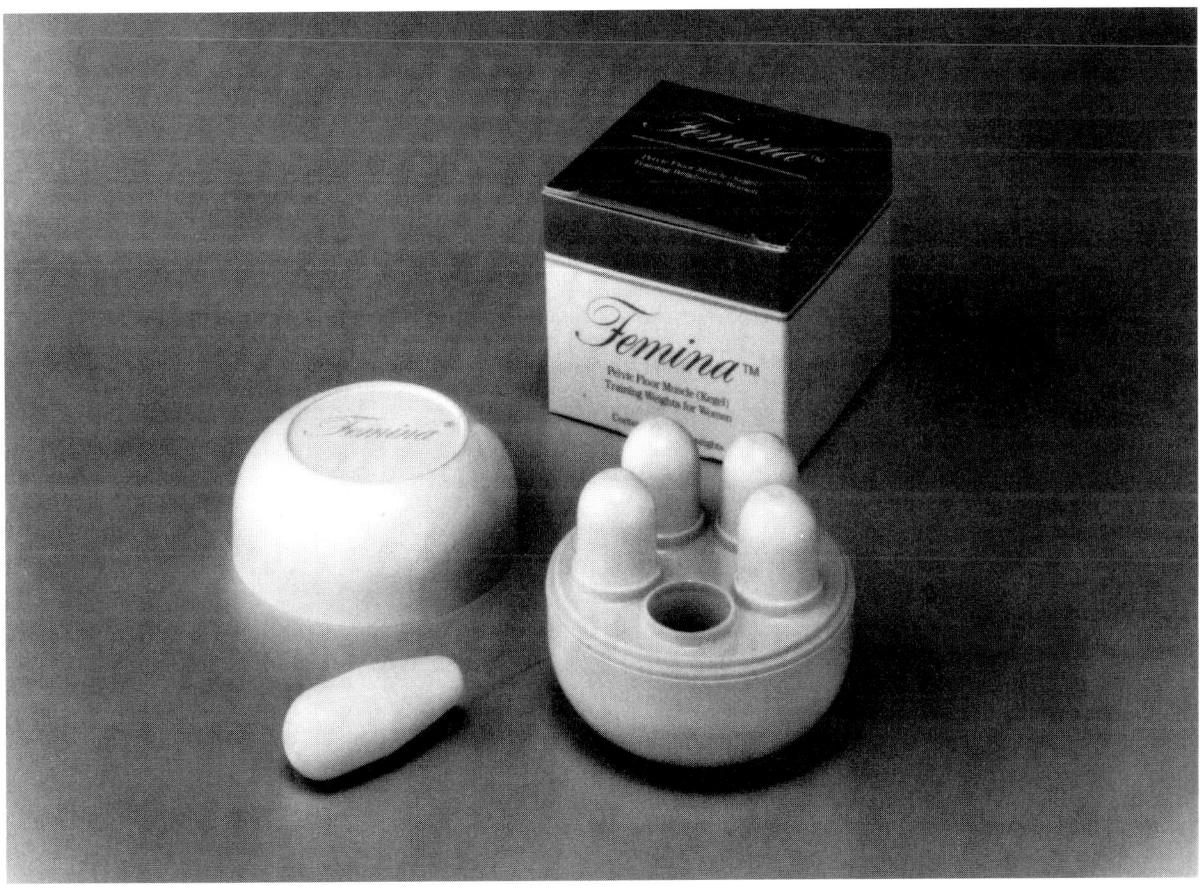

Fig. 8-12. A set of 5 vaginal cones reproduced from Colgate Medical, Berkshire.

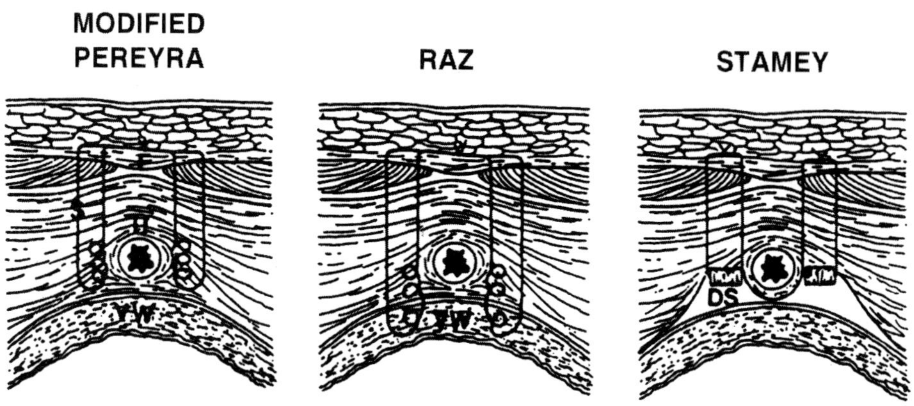

Fig. 18-13. A comparison of the modified Pereyra, Raz and Stamey operations; Coronal section of the bladder neck and surrounding tissues. VW. vaginal wall (From Stanton SL: *Clin Obstet Gynecol* 33:346, 1990.)

Prior to treatment, the general health of the patient has to be considered before the most appropriate type of procedure can be planned. Integrity of the local tissues, particularly around the bladder neck, should also be assessed. In post-menopausal women with atrophied tissues the sutures may tear out. Thus preoperative treatment with estrogens may be indicated. Preoperative voiding function should be assessed because patients with a poor preoperative flow rate are likely to have more postoperative voiding difficulties, irrespective of the cause of their diminished voiding function.

1. Vaginal surgery. The vaginal approach with bladder neck buttress sutures (Kelly plication) is one of the most common operations used by gynecologists. However, because the objective 5-year success rate of this procedure is only 50%, many urogynecologists do not favor it. This operation should be distinguished from anterior colporrhaphy that involves the placement of bladder base buttress sutures for the reduction of a cystocele.

2. Endoscopic needle suspension techniques. The endoscopic needle suspension procedures, such as the Pereyra, Stamey, Raz, and Gittes techniques, all involve the use of a single loop of suture placed on either side of the bladder neck and tied above the rectus sheath (Fig. 18-13). The Pereyra technique employs a single loop of suture that has a tendency to cut out. As the prevesical fascia is not very tough, modifications have been made in these procedures to improve the purchase of the suture at the level of the bladder neck. The popular Stamey procedure has a buffer interposed to mitigate against tearing out. The modified Pereyra procedure involves the use of helical sutures through the deep pelvic fascia, while the modified Raz procedure goes further to include part of the vaginal wall. The Gittes procedure on the other hand uses the full thickness of the vaginal wall and as a result the sutures are exposed to the vaginal environment. However, by 6 weeks postoperatively the vagina has reepithelialized over the sutures. Some authorities are unhappy with this technique as it may result in excessive vaginal discharge in some cases. The overall 5-year success rate for these procedures is about 75%. It is suggested that this procedure be used for older women and those with a narrowed vagina in whom a retropubic procedure might be more difficult.

3. Retropubic procedures. The most commonly performed retropubic procedures are the Marshall Marchetti Kranz (MMK) procedure and the Burch colposuspension. Both involve the use of a Pfannenstiel incision and dissection in the space of Retzius. The bladder is dissected medially off the prevesical fascia and sutures are inserted at the level of the bladder neck. In the MMK procedure, these sutures (one on each side) are then attached to the periosteum of the symphysis pubis and thus elevate the bladder neck by elevating the vagina underneath. Some authorities are concerned with this procedure because of the risk of osteomyelitis of the pubic bone, which is very difficult to treat.

The Burch colposuspension is more popular because, unlike the MMK procedure, the sutures are not placed in the periosteum of the symphysis pubis, but rather into the iliopectineal ligament on either side, thus minimising the risk of osteitis pubis. Because three or four sutures can be used, the Burch colposuspension acts not only as an anti-incontinence procedure, but also can reduce a moderate cystocele or at least can convert a low asymptomatic cystocele to a high symptomatic cystocele. Long term follow up of these cases has shown an increased incidence of enterocele and posterior wall prolapse.[96]

The 5-year success rates for these retropubic procedures is thought to be around 85%, rising to 95% when carried out as a primary procedure. The success rate declines with increasing age of the patient, obesity, and previous surgery.[76]

None of the procedures described so far need to be obstructive to achieve continence. However there is frequently an element of postoperative obstruction to voiding. It is important to emphasize that the probability of success is not dependent upon the probability of inducing obstruction; patients who develop obstruction may not necessarily be continent. In the retropubic procedures, placement of the sutures is crucial. If the sutures are placed too distantly (paraurethral) then the patient is likely to have voiding difficulties, but if placed too proximally (by the side of the bladder), the patient is more likely to experience residual incontinence.

4. Slings. Many different sling procedures have been described. These can be placed either by the vaginal or the abdominal route, though using the vaginal route increases the danger of infection. The material that is used can be endogenous (e.g., rectus fascia), organic (e.g., porcine fascia), or inert (e.g., silastic). Sling procedures are designed to achieve continence by being obstructive; the degree of pull or elevation is crucial to the procedure, and for this reason the success with slings tends to be very operator dependent. The sling should not be used as a primary procedure, but should be reserved for surgical failures where the patient has a "fixed drain pipe" low pressure urethra. In such situations the success rate is not going to be very satisfactory.

5. Periurethral injections. The use of injectibles is an easier option in patients with intrinsic sphincter deficiency in whom a sling procedure would be indicated. Previously materials such as Teflon were injected into the periurethral tissues in order to increase urethral resistance. Complications included urethritis, abscess formation, and even migration of the Teflon particles to the lung and brain. For this reason other materials have been tried and currently GAX collagen shows much promise.[35] The injected material is thought to be replaced by endogenous collagen; therefore not only does it appear safe but also long lasting. Improvement rates for this technique are of the order of 80%. It is thought that these injectibles are ideally suited for patients who do not have bladder neck hypermobility.

6. Artificial sphincters. When all surgical procedures have failed, there is always the option of an artificial sphincter.[71] This is a technique whereby a cuff is placed around the urethra and the control bulb is inserted into the labia majora. By pressing the bulb, it is possible to activate and deactivate the cuff. Most authorities suggest that postoperatively the cuff should not be activated for several weeks until the surgical edema has settled down. As a closed system, if infection has not been introduced at the time of surgery, it is unlikely to develop subsequently. It is usual to deactivate the cuff at night to avoid cuff necrosis. Although expensive, artificial sphincters have transformed the lives of many women.

7. Failures. If all the above procedures fail, there is still a place for urinary diversion or reconstructive surgery. Some patients may not wish to subject themselves to yet another operation, or they may not be fit enough to undergo more surgery. For these patients the conservative option of using diapers and special pants is an option. There have been many advances in absorptive material over the last two decades; it would be advisable to obtain the help of a nurse specializing in palliative care of this sort. Excellent nursing care is essential as excoriation due to urine can be a most irritative and debilitating condition.

Detrusor instability and hyperreflexia

Etiology. Detrusor instability is defined as the occurrence of spontaneous detrusor contractions during the filling phase when the patient is attempting to inhibit micturition.[1] In practice any detrusor activity can be regarded as abnormal if it occurs inappropriately. It is the second most common cause of urinary incontinence in middle-aged women and accounts for about 35% of urogynecologic cases. The incidence increases with age and there appears to be a specific increase after menopause; detrusor instability may well be a condition that is estrogen sensitive.[87] In situations where it is secondary to an upper motor neuron lesion (for example, multiple sclerosis), the condition is known as detrusor hyperreflexia. However, in gynecologic practice the vast majority of cases are idiopathic. Detrusor instability in men is often secondary to outflow obstruction and tends to resolve after the obstruction is relieved, although this may take several months.[61] Outflow obstruction in women is rare. The bladder appears to be sexually differentiated in its response to acute obstruction. In women it tends towards decompensation with the sequel of a big floppy bladder. (See section on overflow incontinence). Some authorities believe that insidious obstruction in women, as in men, can result in detrusor instability. Certainly it is known that after antiincontinence surgery, 18% of women develop detrusor instability who did not have it preoperatively.[12] This may be the bladder's response to outflow obstruction or the operative procedure may have disrupted neural input at the level of the bladder neck.

Diagnosis. By cystometry the condition can be diagnosed during the filling phase if wavelike contractions are seen or if the pressure rise on bladder filling exceeds 15 cm of water. An abnormal detrusor contraction may be provoked when the patient changes posture (e.g., on standing) or following a cough. Some urogynecologists regard idiopathic low compliance as a different entity from detrusor instability; however, the symptoms are similar to detrusor instability as is the treatment. It now transpires that a reduction of the filling rate will exhibit phasic detrusor instability in many patients with idiopathic low compliance. There are a variety of causes for low compliance, including radical pelvic surgery, radiotherapy, recurrent urinary tract infections, and interstitial cystitis.

Although the clinical presentation is varied, frequency, nocturia, urgency, urge incontinence, and enuresis are often the symptoms associated with detrusor instability. Stress incontinence, however, is also a common complaint in patients with detrusor instability. In young women incontinence associated with orgasm is thought to be the result of detrusor instability.

Treatment. The main treatment is behavior modification with the help of pharmacologic agents. There are, however, legions of other treatments available (Table 18-5), but these merely reflect our inadequacy in treating this condition successfully.

Drug therapy. Many different types of drugs have been employed for the treatment of detrusor instability, and they can be broadly classified as in Table 18-5. Any drug, however, may have more than one mode of action. All drugs used in the management of these conditions tend to have side effects, and in particular anticholinergic side effects. Because there is such a high placebo response with this condition (up to 60%), it is very difficult to be certain about the efficacy of many of the agents that are currently used. Oxybutynin chloride is a muscle relaxant, but has anticholinergic properties. It has a short half-life and so has to be administered (3 or 5 mg) every 6 or 8 hours. There is a high incidence of side effects.[78] It is important therefore to raise the dose until a minimum of side effects is experienced by the patient, otherwise an inadequate dose is being administered. As there is so much patient variation, the dosage regimens have to be adjusted to suit each individual. Other useful drugs are emepronium caragenate (300 to 500 mg qid) and dicyclomine hydrochloride (20 mg qid). When nocturnal enuresis is a problem and to avoid side effects during the day, imipramine (50 mg at night) or desmopressin (20 μg at night) can be the drugs of choice. When frequency is the only problem, propantheline bromide (15 to 45 mg qid) can be effective. The use of prostaglandin synthetase inhibitors is less favored because of the high rate of side effects. As none of the available drugs are completely satisfactory, and as pharmacologic therapy is presently inadequate the new generation of calcium-channel blockers is eagerly awaited.

Table 18-5. Treatment of detrusor instability

Psychotherapy	Bladder drill Biofeedback Hypnotherapy

Drug therapy	Inhibit bladder contractions:
	  Anticholinergic agents
	  Muscle relaxants
	  Calcium channel blockers
	  Tricyclic antidepressants
	  Prostaglandin synthetase inhibitors
	Increase outlet resistance:
	  Alpha-adrenergic stimulants
	Local tissues:
	  Estrogens
	Reduce urine production:
	  Synthetic vasopressin

Denervation	Vaginal denervation Sacral neurectomy
Surgery	Bladder transection "Clam" ileocystoplasty Cystectomy and neo-bladder construction Urinary diversion

While rigorous proof demonstrating the validity of estrogen replacement therapy in postmenopausal women with urgency, frequency, and nocturia is lacking, it is thought that estrogen supplementation may raise the sensory threshold of the bladder.[24]

Behavior therapy. There is no evidence that long-term drug therapy is detrimental, but most patients prefer to take medication for only a short time. Thus the main treatment remains behavior modification in the form of bladder drill.[27] By examining the voiding diary, it is possible to determine what the average intervoid time is for any given patient. The patient is then instructed to increase this time even at the risk of incontinence. As the intervoid time increases so does the voided volume, and the result is the reduction in symptoms of detrusor instability. Indeed cystometry carried out after bladder drill shows that there is either reduction in the degree of instability or resolution of the condition. Such bladder training is more easily accomplished on an inpatient basis; even though less successful in the authors' experience, costs dictate that this should be carried out on an ambulatory basis.[28] The key to success lies in the relationship developed between the patient and the trainer, be it a nurse or a physician. Motivation is crucial as is constant encouragement and positive feedback.

Another successful treatment for detrusor instability is biofeedback.[58] This is a situation where the patient is catheterized and her bladder pressure is displayed to her numerically or graphically. Thus she is able to monitor the strength of her own detrusor contractions and is asked to try to inhibit them. While patients may not know how they achieve this, they certainly are able to do so with some practice. Unfortunately, as with other behavior modification techniques, it is time consuming and there is a significant relapse rate; patients need to reinforce this kind of feedback intermittently. Similarly hypnotherapy has had some success but needs reinforcing.[26]

Electrical stimulation. Intravaginal electrical stimulation results in activation of inhibitory nerve fibers in the sympathetic hypogastric nerve and reflex inhibition of detrusor contractility.[51] There have been some clinical reports suggesting that this method is useful in patients with detrusor instability.[23] However, given that the condition tends to fluctuate temporally and there is a high placebo response, larger, well-controlled trials are needed before this method is widely accepted.

Surgery. If the above measures have failed then surgery is an option, although this should not be taken lightly. It is only applicable to a small number of women who have failed to respond to conventional conservative therapy; many of these patients will have a significant neurologic abnormality. These patients should be treated at a tertiary referral center. The surgical options can be divided into those involving denervation and those requiring bladder augmentation.

Denervation. A large number of procedures have been devised including bladder distension, subtrigonal phenol injection, selective sacral nerve blockade, sacral neurectomy, and transvaginal bladder denervation. The postganglionic soma of the parasympathetic nerves supplying the bladder are located in the bladder wall. Bladder distention and phenol injections are likely to disrupt both preganglionic and postganglionic fibers. Other procedures designed to denervate the bladder effectively cause preganglionic section. This will result in a transient decrease in postganglionic activity and thus a reduction in detrusor instability. However, following recovery the situation may be worse than it was before. It is for this reason that denervation procedures are less favored.

Bladder transection. Transection of the bladder (either at laparotomy or via the cystoscope) above the level of the trigone has been advocated on the basis that the neuronal supply enters the bladder in conjunction with the inferior vesical artery. Thus circumferential transection should interrupt the distribution of neuronal supply while leaving sensation intact at the trigone.[80] A study has been reported indicating reasonably good results with this technique.[59]

Augmentation. The rationale for this is that by increasing bladder capacity and interposing a segment of bowel, the effect of detrusor activity is dampened. The most common and successful type of bladder augmentation is the "clam" ileocystoplasty.[60] This is a technique whereby the bladder is transected transversely so that it opens like a clam and a portion of detubularized ileum on its pedicle is sutured onto the defect. This has the effect of limiting the symptoms of detrusor instability but unfortunately these patients tend to have voiding dysfunction; intermittent self-catheterization often needs to be used as adjunctive therapy.

Urinary diversion. When all else fails, patients prefer urinary diversion to being a "bladder cripple" with all the social and medical consequences. These urinary diversion methods can be incontinent (ileal conduit) or continent. The latter involves the creation of an intraabdominal reservoir made from a portion of bowel that is emptied by intermittent catheterization.[33] The simplest form of a continent diversion is the Mitrofanoff procedure; the appendix or a portion of ureter is used as the catheterizable channel with a flap-valve type of continent mechanism interposed between it and the reservoir.

Mixed incontinence

Genuine stress incontinence and detrusor instability. There are some women with both detrusor instability and genuine stress incontinence—they pose a particular problem.[43] The overall cure rate for surgery in this group is of the order of 50%; pharmacological agents are successful in about a third of the cases. Added to these figures would be a small percentage of cases where there is significant improvement without a cure. The physician has to decide on the predominant condition and tailor therapy towards that. However, when it is difficult to decide, the safer approach is to treat the detrusor instability medically, and only resort to surgery when the residual incontinence is intolerable. Patients need counseling prior to such surgery and understand that bladder neck surgery may result in a competent sphincter, but that the detrusor instability may be aggravated by surgery.

Genuine stress incontinence and voiding dysfunction. Bladder neck surgery in these cases will lead to a worsening of voiding function postoperatively. For this reason pelvic floor exercises should be the first line of therapy. If this fails and surgery is contemplated, the patient should be taught clean, intermittent self-catheterization before operation. Surgery should only be performed if the patient accepts that indefinite self-catheterization may be the price for continence.

Detrusor instability and voiding dysfunction. If the voiding difficulty is due to detrusor dysfunction, bladder drill should be encouraged. If anticholinergic agents are used, the patient may develop retention and then have to resort to self-catheterization. If the voiding dysfunction is due to outflow obstruction, relief of the obstruction by urethrotomy may make the incontinence worse.

Overflow incontinence

Etiology. Overflow incontinence is defined as "any involuntary loss of urine associated with overdistention of the bladder[1]". Overdistention of the bladder may result from dysfunction of either the detrusor muscle or the urethral sphincter. Many etiologies are described and they may result in either acute or chronic symptoms.

Urinary retention because of detrusor dysfunction results from hyporeflexia or atony of the detrusor muscle. It is usually due to a lesion in the lower motor neurons supplying the bladder. Conditions associated with neurogenic urinary retention include cerebrovascular accident, multiple sclerosis, spinal cord injury, cauda equina tumors, diabetic neuropathy, AIDS peripheral neuropathy, and pelvic nerve damage secondary to radical pelvic surgery.[34] Detrusor dysfunction may also result from local inflammation, pharmacologic agents, and psychogenic causes.

Urethral obstruction can also cause overdistention of the bladder. Compromise of the outflow tract is common in men with prostatic hypertrophy, but may also occur in women from other causes. Obstruction in women may result from periurethral edema due to trauma, labor, or vaginal surgery. Occasionally a severe cystocele or uterine procidentia causes kinking and obstruction of the proximal urethra. Neurologic conditions can result in failure of the sphincter to relax appropriately during the micturition reflex. Such detrusor-sphincter dyssynergia may occur with upper motor neuron lesions such as cord section or Parkinson's disease.[34]

Diagnosis. The symptoms of overflow incontinence may be difficult to differentiate from stress incontinence. Typically leakage occurs with stress; patients may also complain of dribbling, hesitancy, and prolonged voiding. The physical examination will confirm the distended bladder and may provide evidence of a local cause. A careful neurologic examination of the sacral dermatomes, lower extremity motor function, and perineal reflexes should be performed and consultation sought for any abnormality. The diagnosis is confirmed by identifying an excessive postvoid residual volume by catheterization or ultrasound imaging. A cystometrogram will provide information about bladder sensation and bladder capacity. Voiding studies may assist in differentiating obstruction (high bladder pressure with low flow rate) from detrusor hyporeflexia (low bladder pressure with low flow rate).

Treatment. The treatment of overflow incontinence depends on the cause, although initial management will include drainage by catheterization. If retention is acute and due to a self-limited etiology, then continuous bladder drainage for 24 to 48 hours will suffice. Underlying conditions should be sought and treated. Pharmacologic agents such as muscle relaxants for outflow obstruction and cholinomimetic agents for hyporeflexia are not always successful.[95] Most cases of chronic retention will require management by intermittent self-catheterization.

Genitourinary fistula

A fistula that bypasses the normal sphincter mechanism may result in total incontinence. Worldwide, most fistulae are due to obstetrical trauma, either from necrosis secondary to prolonged pressure of the fetus in the birth canal or to operative intervention. Other causes include surgical trauma, malignancy, and irradiation.

Symptoms include the continuous loss of urine, vulvar irritation, passage of urine from the vagina, and recurrent infections. A large fistula will be visible on examination, but smaller tracts may be difficult to localize. Urinary dyes such as oral phenazopyridine (pyridium) may be helpful. Endoscopic and radiographic studies are necessary to determine if multiple tracts are present and to delineate the location of the fistula relative to the trigone and urethral sphincter.

Treatment of genitourinary fistulae is usually surgical but small lesions may heal spontaneously with long term drainage. Successful repair requires strict adherence to basic surgical principles. The fistulous tract must be identified and excised including all surrounding scar tissue. Wide mobilization of the tissue layers is necessary to assure reconstruction of normal anatomy without tension on the suture lines. If the blood supply is compromised, a vascular tissue pedicle such as the Martius labial-fat-pad graft may be interposed between the tissue layers.[21] Catheterization to divert the urinary stream and to prevent distention and stress on the suture lines is necessary during healing.

URETHRAL DIVERTICULUM

A urethral diverticulum is a saclike herniation of urethral mucosa through a defect in the muscular layer of the urethral wall. The cavity of the sac is connected to the urethral lumen by one or more small ostia. The true incidence of occurrence in the female population is not known. The reported incidence varies between 1% and 4%.[29] Increasing awareness of the condition among clinicians probably increases the frequency with which it is diagnosed. Diverticula occur most frequently in women between the ages of 30 to 50 years and may occur with a higher frequency in African-Americans.[14]

Diagnosis

Urethral diverticula are occasionally diagnosed in children suggesting a congenital etiology. These diverticula may arise from an inherent weakness in the urethral wall or from persistent mesonephric cell rests.[14] However, most diverticula are probably acquired lesions. One theory proposes that traumatic injury as occurs in childbirth, may disrupt the integrity of the urethral wall. However, the condition generally is not associated with increasing parity.[64] Others have suggested postinflammatory obstruction of the paraurethral glands as an etiology. An abscess cavity forms proximal to the obstruction and subsequent rupture into the lumen of the urethra results in a diverticulum. It is likely that inflammation is the commonest cause.[29]

The classic triad of symptoms associated with urethral diverticula consists of dysuria, dyspareunia, and postvoid dribbling. Other symptoms may be related to a urinary tract infection that is often associated. Included in this group are frequency, urgency, and hematuria. Occasionally a patient may complain of the presence of a palpable mass lesion. A significant number of patients are asymptomatic, and the condition is then diagnosed on the basis of physical findings.

Diverticula are differentiated from other vaginal cystic masses primarily by their location. A palpable mass in the anterior vaginal wall suggests a urethral diverticulum. Most diverticula are 1 to 3 cm in diameter and are located in the distal or middle third of the urethra.[4] The ostium almost always occurs on the posterior urethral wall and the mass is often tender. On palpation of the urethra, pus or urine may be expressed from the meatus.

Confirmation of the diagnosis is by imaging and endoscopic methods. A voiding cystourethrogram may demonstrate filling of the diverticulum with contrast media. If not, the urethra is filled under positive pressure using a special double-ballooned catheter. The balloons obstruct both the external meatus and the urethrovesical junction; contrast media can thereby be forced into even a narrow-necked diverticulum sac. Ultrasound imaging has been used successfully to delineate these lesions.[44] Urethroscopy allows direct visualization of the ostium and occasionally demonstrates more than one opening.

Treatment

Several surgical procedures have been recommended for the treatment of symptomatic urethral diverticula. In the setting of acute infection with cellulitis, simple incision and drainage is appropriate.[29] In a subacute situation, excision of the diverticulam sac through a vaginal incision is most often performed.[94] A small probe, a Fogarty balloon catheter, or dye may be placed in the sac to assist the dissection.[47] Care should be taken not to excise normal urethral tissue along with the sac. The defect is closed in several layers using fine suture material and without tension on the suture lines. Catheter drainage of the bladder is maintained for several days. If the diverticulum is located in the distal urethra, marsupialization can be performed.[73] An incision is made from the external meatus to the diverticular sac through the vaginal mucosa and urethral wall. The redundant tissue from the wall of the diverticulum is excised. The urethral mucosa is sewn to the vaginal mucosa to create a new urethral meatus, but this can result in spraying during micturition. This procedure can also result in iatrogenic incontinence if the incision includes the urethral sphincter mechanism. Other complications of diverticular surgery include urethral strictures, fistula formation, and recurrence of diverticula.

URINARY TRACT INFECTIONS

Etiology

The most common organism causing symptomatic or asymptomatic bacteriuria is *Escherichia coli. Proteus mirabilis* and other coliform organisms are also common pathogens. It is now recognized that coagulase-negative staphylococci are a cause of infection in young women. Less commonly *Klebsiella aerogenes* and *Pseudomonas* organisms along with *Streptoccus faecalis* can be urinary pathogens although such pathogens are usually nosocomial rather than primary domiciliary infective agents. Some organisms are difficult to isolate and special culture conditions are required for their identification. Examples of this are lactobacilli, corynebacteria and *Streptococcus milleri*. Similarly *Chlamydia trachomatis* may be a cause of "sterile" infection.

The best indication of a urinary tract infection is pyuria. However, it is possible to have this in the absence of bacteriuria as in patients with stones or papillary necrosis. Conversely many patients with bacteriologically proven infection do not have pyuria. Thus the diagnosis of a urinary tract infection is based on the demonstration of bacteriuria by microbiologic methods. Significant bacteriuria is taken to mean the presence of 100,000 organisms of the same type per mL of freshly plated urine. Counts below 10,000 per mL especially if mixed organisms are present, generally indicate contamination of urine rather than an infection. Counts in the region of 10^4 to 10^5 per mL are equivocal and require a repeat assessment. If diagnosis is difficult, it is best to obtain an early morning urine sample as stasis during the night results in a greater yield. Samples should be taken prior to instituting antibiotic therapy as this will confound the results of culture. If repeated urine samples are contaminated then recourse to suprapubic aspiration is justifiable.[50] This is rarely necessary if patients are carefully and thoroughly instructed on how to obtain a clean catch, mid-stream urine sample. Urethral catheterization for the purpose of obtaining a urine sample for bacteriologic examination is also possible. While a midstream specimen of urine examined and plated out for culture is the standard test for diagnosing a urinary tract infection, the recently introduced dip stick and other chemical methods are usually adequate for screening purposes. Nevertheless, as with all screening techniques, the false-negative rate has to be acceptably low.

Clinical picture

The prevalence of urinary tract infections increases with age, rising from 1% to 2% in schoolgirls to 5% in women of reproductive age; urinary infections become more common with increasing parity. The prevalence rates are found to increase dramatically in the elderly and are reported as over 40% in 90 year olds.[10,11] Recurring urinary tract infections do not necessarily result in pyelonephritis as ascending infections depend upon the presence of a vesico-ureteric reflux. In women with normal urinary tracts this is uncommon.

The vast majority of infections are single isolated episodes that either resolve spontaneously or are readily treated with antibiotics with no recurrence. Half of all women have experienced a urinary infection at least once. Some patients, however, have a predisposition to relapse despite sterilization of the urine by antibacterial treatment; there can be a recurrence of the disease within 7 to 14 days. This usually occurs in patients with stones and in those with scarred, damaged, or cystic kidneys, and occasionally in those patients with diverticula or ureteric stumps. Recurring infections, however, are more commonly the result of reinfection. Treatment failure may be due to inappropriate therapy, noncompliance, or poor absorption due to vomiting.

The pregnant woman is not more likely to harbor asymptomatic bacteriuria than her nonpregnant counterpart. The prevalence rates increase with age and parity, but may also be higher in lower socioeconomic groups. However, women with asymptomatic bacteriuria in early pregnancy have a low spontaneous clearance rate and a very high incidence of acute symptomatic urinary tract infections later in pregnancy. Also, while pregnant women may not be more susceptible to acquisition of infection, they do have a greater predisposition to upper tract infection, which is more serious. Thus a patient diagnosed with asymptomatic bacteriuria in early pregnancy should be treated promptly with antibiotics.

Investigation

In patients with recurring urinary tract infections, an anatomical cause should be sought. An intravenous urogram will detect anatomical or functional abnormalities of the upper tracts that may be correctable. Function of the lower urinary tract can be simply assessed by uroflowmetry and postmicturition ultrasound to detect the presence of a residual. If voiding difficulties are diagnosed (peak flow rate of <15 mL/second and a residual of >100 mL), then cystometry is indicated to determine whether the cause is due to outflow obstruction or poor detrusor contractility. Although providing a greater yield in the elderly, cystoscopy is nonetheless indicated in younger patients with recurring urinary tract infections.

Treatment

Primary infection. Prior to treatment, a midstream specimen of urine should be sent for culture and sensitivity, but treatment can be started while waiting for the bacterial sensitivities. The patient should be encouraged to have a high fluid intake (four pints a day) and the "best guess" antibiotics are co-trimoxazole (trimethoprim 160 mg + sulphamethoxazole 800 mg bid), ampicillin (500 mg tid) or nitrofurantoin (100 mg tid). In pregnancy co-trimoxizole and nitrofurantoin should be avoided. Concomitant treatment with potassium citrate can also be symptomatically helpful. Antibiotic therapy should take place for 5 to 7 days though there is evidence that a 3 day course of therapy may be adequate and even a single large dose (3 g) of amoxicillin gives a high cure rate in uncomplicated cases.[6] Symptoms should usually improve in 48 hours, but if not, the pretreatment urine culture sensitivity should be rechecked.

Recurrent infection. These patients should have a more prolonged antibiotic course of 10 to 15 days and if relapse still occurs then special investigations are indicated. Reinfection on the other hand is much more common and this is best treated by explaining prophylaxis to the patient. She should be encouraged to have a high fluid intake and to void every 2 to 3 hours. If there is evidence of reflux, then the patient should be encouraged to practice double or triple micturition. If postcoital infection is a problem then patients should be encouraged to void immediately after sexual intercourse.[49] For those women in whom postcoital infection is common, prophylaxis with a single dose of antibiotic following coitus is often helpful. In some cases long term low-dose antibiotic prophylaxis may be indicated. The drugs of choice are nitrofurantoin (50 to 100 mg) or trimethoprim (100 mg) last thing at night. Treatment can be continued for as long as 12 months.

Patients with urinary catheters are more prone to infection although those with a urethral catheter are twice as likely to have an infection as those with a suprapubic catheter.

Patients with an ileal conduit, a neurogenic bladder, or multiple calculi are likely to have frequent infections. Such patients should only be treated when they become symptomatic as frequent, multiple antibacterial therapy in these patients will only result in the emergence of polyresistant recalcitrant strains of bacteria which will be very difficult to treat.

In postmenopausal women there is some evidence to suggest that hormone replacement therapy reduces the incidence of urinary tract infections.[13,68]

REFERENCES

1. Abrams P et al: The standardization of terminology of lower urinary tract function, *Br J Obstet Gynaecol* 97 (suppl 6):1-16, 1990.
2. Ahlstrom K et al: Effect of combined treatment with phenylpropanolamine and estriol compared with estriol treatment alone, in postmenopausal women with stress urinary incontinence, *Gynecol Obstet Invest* 30:37, 1990.
3. Allen RE et al: Pelvic floor damage and childbirth: a neurophysiological study, *Brit J Obstet Gynaecol* 97:770-779, 1990.
4. Andersen MJF: The incidence of diverticula in the female urethra, *J Urol* 98:96-98, 1967.
5. Asmussen M, Ulmsten U: Simultaneous urethrocystometry and urethral pressure profile measurement with a new technique, *Acta Obstet Gynaecol Scand* 54:385-388, 1975.
6. Bailey RR, Abbott GD: Treatment of a urinary tract infection with a single dose of amoxicillin, *Nephron* 18:316-318, 1977.
7. Bonney V: On diurnal incontinence of urine in women, *J Obstet Gynaecol Br Emp* 30:358-365, 1923.
8. Bradley WE et al: Neurology of micturition, *J Urol* 115:481-486, 1976.
9. Brocklehurst JC: Urinary incontinence in the community—an analysis of a MORI poll, *Br Med J* 306:832-834, 1993.
10. Brocklehurst JC et al: The prevalence and symptomatology of urinary infection in an aged population, *Geront Clin* 10:242-253, 1968.
11. Brocklehurst JC et al: Urinary infections and symptoms of dysuria in women aged 45-64 years: their relevance to similar findings in the elderly, *Age Aging* 1:41-47, 1972.
12. Cardozo LD, Stanton SL, Williams JE: Detrusor instability following surgery for genuine stress incontinence, *Br J Urol* 51: 204-207, 1979.
13. Cardozo L, and Versi E: Estrogens and the lower urinary tract. In Asch RH and Studd JWW editors: *Annual progress in reproductive medicine*, Carnforth, UK, 1993, Parthenon Publishing Group.
14. Coddington CC, Knab DR: Urethral diverticulum: a review, *Obstet Gynecol Surv* 38:357-364, 1983.
15. Crelin ES: Normal and abnormal development of ureter, *Urology* 112:2-7, 1978.
16. DeLancey JOL: Anatomy and embryology of the lower urinary tract, *Obstet Gynecol Clin NA* 16:717-731, 1989.
17. DeLancey JOL: Anatomy and physiology of urinary incontinence, *Clin Obstet Gynaecol* 33:298-307, 1990.
18. deMartino C, Zamboni L: A morphologic study of the mesonephros of the human embryo, *J Ultrastuct Res* 16:399-427, 1966.
19. Dixon JS, Gosling JA: The role of the pelvic floor in female urinary incontinence, *Int Urogynecol J* 1:212-217, 1990.
20. Drutz HP: Neurophysiology and neuropharmacology of the lower urinary tract, *Int Urogynecol J* 1:91-99, 1990.
21. Elkins TE, DeLancey JOL, McGuire EJ: The use of modified Martius graft as an adjunctive technique in vesicovaginal and rectovaginal fistula repair, *Obstet Gynecol* 75:727-733, 1990.
22. Enhorning G: Simultaneous recording of the intravesical and intraurethral pressures, *Acta Obstet Gynecol Scand* 276 (suppl):1-68, 1961.
23. Fall M: Does electrostimulation cure urinary incontinence? *J Urol* 131:664, 1984.
24. Fantl JA et al: Postmenopausal urinary incontinence: comparison between nonestrogen supplement and estrogen-supplemented women, *Obstet Gynecol* 71:823-826, 1988.
25. Farquharson DM et al: The short-term effect of radical hysterectomy on urethral and bladder function, *Br J Obstet Gynaecol* 94:341-347, 1987.
26. Freeman RM, Baxby K: Hypnotherapy for incontinence caused by the unstable detrusor, *Br Med J* 1:1831, 1982.
27. Frewen WK: An objective assessment of the unstable bladder of psychosomatic origin, *Br J Urol* 50:246, 1978.
28. Frewen WK: A reassessment of bladder training in detrusor dysfunction in the female, *Br J Urol* 54:372, 1982.
29. Ginsburg DS, Genadry R: Suburethral diverticulum in the female, *Obstet Gynecol Surv* 39:1-7, 1984.
30. Gosling JA et al: A comparative study of the human external sphincter and periurethral levator ani muscles, *Brit J Urol* 53:35-41, 1981.

31. Gosling JA, Dixon JS, Lendon RG: The autonomic innervation of the human male and female bladder neck and proximal urethra, *J Urol* 118:302-305, 1977.
32. Grobstein C: Inductive interaction in the development of the mouse metanephros, *J Exp Zool* 130:319-335, 1955.
33. Hendren WH: Urinary tract undiversion. In Welch KJ et al, editors: *Paediatric surgery*, ed 4, Chicago, 1986, Yearbook Medical.
34. Herbaut AG: Neurogenic urinary retention, *Int Urogynecol J* 4:221-228, 1993.
35. Herschorn S, Steele D, Radomski S: Intraurethral collagen for female stress incontinence, *Neurourol Neurodynam* 12:437-439, 1993.
36. Hofmeister FJ: Pelvic anatomy of the ureter in relation to surgery performed through the vagina, *Clin Obstet Gynecol* 25:821-830, 1982.
37. Hu TW: Impact of urinary incontinence on health care costs. In NIH Consensus Development Conference: *Urinary Incontinence in Adults*, National Institute of Health, 1988.
38. Huffman JW: The detailed anatomy of the paraurethral ducts in the adult human female, *Am J Obstet Gynecol* 55:86-100, 1948.
39. Hurt WG: Histology of the urinary bladder and urethra in the female, *AUGS Quarterly Report* 6 (1), 1988.
40. Jarvis GJ et al: An assessment of urodynamic examination in incontinent women, *Br J Obstet Gynaecol* 87:893-896, 1980.
41. Jolleys JV: Reported prevalence of urinary incontinence in women in general practice, *Br Med J* 296: 1300-1302, 1988.
42. Karram MM, Bhatia NN: The Q-Tip test: standardization of the technique and its interpretation in women with urinary incontinence, *Obstet Gynecol* 71:807-811, 1988.
43. Karram MM, Bhatia NN: Management of coexistent stress and urge urinary incontinence, *Obstet Gynecol* 73:4-7, 1989.
44. Keefe B et al: Diverticula of the female urethra: diagnosis by endovaginal and transperineal sonography, *Am J Roentgenol* 156: 1195-1197, 1991.
45. Kegel AH: Progressive resistance exercise in the functional restoration of the perineal muscles, *Am J Obstet Gynecol* 56:238-248, 1948.
46. Kelleher CJ, Khullar V, Cardozo LD: Psychoneuroticism and quality of life impairment in healthy incontinent women, *Neurourol Urodynam* 12: 393-394, 1993.
47. Kohorn EI, Glickman MG, Technical aids in investigation and management of urethral diverticula in the female, *Urol* 40:322-325, 1992.
48. Kondo A et al: Prevalence of hand-washing incontinence in healthy subjects in relation to stress and urge incontinence, *Neurourol Urodynam*, 11:519-523, 1992.
49. Kunin CM: Sexual intercourse and urinary infection, *N Eng J Med* 278:336-338, 1978.
50. Kunin CM: Detection, prevention and managment of urinary tract infections, ed 3, Philadelphia, 1979, Lea & Febiger.
51. Lindstrom S et al: The neuro-physiological basis of bladder inhibition in response to electrical stimulation, *J Urol* 129:405-410, 1983.
52. Lose G, Versi E: Pad-weighing tests in the diagnosis and quantification of urinary incontinence, *Int Urogynecol J* 3:324-328, 1992.
53. Magee MC, Lucey DT, Fried FA: A new embryologic classification for urogynecologic malformations: the syndromes of mesonephric duct induced müllerian deformities, *J Urol* 121:265-267, 1979.
54. Mantle J, Versi E: Physiotherapy for stress urinary incontinence: a national survey, *Br Med J* 302:753-755, 1991.
55. Minaire P, Buzelin JM: Epidemiology of urinary incontinence. In Stag A, editor: *Urinary incontinence,* Edinburgh, 1992, Churchill Livingstone.
56. Minaire P, Jacquetin B: La prevalence de l' incontinence urinare feminine en medicine generale, *J Gynecol Obstet Biol Repro* 26:731-738, 1992.
57. Molander U et al: An epidemiological study of urinary incontinence and related urogenital symptoms in elderly women, *Maturitas* 12:5160, 1990.
58. Moore KM et al: One-shot biofeedback in relation to psychoneurotic status and treatment response in detrusor instability, *Neurourol Urodynam* 11:365-366, 1992.
59. Mundy AR: Long-term results of bladder transection for urge incontinence, *Br J Urol* 55:642, 1983.
60. Mundy AR: The surgical approach to the treatment of incontinence due to drug resistant detrusor instability with particular reference to "clam" ileocystoplasty, *World J Urol* 4:45, 1986.
61. Mundy AR: The aetiology of detrusor instability. In Drife Jo, Hilton P, Stanton SL, editors: *Micturition*, London, 1990, Springer-Verlag.
62. Norton P, Boyd C, Deak S: Collagen synthesis in women with genital prolapse or stress urinary incontinence, *Neurourol Urodyn* 11:300-301, 1992.
63. Oelrich TM: The striated urogenital sphincter muscle in the female, *Anat Rec* 205:223-232, 1983.
64. Pathak U, House M: Diverticulum of the female urethra, *Obstet Gynecol* 36:789-794, 1970.
65. Peattie AB, Plevnik S, Stanton SL: Vaginal cones: a conservative method of treating genuine stress incontinence, *Br J Obstet Gynaecol* 95:1049-1053, 1988.
66. Quinn MJ. Vaginal ultrasound and urinary stress incontinence. In Drife Jo, Hilton P, Stanton SL, editors: *Micturition*, London, 1990, Springer-Verlag.
67. Rai R, Versi E: Alternatives to surgery for stress incontinence. In Studd EJ, editor: *Progress in obstetrics & gynaecology*, vol 10, 1993, Churchill Livingstone.
68. Raz R, Stamm A: A controlled trial of intravaginal estriol in post menopausal women with recurrent urinary tract infections, *N Eng J Med* 329:753-756, 1993.
69. Rud T et al: Factors maintaining the intraurethral pressure in women, *Invest Urol* 17:343-347, 1980.
70. Sand PK, Hill RC, Ostergard DR: Incontinence history as a predictor of detrusor instability, *Obstet Gynecol* 71:257-260, 1988.
71. Scott FB, Bradley WE, Timm GW: Treatment of urinary incontinence by an implantable prosthetic sphincter, *Urology* 1:252-259, 1973.
72. Shepherd AM, Powell PH, Ball AJ: The place of urodynamic studies in the investigation and treatment of female urinary tract symptoms, *J Obstet Gynaecol* 3:123-125, 1982.
73. Spence H, Duckett J: Diverticulum of the female urethra: clinical aspects and presentation of simple operative technique for cure, *J Urol* 104:432-437, 1970.
74. Stanton SL: Classification of incontinence. In Stanton SL, editor: *Clinical gynecologic urology*, St. Louis, 1984, CV Mosby.
75. Stanton SL. Surgical management of urethral sphincter incompetence. In Norton PA, editor: Urinary incontinence, *Clinical Obstetrics and Gynecology* 1990; 33:346-357.
76. Stanton SL, Cardozo LD: Results of colposuspension operation for incontinence and prolapse, *Br J Obstet Gynaecol* 86:693-697, 1979.
77. Tanagho EA, Smith DR: Mechanism of urinary incontinence. 1. Embryologic, anatomic, and pathologic considerations, *J Urol* 100:640-646, 1968.
78. Tapp AJS et al: The treatment of detrusor instability in postmenopausal women with oxybutynin chloride: a double blind placebo controlled study, *Br J Obstet Gynaecol*, 97:521-526, 1990.
79. Thomas TM et al: Prevalence of urinary incontinence, *Br Med J* 281:1243-1245, 1980.
80. Turner-Warwick RT, Ashken MH: The functional results of partial, subtotal, and total cystoplasty with special reference to ureterocystoplasty, selective sphincterotomy, and caecocystoplasty, *Br J Urol* 39:3-12, 1967.
81. Urinary Incontinence Guideline Panel: *Urinary incontinence in adults: clinical practice guidelines*, AHCPR Pub. No. 92-0038. Rockville, MD: Agency for Health Care Policy and Research, Public Health Service, U.S. Department of Health and Human Services, March, 1992.

82. Vaughn ED, Middleton GW: Pertinent genitourinary embryology: review for the practicing urologist, *Urol* 6:139-149, 1975.
83. Vellas B, Sedeuilh M, Albarede JL: Urinary incontinence: epidemiological consideration. *Danish Medical Bulletin* (Suppl 8) 3-9, 1989.
84. Versi E: Effect of hysterectomy on bowel function, *Br Med J* 299:680, 1989.
85. Versi E: Discriminant analysis of urethral pressure profilometry data for the diagnosis of genuine stress incontinence, *Br J Obstet Gynaecol* 97:251-259, 1990.
86. Versi E: The significance of an open bladder neck in women, *Br J Urol* 61:42-43, 1991.
87. Versi E: The bladder in menopause: lower urinary tract dysfunction during the climacteric, *Curr Probl Obstet Gynecol Fert* 17:193-232, 1994.
88. Versi E, Cardozo LD. Urethral instability: diagnosis based on variations in the maximum urethral pressure in normal climacteric women, *Neurourol Urodynam* 5:535-542, 1986.
89. Versi E, Cardozo LD: Urodynamics. In Studd JWW, editor: *Progress in obstetrics and gynaecology,* vol 8, 1990, Churchill Livingstone.
90. Versi E et al: Symptoms analysis for the diagnosis of genuine stress incontinence, *Br J Obstet Gynaecol* 98:815-819, 1991.
91. Versi E, Cardozo L, Cooper DJ: Urethral pressures: analysis of transmission pressure ratios, *Br J Urol* 68: 266-270, 1991.
92. Versi E, Cardozo LD, Studd J: Distal urethral compensatory mechanisms in women with an incompetent bladder neck who remain continent, *Neurourol Urodynam* 9:579-590, 1990.
93. Versi E et al: Internal urinary sphincter in maintenance of female continence, *Br Med J* 292: 166-167, 1986.
94. Ward J, Draper J, Tovell H: Diagnosis and treatment of urethral diverticula in the female, *Surg Gynecol Obstet* 125:1293-1300, 1967.
95. Wheeler JS, Walter JS: Urinary retention in females: a review, *Int Urogynecol J* 3:137-142, 1992.
96. Wiskind AK, Creighton SM, Stanton SL: The incidence of genital prolapse following the Burch colposuspension operation, *Neurourol Urodynam* 10:453-454, 1991.
97. Woodburne RT: Anatomy of the bladder and bladder outlet, *J Urol* 100:474-487, 1968.
98. Zornow DH: Embryology of urinary incontinence, *Urol* 10:293-300, 1977.

Chapter 19

MENOPAUSE

Brian W. Walsh

Menopause is defined as the permanent cessation of menses. This is only one aspect of the climacteric, during which time women undergo endocrine, somatic, and psychologic changes that span several years. Because these changes are related both to aging and to estrogen depletion, it is difficult to quantify the respective effects of each. This chapter addresses the consequences of declining estrogen production in postmenopausal women and the risks and benefits of hormonal replacement therapy.

AGING OF THE OVARY

The mean age of women at menopause is 51 years; approximately 4% of women undergo a natural menopause before 40 years of age (Fig. 19-1).[119] The age at which menopause occurs is *not* influenced by prolonged periods of hypothalamic amenorrhea, number of pregnancies, or oral contraceptive use. Although life expectancy has risen considerably during the twentieth century, the average age at menopause has not changed since antiquity.[3] Thus women in industrialized countries today will spend one third of their life span after ovarian failure.

The aging process of the ovary appears to begin during fetal development. Although 7 million oogonia are present at 20 weeks' gestation, only 700,000 remain at birth.[146] Following birth, the number of oocytes continues to decline even before the onset of puberty.

For several years prior to menopause, estradiol and progesterone production decline despite the occurrence of ovulatory cycles.[150] This waning of ovarian follicular activity reduces the negative feedback inhibition of estradiol on the hypothalamic-pituitary system, resulting in a gradual rise in follicle-stimulating hormone (FSH). The remaining ovarian follicles are increasingly those which are less responsive to FSH; menopause occurs when the residual follicles are refractory to elevated concentrations of FSH.

Estrogen production by the postmenopausal ovary is minimal (Fig. 19-2). The major source of postmenopausal estrogens is adrenal androgens, particularly androstenedione, which undergoes aromatization by peripheral tissues to

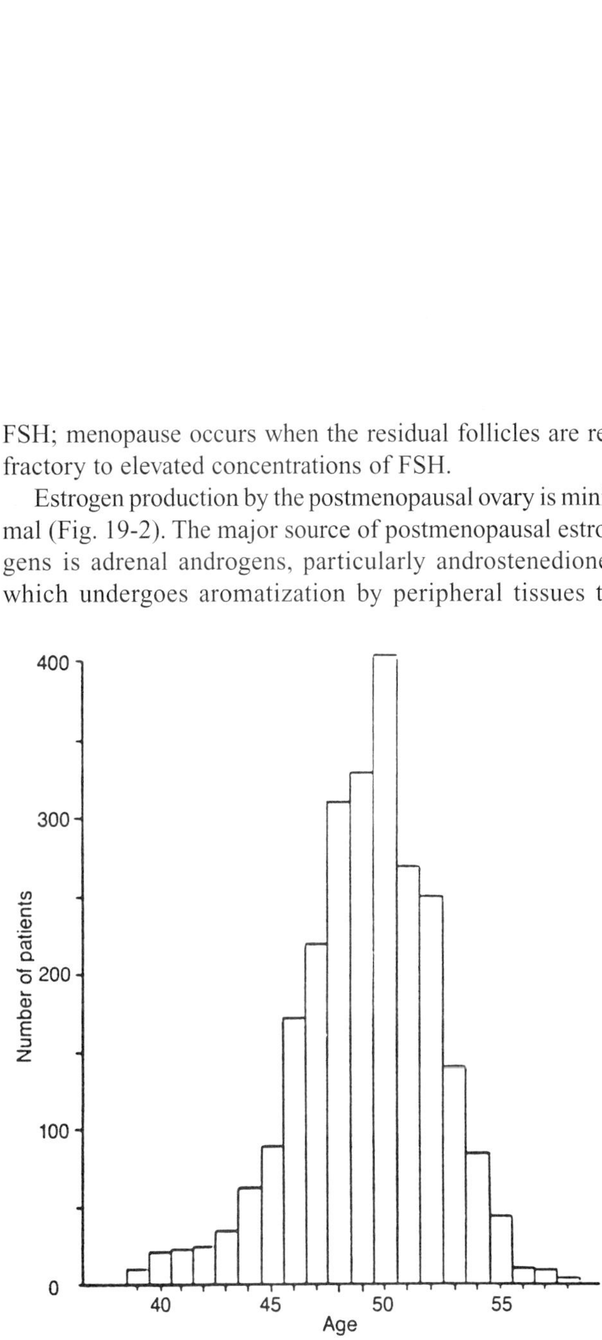

Fig. 19-1. Age of menopause in 2000 women during a natural menopause. (From Gambrell RD Jr: The menopause: benefits and risks of estrogen-progesterone replacement therapy, *Fertil Steril* 32:457, 1982.)

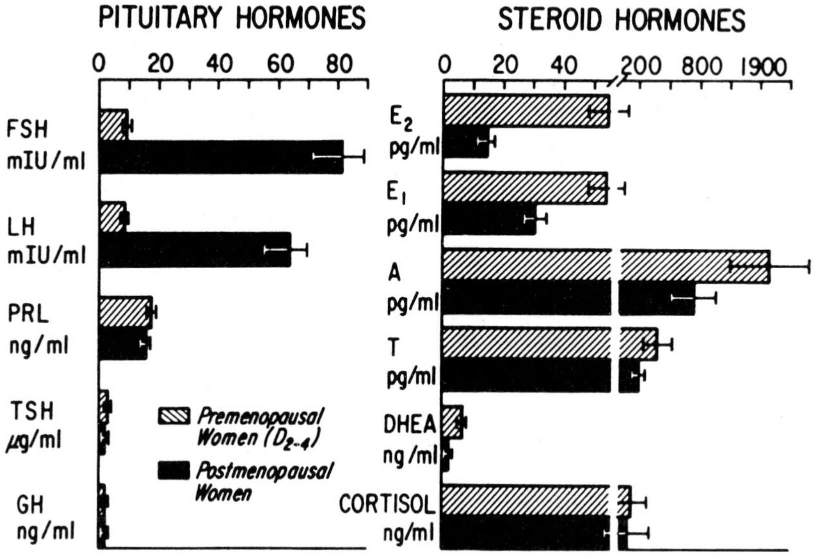

Fig. 19-2. Circulating concentrations of pituitary and steroid hormones in premenopausal (menstrual cycle day 2-4) and postmenopausal women. (From Yen SSC: The biology of menopause, *J Reprod Med* 18:28, 1977.)

estrone. Typically 2.8% of androstenedione is converted to estrone, but higher rates are seen in obese women who have more adipose tissue to aromatize androgens.[68] This explains in part why obese women have fewer menopausal symptoms compared with thin women.[50] The mean postmenopausal concentration of estrone (35 pg/mL) is higher than the mean concentration of estradiol (13 pg/mL).[175] This estradiol is produced by conversion from estrone.

The postmenopausal ovary continues to produce testosterone and androstenedione primarily from stromal and hilar cells (Fig. 19-3). The mean concentration of testosterone in postmenopausal women (approximately 250 pg/mL) is slightly lower than that of premenopausal women. In contrast, the mean postmenopausal concentration of androstenedione (850 pg/mL) is approximately half that of premenopausal women (1500 pg/mL).[175] Because these postmenopausal androgens are no longer opposed by estrogens, they may lead to increased hair growth on the upper lip and the chin.

VASOMOTOR FLUSHES

Vasomotor flushes are one of the most frequent and troublesome symptoms for women at the climacteric; approximately 80% of women experience hot flashes within 3 months of a natural or a surgical menopause. Of these women 85% have them for more than 1 year and 25% to 50% for up to 5 years.[171] For most women the onset of hot flashes occurs

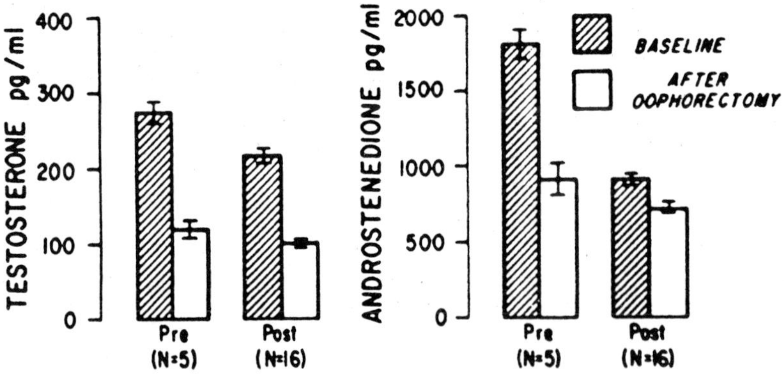

Fig. 19-3. Serum testosterone and androstenedione levels before and 6 to 8 weeks after bilateral oophorectomy. Five premenopausal (Pre) and 16 postmenopausal (Post) women were studied. (From Judd HL, Lucas WE, Yen SSC: Effect of oophorectomy on tetosterone and androstenedione levels, *Am J Obstet Gynecol* 118:793, 1974.)

before the final menstrual period. Ultimately hot flashes lessen in frequency and intensity with advancing age, unlike other sequelae of the menopause that progress with time.

Definitions and pathophysiology

Hot flashes are the subjective sensation of intense warmth of the upper body and range in duration from 30 seconds to 5 minutes but typically last for 4 minutes.[24] They frequently follow a prodrome of palpitations or a sensation of pressure within the head and may be accompanied by weakness, faintness, or vertigo. They usually end in sweating and a cold sensation.

The frequency of hot flashes varies from several per year to many per day. They tend to occur more frequently at night and may awaken the woman. This was shown by Erlik, who monitored the stages of sleep using the sleep polygraph (electroencephalogram, electromyelogram, and electrooculogram) while he simultaneously recorded finger temperature and skin resistance as objective indices of vasomotor flushes (Fig. 19-4).[52] The waking episodes were indeed temporally associated with the occurrence of hot flashes. The resultant poor quality of sleep may lead to chronic fatigue, characterized by symptoms such as irritability, poor concentration, and impaired memory.

A *vasomotor flush* is the objective component of this phenomenon and is characterized by a visible ascending flush of the thorax, neck, and face. First peripheral blood flow increases, particularly to the fingers, and skin temperature reaches a maximum 5 minutes later. This increase in blood flow appears to be limited to the cutaneous vasculature and does not involve blood flow to muscle; thus blood pressure remains stable during a flush. The loss of body heat through the skin causes the core body temperature to fall.[111] The final event occurs when the plasma luteinizing hormone (LH) level rises and reaches its peak 12 minutes after the flush begins.

Etiology

Hot flashes result from the withdrawal of estrogens, not from hypoestrogenism *per se*. They therefore accompany the menopause, whether it be natural, surgical, or "medical" (i.e., hypoestrogenism induced by the use of long-acting gonadotropin-releasing hormone agonists, or by danazol). The discontinuation of exogenous estrogens may precipitate flashes; for example, women with Turner's syndrome, who are hypoestrogenic, do not have hot flashes unless exogenous estrogens have been prescribed and later are withdrawn.[188]

Obese women tend to be less troubled by hot flashes; those who experience minimal symptoms at the menopause weigh considerably more than those who are severely symptomatic.[50] Obese women are relatively "protected" from hot flashes since they are functionally less hypoestrogenic for

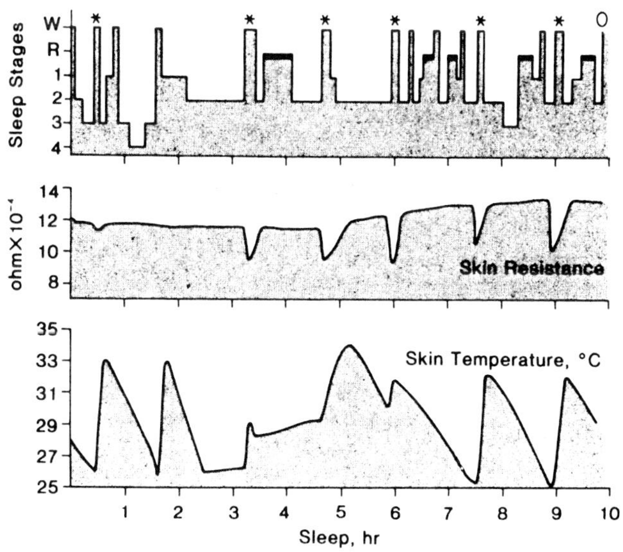

Fig. 19-4. Sleepgram and recordings of skin resistance and temperature in a postmenopausal subject with severe hot flashes. Asterisks denote objectively measured hot flashes. (From Erlik Y et al: Association of waking episodes with menopausal hot flushes, *JAMA* 245:1741, 1981b.)

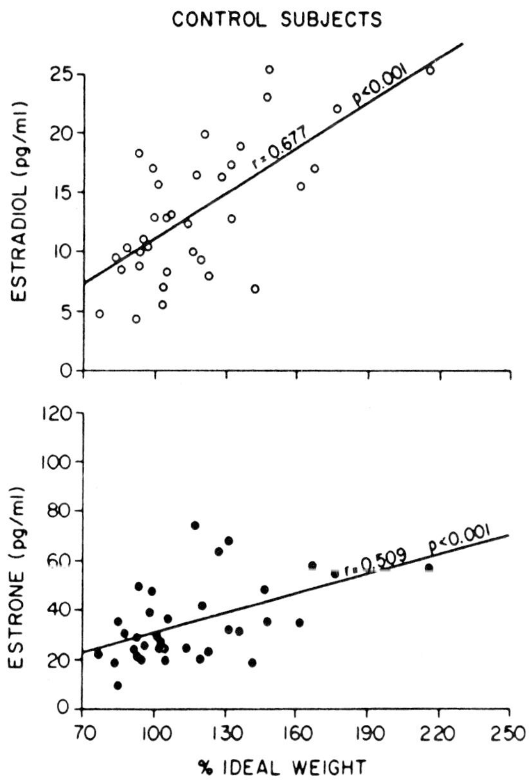

Fig. 19-5. Correlation of plasma estradiol and estrone levels with percentage of ideal weight in postmenopausal women. (From Judd HL et al: Serum androgens and estrogens in postmenopausal women, *Am J Obstet Gynecol* 136:859, 1980.)

the two following reasons: (1) their increased adiposity allows for greater peripheral conversion of adrenal androgens into estrogens,[68] and (2) their sex hormone-binding globulin levels are typically lower, and as a result a greater proportion of their estrogens are unbound and are free to act on target tissues (Fig. 19-5).[39]

Men also may have hot flashes, but these are a consequence of testosterone withdrawal. They develop in 77% of men treated with long-acting GnRH agonists, which lower serum testosterone to castrate levels.[156] Similarly, 62% of men developing testicular insufficiency have flashes, which are considerably alleviated by testosterone replacement.[127] Approximately 76% of men who undergo orchiectomy for prostatic cancer will have flashes.[26] Treatment with estrogens will provide relief, but symptoms may return when estrogen treatment is discontinued.[80] Androgens do not need to be converted to estrogen to suppress hot flashes because a nonaromatizable androgen, fluoxymesterone, effectively relieves them.[41]

Vasomotor flushes are caused by an acute lowering of the set point of the thermoregulatory center located in the hypothalamus which is precipitated by estrogen withdrawal. The presence of estrogen may serve to "stabilize" the thermoregulatory center by maintaining hypothalamic opioid activity. The loss of estrogen at menopause may cause a hypothalamic "opioid withdrawal", leading to thermoregulatory instability. This hypothesis is supported by the observation that estrogen prescribed in physiologic amounts induces hypothalamic opioid activity.[38]

Estrogen's stabilizing effect on the hypothalamic thermoregulatory center can be mediated by neurotransmitters such as norepinephrine (NE). As shown in Fig. 19-6,[13] the intraneuronal level of NE is regulated by the balance between the enzymes tyrosine hydroxylase (the rate-limiting step of NE synthesis from tyrosine) and monoamine oxidase (which irreversibly degrades NE to inactive metabolites). After synthesis, NE is stored in prejunctional vesicles; when released into the synaptic cleft, it binds to postjunctional receptors to propagate a response, either excitatory or inhibitory. This action is terminated by the rapid reuptake of NE back into the postjunctional neuron.

In animals, estrogen has multiple effects on NE neurons. It stimulates tyrosine hydroxylase activity,[11] thereby increasing NE synthesis. In addition, estrogen reduces monoamine oxidase activity,[105] and so retards NE degradation. Both of these actions increase the intraneuronal level of NE. Estrogen also augments NE release[131] and inhibits NE reuptake,[126] thereby potentiating its effect on postjunctional receptors. Finally estrogen appears to increase the number of hypothalamic α_2 postsynaptic receptors.[85] All of these actions enhance α_2 adrenergic activity. Since this work was performed on animals, it is not definitively known if estrogen has the same effects in humans. Nevertheless, these findings suggest that estrogens enhance α_2 adrenergic activity, and that estrogen withdrawal may lead to vasomotor flushes as a result of reduced α_2 adrenergic activity.

This hypothesis is further supported by the finding that α_2 agonists, such as clonidine,[32] aldomet (after conversion to

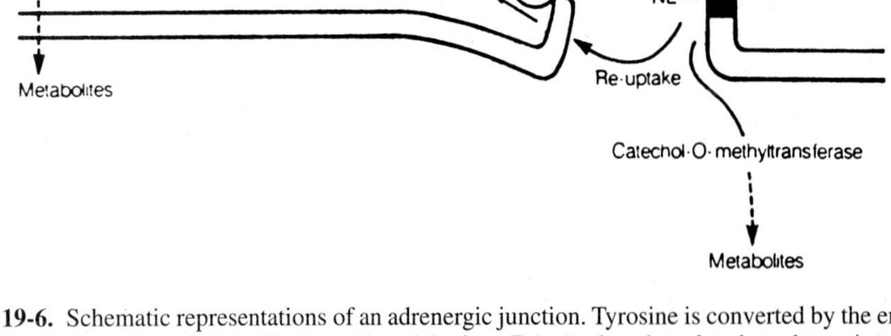

Fig. 19-6. Schematic representations of an adrenergic junction. Tyrosine is converted by the enzyme tyrosine hydroxylase to 3,4-dihydroxyphenylalanine (Dopa), decarboxylated to dopamine (DA), hydroxylated to form norepinephrine (NE), and stored in vesicles. On release, NE interacts with adrenergic receptors. This action is terminated by reuptake of NE back into the prejunctional neurons. NE is degraded into inactive metabolites by monoamine oxidase (MAO) and catechol-O-methyltransferase. (From Berkow R, editor: *The Merck manual of diagnosis and therapy,* Rahway, NJ, 1987, Merck, Sharp & Dohme Research Laboratories, p 2474.)

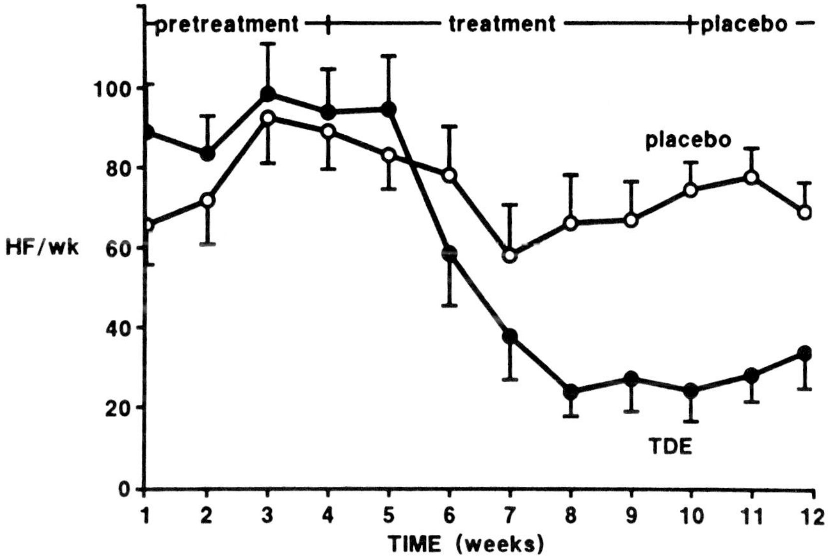

Fig. 19-7. Change in subjective hot flushes (HF) recorded by postmenopausal women treated with transdermal estrogen (TDE) and placebo. (From Haas S et al: The effect of transdermal estradiol on hormone and metabolic dynamics over a 6-week period, *Obstet Gynecol* 1988; 71:671, 1988)

its active form, methylnorepinephrine),[70] and lofexidine,[86] all suppress hot flashes. This is consistent with the observation that yohimbine, which inhibits presynaptic α_2 receptors, provokes hot flashes.[58] This further explains why estrogen treatment must be given for 2 to 4 weeks before hot flashes are maximally relieved[69] because they do not act directly but must alter central NE metabolism. This alteration of NE metabolism may persist for a short time after estrogen withdrawal, explaining why relief of hot flashes continues for a few weeks after estrogens are discontinued.

Diagnosis

The history and physical examination should be sufficient both to make the diagnosis and exclude other conditions that may resemble hot flashes such as thyrotoxicosis, carcinoid tumor, pheochromocytoma, anxiety, diabetic insulin reaction, alcohol withdrawal, and diencephalic epilepsy. Any drug or process that releases histamine, vasoactive peptide (substance P), or prostaglandin may induce flushes; these include nitroglycerine, nifedipine, niacin, vancomycin, calcitonin, ethanol, monosodium glutamate, disulfiram, and corticotropin-releasing hormone. Menopause may be confirmed by demonstrating an elevated serum FSH. However, a low serum estradiol level is not diagnostic because premenopausal women frequently have low levels during menses.

Treatment

Estrogens. Because hot flashes result from estrogen withdrawal, the obvious choice for therapy is estrogen replacement; this has greater than 95% efficacy. By relieving hot flashes, particularly those occurring at night, estrogen replacement improves sleep quality; estrogen treatment has been shown to reduce sleep latency and to increase rapid-eye-movement sleep.[142] In a double-blind, placebo-controlled study, estrogen use decreased insomnia, irritability, and anxiety, and improved memory.[20] Thus those symptoms which appear to result from a chronic sleep disturbance are significantly improved by estrogen replacement.

Treatment with estrogen does not produce immediate relief of hot flashes (Fig. 19-7).[69] Hot flash frequency is not reduced until after 2 weeks of treatment and is not maximal until 4 weeks. Thus treatment for 1 month is necessary to evaluate the adequacy of a particular dose in relieving flashes. After 1 month the dose may be increased because there appears to be a dose-response relationship between the dose of estrogen and the degree to which hot flashes are suppressed. For example, 3 weeks of treatment with transdermal estradiol 0.025 mg reduces flashes by 40%, 0.05 mg by 53%, 0.10 mg by 83%, and 0.20 mg by 91%.[162]

Estrogen replacement is not a permanent cure for hot flashes; they return when treatment is discontinued. The patient should be advised of this when terminating estrogen therapy. The return of hot flashes may be minimized by slowly tapering the dose over a period of several weeks or months.

Progestins. Women with endometrial cancer who underwent treatment with depo-medroxyprogesterone acetate (depo-MPA) were incidentally noted to have relief from their hot flashes. A clinical trial later found that depo-MPA has a dose-dependent effect; 50 mg reduced flashes by 60%, 100 mg by 75%, and 150 mg by 85%.[122] The frequency of hot flashes was reduced within 2 weeks following injection, became maximal at 4 weeks, and remained suppressed for the remainder of the 12 weeks of observation. Both the temporal relationship and the dose-dependency in the relief of hot flashes resembles that seen with transdermal estrogens. Unfortunately the use of depo-MPA is associated with a high incidence of irregular vaginal bleeding, and a prolonged but unpredictable duration of action. For this reason, oral MPA, which has a considerably shorter and more predictable half-life than the depot form, is more commonly given. Treatment with 20 mg daily for 1 month reduces flashes by 70%, compared with a 15% reduction with placebo treatment.[144] A lower dose of MPA (10 mg daily) reduces flush frequency by 87% and is better tolerated by patients.[1]

The mechanism of action of progestins is unknown. It has been hypothesized that they too may act via central neurotransmitters because they raise the hypothalamic thermoregulatory set point during the luteal phase of ovulation. Progestins are useful in patients for whom estrogen is contraindicated but they may cause irregular vaginal bleeding, abdominal bloating, constipation, breast tenderness, and mood changes.

α-adrenergic agonists. Women treated with antihypertensive medicines were noted to have fewer hot flashes. It is hypothesized that these drugs alter hypothalamic neurotransmitters, thereby "stabilizing" the thermoregulatory center. They may also act directly on the peripheral vasculature to block cutaneous vasodilation. Clonidine, an α-adrenergic agonist, is known to significantly reduce hot flash frequency by 30% to 40% when used at doses of 0.1 mg and 0.2 mg twice daily. At these doses, patients frequently complain of dizziness and dry mouth.[93] For this reason, the initial dose should be 0.05 mg twice daily and then be increased to 0.1 mg twice daily if hot flashes persist and if there are no side effects. Similarly, another α-adrenergic agonist, lofexidine, was found to reduce hot flashes by as much as 66%.[86] The initial dose of lofexidine (0.1 mg twice daily) was increased by increments of 0.1 mg (up to a maximum of 0.6 mg) every 2 weeks until flashes ceased, or until side effects such as dry mouth, fatigue, and headache were intolerable. Methyldopa (250 mg tid) has also been found to reduce hot flashes by 20%.[70] Because the use of α-adrenergic agonists is limited by their side effects, hypertensive patients are the best candidates for this nonhormonal treatment.

Veralipride. Veralipride, an antidopaminergic drug, has been found to significantly reduce hot flash frequency both in premenopausal women treated with GnRH agonists[174] and in postmenopausal women.[15] The usual dose is 100 mg daily. Both of these studies did not compare veralipride with placebo.

Bellergal. Bellergal, a preparation of ergotamine tartrate, belladonna alkaloids, and 40 mg phenobarbital, is 50% effective when given as one tablet twice daily.[96] Which of the components is responsible for its effect is unknown. This medicine is rarely necessary because it has addictive potential and safer alternative treatments are available.

Other agents such as tricyclic antidepressants and oxazepam have been proposed for the treatment of hot flashes. Because they have not been compared with placebo, their therapeutic efficacy remains unproven. Comparison with placebo is important because many investigators have shown placebo to significantly reduce hot flashes. Nonmedical treatments are being evaluated for the treatment of hot flashes. For example, paced respiration has been found useful in relieving flushes.[57] Also, Chinese herbal teas have been anecdotally noted to reduce hot flashes. This may be due to a common ingredient, ginseng, which is chemically and functionally similar to estrogen.[133]

OSTEOPOROSIS

Definition and etiology

Osteoporosis is the progressive reduction in bone mass without qualitative abnormalities. It affects trabecular bone earlier than cortical bone, and its major consequence is increased risk of fracture. The most frequent sites of fracture are the vertebral bodies, the distal radius, and the femoral neck. Osteoporosis develops when the rate of bone resorption exceeds the rate of bone formation.

Primary osteoporosis results from estrogen deficiency and constitutes 95% of all cases. Since estrogen receptors are present in bone, estrogen may act on bone directly.[90] Estrogen may also act by any of 3 other mechanisms. Firstly, it may decrease the sensitivity of bone to parathyroid hormone (PTH) without changing the amount of circulatory PTH. Secondly, it may increase calcitonin. This is consistent with the following facts: (1) high estrogen states produced by oral contraceptives and pregnancy are associated with elevated calcitonin[102]; (2) men, who have greater bone mass than women, have higher calcitonin levels[76]; and (3) calcitonin levels decline both with age[42] and with menopause and rise with estrogen replacement.[165] Lastly, estrogen may directly increase intestinal calcium absorption.

Secondary osteoporosis constitutes the minority of cases and may result from any of the following: glucocorticoid[114] or heparin use, renal failure, hyperthyroidism (endogenous or iatrogenic),[147] primary hyperparathyroidism, and hyperadrenalism. It also may occur as a result of dietary calcium deficiency or upper intestinal surgery.

Incidence

At all ages women have less bone mass than men. Both sexes achieve peak bone mass at age 30 and progressively lose bone mass at a rate of approximately 1% to 2% per year after age 40.[73] In women this rate increases to 3.9% per year for the 6 years that follow menopause (Fig. 19-8).[79]

Individuals with a lower peak bone mass are more likely to develop significant osteoporosis. Thus women are at a higher risk than men, Caucasians and Orientals more than African-Americans,[155] and thin women more than those who are obese.[173] The greater bone mass of obese women may be due to their increased weight, which mechanically stresses their axial skeleton. Their greater bone mass also may be due to their higher endogenous estrogen levels resulting from

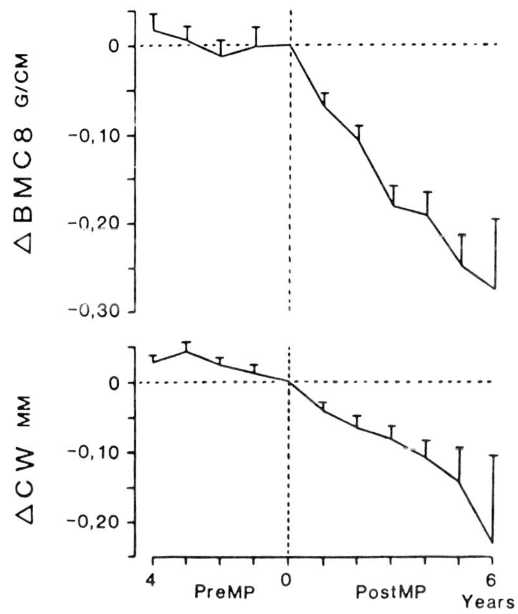

Fig. 19-8. Mean (± SEM) changes in bone mass, measured as bone mineral content (gms/cm^3) of the proximal (BMC8) forearm and mean cortical width (CW) (millimeters) of metacarpals 2, 3, and 4 of both hands. Δ, changes from the last premenopausal (PreMP) year. Broken horizontal line gives values for the last premenopausal year (0), and the broken vertical line indicates the last premenopausal year. (From Falch JA, Oftebro H, Haug E: Early postmenopausal bone loss not associated with decrease in vitamin D, *J Clin Endocrinol Metab* 64:836, 1987.)

the following: (1) increased peripheral aromatization of androstenedione to estrogen,[68] and (2) lower sex hormone-binding globulin levels with greater free estradiol levels.[39] Women with a prior fracture are twice as likely to have subsequent fractures compared to women with the same bone density.[94]

The rate of bone loss varies greatly among individuals. Women who smoke,[78] drink alcohol, are sedentary,[91] or consume two or more cups of coffee per day will lose bone mass more quickly.[10] Also, low calcium consumption[115] and high protein or high phosphate diets accelerate bone loss in women.[98] Family history is also a significant risk factor. This may be due to the presence of one or both alleles for a "low activity" vitamin D receptor protein gene. A study of 117 women, most of whom were Anglo-Irish, found that 74% of those women who did not have this allele had bone density above the "fracture threshold," whereas 61% of women with both of these alleles were below that threshold.[123] Future studies are needed to demonstrate that this allele is a reliable marker for fracture risk.

Twenty-five percent of women beyond age 60 show vertebral fractures on x-ray examination, as do 50% of women beyond age 75.[2,83] Twenty-five percent of women beyond age 80 have a hip fracture[65]; the annual incidence is 1.3% after age 65 and 3.3% after age 85.[99] One out of six women will die within 3 months following hip fracture.[60] The annual health care cost in the United States for these fractures is estimated to be 7 billion dollars.

Diagnosis

Osteoporosis once it has occurred may not be significantly reversed. Unfortunately, known risk factors for osteoporosis (age, weight, calcium, caffeine intake, alcohol and tobacco use, and urinary markers of bone turnover) will not identify 30% of women with low bone mass.[154] Thus a number of radiologic techniques are used to detect early loss of bone mass before significant osteoporosis develops. Early detection provides the opportunity to initiate treatment in women who show early bone loss before fractures occur. Because osteoporosis affects trabecular bone earlier than cortical bone, those modalities which preferentially measure trabecular bone are the most informative.

Single-photon absorptiometry of the distal radius is inexpensive, easy to perform, and requires only 5 mrem of radiation. Because the distal radius consists of 75% cortical bone and only 25% trabecular bone, measurement at this site may not detect early bone loss. In skilled hands it has an accuracy within 5% and a precision of 2% to 4%.[43] Dual-photon absorptiometry of the second to fourth vertebral bodies offers an advantage because this site consists of 60% cortical bone and 40% trabecular bone. It is, however, more expensive, requires 5 to 15 mrem of radiation, and has an accuracy within 5% to 7% with a precision of 2% to 5%.[43]

Computerized tomography of the vertebral body measures 5% cortical bone and 95% trabecular bone, and therefore may detect changes over an interval as brief as 6 months.[21] It has the greatest radiation exposure (200 mrem) and expense, and a precision of 1% to 3%.

The most recent modality to be developed, quantitative digital radiography (QDR), has become the technique of choice. It provides high-resolution images with excellent precision (1% to 2%) and a much lower radiation exposure (1 to 3 mrem).[117] QDR requires less than 8 minutes per study, which is considerably shorter than the 20 to 45 minutes needed for dual-photon absorptiometry.

Ultrasound densitometry is being investigated experimentally as a modality that emits no harmful radiation.[148] Nearly all studies are done using the os calcis (heel) because it is easily accessible and consists of trabecular bone. The precision of this technique and its ability to predict fractures has yet to be established.

Measurement of a woman's bone density today does not predict her bone density in the future. To identify those women who are "fast bone losers" (i.e., greater than 3.1% loss of forearm bone mineral content per year) a nonradiologic method has been proposed.[29] A single measurement of a fasting urinary calcium/creatinine ratio greater than 270 mmole/mole, a fasting urinary hydroxyproline/creatinine ratio greater than 11.2 mole/mole, a serum alkaline phosphatase greater than 120 μ/L, *and* a fat mass index less than 0.222

(calculated from height and weight) correctly identified 79% of the "fast losers" and 78% of the "slow losers." Because the predictive value of a positive test is only 53%, reliance on this method misses a substantial proportion of women who would benefit from estrogen replacement.

Patients who have osteoporosis or osteoporosis-related fractures should undergo careful history and physical examination to exclude an underlying etiology. Measurement of serum calcium, phosphate, alkaline phosphatase, creatinine, sedimentation rate, thyroid studies, or serum protein electrophoresis may assist in identifying any underlying disorder but will be normal in patients with primary osteoporosis.

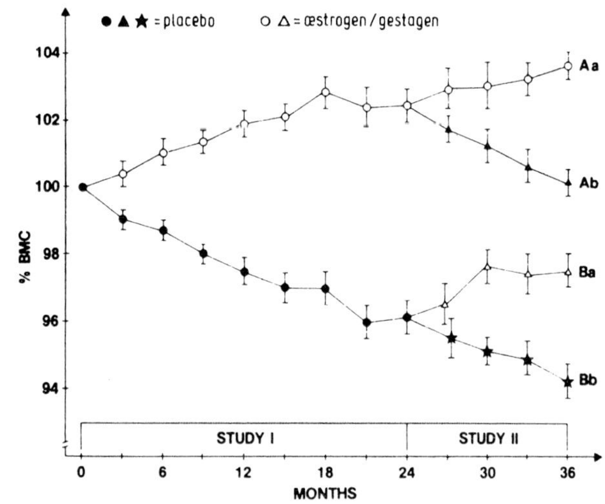

Fig. 19-9. Bone mineral content (BMC) as a function of time and treatment in 94 (study I) and 77 (study II) women soon after menopause. (From Christiansen C, Christiansen MS, Transbol I: Bone mass in postmenopausal women after withdrawal of estrogen/gestagen replacement therapy, *Lancet* 1:459, 1981.)

Treatment

Because established osteoporosis may not be significantly reversed, medical management should emphasize prophylaxis rather than treatment. Stopping smoking, reducing dietary phosphates, and exercising regularly all serve to preserve bone mass.

Estrogens. Estrogens have been clearly shown to prevent the loss of bone mass and thereby reduce the incidence of osteoporotic fractures. They act by decreasing bone resorption (Fig. 19-9),[28] by increasing intestinal calcium absorption, and by reducing renal calcium excretion.[103] Low doses of estrogen appear to be as effective as higher ones; 0.625 mg and 1.25 mg of conjugated equine estrogen (CEE) are equally effective both in preventing bone loss and in reducing the incidence of fractures (Fig. 19-10).[181] Although ethinyl estradiol and mestranol are effective also,[100] conjugated estrogens and estradiol are preferred because they have less impact on the liver.

For those patients who are not candidates for estrogen treatment, "antiestrogens" may be useful. Tamoxifen, 20 mg daily given to 70 postmenopausal women with axillary-node-negative breast cancer for 2 years, was found to preserve lumbar bone density.[104] Whether this treatment prevents fractures remains unknown. Other antiestrogens such as raloxifene are undergoing testing and show promise as antiresorptive agents which do not stimulate endometrial proliferation.[14]

Because bone loss is irreversible, estrogen treatment should be initiated as soon as possible after the menopause to maximize the amount of bone preserved. Treatment should be taken for at least 6 years to substantially reduce the lifetime

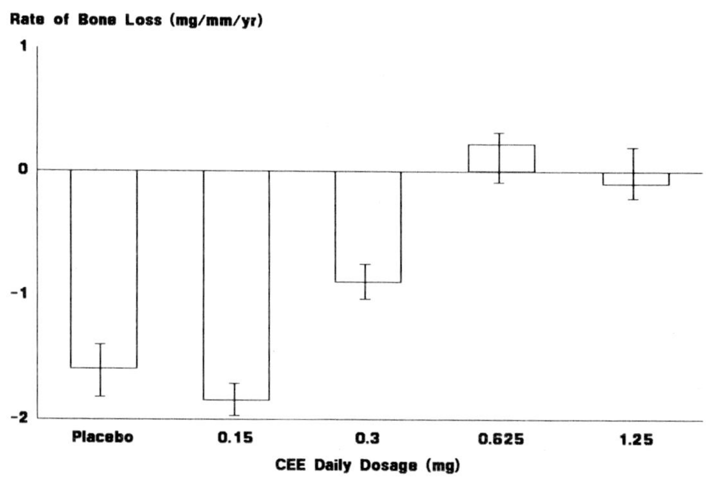

Fig. 19-10. Mean annual change (± SEM) in bone mass in women treated daily with placebo, 0.15, 0.3, 0.625, and 1.25 mg of oral CEE. Bone mineral content measured by single-photon absorptiometry at the midpoint of the third right metacarpal. (From Lindsay R, Hart DM, Clark DM: The minimum effective dose of estrogen for prevention of postmenopausal bone loss, *Obstet Gynecol* 63:759, 1984.)

risk of fracture (Fig. 19-11).[56,181] Because no method identifies all patients who will develop osteoporosis, most postmenopausal women are potential candidates for this therapy. A measurement of baseline bone density may be of help in patients for whom the decision to initiate estrogen replacement is difficult. However, a normal bone density does not rule out the future development of osteoporosis.

Progestins. Progestins used alone do not appear to preserve bone mass; medroxyprogesterone acetate (MPA), 20 mg daily for 2 years, was equivalent to placebo treatment.[59] However, these investigators found that MPA, when combined with estrogen, may act synergistically to conserve bone mass, allowing a lower estrogen dose (e.g., CEE 0.3 mg daily) to be used. A proposed mechanism is that progesterone may block glucocorticoid receptors located on bone,[109] preventing endogenous glucocorticoids from exerting their inhibitory effects on bone metabolism.

Many women cannot or choose not to take hormonal treatment and are therefore at risk for developing osteoporosis. For those women, multiple alternate therapies have been proposed. The following treatments have been evaluated recently for efficacy in preventing or reversing osteoporosis: (1) calcium, (2) fluoride, (3) diphosphonates, (4) calcitonin, (5) vitamin D, and (6) thiazides.

Calcium. The efficacy of calcium in preventing postmenopausal bone loss has been quite controversial. One well-designed study found that oral calcium supplementation in early postmenopausal women with adequate dietary calcium intakes did not prevent bone loss (Fig. 19-12).[136] However, calcium use may prevent bone loss in selected patients as shown in a 2-year clinical trial of 300 healthy postmenopausal women who were given either placebo or 500 mg of calcium carbonate or calcium citrate maleate.[40] Calcium treatment did not prevent bone loss in women who had undergone menopause within the preceding 5 years or in those who consumed more than 400 mg calcium per day. For women who were 6 or more years into menopause *and* who consumed less than 400 mg of calcium, calcium supplementation did prevent bone loss. Calcium citrate maleate was more effective than calcium carbonate, possibly because of better gastrointestinal absorption. Thus it appears that calcium supplementation may reduce "age-related" bone loss in women who are several years after the menopause *and* who have low dietary calcium intakes. Although calcium supplementation cannot prevent "estrogen-related" bone loss occurring shortly after the menopause, it may permit the use of a lower dose of estrogen (e.g., 0.3 mg CEE).[53] Caution should be used in patients with a history of renal stones.

That calcium may prevent "age-related" bone loss was also suggested in a study of 37 healthy premenopausal women between ages 30 and 42.[9] Half of these women were instructed to increase their dietary calcium intake by an average of 610 mg/day; age- and weight-matched controls maintained their usual diets. After 3 years vertebral bone density was unchanged in the women who raised their calcium intake but was 3% lower in controls. It should be noted that the increase in dietary calcium was accompanied by an increased consumption of calories (28%), fat (38%), and protein (60%). In addition, the increased calcium group gained 4.2 kg versus 3.4 kg for the control group over the 3 years. Thus the prevention of age-related bone loss seen in this study may very well be due to increased body fat resulting from a higher caloric consumption. The possibility does exist, however, that increasing dietary calcium after peak bone mass is achieved in the third decade may reduce age-related bone loss and perhaps lessen the incidence of osteoporotic fractures later in life.

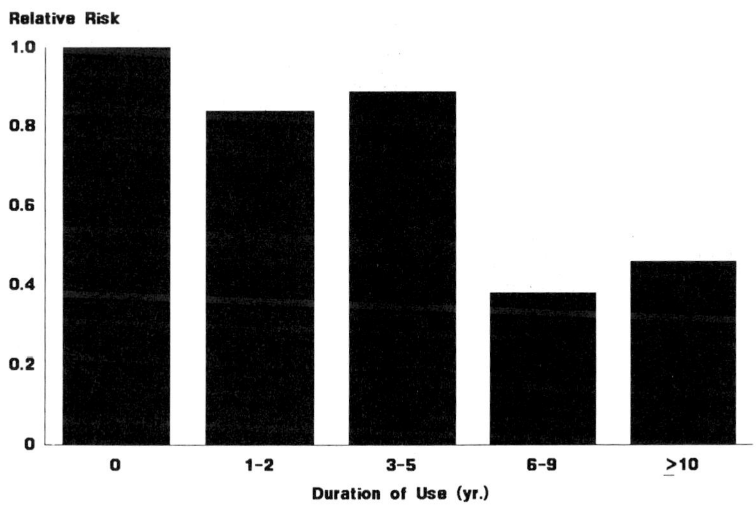

Fig. 19-11. Relative risk for hip or forearm fracture according to duration of postmenopausal estrogen use. (Data from Weiss NS et al: Decreased risk of fractures of the hip and lower forearm with postmenopausal use of estrogen, *N Engl J Med* 303:1195, 1980.)

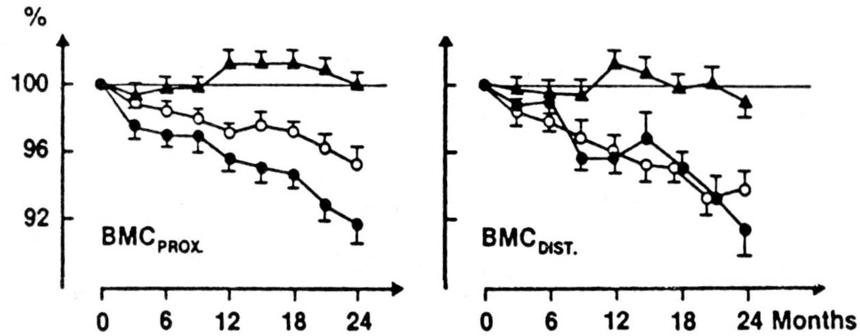

Fig. 19-12. Bone mineral content of the proximal (BMC_{PROX}) and distal (BMC_{DIST}) radius of postmenopausal women treated with percutaneous estrogens (solid triangle), calcium (open circle), and placebo (solid circle). (Data from Riis B, Thomsen K, Christiansen C: Does calcium supplementation prevent postmenopausal bone loss? *N Engl J Med* 316:173, 1987.)

Fluoride. Fluoride stimulates bone formation and increases cancellous bone mass as much as twofold.[16] However, there has been a suspicion that the bone formed is structurally abnormal and weak and more likely to fracture. The effect of fluoride treatment on the incidence of osteoporotic fractures was recently evaluated in 200 osteoporotic postmenopausal women.[135] They were randomized to treatment with sodium fluoride 75 mg per day or to placebo. Although fluoride treatment increased vertebral bone density by 35%, it did not reduce the incidence of vertebral fractures. Most worrisome was that the incidence of nonvertebral fractures was threefold higher in the fluoride group. This was attributed to a fluoride-induced loss of cortical bone suggested by a 4% decrease in density of the radial shaft. Thus fluoride increases cancellous bone at the expense of cortical bone. Not only is the additional cancellous bone structurally weak, which will not prevent vertebral fractures, but the loss of cortical bone increases the risk of fracture of nonvertebral bones. Fluoride does not therefore appear to be effective in the prevention or treatment of osteoporosis.

Bisphosphonates. Etidronate, a bisphosphonate, has been used to treat Paget's disease of the bone because it retards osteoblastic ad osteoclastic activity, which are both abnormally high in this condition. However, when etidronate is given in low doses, the antiosteoclastic activity predominates so that bone mass may increase. Two clinical trials evaluated the effect of etidronate on vertebral bone density and fracture rates.[166, 178] Both studies administered etidronate, 400 mg daily for 2 weeks; this was prescribed four times per year. In both studies etidronate significantly increased vertebral bone density by 2% per year over the 2 to 3 years of observation and substantially decreased the incidence of vertebral fracture. Watts et al[178] found that two years of treatment with etidronate lowered vertebral fracture rates by 50% for the entire cohort and by 70% for women with the least amount of bone mass at the start of treatment. The reduction in vertebral fracture rates continued during a third year of treatment.[72] Storm et al[166] noted that after the first year of treatment the incidence of new vertebral fractures was more than 80% lower in the etidronate users. These studies indicate that short-term, intermittent cyclic therapy with etidronate can reverse postmenopausal vertebral bone loss and the incidence of fractures. The bisphosphonates may offer promise as (1) an alternative to estrogen in the prevention of osteoporosis; (2) as an adjunctive treatment for women who demonstrate bone loss while taking estrogen; (3) and as a primary treatment for women with established osteoporosis. Because the duration of these studies was short (2 and 3 years) and etidronate remains present in bone for many years, the long-term safety and efficacy of etidronate needs to be established prior to routine use. Newer bisphosphonates such as alendronate[71] and risedronate, are being tested for safety and efficacy. They may be superior to etidronate because they appear to be more potent in suppressing osteoclast activity but have less inhibition of bone formation and mineralization.

Calcitonin. Calcitonin is a peptide hormone secreted by the C cells of the thyroid gland. Its main physiologic role is to protect against hypercalcemia, primarily by inhibiting bone resorption. It exerts this action by binding to high-affinity receptors on osteoclasts and markedly inhibiting osteoclastic activity. Treatment with calcitonin has been found to increase bone mass to a variable extent; the greatest increases are seen in women with the highest rates of bone turnover.[31] At present calcitonin is available in the United States only in an injectable form. The usual dose is 50 to 100 units per day or every other day. It appears to have a direct analgesic effect in patients with acute fractures. Approximately 10% to 20% of patients will experience headache, nausea, and flushing. A calcitonin nasal spray has been tested but has not been found to be effective.[27]

Vitamin D. The biologically active form of vitamin D is 1, 25-dihydroxycholecalciferol. Its physiologic action is to increase the efficiency of intestinal calcium absorption and increase osteoblast activity. A clinical trial in 3200 elderly women evaluated the effect of 18 months of treatment with vitamin D, 20 μg (800 IU) per day. Vitamin D significantly decreased the incidence of new hip fractures by 43% and nonvertebral fractures by 32%.[25] Lower doses of vitamin D have been studied in other clinical trials and generally have not been effective. Because higher doses carry a risk of hypercalciuria and even hypercalcemia, this agent should be prescribed with caution.

Thiazide diuretics. Because thiazide diuretics reduce the urinary excretion of calcium, they have been proposed as another modality to prevent osteoporosis. Two studies suggest that thiazides may prevent osteoporotic fractures. Lacroix et al prospectively followed 9500 elderly men and women for 4 years and identified 242 cases of hip fractures.[92] After controlling for the greater body weight and for lower incidence of tobacco use of thiazide users, they found the relative risk (RR) of hip fracture in thiazide users was significantly reduced to 0.68 (CI: 0.49 to 0.94). Dose and duration of thiazide use were not analyzed. Felson et al analyzed 176 cases of hip fracture and 672 age-matched controls from the Framingham Study Cohort.[55] Recent high-dose thiazide use reduced the risk of hip fracture (RR: 0.31; CI: 0.11 to 0.88), but past use has no effect. Surprisingly, low-dose thiazide use appeared to increase the risk of hip fracture (RR: 2.23; CI: 1.26 to 3.94) which may be a spurious finding. Clearly a clinical trial is necessary to define both the optimal thiazide dose and the minimum treatment duration that preserves bone mass and to determine how long the benefit persists after treatment is discontinued. Whether or not thiazides should be used to prevent bone loss must take into account their potentially deleterious effects: (1) increased plasma cholesterol, triglyceride, glucose, and uric acid levels; (2) decreased high-density lipoprotein levels; and (3) potassium depletion which may predispose to arrhythmias. If the efficacy of thiazide diuretics in preventing fractures is confirmed by clinical trials and this benefit outweighs the risks of thiazide use, then thiazides may be particularly useful in the medical treatment of hypertensive postmenopausal women.

GENITAL ATROPHY

Pathogenesis

The tissues of the lower vagina, labia, urethra, and trigone derive from a common embryonic origin, the urogenital sinus, and are all estrogen dependent.[82] Following the loss of estrogen at menopause, the vaginal walls become pale because of diminished vascularity, and thin (typically only 3 or 4 cells thick). The vaginal epithelial cells contain less glycogen, which prior to menopause had been metabolized by lactobacilli to create an acidic pH, thereby protecting the vagina from bacterial overgrowth. Loss of this protective mechanism leaves the thin, friable tissue vulnerable to infection and ulceration. The vagina also loses its rugae and becomes shorter and inelastic.

Patients may complain of symptoms secondary to vaginal dryness, such as dyspareunia and vaginismus, that can compromise sexual satisfaction and lead to diminished libido. Women may also present with symptoms secondary to vaginal ulceration and infection, such as vaginal discharge, burning, itching, or bleeding.

The urethra and urinary trigone undergo atrophic changes similar to that of the vagina. Dysuria, urgency, frequency, and suprapubic pain may occur in the absence of infection. Presumably this occurs because the markedly thin urethral mucosa allows urine to come into close contact with sensory nerves. In addition, the menopausal loss of the resistance to urinary flow by thick, well-vascularized urethral mucosa has been hypothesized to contribute to urinary incontinence.[189]

Diagnosis

Atrophic vaginitis may be diagnosed by its typical appearance. The presence of atrophy may be confirmed, if necessary, by a vaginal cell maturation index, obtained by scraping the lateral vaginal wall at the level of the cervix. The exfoliated cells may then be classified by degree of maturation with a small proportion of superficial cells indicating a high degree of vaginal atrophy. If any atypical lesions are present, they should be biopsied to establish a diagnosis. If a

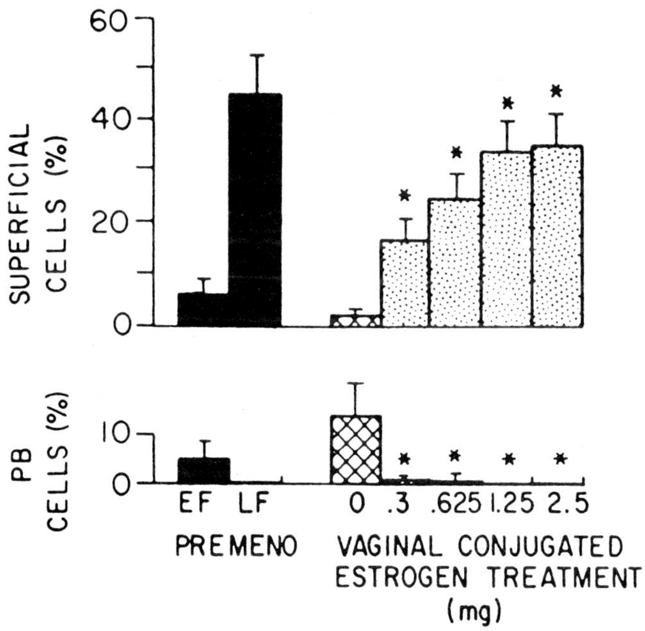

Fig. 19-13. Mean (± SEM) percent superficial and parabasal (PB) cells from vaginal exfoliative cytology. Premenopausal controls in the early follicular (EF) and late follicular (LF) phases of their cycles are compared with postmenopausal women before and after vaginal administration of various doses of conjugated estrogen. *Indicates significant difference (< 0.05) from the untreated postmenopausal value. (From Mandel FP et al: Biologic effects of various doses of vaginally administered conjugated equine estrogens in postmenopausal women, *J Clin Endocrinol Metab* 57:133, 1983.)

discharge is present, it should be evaluated for pathogens such as *Candida*, *Neisseria gonorrhea*, *Chlamydia*, *Trichomonas*, and *Gardnerella*. If *Candida* is found the patient should be screened for diabetes, because the low glycogen content of nonestrogenized vaginal epithelial cells ordinarily will not support its growth.

Atrophic urethritis and/or trigonitis is diagnosed by ruling out the presence of infection. Urethroscopy is usually unnecessary but would reveal a pale, atrophic urethra.

Treatment

Estrogen is the only effective therapy with the dose required generally being lower than that needed to treat hot flashes or osteoporosis. Thus, treatment for these conditions will usually relieve genital atrophy and improve sexual satisfaction.[125] Estrogen treatment has also been found to reduce the incidence of recurrent urinary tract infections.[134] If atrophy is the only indication for estrogen treatment, daily use for a minimum of 2 to 12 weeks is needed to reverse the atrophic changes. Once atrophy is relieved, therapy may be tapered to 2 to 3 times per week. The usual daily oral doses are as follows: (1) CEE 0.3 mg or 0.625 mg; (2) estrone 0.3 mg, 0.625 mg, or 1.25 mg; or (3) micronized estradiol 1 mg or 2 mg.[23] Transdermal estradiol, 50 μg /24° twice weekly, is also effective. Estrogens such as CEE 0.3 mg (Fig. 19-13)[108] or micronized β-estradiol 0.2 mg may also be administered vaginally.[66] Although most of the estrogen acts locally, some of it is rapidly absorbed into the systemic circulation and may stimulate endometrial growth.[145] Thus a progestin should generally be given intermittently with vaginal estrogens for patients with an intact uterus and repeated for as long as the patient has withdrawal bleeding.

If estrogens are contraindicated, synthetic mucopolysaccharides or water-soluble lubricants may relieve dyspareunia. Vaginal stenosis may be improved by the use of graduated vaginal dilators.

ATHEROSCLEROSIS

Cardiovascular disease (CVD) is the leading cause of death among women in industrialized countries; over 50% of postmenopausal women will succumb to CVD. Estrogens have been hypothesized to protect against atherosclerosis because the incidence of CVD is quite low before the menopause. Premenopausal women have approximately one fifth the CVD mortality of men, but after the menopause their mortality rises exponentially to approach that of men (Fig. 19-14).[97] One explanation is that a premenopausal woman's estrogen confers protection that is lost at menopause. This is supported by the observation that women who undergo a premature surgical menopause (i.e., bilateral oophorectomy) and do not use estrogen replacement have twice as much CVD than do age-matched premenopausal controls. If they use estrogen replacement, however, their incidence of CVD is the same as premenopausal women of the same age. Premature natural menopause, in contrast, has not been found to

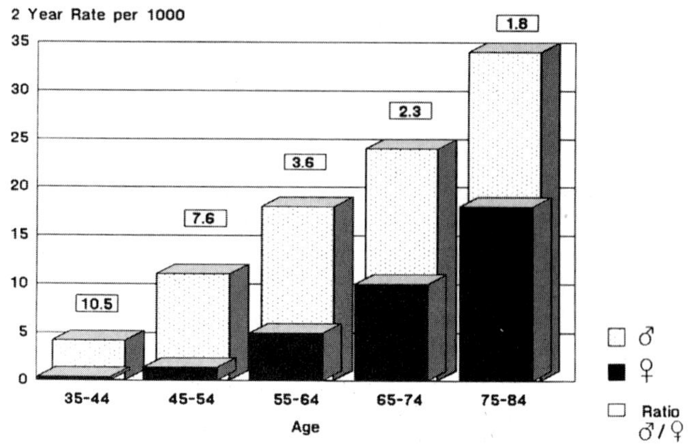

Fig. 19-14. Incidence of myocardial infarctions (MI) by age and sex (female, solid bar; male, stippled bar). Ratio of male to female MIs for each age group is noted at top of graph. (From Lerner DJ, Kannel WB: Patterns of coronary disease morbidity and mortality: a 26-year follow-up of the Framingham population, *Am Heart J* 111:383, 1986.)

increase CVD risk when controlled for age, smoking, and estrogen use.[34]

Epidemiologic studies

Epidemiologic studies have compared the incidence of CVD among postmenopausal estrogen users and nonusers. Retrospective case-control studies provided inconsistent results although most found estrogen use to be associated with less CVD.[7,137] Prospective cohort studies, which have fewer sources of bias, generally showed estrogen use reduces CVD.[18,132] One notable exception, the Framingham Study, found an adverse effect[187] or no effect of estrogen treatment,[47] depending upon how CVD was defined and which multiple regression model was used. In contrast, the Nurses' Health Study,[160] the largest cohort study which followed 48,000 postmenopausal women for up to 10 years, identified 405 cases of nonfatal myocardial infarction (MI) or fatal coronary heart disease. The relative risk of coronary heart disease with estrogen use was significantly reduced to 0.89 (95% CI: 0.78 to 1.0) for "ever" use and 0.56 (CI: 0.40 to 0.80) for current use. Even women at low risk for CVD (nonsmokers without diabetes, hypertension, obesity, or hypercholesterolemia) had significantly less CVD if they used estrogens. Adjustment for a number of cardiovascular risk factors did not alter these findings, arguing against any major physician bias to prescribe estrogens to healthier women.

Additional evidence for the benefit of estrogens was provided by a prospective study of over 8000 postmenopausal women living in a moderately affluent retirement community in Southern California.[75] Over 1400 women died during 7 years of observation. The investigators found that all-cause mortality rates were 20% lower for those women who had ever taken postmenopausal estrogens compared with women who did not (RR of death: 0.80; CI: 0.70 to 0.87). The greatest reductions in mortality rates were seen with current use and with long durations of use; current use for more than 15 years was associated with a 40% lower mortality. This reduction in mortality rates was *not* dependent upon the dose of estrogen used; both high (i.e., ≥ 1.25 mg/day) and low (i.e., ≤ 0.625 mg/day) doses of oral CEE (the most common estrogen used) were associated with nearly equal reductions. This is an interesting observation because 0.625 mg and 1.25 mg of conjugated estrogens produce nearly equal increases in HDL levels and decreases in LDL levels.[177] Because few women in this cohort took progestins or parenteral estrogens, the effect of those hormones on mortality rates cannot be determined from this study. Most of the reduced mortality in estrogen users seen in this study was due to fewer deaths from occlusive arteriosclerotic vascular disease.[75] The study also found that estrogen users had 20% less cancer mortality, which was observed for many malignancies, including those of the breast (RR: 0.81). One possible explanation for this finding is that estrogen users may have had greater health awareness and/or increased medical surveillance and so had less extensive disease at the time of diagnosis. As expected, estrogen users had excess mortality from endometrial cancer (RR: 3.0).

Table 19-1. Relative risks of mortalities from all causes by selected characteristics and history of use of estrogen replacement therapy

Estrogen replacement therapy ever used	No	Yes
Elevated blood pressure		
No	1.00†	0.79‡
Yes	1.54§	1.15
Angina/MI history		
No	1.00†	0.81*
Yes	1.62§	1.02
Smoking		
Never	1.00†	0.74§
Ever	1.28	1.05
Alcohol		
No	1.00†	0.56§
Yes	0.61§	0.39§
Quetelet's index: wt/ht² × 1000		
35	1.14§	0.92
≥ 35	1.00†	0.72‡
Exercise, h/d		
< 0.5	1.00†	0.73§
0.05–0.09	0.67§	0.61§
> 1.0	0.56§	0.43§
Age at last menstrual period		
< 45	1.0†	0.71*
45–54	0.81‡	0.65§
≥ 55	0.75**	0.75**

From Henderson BE, Paganini-Hill A, Ross RK: Decreased mortality in users of estrogen replacement therapy, *Arch Intern Med* 151:75-78, 1991.
†Reference group.
‡ $p < 0.01$, § $p < 0.0001$, * $p < 0.001$, ** $p < 0.05$

Women who underwent menopause before age 45 showed the greatest benefit from estrogen use. For women whose menopause occurred after age 54, estrogen treatment did not reduce mortality. Estrogen use also appeared to reduce mortality rates for women who smoked, had hypertension, or who had a history of angina or MI so that their risk approached that of healthy women who did not use estrogen (Table 19-1). This is a very significant finding; at one time hypertension, tobacco use, and coronary disease were considered to be relative contraindications to estrogen replacement. This was based on the increased incidence of stroke and heart attack in women taking high-dose oral contraceptives and in men taking high-dose conjugated estrogens prescribed as secondary prevention of MI.[35] This does not appear to be a concern with the much lower doses of estrogen prescribed for postmenopausal use.

The findings of these studies argue that nearly all postmenopausal women, particularly those who underwent menopause before age 45, or who are at risk for CVD should be offered estrogen replacement. The results further argue for continuous, long-term treatment because increased durations of treatment are associated with further reductions in mortality. It should be remembered that these studies are epidemiologic observations of estrogen users and nonusers and are *not* clinical trials. Although investigators control for many potential confounding factors, the possibility exists that healthier women are more likely to seek and be prescribed estrogens. Definitive proof of the benefit of estrogen in reducing mortality would require a long-term, large-scale, placebo-controlled clinical trial.

Angiographic studies

Sullivan et al provided evidence that women with preexisting atherosclerosis may benefit from estrogen replacement.[169] These investigators had previously reported that estrogen users undergoing coronary catheterization are less likely to have coronary occlusion, compared with nonusers (RR: 0.44; CI: 0.29 to 0.67).[168] In their most recent study, they retrospectively analyzed the all-cause mortality of women who had undergone catheterization over the preceding 10 years. Unfortunately, relatively few of their subjects were estrogen users, which was defined as those who used estrogen at the time of catheterization (5% of subjects) or began estrogen use sometime thereafter (another 5% of subjects). The adjusted 10-year survival rate of women with severe coronary stenosis who used estrogens was 97% but only 60% for nonusers. For mild to moderate coronary stenosis, the 10-year survival rate was 95% for users and 85% for nonusers. Although these findings suggest that women with coronary atherosclerosis may benefit from estrogen use, it should be recognized that this is a retrospective study with potential bias. The decreased mortality seen in estrogen users may have been in part a self-fulfilling prophecy because estrogen nonusers who lived the longest after catheterization had the greatest opportunity to begin estrogen treatment and be classified as "estrogen users."

Clinical trials

The only clinical trials to reduce CVD by estrogen treatment have all been performed in men. Early studies, enrolling men after an MI, showed that estrogen treatment reduced serum cholesterol but not the incidence of a second event.[159] The Coronary Drug Project, consisting of 1101 MI survivors, was terminated when excess thrombotic events, particularly pulmonary emboli, were seen in the estrogen treated group; the incidence of CVD was not reduced.[35] A similar observation was made in men with prostatic cancer treated with the estrogen, diethylstilbestrol, which increased CVD, possibly by causing excessive fluid accumulation leading to congestive heart failure, or by increasing thromboembolism.[45] This adverse action of estrogen in men may have been the consequence of the highly potent estrogens used and may not reflect the action of estrogen at physiologic levels.

Mechanisms of action of estrogen

Because men and women have an equal incidence of CVD when matched for lipoprotein concentrations,[66] the sex difference in the incidence of CVD may be a consequence of the characteristic sex differences in serum lipoprotein concentrations. Thus premenopausal women appear to be protected against CVD by their typically lower LDL levels and higher HDL levels, compared with men of the same age (Fig. 19-15). However, coincident with the loss of estrogen at menopause, female LDL levels rise to exceed those of men.[116] This loss of estrogen may directly cause the increase in LDL because estrogen replacement lowers LDL levels by 15% to 19% by increasing the clearance of LDL from the circulation (Fig. 19-16).[177] In contrast, HDL levels in women decline by only 5% at menopause.[116] Thus the HDL-raising effect of oral estrogens (typically 16% to 18%)[177] appears to be a pharmacologic action of the high portal estrogen concentrations presented to the liver following intestinal absorption. Therefore, if endogenous estrogens protect against CVD, the likely mechanism is an effect on LDL rather than on HDL. In contrast, the lower incidence of CVD among postmenopausal estrogen users may be due to both increases in HDL levels and decreases in LDL levels. The magnitude of these lipid changes induced by oral estrogen treatment would be expected to lower the incidence of CVD by as much as 40%, using the regression coefficients determined by clinical trials in which cholesterol levels were improved by drug treatment. Reductions of this magnitude have been observed among estrogen users.[75,160] In addition, postmenopausal estrogen treatment has been found to reduce plasma levels of lipoprotein (a), a highly atherogenic particle.[141]

An alternative explanation has been proposed for the sex difference in the incidence of CVD. A semilogarithmic plot of female cardiovascular deaths against age shows that the

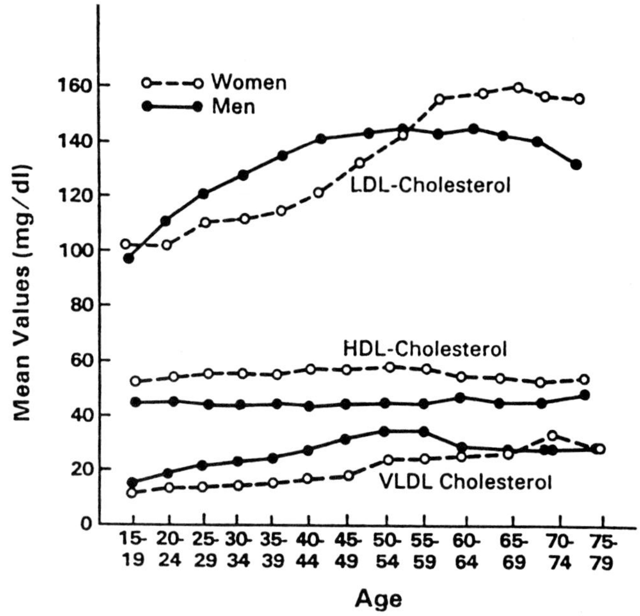

Fig. 19-15. Age and sex trends in lipoprotein cholesterol fractions, Framingham study. (From Kannel WB: Risk factors for coronary disease in women: perspective from the Framingham study, *Am Heart J* 114:413, 1987.)

rate of increase in the rate of CVD is constant throughout a woman's lifetime, and is not accelerated after menopause. In comparison, male CVD shows a decline in the rate of increase after the onset of the "male climacteric," when testosterone levels wane (Fig. 19-17).[74] This decline in androgens therefore may be a major factor responsible for the lower female/male CVD ratio seen with increasing age. Androgens are known to adversely affect serum lipoproteins; both exogenous use (e.g., testosterone enanthate and methyltestosterone) and endogenous increases in androgens (occurring during puberty) have been found to lower HDL levels.[6,88]

Estrogens may also protect against cardiovascular disease independent of their beneficial actions on lipoprotein levels. Estrogens may retard the oxidation of LDL thereby decreasing its atherogenicity. This was demonstrated in healthy postmenopausal women who were infused estradiol intravenously; LDL oxidation was significantly delayed.[140] Estrogens may also suppress the uptake of LDL by blood vessel walls thereby impairing the development of endothelial atheroma.[176] There is also evidence that estrogens act directly to promote vasodilation, as demonstrated in estrogen-treated castrated female monkeys.[186] This may be mediated indirectly by estrogen-induced alterations in prostaglandin metabolism, by increasing the levels of prostacyclin (a vasodilator) and decreasing the levels of thromboxane (a vasoconstrictor).[163] The vasodilatory effect of estrogen may be more direct because estrogen receptors are present throughout the vascular system.[118] The binding of estrogen to endothelial estrogen receptors could stimulate the release of nitric oxide, a potent endogenous vasodilator. This was suggested by work on

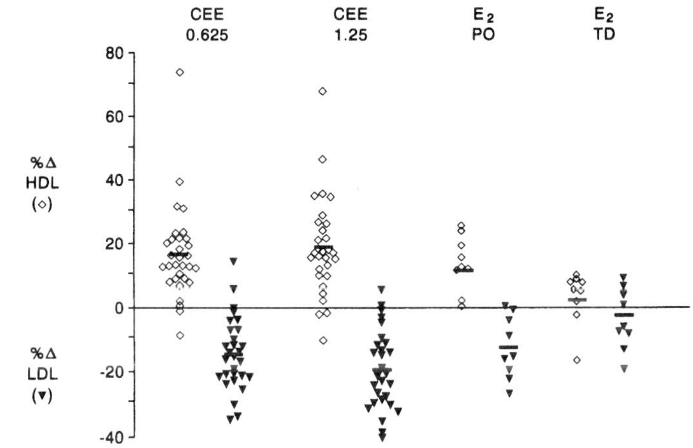

Fig. 19-16. Effect of estrogen treatments on plasma LDL and HDL cholesterol concentrations. Each point represents the individual percentage change with estrogen as compared with placebo. The horizontal bar denotes the mean of the percentage changes. (From Walsh BW et al: Effects of postmenopausal estrogen replacement on the concentrations and metabolism of plasma lipoproteins, *N Engl J Med* 325:1196, 1991.)

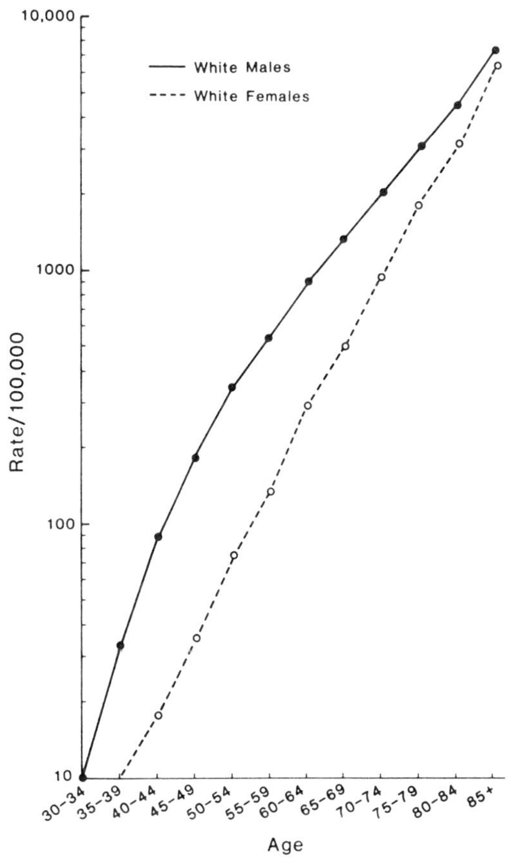

Fig. 19-17. Age-specific mortality rates for ischemic heart disease by sex (Caucasians only, United States, 1977). (From Ross RK, Paganini-Hill A: Estrogen replacement therapy and coronary heart disease, *Semin Reprod Endocrinol* 1:19, 1983.)

female rabbits, in whom endogenous estrogens were found to promote an increase in the basal release rates of nitric oxide.[81]

The preponderance of evidence from epidemiologic studies indicates that estrogen use prevents the development of heart disease. However, at present there are no long-term randomized studies of postmenopausal estrogen replacement that prove this beneficial effect. Such a clinical trial is currently underway and is needed to demonstrate conclusively that postmenopausal estrogen use reduces the incidence of cardiovascular disease. This trial will also determine if the concomitant administration of a progestin detracts from the cardioprotective action of estrogen. There is a concern that progestins, particularly the androgenic 19-nortestosterone derivatives may do so by lowering HDL levels. However, preliminary results from a small trial suggest that combined estrogen and progestin users have as great a reduction in CVD as do estrogen-only users.[54]

ESTROGENS

Pharmacology

Once the decision has been made to treat a postmenopausal woman with estrogen, the next issue is to decide how it should be prescribed. Many preparations are available; conjugated estrogens, synthetic estrogens, and micronized estradiol. All of them may be given orally or parenterally, continuously or cyclically. Because oral estrogens have been prescribed for over 30 years, most of the demonstrated long-term benefits of estrogens are based on experience with oral use. The daily doses of the most common estrogens taken orally are CEE 0.625 mg, micronized estradiol 1 mg, and piperazine estrone sulfate 1.25 mg. These doses are usually effective in relieving menopausal symptoms such as hot flashes and vaginal atrophy and in preventing osteoporosis. Generally CEEs are twice as potent per unit weight compared with pure estrone preparations[113] since up to 50% consists of the potent equine estrogens, equilin, and 17-dihydroequilin sulfates, with the remainder being estrone sulfate. These equine estrogens have a prolonged action, due in part to storage and slow release from adipose tissue. They have been detected in the blood as long as 13 weeks after administration.[185]

Orally administered estradiol is rapidly converted to estrone in the intestinal mucosa. Oral estrogens are then presented to the liver where 30% of an initial dose is conjugated with glucuronide on the first pass.[152] These conjugates undergo rapid renal and biliary excretion. The biliary conjugates are hydrolyzed by intestinal flora, allowing 80% to be reabsorbed and returned to the liver. They may then either be reconjugated and excreted or may enter the systemic circulation. This enterohepatic circulation contributes to the prolonged effect of orally administered estrogens. Thus patients with altered gut flora (e.g., from antibiotic therapy) may not sufficiently hydrolyze these conjugates, thereby preventing reabsorption. As a result, these patients may require higher doses to achieve a therapeutic effect. Also patients chronically maintained on phenytoin have enhanced glucuronidation and will excrete estrogens more rapidly.[49] They too may require higher doses.

Women who smoke may also require a higher estrogen dose. Postmenopausal estrogen users who smoke have one half the serum estrogen levels compared with users who do not smoke.[84] Smoking is believed to stimulate 2-hydroxylation of estradiol, yielding 2-hydroxy estrogens that have minimal estrogenic activity and are rapidly cleared from the circulation.[121] This explains why smokers have a higher incidence of osteoporosis and menopausal symptoms and may require a higher estrogen dose.

The concentration of estrogen in the portal circulation after oral ingestion is 4 to 5 times higher than that in the general circulation. Thus hepatocytes are exposed to higher estrogen levels after oral estrogen administration than are cells of other organs. Estrogens given orally will have a more profound effect on hepatic metabolism than those given parenterally. Although many of these actions on the liver may be potentially deleterious, such as stimulating the production of renin-substrate and coagulation factors, some effects may be beneficial, such as an increased HDL production and an increased LDL catabolism.[177] Both these effects on lipoproteins may reduce cardiovascular risk.

Synthetic estrogens are chemical derivatives of estradiol and are the estrogens currently used in oral contraceptives. Ethinyl estradiol (EE) results from the addition of a 17-ethinyl group, which impedes catabolism by the liver, leading to its long half-life of 48 hours. The other commonly used synthetic estrogen, mestranol, must undergo demethylation by the liver to become EE, its active form. Because this demethylation is only 50% complete, mestranol has only half the potency of EE.[149] These synthetic estrogens when given orally are more than 100 times as potent on a per-weight basis as natural estrogens in stimulating the production of hepatic proteins.[113] Because the minimum dose (10 μg) for therapeutic effect (e.g., to reduce urinary calcium excretion) exceeds the lowest dose which markedly elevates hepatic globulins (5 μg), synthetic estrogens are not recommended for postmenopausal use.[107]

Parenteral estrogens may be given by the vaginal, transdermal, or subcutaneous routes. Vaginal estrogens are absorbed into the systemic circulation and achieve one fourth of the circulatory level of an equal dose given orally.[44] However, they exert a potent local effect; 0.3 mg CEE given vaginally produces the same degree of epithelial maturation as 1.25 mg given orally.[63,108] Continuous vaginal use of estrogen will lead to increased circulatory levels because of enhanced transfer across a healthier, more vascularized epithelium.[152]

Twenty-five milligram subdermal estradiol pellets have been found to be effective but have variable life spans of 3 to 6 months and are difficult to remove. Transdermal skin patches applied twice weekly are more convenient. They provide constant serum estrogen levels; the 50 μg/24° patch produces a mean serum estradiol of 70 pg/mL and an estrone of 50 pg/mL. These levels are usually effective in relieving hot flashes[69] and in preventing bone loss.[164] Whether or not parenteral estrogens reduce the incidence of CVD has yet to be demonstrated.

Possible side effects

Estrogens may cause nausea, mastalgia, headache, and mood changes. More serious risks include the following.

Endometrial neoplasia. Unopposed estrogen use (i.e., without the addition of a progestin) may induce endometrial hyperplasia and ultimately adenocarcinoma. Retrospective case-control studies have found that unopposed estrogen use increases the risk of endometrial cancer 2- to 4-fold, from a baseline incidence of 1/1000 women (ages 50 to 74) per year

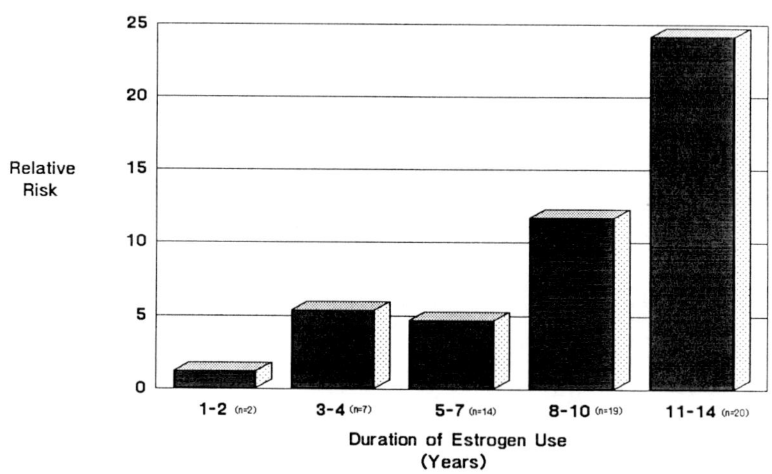

Fig. 19-18. Relative risk of endometrial cancer according to duration of postmenopausal estrogen use. (From Weiss NS et al: Endometrial cancer in relation to patterns of menopausal estrogen use, *JAMA* 242:261, 1979.)

to 4/1000 women per year. The increase in risk appears to be related to both the dose and duration (minimum 1 to 2 years) of estrogen use (Fig. 19-18).[180] The relative risk of endometrial cancer is 1.2 with 0.625 mg of conjugated estrogens daily and is 3.8 with 1.25 mg daily.[138] This elevated risk persists for more than 6 years after therapy is discontinued. Women who use oral contraceptives for more than 12 months and later take unopposed postmenopausal estrogens do not have an increased risk of developing endometrial cancer compared with nonusers. Thus the risk of endometrial cancer associated with unopposed estrogen use is low for women using 0.625 mg CEE, particularly if they previously used oral contraceptives.[138]

Most of the carcinomas associated with estrogen use are of early stage and low grade and have not deeply invaded the myometrium.[30] The adjusted 5-year survival for estrogen users with endometrial cancer is 94% compared with 81% for estrogen nonusers,[48] possibly due to one or more of the following: (1) women prescribed estrogens generally are in better health than nonusers, (2) they are evaluated more frequently allowing for earlier diagnosis, or (3) only well-differentiated endometrial neoplasms retain estrogen receptors by which exogenous estrogens can provide a stimulus.

Progestins can both prevent and reverse endometrial hyperplasia. Studd et al, following 855 women with annual endometrial biopsies for up to 5 years, found an annual incidence of hyperplasia of 15% among women taking 1.25 mg of unopposed conjugated estrogen.[167] The addition of a progestin for 7 days per month reduced this incidence to 3%. Ten days of progestin treatment per month lowered the incidence to 2%, and 13 days treatment reduced this to essentially zero (Fig. 19-19). Based on these data, progestins are typically given for 13 days per month. Progestin treatment has also been successful in completely reversing established endometrial hyperplasia in 94% of 258 women with hyperplasia.[62] Women who use estrogens combined with progestins have a significantly lower incidence of endometrial cancer (71 per 100,000) than women who use estrogens alone (434 per 100,000) or women who use no hormones (242 per 100,000).[61] Thus women who use both estrogens and progestins are considered not to be at an increased risk for endometrial cancer.

Whitehead et al provided biochemical and histologic evidence for the antihyperplastic effect of progestins on the endometrium.[184] They found that numerous progestins reverse the induction of estradiol and progesterone receptors produced by estrogen. Progestins, in addition, increase the activity of estradiol and isocitric dehydrogenases of the endometrium, thereby inactivating estradiol. The magnitude of these effects was more dependent on the duration of progestin therapy rather than on the dose. Whitehead et al found that the minimum effective dose is 1 mg for norethindrone and 0.15 mg for norgestrel.

Ovarian neoplasia. Estrogen replacement may possibly increase the risk of endometriod cancer of the ovary, which comprises 10% to 20% of all ovarian malignancies. This has *not* been conclusively established.[179] It is not known if progestin use will reduce this risk if it indeed exists.

Breast Neoplasia. Whether or not postmenopausal estrogen use increases the risk of breast cancer has been actively debated. There has been a suspicion, based on theoretical grounds, that estrogen use increases the risk of breast cancer for the following reasons: (1) breast cancer can be an estrogen-sensitive tumor, (2) estrogens can induce mammary tumors in rodents, and (3) women with prolonged endogenous estrogen exposure (e.g., early menarche, late menopause, nulliparity) are at increased risk of breast malignancies. For these reasons more than 20 studies have been conducted to

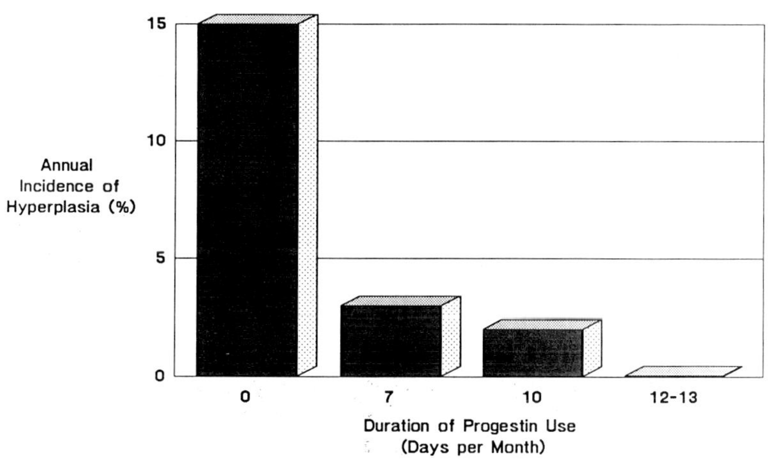

Fig. 19-19. Annual incidence of endometrial hyperplasia according to duration of progestin use per month. (From Studd JWW et al: The prevention and treatment of endometrial pathology. In Pasetto N, Paoletti R, Ambrus JL, editors: *The menopause and postmenopause*, Lancaster, England, 1980, MTP Press, p 127.)

resolve this issue. Nearly all of these studies found that postmenopausal estrogen replacement does not substantially increase the risk of developing breast cancer. The largest epidemiologic study consisted of 1960 cases of breast cancer with 2258 matched controls, identified through a breast screening program with 280,000 participants.[17] The relative risk (RR) of breast cancer for all postmenopausal estrogen users (1.03) was not increased. However, there was a statistically significant increase in breast cancer risk with increasing duration of estrogen use. Exposures of 10 to 14 years had an RR of 1.28. For exposures greater than 20 years the RR was 1.47. This increase is relatively small, and averages approximately 2% per year of estrogen use.

One study which has *not* found duration of estrogen treatment increases the risk of breast cancer is the Nurse's Health Study.[33] It observed 722 cases of breast cancer in 23,000 postmenopausal women prospectively followed for up to 10 years. Past estrogen use, even for as long as 10 years, did not increase the risk of breast cancer, but use within the preceeding year modestly increased the risk of breast cancer (RR: 1.36; CI: 1.11 to 1.67) compared with women who had never used estrogens. This risk was not altered by the dose or duration of estrogen use. In particular, this elevated risk among current estrogen users was confined to those women who regularly consumed alcohol; current estrogen users who did not consume alcohol were *not* at increased risk. This raises the possibility that women who use postmenopausal estrogens may benefit from reducing their alcohol consumption. Of note is that estrogen users were more likely to have their cancer detected by mammography (41% versus 33%) and were 20% less likely to die from their cancer. Unfortunately, there were not enough progestin users to analyze the effect of this hormone on breast cancer risk. These results suggest that long-term past use of postmenopausal estrogens does not increase the risk of breast cancer but that current use may modestly increase the risk. For women currently taking estrogens, self-breast examination and mammography are especially important. Because death rates from CVD are more than four times that of endometrial and breast cancer combined, any adverse carcinogenic effect of estrogen would be far outweighed by its reduction of CVD.

There is the possibility that the addition of a progestin may protect the breast, as it does the endometrium. Gambrell analyzed 69 cases of breast cancer, 11 of which were among combined estrogen and progestin users (incidence 66.8 per 100,000 women-years), and 28 of which were among estrogen-only users (incidence 142 per 100,000 women-years).[62] This difference was *not* statistically significant ($p = 0.08$). Thus the benefit of progestins in preventing breast cancer remains unproven. Moreover, this hypothesis is contrary to the fact that the mitotic activity of the breast increases during the luteal phase (peak endometrial mitosis is during the follicular phase)[4] and that progesterone induces mammary ductal growth in rodents.[46] Because there is no good evidence that progestins will reduce the risk of breast cancer, and because they may adversely affect lipoproteins and thus increase cardiovascular mortality, the use of progestins in women without a uterus is unnecessary and possibly detrimental.

Gallbladder disease. During the first year of use, estrogen treatment increases the risk of cholelithiasis by 20% (95% CI: 0.7 to 2.1).[87] Cholelithiasis occurs probably because estrogens increase the hepatic excretion of LDL cholesterol.[177] Also estrogens reduce the amount of chenodeoxycholic acid in bile, which keeps cholesterol in aqueous solution.[12]

Thromboembolic disease. Estrogen replacement increases the activity of the coagulation and fibrinolytic systems.[19] This may be clinically relevant only to women taking oral contraceptives, particularly those with the highest estrogen content, which are associated with increased risk of thromboembolic disease.[161] This appears to be a dose-response relationship because the incidence of thromboembolic disease is not increased by estrogen replacement.[161]

Hypertension. Estrogen replacement in general may modestly lower blood pressure in many women,[112] but may induce or exacerbate hypertension in others.[36] This idiosyncratic reaction to oral estrogens may be mediated by an increase in the hepatic production of renin substrate or by the production of an aberrant form.[151] In any case, this elevation in blood pressure is usually reversible upon discontinuation of estrogen.

Glucose tolerance. Although oral contraceptives are associated with impaired carbohydrate metabolism,[157] the lower doses used for estrogen replacement have not been linked to impaired glucose tolerance.[158] Postmenopausal estrogen users do not appear to be more likely to develop diabetes than estrogen nonusers.[110] Postmenopausal women with diabetes show no change or show an improvement of their disease with estrogen use, as evidenced by lower glucose levels or reduced insulin requirements.[22] This is consistent with the observation that estrogen appears to increase the binding of insulin to its receptor.[8] Moreover, animal models have shown that estrogen improves experimentally-induced hyperglycemia.[130]

Contraindications

Absolute contraindications to postmenopausal estrogen replacement are as follows:

1. Known or suspected breast cancer. However, women with breast cancer may be treated with tamoxifen citrate, which has been found to conserve bone mass,[104] induce a beneficial lipoprotein profile,[170] and reduce the incidence of cardiac morbidity by 31%.
2. Endometrial carcinoma, if it has spread beyond the uterine corpus. Postmenopausal women with stage I endometrial cancer who take estrogens have been found to have a higher 5-year survival rate compared to women who do not.[37] For this reason, women who have had endometrial cancer confined to the uterus at the time of diagnosis and who remain disease free for a minimum of 2 years may potentially be considered for estrogen treatment if sufficient benefits exist.

3. Undiagnosed genital bleeding.
4. Active liver disease.
5. Active thromboembolic disease or a history of estrogen-related thromboembolic disease.

Relative contraindications are as follows:

1. Chronic liver dysfunction. Impairment of the liver's ability to metabolize estrogen leads to excessive levels of estrogen. This may be compensated for by using smaller and less frequent doses.
2. Poorly-controlled hypertension.
3. History of thromboembolic disease. Although postmenopausal estrogens have not been found to cause thrombosis, the possibility exists that they may do so in this group at increased risk for having a thrombotic event. If estrogen treatment would confer significant benefits, it may be prescribed transdermally, which would not be expected to stimulate the hepatic production of coagulation factors.
4. Preexisting uterine leiomyomata or active endometriosis. Estrogen use may prevent the involution of these conditions which occurs after menopause. Estrogen treatment may be initiated after waiting a short interval (i.e., 3 to 12 months). However, patients who have submucous leiomyomata may experience heavy and/or irregular bleeding with hormone replacement.
5. Acute intermittent porphyria; estrogens may precipitate attacks.

PROGESTOGENS

Progestins are used to prevent endometrial stimulation which may be induced by estrogen treatment. They may also be used to relieve hot flashes in patients who are not candidates for estrogen replacement.

Available preparations

Progesterone and its derivatives are absorbed by the oral, vaginal, rectal, and intramuscular routes. Although convenient, oral absorption is highly variable with as much as a threefold difference between patients.[183] For this reason, variable clinical effects may be seen in patients given the same oral dose. Following absorption, oral progestins are presented to the liver in high concentrations where they may alter the hepatic metabolism of serum lipoproteins and in particular may lower HDL cholesterol levels. Progestins are then rapidly metabolized by the liver to deoxycorticosterone.[128]

Medroxyprogesterone acetate (MPA), 10 mg, is the most commonly used progestin in the United States and is effective against hyperplasia, with modest effects on serum lipids. For those patients unable to tolerate this dose, 5 mg may be used. The 5-mg dose in most cases will offer similar protection against hyperplasia except in individuals who poorly absorb oral MPA.[64] MPA given intramuscularly as its depot form is well absorbed but has a highly variable duration of effectiveness and frequently causes irregular vaginal bleeding. The usual dose is 50 to 150 mg IM every 1 to 3 months (the 50-mg dose is sufficient to relieve hot flashes).[122] Alternatively megestrol acetate 40 to 80 mg daily or micronized progesterone 200 to 300 mg daily may be substituted for MPA. Micronized progesterone offers promise as an "ideal" progestin because it is active against hyperplasia without significantly altering serum lipid levels.[182]

The 19-nortestosterone derivatives are the potent progestins used in oral contraceptives. They have partial androgenic properties and lower HDL cholesterol levels. They are currently available in the United States in low doses only in the form of progestin-only oral contraceptives. Norethindrone is available as either Micronor or Nor-QD, which contain 0.35 mg norethindrone. Typically, three tablets daily are needed to protect against hyperplasia. Norgestrel is available as Ovrette, which contains 0.075 mg; two tablets daily are needed for endometrial protection.[184] The following three less-androgenic 19-nortestosterone–derived progestins currently used in Europe will soon become available in the United States for postmenopausal use: desogestrel, norgestimate, and gestodene.

Adverse effects

Progestins may produce abdominal bloating, mastalgia, headaches, mood changes, and acne. More importantly, all progestins, particularly the 19-nortestosterone derivatives (e.g., norgestrel and norethindrone), negatively affect serum lipids, primarily by lowering HDL levels. HDL levels are lowered by 9% to 16% with 10 mg of medroxyprogesterone acetate daily,[153,172] by 17% to 20% with 0.5 mg of norgestrel daily,[77,129] and by 20% to 36% with 10 mg of norethindrone daily.[77,153] These doses of norgestrel and norethindrone are higher than necessary because 0.15 mg of norgestrel and 1 mg of norethindrone are as effective against hyperplasia as are the higher doses.[184] The effect of these lower doses on lipids in unknown.

The net effect of a hormonal regimen on lipids depends upon the particular estrogen and progestin used as well as the dose, route, and frequency of administration. In general progestins may negate in whole or in part the beneficial effect of estrogen on HDL and LDL. This may compromise the possible reduction in CVD observed with estrogen replacement. Moreover the protective effect of progestins against breast cancer is unproven. Therefore the use of progestins may be justified only for those women with an intact uterus for whom prevention of endometrial cancer is needed.

TREATMENT REGIMENS

Prior to initiating hormonal therapy, the patient should be evaluated by taking a detailed history and conducting a physical examination, including blood pressure, breast and pelvic examination, stool guaiac, and Pap smear. Mammography should be performed to prevent prescribing estrogens to a patient with preexisting subclinical cancer of the breast; this examination should be repeated annually. Serum cholesterol should be measured at least once every 5 years, provided it remains below 200 mg/dL; if serum cholesterol exceeds this level or if HDL cholesterol is below 35 mg/dL, follow-up should be arranged as outlined in Tables 19-2 and 19-3. An endometrial biopsy should be performed prior to treatment if there is a history of abnormal vaginal bleeding or if the patient is at increased risk of having a preexisting endometrial hyperplasia. This may be accomplished either by endometrial aspiration if technically feasible or by fractional dilation and curettage. Before instituting therapy, a biopsy should be performed on patients receiving unopposed estrogens for an extended period of time, regardless of bleeding; biopsy should be repeated every year since the annual incidence of hyperplasia is 30%.[143]

The most commonly used schedule of hormone replacement in the United States for women with intact uteri is cyclic, with CEE 0.625 mg given daily and MPA 10 mg given for the first 13 calendar days of each month. The majority of patients on this regimen will demonstrate withdrawal bleeding typically during the tenth and twentieth days of the month.[5] If bleeding occurs at any other time an endometrial biopsy should be performed. For those patients who have previously undergone hysterectomy, no progestin is needed.

The above schedule may be modified by substituting another estrogen for CEE and/or another progestin for MPA. Appropriate doses of other oral estrogens are 1 mg of micronized estradiol and 1.25 mg of piperazine estrone sulfate. Parenteral estrogens (e.g., transdermal estradiol) are particularly useful for women such as those with a prior history of hepatic dysfunction, thrombosis, or hypertension, whom one wishes to "bypass" the hepatic effects of oral estrogens. The typical starting dose of transdermal estradiol is 0.05 mg applied twice weekly; this may be increased to 0.10 mg after 1 month, if necessary.

To avoid withdrawal bleeding, continuous rather than cyclic hormonal treatment is used. A typical regimen is 0.625 mg CEE daily with 2.5 or 5 mg MPA daily. Over half of the patients will have irregular vaginal bleeding initially, but within 1 year 75% to 85% will be amenorrheic.[5] Women most likely to become amenorrheic are those who are many years beyond the menopause or who are given the higher progestin dose. Alternatively, norethindrone (a progestin-only oral contraceptive) 0.35 to 1.05 mg daily, may substitute for MPA. If a patient develops vaginal bleeding after being amenorrheic on this regimen, an endometrial biopsy should be performed; 2 of 41 women who developed irregular bleeding after several years of continuous estrogen and progestin treatment were found to have endometrial adenocarcinoma.[95]

Transvaginal ultrasound monitoring has been used recently to screen postmenopausal women for endometrial pathology. This technique uses a high-frequency ultrasound transducer placed in the vagina where it is in close anatomic proximity to the uterus and provides high-resolution imaging. This method is superior to transabdominal scanning because it overcomes the difficulties encountered in scanning women who are obese, have excessive bowel gas, or have inadequate

Table 19-2. Initial classification and recommended follow-up based on total cholesterol in adults without CHD.*

Cholesterol (mg/dL)	Classification	Follow-up
< 200	Desirable	Repeat within 5 years**
200 to 239	Borderline-high	With fewer than two CHD risk factors: repeat in 1-2 years** With two CHD risk factors: do lipoprotein analysis (Go to Table 19-3)
≥ 240	High	Do lipoprotein analysis (Go to Table 19-3)

* CHD, coronary heart disease; LDL, low-density lipoprotein; HDL, high-density lipoprotein.
** Do lipoprotein analysis if HDL < 35 mg/dL
Risk factors: male gender, postmenopausal female not taking estrogen, family history of premature CHD, cigarette use, hypertension, diabetes mellitus, HDL cholesterol < 35 mg/dL.
From the Report of the National Cholesterol Education Program Expert Panel on Detection, Evaluation, and Treatment of High Blood Cholesterol in Adults, *JAMA* 269(23):3015-3023, 1993.

Table 19-3. Classification and treatment decisions based on LDL-cholesterol*

Classification		
< 130 mg/dL	Desirable LDL-cholesterol	
130 to 159 mg/dL	Borderline-high-risk LDL-cholesterol	
≥ 160 mg/dL	High-risk LDL cholesterol	
	Initiation level mg/dL	**Minimal goal mg/dL**
Dietary Treatment		
WithoutCHD and with fewer than two other risk factors	≥ 160	< 160
Without CHD and with two or more risk factors	≥ 130	< 130
With CHD	> 100	≤ 100
Drug Treatment		
Without CHD and with fewer than two other risk factors	≥ 190	< 160
Without CHD and with two or more risk factors	≥ 160	< 130
With CHD	≥ 130	≤ 100

*LDL, low density lipoprotein; CHD, coronary heart disease
From the Report of the National Cholesterol Education Program Expert Panel on Detection, Evaluation, and Treatment of High Blood Cholesterol in Adults, *JAMA* 269(23):3015-3023, 1993.

bladder filling as a result of discomfort or incontinence.[120] Ultrasonography accurately measures endometrial thickness within 1 mm of actual thickness seen on pathologic examination.[124] Two large series evaluated postmenopausal vaginal bleeding by transvaginal ultrasonography prior to diagnostic D&C in 205 and 215 women.[67,89] The endometrial thickness in women with endometrial cancer was 18±16 mm; in women with endometrial atrophy, 3±1 mm. Both studies found no cases of endometrial cancer in women with endometrial thickness less than 8 mm. Because 70% of women with postmenopausal vaginal bleeding have an endometrium less than 5 mm thick, a substantial number of D&Cs can be avoided. Additional long-term studies are necessary before this technique can replace endometrial biopsies.

Conclusions

Estrogen replacement offers significant benefits to many postmenopausal women, especially to those whose menopause occurred before age 45. In addition, women at high risk for atherosclerosis or who already have CVD would particularly benefit from estrogen use. The increased risk of endometrial and breast cancer seen with estrogen replacement appears to be small in comparison with its protective effect against cardiovascular disease. The benefits and risks as they pertain to each individual patient should be reviewed with her in detail. Ultimately, she must decide whether or not to initiate therapy and give her informed consent.

REFERENCES

1. Albrecht BH et al: Objective evidence that placebo and oral medroxyprogesterone acetate therapy diminish menopausal vasomotor flushes, *Am J Obstet Gynecol* 139:631, 1981.
2. Alffam PH: An epidemiologic study of cervical and intertrochanteric fractures of the femur in suburban population, *Acta Orthop Scand* 65:1, 1964.
3. Amundsen DW, Diers CJ: The age of menopause in classical Greece and Rome, *Hum Biol* 42:79, 1970.
4. Anderson JJ, Ferguson DJP, Raab GM: Cell turnover in the resting human breast: influence of parity, contraceptive pill, age, and laterality, *Br J Cancer* 46:376, 1982.
5. Archer DF, Pickar JH, Bottiglioni F: Bleeding patterns in postmenopausal women taking continuous combined or sequential regimens of conjugated estrogens with medroxyprogesterone acetate, *Obstet Gynecol* 83:686-92, 1984.
6. Bagatell CJ et al: Physiologic testosterone levels in normal men suppress high-density lipoprotein cholesterol levels, *Ann Intern Med* 116:(12 pt 1):967-973, 1992.
7. Bain C et al: Use of postmenopausal hormones and risk of myocardial infarction, *Circulation* 64:42, 1981.
8. Ballejo G et al: The effect of sex steroids on insulin-bindıng by target tissues in the rat, *Contraception* 28:413, 1983.
9. Baran D et al: Dietary modification with dairy products for preventing vertebral bone loss in premenopausal women: a 3-year prospective study, *J Clin Endocrinol Metab* 70:264-270, 1990.
10. Barrett-Connor E, Chang JC, Edelstein SL: Coffee-associated osteoporosis offset by daily milk consumption, *JAMA* 271:280-283, 1994.
11. Beattie CW, Rodgers CH, Soyka LF: Influence of ovariectomy and ovarian steroids on hypothalamic tyrosine hydroxylase activity in the rat, *Endocrinology* 91:276, 1972.
12. Bennion LJ: Changes in bile lipids accompanying oophorectomy in premenopausal women, *N Engl J Med* 297:709, 1977.
13. Berkow R, editor: *The Merck manual of diagnosis and therapy*, Rahway, NJ, 1987, Merck, Sharp & Dohme Research Laboratories.
14. Black LJ et al: Raloxifene (Ly139481 HCI) prevents bone loss and reduces serum cholesterol without causing uterine hypertrophy in ovariectomized rats, *J Clin Invest* 93(1):63-69, 1994.
15. Boukobza G: Efficacy and tolerance of veralipride in the treatment of flushing in the menopause, *Rev Fr Gynecol Obstet* 81:413-417, 1986.
16. Briancon D, Meunier PJ: Treatment of osteoporosis with fluoride, calcium, and vitamin D, *Orthop Clin North Am* 12:629-648, 1981.
17. Brinton LA, Hoover R, Fraymeni JF: Menopausal oestrogens and breast cancer risk: an expanded case-control study, *Br J Cancer* 54:825, 1986.
18. Bush TL, Cavan LD, Barrett-Connor E: Estrogen use and all-cause mortality, *JAMA* 249:903, 1983.
19. Caine YG et al: Coagulation activation following estrogen administration to postmenopausal women, *Thromb Haemost* 68(4):392-395, 1992.
20. Campbell S, Whitehead M: Estrogen therapy and the postmenopausal syndrome, *Clin Obstet Gynecol* 4:31, 1977.
21. Cann CE, Genant HK, Ettinger B: Spinal mineral loss in oophorectomized women: determination by quantitative computer tomography, *JAMA* 244:2056, 1980.
22. Cantilo E: Successful responses in diabetes mellitus of the menopause provided by the antagonistic action of sex hormones on pituitary activity, *Endocrinology* 28:20, 1941.
23. Carr BR, MacDonald PC: Estrogen treatment of postmenopausal women, *Adv Intern Med* 28:491, 1983.
24. Chang RJ, Judd HL: Elevation of skin temperature of the finger as an objective index of postmenopausal hot flushes: standardization of the techniques, *Am J Obstet Gynecol* 135:713, 1979.
25. Chapuy MC et al: Vitamin D_3 and calcium to prevent hip fractures in elderly women, *N Engl J Med* 327:1637-1642, 1992.
26. Charig CR, Rundle JS: Flushing: long-term side effect of orchiectomy in treatment of prostatic carcinoma, *Urology* 33:175-178, 1989.
27. Chestnut CH III et al: Lack of efficacy of nasal spray calcitonin in early postmenopausal women, *J Bone Miner Res* (8Suppl1)S:249, 1993.
28. Christiansen C, Christiansen MS, Transbol I: Bone mass in postmenopausal women after withdrawal of estrogen/gestagen replacement therapy, *Lancet* 1:459, 1981.
29. Christiansen C, Riis BJ, Rodbro P: Prediction of rapid bone loss in postmenopausal women, *Lancet* 1:1105. 1987.
30. Chu J, Schweid AI, Weiss NS: Survival among women with endometrial cancer: a comparison of estrogen users and nonusers, *Am J Obstet Gynecol* 143:569, 1982.
31. Civitelli R et al: Bone turnover in postmenopausal osteoporosis: effect of calcitonin treatment, *J Clin Invest* 82:1268, 1988.
32. Clayden JR, Bell JW, Pollard P: Menopausal flushing: double-blind trial of a nonhormonal medication, *Br Med J* 1:409, 1974.
33. Colditz GA et al: Prospective study of estrogen replacement therapy and risk of breast cancer in postmenopausal women, *JAMA* 264:2648-2653, 1990.
34. Colditz GA et al: Menopause and the risk of coronary heart disease in women, *N Engl J Med* 316:1105, 1987.
35. The Coronary Drug Project Research Group: Findings leading to discontinuation of the 2.5 mg/day estrogen group, *JAMA* 226:652, 1973.
36. Crane MG, Harris JJ, Windsor W: Hypertension, oral contraceptive agents, and conjugated estrogens, *Ann Intern Med* 74:13, 1971.
37. Creasman WT et al: Estrogen replacement therapy in the patient treated for endometrial cancer, *Obstet Gynecol* 67(3):326-330, 1986.

38. D'Amico JF et al: Induction of hypothalamic opioid activity with transdermal estradiol administration in postmenopausal women, *Fertil Steril* 55:754, 1991.
39. Davidson BJ, Gambone JC, Lagasse LD: Free estradiol in postmenopausal women with and without endometrial cancer, *J Clin Endocrinol Metab* 52:404, 1981.
40. Dawson-Hughes B et al: A controlled trial of the effect of calcium supplementation on bone density in postmenopausal women, *N Engl J Med* 323:878-883, 1990.
41. DeFazio J et al: Direct action of androgen on hot flashes in the human male, *Maturitas* 6:8, 1984.
42. Deftos LJ et al: Influence of age and sex on plasma calcitonin in human beings, *N Engl J Med* 302:1351, 1980.
43. Dequeker JV, Johnston CC, editors: *Noninvasive bone measurements*, Oxford, 1981, IRL Press.
44. Deutsch S, Ossowski B, Benjamin I: Comparison between degree of systemic description of vaginally and orally administered estrogens at different dose levels in postmenopausal women, *Am J Obstet Gynecol* 139:967, 1981.
45. DeVogt HJ et al: Cardiovascular side effects of diethylstilbestrol, cyproterone acetate, and medroxyprogesterone acetate used for treatment of prostatic cancer, *J Urol* 135:303, 1986.
46. Dulbecco R, Henahan M, Armstrong B: Cell types and morphogenesis in the mammary gland, *Proc Natl Acad Sci USA* 79:7346, 1982.
47. Eaker ED, Castelli WP: Coronary heart disease and its risk factors among women in the framingham study. In: *Coronary heart disease in women*, New York, 1987, Haymarket Doyma.
48. Elwood JM, Boyes DA: Clinical and pathologic features and survival of endometrial cancer patients in relation to prior use of estrogens, *Gynecol Oncol* 10:173, 1980.
49. Englund DE, Johansson EDB: Plasma levels of oestrone, oestradiol, and gonadotropins in postmenopausal women after oral and vaginal administration of conjugated equine estrogens, *Br J Obstet Gynaecol* 85:957, 1987.
50. Erlik Y, Meldrum DR, Judd HL: Estrogen levels in postmenopausal women with hot flushes, *Obstet Gynecol* 59:403, 1982.
51. Erlik Y et al: Effect of megestrol acetate on flushing and bone metabolism in postmenopausal women, *Maturitas* 3:167, 1981a.
52. Erlik Y et al: Association of waking episodes with menopausal hot flushes, *JAMA* 245:1741, 1981b.
53. Ettinger B, Cann L, Genant K: Menopausal bone loss: effects of conjugated estrogen and/or high calcium diet, *Maturitas* 6:108, 1984.
54. Falkeborn M et al: The risk of acute myocardial infarction after oestrogen and oestrogen-progestogen replacement, *Br J Obstet Gynaecol* 99(10):821-8, 1992.
55. Felson DT et al: Thiazide diuretics and the risk of hip fractures: results from the Framingham study, *JAMA* 165:370-373, 1991.
56. Felson DT et al: The effect of postmenopausal estrogen therapy on bone density in elderly women, *N Engl J Med* 329(16):1141-1146, 1993.
57. Freedman RR, Woodward S, Sabharwal SC: Alpha 2-adrenergic mechanism in menopausal hot flushes, *Obstet Gynecol* 76:573, 1992.
58. Freedman RR and Woodward S: Behavioral treatment of menopausal hot flushes: evaluation by ambulatory monitoring, *Am J Obstet Gynecol* 167:436-439, 1992.
59. Gallagher JC, Kable WT, Goldgar D: Effect of progestin therapy on cortical and trabecular bone: comparison with estrogen, *Am J Med* 90:171-178, 1991.
60. Gallagher JC, Nordin BEC: Oestrogens and calcium metabolism, *Front Horm Res* 2:98, 1973.
61. Gambrell RD: Clinical use of progestins in the menopausal patient, *J Reprod Med* 27:531, 1982a.
62. Gambrell RD, Massey FW, Castaneda TA: The use of the progestagen challenge test to reduce the risk of endometrial cancer, *Obstet Gynecol* 55:732, 1980.
63. Geola FL et al: Biological effects of various doses of conjugated equine estrogens in postmenopausal women, *J Clin Endocrinol Metab* 51:620, 1980.
64. Gibbons WE et al: A comparison of biochemical and morphological events mediated by estrogen and progestin on the endometrium of postmenopausal women, *Am J Obstet Gynecol* 154:456, 1986.
65. Gordon G, Vaughan C: *Clinical management of the osteoporoses*, Acton, MA, 1976, Publishing Sciences Group.
66. Gordon T et al: High density lipoprotein as a protective factor against coronary heart disease, *Am J Med* 62:707, 1977.
67. Grandberg S et al: Endometrial thickness as measured by endovaginal ultrasound for identifying endometrial abnormality, *Am J Obstet Gynecol* 164(1 Pt 1):47-52, 1991.
68. Grodin JM, Siiteri PK, MacDonald PC: Source of estrogen production in postmenopausal women, *J Clin Endocrinol Metab* 36:207, 1973.
69. Haas S et al: The effect of transdermal estradiol on hormone and metabolic dynamics over a six-week period, *Obstet Gynecol* 71:671, 1988.
70. Hammond MG, Hatley L, Talbert LM: A double-blind study to evaluate the effect of methyldopa on menopausal vasomotor flushes, *J Clin Endocrinol Metab* 58:1158, 1984.
71. Harris ST et al: The effect of short-term treatment with alendronate on vertebral density and biochemical markers on bone remodeling in early postmenopausal women, *J Clin Endocrinol Metab* 76:1399-1406, 1993.
72. Harris ST et al: Four year study of intermittent cyclic etidronate treatment of postmenopausal osteoporosis: three years of blinded therapy followed by one year of open therapy, *Am J Med* 95(6):557-567, 1993.
73. Heanly RP: Estrogens and postmenopausal osteoporosis, *Clin Obstet Gynecol* 19:791, 1976.
74. Heller RF, Jacobs HS: Coronary heart disease in relation to age, sex, and the menopause, *Br Med J* 1:472, 1978.
75. Henderson BE, Paganini-Hill A, Ross RK: Decreased mortality in users of estrogen replacement therapy, *Arch Intern Med* 151:75-78, 1991.
76. Hillyard CJ, Stevenson JC, MacIntyre I: Relative deficiency of plasma calcitonin in normal women, *Lancet* 1:961, 1978.
77. Hirvonen E, Malkonen M, Manninen V: Effects of different progestins, *N Engl J Med* 304:560, 1981.
78. Hopper JL, Seeman E. The bone density of female twins discordant for tobacco use, *N Engl J Med* 330:387-392, 1994.
79. Horsman A, Simpson M, Kirby PA: Nonlinear bone loss in oophorectomized women, *Br J Radiol* 50:504, 1977.
80. Huggins C, Stevens RE, Hodges CU: Studies of prostatic cancer. II. The effects of castration in advanced carcinoma of the prostate, *Arch Surg* 43:209, 1941.
81. Hyashi T et al: Basal release of nitric oxide from aortic rings is greater in female rabbits than in male rabbits: implications for atherosclerosis, *Proc Natl Acad Sci USA* 89(23): 11259-11263, 1992.
82. Iosif CS et al: Estrogen receptors in the human female lower urinary tract, *Am J Obstet Gynecol* 141:817, 1981.
83. Iskrant AP: The etiology of fractured hips in females, *Am J Public Health* 58:485, 1968.
84. Jensen J, Christiansen C, Rodbro P: Cigarette smoking, serum estrogens, and bone loss during hormone-replacement therapy early after menopause, *N Engl J Med* 313(16):973-975, 1985.
85. Johnson AE et al: Estradiol modulation of noradrenergic receptors in the guinea pig brain assessed by tritium-sensitive film autoradiography, *Brain Res* 336:153, 1985.
86. Jones KP, Ravnikar VA, Schiff I: Effect of lofexidine on vasomotor flushes, *Maturitas* 7:135, 1985.
87. Kakar F, Weiss NS, Strite SA: Noncontraceptive estrogen use and risk of gallstone disease in women, *Am J Public Health* 78(5):564, 1988.

88. Kirkland RT et al: Decrease in plasma high-density lipoprotein cholesterol levels at puberty in boys with delayed adolescence: correlation with plasma testosterone levels, *JAMA* 257:502, 1987.
89. Klug PW, Leitner G: Comparisons of vaginal ultrasound and histologic findings of the endometrium, *Geburtshilfe Frauenheilkd* 49(9):797-802, 1989.
90. Komm BS et al: Estrogen binding, receptor mRNA, and biologic response in osteoblast-like osteosarcoma cells, *Science* 241:81, 1988.
91. Krall EA, Dawson-Hughes B: Walking, bone mineral density and bone loss, *J Bone Miner Res* 8(Suppl 1):S150, 1993.
92. Lacroix AZ et al: Thiazide diuretic agents and the incidence of hip fracture, *N Engl J Med* 322:286-290, 1990.
93. Laufer LK et al: Effect of clonidine on hot flashes in postmenopausal women, *Obstet Gynecol* 60:483, 1982.
94. Lauritzen JB et al: Radial and humeral fractures as predictors of subsequent hip, radial or humeral fractures in women and their seasonal variation, *Osteoporosis Int* 3:133-137, 1993.
95. Leather AT, Savvas M, Studd JW: Endometrial histology and bleeding patterns after 8 years of continuous combined estrogen and progestogen therapy in postmenopausal women, *Obstet Gynecol* 78(6):1008-1010, 1991.
96. Lebherz TB, French LT: Nonhormonal treatment of the menopausal syndrome: a double-blind evaluation of an autonomic system stabilizer, *Obstet Gynecol* 33:795, 1969.
97. Lerner DJ, Kannel WB: Patterns of coronary disease morbidity and mortality: a 26-year follow-up of the Framingham population, *Am Heart J* 111(2):383, 1986.
98. Licata AA et al: Acute effects of dietary protein on calcium metabolism in patients with osteoporosis, *J Gerontol* 36:14, 1981.
99. Lindsay R et al: Incidence, cost and risk factors of fracture of the proximal femur in the USA. In Christiansen C et al, editors: *Osteoporosis*, Denmark, 1984, Aalborg Stoftsbogturkkeri.
100. Lindsay R et al: Long-term prevention of postmenopausal osteoporosis by estrogens, *Lancet* 1:1038, 1976b.
101. Lindsay R et al: Comparative effects of oestrogen and a progestagen on bone loss in postmenopausal women, *Clin Sci Mol Med* 54:193, 1978.
102. Lindsay R, Sweeney A: Urinary cyclic AMP in osteoporosis, *Scott Med J* 21:231, 1976a.
103. Lobo RA, Brenner PF, Mishell DR: Metabolic parameters and steroid levels in postmenopausal women receiving lower doses of natural estrogen replacement, *Obstet Gynecol* 62:94, 1983.
104. Love RR et al: Effects of tamoxifen on bone mineral density in postmenopausal women with breast cancer, *N Engl J Med* 326:852-856, 1992.
105. Luine VN, McEwen BS: Effect of estradiol on turnover of type A monamine oxidase in brain, *J Neurochem* 28:1221, 1977.
106. Mandel FP et al: Effect of progestins on bone metabolism in postmenopausal women, *J Reprod Med* 27 (Suppl 8):511, 1982.
107. Mandel FP et al: Biologic effects of various doses of ethinyl estradiol in postmenopausal women, *Obstet Gynecol* 59:673, 1982b.
108. Mandel FP et al: Biologic effects of various doses of vaginally administered conjugated equine estrogens in postmenopausal women, *J Clin Endocrinol Metab* 57:133, 1983.
109. Manolagas SC, Anderson DG: Detection of high-affinity glucocorticoid binding in rat bone, *J Endocrinol* 76:379, 1978.
110. Manson JE et al: A prospective study of postmenopausal estrogen therapy and subsequent incidence of non-insulin-dependent diabetes mellitus, *Ann Epidemiol* 2(5):665-673, 1992.
111. Mashchak CA et al: The relation of physiological changes to subjective symptoms in postmenopausal women with and without hot flushes, *Maturitas* 6:301, 1985a.
112. Mashchak CA, Lobo RA: Estrogen replacement therapy and hypertension, *J Reprod Med* 30(Suppl):805, 1985b.
113. Mashchak CA et al: Comparison of pharmacodynamic properties of various estrogen formulations, *Am J Obstet Gynecol* 144:511, 1982.
114. Mateo L et al: Bone mineral density in patients with temporal arteritis and polymyalgia rheumatica, *J Rheumatol* 20:1369-1373, 1993.
115. Matkovic V et al: Bone status and fracture rates in two regions of Yugoslavia, *Am J Clin Nutr* 32:540, 1979.
116. Matthews KA et al: Menopause and risk factors for coronary heart disease, *N Engl J Med* 321:641-646, 1989.
117. Mazess RB et al: Enhanced precision with dual-energy x-ray absorptiometry, *Calcif Tissue Int* 51:14-17, 1992.
118. McGill HC: Sex steroid hormone receptors in the cardiovascular system, *Postgrad Med* 64-68, April 1989.
119. McKinlay S, Jeffreys M, Thompson B: An investigation of the age of menopause, *J Biosoc Sci* 4:161, 1972.
120. Mendelson EB et al: Endometrial abnormalities: evaluation with transvaginal sonography, *Am J Roentgenol* 150(1):139-142, 1988.
121. Michnovicz JJ et al: Increased 2-hydroxylation of estradiol as a possible mechanism for the anti-estrogenic effect of cigarette smoking, *N Engl J Med* 315(21):1305-1309, 1986.
122. Morrison JC et al: The use of medroxyprogesterone acetate for the relief of climacteric symptoms, *Am J Obstet Gynecol* 138:99, 1980.
123. Mundy GR: Osteoporosis: boning up on genes, *Nature* 367(6460):216-217, 1994.
124. Nasri MN, Coast GJ: Correlation of ultrasound findings and endometrial histopathology in postmenopausal women, *Br J Obstet Gynecol* 96(11):1333-1338, 1989.
125. Nathorst-Boos J et al: Is sexual life influenced by transdermal estrogen therapy: a double blind placebo controlled study in postmenopausal women, *Acta Obstet Gynecol Scand* 72(8):656-660, 1993.
126. Nixon RL, Jamowsky DS, David JM: Effects of progesterone, estradiol, and testosterone on the uptake and metabolism of ^{3}H-norepinephrine, ^{3}H-dopamine, and ^{3}H-serotonin in rat synaptosomes, *Res Commun Chem Pathol Pharmacol* 7:233, 1974.
127. Norcross WA and Schmidt JD: Hot flashes in men with testicular insufficiency, *West J Med* 145:515-516, 1986.
128. Ottosson UB et al: Conversion of oral progesterone into deoxycorticosterone during postmenopausal replacement therapy, *Acta Obstet Gynecol Scand* 63:577, 1984.
129. Ottosson UB, Johanson BG, Schoultz B: Subfraction of high-density lipoprotein cholesterol: a comparison between progesterone and natural progesterone, *Am J Obstet Gynecol* 151:746-750, 1985.
130. Paik SG et al: Induction of insulin-dependent diabetes by streptozotocin: inhibition by estrogens, potentiation by androgens, *Diabetes* 31:724, 1982.
131. Paul SM et al: Estrogen-induced efflux of endogenous catecholamines from the hypothalamus in vitro, *Brain Res* 178:499, 1979.
132. Petitti DB et al: Risk of vascular disease in women: smoking, oral contraceptives, noncontraceptive estrogens and other factors, *JAMA* 242:1150, 1979.
133. Punnonen R, Lukola A: Oestrogen-like effect of ginseng, *Br Med J* 281(6248):1110, 1980.
134. Raz R, Stamm WE: A controlled trial of intravaginal estriol in postmenopausal women with recurrent urinary tract infections, *N Engl J Med* 329:753-756, 1993.
135. Riggs BL et al: Effect of fluoride tretment on the fracture rate in postmenopausal women with osteoporosis, *N Engl J Med* 322:802-809, 1990.
136. Riis B, Thomsen K, Christiansen C: Does calcium supplementation prevent postmenopausal bone loss? *N Engl J Med* 316:173, 1987.
137. Ross RK et al: Menopausal estrogen therapy and protection from death from ischemic heart disease, *Lancet* 1:858, 1981.
138. Rubin GL: Estrogen replacement therapy and the risk of endometrial cancer: remaining controversies, *Am J Obstet Gynecol* 162:148-154, 1990.
139. Rutqvist LE, Anders Mattsson A: Cardiac and thromboembolic morbidity among postmenopausal women with early-stage breast cancer in a randomized trial of adjuvant tamoxifen, *J of Nat Cancer Inst* 85:1398-1406, 1993.

140. Sack MN, Rader DK, Cannon RO: Oestrogen and inhibition of oxidation of low-density lipoproteins in postmenopausal women, *Lancet* 343(8892):269-270, 1994.
141. Sacks FM, McPherson R, Walsh BW: Effect of postmenopausal estrogen replacement of plasma lipoprotein (a) concentrations, *Arch Intern Med* 154:1106-1110, 1994.
142. Schiff I et al: Effects of estrogens on sleep and psychological state of hypogonadal women, *JAMA* 242:2405, 1979.
143. Schiff I et al: Endometrial hyperplasia in women on cyclic or continuous estrogen regimens, *Fertil Steril* 37:79, 1982.
144. Schiff I et al: Oral medroxyprogesterone acetate in the treatment of postmenopausal symptoms, *JAMA* 244:1443, 1980.
145. Schiff I, Tulchinsky D, Ryan KJ: Vaginal absorption of estrone and 17α-estradiol, *Fertil Steril* 28:1963, 1977.
146. Schiff I, Wilson E: Clinical aspects of aging of the female reproductive system. In Schneider EL, editor: *The aging reproductive system*, New York, 1978, Raven Press.
147. Schneider DL, Barrett-Connor EL, Morton DJ: Thyroid hormone use and bone mineral density in elderly women, *JAMA* 271(16):1245-1249, 1994.
148. Schott AM et al: Ultrasound measurements on os calcis: precision and age-related changes in a normal female population, *Osteoporosis Int* 3:249-254, 1993.
149. Schwartz U, Hammerstein J: The estrogenic potency of ethinyl estradiol and mestranol—a comparative study, *J Acta Endocrinol* 72:118, 1973.
150. Sherman BW, West JH, Korenman SG: The menopausal transition: analysis of LH, FSH, estradiol, and progesterone concentrations during menstrual cycles of older women, *J Clin Endocrinol Metab* 42:629, 1976.
151. Shionoiri H et al.: An increase in high-molecular weight renin substrate associated with estrogenic hypertension, *Biochem Med* 29:14, 1983.
152. Siddle N, Whitehead M: Flexible prescribing of estrogens, *Contemp Ob Gyn* 22:137, 1983.
153. Silfverstolpe G et al: Lipid metabolic studies in oophorectomized women: effect on serum lipids and lipoproteins of three synthetic progestagens, *Maturitas* 4:103, 1982.
154. Slemenda CW et al: Predictors of bone mass in perimenopausal women: a prospective study of clinical data using photon absorptiometry, *Ann Intern Med* 112:96-101, 1990.
155. Smith DM, Nance WE, Kang KW: Genetic factors in determining bone mass, *J Clin Invest* 52:2800, 1973.
156. Smith JA: Androgen suppresion by a gonadotropin releasing hormone analogue in patients with metastatic carcinoma of the prostate, *J Urol* 131:110, 1984.
157. Spellacy WN: Carbohydrate metabolism in male infertility and female fertility-control patients, *Fertil Steril* 27:1132, 1976.
158. Spellacy WN, Butri WC, Birk SA: Effect of estrogen treatment for one year on carbohydrate and lipid metabolism in women with normal and abnormal glucose tolerance test results, *Am J Obstet Gynecol* 131:87, 1978.
159. Stamler J et al: Effects of long-term estrogen therapy on serum cholesterol-lipid-lipoprotein levels and mortality in middle aged men with previous myocardial infarction, *Circulation* 22:658, 1980.
160. Stampfer MJ et al: Postmenopausal estrogen therapy and cardiovascular disease: ten-year follow-up from the Nurses' Health Study, *N Engl J Med* 325:756-762, 1991.
161. Stampfer MJ et al: A prospective study of exogenous hormones and risk of pulmonary embolism in women, *Circulation* 86(4):1-676, 1992 (abstract 2689).
162. Steingold KA et al: Treatment of hot flashes with transdermal estradiol, *J Clin Endocrinol Metab* 61:627, 1985.
163. Steinleitner A et al: Decreased in vitro production of 6-keto prostaglandin by uterine arteries from postmenopausal women, *Am J Obstet Gynecol* 161:1677-1681, 1989.
164. Stevenson JC et al: Calcitonin and the calcium-regulating hormones in postmenopausal women: effect of estrogens, *Lancet* 1:693, 1981.
165. Stevenson JC et al: Effects of transdermal versus oral hormone replacement therapy on bone density in spine and proximal femur in postmenopausal women, *Lancet* 336:256-269, 1990.
166. Storm T et al: Effect of intermittent cyclical etidronate therapy on bone mass and fracture rate in women with postmenopausal osteoporosis, *N Engl J Med* 322:1265-1271, 1990.
167. Studd JWW et al: The prevention and treatment of endometrial pathology. In Pasetto N, Paoletti R, Ambrus JL, editors: *The Menopause and postmenopause*, Lancaster, England, 1980, MTP Press.
168. Sullivan JM et al: Postmenopausal estrogen use and coronary atherosclerosis, *Ann Intern Med* 108:358-363, 1988.
169. Sullivan JM et al: Estrogen replacement and coronary artery disease, *Arch Intern Med* 150:2557-2562, 1990.
170. Thangaraju M et al: Effect of tamoxifen on plasma lipids and lipoproteins in postmenopausal women with breast cancer, *Cancer* 73(3):659-663, 1994.
171. Thompson B, Hart SA, Durno D: Menopausal age and symptomatology in general practice, *J Biol Sci* 5:71-82, 1973.
172. Tikkanen MJ et al: Different effects of two progestins on HDL, *Atherosclerosis* 40:365, 1981.
173. Tremollieres FA, Pouilles JM, Ribot C. Vertebral postmenopausal bone loss is reduced in overweight women: a longitudinal study in 155 early postmenopausal women, J Clin Endocrinol Metab 77 (3):683-686, 1993.
174. Vercellini P et al: Veralipride for hot flushes during gonadotropin-releasing hormone agonist treatment, *Gynecol Obstet Invest* 34:102-104, 1992.
175. Vermeulen A: The hormonal activity of the postmenopausal ovary, *J Clin Endocrinol Metab* 42:247, 1976.
176. Wagner JD et al: Estrogen and progesterone replacement therapy reduces low density lipoprotein accumulation in the coronary arteries of surgically postmenopausal cynomolgus monkeys, *J Clin Invest* 88(6):1995-2002, 1991.
177. Walsh BW et al: Effects of postmenopausal estrogen replacement on the concentrations and metabolism of plasma lipoproteins, *N Engl J Med* 325:1196-1204, 1991.
178. Watts NB et al: Intermittent cyclical etidronate treatment of postmenopausal osteoporosis, *N Engl J Med* 323:73-79, 1990.
179. Weiss NS et al: Noncontraceptive estrogen use and the occurrence of ovarian cancer, *J Natl Cancer Inst* 68:95, 1982.
180. Weiss NS et al: Endometrial cancer in relation to patterns of menopausal estrogen use, *JAMA* 242:261, 1979.
181. Weiss NS et al: Decreased risk of fractures of the hip and lower forearm with postmenopausal use of estrogen, *N Engl J Med* 303:1195, 1980.
182. Whitehead MI et al: The pharmacology of progestogens. In Mishell DR, editor: *Menopause, physiology and pharmacology*, Chicago, 1987, Year Book Medical p 326.
183. Whitehead MI et al: Absorption and metabolism of oral progesterone, *Br Med J (Clin Res)* 280:825, 1980.
184. Whitehead MI et al: Effects of estrogens and progestins on the biochemistry and morphology of the postmenopausal endometrium, *N Engl J Med* 305:1599, 1981.
185. Whittaker PG, Morgan MR, Dean PD: Serum equilin, estrone, and estradiol levels in postmenopausal women receiving conjugated equine estrogens, *Lancet* 1:14, 1980.
186. Williams JK et al: Short-term administration of estrogen and vascular responses of atherosclerotic coronary arteries, *J Am Coll Cardiol* 20(2):452-457, 1992.
187. Wilson PWF, Garrison RJ, Castelli WP: Postmenopausal estrogen use, cigarette smoking, and cardiovascular morbidity in women over 50, *N Engl J Med* 313:1038, 1985.
188. Yen SSC: The biology of menopause, *J Reprod Med* 18:28, 1977.
189. Zinner NN, Sterling AM, Ritter RC: Role of urethral softness in urinary incontinence, *Urology* 16:115, 1980.

Chapter 20

MEDICAL GENETICS

Louise Wilkins-Haug

The realization that an orderly progression of human fetal development occurs simultaneously with the emergence of unique, individual traits has perplexed philosophers and scientists for centuries. The ancient Greeks recognized the passage of both desirable and undesirable traits from one generation to another. Hippocrates has been credited with the saying:

> ...when as a rule, baldheaded beget baldheaded, blue-eyed beget blue-eyed and squinting, squinting; and when for other maladies, the same law prevails, what should hinder that longheaded are begotten by longheaded?[139]

Speculation regarding inheritance remained in the realm of philosophy without receiving closer scientific scrutiny until the nineteenth century. In the late 1700s and early 1800s numerous medical accounts of "inherited" disorders in families appeared. Decades before Gregor Mendel's 1865 publication on the laws of inheritance, human examples of genetic inheritance were observed and theories were postulated. Based on the transmission of specific characteristics within families, Joseph Adams in 1814 published guidelines for genetic counseling. Among these were a recognition of recessive ("familial") and dominant ("hereditary") conditions, the effects of consanguinity and inbreeding, the reduced reproductive capacity of affected individuals, and the premise of new mutations.[139]

Although inheritance of specific diseases was recognized in nineteenth century medical writings, a scientific approach to inheritance was established only with the work of Gregor Mendel. In 1865 his quantitative analysis of matings between various pea strains provided a statistical basis for his three laws of inheritance: (1) the law of uniformity—crosses between two homozygotes of differing types result in offspring that are identical and heterozygotic; (2) the law of segregation—intercrosses between heterozygotes result in offspring in ratios of 1:2:1 with respect to homozygosity and heterozygosity, while backcrosses of heterozygotes and homozygotes produce 1:1 ratios of offspring; and (3) the law of independence—traits are segregated independently from one another. Concurrently during the mid 1800s, researchers identified and established the *cell to cell transmission* of chromosomes, a term coined by Waldeyer in 1888. Chromosomes, the carriers of the genetic material integral to Mendel's laws, were independently proposed by three investigators in 1900—Correns, Tschermark and deVries.[139]During the twentieth century, genetics has focused on the identification and visualization of human chromosomes, the delineation of DNA as the functional component of the gene, and the unraveling of defects at the molecular level. The late twentieth century has seen attempts to treat inherited disorders with the correction of DNA defects at the molecular level. The efforts of the Human Genome project that was initiated in 1990 to map the entire genetic material of the human cell are anticipated to take 15 years. The results should further advance our understanding of DNA at the molecular level and should provide a foundation for disease detection and gene therapy.

This chapter lays out the current understanding of various aspects of inheritance including chromosomal, single gene Mendelian, multifactorial, and mitochondrial. It also explores newer theories of unstable DNA, uniparental disomy, and imprinting. The role of sexual differentiation, inherited gynecologic abnormalities, and preconceptional risk counseling for inherited disorders is also covered and will be of specific interest to gynecologists.

GENERAL PRINCIPLES

Cytogenetic inheritance

Each human cell is estimated to contain 5 to 6 million genes representing a total of 2 million meters of DNA.[121] Because each gene is comprised of a unique sequence of approximately 1000 nucleotide pairs, the physics of transcription, replication, and storage of the human genome within each cell are complex. Initiation of specific genes determines that cell's eventual function in relationship to surrounding cells. Alternatively, gene suppression is thought to be governed by methylation, although the sequence of events remains under debate. Once initiated, gene action is accomplished through a multistage process beginning with transcription—the transference of the genetic code from the DNA to the RNA. Subsequent translation—interaction of the messenger RNA with transfer RNA—culminates in the production of amino acids and functional proteins.

Currently at least three types of DNA are recognized: (1) unique DNA possessing only a single copy of the nucleotide sequence coding for a particular protein; (2) highly repetitious DNA responsible for packaging; and (3) moderately repetitive DNA that codes for histones or ribosomes.[133] Unique, coding sequences (exons) are separated from one another by noncoding sequences called introns. Proteins are thus constructed by a discontinuous sequence of unique DNA, interrupted by intron sequences with a role in the proper positioning of the DNA (Fig. 20-1).

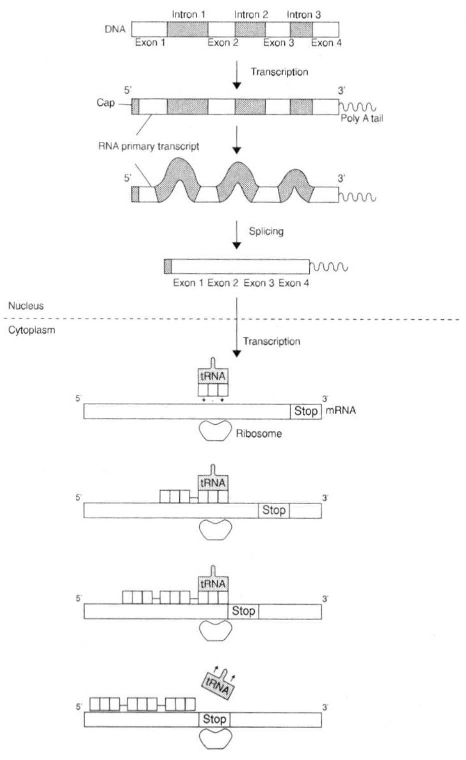

Fig. 20-1. Transcription, RNA processing, and translation. (From Friedman JM et al: *Genetics*, Baltimore, 1992, Williams and Wilkins, p 6.)

Packaging of the human genome into discrete units, the chromosomes, facilitates the orderly replication and passage of DNA from one generation to the next. Each chromosome is comprised of a continuous double strand of DNA containing 1000 to 2000 genes and associated proteins, the histones. Five subtypes of histones bind at regularly spaced intervals coiling the double stranded DNA into subunits known as nucleosomes. Nucleosomes, depicted in Fig. 20-2, play a critical role in the condensation of chromosomes at times of replication and division and also may play a role in the control of gene transcription.[133]

Chromosomes were first described in 1870, although they were not accepted as the packaging unit for genetic material until the early 1900s. In humans the exact number of chromosomes per cell was not established until 1956. Before this

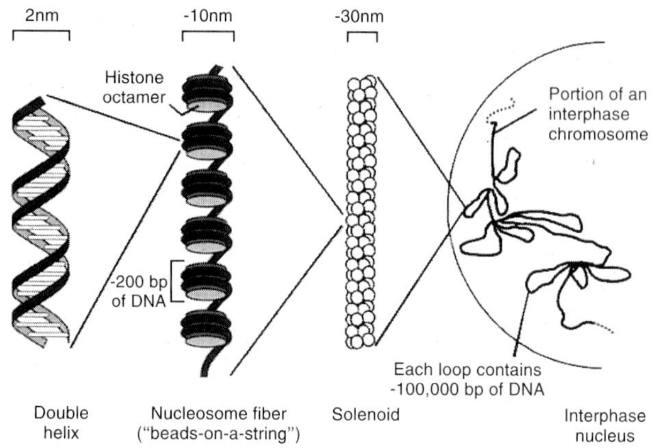

Fig. 20-2. Hierarchical levels of chromatin packaging in a human chromosome. (From Thompson MW, McInnes RR, Willard HF: *Thompson and Thompson: genetics in medicine*, ed 5, Philadelphia, 1991, WB Saunders, p 35.)

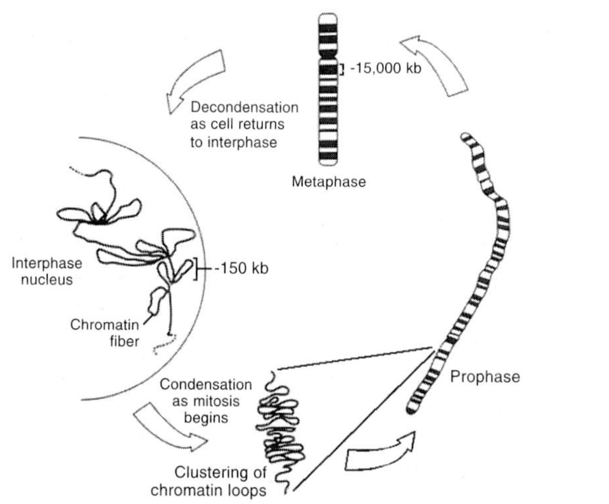

Fig. 20-3. Cycle of condensation and decondensation as a chromosome proceeds through the cell cycle. (From Thompson MW, McInnes RR, Willard HF: *Thompson and Thompson: genetics in medicine*, ed 5, Philadelphia, 1991, WB Saunders, p 36.)

time, 48 chromosomes instead of 46 were identified in human cells.[61] As shown in Fig. 20-3, chromosomes are best visualized during metaphase, the stage during cell division when the DNA is condensed. Metaphase spreads can be obtained from any cell with a nucleus (e.g., peripheral blood lymphocyte, bone marrow, amniotic fluid, chorionic villi, skin fibroblast). Few cell lines have a large percentage of cells spontaneously dividing. However, cell division can be induced in metaphase by phytohemagglutinin and halted in metaphase by the use of colcemid, a spindle poison. Cells that are rapidly dividing from bone marrow or chorionic villi, do not require induction of division, thus the time needed to obtain an analysis is markedly decreased.

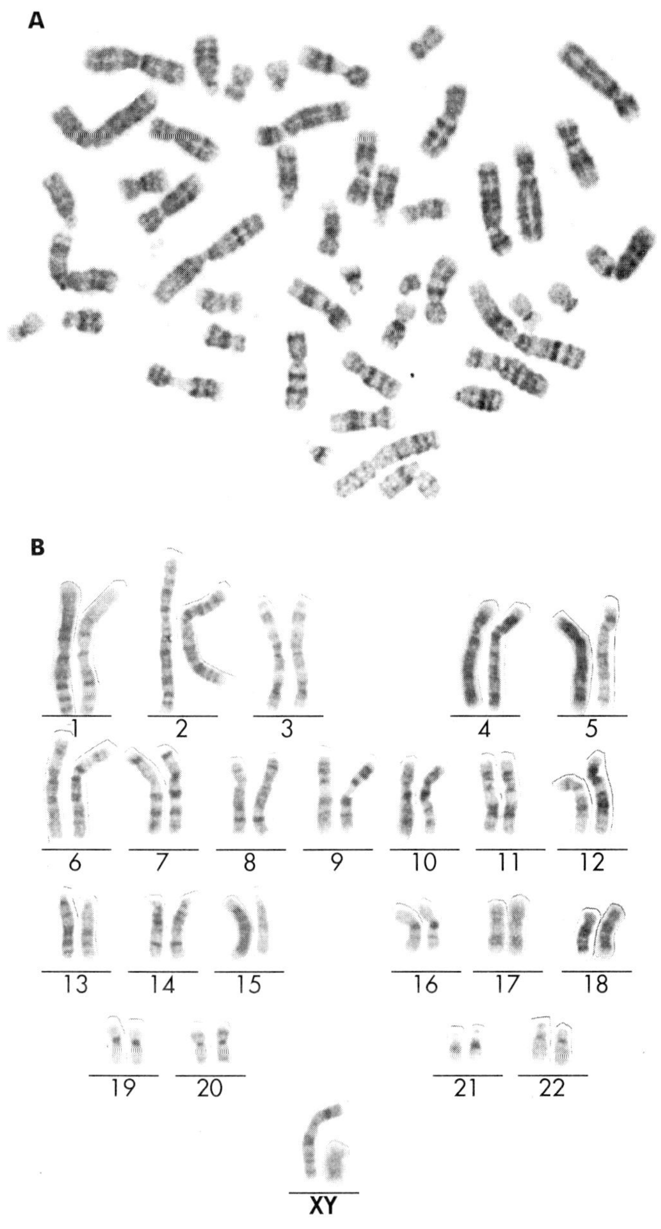

Fig. 20-4. A, Human chromosomes from a peripheral blood lymphocyte culture arrested in metaphase and stained with Giemsa banding technique. **B,** Chromosomes placed in groups by size and position of centimere and displayed as a karyotype. (Courtesy CC Morton, Cytogenetics, Department of Pathology, Brigham and Women's Hospital.)

Karyotype analysis. Chromosomes are traditionally displayed as a karyotype, with the 23 pairs of chromosomes aligned from largest to smallest (Fig. 20-4). Recognition of a specific chromosome is dependent upon its size, shape, and unique banding characteristics. Before banding techniques, chromosomes could be recognized only by their size and shape (Denver nomenclature) and were subdivided into groups (A to G). Subsequently in 1968 Caspersson introduced techniques to produce discrete light and dark banding patterns in metaphase chromosomes by exposure to quinacrine mustard which permitted identification of each individual chromosome.[32]

Each chromosome has a unique pattern of darkly and lightly stained regions or "bands" that can be elicited with various stains. These banding patterns are delineated by a standardized nomenclature, allowing precise identification of specific regions of a chromosome. Based upon the Paris conference in 1971, the short arm of the chromosome is "p" and the long arm is "q". Specific regions of either arm are then delineated by a standardized numeric nomenclature. Separating the short and long arms is the centromere, the site at which the two sister chromatids are joined at metaphase. Metacentric chromosomes have a centromere separating arms of equal lengths, submetacentric chromosomes have short and long arms, and acrocentrics have markedly diminished short arms (Fig. 20-5).

Table 20-1. List of abbreviations according to the International System for Human Cytogenetic Nomenclature (ISCN) 1985

A-G	Chromsome groups
1-22	Autosome numbers
X,Y	Sex chromosome
del	Deletion
der	Derivative chromosome
dic	Dicentric
dup	Duplication
fra	Fragile site
i	Isochromosome
ins	Insertion
inv	Inversion
mar	Marker chromosome
mat	Maternal origin
mos	Mosaic
p	Short arm of chromosome
pat	Paternal origin
q	Long arm of chromosome
r	Ring chromosome
rcp	Reciprocal
rec	Recombinant chromosome
rob	Robertsonian translocation
t	Translocation
ter	Terminal (end of chromosome)

Table 20-2. Commonly encountered karyotypes and their interpretation based on ISCN nomenclature (1985)

Karyotype	Interpretation
45,X/46,XY	A mosaic with two cell lines, one with 45 chromosomes and a single X, the other with 46 chromosomes and XY sex chromosomes.
46,XX,r(16)	Female karyotype with 46 chromosomes, including a ring chromosome 16.
46,X,i(Xq)	Female karyotype with 46 chromosomes, including one normal X chromosome and one chromosome represented by an isochromosome for the long arm of the X.
46,XX,del(1)(q21) or 46,XX,del(1)(pter→q21:)	The single colon (:) indicates a break at band lq21 and deletion of the long-arm segment distal to it. The remaining chromosome consists of the entire short arm of chromosome 1 and part of the long arm lying between the centromere and band lq21.
46,XY,inv(2)(p13p24) or 46,XY,inv(2)(pter→p24:: p13→p24::p13→qter)	Breakage and reunion have occurred at bands 2p13 and 2p24 in the short arm of chromosome 2. The segment lying between these bands is still present but inverted.
46,XY,inv(2)(p21q31) or 46,XY,inv(2)(pter p21: :q31 p21::q31 qter)	Breakage and reunion have occurred at band 2p21 in the short arm and 2q31 in the long arm of chromosome 2. The segment lying between these bands is inverted.
46,XY,t(2;5)(q21;q31)	Breakage and reunion have occurred atbands 2q21 and 5q31 in the long arm of chromosome 2 and 5, respectively. The segments distal to these bands have been exchanged between the two chromosomes.
45,XX,t(13q14q)	A female carrier of a Robertsonian translocation. The rearranged chromosome has the long arms of both chromosomes separated by a centromere. Both short arms have been lost.
46,XX,-13,+t(13q21q)	A female affected with Down's syndrome. A normal number 13 is replaced by a Robertsonian translocation involving 13 and 21, 2 normal number 21 chromosomes are presumed present.

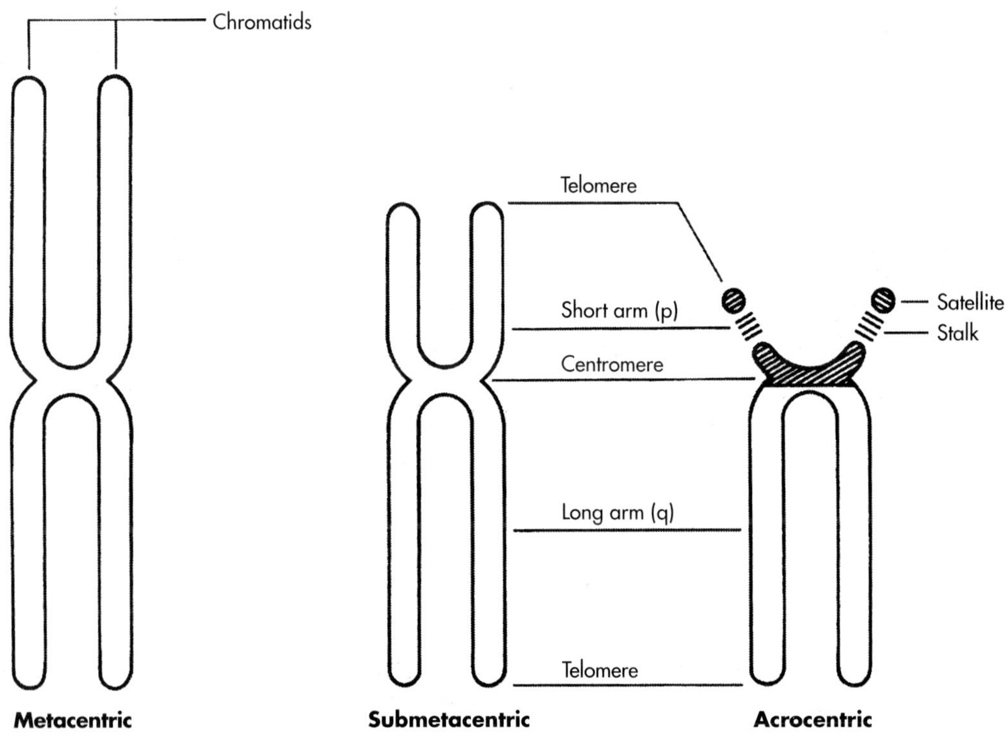

Fig. 20-5. Human chromosome morphology with delineation of landmarks. (From Thompson MW, McInnes RR, Willard MF. *Thompson and Thompson: genetics in medicine*, ed 5, Philadelphia, 1991, WB Saunders, p 15.)

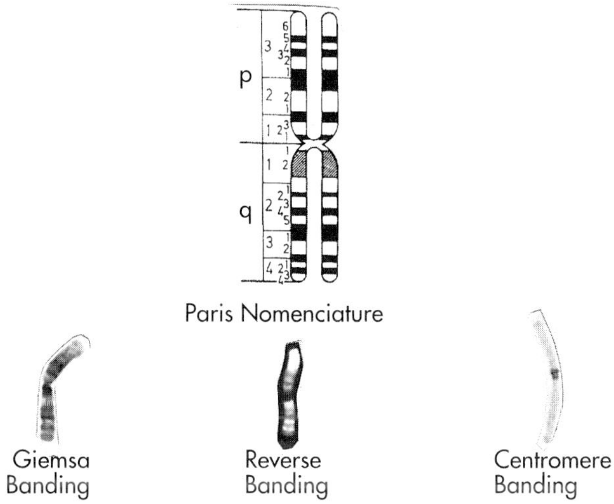

Fig. 20-6. Chromosome 1 displayed with ideogram and various staining technologies. (Courtesy CC Morton, Cytogenetics, Brigham and Women's Hospital.)

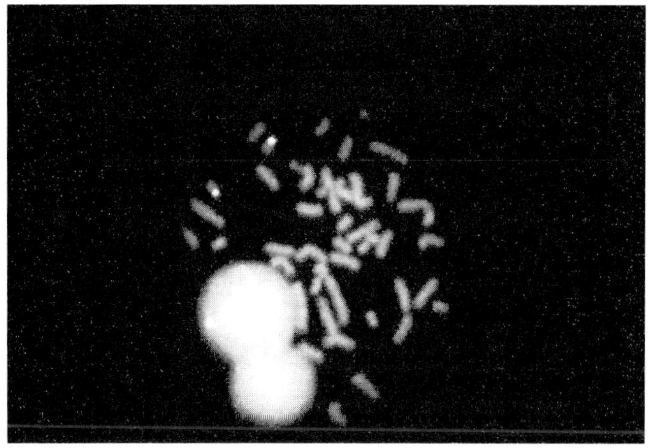

Fig. 20-7. Fluorescence in situ hybridization (FISH) of interface nucleus as well as metaphase spread with a probe derived from an alpha repeat of chromosome 18. (Courtesy CC Morton, Cytogenetics, Brigham and Women's Hospital.)

When describing the chromosomal complement of a cell, the following convention is followed:

- number of chromosomes
- sex chromosome pair
- abnormal chromosome

Structurally aberrant chromosomes are designated with standardized abbreviations (Table 20-1). Delineation of a specific breakpoint is done with a numbering system, extending from the centromere to the distal end of either arm, with further subdivisions designated after a period.[52] Commonly encountered karyotypes are indicated in Table 20-2.

A routine staining technique produced by Giemsa treatment of the chromosomes after exposure to trypsin produces 'G' bands. 'Q' banding patterns are similar, though they require quinacrine mustard for staining and a fluorescence microscope for detection. 'R' bands produced by denaturation of the chromosomes result in a pattern opposite to G or Q banding. 'T' and 'C' bands are specific to telomeres (ends of chromosomes) and centromeres, respectively (Fig. 20-6). Stains specific to an individual chromosome, such as the DAPI stain and chromosome 15, can further assist in delineation of a chromosome that is not recognizable by the more commonly applied banding techniques.

In addition to providing a fingerprint of the individual chromosomes, the banding patterns obtained by the various staining techniques represent differences in DNA content and probable function. Giemsa (G) and quinacrine (Q) positive regions contain moderately or highly repetitive DNA rich in AT sequences. Reverse (R) positive regions are enriched with guanine and cytosine base pairs and represent unique sequence DNA.[133] Clinical correlations with these banding patterns indicate alterations in R positive bands—those regions with unique sequences that carry greater clinical consequences than aberrations in repetitious DNA, the regions with positive G and Q bands.[121]

Fluorescence in situ hybridization (FISH) offers another means of chromosome identification. Using the innate property of double stranded denatured DNA to hybridize preferentially to complementary DNA, chromosome identification is based on whether a specific probe of known origin is able to hybridize when provided with the appropriate conditions.[94] Denaturating of the DNA can be accomplished in situ on a microscopic slide without disrupting the chromosomes. Repetitive DNA labeled with a tag and derived from a specific site on a known chromosome can be supplied as the probe for the hybridization. As with denaturating, the hybridizing occurs in situ without disrupting the integrity of the microscopic preparation (Fig. 20-7). Applications of FISH continue to be published and include the identification of segments of chromosomes unrecognizable by conventional banding,[110, 152] identification of chromosomes during interphase,[41] and identification of chromosomes in tissues from which cultured cells can not be obtained (paraffin embedded pathology sections).

Abnormalities of chromosomal inheritance

Meiosis/Mitosis. Delineation of the abnormalities of chromosomal inheritance requires an understanding of mitosis and meiosis. While mitosis represents a process in which the nuclear DNA is copied and passed to a daughter cell, meiosis allows for two related events: (1) recombination of genes with respect to their locations on maternally and paternally derived chromosomes, and (2) the halving of the diploid (2N) DNA content to produce a gametic cell with a haploid complement (N).

During meiosis I (reduction division), each chromosome replicates its DNA and the two sister chromatids are joined

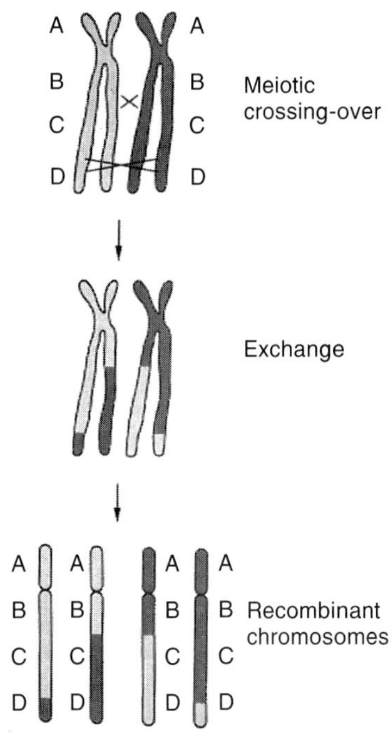

Fig. 20-8. Crossing over between homologous chromosomes during meiosis. (From Thompson MW, McInnes RR, Willard HF: *Thompson and Thompson: genetics in medicine*, ed 5, Philadelphia, 1991, WB Saunders, p 178.)

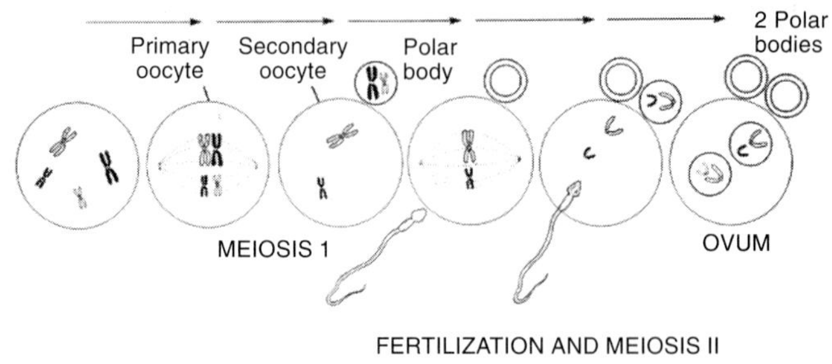

Fig. 20-9. Illustration of human oogenesis and fertilization in relation to meiosis I and II. (From Thompson MW, McInnes RR, Willard HF: *Thompson and Thompson: genetics in medicine*, ed 5, Philadelphia, 1991, WB Saunders, p 29.)

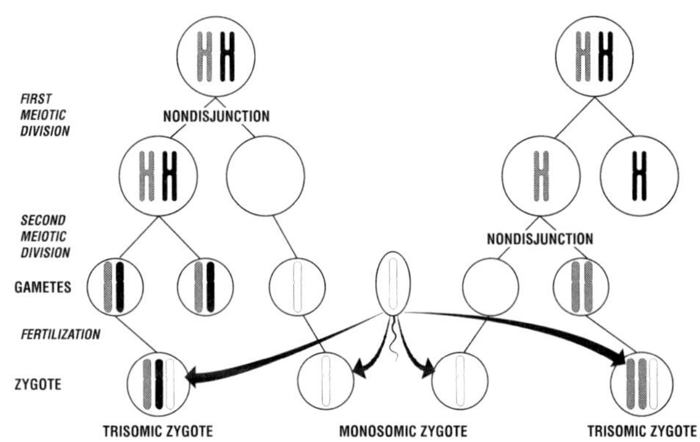

Fig. 20-10. Consequences of nondisjunction occurring in the first or second meiotic division. (From Gelehrter TD, Collins FS: *Principles of Medical Genetics*, Baltimore, 1990, Williams and Wilkins, p 165.)

at the centromere. In females a suspended stage of meiosis 1 (dictyotene) ensues for decades until ovulation occurs. As meiosis continues, the homologous pairs align during the diplotene stage and an exchange of chromatid segments between the homologous chromosomes can occur at crossing-over sites, the chiasmata. For any chromosome pair, crossing over serves to redistribute the genetic material between both members (Fig. 20-8). The chromosomes then separate, undergoing disjunction, and each are distributed to one of the two daughter cells. Throughout meiosis I the centromeres remain intact. Meiosis II is not preceded by DNA synthesis. The chromosomes (now 23 joined sets of sister chromatids per cell) each separate at their centromeres, with 23 chromosomes remaining and 23 distributed to the second polar body. In the female, meiosis II is initiated by fertilization and entry into the ovum of the sperm nucleus (Fig. 20-9).

Abnormalities of chromosome number. Numeric chromosome abnormalities can involve either *aneuploidy* or *polyploidy*. Aneuploidy refers to the addition or loss of a single chromosome with a resulting alteration in the diploid (2N) complement by one. As shown in Fig. 20-10, an additional chromosome can arise through *nondisjunction,* the failure of the chromosomes to segregate to the proper daughter cells during either meiosis I or meiosis II. The loss of a chromosome can occur through *anaphase lag*, the failure to include a chromosome during the anaphase stage of meiotic cell division. In humans, cells with 47 chromosomes, (2N + 1) are designated as trisomies and cells with 45 chromosomes (2N − 1) are considered monosomic. Both Down's and Turner's syndromes are representative of aneuploidies, trisomy 21 and monosomy X respectively. In polyploidy, human cells contain one or more copies of each of the 23 chromosomes (2N + N). Partial molar gestations with triploidy (69 chromosomes) in each cell are an example of polyploidy.

The mechanisms responsible for either aneuploidy or polyploidy remain unclear, although several theories have been postulated. The association of Down's syndrome with increasing maternal age was first noted by Penrose in 1933. As shown in Table 20-3, the incidence of trisomy 21 (and all chromosomal trisomies) rises with increasing maternal age, although the exact phenomena that increase the rate of nondisjunction in the older women remain unknown. Postulates have included a reduction in crossing over (chiasmata) at meiosis I; an age-related increase in background exposures to environmental agents such as radiation; factors intrinsic to the aging ovum involving the integrity of the spindle formation, and a genetic predisposition to nondisjunction. Recent studies with DNA polymorphisms have revealed that at least 90% of trisomy 21 originates from a maternal nondisjunction,[115] and have dispelled an earlier theory of decreased recognition and loss of chromosomally abnormal fetuses in older mothers.[51]

Table 20-3. Maternal age and chromsome abnormalities in liveborns

Maternal age	Risk for Down's syndrome	Total risk for chromosomal abnormalities*
20	1/667	1/526
21	1/667	1/526
22	1/1429	1/500
23	1/1429	1/500
24	1/1250	1/476
25	1/1250	1/476
26	1/1176	1/476
27	1/1111	1/455
28	1/1053	1/435
29	1/1000	1/417
30	1/952	1/417
31	1/909	1/385
32	1/769	1/322
33	1/602	1/286
34	1/485	1/238
35	1/378	1/192
36	1/289	1/156
37	1/224	1/127
38	1/173	1/102
39	1/136	1/83
40	1/106	1/66
41	1/82	1/53
42	1/63	1/42
43	1/49	1/33
44	1/38	1/26
45	1/30	1/21
46	1/23	1/16
47	1/18	1/13
48	1/14	1/10
49	1/11	1/8

*Data not available for 47,XXX at ages 20 to 32.
(From Hook EB: Rates of chromosomal abnormalities at different maternal ages, *Obstet Gynecol* 58:282, 1981.)

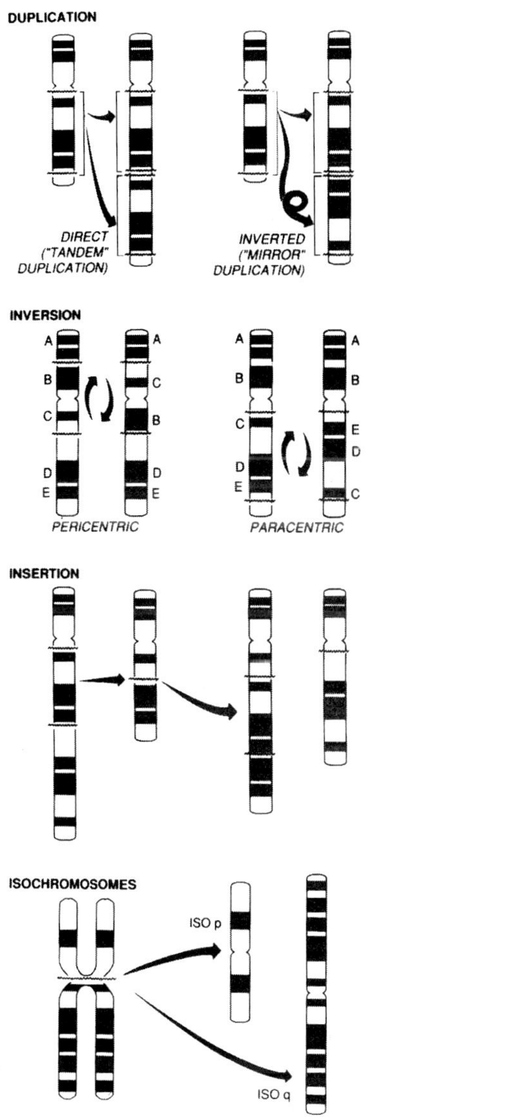

Fig. 20-11. Structural abnormalities of chromosomes depicted by ideograms. (From Gelehrter TD, Collins FS: *Principles of Medical Genetics*, Baltimore, 199, Williams and Wilkins, p 166.)

These studies suggest that the aneuploidy/maternal age association is secondary to an ovarian nondisjunctional event during meiosis.[121] By contrast, most cases of polyploidy, especially triploidy, contain an extra set of paternal chromosomes. The most common mechanism in these cases is fertilization of a normal ovum by two sperm (dispermy).[58]

The clinical impact of an additional autosomal chromosome is determined by its size and the specific genes located on that chromosome. In general, full trisomies of only the smaller chromosomes are seen in liveborns with Down's syndrome (trisomy 21) the most common (1 in 600). Although trisomies of the larger chromosomes (numbers 2 to 12) can be seen in spontaneous abortions, documentation of their existence in liveborns is rare. Trisomy of the largest chromosome, number 1, appears to be incompatible with development, having been reported in a only a single case of a six cell embryo and not in either spontaneous abortions or the liveborns.[121]

Although monosomies of the autosomes are rare among liveborns and spontaneous abortions, monosomy X is the most frequently noted chromosomal aberration among spontaneous abortions. Monosomy X (Turner's syndrome) occurs at a rate of 1:5000 female births, and X trisomy (47,XXX) occurs with a relative greater frequency of 1:1000 female births. Additionally, numeric alterations of the X chromosome are usually associated with delayed mental development that is typical of autosomal trisomies. The role of X-inactivation and the phenotypes of sex chromosomal abnormalities will be addressed under a discussion of X-linked inheritance and disorders of sex chromosomes.

Abnormalities of chromosome structure. Alterations in both chromosome size and shape can occur (Fig. 20-11). Not all structural abnormalities are associated with clinically

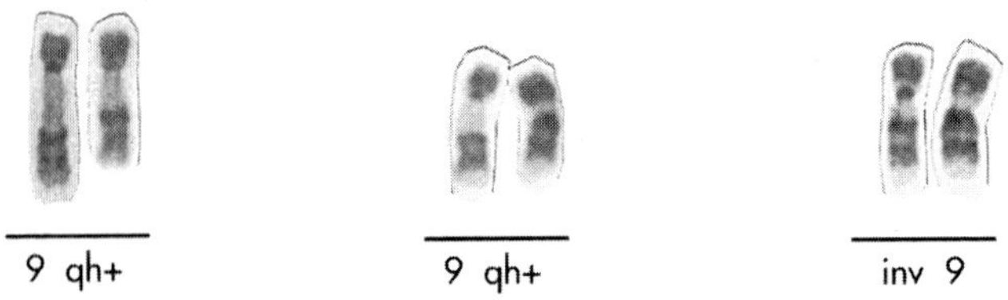

Fig. 20-12. Heterochromatin variants of chromosome 9 (Courtesy CC Morton, Cytogenetics, Brigham and Women's Hospital).

significant changes in an individual's physical or mental development (the *phenotype*). Particular regions of some chromosomes contain heterochromatic, highly repetitive DNA, and variations in size are common. Known as polymorphisms, alterations in size and shape of chromosomes 1, 9, and 16 and the satellite regions of the acrocentric chromosomes can be useful in tracking the segregation of a particular chromosome (Fig. 20-12).

Similarly the overall shape of a chromosome can be changed by centromere relocation as the result of an *inversion*. Inversions require two breaks within a chromosome, with a subsequent 180° rotation of the intervening chromosomal segment. Inversions occurring on either side of a centromere (pericentric) alter the shape of the chromosome, while inversions not involving the centromere (paracentric) alter the banding pattern (Fig. 20-11). If genetic material is not lost in the process, the inversion itself can occur without phenotypic impact. However, because of meiotic cross overs, inversion carriers are at greater risk for unequal chromosomal distribution and clinical abnormalities in their offspring. This risk is greatest for maternal inversions ascertained through an affected individual. In these cases the risk of a subsequent liveborn with an unbalanced complement is approximately 8%. Male inversion carriers face a 4% risk of an abnormal liveborn.[4] A recent series found a 3.3% risk of an abnormal outcome for maternal carriers and no increased paternal risk, though the size of the inversion may play a role.[16] By contrast, inversions ascertained through clinically unaffected individuals may not represent any increased risk for an abnormal liveborn. Inversions identified during prenatal testing should be compared to the parental chromosome complements. If these are identical in size and in banding pattern to the parental inversion, the fetus is considered to have a balanced complement. Although the number of cases for study are small, de novo inversions detected only in the fetus with normal parental karyotypes face an approximately 10% risk of phenotypic abnormality.[145]

Alterations in chromosome structure involving two chromosomes are referred to as *translocations*. Two broad categories of translocations exist: (1) *reciprocal translocations* involving exchange of chromosomal segments between two chromosomes; and (2) *Robertsonian translocations* involving joining of two chromosomes into one. Fig. 20-11 depicts schematically the different origins of these translocations.

In reciprocal translocations the break and exchange of material can occur between any two chromosomes of the complement. If genetic material is not lost during this exchange, the individual has a normal phenotype and the

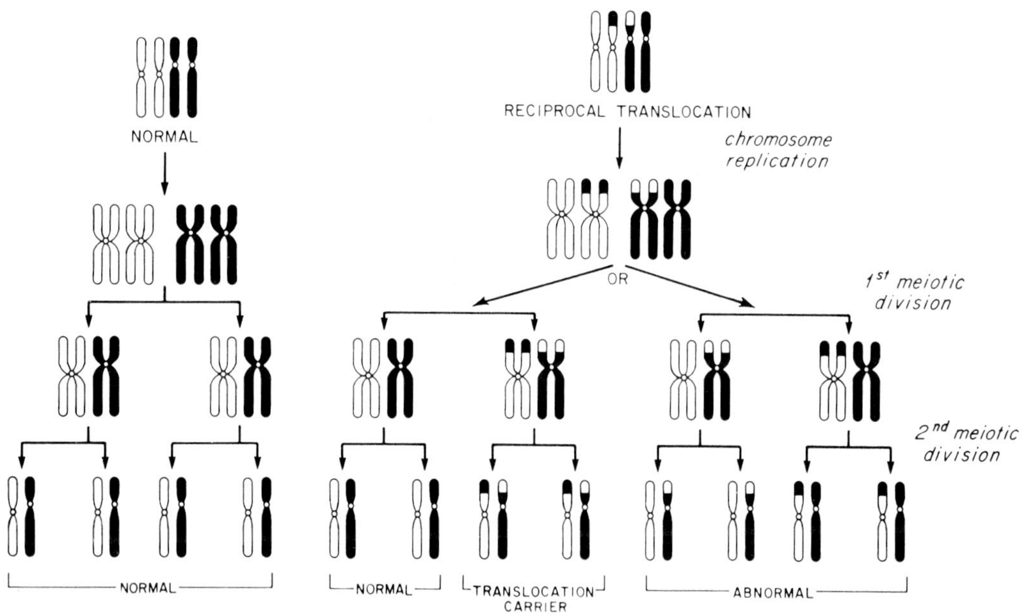

Fig. 20-13. Meiotic division of normal chromosomes and of chromosomes with reciprocal translocation. Shown are two of the four possible abnormal chromosomal complements resulting from random segregation of reciprocally translocated chromosomes.

genetic complement is considered balanced. However, the presence of the exchanged genetic material creates malalignments at meiosis, and distribution of balanced and unbalanced chromosomal complements to the offspring are possible (Fig. 20-13). Because not all combinations are compatible with a liveborn infant, the risk of an unbalanced liveborn is actually less than depicted in Fig. 20-13. The frequency of unbalanced segregation is influenced by the size of the rearrangement, the sex of the parental carrier, and the method of ascertainment of the translocation. With some rearrangements, the risk may be minimally increased; for others, a substantial risk exists. As shown in Table 20-4, the method of ascertainment of the reciprocal translocation markedly alters the risk for unbalanced conceptions at amniocentesis in subsequent pregnancies.[16] When a reciprocal translocation is detected de novo from amniotic fluid, given a possible submicroscopic loss of DNA, even apparently balanced rearrangements are associated with a 10% risk of a phenotypic abnormality.[145]

Robertsonian translocations are unique in their involvement of only the D and G group chromosomes that are acrocentrics possessing minimal short arms. Balanced Robertsonian translocations are generally created by centromere to centromere fusion of two acrocentric chromosomes (Fig. 20-14). Similar to reciprocal translocations, alterations in chromosome structure create aberrations in meiotic pairing, leading to unbalanced segregation of the involved chromosomes. Because two of the three most common autosomal trisomies in liveborns involve acrocentric chromosomes (trisomy 21 and 13), unbalanced segregants from a balanced Robertsonian translocation can result in liveborns with trisomy 21 or 13. Maternal carriers of a Robertson translocation can face a 10% to 25% risk of an unbalanced offspring, depending upon the chromosomes involved. In contrast, paternal carriers of Robertsonian translocations have not been clearly shown to be at increased risk for unbalanced segregants.[121] Carriers of Robertsonian translocations involving both members of a chromosome pair (t21q21) face an essentially 100% recurrence risk for an unbalanced, trisomy 21 offspring. A rare case of a maternal 21q21q translocation producing an offspring with the Robertsonian translocation without trisomy 21 does exist. The mechanism postulated involves subsequent loss of the paternal number 21 or the fertilization of the 21q21q containing ovum with a sperm nullisomic the number 21 chromosome. This phenomenon is rare, and in situations in which a Robertson translocation involving the same chromosome is identified, counseling should be considered regarding either ovum or sperm donor gametes. Though often impaired in such individuals, fertility is still possible. To avoid recurrence of abnormal segregants in offspring, sterilization should be offered.[119]

Other structural abnormalities associated with abnormal phenotypes include *deletions* such as those of the short arm of chromosome 5 (Cri du Chat syndrome). Although some deletions occur as a result of an unbalanced segregation from a reciprocal translocation, the majority of chromosomal deletions arise de novo in the affected individual. Loss of genetic material from any of the autosomes is characteristically associated with delays in both physical and mental development in the offspring. Agents capable of breaking chromosomes in vitro (clastogens) include radiation, viruses, and some chemicals. However, among liveborns with chromosomal breaks and deletions, an etiologic agent has been difficult to establish.

When centromeres divide horizontally rather than longitudinally, the resulting chromosome contains mirror images of only one arm. Known as *isochromosomes*, these structurally abnormal chromosomes contain duplication of one arm and deficiency of the other arm. The most common example of this rearrangement is an isochromosome of the X chromosome.[121]

In general, aberrations of autosomes, whether trisomies, deletions, or duplications, are associated with significant disorders in the development of the fetus. To varying degrees, the autosomal chromosome abnormalities have in common mental retardation, somatic growth delay, an increase in structural malformations, and alterations of craniofacial

Table 20-4. Amniocentesis results for reciprocal translocation carriers by parental origin and method of ascertainment

	Maternal origin % Outcomes in subsequent pregnancies			Paternal origin % Outcomes on subsequent pregnancies		
	Balanced	**Normal**	**Unbalanced**	**Balanced**	**Normal**	**Unbalanced**
Ascertainment of rearrangement						
Term, unbalanced infant	41.2	38.9	19.8	40.3	37.5	27.2
Recurrent miscarriages	54.5	40.7	4.8	55.4	43.2	1.4

Daniel A, Hook EB, Wulf G:Risks of unbalanced progeny at amniocentesis to carriers of chromosome rearrangements: data from United States and Canadian Laboratories, *Am J Med Genet* 31:14, 1989.

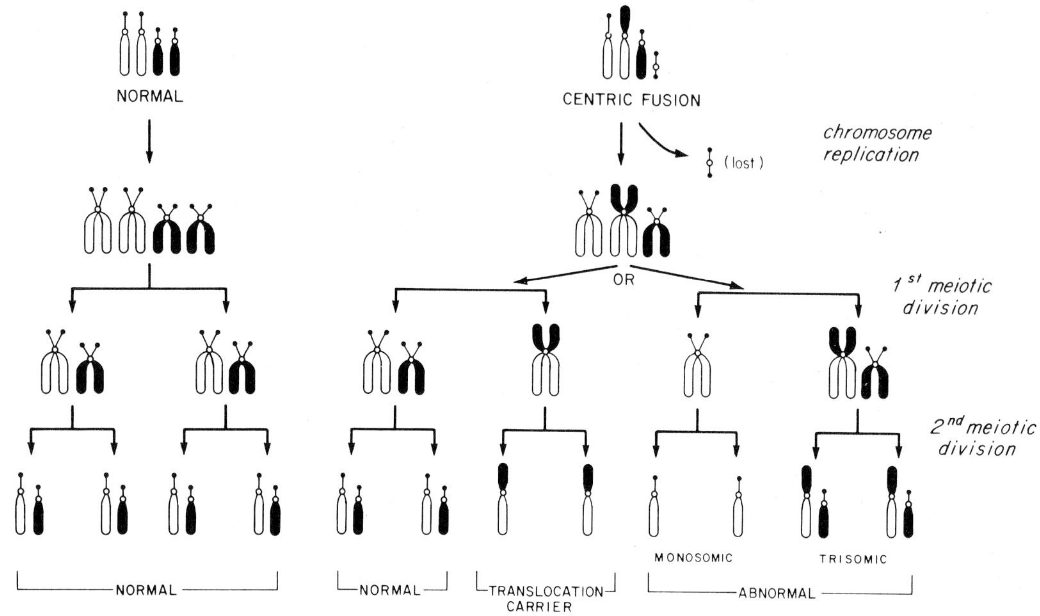

Fig. 20-14. Meiotic division of normal chromosomes and Robertsonian translocation. As in Fig. 20-13, two of the four possible abnormal chromosomal complements are illustrated.

development, leading to various degrees of dysmorphology. Despite these shared characteristics, individuals with the same chromosomal abnormalities also possess remarkable similarity among themselves, leading to specific recognizable phenotypes. Numerous descriptions of the various autosomal chromosomal syndromes are available.[56, 156] Abnormalities of the sex chromosomes will be discussed in detail with regard to disorders of sexual differentiation.

Mendelian inheritance

Specific diseases have been ascribed to abnormal genes since Garrod's description of "inborn errors of metabolism" in the 1860s. Only since 1944, however, has DNA been recognized as the transmitter of inherited traits on the molecular level.[121] For numerous genetic disorders, the association of disease symptoms with an abnormal protein was followed by sequencing of the responsible gene and identifying the DNA mutation. The advancements in sickle cell disease are representative of such progress. Pauling in 1949 identified an abnormal hemoglobin in persons with sickle cell disease. Ingram in 1957 followed with a report of abnormal electrophoretic migration of sickle hemoglobin as indicative of a change in amino acid sequence and hemoglobin configuration. The specific alteration of the amino acid sequence was identified in 1961 as a point mutation in the gene for beta globin.[139] Prenatal diagnosis of sickle cell disease by analysis of DNA polymorphisms closely linked to the site of mutation occurred in 1978.[60] Specific restriction enzymes cleaving within the sickle cell gene now provide direct DNA diagnosis of sickle cell disease.[11]

Diagnostic technologies. The tools of molecular genetics have allowed researchers of inherited diseases to move from an analysis of abnormal protein production to the examination of DNA sequences. Although the ability to isolate DNA from human cells has existed for several decades, the capability to reproducibly fractionate a vast quantity of DNA into smaller, more easily analyzed segments has only recently been achieved. Integral to the study of genetics at the DNA level was the identification of restriction endonucleases, bacterial enzymes with the ability to cleave DNA at specific sites. Different restriction enzymes are unique not only in the sequence of bases they recognize but also in their ability to reproducibly recognize the same sequences. Using techniques developed by Southern, DNA, once extracted, can be cleaved with specific restriction endonucleases into smaller segments that can be separated from one another by agarose gel electrophoresis.[133]

Indirect methodologies. The ability both to identify and to retrieve specific sequences of DNA within segments produced by restriction endonucleases evolved with the development of DNA probe technology. When DNA is denatured, double strands are separated into single strands. If appropriate conditions are provided, DNA will hybridize, or re-form double strands with any available complementary DNA (Fig. 20-15). Under appropriate conditions, *DNA probes* (DNA segments of known human genome map location, and in some cases actually sequenced) can serve as complimentary DNA for the hybridization process. DNA probes are tagged with a marker to allow their visual identification usually by radioactivity or by fluorescence. As shown in Fig. 20-16, genomic

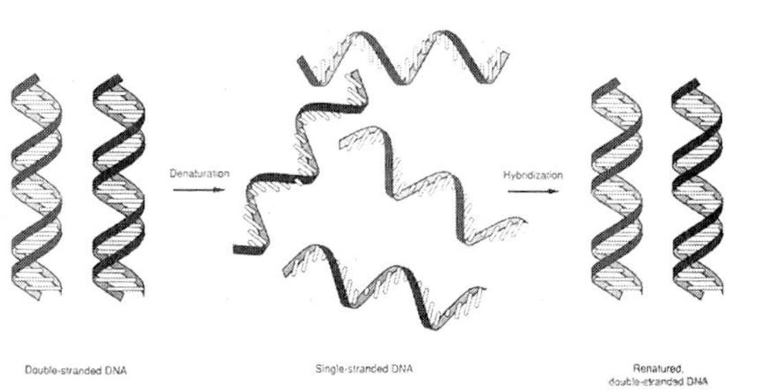

Fig. 20-15. The principal of nucleic acid hybridization. (From Thompson MW, McInnes RR, Willard HF: *Thompson and Thompson: genetics in medicine*, ed 5, Philadelphia, 1991, WB Saunders, p 105.)

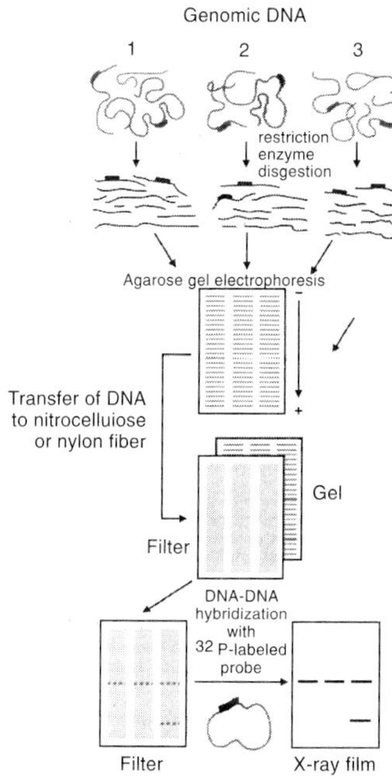

Fig. 20-16. The southern blotting procedure for analyzing specific DNA sequences in a complex mixture of different sequences such as normal DNA. (From Thompson MW, McInnes RR, Willard HF: *Thompson and Thompson: genetics in medicine*, ed 5, Philadelphia, 1991, WB Saunders, p 107.)

DNA can be fragmented with restriction endonucleases, undergo denaturation, the single strands transferred from gel to filter paper, and hybridized with known probes in a search for a particular gene sequence.[121]

An extension of the above concept of endonuclease restriction enzymes and probe identification involves the production of *restriction fragment length polymorphisms (RFLPs)*. In the noncoding regions of DNA, base sequence variation occurs that can alter the sites of specific restriction endonucleases action. The first RFLP was identified in 1978,[153] and such variations are estimated to occur once in every 200 base pairs.[53,54] When changes in base sequence involve a restriction endonuclease site, the DNA fragments resulting after enzyme cleavage are altered in size and thus in gel mobility. Useful RFLPS are highly variable (polymorphic); the chances of two individuals sharing the same variation at a specific restriction endonuclease site is extremely rare. For genetic diseases in which the DNA sequence has not been determined, RFLP analysis of affected individuals and other family members may provide an indirect method of tracking the abnormal gene through a family. As with genetic linkage analysis involving segregation of associated traits for tracking an inherited disease, RFLP analysis can be confounded by crossing over between the gene in question and the RFLP, and the need for multiple informative members from a family.

Direct methodologies. Detection of a genetic disorder by direct analysis of the abnormal gene is the most straightforward approach but remains the most difficult to achieve. Initially, disorders secondary to a deletion of DNA (α-thalessemia, Duchenne and Becker muscular dystrophy, cystic fibrosis and growth hormone deficiency) were detected by direct DNA analysis.[82] In these disorders the detection of deleted DNA was possible through the introduction of the polymerase chain reaction (PCR) technology. PCR is unique in its ability to amplify a predetermined segment of DNA selected by knowledge of unique oligonucleotide primers (short sequences of DNA) flanking opposite sides of the DNA under study.[106] Quantities of DNA previously considered inaccessible can be investigated through a PCR reaction. Even DNA from a single cell, such as would be needed for preimplantation diagnosis can be amplified though modifications of the PCR protocols.

Direct detection of the DNA mutation can be accomplished also by allele specific oligonucleotides (ASO) analysis. Again, PCR directed amplification of the target DNA is required. However, in diseases in which the abnormal amplified DNA is not altered in size by a deletion or insertion, recognition of a change in the DNA sequence requires additional steps. Provided the DNA mutation has been sequenced, allele-specific probes can be developed and suspect DNA can be tested for the pattern of hybridization to the normal and mutant alleles. In this fashion, direct DNA diagnosis for Tay Sachs disease,[85] α- and β-thalassemia,[62] cystic fibrosis,[63] and phenylketonuria are possible.[20]

While direct DNA diagnosis requires knowledge of the mutated sequence, in some cases this has been obtained without knowledge of an associated abnormal protein or how the disease symptoms are produced. Known as positional cloning (or reverse genetics), the abnormal sequence can initially be localized to a chromosome through somatic cell hybrids—cells which can be created to replicate with individual human chromosomes. In addition, gene mapping to areas of the karyotype can be accomplished with naturally occurring structural chromosome rearrangements and RFLPS. The DNA sequence in question can then be isolated through yeast artificial chromosomes (YACs).[133] This allows the eventual isolation and direct sequencing of the DNA under

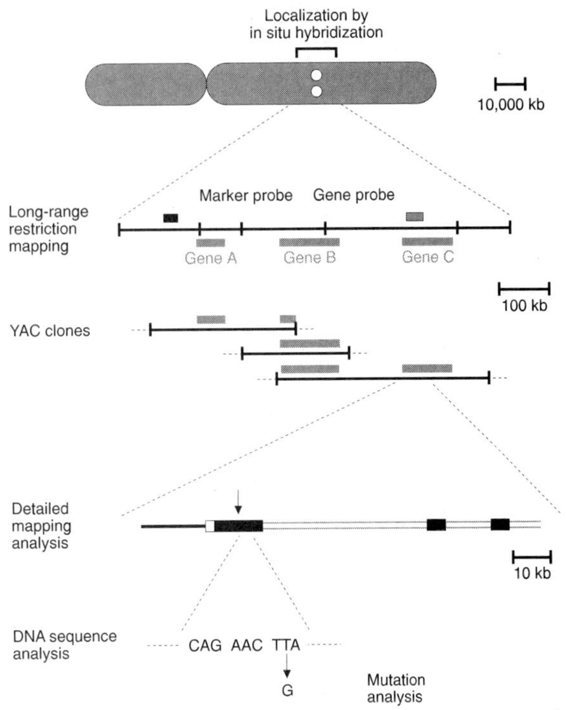

Fig. 20-17. Reversed genetics for cloning analysis of a hypothetical disease gene. (From Thompson MW, McInnes RR, Willard HF: *Thompson and Thompson: genetics in medicine*, ed 5, Philadelphia, 1991, WB Saunders, p 177.)

investigation (Fig. 20-17). Candidate genes for Duchenne muscular dystrophy, cystic fibrosis, and myotonic dystrophy have been sequenced in this fashion.

For many genetic disorders inherited in a Mendelian fashion, DNA sequencing has revealed not one but several mutations in a specific gene locus. The molecular genetics of cystic fibrosis (CF) emphasize this concept. Sequencing of the DNA responsible for the abnormal protein associated with cystic fibrosis (CFTR) has revealed numerous possible sites of mutation, all of which culminate in the symptoms of cystic fibrosis. A DNA change at the delta 508 position, the loss of three bases, is the most common cause of an abnormal CFTR protein among the Caucasian population. In persons with a northern European heritage, 76% of the cystic fibrosis mutations are delta 508. The remaining 24% of CF mutations in a Caucasian population result from other abnormalities in this gene. Currently, 140 additional mutations have been identified, each of which are noted in only a minority of CF cases.[82] When all probes are analyzed, about 90% of CF mutations can be identified. Given the laws of segregation of genes within a population, these estimates are applicable only to the population from which they are derived, generally a northern European Caucasian population. Researchers are currently establishing the frequencies of these mutations in other populations in which cystic fibrosis is less common.

Patterns of inheritance. Traits and diseases passed from one generation to another often follow predictable patterns. Gregor Mendel in the late nineteenth century identified various patterns of inheritance that have remained true for many genetic diseases. For an increasing number of inherited conditions, the abnormal protein and even the DNA mutation responsible have been identified. However, for the majority of genetic diseases the underlying protein abnormality remains undetected and the exact DNA mutation is unknown. In these cases, an individual's chance of inheriting a specific familial condition can be predicted based upon Mendel's segregation laws of autosomal recessive, autosomal dominant, sex-linked recessive, or sex-linked dominant inheritance.

A gene locus, the DNA sequence responsible for encoding a specific protein, is comprised of two alleles—the DNA sequence on the maternal chromosome and the companion DNA sequence on the paternal chromosome. In general, both alleles need to be present for gene function to proceed normally. The production of disease by the presence of two mutated alleles as opposed to one mutated allele determines whether the gene has characteristics of recessive or dominant inheritance. The presence of the alleles on sex chromosomes as opposed to the autosomes governs some of the intricacies of trait expression based upon the sex of the individual.

Autosomal recessive. *Autosomal recessive* disease results when alleles at a gene locus are both homozygotic and abnormal (aa). Homozygosity for the normal allele (AA) does not lead to the disease state. Generally the abnormal protein produced in autosomal recessive disease results in a metabolic disorder, most often manifesting during infancy or childhood. Given the early presence of the disease state, the affected individual's reproductive fitness and thus capacity to pass mutated alleles to offspring often is limited. The vast majority of mutated alleles inherited in an autosomal recessive fashion exist in a population in asymptomatic heterozygotic carriers (Aa). Population studies have shown all individuals carry 2 to 6 recessive, deleterious genes in the heterozygotic state.[121] Autosomal recessive diseases are further characterized by full expression of the disease state in affected individuals, or full *penetrance*. Additionally, since the gene locus resides on one of the 22 autosomal chromosomes, the ratio of affected males to females is equal.

With a normal and abnormal allele at the gene locus in question, matings between heterozygotic individuals have a 25% chance of an affected homozygotic offspring and a 75% chance of a clinically asymptomatic offspring. Among the asymptomatic siblings of an affected individual, one of three will be homozygotic normal alleles (AA) and two of three will be heterozygotic carriers (Aa) (Fig. 20-18). Before testing, an unaffected sibling of an individual with an autosomal recessive disease thus has a 2:3 (66%) chance of being a carrier. The parents of the affected individual are obligate heterozygotic carriers.

In any population, the probability that two random individuals carry abnormal alleles at the same gene locus is a governed by two parameters. First, if the individuals are related (*consanguinous*), a portion of their DNA is the same, depending on how many generations have intervened between their common ancestor. Brothers and sisters share 50% of their gene loci given their common parents, while uncles and nieces share 25% of their DNA and 1st cousins share 12.5%. More often seen in families of homozygotic-affected offspring, consanguinity markedly restricts the gene pool, thus increasing the chances of matings between heterozygotic carriers for the same recessive alleles. Secondly, the gene frequency within a specific ethnic population influences the chances of any two individuals who are heterozygotic for the same recessive allele. Within any population, offspring are more commonly produced by individuals of the same ethnic or racial groups than by partners from different populations. This serves to contain and redistribute genes within the same pool or population. For some recessive disorders, the gene may be very common in one population and thus the carrier frequency relatively high. In another population the same gene may have a frequency that is negligible. Matings between members of the same population would have a greater random chance of both individuals being carriers, while matings between populations would be at lower risk.

With regard to populations, the Hardy Weinberg equation is helpful for determining the distribution of carriers and affected individuals based upon gene frequencies. This equation was introduced in 1908 by the independent investigators Hardy, a British mathematician, and Weinberg, a German physician.[121] Calculations are based upon expectations regarding the quantitative distribution of a gene in a population:

1. the normal allele (A) has a frequency = p
2. the abnormal allele (a) has a frequency = q
3. each allele frequency represents a portion of unity ($p + q = 1$)
4. the frequencies of AA (normal) individuals, Aa individuals (carriers), and aa individuals (affected) are proportions of unity ($p2 + 2pq + q2 = 1$)
5. for rare disorders, p is equal to 1 so that $2pq = 2q$

The Hardy Weinberg formula can be solved to determine the carrier frequency if a disease frequency is known, the disease frequency given the mutant allele frequency, or disease frequency if carrier frequency is established.

Autosomal dominant. A trait or abnormality produced by the presence of only one mutated allele at a gene locus is governed by autosomal dominant inheritance. As each person with the trait has a normal and an abnormal allele at that locus, the affected individual has a 50% chance of segregating the abnormal allele to their offspring and a 50% chance of segregating the normal allele. Because the gene locus resides on an autosome, males and females have an equal chance of inheriting the abnormal allele and being affected.

Several characteristics of autosomal disorders can confound the interpretation of a pedigree. Autosomal dominant disorders may not display characteristics of the disease until after reproductive age. Additionally, many autosomal disorders have reduced penetrance such that not all persons carrying the same mutated allele display the same characteristics. A minimally affected parent can have a severely affected child. These attributes of autosomal dominant inheritance can convey the impression of a disorder skipping a

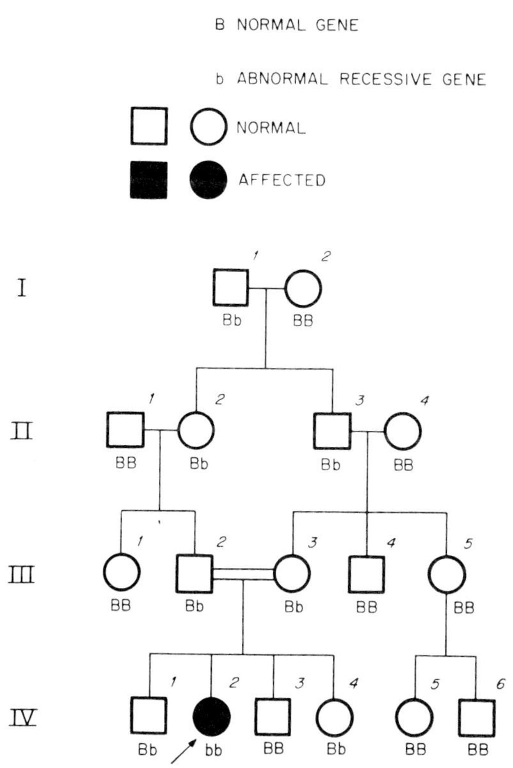

Fig. 20-18. Pedigree illustrating autosomal recessive inheritance.

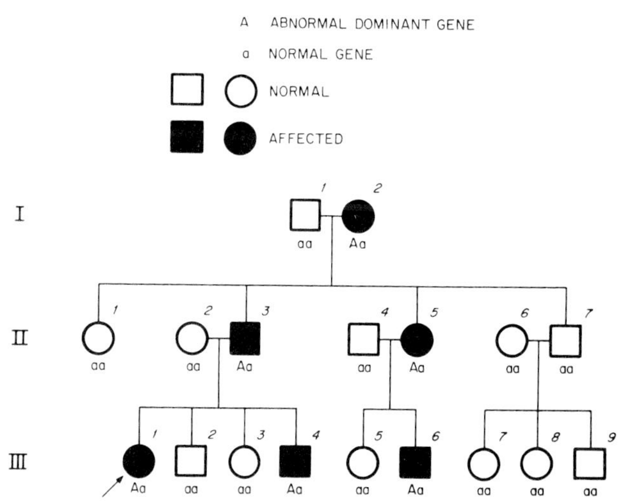

Fig. 20-19. Pedigree illustrating autosomal dominant inheritance.

generation. In such instances the intervening person may express minimal symptoms or die from unrelated causes prior to the development of symptoms. Rarely are dominant pedigrees as clear cut as Fig. 20-19.

X-linked recessive. The intricacies of gene segregation on the sex chromosomes are governed by the properties of X chromatin inactivation and the *Lyon hypothesis*. With only one active X chromosome in any cell, the inactivation of X chromosome gene loci when more than one X is present (as in normal females, 46,XX) is governed by several principles.[75] Inactivation occurs around the time of implantation, and in the majority of cells random variability determines whether the maternally or paternally derived X is inactivated. All daughter cells, however, maintain the original inactivation. In addition, inactivation of the loci appears to be selective with most but not all X chromosome loci involved. Loci for steroid sulfatase and ovarian maintenance determinants located on the distal short arm are not inactivated.[121] Furthermore X-inactivation appears to be influenced by the tissue in which the cells reside. X-inactivation does not occur in fetal germ cells and in extraembryonic tissues[34]; X-inactivation is not random with preferential inactivation of the paternal X in cytotrophoblastic cell lines.[44]

X-inactivation may be controlled by methylation although the details have not been fully elucidated. The physical representation of X-inactivation is the Barr body, also known as the sex chromatin. As the last chromosome to replicate in DNA synthesis, the extensive heterochromatin of the inactivated X chromosome remains visible in interphase cells (Fig. 20-20). Barr bodies reflect the number of X chromosomes present plus one (46,XX—one Barr body; 47,XXX—two Barr bodies).

Segregation of X-linked recessive diseases also reflects the unique dissimilarity of the sex chromosome pair. While the 22 autosomal pairs are comprised of matching members, the sex chromosome pair can be either the same chromosomes, XX (a female) or dissimilar XY (a male). In males with only one X chromosome, abnormal alleles located on the X chromosome are expressed; in females the two X chromosomes result in the carrier state. In general, carrier females are not affected, although in some instances X-inactivation on a random basis results in a predominance of cells with the active X possessing the abnormal allele.

Females who are heterozygotic carriers for an X-linked recessive allele face one of two segregations when forming gametes. Half of the gametes receive the X with the abnormal allele, and half the X chromosome with the normal allele. The contribution by the sperm of either an X, resulting in a XX (female zygote), or a Y (male zygote) will determine if the abnormal allele results in the carrier state or an affected individual, respectively. Males with only one X are considered *hemizygous* and X-linked disorders will be expressed (Fig. 20-21).

In X-linked recessive disorders, new mutations are fairly common. For an isolated case of an X-linked disorder, the mutation may have occurred at one of three sites—on the X of the affected male or on one of the two maternal X chromosomes. Without diagnostic testing, the mother of a son with a new mutation X-linked disorder faces a two-thirds chance of being a carrier and a one-third chance that the mutation arose in her son. These numbers can be incorporated in a Bayesian calculation when empirically establishing the risk of carrier status for other female relatives. In situations in which two males in a family are affected, the intervening females are by definition obligate carriers with a 50% chance of affected sons and 50% chance of carrier daughters.

X-linked dominant. Rarely, X-linked dominant traits have been described. In these situations, females with one abnormal allele would also express the disease. In two disorders, Rett syndrome and ornithine transcarbamylase deficiency,

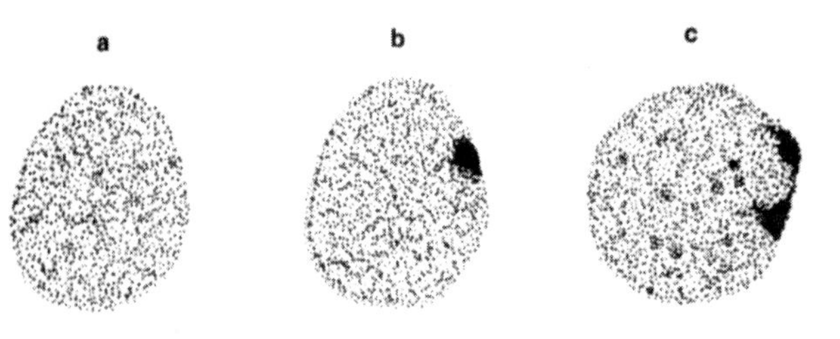

Fig. 20-20. Sex chromatin (Barr body). **A,** The nucleus of a cell with no sex chromatin (usually a male). **B,** 1 Barr body (usually a female). **C,** 2 Barr bodies (as found in individuals with 3 X chromosomes) (From Cavalli-Sforza, *Elements of Human Genetics*, Monto Park CA, 1977, WA Benjamin, p 38.)

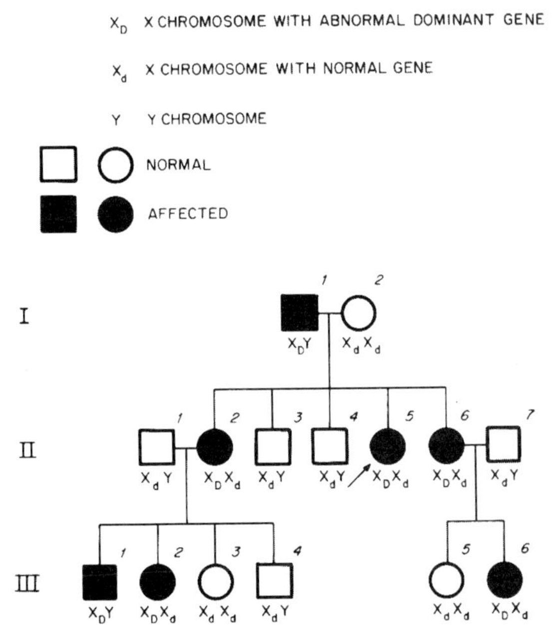

Fig. 20-21. Pedigree illustrating X-linked recessive inheritance.

severely affected males generally die shortly after birth.[133] Vitamin D-resistant rickets, also inherited as an X-linked dominant, while not leading to neonatal demise, displays a more severe disease in males than females (Fig. 20-22).

Multifactorial and polygenic inheritance

Many birth defects, while not attributable to a specific Mendelian disorder or chromosomal abnormality, display a marked familial clustering. While exposure to a common environment, especially prenatally, is sometimes invoked when several family members have children with the same nonMendelian birth defect, the genetic constitution of the child also plays a role. Such disorders, referred to as *multifactorial,* include a great number of the isolated structural defects present at birth (Table 20-5).

For multifactorial disorders, twin studies have been useful for examining the role of environmental exposure and genetically determined thresholds (Fig 20-23). Twins, given their shared prenatal environment are exposed to the same background of possible deleterious environmental agents. For birth defects in which a genetically determined threshold plays a role, identical (monozygotic) twins would be expected to more often be similarly affected than nonidentical (dizygotic) twins. In general, multifactorial traits with an incidence in livebirths of approximately 1 in 1000 have an average recurrence risk percentage of 1 to 5 for both a similarly affected offspring or for an affected parent to have an affected offspring. For traits that are more common in one of the sexes, an affected offspring of the less commonly affected sex carries a higher recurrence risk.[121]

Polygenic inheritance, distinct from multifactorial, refers to the inheritance of continuously distributed traits controlled by multiple rather than a single gene locus. Height, weight, blood pressure, age at menarche, and IQ are all thought to be

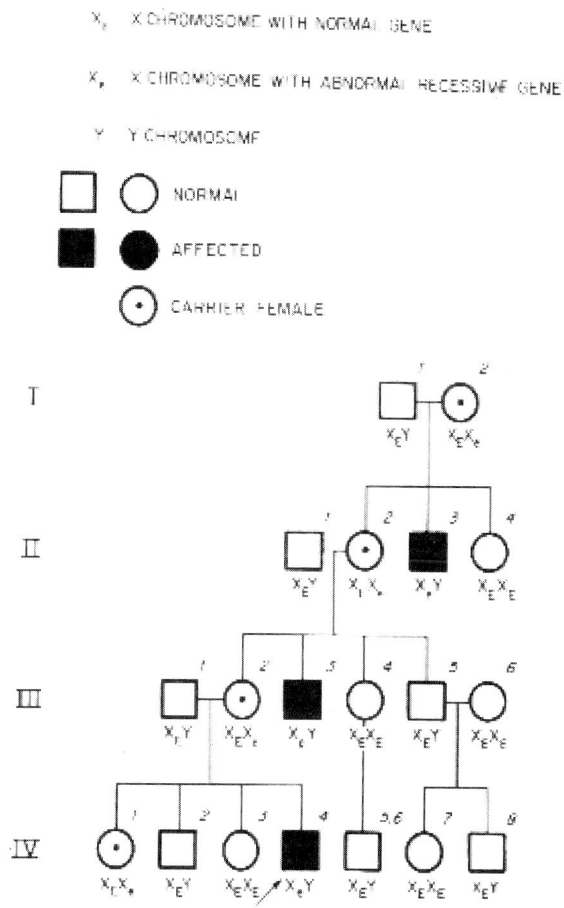

Fig. 20-22. Pedigree illustrating in X-linked dominant inheritance.

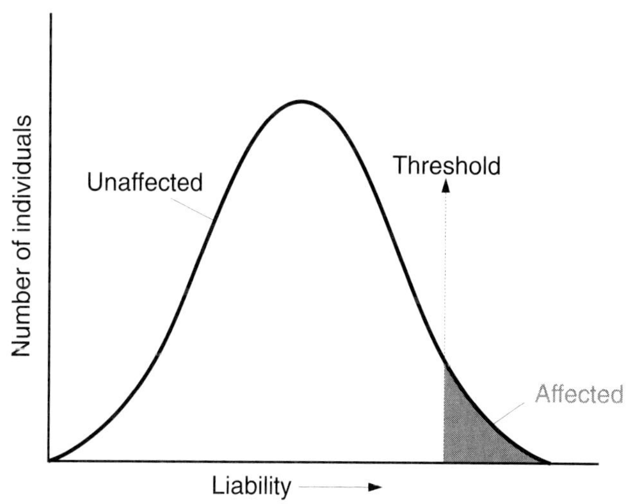

Fig. 20-23. Multifactorial threshold model. Liability to a trait is distributed normally with a threshold dividing the population into unaffected and affected classes. (From Thompson MW, McInnes RR, Willard HF: *Thompson and Thompson: genetics in medicine,* ed 5, Philadelphia, 1991, WB Saunders, p 352.)

Table 20-5. Polygenic/multifactorial traits

Neural tube defects (anencephaly, spina bifida, encephalocele)
Hydrocephaly (except some cases of aqueductal stenosis and some cases of Dandy-Walker syndrome)
Cleft lip, with or without cleft palate
Cleft lip (alone)
Cardiac defects (most types)
Diaphragmatic hernia
Omphalocele
Renal agenesis
Ureteral anomalies
Hypospadias (most forms)
Posterior urethral valves
Uterine (müllerian fusion) defects
Hip dislocation
Limb reduction defects (most forms)
Talipes equinovarus (clubfoot)

Simpson JL, Golbus MS: *Genetics in obstetrics and gynecology,* ed 2, Philadelphia, 1992, WB Saunders.

governed by polygenic inheritance. Embryonic control of cell growth and differentiation is likely to be polygenic with alterations in the timing of cell division under genetic control. Familial tendencies for many continuous traits, such as height and weight, may reflect polygenic inheritance. An overlap of polygenic and multifactorial inheritance of noncontinuous traits (such as the birth defects in Table 20-5) may occur if genetically controlled timing of cell differentiation alters a fetus' susceptibility to environmental teratogens, which themselves produce damage only at particular stages.[121]

Mitochondrial inheritance

Although the majority of cellular DNA is contained within the nucleus, DNA also exists in the mitochondria. Mitochondrial DNA is circular and has been shown to code for several proteins. Unique to mitochondrial DNA is a paucity of noncoding sequences. Thirteen structural genes have been located in the mitochondria. Cytoplasmic mitochondria segregate in conjunction with the nucleus of an ovum but not with the nucleus of a sperm. Thus mitochondrial genes are passed only from mother to offspring. Several diseases including Leber hereditary optic neuropathy, Leigh's disease, and myoclonic epilepsy with ragged red fibers have been mapped to the mitochondrial DNA.[133] Inheritance in families is consistent with a cytoplasmic passage from only the mother to her offspring.

New theories of inheritance

While many diseases result from a single gene defect that segregates in a stable fashion, in other disorders familial clustering is recognized but a clear pattern of inheritance cannot be established. The presumed genetic defect may skip generations or have wide variability in expression. Newly recognized patterns of gene transmission and expression including unstable DNA, uniparental disomy, and imprinting provide insight into these previously unexplained pedigrees.

Unstable DNA. The transmission of DNA from parent to offspring has traditionally been viewed as a stable process. Alterations in DNA structure were considered rare and once they occur, were thought to be stable. Increases or decreases in DNA were not considered possible. Recent investigations in fragile X syndrome suggest DNA instability may represent a means of regulating gene expression.

Fragile X syndrome. Males affected fragile X syndrome, the most common cause of familial mental retardation, are characterized by large ears and testes, a prominent jaw, and moderate to severe mental retardation.[135, 147] The syndrome is associated with an X chromosome fragile site (Xq27.3) that can be induced under folate deficient culture conditions (Fig. 20-24). In both affected males and carriers, evidence of the fragile site is variable with a wide range of cells (5% to 60%) displaying a break on the long arm of the X chromosome.[131]

Though involving a locus mapped to the X chromosome, transmission of this syndrome deviates from accepted theories of X-linked inheritance. Family studies reveal that inheritance is passed through normal transmitting males (NTM) who are neither symptomatic nor have any cytogenetic evidence of a fragile site. In contrast to most X-linked disorders, carrier females also can be affected so that up to 35% may have mental retardation. The concept that within a family the same X chromosome mutation in a NTM, carrier female, or affected male can produce widely variable phenotypic effects is known as *Sherman's paradox*.[113, 114]

In 1991 the gene responsible for the phenotype, FMR-1, was partially sequenced. Initial investigations found the fragile site was hypermethylated in affected males but not in normal transmitting or unaffected males.[3, 88, 138] Sequencing of this region revealed an abundance of cytidine phosphate guanosine (CpG) dinucleotides that when methylated halted the expression of adjacent genes.[134]

Abnormal methylation of the fragile site was only one piece of the puzzle. Sequencing within the region of the fragile X identified tandemly arranged arrays of trinucleotides (p[CGG]n) of variable length.[66] Direct DNA analysis of families with the fragile X found the largest trinucleotide fragments were associated with the abnormal methylation and full fragile X phenotype. Smaller increases in the fragment length, (premutations) were identified in normal transmitting males who had normal methylation patterns and only

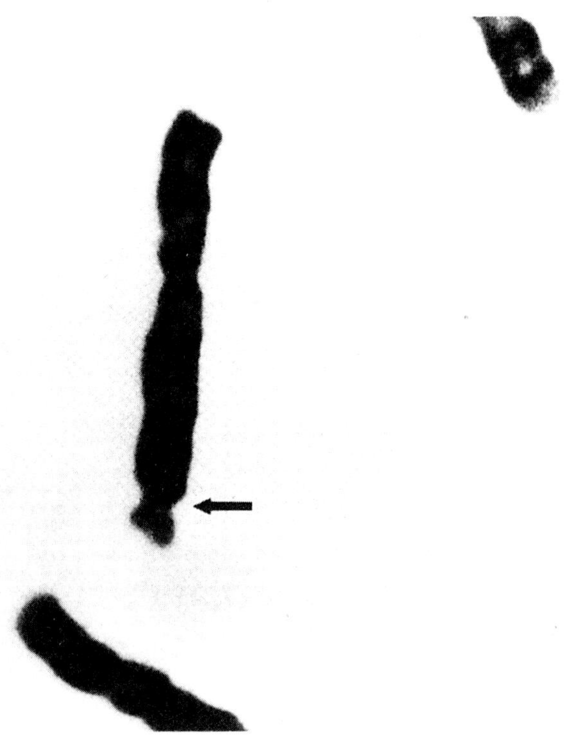

Fig. 20-24. Fragile X site produced under folic acid deficient media conditions. (From Friedman JM et al: *Genetics*, Baltimore, 1992, Williams and Wilkins, p 41.)

rare instances of mental retardation. In females, carriers of the premutation had a 3% incidence of mental retardation; those carrying the full mutation had a 50% frequency of mental retardation.[103] Predictions as to the degree of phenotypic expression of the full mutation in females are confounded by X-inactivation.

Uniparental disomy. Uniparental disomy, the presence of both members of a chromosome pair originating from one parent, was originally proposed by Engel in 1980. Uniparental disomy establishes the potential for single parent contribution of both alleles at a given locus. Because this theory was a radical departure from Mendelian biparental inheritance, Engel's theory received little attention until a decade later when polymorphic DNA probes discerned the parental origin of chromosomes and cases of uniparental inheritance were reported.[25]

Mechanisms producing uniparental disomy are currently unclear. Uniparental origin of a chromosome pair could occur through gamete complementation (fertilization of gametes with complementary loss and gain involving the same chromosome pair), monosomic duplication, or in an initially trisomic conceptus. With reference to the latter, postzygotic loss of a chromosome in an originally trisomic conceptus is supported by the identification of uniparental disomy for chromosome 15 in a diploid individual. In this individual, trisomy 15 was originally detected on chorionic villus sampling.[99, 127]

A further level of complexity, and clinically a source of variability in uniparental disomic gene inheritance also should be considered. Within a uniparental chromosome pair, each chromosome can be genetically identical (*isodisomy*) or dissimilar (*heterodisomy*), depending upon when the nondisjunctional event occurs during meiosis. Heterodisomy would result from a nondisjunctional event during the first meiotic division; isodisomy could be produced either by a second meiotic division or postzygotic nondisjunctional.[127] Thus in cases of uniparental disomy, the two alleles are contributed from only one parent and furthermore, in the cases of isodisomy the genomic content may be identical.

The clinical implications of uniparental disomy have been far reaching. As postulated by Engel, clinical situations that defy Mendelian theory and that possibly are explained by uniparental disomy include the following:

1. Autosomal recessive disorders in the offspring of couples in which only one parent is a heterozygotic carrier—two cases of uniparental isodisomy for chromosome 7 resulting in cystic fibrosis in an offspring with only one carrier parent.[127, 140]
2. Transmission of an X-linked disorder from a father to a son as a result of uniparental inheritance of both the X and Y from the father—one case of hemophilia A in a father and son.[137]
3. Expression of X-linked disorders in females as a result of inheritance of both X chromosomes from a carrier mother.

Additionally, syndromes classically produced by deletion of chromosomal material are now known also to be produced by uniparental disomy. In Prader Willi syndrome (PWS), the most common dysmorphic form of obesity, deletions of the paternally derived chromosome 15 are present in the majority of individuals. In nondeletion cases, maternal uniparental disomy is an alternative mechanism producing only maternal alleles (and thus no paternal alleles) at the critical site.[79,86] Both maternal heterodisomy (two different number 15 homologues from the mother) and maternal isodisomy (identical number 15 homologues from the mother), have been reported which argues against the phenotype resulting solely from uniparental isodisomy of a recessive gene. More likely, the critical region in PWS is involved in imprinting, the inactivation of one set of alleles resulting in functional hemizygosity. The characteristic Prader Willi phenotype results from the lack of paternal alleles at a specific region (15q11q13), either through the presence of a visible or microscopic deletion of the paternal number 15, or through the presence of two copies of the maternal number 15 as a result of uniparental disomy.

Similar investigations in Angelman syndrome (AS) have also revealed uniparental disomy.[77] Characterized by dysmorphia, severe mental retardation, paroxysms of laughter, and seizures, AS is phenotypically distinct from PWS, although almost half of the patients possess a karyotypically identical deletion of chromosome 15.[64, 150] However, in contrast to the paternal origin of the deletion in PWS, in AS the maternally inherited number 15 is consistently deleted. The phenotype of AS arises from the lack of maternal genes at a critical region—a region in close proximity to that involved in PWS.[77] In addition, similar to the Prader Willi investigations, in cases of AS without recognized deletion at 15q11q13, paternal uniparental disomy, and thus functional maternal nullisomy at this region, has now been reported.[77, 86]

While the number of syndromes recognized as resulting from uniparental disomy is limited, the identification of this form of inheritance is far reaching. Evidence for uniparental disomy involving ten chromosomes has been cited.[43] At present, the full clinical impact of uniparental disomy remains unknown.

Imprinting. At some loci, alterations in gene expression occur not by structural changes in the DNA but as a result of transient silencing of gene function. When this process occurs during gametogenesis, such modifications are known as imprinting. Clinically, imprinted genes result in differences in gene expression, depending upon the parent of origin. Much of our current knowledge of imprinting has stemmed from extensive animal studies. In mice, imprinted loci appear to undergo selective suppression during oogenesis and spermatogenesis which can be reversed in somatic cells.[9] While the molecular basis underlying imprinting is not yet understood, methylation may play a role.[132] At least one quarter of the mouse genome appears to undergo imprinting.[108]

In humans, imprinted genes are now being recognized by the different phenotypic effects produced, which are dependent upon whether the gene is inherited from the mother or from the father. Uniparental disomy, as described in the preceding section, is one mechanism by which imprinted genes may be revealed and play a role in the production of pathologic states. The different phenotypic expressions of maternally versus paternally derived disomies in Prader Willi and Angelman syndromes may reflect uncovering of imprinted genes in the 15q11q13 region. Based upon the known location of imprinted genes in the mouse genome and established homologies between the karyotypes from mouse and man, a role for imprinting has been postulated for several human disease states.[112]

Evidence is accumulating that imprinting is not only responsible for some pathologic states but also may play a fundamental role in human growth potential and survival. In animals, imprinting at certain loci is a critical process for the balanced expression of genes affecting cell growth and differentiation.[129]

Beckwith-Wiedemann syndrome (BWS), characterized by overgrowth of various organs resulting in gigantism, macroglossia, hemihypertrophy, and visceromegaly may provide some clues to imprinting and control of cell growth in humans. BWS has been mapped to 11p15.5, a region containing insulin-like growth factor 2 (Igf/2) that plays a role in maintaining the proper control of cell growth. Overproduction of Igf/2 has been proposed as an etiologic mechanism for the excessive growth noted in BWS.[72] Igf/2 has recently been recognized as an imprinted gene with only the paternally derived allele expressed, even though alleles from both parents are present. Paternal uniparental disomy of region 11p15.5 in three eighths of BWS cases supports an overexpression of the paternally imprinted Igf/2 as instrumental in the overgrowth noted in this syndrome.[46]

GENETICS IN GYNECOLOGIC PRACTICE

Disorders of sexual differentiation

Embryology. Determination of sexual development is dependent upon two factors: (1) the composition of the sex chromosome pair, and (2) the proper functioning of autosomal genes controlling sex differentiating hormones. Sexual differentiation follows an orderly sequence of events. At six weeks of development, genital cells migrate from an extraembryonic location to the gonadal ridges and become surrounded by sex cords to form primitive gonads.[133] Further differentiation of the bipotential gonad is directed by a testes determining factor (TDF)—most likely a single gene

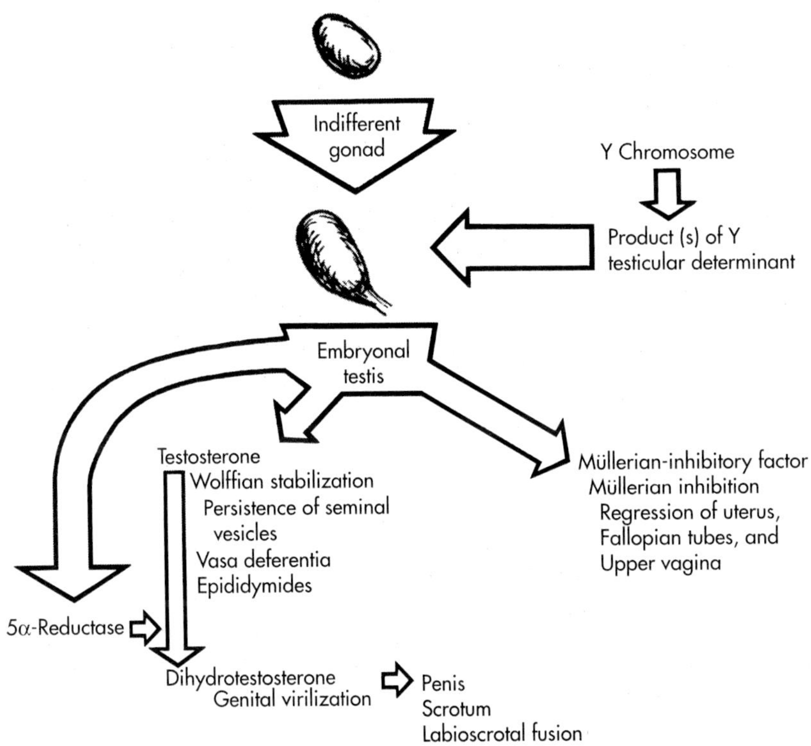

Fig. 20-25. Schematic diagram of normal male differentiation. (From Simpson JL and Golbus M: *Genetics in obstetrics and gynecology*, ed 2, Philadelphia, 1992, WB Saunders, p 137).

product. Without functional TDF, the gonad differentiates as an ovary. The H-Y antigen on the long arm of the Y chromosome was initially proposed as the TDF. However, current investigation supports the sex determining region (SRY) on the short arm of the Y chromosome as the site for the TDF.[121] TDF does not operate alone as genes on both the X chromosome and autosomes are crucial in differentiation of the testes (Fig. 20-25).

Without TDF the undifferentiated gonad at 6 weeks differentiates into an ovary by 8 weeks (Fig. 20-26). The development of the ovary and its germ cells results not from the presence of the two X chromosomes but from the lack of the Y chromosome short arm and TDF. In Turner fetuses with only one X chromosome, ovaries with germ cells develop only to undergo attrition prior to birth, resulting in gonadal. Thus while two X chromosomes are not needed to initiate and accomplish ovarian differentiation, they are required for maintenance of ovarian differentiation. Gene loci for ovarian maintenance are located on both the short and long arms of the X chromosome and on an autosome.[117]

Concomitant with germ cell migration, orderly thickening of the genital ridges occurs forming the mesonephric (wolffian) and paramesonephric (müllerian) ducts. In the male, the differentiation of seminiferous tubules and Leydig cells is governed by genes separate from those that control gonadal differentiation.[90] Progression of the wolffian ducts into the tubular structures of the testes (vasa deferentia, epididymides, and seminal vesicles) is initiated by the production of testosterone by the fetal Leydig cells. Leydig cell testosterone production is triggered by placental human chorionic gonadotropin. Exogenous testosterone at this gestational age will result in male tubular differentiation also regardless, of the sex chromosome complement. Simultaneous resolution of the müllerian structures (precursors of the uterus and fallopian tubes) is governed by antimüllerian glycoprotein from the Sertoli cells. This glycoprotein is controlled by a gene located on an autosome.[121] Without testosterone and the antimüllerian glycoprotein of the Sertoli cells, and in fact in the complete absence of gonadal development, the fetus develops ductal and genital structures along a female line.

Clinical disorders of sexual differentiation. Disorders of sexual differentiation are numerous and may present with a variety of external genitalia including normal male, normal female, or ambiguous genitalia. For the practicing gynecologist, disorders of sexual differentiation are generally encountered in women with primary amenorrhea. Evaluations for primary amenorrhea will most likely uncover women with gonadal dysgenesis (45,X, 46,XX or 47,XY),

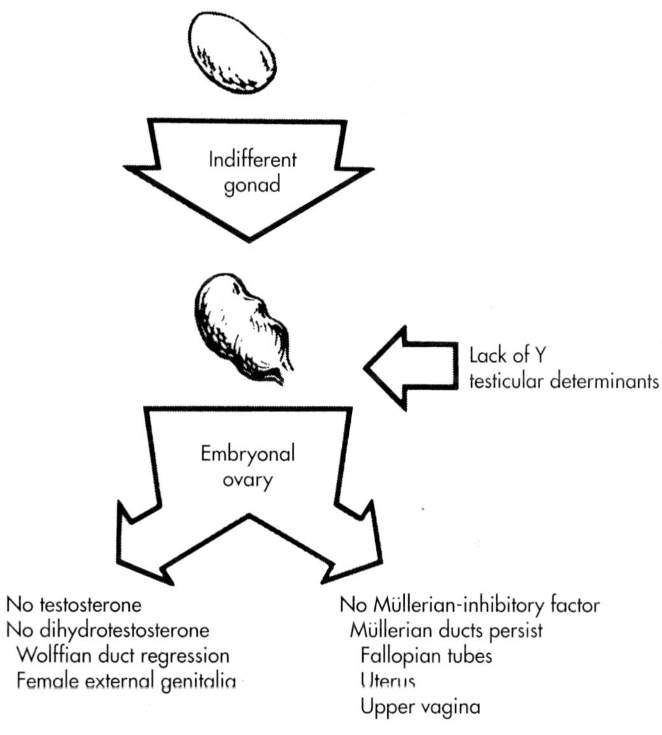

Fig. 20-26. Schematic diagram of normal female differentiation. (From Simpson JL and Golbus M, ed 2, *Genetics in obstetrics and gynecology*, ed 2, Philadelphia, 1992, WB Saunders, p 138).

male pseudohermaphroditism, or rare sex chromosome aneuploidies. Less commonly the gynecologist will need to be familiar with disorders of newborn or childhood genital ambiguity, and in some instances of infertility evaluations, the disorders of sexual differentiation presenting with male genitalia. The following sections present the mechanisms, clinical characteristics, and variable expressions of these disorders. In depth reviews can be found in Simpson[117, 121] and the multiple malformation syndromes involving ambiguous genitalia are delineated in Jones.[56]

Gonadal dysgenesis. Replacement of the gonads by fibrous tissue devoid of germ cells (streak gonads) occurs with 45,X, 46,XX, and 46,XY karyotypes. When identified during evaluation for primary ammenorrhea, gonadal dysgenesis is due to 45,X in 40% of cases, 40% have 46,XX or 46,XY complements, and the remaining 20% possess structural rearrangements of the X chromosome.[117] Common to all cases of gonadal dysgenesis, regardless of the karyotype, is the development of female external genitalia, uterus, and fallopian tubes. As all lack the development of gonadal tissue, elevated levels of gonadotropins are present. Somatic variations in the associated structural abnormalities and phenotypes reflect the differing karyotypes.

The *Turner, 45,X* phenotype, depicted in Fig. 20-27, is characterized by short stature, amenorrhea, and usually normal intelligence. Additional features are presented in Table 20-6. The basis for the short stature of Turner's females remains unknown, although loci on a homologous region of the short arms of the X and Y chromosomes may play a role. Because this region does not undergo X-inactivation, monosomy X individuals have half the usual number of alleles at this locus.[30] Recently children with monosomy X have been treated with human recombinant DNA-derived growth factor in an effort to increase their average adult height. However, an underlying abnormality in their epiphyseal plates may limit their eventual adult heights.[121] Most individuals with monosomy X have normal intelligence, though many score poorly on spatial visual testing. Adult diseases such as hypertension (in one third of adults with monosomy X) and diabetes should be considered in the long term health management of these individuals.

Generally, ovarian function in Turner's sydrome is absent with markedly decreased estrogen and androgen production in the presence of elevated gonadotropins. Without estrogen stimulation at puberty, several somatic features of Turner's syndrome are predictable, including decreased quantities of pubic and axillary hair, scant breast tissue with pale areolae and failure of the müllerian derivatives and external genitalia to differentiate from infantile to adult states.[14,121]

Ovarian function as reflected by menstruation and breast development in monosomy X individuals is rarely reported (<5%). In such cases undetected mosaic cell lines with a normal female complement (46,XX) are proposed but usually

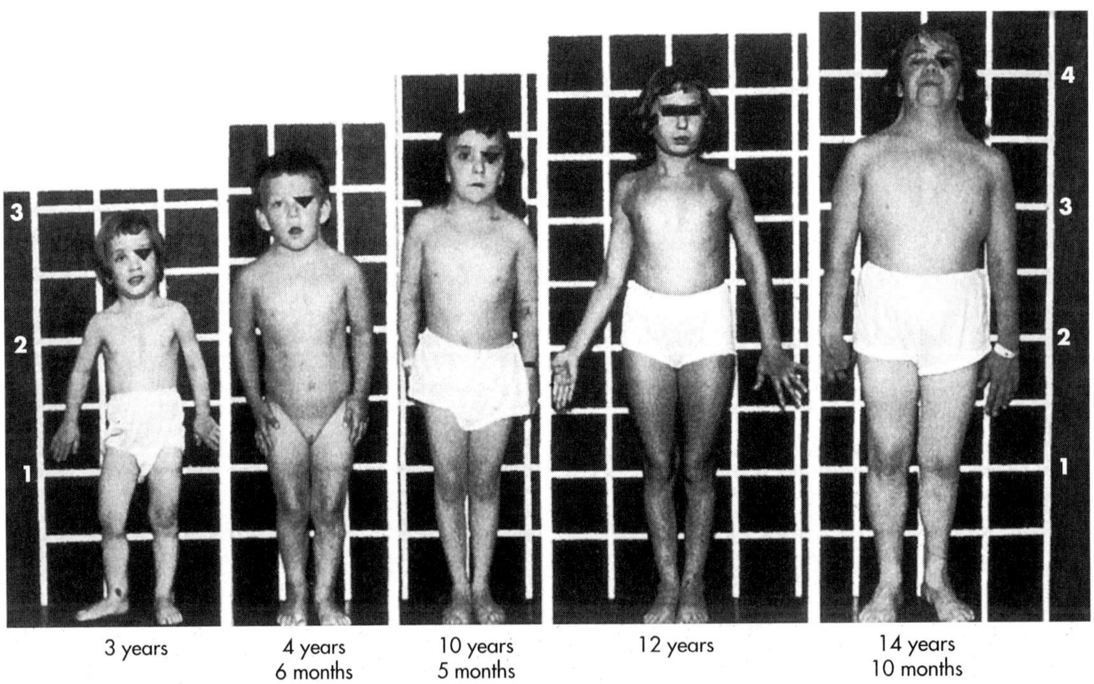

Fig. 20-27. Five girls with Turner's syndrome. Note the variability of such features as webbed neck and broad chest. (From Jones KL: Smith's recognizable pattern of malformation, ed 4, Philadelphia, 1988, WB Saunders, p 78.)

not documented. Women with a known combination of 46,XX and 45,X cells (mosaics) have been shown to have a greater chance of menstruating (12%) with a taller adult height and fewer somatic anomalies.[121] In nonmosaic 45,X, without assisted reproduction, pregnancy rarely occurs. Whether the incidence of chromosomally abnormal offspring is increased remains unclear because few cases have been studied.[19,121] Alternatively, estrogen and cyclic progesterone replacement at puberty can lead to a normal uterine size and pregnancies have been reported with donor oocytes.[14]

While a 45,X karyotype results in the full phenotype of Turner's syndrome with gonadal dysgenesis and a characteristic constellation of somatic changes (Fig. 20-27), structural abnormalities of the X chromosome can produce some or all of the features of Turner's syndrome. Comparison of these various structural changes in the X chromosome have enabled delineation of the determinant regions for both ovarian maintenance and structural growth (Fig 20-28).[154] Individuals with deletions of the X chromosome short arm (46,X,del[X]p or 46,X,i[Xq]) generally present with a combination of gonadal dysgenesis, short stature, and Turner phenotype. Various deletions of the long arm of the X chromosome suggest an additional site of ovarian function determination with affected individuals presenting with either gonadal dysgenesis or premature ovarian failure although often in the setting of normal height.[121]

Familial gonadal dysgenesis, XX type, presents in karyotypically normal females (46,XX). As in Turner's syndrome and other forms of gonadal dysgenesis, affected individuals have streak gonads and a lack of estrogenization of both the external female genitalia and the müllerian derivatives. Inherited in an autosomal recessive fashion, presentation is usually with primary amenorrhea as their normal height and lack of somatic anomalies fails to suggest an earlier diagnosis.[99, 117] Autosomal recessive inheritance suggests additional non-X chromosome gene locations governing ovarian maintenance. 46,XX gonadal dysgenesis also may be seen as a component of more complex syndromes such as neurosensory deafness (Perrault's syndrome),[87] with myopathy,[73] with cerebellar ataxia,[122] and with microcephaly/arachnodactyly.[80]

Gonadal dysgenesis in the setting of a male karyotype (*Swyer syndrome, 46,XY)* also presents with features previously described as common to gonadal dysgenesis. Because these individuals do not have associated somatic anomalies, at their presentation for primary amenorrhea they are clinically and biochemically indistinguishable from 46,XX gonadal dysgenesis. Loss of testicular tissue before 7 to 8 weeks gestation appears to be the underlying pathology. Various modes of inheritance have been proposed, including X-linked recessive and autosomal recessive.[13, 26, 121] The initial differentiation of testicular tissue in the gonad, although replaced by fibrosis, places these individuals at increased risk (20% to 30%) for dysgerminoma or gonadoblastoma. Although an association between the presence of HY antigen and the development of neoplasia has been noted,[141] all 46,XY gonadal dysgenesis patients should be counseled regarding

Table 20-6. Turner phenotype: major features and their incidence

Feature	Incidence (%)
Small stature, often noted at birth	100
Ovarian dysgenesis with variable degree of hypoplasia of germinal elements	90+
Transient congenital lymphedema, especially notable over the dorsum of the hands and feet	80+
Shield-like, broad chest with widely spaced, inverted, and/or hypoplastic nipples	80+
Prominent auricles	80+
Low posterior hairline, giving the appearance of a short neck	80+
Webbing of posterior neck	50
Anomalies of elbow, including cubitus valgus	70
Short metacarpal and/or metatarsal	50
Narrow, hyperconvex, and/or deepset nails	70
Renal anomalies	60+
Cardiac anomalies (coarction of the aorta in 70% of cases)	20+
Perceptive hearing loss	50

Jones OW, Cahill TC: Basic genetics and patterns of inheritance. In Creasy RK, Resnick R, editors: *Maternal fetal medicine*, Philadelphia, 1994, WB Saunders, p32.

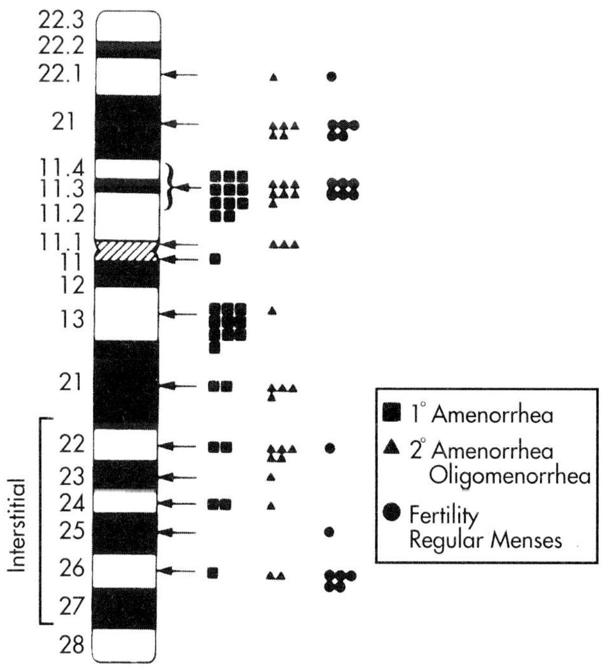

Fig. 20-28. Schematic diagram of X-chromosome showing ovarian function by site of structural abnormalities (From Simpson JL: *Disorders of sexual differentiation: etiology and clinical delineation*, New York, 1976, Academic Press, p 136).

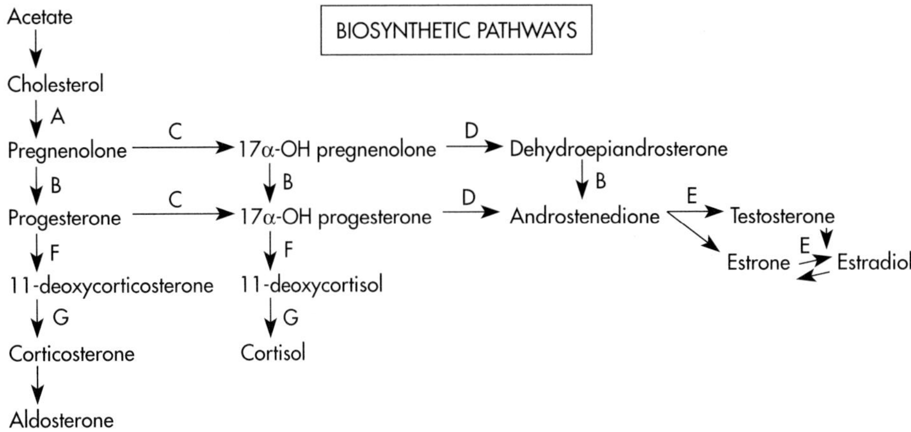

Fig. 20-29. Important adrenal and gonadal biosynthetic pathways. Letters designate enzymes required for the appropriate conversions; A, 20 alpha-hydroxylase, 22 alpha-hydroxylase and 20,22-desmolase; B, 38 beta-ol-dehydrogenase; C, 17 alphahydroxylase; D, 17, 20-desmolase; E, 17-ketosteroid reductase; F, 21-hydroxylase; G, 11-hydroxylase. (From Simpson JL: disorders of sexual differentiation: etiology and clinical delineation, New York, Academic Press, 1976, page 145 reproduced with permission.)

gonadectomy, although retention of the uterus and tubes will allow for future reproductive function by assisted reproductive technologies.[14]

Female pseudohermaphroditism. Presenting as a discordancy between the external genitalia and well-differentiated internal gonadal structures, female pseudohermaphrodites have a 46,XX karyotype, masculinized external genitalia, and differentiated ovaries. In general, the karyotype and internal ductal structures correspond to the gonad: female pseudohermaphrodites possess ovaries and paramesonephric derivatives (uterus, tubes, upper vagina), regardless of their external genitalia. With some exceptions, female pseudohermaphrodites typically are diagnosed during the newborn or infancy period when partial virilization of the external genitalia results in an ambiguous sexual identification.

Female pseudohermaphroditism with virilization of external genitalia and normal ovarian development can occur from exposure to testosterone or its derivatives, either endogenously through a hormonal abnormality or exogenously through ingested hormones. In such cases the development of normal ovaries in conjunction with müllerian structures argues against an underlying sex chromosome abnormality. Clinically the genitalia are characterized by clitoromegaly, displacement of the urethra, and labial fusion.

The most common hormonal imbalances producing increased testosterone and thus virilization in affected females are the *adrenogenital sydromes*. Multiple inherited enzyme abnormalities along the pathway of cortisol production from cholesterol can occur. The specific enzyme defect will determine if other metabolic perturbations are also present (Fig. 20-29). The two most common deficiencies, 21-hydroxylase and 11 β-hydroxylase account for 90% and 5% of congenital adrenal hyperplasia (CAH) cases.[69] Although the enzyme deficiencies of the adrenogenital syndrome are inherited in an autosomal recessive fashion with both male and females equally affected, only females exhibit evidence of testosterone excess as newborns (Table 20-7). Production of the adrenal enzymes begins by 8 to 9 weeks gestation so that elevated quantities of testosterone in utero can result in a virilized female newborn with intact müllerian structures and ovaries. While a few males may be detected at birth by the increased pigmentation that results from the melanocyte stimulating properties of ACTH, in males without complications of salt wasting, the diagnosis may be otherwise unsuspected.[121]

Table 20-7. Types of congenital adrenal hyperplasia

Form	Genitalia	Androgens	Other
21-OH deficiency	Virilized ♀	↑↑	±Salt-losing, most common
11-OH deficiency	Virilized ♀	↑↑	Hypertension
Cholesterol desmolase	Ambiguous ♂	N/A	Salt-wasting
3- β-OH steroid	Ambiguous ♂	↑↑	Lethal
17-OH deficiency	Ambiguous ♂	↓	Hypertension
17,20-lyase	Ambiguous ♂	↓	Isolated defect

Note: ↑=increase, ↓=decrease, ±=with or without, ♂= male, ♀= female
From Friedman JM et al: *Genetics*, Baltimore, 1992, Williams and Wilkins, p 138.

The prenatal diagnosis of 21-hydroxylase deficiency is possible using a combination of HLA linkage analysis and DNA studies. With a 25% recurrence risk, prenatal diagnosis of 21-hydroxylase deficiency allows for the detection and potential treatment of affected females to prevent virilization. In such cases, maternal dexamethasone to suppress the fetal pituitary-adrenal axis would be needed by 5 weeks' gestation. Either CVS or amniocentesis could then establish the fetal sex and 21-hydroxylase status. Affected females would need to be maintained on maternal dexamethasone therapy. Reported series of such treatment plans have yielded variable results. In approximately two thirds of cases, virilization has been prevented or reduced. However, in one third of cases virilization was not abated because of differences in dosing regimens, interruptions in medication, delay in treatment, or variability in maternal steroid metabolism.[69] Additionally, dexamethasone therapy requires appropriate surveillance for maternal side effects and the long term consequences for the fetus remain unexplored. At present the prenatal treatment of 21-hydroxylase deficiency remains to be fully evaluated.

Exogenous ingestion of masculinizing substances can produce female pseudohermaphroditism. During prenatal development, maternally administered synthetic progestins will result in virilization of the female fetus.[39] Testosterone, ethinyl testosterone, norethindrone acetate and norethindrone, (the latter two are components of several oral contraceptives) may produce virilization depending upon the dose and timing of exposure. Rarely associated with virilization are norethynodrel, medroxyprogesterone and 17α-OH-progesterone caproate.[121] Rarely will virilizing maternal tumors virilize a female fetus because affected women seldom become pregnant.

Male pseudohermaphrodites. Possessing a 46,XY karyotype, testes, and female external genitalia, male pseudohermaphrodites also have tubular derivatives corresponding to their internal gonad. In general, their well-differentiated testes are accompanied by mesonephric derivatives (vasa deferentia, epididymides, and seminal vesicles). Rarely presentation may be in the newborn with ambiguous genitalia. More commonly, male pseudohermaphrodites present with primary amenorrhea with normal female or ambiguous genitalia but lack evidence of müllerian structures.

Complete androgen insensitivity (*complete testicular feminization*) represents a form of male pseudohermaphroditism. During an evaluation for primary amenorrhea, affected individuals can be identified by their lack of müllerian derivatives (absent uterus, tubes, and upper vagina). Their female appearance is characterized by breast development, although the areola is pale, pubic and axillary hair is scant, and the vaginal pouch is shortened. Testes can be documented abdominally in the inguinal canal or in the labia. An increased risk of 5% exists for testicular carcinomas, which typically present in the second or third decade.[118] Complete testicular feminization syndrome results from end-organ insensitivity to androgens in the presence of normal testosterone levels. In the majority of cases, androgen receptors are absent, while less often a nonfunctional receptor is present. The testosterone receptor gene is located on the X chromosome, and several mutations within this gene are described.[96] Inherited in an X-linked recessive fashion, affected males display complete testicular feminization while carrier females generally do not have discernible clinical abnormalities.

Mutations in other regions of the androgen-binding gene can produce partial androgen insensitivity. Also inherited as an X-linked recessive condition, *partial testicular feminization* is characterized by initially male or ambiguous genitalia that then undergoes feminization along with breast development at puberty. As with complete feminization, testes are present though often not descended, müllerian derivatives are absent, and pubertal virilization with development of the secondary-sex characteristics fails to occur. Either decreased numbers of androgen receptors or qualitative abnormalities of the receptors have been proposed.[95]

Less common in office gynecology but encountered in newborns with ambiguous genitalia is male pseudohermaphroditism caused by *5α-reductase deficiency*. While external genitalia may be ambiguous at birth and even a perineal opening resembling a vaginal dimple may exist, müllerian structures are lacking and at puberty normal virilization occurs. Gynecomastia is absent in contrast to other forms of male pseudohermaphroditism. Inherited in an autosomal recessive fashion, individuals have a deficiency of 5α-reductase, the enzyme needed in the conversion of testosterone to dihydrotestosterone. Lack of dihydrotestosterone leads to poor virilization of the fetal external genitalia, although testosterone alone is sufficient for maintenance of the wolffian structures. At puberty the increases in testosterone result in subsequent virilization even in the absence of adequate levels of dihydrotestosterone.[92, 121]

True hermaphroditism. The presence of both ovarian and testicular tissue and variable external genitalia characterizes true hermaphroditism. With either a separate ovary and testes or combined in an ovotestes, the majority have a normal female karyotype (46,XX); others possess various combinations of both XY and XX cell lines. Chimerism, the presence of two-cell lines as a result of fusion between two zygotes, has been documented in human twin pairs of opposite sexes and may represent one etiology of true hermaphroditism. Individuals in whom only XX cell lines are recovered could represent either undetected chimerism, possess the TDF of the Y chromosome translocated to an autosome, or express autosomal genes controlling sex reversal.[18]

A diagnosis of true hermaphroditism occurs only after the exclusion of pseudohermaphroditism. Generally a uterus is present although anomalies of uterine horn development are common. In these patients an absent uterine horn is often associated with a testes or ovotestes. Sufficient normal ovarian tissue may exist to produce estrogen for breast development, menstruation, and ovulation. Conversely, although the testicular tissue produces testosterone and virilization of the external genitalia, it is generally devoid of spermatozoa.

Aneuploidies of sex chromosomes. Individuals with *45,X/46,XY* mosaicism may present with Turner phenotypes, ambiguous genitalia, or as a normal male. In 45,X/46,XY individuals with Turner stigmata, given the presence of the 46,XY cell line, the streak gonads are at risk for development of carcinoma. Occurring in 15% to 20% of cases, the neoplasia develops during the first and second decade. Gonadectomy with retention of müllerian structures to aid in assisted reproduction potential is recommended.[121] 45,X/46,XY may also present as mixed gonadal dysgenesis with the presence of a streak gonad and dysgenic testes. Especially among prenatally diagnosed cases, the most common outcome of 45,X/46,XY is a normal male phenotype. The risk of gonadal carcinoma in these individuals is markedly less; gonadectomy is generally not suggested unless a close clinical evaluation of intrascrotal testes can be performed.[121]

Polysomy of the X chromosome *(47,XXX)* presents most often in individuals with normal female genitalia. The presence of an additional X chromosome allows proper ovarian maintenance through embryonic and fetal development, although delayed menarche and premature ovarian failure are common. Polysomy of the X chromosome is associated with mental retardation of varying degrees. 47,XXX individuals appear to be at some risk for IQ levels slightly lower than unaffected siblings. With additional X chromosomes (48,XXXX), the prevalence of mental retardation increases; mental delay is always present in individuals with 49,XXXXX.[100]

Sex chromosome abnormalities presenting with normal or near normal male external genitalia include Klinefelter's syndrome (47,XXY). Uncommonly encountered by gynecologists, this condition occurs in 1 in 1000 male livebirths and is identified in 1 in 10 azoospermic males. Klinefelter's syndrome is characterized generally by normal male external genitalia in the presence of poorly developed facial hair, female distribution of body fat, and a height slightly taller than average (Fig. 20-30). Mental retardation and additional somatic anomalies may be present in some but not all individuals. Two thirds of XXY individuals are thought to have learning disabilities. Low levels of testosterone are characteristic with seminiferous tubule degeneration leading to small testes.

Similarly, individuals with *47,XYY* also present with normal male external genitalia, taller than average height, and often azoospermia in the presence of normal testosterone levels. Intelligence may be decreased. The relationship of XYY to mental retardation, mental illness, and antisocial behavior continues to be debated. While the risk of abnormal behavior is not as high as originally estimated,[52] the rate of incarceration of XYY males continues to be ten times greater than for 46,XY males.[121] However when XYY males were compared to XY males of comparable reduced intelligence, the criminal rate was not found to be different.[151]

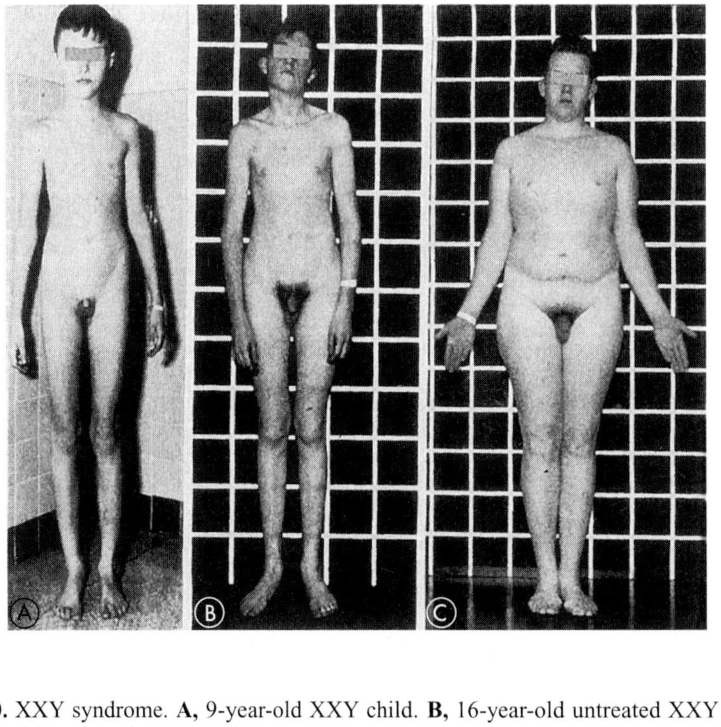

Fig. 20-30. XXY syndrome. **A,** 9-year-old XXY child. **B,** 16-year-old untreated XXY adolescent. **C,** 21-year-old untreated XXY adult. (From Jones KL: *Smith's recognizable pattern of malformation*, ed 3, Philadelphia, 1988, WB Saunders, p 68.)

Reproductive loss

Spontaneous miscarriage. Recent studies show that almost a third (31%) of all pregnancies are lost in the first trimester. In a group of women followed with serial human chorionic gonadotropin measurements from the time of implantation, a 22% rate of loss prior to clinical recognition of the pregnancy and a 9% loss rate thereafter was documented.[149] Researchers have long appreciated that chromosomal abnormalities are present in at least 50% of the latter subgroup of clinically recognized pregnancies lost in the first trimester.[5, 60] Among those losses prior to the clinical recognition of pregnancy, the frequency of chromosomal abnormalities has been more difficult to establish. The classic studies of Hertig and Rock which noted a high frequency of morphologic abnormalities among preimplantation embryos would suggest an associated high frequency of chromosomal abnormalities.[47] Karyotype analysis of 2 to 8 cell human embryos obtained by in vitro fertlization also supports a high rate of chromosomal abnormalities in prerecognition losses, although the exact numbers remain unclear.[97]

Autosomal trisomies represent the most frequent class of karyotypically abnormal first trimester miscarriages (50%), with trisomy 16 being the most common individual trisomy (Table 20-8). The most common single abnormality is 45,X and is identified in 20% of losses.[133] Based upon the rate of Turner's syndrome among liveborns, over 90% of 45,X conceptuses are lost as spontaneous abortions. Characteristically, first trimester 45,X losses exhibit lack of embryonic development with the placenta containing thrombi and hypoplastic villi.[49] Losses of Turner's syndrome, later in gestation are characterized by fetal cystic hygromas and edema. Advanced maternal age is not a feature of Turner's syndrome, with monosomy X usually resulting from the loss of the paternal X.[10]

Table 20-8. Relative frequencies of aberrations in chromosomally abnormal abortuses

Type	Frequency (approximate) Percent (%)
Aneuploidy	
45,X	20
Autosomal monosomy	<1
Autosomal trisomy	
Total	52
Trisomy 16	16
Trisomy 18	3
Trisomy 21	5
Trisomy 22	5
Other trisomies	23
Triploidy	16
Tetraploidy	6
Structural Rearrangements	4

Data chiefly from Boue J, Gropp A: Cytogenetics of pregnancy wastage, *Ann Rev Genet* 14:1-57, 1985.
From Thompson MW, McInnes RR, Willard HF. In Thompson and Thompson, editors: *Genetics in medicine*, ed 5, Philadelphia, 1991, WB Saunders, p 216.

Pregnancy losses with a triploid complement typically result from dispermy, the fertilization of a normal ovum with two sperm. However, meiotic nondisjunction in either parent may also occur, with cells of the resulting embryo containing 69 chromosomes. The placenta in triploids with an additional paternal complement is generally hydropic with cystic degeneration. Association of a fetus with a focally hydropic placenta with focal trophoblastic hyperplasia constitutes a partial mole, and the current management for gestational trophoblastic disease is recommended. In triploidy resulting from an additional maternal complement, severe growth retardation with a small, poorly formed placenta has been seen.[81] These differences between paternally as opposed to maternally derived triploids suggest a human example of the imprinting phenomena observed in mice. Following a triploid conception, an increased risk for a chromosomally abnormal fetus in a subsequent pregnancy has been suggested by some but not all investigators. While recurrence within a family of liveborn triploid infants has not been reported, an increased rate of aneuploidy both before and after a triploid conception has been noted.[136] In addition, karyotypic studies of serial pregnancy losses suggest an increase in both trisomic and triploid conceptions following an initial triploid spontaneous loss.[2, 45] The contribution of increasing maternal age to the higher risk of aneuploidy following a triploid conceptus in these studies may provide a partial explanation.[146]

Karyotype analysis of a spontaneous loss often reveals a karyotype abnormality. In the rare situations when an unbalanced structural rearrangement is detected (1.5%), further evaluation of the couple may reveal a balanced translocation carrier. In these cases, recurrence risk counseling based on empiric data regarding the translocation can be provided. However, more often a trisomic conceptus is discovered. For these couples the risk for a subsequent livebirth with a karyotype abnormality continues to be debated. Initially, studies of women with a karyotypically abnormal spontaneous loss followed by a second spontaneous loss were interpreted as showing an 80% likelihood that a second loss would be karyotypically abnormal as well.[45] Reanalysis with adjustment for maternal age at the second miscarriage refuted the significance of this earlier finding.[146]

Several investigators, however, support a recurrence for aneuploidy once an aneuploid conceptus, either spontaneous miscarriage or livebirth, is documented. A 1% risk for a liveborn trisomy 21 after an aneuploid spontaneous loss has been documented in one series.[2a] In addition, after a livebirth of a child with trisomy 21, a women under the age of 30 years has a 1% risk for a subsequent liveborn with a nondisjunction event. This risk includes the same trisomy as the original liveborn and other common aneuploidies.[128] Parallel evidence has been derived from couples with two spontaneous losses and normal parental karyotypes who at amniocentesis were found to have a 1.6% risk of a fetus with nondisjunction versus a 0.3% risk for maternal age matched controls.[21] Underlying mechanisms such as gonadal mosaicism or an inherited tendency to nondisjunction through action on the spindle fibers have been proposed.

Recurrent spontaneous abortions. Among couples experiencing repeated spontaneous abortions, balanced translocations are identified in approximately 3% of females and 2% of males. This rate is slightly lower if only couples without a liveborn are considered (females 2.4% and males 1.6%). Of note, if multiple miscarriages occur in conjunction with a stillbirth or a prior abnormal liveborn, the frequency of translocations increased in one study to 16.7%.[111] A recent review of over 22,000 couples with two or more spontaneous losses found balanced structural rearrangements in 4.7%.[17]

Common gynecologic variants and disorders

Physiologic variants. Polygenic inheritance, in which multiple gene loci function to control a continuous trait, may play a role in the inheritance of the age of menarche. Twin studies have shown identical twins are more similar (concordant) in their menarche age than are nonidentical twins. Elaborate quantitative twin studies have demonstrated that 65% of the variation in timing of menarche is due to genetic influence.[121]

Müllerian abnormalities. As a result of altered timing of mesonephric duct formation, abnormalities in the development of the müllerian system can occur. As the defect involves only the fusion of the tubules to form the uterine body, cervix, and upper vagina, normal development is seen in the ovaries and the fallopian tubes, and the external genitalia are feminized. Defects include aplasia, duplication, and incomplete fusion, which can be present as an isolated defect or as a component of several dysmorphology syndromes.[121]

True müllerian aplasia *(Rokitansky-Kuster-Hauser syndrome)* results in absence of the upper vagina, cervix, and uterus, with normal ovaries, remnant uterine cords, and feminized external genitalia with a blind vaginal pouch. Renal anomalies such as pelvic kidney, and unilateral aplasia, are present in 40% of patients[7] and vertebral anomalies are common. This disorder may be inherited in a polygenic fashion. Autosomal recessive and X-linked dominant theories have been proposed but generally not accepted for all families.[121]

True duplication of the müllerian system is rare and involves two separate uteri each of which possess two fallopian tubes. More commonly, incomplete fusion of the müllerian system gives rise to two uterine horns, each with only one fallopian tube. In general, if renal anomalies occur, they are seen on the ipsilateral side with the atretic horn. Incomplete fusion anomalies occur in 1 in 1000 females and a polygenic inheritance pattern seems likely.

Endometriosis. While studies of endometriosis have been complicated by biases of ascertainment, difficulty in diagnosis, and population specificities, an inherited tendency to this disease process has been suspected.[33] Multifactorial inheritance has been suggested by a 7% recurrence rate among first degree relatives of affected individuals, although incomplete penetrance with a Mendelian inheritance pattern has not been excluded.[120] Similarly, concordance in severity among affected individuals supports an inherited disease process.[78]

Polycystic ovary syndrome (PCO). While the diagnosis of PCO often represents a heterogeneous collection of women, several of the adrenal cortical enzyme abnormalities can present with a PCO-like clinical picture. Adult onset 21-hydroxylase deficiency, partial 17α-hydroxylase and 3β-ol-dehydrogenase may each present with PCO symptomatology. In essential PCO, a dominant inheritance pattern, either autosomal or X-linked, has been proposed by some investigators.[121] Further studies with control of population characteristics, diagnostic parameters, and biases will be needed.

Premature ovarian failure (POF). Structural abnormalities of the X chromosome andrare cases of XX gonadal dysgenesis can present with POF. In addition, familial aggregates of POF without chromosome abnormalities exist.[121]

Gynecologic cancers

The role of inheritance in gynecologic cancers reflects two principles of cancer genetics: (1) Knudson's "two hit" hypothesis, and (2) the identification of cancer genes. The role of each of these two principles in cancer families has been extensively investigated over the past twenty years. While familial aggregates of various cancers, including those of the gynecologic system, have been recognized for decades, the contribution of environmental exposures versus inherited tendencies has yet to be resolved. Only in rare situations, such as retinoblastoma, and currently in no cancers involving the reproductive system, can the inheritance of a cancer be clearly delineated as segregating in a Mendelian fashion.

The majority of cancers are clonal in origin, arising from a single cell.[28] With reference to gynecologic neoplasms, both carcinoma of the cervix and leiomyomata have been shown to result from multiple divisions of one cell. Given the premise of single cell origin of neoplasms, Knudsen proposed a two-step process of DNA mutation leading to uncontrolled cell division.[65] In families with aggregates of cancer, the first step most likely is an inherited mutation. In isolated cases of cancer, the first step probably occurs as an acquired mutation from exposure to known oncogens such as radiation, viruses, or chemicals. In both situations, the second step, or mutation, was thought to be acquired. In familial cancers, while the mutation (Knudson's first step) may be inherited in a Mendelian fashion, the development of cancer remains dependent upon a second mutational event (Fig. 20-31). This theory is also applicable to families with multiple members with different cancers.[121, 133]

A second principle integral to the understanding of inherited cancers has been the recent identification of cancer genes,

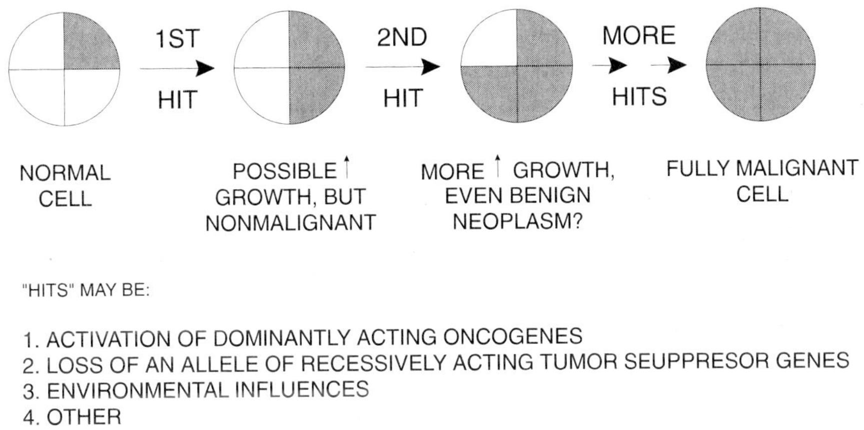

Fig. 20-31. Diagram of multistep origin of cancer. (From Gelehrter TD, Collins FS: *Principles of Medical Genetics*, Baltimore, 1990, Williams and Wilkins, p 165.)

both *oncogenes* and *tumor suppressor genes*. Oncogenes, genomic sequences known to transform normal cells to tumor cells, initially were identified in viruses. Also found in the human genome, oncogenes have close sequence homology to genes normally controlling growth and embryonic development. *Protooncogenes* are genomic sequences that become functional oncogenes (c-onc) through several mechanisms. Physical relocation of protooncogenes involving a chromosome translocation may result in release of surrounding regulatory controls.[40] Alternatively, incorporation into the human genome of a viral oncogene may trigger protooncogene transformation to a c-onc. Additionally, long terminal repeat sequences (LTRS) have been identified and proposed as triggering factors if inserted near a protooncogene.[109] Oncogenes have been reported in association with embryonal ovarian carcinoma, squamous cervical carcinoma, endometrial adenocarcinoma, ovarian epithelial carcinoma, and choriocarcinoma.[121]

Tumor suppressor genes play a role in cancer through regulation of genes controlling cell growth. Normally responsible for blocking cell growth, loss of function of tumor suppressor genes can contribute to malignancy through uninhibited cell growth. Currently the role of tumor suppressor genes in gynecologic cancers is unknown with the majority of support for these genes found in familial colon cancers, Wilms tumor, and neurofibromatosis (type 1).[133]

Ovarian carcinoma. With regard to specific cancers, the strongest evidence for genetic predisposition to a gynecologic cancer occurs with ovarian epithelial carcinoma. Among all individuals with ovarian epithelial carcinoma, serous and mucinous are the most common, while the endometrial is rarely encountered. However, among familial aggregates of ovarian cancer, serous or undifferentiated predominate.[121] Also supporting an inherited component in familial cases are a younger age of onset and an increased bilaterality of disease.[31]

Chromosomal abnormalities with the potential for translocation of a protooncogene site and thus activation to an oncogene are commonly seen in transformed ovarian tissue.[142] A t(6:14)(q21;q24) translocation has been the most frequently reported. Evidence exists as well for alteration of several specific oncogenes, c-myc and c-K-ras2.[29]

Given the limited means for prospective clinical surveillance, the poor response to therapy, and the significant mortality associated with ovarian carcinoma, determination of the risk faced by additional female family members of an individual with ovarian carcinoma continues to be pursued. Epidemiologic studies have proposed 5% to 10% of ovarian cancers have a hereditary basis.[74] Registries of ovarian cancer families are now being compiled and the current recommendation to female relatives of an individual with ovarian carcinoma includes consideration of prophylactic oophorectomy if multiple, first-degree female relatives have been diagnosed with serous ovarian carcinoma.[121]

For the nonepithelial ovarian carcinomas, limited evidence exists to support an inherited etiology with two exceptions, benign cystic teratoma and ovarian stroma neoplasias (granulosa cell, Sertoli/Leydig and fibromas). With regard to benign cystic teratoma (dermoids), their bilaterality suggests an inherited predisposition and reports of multiple affected family members exist.[116] Teratomas originate through parthenogenesis, development from a single germ cell that then undergoes self replication. Analysis of chromosome markers has shown dermoids most likely originate either from a lack of second polar body formation or reincorporation of the second polar body.[70]

Gestational trophoblast disease (GTD). As a group, GTD include the entities of hydatidiform mole, invasive mole, and choriocarcinoma. Hydatidiform mole includes both partial mole, in which fetal parts can be identified with a cystic placenta, and complete mole, in which only hydropic placenta is identified. Whether partial or complete, hydatidiform moles are characterized by avascular hydropic villi and are considered a benign form of gestational trophoblastic disease. However, 15% complete moles and 4% of partial moles develop persistent gestational trophoblastic tumor. As described with regards to pregnancy loss, partial moles are characteristically triploid (total chromosome count 69) and almost invariably have inherited the additional haploid set of chromosomes from the father. Triploid fetuses with the additional complement derived from the mother do not display molar changes but are characterized by severe fetal growth retardation.[81]

In contrast, although complete moles are characteristically diploid, they do not possess a normal biparental contribution of chromosomes. The completely paternal origin of the diploid complement in complete moles usually arises from fertilization of an ovum devoid of maternal DNA. Despite the appropriate number of chromosomes, the lack of biparental contribution of the genome, and specifically the lack of maternally imprinted chromosomes, leads to the production of hydropic villa and lack of fetal development. These findings are analogous to the classic murine studies in which androgenically produced mice—those created by duplication of the paternal genome without maternal chromosomal contribution—fail to form an organized fetus.[130]

The recurrence of GTD, whether hydatidiform mole, invasive mole, or choriocarcinoma, appears to be increased over the general population. Both recurrent complete moles and partial moles have been reported.[48, 50] The risk of recurrence has been estimated at 1.3%, although possible bias favoring repetitive cases may exist.[107] Additional studies have shown a recurrence of 28% after two pregnancies complicated by a gestational trophoblast neoplasm.[121] More than one family member has been reported with GTD though the significance of these family aggregates has not been studied in a consistent fashion.[68]

Preconception counseling

Gynecologists are often provided with an ideal opportunity to undertake preconception counseling with their patients. While many women seek birth control, this is often temporary with a pregnancy planned in the future. Additionally some women may currently be attempting a pregnancy or undergoing infertility evaluations. All of these settings provide an opportunity to review both the woman's and her partner's family, medical, and social histories to determine if genetic preconception counseling is needed. Whether counseling is undertaken by the gynecologist or assisted by referral to a geneticist or genetic counselor, the ability to identify the woman at risk is essential. For the specific techniques and risks of prenatal diagnostic testing, the reader is referred to several comprehensive reviews.[15, 27, 82]

Risk of chromosomal disorders. The association of advanced maternal age with chromosomal abnormalities has long been recognized. While a risk for a chromosomally abnormal infant exists at all ages, at maternal age 35 the risk of trisomy 21 at midtrimester is 1 in 260, approximately equal to the 1 in 200 to 400 risk of pregnancy loss after a midtrimester amniocentesis. If all chromosomal disorders are considered, at maternal age 32 years, the risk for a chromosomally unbalanced fetus is 1 in 280. Multiple gestations per se are not associated with an increased risk of chromosome abnormalities. However, with dizygotic twins, the woman faces the risk of two infants with trisomy 21 so that mathematically the chance either twin will have trisomy 21 (or rarely both) is 1 in 270 at a maternal age of 32 years.[101]

In some situations women will be at an increased risk for a chromosome abnormality because of their past obstetric history. For women with a prior liveborn with a nondisjunctional event, or if a parental balanced translocation has been identified, an increased risk for a chromosomally abnormal offspring exists. In other situations, controversy remains about whether a woman is at increased risk for an aneuploid infant. A history of two prior miscarriages even with normal parental karyotypes, a history of a triploid fetus, a history of a prior macerated stillbirth without karyotype obtained, and a history of a chromosomally abnormal spontaneous abortion each have been associated with a greater than general population risk for an aneuploid fetus in a subsequent pregnancy. Studies supporting as well as refuting the increased risk in these situations are discussed elsewhere in this chapter.

For women under the age of 35, maternal serum analysis of α-fetoprotein (AFP), β-human chorionic gonadotropin (β-hCG), and estriol (UE3) provides a screening method for identifying women with an increased risk of an infant with trisomy 21. Prospective studies of maternal serum screening have shown that approximately 60% of trisomy 21 cases in younger women can be found among those with positive triple panel screens (Table 20-9). By comparison, amniocentesis of women 35 or older at delivery will detect only 20% of Down's syndrome infants. Application of the serum screening programs to women over the age of 35 theoretically should be possible. Careful counseling is essential, however, as the maternal serum screen does not detect all cases of Down's syndrome. In an estimated 20% of Down's syndrome cases born to women over 35, the serum screen will be normal.[144] In addition, other chromosomal abnormalities are also associated with an increase in maternal age, and their detection by the serum panel is less well defined. Currently only analysis of the fetal chromosomes either by CVS or amniocentesis will provide complete detection of all chromosome abnormalities to women aged 35 years or older at delivery.

Women at risk for Mendelian disorders. With regard to X-linked recessive disorders, the gynecologist should be familiar with the more common disorders inherited in this fashion, such as Duchenne and Becker muscular dystrophy and the hemophilias. Though a close relative such as a brother or uncle may have been affected, often a woman does not realize she is at risk because this information may have been inadequately conveyed or understood. In addition, given the rapid advances in genetic testing with DNA analysis, carrier

Table 20-9. Prospective studies of maternal serum triple panels for trisomy 21 (Down's syndrome)

Author	N	Initial positive screen	Positive after ultrasonography†	% of trisomy 21 detected	PPV*
Haddow[42]	25,207	6.6%	3.8%	58%	2.6%
Wald[143]	11,993	4.9%	3.3%	39%	1.7%
Phillips[93]	9,993	7.0%	3.2%	57%	1.9%

*PPV=Positive predictive value at amniocentesis. †Confirmation of gestational age.

testing may have employed older technologies; tests should be repeated. Additionally, while direct DNA studies are available for some X-linked disorders, in many situations linkage with RFLPs may need to be performed. Especially when analyzing multiple family members, initiation of such carrier testing before a pregnancy is advantageous.

For autosomal recessive diseases, only in rare situations is an abnormal gene known to be segregating in a family as evidenced by a prior homozygotic affected child. The overwhelming majority of children with autosomal recessive disorders are born to couples in which neither is known to be a carrier, no family history of a similarly affected child exists, and there is no evidence of consanguinity in the family. To this end, it is reasonable to screen persons for autosomal recessive alleles known from population studies to have increased prevalence in their specific ethnic or racial population. Currently populations at risk for sickle cell, thalassemia, and Tay Sachs disease are offered screening as their carrier frequencies are on the order of 1:10 to 1:30 persons (Table 20-10). With a carrier frequency of 1:10, the chance of two random individuals being carriers is small (1:10 x 1:10 = 1:100) but possible.

With regard to cystic fibrosis screening, the less than 100% detection of mutations leading to cystic fibrosis has played a limiting role in efforts to offer population screening to Caucasians. Unless all mutations producing the cystic fibrosis disease are identified, couples in which one individual carries a mutation and the other has a negative mutation panel, continue to face a risk, although reduced, of an offspring with cystic fibrosis. In these situations, further prenatal diagnosis would not be able to distinguish carrier from affected fetuses. Currently until a greater number of the mutations can be detected, the position of the American Society of Human Genetics is to offer cystic fibrosis screening only to individuals with a family history.[8] As genetic technology advances, it may soon be feasible to offer cystic fibrosis screening to all Caucasians of northern European ancestry.

For many autosomal dominant disorders, disease manifestation often occurs later in life. For this reason, a careful family history is needed to ascertain individuals who may be carrying a dominant mutation and as yet are unaffected. Such individuals may benefit for two reasons: (1) the disease itself may pose additional risk during pregnancy, and (2) a 50% risk of an affected offspring exists. Family studies with linked markers may be available, or in an increasing number of cases, direct DNA diagnoses can be offered. Dominant disorders that may be encountered by the gynecologist include Marfan syndrome, myotonic dystrophy, Huntington's disease, and adult onset polycystic kidney disease.

Women at risk for multifactorial diseases. In general, if a couple has experienced one child with a multifactorial birth defect, or if the parents themselves are affected, the

Table 20-10. Diseases with increased prevalence in specific populations

Disease	Population at increased risk	Carrier test
Tay-Sachs	Ashkenazic Jewish French Canadians	Serum hexosaminidase A
Sickle Cell	Black African Mediterranean (Greek, Italian) Arabic, Indian, Pakistani Caribbean (Cuban, Puerto Rican, Haitian) Hispanic, Central American	Sickle dex for hemoglobin S Hemoglobin electrophoresis for variants
Thalassemia	Mediterranean (Greek, Italian) Southeast Asian (Vietnamese, Laotian, Cambodian, Filipino) Southern Chinese North African Pakistani, Indian	Hematocrit and MCV
Cystic Fibrosis	Caucasian-Northern European ancestry	DNA analysis

chances a subsequent offspring will be similarly affected is approximately 3%. This risk estimate can be refined, however, for specific conditions based on further knowledge of the defect. (Table 20-11)

Neural tube defects (NTD). While the majority of NTDs are presumed to be multifactorial in nature with an associated 3% recurrence, a small portion are seen in conjunction with a chromosomal etiology. Attempts should be made to obtain the karyotype and autopsy results on previously affected infants.

A recent randomized, double-blinded study has demonstrated maternal folic acid supplementation can lower the recurrence risk for neural tube defects in women with a previously affected infant. Initiated preconceptionally, ingestion of 4 mg of folic acid per day decreased the chances for recurrence by 72%.[84] Multivitamins with a lower dose of folic acid (0.36 mg/day) similarly were found to be effective in reducing the risk of NTDs in women with and without a history of a previously affected infant.[83] Expansion of folic acid supplementation, on the order of 0.4 to 1 mg per day for all pregnant women has been proposed.[83] Given the early gestational timing of neural tube development, folic acid supplementation needs to be initiated preconceptionally. Presently, long term ingestion of folic acid at either the 1 or 4 mg per day levels has not been fully evaluated. However, with the exception of women with unrecognized B_{12} deficiency, supplementation is not thought to be associated with maternal side effects.[83] Preconceptional prophylaxis for the woman with a prior NTD child should include folic acid supplementation. Also, the availability of ultrasonography and amniocentesis for detection of an affected offspring in a subsequent pregnancy should be discussed.

Women at risk for teratogen exposure

Maternal diseases. Women contemplating pregnancy who have an ongoing medical illness can face an increased risk for a child with a congenital anomaly either because of the disease process or secondary to teratogenic effects of medications needed for the disease state.

Insulin dependent diabetes (IDDM) is one disorder in which a teratogenic risk is associated with the disease process itself. A twofold to threefold increase in congenital malformations among the children of women with IDDM has been noted since the mid 1960s. Subsequently, several investigators have shown that poorly controlled IDDM patients, as reflected by increased hemoglobin A_{1C} levels, have the highest rates of malformations (Table 20-12).[36,155] However, a recent large multicenter study was unable to document an association between the incidence of congenital malformations and hemoglobin A_{1C} possibly because of the paucity of patients who were poorly controlled. The mechanism of teratogenicity in poorly controlled IDDM patients remains unclear. Insulin is not considered to be teratogenic and hyperglycemia alone does not appear to be the sole mechanism. Interactions with other metabolites have been postulated.[104, 105] While a range of anomalies can be seen, specific malformations such as caudal regression, situs inversus, and NTDs are increased 30- to 200-fold.[67] Because these anomalies would require a teratogenic insult by 6 weeks postovulation, attempts to lower the rate of malformations have centered on preconception tightening of glycemic

Table 20-11. Recurrence risks in cardiac anomalies

Anomaly	Normal parents and one affected offspring (%)	Affected parent and no previously affected offspring: Affected mother (%)	Affected parent and no previously affected offspring: Affected father (%)
Ventricular septal defect	4.4	9.5	2.1
Patent ductus arteriosus	3.4	4.1	2.3
Tetralology of Fallot	2.7	2.6	1.4
Atrial septal defect	3.2	4.6	1.5
Pulmonic stenosis	2.9	6.5	1.8
Aortic stenosis, valvular	2.2	17.9	2.8
Aortic coarction	1.8	4.1	1.9
Transposition of the great vessels	1.9		
Atrioventricular canal anomaly (endocardial cushion defect)	2.6		
Tricuspid valve	1.0		
Tricuspid valve, Ebstein anomaly	1.1		
Truncus arteriosus	1.2		
Pulmonic atresia	1.3		
Endocardial fibroelastosis	3.8		

Nora JJ: Etiologic factors in congenital heart disease, *Pediatr Clin North Am* 18:1059, 1971; and Nora JJ, Nora AH: *Genetics and counseling in cardiovascular diseases*, Springfield, 1978, Charles C Thomas. Recurrence risk is applied to offspring in this tabulation.
From Simpson JL, Golbus MS: *Genetics in obstetrics and gynecology*, ed 2, Philadelphia, 1992, WB Saunders, p 83.

control. Multiple investigators have now shown that preconception counseling and glycemic control can result in a lower rate of malformations (0.8% to 1.6%).[38]

Exposure to medications with proposed or proven teratogenic effects can sometimes be avoided by patient education and change of medications if a pregnancy is contemplated. Phenytoin (hydantoin) is a recognized teratogen associated with a twofold increase in major and minor malformations, specifically developmental delay, skeletal anomalies, cardiac defects, and cleft lip and/or palate. Other anticonvulsants have teratogenic effects also. Valproic acid has been associated with a characteristic facial dysmorphia, cardiovascular anomalies, and neural tube defects. Carbamazepine recently has been associated with facial dysmorphia and neural tube defects.[57,102] A common pathway for the association of birth defects with many of the anticonvulsants may be their involvement in the epoxide pathway. Epoxide itself rather than the specific anticonvulsant may be the teratogenic agent. In one study infants with deficiencies of the epoxide hydrolase enzyme, who were taking anticonvulsants also were shown to have the highest rate of fetal hydantoin syndrome. Infants with normal epoxide hydralase activity exposed to anticonvulsants did not manifest malformations.[6] Changes or discontinuations of anticonvulsants are best attempted prior to a pregnancy; discontinuation should be considered if feasible. If discontinuation is not feasible, a change to an agent with a lesser rate of congenital malformations may be possible.

Other disorders in which commonly used medications carry a teratogenic potential are indicated in Table 20-13. While the majority of teratogenic medications are often revealed during a routine history of illness, others such as isotretinoin, an acne medication with known teratogenic potential, may require more specific questioning. Discontinuing or altering potentially teratogenic medications may

Table 20-12. Major malformations in IDDM offspring according to HB A_{1c}

HB A_{1c}	Major malformation	Nonmalformed	%
< 7.9	2	61	3.1
8.0 - 9.9	5	57	8.1
> 10.0	4	13	23.5
TOTAL	11	131	7.7

Ylinen KE: Risk of minor and major fetal malformations in diabetics with high hemoglobin A_{1c} values in early pregnancy, *Br Med J* 289:345-346, 1984.

Table 20-13. Chemical teratogens

Definite relationship to fetal abnormalities
Alcohol
Diphenylhydantoin
Folic acid antagonists
Inorganic iodides
Lithium
Organic mercury
Retinoic acid and related compounds
Sex steroids (virilization of male fetuses)
Streptomycin
Tetracyclines
Thalidomide
Thiourea compounds
Trimethadione
Valproic acid
Warfarin

Probable relationship to fetal abnormalities
Alkylating agents
Carbamazepine
Chlorobiphenyls
Aminoglycosides (kanamycin, gentamycin, neomycin)
Methimazole

Possible relationship to fetal abnormalities (unproven claims)
Amphetamines
Chlordiazepoxide
Cigarette smoking
Clomiphene
Diazepam
Diphenydramine
Ethionamide
General anesthesia (chronic exposure)
Meprobamate
Metronidazole
Oral hypoglycemic agents
Penicillamine
Phenothiazines
Quinine

No relationship to fetal abnormalities (proven safety)
Bendectin
Corticosteroids
General anesthesia (short time exposure)
Heparin
Isoniazid
Meclizine
Penicillin
Phenobarbitol
Sulfonamides
Sex steroids (nongenital anomalies)

Simpson JL, Globus MS: *Genetics in obstetrics and gynecology*, ed 2, Philadelphia, 1992, WB Saunders, p 260.

be appropriate if a pregnancy is planned. In other situations, specific attention to the continued use of a reliable method of birth control is needed for the duration of medication exposure.

Recreational exposures. In conjunction with current medication use, recreational drug abuse may also place a woman at increased risk for congenital anomalies. A specific dysmorphology, congenital defects, and growth and developmental delay are now being appreciated with the use of cocaine. One theorized mechanism involves the impact on embryonic structures of interrupted vascular supply. Chasnoff first noted congenital anomalies in cocaine-exposed infants in 1985, and while an association remains controversial, genitourinary, cardiovascular, and central nervous system anomalies appear more frequent.[12, 71]

Maternal ingestion of alcohol represents the most frequent teratogen to which fetuses are exposed. Fetal alcohol syndrome (FAS) was initially estimated to occur in 1 in 250 to 1 in 500 livebirths.[123] Recently in the western world FAS rates have been estimated at 1 in 3000 livebirths.[1] An estimated 10% to 20% of mental deficiency in the 50 to 80 IQ range has been attributed to fetal alcohol exposure.[89] Fetal alcohol syndrome is characterized by prenatal and postnatal growth deficiency, developmental delay/mental retardation, microcephaly, facial dysmorphia, and minor skeletal malformations (Fig 20-32).[56] An overall relationship between the quantity of alcohol consumed and the appearance of FAS has emerged. With two drinks a day, lowered birth weight is apparent. With 4 to 6 drinks (5 oz absolute alcohol) a day, other clinical features can be detected, and with 8 to 10 drinks a day, 30% to 50% of the exposed offspring will display some manifestation of FAS, usually mental retardation.[56] Despite recommendations from the Surgeon General in 1981 that the safest approach to alcohol during pregnancy was abstinence, the National Natality Survey from 1985 demonstrated 39% of women continued to consume alcohol during pregnancy.[98] Heavy alcohol consumption during pregnancy has a prevalence of 6% to 11%.[124] At preconception evaluations, identification of women with evidence of alcohol abuse should be sought. The majority of these women remain undetected and screening with a brief questionnaire to identify such women may be appropriate.[125]

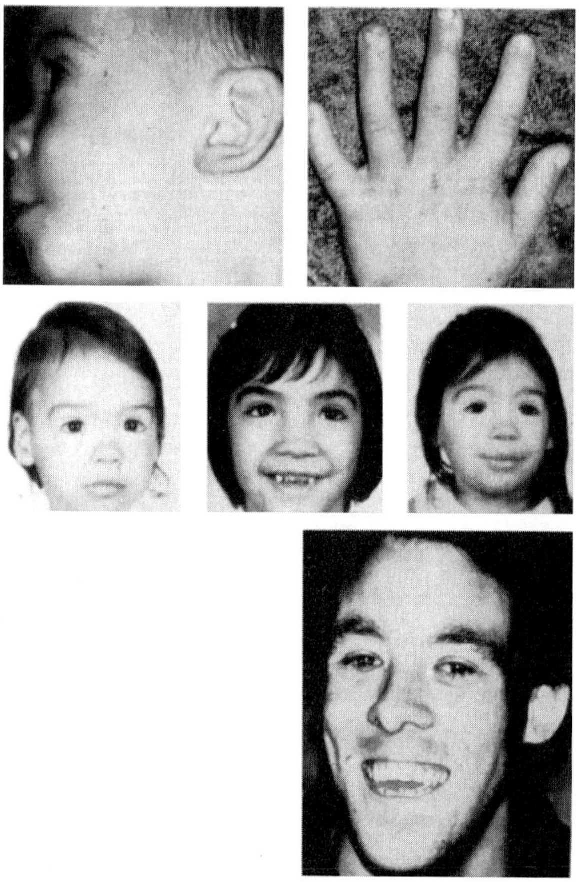

Fig. 20-32. Fetal alcohol effects. Change in the faces in the same child from 18 months to 2 and 1/2 years to 7 years of age. (From Jones KL: Smith's Recognizable Pattern of Malformation, ed 4, Philadelphia, 1988, WB Saunders, p 493.)

REFERENCES

1. Abel EL, Sokol RJ: A revised conservative estimate of the incidence of FAS and its economic impact, *Alcohol Clin Exp Res 15:514, 1991.*
2. Alberman ED et al: Previous reproductive histories in mothers presenting with spontaneous abortions, *Br J Obstet Gynaecol* 82:366, 1975.

2a. Alberman ED: The abortus as a predictor of future trisomy 21. In De la Cruz F, Gerald P, editors: *Trisomy 21 (Down Syndrome)*, Baltimore, 1981, University Park Press.

3. Bell M et al: Physical mapping across the fragile X: hypermethylation and clinical expression of the fragile X syndrome, *Cell* 64:861-866, 1991.
4. Bové A, Gallano P: A collaborative study of the segregation of inherited chromosome structural rearrangements in 1356 prenatal diagnoses, *Prenat Diagn* 4:45, 1984.
5. Boué J et al. Phenotypic expression of lethal chromosomal anomalies in human abortuses, *Teratology* 14:3, 1976.
6. Buehler BA et al: Prenatal prediction of risk of the fetal hydantoin syndrome, *N Engl J Med* 322:1567, 1990.
7. Carson SA et al. Heritable aspects of uterine anomalies II. Genetic analysis of mullerian aplasia, *Fertil Steril* 40:86, 1983.
8. Caskey CT et al: The American Society of Human Genetics on cystic fibrosis screening, *Am J Hum Genet* 46:393, 1990.
9. Cattanach B, Kirk M: Differential activity of maternally and paternally derived chromosome regions in mice, *Nature* 315:496-498, 1985.
10. Chandley AC: The origin of chromosome aberrations in man and their potential for survival and reproduction in the adult human population, *Ann Genet* 24:55, 1981.
11. Chang JC, Kan YW: A sensitive new prenatal test for sickle cell anemia, *N Engl J Med* 307:30, 1982.
12. Chasnoff IJ et al: Cocaine use in pregnancy, *N Engl J Med* 313:666, 1985.
13. Chemke J et al: Familial XY gonadal dysgenesis, *J Med Genet* 7:105, 1970.
14. Cornet D et al. Pregnancies following ovum donation in gonadal dysgenesis, *Hum Reprod* 5:291, 1990.
15. D'Alton ME, DeCherney AH: Prenatal diagnosis, *N Engl J Med* 328:114, 1993.
16. Daniel A, Hook EB, Wulf G: Risks of unbalanced progeny at amniocentesis to carriers of chromosome rearrangements: data from United States and Canadian Laboratories, *Am J Med Genet* 31:14, 1989.

17. De Braekeleer M, Dao T-N: Cytogenetic studies in couples experiencing repeated pregnancy losses, *Hum Reprod* 5:519, 1990.
18. de la Chapelle A: The complicated issue of human sex differentiation, *Am J Hum Genet* 43:1, 1988.
19. Dewhurst J: Fertility in 47,XXX and 45,X patients, *J Med Genet* 15:132, 1978.
20. Dilella AG, Huang WM, Woo SL: Screening for phenylketonuria mutations by DNA amplification with the polymerase chain reaction, *Lancet* 5:497, 1988.
21. Drugan A et al: Prenatal genetic diagnosis following recurrent early pregnancy loss, *Obstet Gynecol* 75:381, 1990.
22. Dutrillaux B, Couturier J: Chromosome imbalances in endometrial adenocarcinomas: a possible adaptation to abnormal metabolic pathways, *Ann Genet* 29:76, 1986.
23. Dutrillaux B, Prieur M, Aurias A: Theoretical study of inversions affecting human chromosomes, *Ann Genet* 29:184, 1986.
24. Engel E: A new genetic concept: uniparental disomy and its potential effect, isodisomy, *Am J Med Genet* 6:137-43, 1980.
25. Engel E, DeLozier-Blanchet D: Uniparental disomy, isodisomy, and imprinting: probable effects in man and strategies for their detection, *Am J Med Genet* 40:432-439, 1991.
26. Espiner EA et al: Familial syndrome of streak gonads and normal male karyotype in five phenotypic females, *N Engl J Med* 283:6, 1970.
27. Evans MI, Drugan A, Koppitch FC: Genetic diagnosis in the first trimester: the norm for the 1990s, *Am J Obstet Gynecol* 160:1332, 1989.
28. Fialkow PJ: Use of genetic markers to study cellular origins and development of tumors in human females, *Cancer Treat Rev* 15:191, 1972.
29. Filmus JE, Buick RN: Stability of C-K-ras amplification during progression in a patient with adenocarcinoma of the ovary, *Cancer Res* 45:4486, 1985.
30. Fisher EMC et al: Homologous ribosomal protein genes on the human X and Y chromosomes: escape from X inactivation and implications for Turner syndrome, *Cell* 63:1205, 1990.
31. Franceschi S, La Vecchia C, Mangioni C: Familial ovarian cancer: eight more families, *Gynecol Oncol* 13:31, 1982.
32. Friedman JM et al: *Genetics*, Baltimore, 1992, Williams and Wilkins.
33. Gardner GH, Greene RR, Ranney B: The histogenesis of endometriosis, *Obstet Gynecol* 1:615, 1953.
34. Gartler SM et al: Evidence of two functional X chromosomes in human oocytes, *Cell Differ* 1:215, 1972.
35. Gelehrter TD, Collins FS: *Principles of medical genetics*, Baltimore, 1990, Williams and Wilkins.
36. Greene MF et al: First-trimester hemoglobin A_1 and risk for major malformation and spontaneous abortion in diabetic pregnancy, *Teratology* 39:225-231, 1989.
37. Gregory R et al: Maternal serum alpha-fetoprotein levels in diabetic pregnancies, *Lancet* 2:345-346, 1988.
38. Gregory R, Tattersall RB: Are diabetic pre-pregnancy clinics worth while? *Lancet* 340(8820):656, 1992.
39. Grumbach MM, Ducharme JR, Moloshok RE: On the fetal masculinizing action of certain oral progestins, *J Clin Endocrinol Metab* 19:1369, 1959.
40. Guy K et al: Recurrent mutation of immunoglobulin and c-myc genes and differential expression of cell surface antigens occur in variant cell lines derived from a Burkitt lymphoma, *Int J Cancer* 45:109, 1990.
41. Guyot B et al: Prenatal diagnosis with biotinylated chromosome specific probes, *Prenat Diagn* 7:485, 1988.
42. Haddow JE et al: Prenatal screening for Down's syndrome with use of maternal serum markers, *N Engl J Med* 327(9):588, 1992.
43. Hall J: Genomic imprinting and its clinical implications, *N Engl J Med* 326:827-829, 1992.
44. Harrison KB: X-chromosome inactivation in the human cytotrophoblast, *Cytogenet Cell Genet* 52:37, 1989.
45. Hassold TJ: A cytogenetic study of repeated abortions, *Am J Hum Genet* 32:723, 1980.
46. Henry I et al: Uniparental disomy in a genetic cancer-predisposing syndrome, *Nature* 351:665-667, 1991.
47. Hertig AT, Rock J: Searching for early human ova, *Gynecol Obstet Invest* 4:121, 1973.
48. Honore' LH: Recurrent partial hydatidiform mole: report of a case, *Am J Obstet Gynecol* 156:922, 1987.
49. Honore' LH, Dill FJ, Poland BJ: Placental morphology in spontaneous human abortuses with normal and abnormal karyotypes, *Teratology* 14:151, 1976.
50. Honore' LH, Lin EC, Morrish DW: Recurrent partial mole, *Am J Obstet Gynecol* 158:442, 1988.
51. Hook EB, Cross PK, Schreinemachers DM: Chromosome abnormality rates at amniocentesis and in liveborn infants, *JAMA* 249:2043, 1983.
52. Jacobs PA et al: Aggressive behavior, mental subnormality, and XYY male, *Nature* 208:1351, 1965.
53. Jeffreys AJ: DNA sequence variants in the y,ó, and ß globin genes of man, *Cell* 18:1, 1979.
54. Jeffreys JA: DNA sequence variation in the G gamma, A gamma, delta and beta globin genes of man, *Cell* 18:131, 1979.
55. Jeffreys AJ, Wilson V, Thein SL: Hypervariable minisatellite regions in human DNA, *Nature* 314:67, 1985.
56. Jones KL: *Smith's recognizable pattern of malformation*, ed 4, Philadelphia, 1988, WB Saunders.
57. Jones KL et al: Patterns of malformations in the children of women treated with carbamazepine during pregnancy, *N Engl J Med 320:1661, 1989.*
58. Kajii T, Nikawa N: Origin of triploidy and tetraploidy in man: cases with chromosome markers, *Cytogenet Cell Genet* 18:109, 1977.
59. Kajii T et al: Banding analysis of abnormal karyotypes of spontaneous abortions, *Am J Hum Genet* 25:539, 1973.
60. Kan YW, Dozy AM: Antenatal diagnosis of sickle cell anemia by DNA analysis of amniotic fluid cells, *Lancet* 2:910, 1978.
61. Kan YW, Dozy AM: Antenatal diagnosis of sickle cell anemia by DNA analysis of amniotic fluid cell, *Am J Hum Genet* 25:539, 1973.
62. Kazazian HH Jr, Boehm CD: Molecular basis and prenatal diagnosis of beta-thalassemia, *Blood* 72:1107, 1988.
63. Kerem B-S et al: Identification of the cystic fibrosis gene: genetic analysis, *Science* 245:1073, 1989.
64. Knoll J et al: Angleman and Prader-Willi syndromes share a common chromosome 15 deletion but differ in parental origin of the deletion, *Am J Med Genet* 32:285-90, 1989.
65. Knudson AG, Strong LC, Anderson DE: Heredity and cancer in man, *Prog Med Genet* 9:113, 1973.
66. Kremer E et al: Mapping of DNA instability at the fragile X to a trinucleotide repeat sequence p(CGG)n, *Science* 252:1711-1714, 1991.
67. Kucera J: Rate and type of congenital anomalies among offspring of diabetic women, *J Repro Med* 7:61-70, 1971.
68. LeVecchia C et al: Gestational trophoblastic neoplasms in monozygous twins, *Obstet Gynecol* 60:250, 1982.
69. Levine LS, Pang S: Prenatal diagnosis and treatment of congenital adrenal hyperplasia. In Milunsky A, editor: *The fetus*, Baltimore, 1993, John Hopkins University Press.
70. Linder D, McGaw BR, Hecht F: Parthenogenic origin of benign ovarian teratomas, *N Engl J Med* 292:63, 1975.
71. Little BB, Snell LM: Cocaine use during pregnancy and congenital anomalies: further study, *Am J Obstet Gynecol* 164:350, 1991b.
72. Little M, Van Heyningen V, Hastie N: Dads and disomy and disease, *Nature* 351:609-610, 1991.

73. Lundgren PO: Hereditary myopathy, oligoophrenia, cataract, skeletal abnormalites and hypergonadotrophic hypogonadism: a new syndrome, *Eur Neurol* 10:261, 1976.
74. Lynch HT et al: Hereditary ovarian cancer clinical and biomarker studies. In Lynch HT, Kullander S, editors: *Cancer genetics in women*, Boca Raton, 1987, CRC Press.
75. Lyon MF: Sex chromatin and gene action in the mammelian X-chromosome, *Am J Human Genet* 14:135, 1962.
76. Magenis R et al: Comparison of the 15q deletions in Prader-Willi and Angelman syndromes: specific regions, extent of deletions, parental origin, and clinical consequences, *Am J Med Genet* 35:333-49, 1990.
77. Malcolm S et al: Uniparental disomy in Angleman's syndrome, *Lancet* 337:694-697, 1991.
78. Malinak LR et al: Heritable aspects of endometriosis II. Clinical characteristics of familial endometriosis, *Am J Obstet Gynecol* 137:332, 1980.
79. Mascari M et al: The frequency of uniparental disomy in Prader-Willi syndrome, *N Eng J Med* 326:1599, 1992.
80. Maximilian C, Ionescu B, Bucur A: Deux soeurs avec dysgenesie gonadique majeure, hypotrophic staturale, microcephalie, arachnodactylie et carotype 46,XX, *J Genet Hum* 18:365, 1970.
81. McFadden DE, Kalousek DK: Two different phenotypes of fetuses with chromosomal triploidy: correlation with parental origin of the extra haploid set, *Am J Med Genet* 38:535, 1991.
82. Milunsky A: *Genetic disorders and the fetus*, ed 3, New York, 1993, Plenum Press.
83. Milunsky A et al: Multivitamin/folic acid supplementation in the earliest weeks of pregnancy reduces the prevalence of neural tube defects, *JAMA* 262:2847, 1989.
84. MRC Vitamin Study Research Group: prevention of neural tube defects: results of the Medical Research Council Vitamin Study, *Lancet* 228:131, 1991.
85. Myerowitz R: Splice junction mutation in some Ashkenazi Jews with Tay-Sachs disease: evidence against a single defect within this ethnic group, *Proc Natl Acad Sci USA* 85:3955, 1988.
86. Nicholls R et al: Genetic imprinting suggested by maternal heterodisomy in nondeletion Prader-Willi syndrome, *Nature* 342:281-285, 1989.
87. Nishi Y et al: The Perrault syndrome: clinical report and review, *Am J Med Genet* 31:623, 1988.
88. Oberle I et al: Instability of a 550-base pair DNA segment and abnormal methylation in fragile X syndrome, *Science* 252:1097, 1991.
89. Olegaard R et al: Effects on the child of alcohol abuse during pregnancy, *Acta Paediat Scand* 275:112, 1979.
90. Patsavoudi E et al: Dissociation between testicular morphogenesis and functional differentiation of Leydig cells, *J Endocrinol* 105:235, 1985.
91. Perez-Ballester B, Greenblatt RB, Byrd JR: Familial gonadal dysgenesis, *Am J Obstet Gynecol* 15:1262, 1970.
92. Peterson RE et al: Male pseudohermaphroditism due to steroid 5-a-reductase deficiency, *Am J Med Genet* 62:170, 1977.
93. Phillips OP et al: Maternal serum screening for fetal Down's syndrome in women less than 35 years of age using alpha-fetoprotein, hCG, and unconjugated estriol: a prospective 2-year study, *Obstet Gynecol* 353, 1992.
94. Pinkel D et al: Fluorescence in situ hybridization with human chromosome specific libraries: detection of trisomy 21 with translocations of chromosome 4, *Proc Natl Acad Sci USA* 85:9138, 1988.
95. Pinsky L, Kaufman M: Genetics of steroid receptors and their disorders, *Adv Hum Genet* 16:299, 1985.
96. Pinsky L, Kaufman M, Killinger DW: Impaired spermatogenesis is not an obligate expression of receptor defective androgen resistance, *Am J Hum Genet* 32:100, 1989.
97. Plachot M et al: Chromosome investigations in early life: human preimplantation embryos, *Hum Reprod* 2:29, 1987.
98. Prager K et al: Smoking and drinking behavior before and during pregnancy of married mothers of liveborn infants and stillborn infants, *Public Health Rep* 99:117, 1985.
99. Purvis-Smith S et al: Uniparental disomy 15 resulting from "correction of an initial trisomy 15", *Am J Hum Genet* 50:1348, 1992.
100. Robinson A, Lubs HA, Bergsma D: Sex chromosome aneuploidy: prospective studies on children, *Birth Defects* 15(1):1, 1979.
101. Rodis JF et al: Calculated risk of chromosomal abnormalities in twin gestations, *Obstet Gynecol* 76:1037, 1990.
102. Rosa FW: Spina bifida in infants of women treated with carbamazepine during pregnancy, *N Engl J Med* 324:674, 1991.
103. Rousseau F et al: Direct diagnosis by DNA analysis of the fragile X syndrome of mental retardation, *New Eng J Med* 24:1673-1681, 1991.
104. Sadler TW: Effects of maternal diabetes on early embryogenesis I. the teratogenic potential of diabetic serum, *Teratology* 21(3):339, 1980.
105. Sadler TW, Horton WE Jr: Effects of maternal diabetes on early embryogenesis: the role of insulin and insulin therapy, *Diabetes* 32(11):1070, 1983.
106. Saiki RK et al: Enzymatic amplification of beta globin genomic sequences and restriction site analysis for diagnosis of sickle cell anemia, *Science* 230:1350, 1985.
107. Sand PK, Lurain JR, Brewer JI: Repeat gestational trophoblastic disease, *Obstet Gynecol* 63:140, 1984.
108. Sapienza C: Genome imprinting and dominence modification, *Ann NY Acad Sci* 564:24-38, 1989.
109. Savard P et al: Important role of the long terminal repeat of the helper Moloney murine leukemia virus in Abelson virus-induced lymphoma, *J Virol* 61:3266, 1987.
110. Schad C et al: Use of fluorescent in situ hybridization for marker chromosome identification in congenital and neoplastic disease, *Am J Clin Pathol* 96:203, 1991.
111. Schwartz S, Palmer C: Chromosomal findings in 164 couples with repeated spontaneous abortions: with special consideration to prior reproductive history, *Hum Genet* 62:28, 1983.
112. Searle G et al: Chromosome maps of man and mouse IV, *Ann Hum Genet* 53:89-140, 1989.
113. Sherman S et al: Further segregation analysis of the fragile X syndrome with special reference to transmitting males, *Hum Genet* 69:289-299, 1985.
114. Sherman S et al: The marker (X) chromosome: a cytogenetic and genetic analysis, *Ann Hum Genet* 48:21-37,1984.
115. Sherman SL et al: Trisomy 21: association between reduced recombination and nondisjunction, *Am J Hum Genet* 43:A97, 1990.
116. Simon A et al: Familial occurrence of mature ovarian teratomas, *Obstet Gynecol* 66:278, 1985.
117. Simpson JL: *Disorders of sexual differentiation: etiology and clinical delineation*, New York, 1976, Academic Press.
118. Simpson JL: Genetic control of sexual development. In Teoh ES, Ratnam SS, Goh VHH, editors: *Advances in fertility and sterility: releasing hormones and genetics and immunology in human reproduction, vol 3*, Lancaster, UK, 1987, Parthenon.
119. Simpson JL: Maternal serum screening for fetal Down's syndrome in women less than 35 years of age using alpha-fetoprotein, hCG, and unconjugated estriol: a prospective 2-year study, *Obstet Gynecol* 353, 1992.
120. Simpson JL: Genetic control of sexual development. In Teoh ES, Ratnam SS, Goh VHH, editors: *Advances in Fertility and Sterility: Releasing Hormones and Genetics and Immunology in Human Reproduction* (Vol 3), Pathenon, Lancester, UK 1987b, p 165.
121. Simpson JL, Golbus MS: *Genetics in obstetrics and gynecology*, ed 2, Philadelphia, 1992, WB Saunders.
122. Skre H et al: Cerebellar ataxia and hypergonadism in the two kindreds: chance occurrence, pleiotropism or linkage? *Clin Genet* 9:234, 1976.
123. Smith DW: The fetal alcohol syndrome, *Hosp Pract* 297:1204, 1979.

124. Sokol RJ: Alcohol and abnormal outcomes of pregnancy, *Can Med Assoc J,* 125(2):143, 1981.
125. Sokol RJ, Miller SI: Identifying the alcohol-abusing obstetric/gynecologic patient: a practical approach, *Alcohol Health Res World* 4:36, 1980.
126. Sokol RJ, Miller SI, Debanne S, et al: The Cleveland/NIAA prospective alcohol-in-pregnancy study: the first year, *Neurobehav Toxicol Teratol* 3:203, 1981.
127. Spence J et al: Uniparental disomy as a mechanism for human genetic disease, *Am J Hum Genet* 42:217-226, 1988.
128. Stene J, Mikkelsen M: Risk for chromosomal abnormality at amniocentesis following a child with a noninherited chromosome aberration, *Prenatal Diag* 4:81, 1984.
129. Surani M: Influence of genome imprinting on gene expression, phenotypic variations and development, *Hum Repro* 6:45-51, 1991.
130. Surani MA, Barton SC, Norris ML: Development of reconstituted eggs suggests imprinting of the genome during gametogenesis, *Nature* 308(5959):548, 1984.
131. Sutherland G: Fragile sites on human chromosomes: demonstration of their dependence on the type of tissue culture medium, *Science* 197:265-266, 1977.
132. Swain J, Stewart T, Leder P: Parental legacy determines methylation expression of an automsome transgene: a molecular mechanism for parental imprint, *Cell* 50:719-727, 1987.
133. Thompson MW, McInnes RR, Willard HF: *Thompson and Thompson: genetics in medicine, ed 5,* Philadelphia, 1991, WB Saunders.
134. Toniolo D et al: Expression of the G6PD locus on the human X chromosome is associated with demethylation of three CpG islands within 100 kb of DNA, *Embo J* 7:401-406, 1988.
135. Turner G et al: Preventive screening for the fragile X syndrome, *N Engl J Med* 315:607-609, 1986.
136. Uchida IA, Freeman VC: Triploidy and chromosomes, *Am J Obstet Gynecol* 151(1):65, 1985.
137. Vidaud D et al: Father-to-son transmission of hemophilia A due to uniparental disomy, *Am J Hum Genet* 45(s):A226, 1989.
138. Vincent A et al: Abnormal pattern detected in fragile-X patients by pulsed-field gel electrophoresis, *Nature* 349:624-626, 1991.
139. Vogel F, Motulsky AG: *Human genetics problems and approaches,* ed 3, Berlin, 1986, Springer-Verlag.
140. Voss R et al: Isodisomy of chromosome 7 in a patient with cystic fibrosis: could uniparental disomy be common in humans? *Am J Hum Genet* 45:373-380, 1989.
141. Wachtel SS: *H-Y antigen and the biology of sex determination,* New York, 1983, Grune & Stratton.
142. Wake N et al: Specific cytogenetic changes in ovarian cancer involving chromosomes 6 and 14, *Cancer Res* 40:4512, 1980.
143. Wald NJ et al: Maternal serum screening for Down's syndrome in early pregnancy, *Br Med J* 297:883, 1988.
144. Wald NJ et al: Antenatal maternal serum screening for Down's syndrome: results of a demonstration project, *Br Med J* 305(6850):391, 1992.
145. Warburton D: De novo balanced chromosome rearrangements and extra marker chromosome identified at prenatal diagnosis: clinical significance and distribution of breakpoints, *Am J Hum Genet* 49:995, 1991.
146. Warburton D et al: Does the karyotype of a spontaneous abortion predict the karyotype of a subsequent abortion? *Am J Hum Genet* 41:465, 1987.
147. Webb T: The epidemiology of the fragile X syndrome. In Davies KE, editor: *The fragile X syndrome,* Oxford, England, 1989, Oxford University Press.
148. West JD et al: Sexing the human pre-embryo by DNA-DNA in situ hybridization, *Lancet* 8546:1345, 1987.
149. Wilcox AJ et al: Incidence of early pregnancy loss, *N Engl J Med* 319:189, 1988.
150. Williams C et al: Incidence of 15q deletions in the Angleman syndrome: a survey of twelve affected persons, *Am J Med Genet* 32:339-345, 1989.
151. Witkin HA et al: Criminality in XYY and XXY men, *Science* 13:547, 1976.
152. Wolff DJ, Scwhartz S: Characterization of Robertsonian translocation by using fluorescence in situ hybridization, *Am J Hum Genet* 50:174, 1992.
153. Wyman AR, White R: A highly polymorphic locus in human DNA, *Proc Natl Acad Sci USA* 77:6754, 1980.
154. Wyss D et al: Structural anomalies of the X chromosome: personal observation and review of non mosaic cases, *Clin Genet* 21:145, 1982.
155. Ylinen K et al: Risk of minor and major fetal malformations in diabetics with high haemoglobin A_{1c} values in early pregnancy, *Br Med J* 289:345-346, 1984.
156. Yunis JJ: *New Chromosomal Syndromes,* New York, 1977, Academic Press.

Chapter 21

GYNECOLOGIC INFECTIONS

Ruth Tuomala

In this chapter infectious diseases that affect the female genital tract are discussed, with emphasis on clinical diagnosis and management. The specific diseases that are presented were chosen on the basis of prevalence, the importance of sequelae, or in some cases because they are considerations in the differential diagnosis of more common entities.

PELVIC INFLAMMATORY DISEASE

Pelvic inflammatory disease (PID) affects the upper genital tract and is characterized primarily by infection of the endosalpingeal cells that line the fallopian tubes. Infection may be confined to the tubes (salpingitis) or may involve the ovaries (salpingo-oophoritis). Occasionally, either the endometrium (endometritis) or ovary (oophoritis) may be the sole focus of infection. Infection involves disruption and destruction of normal architecture on a microscopic or macroscopic level. Even apparently mild disease can lead to functional impairment. Marked inflammation resulting in the involvement of contiguous intraperitoneal structures in inflammatory processes and massive suppuration leading to tuboovarian abscess (TOA) formation can totally destroy normal architecture and function.

Pelvic inflammatory disease is a disease of sexually active, menstruating women. It is rare during pregnancy and in premenarchal, postmenopausal, and celibate women. When it occurs in these groups of women, it is often secondary and has spread from other foci of intraabdominal sepsis, such as a ruptured appendiceal abscess. The exact incidence of PID in the United States is unknown, although estimates suggest that it accounts for 400,000 outpatient visits per year for a first diagnosis of PID and 5% to 20% of all gynecologic hospital admissions.[201] In 1990 the total direct and indirect costs of diagnosing and treating PID were estimated to be $4.2 billion.[270]

Most cases of PID are thought to be caused by microorganisms that ascend from the lower genital tract through the cervix, along the endometrium to the normally sterile tubes.[53] Infection also may spread to the tubes and ovaries via the parametrium from cervical vessels and lymphatics. Pelvic inflammatory disease is a polymicrobial infection.[53] Organisms that are sexually transmitted and organisms that are part of the normal, endogenous flora of the lower genital tract are both participants in PID. Sexually transmitted organisms such as *Neisseria gonorrhoeae* and *Chlamydia trachomatis* may be the sole pathogens in cases of PID or they may be found along with other nonsexually transmitted organisms. Current estimates are that in the United States 25% to 80% of cases of PID involve the gonococcus. There is a wide range of prevalence of gonorrhea related to population variations. It has been suggested that cases of PID diagnosed in emergency rooms are likely to be those associated with higher rates of gonorrhea.[228] *C. trachomatis* is isolated in 10% to 40% of cases of PID and may be of particular importance in the adolescent population. *Mycoplasma* species are recovered from sites of pelvic infection, but their role as a major contributor in causing infection has not been demonstrated.[146]

Multiple species of aerobic and anaerobic bacteria normally found in the lower genital tract of asymptomatic women can be found at the site of upper genital tract infection both in the presence of and in the absence of sexually transmitted organisms. PID may be purely aerobic, purely anaerobic, or a mixed aerobic-anaerobic infection. In approximately two thirds of cases, anaerobes are involved. Aerobic endogenous bacteria that are associated with PID include the enterobacteriaceae, particularly *Escherichia coli*, staphylococcal species, and streptococcal species, including the enterococci. Anaerobes that are associated with PID include peptococci, peptostreptococci, anaerobic streptococci, and bacteroides species, including *B. fragilis* and *B. melaninogenicus* and *B. bivius*.

Key organisms are likely responsible for the initial invasion of the upper genital tract, and other organisms probably become involved in infection under altered conditions and structure of the upper genital tract.[53, 75] The exact microbial and host factors responsible for tissue invasion and infection are currently the subject of much ongoing research.

The exact organisms involved in a particular infection can be ascertained only by direct culture of the infected site. In PID this involves culture of tubal exudate, or tubal biopsy specimens, or of cul-de-sac fluid obtained at the time of laparoscopy or laparotomy. Cultures of the lower genital tract do not accurately reflect the organisms that are present in an upper genital tract infection. Contamination by lower genital tract flora of peritoneal fluid cultures obtained by culdocentesis render these specimens unacceptable. Although endometrial cultures also suffer from a high degree of lower genital tract contamination, particularly by low virulence pathogens, endometrial cultures specifically for *C. trachomatis* may be helpful. In addition, cervical culture for *N. gonorrhoeae* and cervical assessment for *Chlamydia* is always appropriate. The presumed microbiology of individual infections is largely an estimation based on usual organism involvement and to some extent on differential clinical presentation.

Diagnosis

The clinical diagnosis of PID is inexact. There are multiple potential symptoms and signs ascribable to PID as predicted by areas of inflammatory involvement. No symptoms or signs are pathognomonic for PID.

Reports in which all clinical diagnoses of PID are confirmed by laparoscopy suggest that in one third of cases, the clinical diagnosis of PID is in error.[104, 249] Other conditions that may be diagnosed as PID include appendicitis, ectopic pregnancy, endometriosis, adhesions, and adnexal tumors including ruptured or hemorrhagic functional ovarian cysts. In addition, 10% to 15% of cases of PID are diagnosed initially as another condition.

For the majority of cases in which PID is erroneously diagnosed, no pelvic pathologic features can be defined by laparoscopy. Without treatment for PID, symptoms in these women resolve and long-term sequelae associated with PID do not ensue. A portion of disease in this group with normal visual findings may be infection confined to the lower genital tract or endometrium, and a portion may involve disease of other organ systems.

The largest such laparoscopy series which has been conducted on an ongoing basis was reported initially by Jacobson and Westrom in Sweden in 1969,[104] and periodically was updated by Westrom and others.[277] When these investigators compared the incidence of various symptoms and signs between women with PID and women with a laparoscopically normal pelvis, very few symptoms and signs were seen more frequently in the group of women with PID (Table 21-1). Although seen in a minority of cases, multiple signs and symptoms present in one person confer the greatest accuracy of clinical diagnosis.

Traditional laboratory studies do little to improve the accuracy of a diagnosis of PID. The white blood cell (WBC) count is elevated both in women with PID and in women without the disease. The erythrocyte sedimentation rate (ESR) is often elevated in women with PID and may be helpful in judging response to therapy, but this test is nonspecific. The ESR may be elevated in a large number of women without PID. Ultrasonography and computed tomography (CT) may aid in detecting the presence of and in following the resolution of TOAs but cannot accurately differentiate abscess formation from other causes of pelvic masses.

Virtually all women who have PID have WBCs present in lower genital tract discharge. If WBCs are not present in this discharge, the diagnosis of PID is unlikely. A Gram stain of cervical discharge that is positive for intracellular gram-negative diplococci supports but does not confirm and is not necessary for a diagnosis of gonococcal PID. A positive Gram stain, however, can be helpful in determining therapy.

Normal cul-de-sac fluid contains 1500 WBCs/mm^3. The majority of cul-de-sac samples taken by culdocentesis from women with PID contains 15,000 to 30,000 WBCs/mm^3. Though rarely helpful for culture, culdocentesis can be helpful in establishing a clinical diagnosis of PID.

Diagnostic laparoscopy should be performed when the differential diagnosis of pelvic pain is between PID and a

Table 21-1. Symptoms and signs seen significantly more often in patients with pelvic inflammatory disease than in those with laparoscopically normal pelvic findings

	PID (%)	Visually normal (%)
Symptoms		
Fever and chills	41.0	20.0
Proctitis	6.9	2.7
Signs		
Adnexal tenderness	92.0	87.0
Palpable mass or swelling	49.4	24.5
Erythrocyte sedimentation rate (ESR) > 15 mm/hr	75.9	52.7
Abnormal discharge	63.2	40.2
Temperature > 38° C	32.9	14.1

From Jacobson L, Weström L: Objectivized diagnosis of acute pelvic inflammatory disease: diagnostic and prognostic value of routine laparoscopy, *Am J Obstet Gynecol* 105:1088, 1969.

surgical condition, and in cases of nonresponse or recurrent clinical disease not associated with an obvious precipitating cause. The use of laparoscopy in other cases should be individualized, although some investigators suggest that extending the use of laparoscopy to all may prove to be cost effective. Laparoscopic criteria for the diagnosis of PID are listed in Table 21-2.

Endometritis is seen in association with salpingitis in up to 70% to 85% of selected cases. In addition, women with signs and symptoms of PID without laparoscopic evidence of the disease may have endometritis.[173, 287] Endometritis is assumed to be responsible for symptomatology in these cases. The overlap in symptoms between women with laparoscopically documented PID and those with endometritis is such that differential diagnosis by any specific clinical criteria is not possible. Endometritis is strongly associated with the presence of *C. trachomatis* isolated from the cervix, from both the cervix and the endometrium, or from the endometrium alone. To a lesser extent it is associated with *N. gonorrhoeae*. A large number of women with clinically apparent cervicitis may also have endometritis found on biopsy. The majority of cases show histopathologic evidence of plasma cell endometritis, although severe endometritis including even microabscesses has been described. There is no correlation between the histopathologic severity of endometritis described and the degree of tubal damage in cases of coincidental PID. The discovery of the association between cervicitis, endometritis, and PID and the overlap in symptomatology supports the ascending theory of infection. An endometrial biopsy diagnostic of endometritis can be helpful in establishing the diagnosis of infection in women with pelvic pain in whom a diagnosis of PID is considered.

Table 21-2. Laparoscopic criteria for acute pelvic inflammatory disease

Minimum criteria
Erythema of fallopian tubes
Edema and swelling of fallopian tube
Exudate from fimbria or on serosa of fallopian tube
Scoring
Mild: minimum criteria, tubes freely movable and patent
Moderate: more marked, tubes not freely movable, patency uncertain
Severe: inflammatory mass

From Jacobson L: Differential diagnosis of acute pelvic inflammatory disease, *Am J Obstet Gynecol* 138:1006-1011, 1980.

Table 21-3. Salpingitis: clinical criteria for diagnosis

Criteria	
Abdominal direct tenderness, with or without rebound tenderness Tenderness with motion of cervix and uterus Adnexal tenderness	All three necessary for diagnosis
	Plus
Gram stain of endocervix—positive for gram-negative, intracellular diplococci Temperature (38° C) Leukocytosis (>10,000/mm^3) Purulent material (WBCs present) from peritoneal cavity by culdocentesis of laparoscopy Pelvic abscess or inflammatory complex on bimanual examination or by sonography	One or more necessary for diagnosis

Hager et al: Criteria for diagnosis and grading of salpingitis, *Obstet Gynecol* 61:114, 1983.

To establish at least minimal criteria for the diagnosis of PID and to better compare data between institutions, Hager et al proposed baseline criteria for a clinical diagnosis of PID. These criteria are listed in Table 21-3. In addition, classifying disease according to severity either by clinical or laparoscopic criteria may be useful in predicting the duration of therapy and the prognosis in regard to sequelae, and in developing comparative data bases.[227] Any grading system should emphasize sensitivity in diagnosing mild disease to minimize adverse outcome of PID.

Approximately 5% of women with PID have an associated syndrome of perihepatitis called the Fitz-Hugh-Curtis syndrome. This syndrome is an inflammatory, fibrinous perihepatitis associated with right upper quadrant pain, tenderness, and mildly deranged liver function tests. Eventual scarring results in the classic fibrous "violin string" adhesions between the dome of the liver and the diaphragm. This process is associated with both gonococcal and chlamydial PID.[45, 164] Laparoscopic assessment of women with either acute or chronic pelvic pain should include an assessment of the right upper quadrant if a diagnosis of acute or past PID is considered.

Some risk factors for the occurrence of PID have been delineated and should be considered when a history is taken from a woman who presents with pelvic pain. These risk factors include those related to sexual activity, age, and contraceptive practices. In addition, recent epidemiologic studies suggest an association between smoking and douching and the occurrence of PID.[144, 217, 286]

A history of sexual activity is necessary to seriously consider the diagnosis of PID. The risk is probably largely confined to women who are heterosexually active. Young age at first intercourse, multiple partners, a recent new sexual partner, and frequency of intercourse even within a monogamous relationship all increase risk.[131] Prior or concomitant documented sexually transmitted disease, including prior PID and gonorrhea, increase the risk of PID. Some recent studies strongly suggest that the presence of bacterial vaginosis increases risk of primary and recurrent PID.[128]

Age is an important risk factor in PID. Peak incidence of PID in the United States is in the 15- to 24-year age group. After age 25 years, and particularly after age 30 years, the incidence of PID markedly declines. It is unclear whether age-related risk is associated with sexual habits, with the development of protective antibodies at the cervical level, or with other factors.

Contraceptive practices influence the risk of PID,[51, 116, 205] although exact risks are skewed by the fact that the bulk of data is based on PID cases requiring hospitalization. Oral contraceptives and barrier methods decrease the risk of PID compared with no contraceptive method. Although use of oral contraceptives confers a greater risk of *C. trachomatis*, the risk of upper tract infection in women with lower genital tract chlamydial infection is decreased in those women who take oral contraceptives.[287] In addition, women with PID who use oral contraceptives appear to have milder disease. The presence of an intrauterine device (IUD) increases the risk of PID above that of women who use no contraception. This risk is greatest for the Dalkon shield but exists for all types of IUDs, and it does not differ appreciably among the other types. The risk of PID is the greatest immediately after IUD insertion.[55] Thereafter there is a small increase in risk of PID regardless of duration of IUD use, of socioeconomic status, and of parity. Nulliparous women may be at a greater risk of IUD-associated PID than multiparous women, and they also appear to be at greater risk of tubal factor infertility associated with the IUD. Recent studies suggest that the risk of IUD-associated PID is not as large as previously stated but instead is largely related to the baseline risks for acquisition of sexually transmitted diseases in individual IUD users.[130]

Unilateral TOA formation was formerly thought to be highly associated with IUD use. Also, it presumably occurred because of parametrial spread of infection secondary to erosion of the endometrium by the IUD. More recent studies have documented that approximately 60% of all TOAs are unilateral and that this percentage is constant regardless of whether or not an IUD is present.[77, 221]

All invasive gynecologic procedures are associated with a risk for upper genital tract infection. Such procedures include tubal lavage, hysterosalpingograms, endometrial biopsies, and dilatation and curettages (D&Cs) performed either for diagnosis or for therapeutic abortion. Such iatrogenic infections may be associated with either endogenous flora or with sexually transmitted organisms. It has been suggested that the presence of *C. trachomatis* in the cervix increases the risk of postabortal PID. It is not clear whether or not prophylactic antibiotics prevent pelvic infections associated with gynecologic procedures or if they are appropriate in these varied settings. Whether or not the widespread use of antimicrobial prophylaxis for such procedures is cost effective also remains uncertain.

The clinical presentation of PID may differ, depending on the primary pathogens involved.[250] Gonococcal PID usually presents acutely within 48 hours of onset of multiple symptoms and signs, including high fever, peritoneal signs, and purulent vaginal discharge. It often presents as an initial episode of PID. Abscess formation is less frequent with gonococcal PID, and therapeutic response is usually prompt. In contrast, chlamydial PID usually presents with moderate symptoms and follows a protracted course. Chronic, low-grade pelvic pain, irregular bleeding, subtle signs on physical examination but an elevated ESR, and severe inflammatory changes identified by laparoscopic examination with a high percentage of tubal scarring all may be features of chlamydial infection. *C. trachomatis* and *N. gonorrhoeae* often are found together in cases of PID, and many of their symptoms overlap. Therefore treatment of both organisms is standard as opposed to treatment of differential clinical features.

Nongonococcal, nonchlamydial PID is often recurrent and follows a semiacute course. Unlike PID associated with either gonorrhea or chlamydia, in which symptoms usually begin within 7 days of the menses, symptoms in other cases of PID frequently occur more than 14 days after menses. After having symptoms for 5 to 7 days, patients seek medical attention but do not look acutely ill. Fever and peritoneal signs

Table 21-4. Summary of long-term sequelae seen in 415 cases of laparoscopically documented pelvic inflammatory disease and in 100 controls with laparoscopically normal pelvic findings

Sequelae	Normal pelvis	PID
Chronic abdominal pain > 6 mo	5.0%	18.1%
Ectopic/intrauterine pregnancy	1/417	1/24
Involuntary infertility related to tubal factor	0%	17.3%

Infertility-related episodes of PID		Infertility related to severity of PID (first episode only)	
No. of episodes	**% Infertile**	**Severity of episodes**	**% Infertile**
1	12.8	Mild	2.6
2	35.5	Moderate	13.1
3+	75.0	Severe	28.6

From Weström L: Effect of acute pelvic inflammatory disease on fertility, *Am J Obstet Gynecol* 121:707, 1975.

are not prominent, but ESRs often are elevated, abscess formation is frequent, and response to therapy often is not dramatic. Anaerobic organisms, particularly bacteroides species, are of concern in multiple recurrences, in women more than 30 years of age, and when abscesses are present.

The four well-documented long-term consequences of PID are as follows: (1) disease recurrence, (2) pelvic pain, (3) infertility, and (4) ectopic pregnancy. Approximately one fourth of all women who have had PID suffer from one or more of these sequelae. Women who have had PID are admitted to hospital more frequently for abdominal and pelvic pain, hysterectomy, and ectopic pregnancy than women who have never had PID.[277] As previously mentioned, PID is a recurrent disease despite apparently adequate therapy. Whether or not aggressive attempts at elucidating and eradicating the microbiologic pathogens and treatment of sexual partners appreciably decrease the rates of recurrence of upper genital tract infections remains to be seen.

Approximately 20% of all women who have had documented PID have some type of chronic pelvic pain. This may be sporadic or cyclic or may be constant and debilitating. This sequela often eventuates in hysterectomy[21]; PID and its sequelae are responsible for approximately 25% of abdominal hysterectomies performed in the United States each year.

Women who have had PID are at an increased risk of infertility because of tubal obstruction. Approximately 20% to 30% of cases of infertility are thought to result from fallopian tube obstruction, most often a consequence of PID. The risk of infertility is related both to the number of episodes of infection and to the severity of these episodes (Table 21-4).[276] Infertility risk also is associated with a young age at first intercourse[208] and is increased in diseases that involve either *C. trachomatis* or a tuboovarian abscess.[19, 85] If pregnancy is achieved after PID, there is an increased incidence of ectopic pregnancies. PID is thought to increase the risk of ectopic pregnancies up to 10 times and is a major factor in the increasing incidence of ectopic pregnancies in the United States. The sequelae of both infertility and ectopic pregnancy are increased with a longer duration of symptoms before therapy. At least one study has suggested that prompt evaluation and treatment of PID associated with chlamydia results in fewer long term sequelae.[91]

Treatment

To date, there are no large-scale comparative trials that support any therapeutic regimen as the most efficacious for the treatment of PID. Essential components of adequate therapy are frequent observation for response, thoughtful use of antibiotics, and contact tracing and treatment of sexual partners for *N. gonorrhoeae* and *C. trachomatis*.

Currently suggested antibiotic treatment regimens outlined by the Centers for Disease Control (CDC) are presented in Table 21-5. The microbiologic rationale for their selection is sound, but these regimens are not considered to be exclusive. Most authorities support the need for multiple drug regimens for either inpatient or outpatient therapy of PID.[24] Failure rates for single-drug therapy of 15% to 20% are documented and are unacceptably high. The appropriate length of time for adequate antimicrobial therapy, the need for protracted oral therapy in the follow-up of parenteral therapy, and the correlation between resolution of symptoms and length of therapy have not been determined. Antimicrobial regimens that have been studied have clinical cure rates of 75% to 94% and microbiologic cure rates of 71% to 100%.[266] It has been suggested that hospitalized patients receive at least 4 to 7 days of parenteral therapy and subsequent outpatient therapy of 14 to 21 days.[251]

Hospitalization for the treatment of PID with parenteral antibiotics and close observation is suggested for all patients with severe disease as defined by peritoneal signs or abscess formation. In addition, hopitalization is indicated for the following reasons: (1) when the diagnosis is in doubt; (2) the outpatient cannot take oral antibiotics for any reason; (3) the initial course of oral therapy has failed; (4) close observation of an outpatient for monitoring response is difficult; and (5) suspected pregnancy. PID during pregnancy is quite rare. However, when it occurs it can be particularly virulent, resulting in severe morbidity and in high rates of pregnancy loss and requires close observation and aggressive antibiotic therapy. Many authorities believe that

Table 21-5. Recommendations of the Centers for Disease Control for treatment of PID

Inpatient therapy
- A. Uncomplicated acute salpingitis
  - cefotetan, 2 g IV q12h
  - or
  - cefoxitin, 2 g IV q6h
  - plus
  - doxycycline,* 100 mg IV or PO q12h
- B. Complicated salpingitis (tuboovarian abscess or inflammatory complex)
  - clindamycin, 900 mg IV q8h
  - or
  - metronidazole, 500 mg IV q8h
  - plus
  - gentamicin, 2 mg/kg IV loading dose followed by 1.5 mg/kg IV q8h

Outpatient therapy
- ceftriaxone, 250 mg IM
- or
- cefoxitin, 2 g IM
- plus
- doxycycline,** 100 mg PO bid

Alternative:
- ofloxacin,** 400 mg PO bid
- clindamycin,** 450 mg PO qid
- metronidazole,** 500 mg PO bid

*Should be given for 14 days
**To be given for 10-14 days

all adolescents with PID should be hospitalized because of concerns regarding compliance with medical care and the grave long-term consequences of a lack of such compliance.[232] Some authorities additionally would hospitalize all women with PID who desire future childbearing. Hospitalization for treatment of PID can also provide an opportunity to educate patients about the pathogenesis of PID, thereby reducing risky behaviors and promoting recognition of early signs and symptoms of acute disease. This is particularly important in the successful longterm treatment of adolescents and in the preservation of fertility.

The best way to treat IUD-associated PID has not been determined. The need for IUD removal to effect clinical cure has not been proved, but the resolution of disease may be slower and less complete if an IUD is left in situ. Therefore it is common practice to remove an IUD when associated PID is treated.

TOAs deserve a trial of medical therapy because 75% to 80% of cases may respond to antibiotic therapy.[125, 196] The majority of abscesses of less than 8 cm respond to medical therapy on an acute basis. Ruptured TOAs, TOAs that do not respond to medical therapy within 4 to 5 days, and TOAs that result in chronic pain require surgical extirpation.[256] While under observation, 3% of TOAs rupture and require immediate surgical intervention. Rates of "late failures" requiring surgical intervention to cure persistent abscesses or to handle sequelae of persistent pain may be as high as 30%. Because successful pregnancy rates after TOA are only 4% to 15% and because of the potential need for later surgery to deal with persistent symptoms, some authorities advocate more aggressive surgical management of the acute disease. There is no strong evidence that operative complication rates are dependent on the time between onset of medical therapy and surgical intervention. For these reasons, decisions regarding medical and surgical management of TOA should be individualized.

The approach of total abdominal hysterectomy with bilateral salpingo-oophorectomy as the sole surgical therapy for TOA is now outmoded. Although necessary or desired in some cases, greater conservation is appropriate for the majority of patients. In particular, unilateral adnexectomy with continued medical management is an accepted surgical treatment of unilateral TOA. Some advocate simple drainage of abscess collections with aggressive medical therapy as the best way to maximize ovarian conservation for future reproduction. Laparoscopic and pelviscopic drainage of abscess collections and of pyosalpinxes is increasingly used. After cure of acute PID complicated by TOA, there is increasing justification for fertility surgery and treatment with procedures aimed at optimizing either natural or in vitro fertilization techniques.

Finally, evaluation of and therapy for both symptomatic and asymptomatic male partners is an integral part of treatment of PID.[112] Assessment of male partners should take into account the reservoir of asymptomatic males who harbor gonorrhea and chlamydia, regardless of the organisms isolated from their female partners with PID.[74] At a minimum, all sexual partners should be assessed for the presence of these organisms. Some authorities advocate presumptive therapy for all sex partners of women with newly diagnosed PID.

It must be remembered that PID is intimately associated with other sexually transmitted diseases. To achieve a decrease in the incidence of PID, successful strategies to decrease the incidence of both *N. gonorrhoeae* and *C. trachomatis* must be developed. Women diagnosed with PID should be evaluated for other sexually transmitted diseases (STDs). Serosurveys of patients hospitalized with PID suggest rates of human immunodeficiency virus (HIV) positivity of 6% to 20.9%.[93, 207]

GONORRHEA

Gonorrhea is one of the most prevalent sexually transmitted diseases in the United States today. More than 1 to 1.5 million cases are reported each year. From 1986 to 1989, the incidence of gonorrhea decreased 22%.[73] This reduction continued through 1992, except for adolescents, whose rate increased or remained stable depending on the year and the community. Between 1981 and 1991, 24% to 30% of the gonorrhea in the United States occurred in adolescents.[271] In addition to its association with younger age, gonorrhea is more common in the following: (1) urban populations, (2) lower socioeconomic groups, (3) those with multiple sexual partners, (4) those who experienced first intercourse at a young age, and (5) those women who have a sex partner with a urethral discharge or diagnosed gonorrhea.

Gonorrhea may present as a localized infection of the lower genital tract, an invasive infection of the upper genital tract, a disseminated disease with systemic manifestations, or it may be asymptomatic. The causative organism of gonorrhea is *N. gonorrhoeae*, a Gram-negative aerobic diplococcus that grows best in carbon dioxide and is very sensitive to drying and to extremes in temperature. The organism commonly infects columnar and transitional cells.

The majority of gonorrhea cases are transmitted through sexual activity. An infected male partner transmits infection through vaginal intercourse with approximately 50% efficiency. The incubation period is approximately 3 to 5 days in cases in which symptoms are recognizable. In women, *N. gonorrhoeae* is harbored chiefly in the endocervix. It is also found in the urethra, rectum, and oropharynx and occasionally is found in one of these locations in the absence of cervical gonorrhea. Infection of multiple sites occurs in more than 20% of cases.

The manifestations of gonorrhea in women most often are subtle. Gonorrhea presents much more frequently without symptoms in women as opposed to men. STD clinics report that the prevalence of gonorrhea is higher in those attending as contacts as opposed to those attending with symptoms.[174] Endocervical gonorrhea is associated with a purulent cervical discharge, which may or may not be noticed as abnormal. Occasionally irregular vaginal bleeding is noted. Urethral gonorrhea or involvement of Skene's glands may be associated with symptoms of lower urinary tract infection, such as dysuria and frequency of urination. Rectal gonorrhea often causes no symptoms. *N. gonorrhoeae* present in the oropharynx may cause acute pharyngitis but usually is asymptomatic. Because colonization with *N. gonorrhoeae* produces either no symptoms or vague ones in 80% of cases,[290] women do not seek medical attention and form a major reservoir of disease transmission. Interpretation of symptoms and diagnosis of gonorrhea may be further complicated by coinfection by other sexually transmitted diseases, particularly *C. trachomatis* and *Trichomonas vaginalis*.

Lower genital tract gonorrhea can lead to infection of the Bartholin's glands and the formation of Bartholin's abscesses. Bartholin's abscesses associated with gonorrhea most often are unilateral, acutely suppurative, and painful. They may spontaneously drain, require incision and drainage, or on occasion they may spontaneously resolve.

Ten percent to 20% of women with endocervical gonorrhea develop acute salpingitis. *N. gonorrhoeae* can invade and infect the upper genital tract as a solitary pathogen or as a part of a polymicrobial infection. Some strains of *N. gonorrhoeae* are more pathogenic for the upper genital tract than others. A lipopolysaccharide endotoxin is responsible both for local cytotoxicity and inflammation and for fever and systemic toxicity. Furthermore, outer membrane pili proteins and IgA protease facilitate attachment of the gonococcus to host cells. In addition, certain risk factors in the host that predispose to salpingitis have been previously outlined. The exact microbial and host factors that lead to invasion and to infection of the upper genital tract by *N. gonorrhoeae* are incompletely understood. In the United States estimates of the incidence of gonococcal salpingitis range from 25% to 80% of all cases of salpingitis.

Although up to 40% of rectal cultures obtained from women with gonorrhea are positive, some of these cultures are positive because of perineal contamination and do not reflect true rectal colonization. Rectal colonization may produce symptoms of discharge, bleeding, pain, tenesmus, constipation, and signs such as exudate or mucosal bleeding. However, rectal gonorrhea is most frequently asymptomatic. Rectal gonorrhea is more likely to be ineffectively treated by tetracycline therapy. In addition, since 30% of treatment failures in women are discovered only by posttreatment rectal culture, some authorities suggest that posttreatment cultures should always include a rectal culture.

Pharyngeal carriage of *N. gonorrhoeae* is most often asymptomatic. It can occasionally be associated with an acute, exudative pharyngitis. Pharyngeal gonorrhea is thought to be almost exclusively a result of fellatio with an infected male partner. Largely asymptomatic, pharyngeal gonorrhea is not thought to be very contagious or to be a major reservoir of disease transmission. There is evidence that without treatment spontaneous remission may occur over a 10- to 12-week period. However, there may be a greater tendency for pharyngeal gonorrhea to disseminate because the number of cases of disseminated gonococcal infection (DGI) associated with pharyngeal gonorrhea appears to be disproportionately high. Also, pharyngeal gonorrhea is more resistant to therapy with standard antimicrobial regimens.

The incidence of DGI in all persons with gonorrhea is approximately 5%. Exact risk factors are unknown, although pregnancy may predispose to DGI. Twenty-eight percent to 42% of cases of DGI in some series have been in pregnant women.

DGI usually presents in one of two distinct forms.[95] It may present as a systemic illness associated with chills, fever, malaise, asymmetric polyarthralgias, and painful skin lesions. The fingers, toes, hands, wrists, knees, and ankles are most frequently involved in what appears to be a tenosynovitis and rarely, a frank, suppurative arthritis. Skin lesions classically appear as a slightly raised, erythematous base with a necrotic center but may be petechial, papular, pustular, and hemorrhagic, and occasionally may be bullous. These lesions are lightly scattered about the body, are usually fewer than 20, and often are on the extremities. An average of 10% to 30%, though up to 50%, of acutely symptomatic patients with DGI may have positive blood cultures.

The second common clinical syndrome of DGI is that of a septic, monoarticular arthritis. *N. gonorrhoeae* may be the most common cause of septic arthritis in patients younger than 30 years of age. Knees are most frequently involved although elbow, ankle, and wrist involvement is also seen. Joint effusion is exudative, often purulent, with the gonococcus identified by a Gram stain or by a routine culture in approximately 50% of cases. Culture positivity is proportional to the WBC count in the joint fluid. Blood cultures are not positive.

Disseminated *N. gonorrhoeae* may rarely cause endocarditis, myocarditis, pericarditis, hepatitis, or meningitis.

People with DGI often lack typical local symptoms of gonorrhea. If DGI is suspected, all common sites for gonococcal colonization should be cultured. The need to hospitalize everyone with DGI is unclear; however, close observation for the first 48 hours of treatment to judge early therapeutic response and to rule out serious complications is prudent.

Diagnosis

The diagnosis of gonorrhea is most accurately made by a culture of the organism on selective media such as modified Thayer-Martin agar. This is a chocolate-based agar modified by the addition of antibiotics to inhibit the growth of organisms from sites commonly contaminated by polymicrobial growth, such as the cervix or rectum. The specimen should be plated directly on warmed media and incubated in CO_2 without delay to minimize false-negative results from improper handling. Growth markedly decreases after 3 hours if the specimen is improperly handled.

Obtaining specimens from multiple sites increases the yield of cultures for suspected gonorrhea. The endocervix is the site that most frequently produces positive cultures in women and should always be sampled. Cultures from the urethra, rectum, and pharynx may be positive despite negative cervical cultures and should be performed when indicated by history, strong clinical suspicion of gonococcal disease, and in all cases of recurrent disease.

A Gram stain may help in making a tentative diagnosis of gonorrhea in patients who are symptomatic or who have a history of contact with known gonorrhea. A Gram stain is considered to be positive if intracellular Gram-negative diplococci are seen in a minimum of three polymorphonuclear leukocytes per high-power field (HPF). Sensitivity and specificity vary by site of isolation. Up to two thirds of women with endocervical gonorrhea have suggestive Gram stains, but specificity in asymptomatic women is as low as 40% to 70%.

Rapid diagnosis by fluorescent monoclonal antibody slides or enzyme assays are of limited value in asymptomatic and low-risk individuals. Chemiluminescent DNA probe assays are reported to be highly specific, have high positive predictive values, and have a sensitivity of 90%.[78, 176] DNA probes may be used for diagnosis of rectal and pharyngeal gonorrhea and have the additional advantage of concomitant assessment for chlamydia.[133]

Treatment

Treatment of gonorrhea in the United States has been modified by the two following factors: (1) the emergence of resistant strains of *N. gonorrhoeae,* and (2) the need to provide concomitant treatment for *C. trachomatis* when gonorrhea is treated.

The majority of *N. gonorrhoeae* organisms in the United States is sensitive to high-dose penicillin. However, a penicillin resistance at rates of > 3% in most communities has changed the recommendations for therapy.[31, 37] First recognized in 1976, a plasmid-mediated β-lactamase or penicillinase is responsible for most gonococcal resistance. Initially confined to defined urban areas, particularly those in California, New York, and Florida, most cases of penicillinase-producing *N. gonorrhoeae* (PPNG) in other geographic areas were related to travel to the high-risk areas. Currently more than 75% of reported cases of PPNG are associated with endemic contact. Two other forms of resistant *N. gonorrhoeae* exist. A chromosomally mediated resistant *N. gonorrhoeae* strain that is resistant to penicillin, tetracycline, and other antibiotics is recognized but is not yet widespread. Also, plasmid-mediated tetracycline-resistant *N. gonorrhoeae* has recently been reported. Spectinomycin is effective against virtually all PPNG strains, and ceftriaxone is effective against all resistant strains.

In women, *C. trachomatis* is isolated from 30% to 50% of those from whom the gonococcus is isolated. Studies of single-drug therapy for gonorrhea show that the rates of post-treatment isolation of *C. trachomatis* and the occurrence of PID are high if a penicillin, a penicillin derivative, or a cephalosporin are used but are low if a tetracycline is used. However, up to 10% of cases of gonorrhea are not cured if tetracycline is the sole treatment. Therefore, multiple drug therapies for treatment of gonorrhea that take into account chlamydia are standard now.[242]

Proper treatment for gonorrhea factors in resistance and likely sites of infection. While penicillin is the treatment of choice if rates of resistance are less than 1%, nonpenicillin alternatives are preferred if rates of resistant strains are more than 1%. Spectinomycin is less effective for pharyngeal gonorrhea but is an excellent drug for rectal gonorrhea. Penicillin and probably most cephalosporins eradicate incubating syphilis; however, spectinomycin is ineffective for this indication. Current guidelines for treatment of gonorrhea are as outlined in Table 21-6.

Table 21-6. Treatment of gonorrhea

Condition	Treatment
Uncomplicated urethral, endocervical, or rectal infection	*Parenteral regimens**
	Ceftriaxone, 125 mg IM × 1 dose**
	Cefotaxime, 500 mg × 1 dose
	Cefotetan, 1 g IM × 1 dose
	Cefoxitin, 2 g IM × 1 dose
	Ceftizoxime, 500 mg IM × 1 dose
	*Oral regimens**
	Cefixime, 400 mg × 1 dose**
	Cefuroxime axetil, 1 gm plus 1 g probenecid
	Ciprofloxacin, 500 mg × 1 dose
	Norfloxacin, 400 mg × 1 dose
	Tetracycline, 500 mg qid × 7 days
	Doxycycline, 100 mg bid × 7 days
Pharyngitis	Ceftriaxone, 125 mg IM × 1 dose
	Cefixime, 400 mg PO × 1 dose
	Ciprofloxacin, 500 mg PO × 1 dose
	Ofloxacin 400 mg PO × 1 dose
Disseminated gonococcal infection†	
	Ceftriaxone, 1 g IM or IV every 24 hours
	Ceftizoxime, 1 g IV every 8 hours
	Cefotaxime, 1 g IV every 8 hours
	Spectinomycin, 2 g IM every 12 hours

* All single-dose parenteral and oral regimens for gonorrhea should be followed by doxycyline, 100 mg orally twice daily, to provide coverage for possible concurrent infection with *Chlamydia*. In pregnant women, erythromycin base, 500 mg PO four times daily for 7 days, or azithromycin, 1000 mg PO in a single dose, should be substituted for doxycycline.

** Drugs of choice.

† Parenteral therapy should be continued until the patient has been afebrile and asymptomatic for 24 to 48 hours. She then should receive oral antibiotics to complete a total of 1 week of therapy. Appropriate oral antibiotics include cefixime, 400 mg twice daily, or ciprofloxacin, 500 mg twice daily. Ciprofloxacin is contraindicated in pregnant and lactating women and in children less than 17 years of age.

It is important to reculture all pertinent sites for gonorrhea 3 to 7 days after therapy is completed. Most cases of positive gonorrhea cultures after therapy are a result of reinfection from untreated sexual partners. The prevalence of asymptomatic gonorrhea in male partners may be as high as 20% to 30%. Adequate contact tracing remains an integral part of adequate therapy for gonorrhea, as does screening of all populations in which the prevalence of culture positivity is more than 1% to 1.5%.[187] Screening in "high prevalence" populations is justified as cost effective in decreasing adverse disease outcomes. Targeted screening programs based on risk factors among sexually active women are also proposed.[186]

CHLAMYDIA

C. trachomatis is an obligate intracellular bacterial parasite of columnar and transitional epithelial cells. Its role as a pathogen for the genital tract was first recognized as the causative agent of lymphogranuloma venereum (LGV). Non-LGV serotypes of *C. trachomatis* are now associated with asymptomatic carriage in a variety of infections of the female genital tract.

Chlamydia is now thought to be the most prevalent sexually transmitted disease in the United States, with an estimated 3 to 4 million cases yearly. The overall prevalence of *C. trachomatis* in the female genital tract varies by practice site, ranging from 2% to 35% in prenatal clinics and 5% to 23% in family planning clinics. In addition, prevalence increases in those presenting with symptoms. It is most prevalent in those younger than 25 years of age, in nulliparous and unmarried women, in users of nonbarrier contraceptive methods, and in those with recent multiple or new sexual partners. It occurs in a more geographically diverse population than gonorrhea.[290] Chlamydia is frequently associated with gonorrhea; approximately 30% to 50% of the time it is cultured from the genital tract after successful therapy for gonorrhea, and the gonococcus is found in 10% to 50% of women with chlamydia. It is a major pathogen in cases of postgonococcal and nongonococcal urethritis in the male, and female partners of these males are at high risk for chlamydial colonization and disease.

Up to 80% of women colonized with *Chlamydia* are asymptomatic or have mild, unrecognized symptoms. This is one of the problems in controlling chlamydial infection and its sequelae.[29] The majority of chlamydial infections in women are identified through screening or contact tracing, neither of which is universal or routine.

C. trachomatis has been associated with cervicitis, which may or may not cause symptoms.[18] The presence of *C. trachomatis* in the cervix is associated with a cervicitis characterized by a hypertrophic-appearing, friable central eversion or ectopy with mucopus. Endocervical mucus that appears yellow against a cotton-tipped applicator (abnormal Q-tip test result) and microscopic examination that reveals the presence of WBCs signify mucopurulence. If both are present, *Chlamydia* is found in 85% of cases. Cervical erythema and friability also are independently correlated with *Chlamydia*. If signs of cervicitis are seen in a woman with symptoms of PID, chlamydial infection should be suspected.

The female urethral syndrome of dysuria, pyuria greater than 10 WBCs/HPF, and negative bacterial culture are associated with *C. trachomatis* in up to 50% of cases. Therapy with doxycycline results in resolution of symptoms.

C. trachomatis is also implicated as a cause of Bartholinitis and late postpartum endometritis. It can be transmitted to neonates at birth through an infected birth canal and, in neonates, is associated with a distinctive conjunctivitis and pneumonitis.

Chlamydia is associated with up to 30% to 50% of cases of PID,[148] particularly in adolescents. The exact contribution of *Chlamydia* to morbidity and long-term sequelae associated with PID is unclear. If PID is treated with antibiotics, which are not effective against *Chlamydia*, acute symptoms subside, but recurrence of the disease is common. Some cases of chlamydial PID are very subtle clinically yet are associated with unexpectedly severe disease by laparoscopy. The subtle nature of the symptoms possibly contributes to a delay in treatment, which contributes to the high rate of sequelae of infertility seen in some series.

Chlamydia is found by biopsy or by culture in the endometrium of women with intermenstrual spotting or symptoms of PID with or without laparoscopic confirmation of upper genital tract infection.[122, 284] Occasionally it is seen in asymptomatic women with documented clinical disease.[108]

Silent chlamydial infection is implicated in both tubal factor infertility and ectopic pregnancy. Greater presence of and higher levels of antichlamydial antibody titer are linked to both conditions in a population of women the majority of whom have no known history of PID. In addition, these women are more likely to have visible tubal damage than those without antibody titer.[85, 189, 223, 267]

In recognition of the rapidly increasing prevalence of *C. trachomatis* and of the potential reproductive tract sequelae caused by chlamydial infection, strategies to monitor prevalence, control spread, and educate the public have been proposed. These strategies include screening of all groups at risk of the disease,[117, 275] particularly adolescents and those with other STDs. Additional strategies include evaluation of all those with referable symptoms, signs, or exposures, and potential empiric treatment of all females at high risk for chlamydial disease. Suggested risk factors for screening or for presumptive therapy in high prevalence populations include young age, evidence of cervicitis or urethritis, exposure to gonorrhea, new male partners with urethritis, multiple sexual partners within the year, and a sexual partner within the preceding 3 months.[82, 142, 188, 243]

Diagnosis

The presence of *C. trachomatis* is determined most accurately by demonstrating the intracellular organism in cell culture. Direct fluorescent antibody slide staining, enzyme-linked immunosorbent assay (ELISA) techniques, and DNA probe systems have been introduced for rapid chlamydial antigen detection. These tests are more widely available and are less expensive than the presently available culture techniques. However, sensitivity and specificity are less when used in low-prevalence populations and are best in the hands of experienced laboratories with demonstrated ongoing quality control.[135] The use of rapid tests for assessment of cure may result in false positives if they are repeated too soon after successful therapy. False negatives may occur in cases where inappropriate or incomplete therapy temporarily halts organism replication.

Intensive study of cytologic findings associated with *Chlamydia* by routine Papanicolaou smear techniques has revealed certain typical changes. Inflammatory changes, particularly the presence of lymphocytes and histiocytes, plus mild cellular atypia, such as reactive or atypical metaplasia or reactive endocervical cells, have all been correlated with the presence of *Chlamydia*. However, specificity of these findings is 30% to 60% at best, and their presence should prompt no more than further assessment of individual cases. The sensitivity of cytology is too low to be effective as a screening technique. Treatment appropriate for chlamydia can be expected to result in resolution of cytologic abnormalities in cases of true infection.

Invasive infection with *C. trachomatis* produces an immunogenic response, and chlamydial antibodies are measurable using complement fixation, microimmunofluorescence, and ELISA techniques. When a fourfold rise in IgG titer or the presence of specific IgM antibodies is documented, chlamydial disease may be diagnosed. The presence of preexisting antibody, of cross-reactivity of various serotypes of *Chlamydia*, and of the lack of antibody response to some chlamydial carriage limit serologic analysis as a diagnostic tool.

Treatment

The drug of choice for the treatment of chlamydia is tetracycline. The exact duration of therapy necessary to achieve cure is unknown, but 500 mg four times daily for 7 days appears to be adequate. Tetracycline, 250 mg four times daily for 14 days, is also curative. Cephalosporins and penicillin are not effective antichlamydial agents. Ampicillin is well tolerated and curative in compliant populations but is not the drug of choice for chlamydial disease. Newer penicillin derivatives and clindamycin have some antichlamydial spectrum, and in antimicrobial trials of PID therapy they have good cure rates for upper genital tract infection associated with chlamydia. Sulfa drugs and fluoroquinolones both have antichlamydial activity. Azithromycin, a long-acting macrolide, has promise as a single-dose therapy for chlamydia, although current cost issues dictate its use only in noncompliant populations. Current recommendations for treatment of chlamydia are listed in Table 21-7. Treatment to eliminate chlamydia should be based on laboratory documentation. However, when facilities are not available or when testing is impractical, presumptive therapy may be instituted for suspected carriage or disease in a high-risk population. Documentation of organism presence may aid effective education, compliance, and partner treatment.

Table 21-7. CDC recommendations for *C. trachomatis*

Genital Infections	
Tetracycline	250 mg, 4 times/day × 14 days
Tetracycline	500 mg, 4 times/day × 7 days
Erythromycin	500 mg, 4 times/day × 7 days
Doxycyline	100 mg bid × 7 days
Sulfasoxazole	500 mg, 5 times/day × 10 to 14 days
Ampicillin*	500 mg, 4 times/day × 10 days
Azithromycin	1 g orally
Ofloxacin**	300 mg, 2 times/day × 7 days

* May also be effective

** Contraindicated in patients ≤ 17 years of age, in pregnant or lactating women.

Repeat testing after therapy should be performed 3 to 4 weeks after completion of antimicrobial therapy at the earliest. All sexual partners must also be referred for evaluation and treatment. It has been suggested that contact tracing for chlamydial disease is cost effective.

ACTINOMYCOSIS

Infection by *Actinomyces israelii* is an infrequent cause of disease of the upper genital tract. *A. israelii* is a Gram-positive, nonacid-fast anaerobic bacterium with a characteristic radially branching filamentous formation. It is most typically found in the oral cavity. Actinomycosis is a sporadic infection of soft tissues and is characterized by an invasion of areas of trauma, with chronic, suppurative infection. This infection results in tissue destruction, fibrosis, and the formation of draining sinuses. Active actinomycotic infection usually is polymicrobial; other anaerobic organisms frequently are involved.

Actinomycosis is a rare cause of indolent pelvic infection secondary to the seeding of the upper genital tract from other intraabdominal sources or hematogenous dissemination of *Actinomyces*. In addition, ascending pelvic actinomycotic infection is described in the presence of an IUD.[23, 214, 262]

Colonization of the lower genital tract by *Actinomyces* occurs most frequently in IUD users or in the presence of other foreign bodies. The prevalence of colonization increases with the duration of IUD use. A small percentage of women in whom colonization occurs manifests upper genital tract infection with actinomycosis. Irregular vaginal bleeding and mild, chronic, pelvic discomfort may precede this manifestation. By the time of presentation, the pelvic organs may be massively indurated and fibrotic, with near total destruction of anatomy and adherence to surrounding structures. Because *Actinomyces* tends to invade across tissue planes and boundaries, cases of actinomycotic pelvic infection presenting with ureteric obstruction, rectosigmoid stricture, or as a retroperitoneal mass have been reported.[81, 94, 179, 260] Because medical therapy has only a limited chance of restoring structure and function, treatment is frequently surgical removal of affected organs.

Diagnosis

The diagnosis of actinomycosis can be suspected by a suggestive Gram stain. Histologic sections of actinomycotic infections show necrotic debris and inflammation associated with sulfur granules, which are central organisms with branching filaments that stain yellow with a silver stain. Using appropriate anaerobic media and techniques, diagnosis can be confirmed by a culture.

Treatment

When colonization is suspected by a Papanicolaou smear or immunofluorescent slide screening, treatment with antibiotics has not been shown to effectively eliminate *Actinomyces* from the lower genital tract. Current recommendations are to remove IUDs in cases of suspected colonization and to repeat Papanicolaou smears in 3 to 6 months; if the smear is normal, the IUD may be reinserted.

Actinomycosis is sensitive to penicillins, tetracycline, chloramphenicol, and clindamycin. Treatment of infection is with high-dose parenteral antibiotics, typically penicillin. The exact length of required therapy is not established, although the slow growth of these organisms and the extensive involvement of infection usually necessitate a minimum of 6 weeks of therapy. Initial parenteral therapy is often completed orally with doxycycline. Treatment of actinomycotic pelvic infection should cover other organisms typically found in cases of upper genital tract infection, particularly anaerobic organisms. Aggressive medical therapy has resulted in resolution of obstruction and shrinkage of large masses. Medical therapy can facilitate later surgical intervention, which often is required for cure.

GENITAL TRACT TUBERCULOSIS AS AN ETIOLOGIC AGENT FOR PELVIC INFLAMMATORY DISEASE

In developed countries tuberculosis is a rare cause of upper genital tract infection. Today the disease most often presents in older women exposed to tuberculosis before the advent of effective chemoprophylaxis and in younger women who emigrate from countries where tuberculosis is endemic.

Genital tract tuberculosis is usually secondary to hematogenous spread from pulmonary or from other nongenital tract foci. It rarely spreads to the genital tract from other intraperitoneal foci or from male sexual partners with tuberculous epididymitis.

The most frequent sites of tuberculous involvement in the female genital tract are the fallopian tube and endometrium,[1] although the cervix and ovary also can be affected. The vagina and vulva are rarely involved.

Genital tract tuberculosis is an extremely indolent infection. Disease may not become manifest for more than 10 years after the initial seeding of the genital tract. Presenting symptoms may be unusual vaginal bleeding patterns, including altered menses, amenorrhea, and postmenopausal bleeding. Approximately 25% to 35% of women with pelvic tuberculosis may complain of vague, chronic, lower abdominal or pelvic pain. The chief presenting complaint of young women with genital tract tuberculosis is infertility.[1, 170] Occasionally, women with the disease present with tuberculous peritonitis and ascites, although these more frequently are secondary to direct hematogenous seeding of the peritoneum.

Diagnosis

The diagnosis of genital tract tuberculosis may be suspected from medical history, travel history, and a chest roentgenogram with evidence of healed pulmonary tuberculosis. However, a significant portion of women with pelvic tuberculosis may have no history of tuberculosis infection and may present with a normal chest x-ray.[211] Except in debilitated, systemically ill patients, a skin test with a purified protein derivative of tuberculin yields positive findings. A hysterosalpingogram may show characteristic changes suggestive of tuberculous infection, which includes beading, sacculation, sinus formation, and rigid pipestem patterning.

Diagnosis can be confirmed by a histologic examination that reveals typical granulomas or by an acid-fast stain or a culture of surgical specimen or endometrial biopsy tissue. Acid-fast stain is less sensitive than culture and histology. Both endometrial biopsy specimens and menstrual blood collected in a vaginal cup or cervical cup may be submitted for culture. Menstrual fluid is reported to be culture positive more frequently than biopsy.[170]

Treatment

The treatment of genital tract tuberculosis is primarily medical, with administration of two or three antituberculosis drugs for 18 to 24 months. Surgery is indicated if the symptoms or the physical examination suggest a persistence or increase in disease despite adequate therapy, or if culture or biopsy results suggest resistant organisms. Surgical therapy most often consists of total abdominal hysterectomy and bilateral salpingo-oophorectomy. Early, aggressive medical therapy, however, may warrant infertility-related procedures.

GENITAL HERPES

Genital herpes is a sexually transmitted infection of increasing concern for all sexually active women. An estimated 270,000 to 600,000 new cases appear each year, with the peak incidence in the third decade. Up to 46% of women attending an STD clinic and 9% of college students are reported to have antibody evidence of genital herpes. One national survey suggests that 16.4% of persons 15 to 74 years of age in the United States have antibody evidence of genital herpes.[107] Symptomatic genital herpes is the most frequent cause of painful lesions of the lower genital tract of women in the United States. Herpes infection of the lower genital tract has been associated with cervical cancer, although a causative role remains unproven. In addition, contact with genital herpes during passage through the birth canal has been associated with systemic neonatal infection, which carries major risks of serious morbidity and a high mortality rate.

The exact prevalence of genital herpes infection is unknown, since not all people with active infections seek medical care and because there is a relatively high proportion of asymptomatic disease. However, some authorities consider the incidence of herpes to be steadily increasing and genital herpes to be one of the most frequent STDs in the United States today.

Genital herpes is caused by the herpes simplex virus (HSV)—a member of the DNA-containing Herpesviridae family. There are two major types of HSV; type 1 (HSV-1) and type 2 (HSV-2). They are closely related and are homologous for approximately 50% of antigens. Although HSV-2 causes the majority of genital herpes lesions, and HSV-1 primarily causes oral-labial lesions, a significant overlap clearly exists. Approximately 85% to 90% of genital herpes infections are caused by HSV- 2, whereas the remainder are caused by HSV-1. This proportion varies, and up to 50% of genital lesions were caused by HSV-1 according to a survey that took place in England.

Genital herpes is a recurrent infection. Periods of active infection are separated by periods of latency during which the inactive virus resides in the dorsal root sacral ganglia. Under the stimulus of various endogenous and exogenous factors, the virus travels down the sensory nerve root to the lower genital area where it replicates. Outward manifestations of the disease become apparent, and HSV can be identified by culture.

The lesions of genital herpes are typically painful and begin as fluid-filled vesicles or papules, which progress to well-circumscribed, occasionally coalescent, shallow-based ulcers. These ulcers heal by the reepithelialization of mucous membranes or by the crusting over of epidermal surfaces. The virus is shed from active lesions until healing begins, and it can be transmitted during the time of shedding. The clinical presentation and the duration of active infection vary widely and depend on the virus type, location of presentation, preexistence of antibodies, and presentation as initial or recurrent disease.

The initial presentation of genital herpes infection occurs 1 to 45 days (mean 5.8 days) after exposure to the virus. Manifestations of the initial HSV infection are more severe and last longer than those of the recurrent disease. First episodes are more severe in women than in men. Multiple, painful, usually bilateral lesions occur on the external genitalia. Symptoms tend to peak within 8 to 10 days and gradually decrease over the next week. Crops of new lesions form over a mean of 10 days. Ulcers last 4 to 15 days, and the mean time from the onset of the lesions to total healing is 20 to 21 days. The virus is shed from lesions up to the time of crusting over, and the average duration of shedding is 11 days. Most often, local lesions are accompanied by bilateral, tender lymphadenopathy of the inguinal region and sometimes of the femoral and iliac regions. Adenopathy of the deep inguinal nodes can be responsible for severe lower pelvic pain. Adenopathy appears after the onset of lesions and often takes longer to resolve, lasting beyond the period of the lesions themselves.

Local involvement includes urethritis in the majority of cases; 82% of urethral cultures are positive. Urination may be problematic either because of periurethral and vulvar edema or because of intense dysuria resulting from urethral herpetic involvement.

Initial genital herpes infection involves the cervix in more than 80% of cases. Cervical involvement may be clinically apparent with friability of the cervix, ulcerative and occasionally necrotic lesions of the cervix, and a marked increase in cervical discharge. Both the exocervix and endocervix may be involved. In some cases the involvement of the cervix may not be clinically apparent, although the virus can be cultured.

Other genital tract sites may be involved. Vaginal lesions are apparent in 4% of cases. Although HSV has been cultured from the fallopian tube, how often the upper genital tract is involved in initial cases of genital herpes is unclear. At present, this is not believed to be a major clinical problem.

Women develop complications of initial HSV infection more commonly than men. These complications may be due to local spread or to more distant effects of the virus.

Coincident with the initial symptomatic genital herpes infection, symptomatic pharyngitis is reported in approximately 10% of cases.[38] HSV can be isolated from the pharynx of individuals with symptomatic pharyngitis and from those without pharyngeal symptoms. Pharyngitis and pharyngeal viral shedding occur with genital infection with both HSV-1 and HSV-2.

In approximately one fourth of cases, secondary spread of local lesions to other body sites occurs after the onset of lesions and before they have crusted over. Extragenital involvement most often occurs in sites below the waist, such as the buttocks and upper legs. However, involvement of the fingers and eyes also has been reported. The secondary spread is thought to happen primarily because of autoinoculation and most often occurs in the second week of disease.

In one half to two thirds of cases of initial genital herpes infection, systemic symptoms are apparent early in the course of illness. Fever, malaise, headache, and myalgias are common. Other systemic complications include hepatitis, aseptic meningitis, and autonomic nervous system dysfunction.

Hepatitis exhibits a picture typical for hepatocellular necrosis and presents after the onset of local genital lesions. This usually occurs within the first week of illness and is most often accompanied by other systemic symptoms.

Aseptic meningitis is seen more frequently with HSV-2 than with HSV-1 infections. It occurs in up to 36% of initial genital herpes infections. Headache, stiff neck, and photophobia, with or without fever are typical symptoms. It is accompanied by a cerebrospinal fluid pleocytosis consisting largely of lymphocytes. Meningitis is self-limited, requires only supportive care, and resolves without permanent neurologic sequelae. Encephalitis is rarely a complication of genital herpes infection.

Sacral autonomic nervous system dysfunction is an uncommon complication of initial genital herpes infection. Typical symptoms include decreased sensation along the sacral nerve route distribution, inability to void as a result of bladder dysfunction,[26] and constipation because of bowel dysfunction. Nerve dysfunction is confirmed through electromyography and may last 6 to 8 weeks. Occasionally, sensory involvement may take the form of hyperesthesia in a radicular pattern. A presentation of self-limited transverse myelitis with paralysis has been reported.

Recurrent genital herpes infection typically is less severe, is of shorter duration, and is less frequently involved in systemic manifestations than the initial disease. One to 2 days to a few hours before the onset of recurrent lesions, prodromal symptoms may occur.[80] Symptoms are typically described as a tingling sensation, an itching, or a hyperesthesia of the genital area where lesions will occur. The prodrome may also include a sacral dermatomal neuralgia with pain radiating to the buttocks and hips.

Recurrent genital lesions are fewer, smaller, and more often unilateral. Recurrent lesions may not have the typical ulcerative appearance. Instead they may be similar to a fissure or to an excoriation. Recurrences are usually painful and tend to appear in the same location and have the same appearance each episode. Symptoms of recurrent lesions last 4 to 8 days, and there are fewer crops of new lesions. The mean time until recurrent lesions disappear is 9 to 10 days, and viral shedding averages 5 days.

Both urethritis and cervicitis are seen less frequently with recurrent genital infection than with initial infection. Cervicitis is typically manifest solely as virus positivity. Shedding of the virus from the cervix during recurrent disease occurs in 10% to 15% of episodes.[38] Tender local adenopathy may be present but is usually less severe and is of shorter duration. Systemic manifestations are uncommon, and extragenital involvement is seen in less than 5% of cases.

The frequency of recurrent disease and the length of time between recurrences of active infection are highly variable. The average number of recurrences in women who have symptomatic recurrent genital herpes is 5 to 8 per year. Some evidence suggests that the mean time to recurrence is greater from the initial episode to the first recurrence than between subsequent recurrences. Recurrences may be precipitated by an obvious endogenous stimulus, such as cyclic hormonal variation, or they may be precipitated by exposure to HSV through sexual contact with an infected partner. Whether contact with exogenous virus precipitates recurrent infection or whether this is actually reinfection with a different viral strain is unclear. Although the general impression is that the frequency of recurrent disease decreases as time from initial infection increases, recurrent disease may be independent of time for at least the first 3 to 4 years.

Approximately 25% of initial genital herpes infections present in women who have preexisting antibody to HSV. Nonprimary first episodes tend to be less severe with fewer systemic manifestations than true primary episodes in an antibody-negative individual and may actually be recurrent infection in a person with previous asymptomatic HSV-2 infection. In other cases the presence of antibody to HSV-1 of oral-labial origin may serve to ameliorate the clinical expression of genital infection. The initial presentation of both primary and nonprimary disease may be asymptomatic.

Although the initial presentation of genital herpes infection caused by HSV-1 cannot be distinguished from that caused by HSV-2, HSV-1 is less likely to result in recurrent genital infection.[38] Recurrences of infection caused by HSV-1 are much less frequent and also less severe. This difference probably is related to virus type and not to antibody response.

Asymptomatic genital herpes infection is defined by culture-positive viral shedding in the absence of symptoms and lesions. The prevalence of asymptomatic shedding is unknown. Such shedding occurs both from the cervix and from the vulva, probably with approximately equal frequency. The peak in frequency of shedding may be during the first 3 months after a primary lesion. Thereafter shedding appears to be sporadic and of brief duration. In one culture survey of women with known genital herpes, daily cultures were positive for HSV on only 1% of days.[16] Risk factors for asymptomatic shedding are incompletely described; however, shedding is more common with HSV-2 than HSV-1 and is not related to the menstrual cycle.

Both the virus type and the presence of asymptomatic shedding are factors in the transmission of genital herpes. The overall risk of transmission in monogamous relationships when one partner has genital herpes and the other does not is approximately 10% per year, and is probably highest when a male is the infected partner.[20] The risk of seroconversion appears to be higher in partners with no prior history of genital herpes and who also have no preexisting antibody. Transmission is less frequently seen when infected partners have a less symptomatic disease. The majority of transmission occurs during periods of asymptomatic shedding, during the prodromal period, or at the onset of a lesion.[158, 159]

Diagnosis

The diagnosis of genital herpes is often suggested by the characteristic clinical presentation and the appearance of lesions. The most accurate diagnostic test to confirm clinical impression is virus isolation by tissue culture. The virus may be isolated from either the vesicle fluid or the base of a wet ulcer. If vesicles are present, the vesicles should be unroofed and the fluid should be cultured directly. A single virus culture done on an appropriate lesion identifies live virus in 85% to 90% of cases. Virus grown in culture can be typed. Tests less sensitive, but helpful when viral cultures are not available, rely on cytologic methods to identify changes in cells typically produced by the HSV. Scrapings of viral lesions are gathered for fluorescent staining for a Papanicolaou smear or for Tzanck preparation. Genital tract smears appear to be neither sensitive nor specific. A Tzanck smear stained with either Wright's or Giemsa stain is positive if multinucleated giant cells are identified. This occurs in up to 50% of cases. Antibody testing is generally of no value in diagnosing genital herpes infections. Forty percent to 60% of adults have antibodies to HSV-1, and 15% to 35% have antibodies to HSV-2, which represents past exposure that may have resulted in clinically apparent infection or asymptomatic infection. Although it is possible to distinguish HSV-2 antibodies from HSV-1 antibodies, antibody response to type-common antigens leads to a large crossover in identification and to difficulty in detecting new antibody formation in a person with a previous type-common antibody response. Many commercial laboratories have substantial false-positive and false-negative herpes antibody results as well as inaccurate viral typing because of cross reactivity of common antigens.[4] The existence of antibody to HSV at the onset of an initial genital herpes infection may preclude identification of this episode as either a primary infection in a previously antibody-negative host or a recurrent infection in a previously asymptomatic host. In addition, the presence of antibody to HSV at the onset of a herpes genital lesion may identify past exposure to this virus but not, however, identify the etiology of active lesions. Occasionally, if there is no antibody to HSV present at the onset of a suspected primary genital herpes infection, and if antibody develops during the course of illness, antibody testing can be of some value. Because of the variety in expression of the disease, and because of the inherent inaccuracies in diagnosis by antibody assessment, the timing and the sources of specific infection may be difficult if not impossible to determine.

Treatment

There is no therapy that effectively prevents establishment of latency of genital herpes or that eradicates infection. The currently available antiviral agent that most effectively alters the course of genital herpes infection is acyclovir. Acyclovir is available in three forms. Topical application of acyclovir every 4 hours decreases the duration of symptoms and the length of viral shedding for the initial episode of disease. Its use is sometimes limited by the side effect of local irritation. Topical acyclovir is not effective in altering the course of recurrent genital herpes infection. Intravenous acyclovir is used to treat disseminated herpetic infection in immunosuppressed individuals. In addition, both intravenous (IV) and oral acyclovir ameliorate the course of initial episodes of genital herpes.[180] If given within 7 days of onset of a first episode, IV acyclovir decreases the duration of symptoms, lesions, viral shedding, systemic manifestations, and episodes of new vesicle formation. If given within 5 to 6 days of onset of a first episode, oral acyclovir decreases the duration of symptoms, lesions, viral shedding, and new vesicle formation. Both are more effective for primary than for nonprimary first episodes, and neither change the course of subsequent recurrences.

Oral acyclovir can be taken either on a daily basis to suppress recurrent disease or on an acute episodic basis to ameliorate the effects of recurrent disease. Women who take acyclovir daily as suppressive therapy have fewer recurrences, which are less severe and are of shorter duration. Many women have no recurrences, although asymptomatic shedding can occur even in the total absence of recognizable recurrences. There is no evidence that suppression influences the long-term natural history of recurrent disease, and recurrences occur with previous frequency when suppression is discontinued. The length of time one can safely remain on suppressive therapy is unknown, although continued efficacy and no cumulative toxicity is apparent with up to 5 years of use.[76] The possibility of the emergence of a resistant virus remains a concern. Suppressive therapy is currently suggested for those with more than six recurrences yearly, for those with complications associated with recurrent disease, and immunosuppressed individuals. HIV-infected individuals often require high doses of acyclovir for suppression of recurrent disease. Suppressive therapy should be discontinued periodically to assess the frequency of recurrences and the need for further therapy. Episodic oral acyclovir, taken at the earliest sign of a recurrence, decreases the duration of lesions, symptoms, viral shedding, and the formation of new lesions. It does not alter the time period between recurrences.[157]

The mainstay of treatment of genital herpes infections remains the care of local lesions and supportive care through any systemic illness. Local measures should be taken to decrease superinfections of lesions and to increase comfort. The use of an in-dwelling bladder catheter may be necessary in severe cases of herpes urethritis. Hospitalization for observation and supportive care during episodes of aseptic meningitis may be necessary. Finally, because psychologic issues frequently are more debilitating than physical manifestations of genital herpes, appropriate counseling must be provided for the emotional and informational needs of patients in whom genital herpes infection is diagnosed.[27, 118]

SYPHILIS

Syphilis occurs when the causative organism, the spirochete *Treponema pallidum*, is inoculated into mucous membranes. This occurs most frequently during sexual activity. In the United States approximately 20,000 to 30,000 new cases of syphilis are reported each year, predominantly in the 15- to 40-year age group. From 1985 to 1991, reported cases of syphilis and congenital syphilis steadily increased. From 1986 to 1989 cases of primary and secondary syphilis increased 59% but decreased for the first time in 1991.[73, 272,273] The majority of the increase in syphilis in the late 1980s was seen in urban areas, in women, and in minority populations. From 1981 to 1991, 10% to 12% of reported cases occurred in adolescents.[271] The increase in syphilis has been strongly associated with illicit drug use and HIV disease, the latter particularly in women and adolescents.[193]

Syphilis exists in well-described stages defined both by clinical presentation and by time course. The incubation period from the contact to the onset of lesions of primary syphilis ranges from 9 to 90 days, with an average time of 3 weeks. The lesions of primary syphilis are chancres; solitary, painless ulcerations that form at the site of inoculation. A chancre begins as a firm papule and breaks down to become a well-demarcated hard ulcer with a raised, rolled border and a finely granular, erythematous base. The average size of a chancre is 0.5 to 2.0 cm. Most frequently they occur on the labia, the posterior fourchette, the cervix, or the vagina, although pharyngeal and anal chancres also appear. Bilateral, firm, nontender regional adenopathy is common. Because chancres are not painful, they often remain unnoticed and undetected. Spirochetes are found at the base of the ulcer, and chancres are infectious. If untreated, chancres heal spontaneously in 2 to 6 weeks.

Nine to 90 days after chancre formation, or an average of 6 to 12 weeks after exposure, hematogenous dissemination of spirochetes occurs, and the onset of symptoms of secondary syphilis begins. The chancre of primary syphilis still may be present at this time. Secondary syphilis has mucocutaneous and systemic manifestations with multiorgan involvement. The most common manifestations of secondary syphilis are rash, lymphadenopathy, and mucous patches of the mouth or of the genital area. Various types of generalized skin lesions may occur. Usually only one type exists at a time, although lesions may evolve. Macular, maculopapular, or primarily papular generalized skin eruptions are typical. Facial sparing and involvement of the palms and soles is classic. Pustular and discoid lesions as well as alopecia and mucous membrane patches are well-described variants of the mucocutaneous lesions of secondary syphilis. Another classic lesion of secondary syphilis is the condyloma latum, which is a confluence of raised, moist, flat hypertrophic, exuberant granulomatous papular lesions that occur primarily in intertriginous or moist areas. These lesions are infectious.

Generalized, usually nontender, lymphadenopathy may commonly develop with the skin lesions of secondary syphilis. Influenza-type symptoms, such as fever, malaise, headache, sore throat, arthralgias, leukocytosis, anemia, and occasional splenomegaly typify the systemic manifestations of secondary syphilis. Manifestations of involvement of other organ systems, such as hepatitis and meningitis, also occur.

Following resolution of signs of secondary syphilis, the infection enters a latent period. Formerly, latent syphilis of up to 4 years' duration was classified as early latent syphilis, and syphilis of more than 4 years' duration was classified as late latent syphilis. Currently all syphilis of less than 1 year's duration is classified as early syphilis and little distinction is made for all latent syphilis of more than 1 year's duration. Symptoms of secondary syphillis can recur during early syphilis. Otherwise, latent syphilis is asymptomatic and is not infectious.

Manifestations of late syphilis are thought to be largely a result of endothelial damage and of ongoing chronic inflammation. Five to 20 years or more after the initial disease, the consequences of late syphilis present as single-system or as multisystem involvement.

Benign, mucocutaneous, late disease presents with painless, indolent, destructive lesions. The classic skin lesion of late syphilis is the solitary gumma; a progressive, granulomatous, necrotic ulcer. Lesions also may be nodular and multiple. Gummas and destructive lesions of late syphilis may involve visceral organs, long bones, and joints.

Cardiovascular syphilis and neurosyphilis are two other distinct forms of late syphilis. Cardiovascular syphilis prominently involves the aorta, resulting in aortic insufficiency and in thoracic aortic aneurysms. Neurosyphilis may be asymptomatic, may present as acute meningitis, or may be responsible for the gradual deterioration of intellectual and motor capacity. Neurosyphilis is likely prevented through synergy between therapy for early syphilis with penicillin and the immune system. Neurosyphilis is of particular concern in the HIV-infected individual.[96] Even without symptoms, up to 50% of HIV-infected patients with syphilis are estimated to have neurosyphilis. One series showed that 30% of HIV-infected persons with positive serologic testing for syphilis have abnormal cerebral spinal fluid exams.

Syphilis can be transmitted to the fetus at any stage of pregnancy, resulting in deformities, acute neonatal illness, and late manifestations of the disease. Congenital syphilis is prevented or ameliorated by maternal treatment during pregnancy. For this reason, premarital and prenatal screening for syphilis are mandatory. Because of the increase in congenital syphilis during the late 1980s and early 1990s, universal prenatal screening multiple times during gestation is recommended.

Diagnosis

A dark-field examination should be performed on secretions from a cleaned lesion. If spirochetes are demonstrated, a diagnosis of syphilis may be made. A positive dark-field examination is reported in 78% of chancres of primary syphilis.[2] False-negative results of dark-field examinations can occur, particularly when topical or systemic antimicrobial therapy suppresses the numbers of spirochetes.

The diagnosis of syphilis most often is made by serologic methods. Serologic tests for syphilis are of two types; nontreponemal and treponemal tests.

The nontreponemal tests most widely available are the Venereal Disease Research Laboratory (VDRL) slide tests and the rapid plasma reagin circle card test (RPR-CT). These tests detect the presence of cardiolipin, a nonspecific antigen produced during syphilitic infection. These tests are quantitative, and decreasing serial titers may be used to judge therapeutic response. An abnormal nontreponemal test result is suggestive of but not specific for a diagnosis of syphilis. Positive nontreponemal test results for syphilis also are associated with a variety of conditions and disorders, including collagen-vascular diseases, lymphomas, drug abuse, sarcoidosis, and acute infections such as mononucleosis, *Mycoplasma* infections, HIV infection, and other febrile illnesses.

A definitive diagnosis of syphilis is made by testing for the presence of specific antitreponemal antibodies. The fluorescent treponemal antibody absorption test (FTA-ABS) and the microhemagglutination treponemal serology test (MHA-TPS) are the treponemal tests most widely used. These tests confirm a diagnosis of syphilis with a low false-positive rate of 1% to 2%. Once positive, a specific antitreponemal antibody test result will remain positive despite successful therapy.

A serologic test for syphilis predicts the disease in about 75% of cases by the fourth week after exposure. By 6 weeks to 3 months, 99% to 100% of serologic test results are abnormal. Although a chancre may be present before seropositivity, secondary syphilis is usually accompanied by an abnormal serologic test result. If a serologic test result for syphilis remains negative 3 months after suspected exposure, the diagnosis of syphilis is not made. There is no association between the magnitude of antibody titer and the stage of the disease. In the late stages of syphilis, nontreponemal test results for syphilis may be negative in up to 30% of cases. However, the treponemal test result will be positive in virtually 100% of cases.

When results of a serologic test for syphilis are positive, the stage of disease is determined using historical guidelines. If the patient is presently asymptomatic and a serologic test result determined within the preceding year is negative, or if symptoms of primary or secondary syphilis are present within the preceding year, early syphilis is diagnosed. If normal serologic testing within the preceding year is not documented, and if no symptoms of primary or secondary syphilis are documented, syphilis of more than 1 year's duration is presumed. If latent syphilis of prolonged duration is suspected, a lumbar puncture will rule out neurosyphilis. However, the decision to perform this procedure must be individualized.[206] If no neurologic or psychiatric abnormalities exist, and if the treatment is penicillin, a lumbar puncture may be unnecessary because standard penicillin therapy for syphilis of more than 1 year's duration is curative for the majority of cases of asymptomatic neurosyphilis. However, all HIV-infected persons or individuals who are immunosuppressed with newly diagnosed syphilis should have a lumbar puncture performed.

Syphilis is usually diagnosed through screening and contact tracing. In addition to premarital and prenatal screening, it has been suggested that it is cost effective to screen for syphilis in patients in whom other STDs are diagnosed and in areas or populations where syphilis is diagnosed with unusual frequency.[86]

Treatment

Treatment of syphilis will abort acute disease and prevent progression of the disease but will not alter permanent changes produced by tissue destruction. Primary therapy of syphilis is with benzathine penicillin. Penicillin-allergic patients are treated with tetracycline. The length of therapy is determined by the stage of disease. Early syphilis is treated with 2.4 million units of benzathine penicillin G intramuscularly at a single session or 500 mg of tetracycline orally four times daily for 15 days. Syphilis of more than 1 year's duration is treated with the penicillin regimen just described once per week for 3 successive weeks or with tetracycline for 30 days. Penicillin-allergic patients who are pregnant or HIV-infected may need to be hospitalized for desensitization and treatment with parenteral penicillin for optimal therapy.

After successful therapy, nontreponemal serologic test results revert to normal in a large percentage of cases, depending on the duration of disease.[17, 61, 63, 202] Within 1 year 100% of patients with primary syphilis are seronegative. Within 2 years virtually all patients with secondary syphilis have normal nontreponemal serologic test results. Within 5 years approximately 45% of patients with latent syphilis are seronegative. Titers should be followed after therapy until they stabilize or disappear. If titers increase by fourfold, or if symptoms persist or recur, reinfection is presumed and retreatment is indicated.

The Jarisch-Herxheimer reaction is a well-described phenomenon occurring in some patients treated for primary or secondary syphilis. Approximately 12 hours after therapy, skin lesions become more prominent and pronounced systemic symptoms of fever, rigors, headache, myalgias, and arthralgias occur. Presumably either the release of treponemal toxins or the formation of circulating antigen-antibody complexes causes the reaction. Symptoms are self-limited and do not recur, and no specific therapy is indicated.

CHANCROID

Chancroid is a sexually transmitted disease caused by *H. ducreyi*, a short, thick, gram-negative bacillus which is a facultative anaerobe. Chancroid is characterized by painful genital ulcers and suppurative inguinal lymphadenopathy with a lack of systemic signs and symptoms. Chancroid is endemic in tropical and subtropical developing countries. The occurrence of chancroid is associated with illicit drug use, prostitution, lack of cleanliness in uncircumcised male partners, syphilis, and HIV infection. In Africa the presence of chancroid is a major risk factor for heterosexual acquisition of HIV infection. Since 1981, many outbreaks of chancroid in the United States have been documented, usually in urban areas, and are often associated with contact with an infected prostitute.[219] Unlike that of developing countries, control and eradication of outbreaks in the United States largely have been successful.

After an incubation period averaging 3 to 7 days, the genital lesions of chancroid appear as small papules or vesicles, which become pustular. These lesions rupture and form an ulcer within 1 to 3 days of their onset. These ulcers are soft, not indurated, and have irregular, ragged borders with undermined edges. A rim of erythema may surround the ulcer. The base of the ulcer is granulomatous and friable, often covered with gray, adherent, sometimes necrotic, sometimes serosanguinous exudate. Ulcers are painful and tender and may occur individually or in numbers. Contiguous spread results from autoinoculation. Ulcers vary from a few millimeters to 20 millimeters. Most often the labia, the posterior fourchette, and the perianal region are involved, but the cervix, vagina, clitoris, and urethra may be involved. Asymptomatic women can have the organism present in cervical secretions.

Regional lymph nodes are involved in more than 50% of cases. Bilateral involvement of inguinal nodes is common, although if genital lesions are unilateral, lymph node involvement is also unilateral. The lymph nodes are superficially tender, increase in size, and may become matted, suppurate, and fluctuant. Overlying skin becomes thinned and necrotic, leading to spontaneous rupture and drainage. If lymph nodes are indurated and fluctuant, they may be aspirated, and a large, chronic, draining sinus may be prevented.

Diagnosis

The accuracy of a clinical diagnosis of chancroid is approximately 80%.[46, 56] The diagnosis of chancroid is made either by scraping material from the edges of an ulcer or by collecting material from a suppurating lymph node and culturing it on specific media.[109] A Gram stain of this material reveals predominantly gram-negative coccobacillary forms often arranged in a chaining "school of fish" pattern. *H. ducreyi* may be one of many bacterial species present in the lesions of chancroid; the diagnosis in these cases may be more difficult to document. Experience is being gained with both immunofluorescent staining of lesion material and immunobinding serologic testing. The diagnosis of chancroid is often made by clinical presentation and by exclusion of other causes of genital ulceration such as genital herpes, LGV, and syphilis.[162]

Treatment

If untreated, ulcers may persist, increase in size, and form more extensive, erosive lesions. Occasionally, local lesions may run a self-limited course. Treatment classically consisted of administration of sulfa or tetracycline. Tetracycline resistance, however, is now widespread and there are increasing reports of sulfa resistance. Resistance to other antimicrobials is highly variable geographically. Currently recommended therapeutic options include erythromycin, trimethoprim-sulfamethoxazole, fluoroquinolones, and ceftriaxone. Short courses of therapy in the range of 7 to 14 days are curative for chancroid. *H. ducreyi* is rapidly eliminated from lesions and nodes, although healing takes longer, occasionally weeks. Successful therapy is heralded by subjective improvement in pain and tenderness within 2 to 3 days. Fluctuance of lymph nodes can occur despite effective therapy; aspiration of fluctuance should handle this progression. Sexual partners should be treated whether or not they are symptomatic or have visible lesions.

LYMPHOGRANULOMA VENEREUM

Lymphogranuloma venereum is a sexually transmitted disease whose major clinical manifestations result from infection of regional lymph nodes that drain sites of transient local genital infection. The causative organism of LGV is *C. trachomatis*, specifically immunotypes L1, L2, and L3. LGV is rare in North America and other industrialized countries, and is commonly found in tropical and semitropical areas, particularly in developing countries. Because of the increase in immigration from Southeast Asia and South America, the incidence of LGV in the United States is increasing.

The transient mucosal or cutaneous lesion of LGV occurs at the site of inoculation 4 to 21 days after exposure. In women, lesions usually occur individually, although they may occur in numbers. Also, they occur predominantly on the posterior vulva, the urethral meatus, and the medial labia, although the vagina and cervix may be involved. Lesions are small, vesicular, papular, or pustular and are less than 6 mm in diameter. They progress to small, shallow ulcers with irregular borders and an erythematous base. Ulcers usually are not painful and often are not recognized. After a short time, local lesions heal spontaneously, and after variable periods of latency symptoms of local lymphadenitis become manifest.

The symptoms of adenitis vary according to the lymph chains that are involved and the chronicity of infection. The immediate course of lymph node involvement is a 1- to 4-week period, during which multiple nodes become inflamed and suppurate, become fixated to overlying skin, and spontaneously rupture and drain. Chronic inflammation of involved lymphatics may lead to obstruction with retrograde edema and occasional ulceration. Involved tissue is often totally replaced by fibrosis and constriction with scarring. Repeated episodes of spontaneous rupture and drainage may lead to chronically draining sinuses, fistula formation, and scarring.

Initial LGV lesions of the anterior vulva and lower portion of the vagina drain into femoral and inguinal lymphatics, resulting in the inguinal syndrome. Multiple nodes of both inguinal and femoral regions become firm, adhere to each other, and eventfully form buboes that are fluctuant and painful with skin fixation. If both the inguinal and femoral areas are involved, buboes are separated by the inguinal ligament forming the pathognomonic groove sign. Involvement most often is unilateral. Aspiration of fluctuant nodes through normal skin can prevent spontaneous rupture with chronic sinus formation. Chronic inflammation of inguinal lymph nodes can lead to fibrous constriction of the inguinal area, often accompanied by draining sinuses. Hypertrophy and edema of vulvar lymphatic tissues can be marked. This action is called esthiomene and when it occurs is analogous to elephantiasis in men. Overlying vulvar skin may ulcerate. Chronic inflammation in the vaginal and periuretheral area can lead to stricture and fistula formation.

More often in women the perirectal and pelvic lymph nodes are involved, leading to genitorectal manifestations of LGV. This presents as a proctocolitis with bloody diarrhea and perianal discharge or as retroperitoneal lymphadenopathy demonstrated by noninvasive imaging techniques. Fibrosis of edematous mucosa eventually leads to stricture formation, and rectovaginal fistulas are common.

Unlike cases of chancroid, systemic symptoms may be present at the time of presentation of LGV. Approximately 50% of patients have fever, malaise, headache, and anorexia at the time of initial lymphadenitis.

Diagnosis

The diagnosis of LGV is most frequently made by antibody testing. Complement fixation titers to *C. trachomatis* greater than or equal to 1:128 suggest LGV. Antibody testing by microimmunofluorescence may show an increase in specific IgG titers or the presence of specific IgM antibody. Chlamydial organisms occasionally may be isolated from the exudate of fluctuant or draining buboes, or characteristic chlamydial inclusion bodies can be demonstrated by direct fluorescent antibody staining techniques. Histologic examination of involved nodes may show suggestive palisading aggregates of mononuclear cells surrounding the granulomas or the microabscesses but may be fairly nonspecific, and biopsy is not the primary mode of diagnosis.

Treatment

Treatment of LGV is usually with tetracycline continued for at least 2 weeks after the remission of all systemic symptoms and local disease. Alternative therapies include sulfonamides and erythromycin.

DONOVANOSIS

Donovanosis, formerly called granuloma inguinale, is a disease of the lower genital tract and is characterized by slowly progressive, hypertrophic ulceration with tissue destruction. Donovanosis is an STD associated with the encapsulated gram-negative bacillus *C. granulomatis*.

The incubation period of donovanosis may be up to 6 months, although it averages 2 to 4 months. The initial genital tract lesion is a painless, indurated, reddish brown papule, which over a course of days or weeks erodes and ulcerates. Ulcerations have well-defined borders and clean bases with exuberant velvety granulation tissue. Most lesions present on the vulva, are fairly superficial, and spread by contact, autoinoculation, and lymphatic extension. They are not tender unless superinfected. Involved tissue undergoes repeated granulomatous proliferation, ulceration, and scarring with eventual extensive tissue destruction. Although donovanosis most commonly results in genital ulcers, bleeding from the anogenital tract can occur in up to 20% of cases.[9,98] Extension to the inguinal area is associated with subcutaneous induration, swelling, and eventual breakdown with pseudobubo formation. Lymph nodes may be slightly increased in size and occasionally tender, but they do not suppurate. Systemic signs are rare, and when they do occur they are related to extensive disease with secondary infection.

Donovanosis is rare in Europe and North America and is most common in tropical and subtropical countries. It tends to occur in small endemic foci and has been associated with a history of syphilis.

Diagnosis

The diagnosis of donovanosis is established by demonstrating the presence of Donovan bodies in tissue preparations stained with Wright's stain or Giemsa stain. Donovan bodies are mononuclear cells containing large numbers of encapsulated bacilli. The organisms appear in clusters of blue or black, and the Donovan body resembles a safety pin. Scrapings of lesions, crush preparations of tissue, or biopsy samples taken from the edge of an ulcer reveal these characteristic formations.

Treatment

If untreated, lesions of donovanosis appear to undergo periods of spontaneous resolution or healing, with a subsequent relapse of active disease. Active lesions resolve with antibiotic therapy and relapse less frequently. Occasionally, prolonged courses of antibiotics are used to prevent recurrent disease. Doxycycline and tetracycline are the antibiotics of choice although erythromycin, ampicillin, co-trimoxazole, and streptomycin also have been effective.[129]

GENITAL WARTS

Genital warts are caused by the human papillomavirus (HPV), a DNA virus structurally and probably antigenically related to the causative agent of common skin warts. Three percent to 5% of all gynecology patients have a history of or have clinically evident warts.[12] Those with clinically evident lesions are the smaller portion of those infected with HPV. Currently, more than 50 types of HPV have been defined. Genital warts are sexually transmitted and have an incubation period ranging from 3 weeks to 8 months, averaging approximately 3 months. The transmission rate for genital warts is 25% to 60%, and infectivity may be influenced by the number and the age of the lesions. Genital warts of longer duration tend to be less infectious.

Typical genital warts are exophytic growths that appear as papillary, pink to white, frond-like lesions. These lesions are superficial, may be solitary, may occur in clusters, or may coalesce into large cauliflower-like masses. Some gross warts appear as discrete, flat-topped, hyperkeratotic papules. The lesions usually are not painful, although they may be pruritic. When exceptionally large, the warts may become necrotic and secondarily infected, resulting in superficial bleeding, discharge, and a fetid odor.

Any part of the vulva, particularly the posterior fourchette, may involve HPV. The mons, the perineum, and the perianal areas may be involved, as may be the vagina, cervix, and anal canal. If warts are present near orifices, internal involvement is apparent in 50% to 70% of cases. For this reason, all patients with vulvar warts should have a speculum examination, and all patients with perianal warts should have a rectal examination or perhaps anoscopy. Visible warts that occur in the vagina and on the cervix usually appear as flat or papular lesions. The majority of cervical warts are flat and are visible only by acetic acid staining or by colposcopy.

The growth of genital warts is stimulated by heat, moisture, and probably the number, type, and age of the lesions. Autoinoculation may be responsible for contiguous spread. In addition, some genital warts may grow remarkably during pregnancy, only to recede postpartum. Whether this is related to hormonal factors or to changes in local cellular immunity is unclear. The growth of warts tends to slow with time, and up to one third undergo spontaneous remission within 6 to 12 months. Cellular immune mechanisms are thought to partly control HPV. Diabetic individuals, immunosuppressed individuals, and those with systemic illness affecting their cellular immunity often have experienced massive growth of warts that is difficult to control.

Because documentation of only gross disease exists, the prevalence of HPV genital disease is underestimated.[12] By colposcopy, cytologic assessment, and immunoperoxidase and DNA techniques, unapparent viral presence can be documented surrounding gross disease or in multicentric locations along with gross disease. Additionally, viral presence may be found multifocally in the genital tract with no apparent visible foci.

HPV has been associated with dysplasia and with cancer of the lower genital tract, particularly of the vulva and the cervix. Among other evidence, there is a statistical association between cervical warts and cervical dysplasia, and HPV DNA is detected in several types of genital malignancies.[198] Of the multiple types of HPV, certain types more than others are associated with malignancy. For example, HPV types 6 and 11 are seen in most cases of typical genital warts or in association with mild dysplasia. HPV types 16 and 18 are disproportionately associated with severe dysplasia and malignancy of both the cervix and the vulva.

Diagnosis

The diagnosis of genital warts is suggested by a typical gross appearance and by the exclusion of other processes by biopsy. Colposcopic localization of lesions may be of value. Histologic features of genital warts include papilomatosis, acanthosis, and parakeratosis with vacuolization of epithelial cells. Specific HPV detection by DNA probes or immunoblot techniques can help to characterize histologically equivocal lesions. In addition, by revealing characteristic koilocytotic changes, cervical Papanicolaou smears may suggest the presence of HPV in up to 1% to 2% of childbearing women. Typing a virus by DNA probe or by in situ hybridization techniques is in the investigational stage. At present, typing of HPV is not clinically helpful in guiding either prognosis or therapy.

Treatment

Genital warts are commonly treated with either local cytotoxic agents or ablative therapy. Local application of 20% to 25% podophyllin in benzoin, an antimitotic agent that incorporates into the wart, causes sloughing of the tissue within 3 to 4 days. This treatment is slightly less effective for hyperkeratotic warts and may need to be repeated at weekly intervals for resolution of larger warts. Repeated self-application of 0.5% podophyllotoxin, one of the active components of podophyllin, has been reported to be safe and efficacious.[15] Trichloroacetic acid and bichloroacetic acid is of particular value as a treatment for flat warts and for warts on mucosal surfaces.

Cryocautery, laser therapy, and electrocautery all have been used successfully as ablative therapy.[245, 289] During cryocautery, the lesions should be frozen to the base. The blistering and the resolution of the lesions may take place with initial freezing or may require repeated freezings. Laser therapy and electrocautery both attempt to completely remove lesions at the initial therapy. Fewer warts recur after laser therapy if a margin of normal-appearing tissue is also treated.[259] All ablative therapies are associated with recurrences of warts to some degree, probably because of latent HPV infection in surrounding tissues. Recurrences are more common in immunosuppressed individuals. Also, recurrences in these individuals or in women older than 40 years of age may be associated with malignancy, including squamous disease of the lower genital tract and lymphoproliferative disorders.[149] There is no apparent difference in treatment failures according to whether or not male partners are evaluated and treated.[121] Occasionally, large warts require surgical removal. However, electrocautery and surgical removal can be associated with significant blood loss, particularly during pregnancy.

Most studies of interferon suggest that the majority of warts regress with therapy. However, warts often recur when interferon is used alone. Increasing experience with interferon therapy, either systemic, topical, or intralesional, suggests that this may be useful as adjunctive therapy in addition to ablative therapy for treatment of extensive lesions.[273]

Any associated vaginal infections should be treated concomitantly. Any decrease in local moisture can limit the growth of lesions that are present. Occasionally, small lesions may resolve spontaneously with symptomatic therapy. After the initial disappearance or the removal of lesions, follow-up of patients and prompt treatment for new or recurrent lesions is necessary.

Patients with a history of genital warts or those with persistent or atypical genital warts should be followed for the possibility of dysplasia or malignancy. Biopsies of persistent or atypical lesions should be performed.

MOLLUSCUM CONTAGIOSUM

Molluscum contagiosum is a benign viral skin infection caused by a DNA-containing pox virus. This infection is spread by intimate, skin-to-skin contact, by autoinoculation, and occasionally by fomites. Perigenital molluscum contagiosum is sexually transmitted, and at least 10% of women diagnosed with molluscum are diagnosed concomitantly with another STD.[194]

Characteristic molluscum lesions are small (2 to 5 mm), flesh-colored or slightly erythematous, firm papules. They have umbilicated centers and are found on the epidermal surfaces of the extremities, trunk, or genital areas, including the lower abdomen, pubic area, and inner thighs. Lesions appear 2 to 7 weeks after contact and are usually multiple and asymptomatic. Lesions may occur in crops, and often spontaneously resolve. The entire course of the disease lasts 6 to 9 months.

Diagnosis

Diagnosis of molluscum contagiosum is usually made by its clinical appearance. Lesions project into the dermis but do not cross the basement membrane. They can be removed intact, and when crushed onto a slide, Wright's or Giemsa stain reveals molluscum bodies in infected cells. These are ovoid accumulations of replicating virus within the cytoplasm.

Treatment

Most molluscum contagiosum infections resolve, if left untreated. However, to contain the spread of lesions or for cosmetic purposes, treatment may be indicated.[13] Individual lesions can be extracted by curette or by incision. Cryotherapy with liquid nitrogen is effective, comfortable, and widely used. The use of laser has also been described.

Widespread distribution of molluscum-like lesions, giant lesions, and occurrence in atypical locations, such as the face, have occured with severe cellular immunosuppression in association with HIV infection. A biopsy of such lesions is recommended before treatment to rule out fungal skin infection, in particular *Cryptococcus neoformans*.[182, 220]

VAGINITIS

Vaginitis is characterized by abnormal discharge, vulvovaginal discomfort, or both. Many microorganisms, including those associated with vaginitis can be cultured from the vagina of asymptomatic women. Unless symptoms are present, the diagnosis of vaginitis should not be made, and in the majority of cases treatment is not indicated.

An average of four to seven organisms can be found upon routine culturing of the vagina.[7, 70, 71, 127, 136] Both aerobic and anaerobic bacteria are present. Potential pathogens of the upper genital tract such as gram-negative enteric rods, staphylococcus species, streptococci (including enterococci), anaerobic gram-positive cocci, and bacteroides species, are considered to be normal flora of the vagina. In addition, nonpathogens such as lactobacilli and diphtheroids also are frequently found. The normal pH of the vagina is 3.5 to 4.5.[100] The pH of the vagina is influenced by the organic acid by-products of metabolism, which are produced by the predominant species in the vaginal flora. Both vaginal pH and normal vaginal flora must be considered when vaginitis is diagnosed. It is increasingly apparent that lactobacilli are regarded as an important microbial defense. Hydrogen peroxide-producing species appear to be associated with vaginal health, whereas H_2O_2-negative species are associated with infection and vaginitis-associated organisms.[90] Antibiotics, hormonal changes, disease states, immunosuppression, and sexual activity all may have an influence on vaginal microflora.[70, 145, 152, 154] Cervical mucus and normal vaginal discharge must be considered when the symptoms of vaginitis are interpreted.

Three types of infectious vaginitis are recognized (Table 21-8). These are discussed in turn.

Candidiasis. The majority of candidiasis is caused by *Candida albicans*, an organism that can be found in the lower genital tract of 30% to 80% of women with minimal or no symptoms. A small number of fungal vaginal infections are caused by *Candida glabrata* or by other candidal species.

The hallmark of candidiasis is itching, irritation, or both. Itching may be quite severe in either the vaginal or vulvar area and irritation may be associated with dysuria and dyspareunia. Discharge is commonly described as cottage cheesy or thick, white, and clumpy, although it is not always present with symptomatic candidiasis and occasionally may be thin and watery.

Symptoms of candidiasis frequently begin just before the menses. In addition, a number of precipitating factors in symptomatic candidiasis are delineated. *Candida* species frequently may be found in the vagina, and some of the precipitating factors for symptomatic candidiasis are those that foster overgrowth of *Candida*. This overgrowth may occur by the depression of normal bacterial flora, the depression of local cellular immunity, alterations in the metabolic and nutritional milieu of the vagina, and unknown mechanisms. Precipitating factors for symptomatic candidiasis include immunosuppressive or steroid therapy, diabetes mellitus, pregnancy, hormone replacement therapy, oral contraceptive agents, and systemic antibiotics. One study suggested that women treated with systemic antibiotics were 5.5 times more likely to develop symptomatic

Table 21-8. Diagnosis of vaginits

	Typical symptoms	Clinical findings	Discharge	Wet pH	Preparation	Other
Candidiasis	Itching, irritation, dyspareunia	Erythema, edema	White and clumpy, occasionally watery and clumpy, may be none	< 4.5	Potassium hydroxide reveals hyphae, buds	Culture may be of value
Trichomoniasis	Discharge, pain occasionally itching	Strawberry cervix or vagina	Copious, pooling, frothy gray-white to yellow-green	> 5.5	Saline reveals motile *Trichomonas*	> 10 WBCs/HPF
Bacterial vaginosis	Discharge, odor	No mucosal changes	Sticky, homogenous	> 4.7	Saline reveals clue cells	Positive Whiff test; lack of WCBs and lactobacilli

candidiasis within 28 days compared with controls taking no antibiotics.

Candidiasis often presents as apparent vulvitis or vulvovaginitis. Examination reveals well-demarcated erythema of the vulva with satellite lesions surrounding the major rim of erythema. The vulva can be notably edematous. The vagina also may be edematous and erythematous, with erythema extending onto the squamous exocervix. Excoriations and fissures of the vulva and occasionally the vagina are not unusual. Even if discharge has not been described by the patient, an adherent clumpy white discharge may be found in the upper portion of the vagina. The pH of this discharge is most often less than 4.5. When 1 drop of the discharge is mixed with 1 drop of 10% KOH, covered with a coverslip, and examined under the microscope, normal cellular elements are lysed, and the branching hyphae and buds of the *Candida* are visible. In up to 25% to 30% of cases of symptomatic candidiasis, the KOH wet preparation is falsely negative. When candidiasis is suspected from the clinical presentation, diagnostic accuracy can be improved by use of the Gram stain or by culture on specific media. Hyphae and buds are gram-positive; buds are slightly larger than WBCs. Solid media used for specific *Candida* cultures include Nickerson's media and Sabouraud agar.

Initial treatment of candidiasis is with local vaginal antifungal preparations. Nystatin suppositories or cream can be used twice daily for 14 days. Imidazole (miconazole, clotrimazole, butoconazole) and triazole (terconazole) cream or suppositories have slightly higher initial cure rates. Treatment ranges from 1 to 7 days with doses decreasing in strength, and all are approximately equally efficacious. A shorter course of therapy with a higher dose may decrease symptoms more rapidly but may be associated with an increased rate of local hypersensitivity reactions. Miconazole and clotrimazole cream or suppositories are used once daily for 7 days and have a slightly higher initial cure rate. Possibly these preparations may be used for shorter periods of time to achieve acceptable cure rates. Interest has developed in the use of boric acid (600 to 650 mg in a gel capsule used daily for 14 days) to treat candidiasis.[263] Initial results indicate acceptable cure rates, and the lack of compounding chemicals makes this an attractive therapeutic alternative in patients who are hypersensitive to other local antiinfective agents. Gentian violet-impregnated tampons are messy and occasionally irritate but are useful in some patients. Application of gentian violet directly to the vaginal vault each week until symptoms resolve is inconvenient but may be helpful in recurrent cases.

Ketoconazole is a systemic oral antifungal agent that has been efficacious in the treatment of vulvovaginal candidiasis. Whether this therapy is more effective than local preparations is unclear. The exact duration of therapy required to achieve the highest cure rates is unknown. However, 1- to 2-week courses of therapy are probably effective in the majority of cases. With the use of more long-term ketoconazole, the most serious side effect is a reversible but occasionally severe hepatotoxic reaction. Fluconazole is a newer systemic oral antifungal agent that appears to have fewer side effects and is also effective in decreasing symptoms of candidiasis. Oral therapy is not associated with better cure rates for acute infections than local therapies.

Some women develop chronic symptoms or recurrent episodes of candidiasis. Such recurrent vulvovaginitis has been associated with transient suppression of local cell-mediated immunity and, in some cases, with enhanced local allergic responses to *Candida* as well as other locally applied substances.[58, 64, 279-282] Recurrences do not appear to be associated with drug resistance. The risk factors for recurrent candidiasis are poorly understood, but may include oral contraceptives, frequent use of local therapies including douching and spermicides, and multiple antibiotic therapies.[195, 225, 235]

A number of approaches to recurrent candidiasis exist.[225] Longer courses of therapy can be used. Intermittent therapy with agents such as clotrimazole or boric acid over a long term, such as 3 to 6 months, is reported to decrease recurrences.[110] Male sexual partners displaying symptoms can be treated. However, general treatment of all male partners has not been shown to be helpful. Although general dietary changes are not helpful, daily ingestion of yoghurt containing *Lactobacillus acidophilus* appears to decrease candida colonization and symptomatic infections.[88] Long-term, low-dose suppressive ketoconazole decreases multiple recurrences of symptomatic candidiasis in healthy women. Suppressive therapy with fluconazole is used extensively to suppress candidal syndromes in HIV-infected individuals and may prove to be efficacious and well tolerated in others.

Trichomoniasis. Trichomoniasis is caused by the flagellated parasite *T. vaginalis*. Male partners of women with trichomoniasis may harbor *Trichomonas*, and there is a high rate of reinfection of women whose male sexual partners are not treated concomitantly. For this reason, trichomoniasis is considered to be an STD. It is often isolated along with other sexually transmitted organisms, in particular, *N. gonorrhoeae*. Risk factors associated with sexual activity, such as multiple or new partners, increase the chances of contracting trichomonas.[6]

The incubation period for trichomoniasis is approximately 20 days. Symptoms often peak just after the menses. Classic symptoms of trichomoniasis include a copious, frothy discharge and local pain and irritation. Dysuria, dyspareunia, and dull lower abdominal pain may be present. Occasionally, itching is the predominant local symptom.

Examination of the vulva and vagina reveals a copious, frothy discharge that is most often white to greenish yellow. The pH of the discharge is greater than 6.0. A wet preparation made by mixing 1 drop of the discharge with 1 drop of normal saline reveals motile trichomonads in the majority of cases of symptomatic trichomoniasis. These parasites are slightly larger than WBCs, are ovoid, and possess a central undulating membrane and a terminal flagella. In addition, greater than 10 WBCs/HPF are found on wet preparation in the majority of cases. Diagnostic accuracy with normal findings from a wet preparation can be improved by a culture in specific media, such as Diamond medium or Tichosel broth.[65, 123] Papanicolau smears occasionally reveal trichomonads but have a false-positive rate of 30% to 40% in diagnosing trichomoniasis.[274]

Occasionally, the cervix and upper portion of the vagina have raised, punctate erythema. This strawberry appearance is pathognomonic for trichomoniasis but is found in the minority of cases.

The most effective therapy for trichomoniasis currently available in the United States is oral metronidazole. Two dosage regimens have been shown to be effective. A single high-dose therapy with 2 gm of metronidazole effectively eradicates *Trichomonas* in 90% of cases. Particularly when this therapy is taken with other medications, severe nausea and vomiting occasionally preclude effective use. Lower-dose longer-term therapy with 250 mg three times daily for 7 to 10 days or 500 mg twice daily for 5 to 7 days also may be used. Because many women are reinfected by their male sexual partners, common practice is to treat male partners whether or not they are asymptomatic. If metronidazole cannot be used, intravaginal clotrimazole or boric acid may provide relief from symptoms and may be curative in some cases. Trichomonas infections that are relatively resistant to metronidazole occur in a few cases. High-dose therapy repeated for 3 to 5 days, concomitant oral and vaginal therapy, and intravenous metronidazole all have cured resistant trichomoniasis.[163]

Trichomoniasis has been implicated as a risk factor in post-hysterectomy cuff cellulitis, cuff abscess, and adverse outcome of pregnancy. Some authorities have proposed routine screening for and therapy of trichomonas before gynecologic surgery and during prenatal care.

Bacterial vaginosis. Bacterial vaginosis (BV), formerly called *Gardnerella-associated vaginitis* or *nonspecific vaginitis*, is characterized by excessive discharge and odor. Although for many years the exact microbiologic etiology of this infection was unknown, this infection is now regarded as a result of synergism among various bacteria, including *Gardnerella vaginalis*, *Mobiluncus* species, and vaginal anaerobes. *G. vaginalis* is commonly found as part of the vaginal flora in approximately one third of sexually active women. Without a critical concentration of other vaginal bacteria, particularly anaerobes, this organism is not thought to be responsible for symptoms.[234] The effect bacterial synergy has in causing symptoms is shown using gas-liquid chromatography on specimens from patients with symptomatic disease. This process reveals organic acid metabolites of anaerobes and the disappearance of symptoms that correlate with the appearance of metabolites produced by *Lactobacillus* and streptococcal species. The replacement of lactobacilli by *G. vaginalis*, anaerobes such as *Bacteroides* species and *Mobiluncus*, and genital mycoplasms is a characteristic feature of bacterial vaginosis.[233]

BV is more commonly seen in sexually active premenopausal women. It does not appear to be closely associated with sexual activity, and the treatment of male sexual partners is not necessary to cure the majority of cases.

The onset of odor and discharge associated with BV is evenly distributed throughout the menstrual cycle, and local discomfort is rarely a problem.

The diagnosis of BV is made with a high degree of certainty on examination of the patient and of the discharge. Up to 50% of women with BV may be asymptomatic. The discharge of BV is typically homogeneous, grayish white to yellowish white, and partially adherent to the vulva and vaginal walls. Underlying edema or erythema of the vulva or vagina are not typical. The pH of this vaginal discharge is greater than 4.7. When 1 drop of KOH is added to 1 drop of discharge, an intense amine odor produces a positive Whiff test result. Typically this discharge on normal saline wet preparation has a paucity of WBCs and a predominance of clue cells produced by the adherence of *G. vaginalis* to epithelial cells. By wet preparation, clue cells are best identified by a stippled birefringence, which so densely covers the epithelial cell that the normal borders and nuclei are obscured. By Gram stain, clue cells can be identified as epithelial cells almost totally covered by small, gram-negative rods. A paucity of other organisms can be seen in the background. Notably there is an absence of lactobacilli. BV can be diagnosed clinically by the presence of 3 of the following: (1) homogeneous discharge; (2) pH $\geq$ 4.7; (3) positive Whiff test; and (4) clue cells.[255] The single most reliable sign is the presence of clue cells. Laboratory tests that detect the presence of the microbial by-products unique to BV, such as volatile amines by gas-liquid chromatography, proline aminopeptidase by colorimetric assay, and sialidases, are used on a research basis but are not yet clinically applicable.[253] Various scoring systems that assess the presence and concentration of lactobacilli, clue cells, and gram-negative or gram-variable rods or curved organisms consistent with anaerobic *Bacteroides* and *Mobiluncus* species have been proposed.[54, 89, 169] Gram stain assessment may prove to be valuable when immediate microscopy is not available and for greater reproducibility as a research tool. Culture on specific media is rarely useful. BV-associated organisms may be present as part of the normal vaginal flora, although concentrations are typically higher when BV is present.

The most effective treatment for BV is metronidazole.[184] Dose regimens of 2 g per day, 2 g every 2 days, and 250 mg three times a day or 500 mg twice a day for 5 to 7 days appear to be equally effective.[139] Metronidazole is thought to cure this infection because of its effect on the vaginal anaerobes. Increasing experience suggests that vaginal therapy with metronidazole gel or clindamycin cream are also effective.[248] Alternative therapy with oral ampicillin, cephalosporins, or vaginal acidification may be effective in a few cases. Symptoms may recur within 1 month after treatment in up to 15% of cases. The risk factors in recurrence are incompletely understood, but BV may be more commonly seen in users of diaphragms or vaginal contraceptive sponges.

BV has been associated with more invasive infections, including urinary tract infections in diaphragm users, PID, posthysterectomy infection, postpartum endometritis, and intraamniotic infection.[50,54,228, 229, 254] A reduction in these infections by screening for and by treatment of BV has not been demonstrated.

Other causes of vaginitis symptoms. Excessive vaginal discharge may be a manifestation of cervicitis. Organisms associated with cervicitis include *T. vaginalis*, *N. gonorrhoeae*, *C. trachomatis*, and herpes simplex virus. If diagnosed, these conditions should be treated accordingly. In addition, excess vaginal discharge may be associated with cervical ectopy or eversion, with no apparent infectious etiology.

Discharge and odor are associated with the presence of foreign bodies in the vaginal vault. Although this is mainly a concern in pediatric populations, forgotten tampons may also be a source of discharge.

In addition to vulvar dystrophies, dysplasias, and vulvar vestibulitis syndrome, vulvar discomfort may be a result of hypersensitivity reactions. These should be considered in women who have received numerous courses of topical anti-infective therapy.

URINARY TRACT INFECTION

One in 5 women have a urinary tract infection (UTI) at some time, up to 25% of women will experience symptoms of acute dysuria each year, and 3 to 5 million visits to physicians yearly are for the evaluation of UTIs or related symptoms. Although UTI is not a gynecologic infection, symptoms associated with this type of infection occur with various gynecologic disorders and women frequently visit a gynecologist for diagnosis of UTI.

The vast majority of symptomatic UTIs, which are commonly termed cystitis, involve the lower urinary tract. UTIs may present as asymptomatic bacteriuria or acute pyelonephritis. Symptoms suggestive of lower UTIs are also seen with STDs, various noninfectious urethral syndromes, and vaginitis.

Women with lower UTI present with acute symptoms of dysuria, frequency, and urgency. They also experience gross hematuria, suprapubic pain, and flank or back discomfort. Both pyuria and bacteriuria are present in symptomatic lower UTI.

The previously held belief that "significant bacteriuria" necessary for a diagnosis of UTI consists of 100,000 or more organisms/mL is clearly erroneous when referring to lower UTI. Although 50% of women with lower UTI have 100,000 or more organisms cultured from urine, approximately one third of women who present with symptoms of acute dysuria, frequency, and urgency have between 100 and 100,000 organisms by properly obtained culture yet warrant a diagnosis of UTI.[238, 241] Studies of bladder urine specimens obtained by suprapubic aspiration or by transurethral catheterization demonstrated that smaller numbers of organisms in symptomatic women are associated with reproducible bladder bacteriuria, pyuria, and a predictable response to UTI therapy. The concept of significant bacteriuria or a single organism colony count of 100,000 or more organisms/mL is appropriate only when applied to asymptomatic bacteriuria[115] or acute pyelonephritis.

More than 90% of UTIs in women are caused by two organisms, *E. coli* and *Staphylococcus saprophyticus*,[99] with at least 80% caused by *E. coli*.

Approximately 20% of women with UTI have recurrences of symptoms within variable periods of time. Recurrences are most often reinfections, demonstrated by culture negativity between episodes and by the isolation of different organisms as shown by determining the biotype and the sensitivity patterns in each episode. These reinfections rarely represent serious morbidity or renal involvement. Recurrences develop in characteristic clusters of symptomatic UTI, often during 6- to 12-month time periods.

Less frequently, recurrent symptoms result from the persistence of the same organism. In particular, close intervals of 10 to 14 days between symptomatic recurrences may indicate upper tract infection. Persistence of a single organism raises the concern of congenital or acquired structural or functional abnormalities of the urinary tract.

UTIs are dependent both on host factors and the properties of infecting organisms. Bacterial adherence to uroepithelial cells precedes infection. Flora, particularly coliforms, from the GI tract colonize the vaginal introital and periurethral-meatal area and ascend into the bladder, causing both symptomatic and asymptomatic bacteriuria. Various bacterial adhesions, surface receptor sites, and attachment properties of bacteria have been identified.[147, 197] Women susceptible to UTIs demonstrate an increase in the incidence and density of colonization and more sites for bacterial attachment on uroepithelial surfaces compared with women without UTIs. The efficiency of bacterial adherence is probably influenced by genetic, hormonal, and other factors. Natural defenses against the bacterial adherence to and the ascent into the urinary tract may be genetically determined. These defenses include various substances produced by the urinary tract, local immunoglobulins, competitive bacterial flora, and normal voiding patterns.

Among sexually active women, most lower UTIs are associated with sexual intercourse.[59] The largest proportion of susceptible women become symptomatic within a short period of time after intercourse. Intercourse is thought to introduce colonizing bacteria into the bladder and is shown to transiently increase the numbers of bacteria in the urine up to tenfold.

An independent risk factor of UTI is diaphragm use.[60, 247] Compared with nonusers, diaphragm users have two to two and one half times the risk for UTI and have increased vaginal colonization with coliforms. Other risk factors for UTI include a past history of UTI and the failure to void following intercourse. Factors not associated with UTI include perineal hygiene, direction of wiping, tampons, and oral contraceptives.

Two percent to 10% of women have asymptomatic bacteriuria, as defined by the presence of 100,000 or more single pathogens found on more than two midstream, clean, voided specimens. Asymptomatic bacteriuria may be transient or intermittent, and whether or not its natural, long-term course is influenced by treatment is unclear. In nonpregnant, nonimmunocompromised women with normal urinary tracts, asymptomatic bacteriuria does not appear to be associated with UTI or with long-term morbidity and does not require eradication. In conditions that predispose to upper UTI, such as pregnancy, eradication is warranted.

Studies suggest that early infection or colonization of the upper urinary tract occurs in a proportion of women with lower UTI. How many women subsequently develop acute pyelonephritis if left untreated is unclear. However, the majority of women with lower UTI appear not to be predisposed to acute pyelonephritis. The occurrence of pyelonephritis is influenced by pathogenic properties of bacteria and by factors in the host that affect bacterial adherence and ascent. Abnormalities of the urinary tract such as reflux, obstruction or stones, abnormalities in host defenses (e.g., diabetes and immunosuppression), and the introduction of virulent bacteria during catheterization or during other instrumentation all are associated with pyelonephritis. Pyelonephritis causes dysuria, frequency, and urgency in 50% of cases. In addition, fever, chills, malaise, and flank or back (costovertebral angle) pain and tenderness are hallmarks. Pyelonephritis is more morbid than lower UTI; it increases the risk of bacteremia, long-term sequelae and the need for longer treatment.

Women who present with dysuria, frequency, and urgency may not have bacterial infection of the lower urinary tract.[120, 239] Urethritis caused by STDs such as *C. trachomatis*, *N. gonorrhoeae*, *T. vaginalis*, and *Herpes simplex* can cause identical symptoms. Epidemiologic risk factors, sexual history or history of disease in sexual partners, and associated symptomatology may suggest these diagnoses. Symptoms of urethritis typically occur less acutely, and urinalysis reveals pyuria but rarely hematuria. Urethritis is suspected in symptomatic women who have pyuria with negative urine cultures. In particular, *Chlamydia* causes symptoms in one third of women with dysuria, pyuria, and negative urine cultures.

Vaginitis also may cause dysuria and urgency. Although vaginitis classically causes external dysuria and UTI causes internal dysuria, this distinction is unreliable. If a urinalysis is properly obtained, and if bacteriuria and pyuria are not demonstrable, other symptoms and signs of vaginitis should become apparent by direct history and examination.

Diagnosis

The diagnosis of UTI is made by urinalysis and urine culture.

The majority of women with symptomatic UTI who later are documented to have bacteriuria have pyuria with more than 8 to 10 WBCs/mL in unspun urine and 2 to 5 WBCs/HPF in spun urine sediment. Some authorities suggest that the presence of pyuria be used as a screen to determine which urine specimens should be cultured and which women should be treated presumptively for UTI.

A midstream, clean, voided urine sample, cultured using quantitative techniques, is appropriate for the evaluation of asymptomatic bacteriuria, pyelonephritis, and the majority of cases of lower UTI. If lower UTI is associated with bacterial counts between 100 and 100,000 colonies/mL, contamination of specimens with other organisms may confuse the interpretation of culture results. Clarification by culture of suprapubic aspiration or catheterization specimens may occasionally be of value. Urine cultures that reveal 100,000 or more colonies/mL of a single pathogen support the diagnosis of UTI in asymptomatic women; cultures that reveal 100 or more colonies/mL of a single pathogen support the diagnosis of UTI in symptomatic women. Microbiology laboratories should be instructed to identify all bacterial species in cultures obtained from symptomatic women and to quantify and identify all *E. coli* and staphylococcal species in cultures obtained from symptomatic women.

Whether recurrences of infection are episodes of reinfection or are persistent infection should be determined. Persistence of infection despite adequate antibiotic therapy or multiple episodes of reinfection, variably defined as more than three to six episodes in 1 year warrants urologic referral and evaluation for urinary tract abnormality. In addition, episodes of pyelonephritis in nonpregnant women or infections with unusual organisms, such as *Proteus* and other urea splitters associated with stone formation, are indications for urologic consultation.

The majority of symptomatic lower urinary tract reinfections is not associated with urinary tract abnormalities. Women can predict the presence of UTI by symptoms in cases of reinfection with 90% accuracy. With assurance of normalcy of the urinary tract and with known patterns of previous cultures and infections, the institution of therapy without laboratory diagnosis is suggested to be a cost-effective and appropriate alternative.

The proper diagnosis of lower UTI must take into account alternative diagnoses for symptoms of dysuria, frequency, and urgency. In addition to urinalysis and to urine culture, pelvic examination, wet preparations, and STD cultures may be warranted (Table 21-9).

Treatment

Single-dose antimicrobial therapy or standard dosage schedules of antibiotics for periods of 3, 5, 7, or 10 days all are appropriate therapy for lower UTI. Without antibiotic therapy UTI resolves spontaneously in up to 70% of women. However, treatment eliminates symptoms more quickly, may treat unrecognized upper UTI, and may decrease recurrent, symptomatic infection.

Approximately 80% of lower UTI is cured with single-dose therapy.[230] Appropriate single-dose agents include trimethoprim-sulfamethoxazole, trimethoprim, sulfasoxizole, and ampicillin or amoxicillin. Cephalosporins are not effective single-agent choices. Single-dose therapy is not appropriate for children, pregnant women, or women with underlying medical problems. Symptoms often do not disappear for 2 to 3 days and often persist up to this point. This persistence is not a demonstration of failure of single-dose therapy.

Standard antibiotic dosage regimens of 3 to 5 days cure 80% to 90% of lower UTI and result in fewer early recurrences when compared with single-dose therapy. Whether 7- to 14-day courses of antibiotics provide further benefit is unclear. Appropriate standard dosage regimen choices include nitrofurantoin, trimethoprim-sulfamethoxazole, other sulphas, trimethoprim, penicillins, ampicillin or ampicillin combinations, and cephalosporins. The use of the newer quinoline antibiotics should probably be reserved for infection with resistent gram-negative organisms.

Pyelonephritis should be treated with standard antibiotic dosage regimens for at least 10 days. Occasionally hospitalization for IV therapy is chosen because of the degree of illness or fever. In these cases, IV therapy should continue for at least 24 hours of afebrility and a total course of 10 days with oral antibiotics.

The frequency of recurrent symptomatic lower UTI that results from reinfection is decreased by low-dose antibiotics given prophylactically either as a single night-time dose or as a single postintercourse dose. Nitrofurantoin and

Table 21-9. Differential diagnosis of symptoms of dysuria, frequency, and urgency

	Onset	Urinalysis	Urine culture	Causative organisms
Lower UTI	Acute	pyuria, hematuria	$\geq$ 100 organisms/mL	*E. coli, S. saprophyticus*
Pyelonephritis	Subacute (up to 10 days)	pyuria, hematuria, casts	$\geq$ 100,000 organisms/mL	*E. coli*, other gram-negative enterics, enterococci
Urethritis	Acute or subacute	pyuria	—	*C. trachomatis, T. vaginalis, N. gonorrhoeae, H. simplex*
Vaginitis	Acute or subacute	—	—	*T. Vaginalis, C. albicans*
Other lower urinary tract syndromes	Subacute	—	—	—

trimethoprim-sulfamethoxazole demonstrate prophylactic benefit. Therapy should be instituted only after the infection has been cured and should be empirically continued for 6-month periods. Alternatively, self-medication with short-course therapy at the earliest signs of reinfection may be more cost effective and more acceptable to patients than prophylaxis.

POSTOPERATIVE INFECTIONS

Virtually all major and minor surgical procedures of the lower genital tract may result in localized postsurgical infection. The risk of operative site infection most strongly correlates with contamination of the operative site by potential pathogens. Procedures that expose the upper genital tract, the intraabdominal cavity, or any skin wounds to lower genital tract flora may result in significant postoperative infection.

A discussion of the microbiology of the lower genital tract facilitates an understanding of the microbiology of postoperative infection. The vulva, vagina, and cervix normally are colonized with a wide variety of bacteria. The lower genital tract flora is polymicrobial and includes both aerobic and anaerobic organisms. The exact composition of lower genital tract flora varies among individuals and appears to be influenced by age, hormonal status, sexual experience, and possibly immune status. Tissue type may also affect flora, possibly because of differences in bacterial adherence to cell surfaces and differences in cell turnover. Although the vulva, vagina, and cervix are colonized with similar species of organisms, the exact types and the quantities of organisms present in each area may be distinct. Bacteriologic surveys of lower genital tract flora have been performed on various patient populations by several investigators.

The results of prevalence surveys of lower genital tract flora have been compared with infection site cultures. Some species of bacteria frequently are found at sites of infection and are classified as potential pathogens. Other organisms that are part of the normal lower genital tract flora do not commonly cause local or systemic infections and are considered to be of very low pathogenic potential. Certain bacterial species, such as *E. coli* and *B. fragilis*, are underrepresented in the lower genital tract compared with their occurrence at the site of infection. This may represent a propensity of these organisms to invade and to cause infection. The presence of virulence factors in certain organisms may contribute to their pathogenicity; the presence of a polysaccharide capsular antigen that helps to resist phagocytosis and opsonization while enhancing tissue invasiveness is an example of one such factor.

The pathogenic potential of the lower genital tract flora may also be determined by interactions between bacteria. Some organisms may be capable of initially invading tissue and thereby causing inflammation. Other organisms may contribute to the inflammation and may further the process of infection once initial tissue destruction has progressed and once anaerobic conditions are present. Therefore the types and the quantity of organisms present and the proportions of potential pathogens at an operative site all may determine postoperative infection.

The major aerobic pathogens in postoperative infections are enterobacteriaceae, including *E. coli*; streptococci, including *S. viridans*; enterococci; and staphylococci, including *S. aureus*. *S. aureus* and streptococcal species may be the sole pathogens at the site of wound infections, and other organisms may the sole pathogens at the site of postoperative infection. However, most often these organisms are seen in combination with other aerobic or anaerobic organisms. The most numerous anaerobic pathogens are the anaerobic gram-positive cocci, including anaerobic streptococci, peptococci, and peptostreptococci. *Bacteroides* species, including *B. fragilis* and *B. melaninogenicus*, are major anaerobic pathogens of wound and soft tissue infection. *Clostridum perfringens* and other anaerobic bacteria are less prevalent but are potential pathogens.

Cultures of the lower genital tract may not accurately reflect the organisms that are present at the site of postoperative infection. Unless material from postoperative abscesses or from wound infections is obtained for culture, treatment is most often based on the knowledge of which species may be involved in an infection. Aerobic organisms such as the streptococci and coliforms are of particular concern in acute illness. Anaerobes, particularly the *Bacteroides* species, are of concern especially in abscess formation.

The risk of infection after hysterectomy ranges from 7% to 30%. After vaginal hysterectomy, pelvic infections such as cuff cellulitis or pelvic abscess may occur. The risk of both pelvic and abdominal wound infection exists following abdominal hysterectomy. Women with posthysterectomy pelvic cellulitis experience fever and lower pelvic pain 2 to 5 days after surgery. The vaginal cuff is often indurated, warm, and very painful. Postoperative pelvic abscesses of the vaginal cuff, pelvic floor, and side walls at the site of intra-abdominal blood collection or in the adnexal structures usually occur more than 5 days after hysterectomy. Pelvic cellulitis often responds to simple broad-spectrum antibiotic therapy, not including extensive coverage for *B. fragilis*. If the formation of an early abscess is suggested, response to initial therapy is not prompt, or the patient is severely ill, antimicrobial coverage for gram-negative enteric bacilli, streptococci, anaerobic cocci, and *B. fragilis* must be provided. Drainage of the vaginal cuff can be a helpful adjunct to antibiotic therapy. In fact, surgical management of post-operative abscesses must be considered when the response to antibiotic therapy is not prompt and complete.

Postoperative wound infections may present acutely with fever and incisional pain, erythema, induration, warmth, and tenderness. Group A β-hemolytic *Streptococcus* can cause wound infection and high fevers within 24 to 48 hours of surgery. However, a less immediate onset of wound infection is typical. Often a wound infection is the cause of spiking, low-grade fevers, whose source does not become obvious until a collection of pus is discovered through spontaneous drainage or by wound exploration. More than 20% of wound infections become apparent after hospitalization. *S. aureus* and other skin organisms are common causes of postoperative wound infections. Mixed flora may also cause wound infections after genital tract surgery. Because of the unique exposure to mixed aerobic-anaerobic pathogens during surgery, patients are at risk of a distinct but uncommon *synergistic wound infection*. Synergistic wound infections occur when both aerobic and anaerobic organisms invade tissue planes. Some authorities theorize that aerobic organisms cause initial tissue infection and tissue damage and that anaerobic organisms further destroy tissue in an atmosphere of decreased oxygen tension.[155, 244] Diabetes, debilitating disease, obesity, and prior radiation therapy are risk factors for synergistic infections.[45, 156, 168]

Synergistic infections may progress rapidly and necrosis may spread along fascial lines or through the subcutaneous tissue in only a few hours. This progression is called *necrotizing fasciitis*, or *cellulitis*. In such cases fever and signs of systemic sepsis are usually present. Examination of the skin and of the subcutaneous tissue reveals a necrotic eschar formation and underlying crepitance. Cross-table lateral x-ray films may reveal a subcutaneous gas pattern. Necrotizing wound infection that results from *C. perfringens* may also cause a similar occurence.

In other cases synergistic wound infections have a more insidious onset with a lack of systemic signs. Physical pain is often intense, and by the time the characteristic skin changes of central necrosis with surrounding erythema become apparent, the subcutaneous tissue necrosis is more advanced than would be expected. This type of infection is sometimes called *progressive synergistic bacterial gangrene*.

A number of combinations of flora can cause synergistic wound infections. Originally these wound infections were described as mixed aerobic staphylococcal and microaerophilic streptococcal. Combinations of *E. coli* and other gram-negative enteric bacilli or aerobic streptococci with anaerobic cocci and *Bacteroides* species can also be isolated from these types of wound infections. Antibiotic therapy in cases of suspected synergistic wound infections must provide broad-spectrum coverage for both aerobic and anaerobic organisms and must include coverage for clostridial infections. However, antimicrobial therapy alone rarely cures infections. Most often, wide debridement of all affected tissues is necessary. In cases of rapidly progressive disease, prompt debridement may be lifesaving. At surgery the infected tissue appears to undermine the skin and classically is described as gray, stringy, and devitalized with a purulent and fetid discharge. All such devitalized tissue must be totally resected to the point of healthy-appearing, bleeding tissue. Healing should be by secondary intention. Fascial grafting with synthetic grafts may be necessary.

The risk of pelvic infection after vaginal hysterectomy and the risk of pelvic and wound infection after abdominal hysterectomy is significantly reduced by perioperative antimicrobial prophylaxis.[161, 192] Parenteral antibiotics should be used for such prophylaxis, should be administered just before surgery, and should be continued postoperatively for less than 24 hours. There is no benefit in extending the use of preoperative or postoperative antibiotics to prevent infection.[36] Broad-spectrum first-generation antimicrobials such as cefazolin are usually used. More expensive and toxic regimens that provide additional coverage for anaerobes and resistent gram-negative enteric bacilli do not appear to further decrease postoperative infection. In addition to the expense and the toxicity, these regimens may cause superinfection by resistant organisms.

Properly functioning, active intraperitoneal or subperitoneal drains prevent some postoperative infection. Whether these drains are as effective as or are additive to the efficacy of perioperative antimicrobial prophylaxis is unclear. The efficacy of antimicrobial prophylaxis for other gynecologic surgical procedures such as adnexal surgery or infertility surgery is not proved, perhaps because of the inherent very low rate of infection after these procedures.

Antimicrobial coverage for posthysterectomy infections typically consists of broad-spectrum, multiple-drug therapy effective against gram-negative enteric bacilli, gram-positive aerobic cocci, and a variety of anaerobic organisms. Parenteral therapy is usually continued 24 to 72 hours after the fever disappears. Even in cases of collections, surgery is usually not necessary for cure.

TOXIC SHOCK SYNDROME

Toxic shock syndrome (TSS) is a multisystem illness caused by toxin-producing *S. aureus*. Although described as early as 1927, TSS was first characterized by Todd et al in 1978 as a uniform syndrome occurring in a group of children.[257] In 1980 TSS was recognized as occurring in epidemic proportions in menstruating women.[30, 222] Subsequent case reports and mobilization of the epidemiologic and research communities lead to elucidation of pathophysiology and to efforts aimed at disease control. These efforts were somewhat successful in halting the further spread of the epidemic. From 1980 to 1981, TSS occurred in 6 to 6.2 per 100,000 women. Currently the prevalence of this disease is 4 per 100,000 women and nonmenstrual TSS occurs as commonly as menstrual TSS.

Toxic shock syndrome is a dramatic illness that presents acutely and is commonly associated with high fevers, characteristic skin changes, prominent gastrointestinal (GI) manifestations, hypotension, and other systemic effects. The case-fatality ratio is approximately 3%.

The onset of menstrual TSS typically occurs on the third or fourth day of the menses. The earliest manifestation is high fever with a temperature usually in excess of 38.9° C. A diffusely erythematous, finely macular rash that resembles a sunburn in appearance and often in sensation may appear, particularly on the upper trunk, face, or extremities. Profuse diarrhea occurs, and within 2 to 3 days profound hypotension ensues. Virtually any other organ system may become involved, as evidenced by symptoms, signs, or laboratory abnormalities. The almost universal muscle involvement leads to severe myalgias and to tenderness. A more distinctly macular rash may evolve with erythema and some edema of the palms and soles. Eventually, fine desquamation of areas of the rash occurs and by 8 to 12 days, the skin from the palms and soles characteristically sloughs off. This desquamation heals by reepithelialization without scarring.

Full-blown TSS fits the rigid case definition outlined in Table 21-10.[258] Most authorities agree that similar but less dramatic variations of TSS probably occur by similar pathophysiologic mechanisms.

The major long-term effect of TSS is recurrence. TSS recurs during subsequent menses in approximately 30% of cases.[47] Typically, recurrences are milder and may occur over a period of time. Recurrences with up to five subsequent menses have been reported.

The toxin-producing *S. aureus* is associated with TSS.[246] In one series, greater than 90% of women who had TSS had *S. aureus* isolated from the genital tract. In other surveys only approximately 9% of women had *S. aureus* isolated from the vagina or from the cervix. A distinct toxin, TSS toxin-1, is isolated in up to 90% of strains of *S. aureus* associated with TSS.[14] This toxin is presumably responsible for the typical systemic effects in cases of TSS. However, some of the multisystem effects may be secondary to the effects of profound hypotension.

The major factor epidemiologically associated with menstrual TSS is the use of tampons as opposed to the use of sanitary pads. The absorbency of tampons is directly related to the risk for TSS.[11,222] One particular brand of tampon that contained magnesium was particularly associated with TSS, leading to the observation that toxin-producing *S. aureus* has a growth requirement for magnesium. The removal of most tampons that contain magnesium and a general decrease in the absorbency of others has markedly decreased the incidence of menstrual TSS.[218]

Nonmenstrual TSS occurs in a more heterogeneous population and more often with nosocomial infections and prior use of antibiotics.[111] It is associated with a number of staphylococcal infections, including cutaneous and subcutaneous abscesses, osteomyelitis and other deep-seated infections, and staphylococcal superinfections that occur with influenza. Postsurgical wound infections, postpartum infection, gynecologic procedures such as loop electrosurgical excision procedure (LEEP), and vulvar fasciitis all have been reported with TSS. In addition, TSS has been reported with the use of diaphragms and contraceptive sponges.

TSS is diagnosed by the characteristic clinical picture in the absence of documentation, by either culture or serology, of another cause for an acute febrile illness of a similar nature.[222] The differential diagnoses include Kawasaki disease, Rocky Mountain spotted fever, streptococcal scarlet

Table 21-10. Case definitions of toxic shock syndrome

Fever:
- Temperature, $\geq 38.9°$ C

Rash:
- Diffuse macular erythroderma

Desquamation:
- Palms and soles 1–2 weeks after onset

Hypotension:
- Systolic blood pressure < 90 mm Hg, orthostatic drop in diastolic blood pressure >15 mm Hg, or orthostatic dizziness

Multisystem involvement (three or more of the following):
- Gastrointestinal: vomitting or diarrhea at onset
- Muscular: myalgia or elevated creatinine phosphokinase level
- Mucous membrane: vaginal, oropharyngeal, or conjunctival hyperemia
- Renal: elevated serum urea nitrogen or creatinine levels, or aseptic pyuria
- Hepatic: elevated bilirubin, aspartate aminotransferase (AST) (SGOT), or alanine aminotransferase (ALT) (SGPT) levels
- Hematologic: platelets $\leq 100{,}000/mm^3$
- Central nervous system: disorientation or altered consciousness without focal neurologic signs

Negative results for the following, if obtained:
- Blood (except *S. aureus*), throat, or cerebrospinal fluid cultures; rise in titer to Rocky Mountain spotted fever, leptospirosis, or rubeola

fever, and bacteremia. Although in TSS blood cultures are negative for *S. aureus*, supportive evidence for TSS is found by culturing the genital tract, oropharynx, urine, and any referable skin sites for *S. aureus*. Complete laboratory evaluation for multisystem involvement as indicated in Table 21-10 should be performed.

Initial treatment for TSS is supportive care, with attention to aggressive fluid, electrolyte, and blood product replacement. Any tampons, foreign bodies, or collections of purulence present at the onset of symptoms should be removed. The administration of a β-lactamase–resistent antibiotic, such as oxacillin, a cephalosporin, or vancomycin, for 10 days decreases recurrences. In addition, the discontinued use of tampons decreases recurrences.

Although not a common illness, the risk for TSS can be decreased by counseling women to use tampons intermittently as opposed to continually throughout menses and to use the least absorbent tampon that is reasonable.

HUMAN IMMUNODEFICIENCY VIRUS DISEASE, INCLUDING ACQUIRED IMMUNE DEFICIENCY SYNDROME

Acquired immune deficiency syndrome (AIDS) is the most advanced stage in a continuum of clinical syndromes caused by the human immunodeficiency virus (HIV-1). These syndromes are characterized both by the direct effect of this virus on organ systems and the sequelae of profound alterations in normal immune mechanisms that eventually lead to death.

AIDS was first described in populations of the United States, in 1981, although this disease existed and was described in other countries, most notably Africa and the Caribbean, before this time. Infection with HIV is now a major, worldwide epidemic. Unique medical, societal, economical, legal, and other dilemmas are posed by this virus. Its long latency is in part responsible for an incompletely understood pathophysiology and natural history, and its cure remains elusive.

In the United States this epidemic initially occurred largely within the male homosexual and bisexual community. By 1988, reported cases of AIDS in women and the pediatric population accounted for approximately 7% of the total. However, since then this disease has increased most rapidly in women. By 1993, 13% of reported cases of AIDS occurred in women. Currently HIV disease in women is a disease of minority, disadvantaged, and young women, with 70% of AIDS cases reported in African-American or Hispanic women and 80% reported in women of childbearing age. Transmission occurs in association with injection-drug use in approximately 50% of cases and in association with heterosexual activity in other cases.

HIV is a retrovirus that possesses a unique reverse transcriptase that allows its RNA to encode DNA within the infected cell, which then becomes irreversibly incorporated within the host DNA. This intertwining of viral and host genetic structures leads to major alterations in function and to probable destruction of the host cells. It also provides a mechanism for further infection of target cells within the body. The HIV target cell membranes contain a surface molecule, the CD4 receptor. A CD4 envelope protein on the surface of the virus binds to the CD4 receptor. The main target cells for this virus are T_4-helper lymphocytes. The gradual alteration in the function of and the eventual depletion of this subpopulation of T lymphocytes lead to profound effects on cellular immunity characteristic of HIV infection and of associated life-threatening diseases characteristic of AIDS. Infection of macrophages and other monocytes is also central to HIV's pathogenicity. HIV has also been demonstrated in lymph nodes, bone marrow, and spleen, lung, brain, and retinal tissue.

There is a spectrum of HIV disease whose categorization is still evolving. An average of 14 weeks after the initial infection, many people experience a self-limited, febrile, nonspecific mononucleosis-like illness. Following this, HIV infection remains asymptomatic for variable periods of time. Eventually illnesses associated with defects in cellular immunity or with HIV infection of target organs, such as the GI tract or the central nervous system, occur. At any time during the asymptomatic stage or during early manifestations of illness, laboratory abnormalities associated with immune dysfunction such as lymphopenia, thrombocytopenia, and T_4 cell depletion may evolve. Generalized lymphadenopathy, isolated or in conjunction with diffuse, constitutional symptoms, can occur at variable points in the course of the disease.

The last stage of HIV infection is AIDS. The current case definition of AIDS is achieved when one of a list of illnesses associated with immune suppression is diagnosed in a person with no underlying reason, such as age, malignancy, or immunosuppressive medication. Despite maximal efforts at treatment, these associated diseases and conditions ultimately lead to death. These illnesses include key infections such as *Pneumocystis carinii*, disseminated viral infections, unusual protozoal and helminthic infections, and atypical mycobacterial infections. They also include atypical malignancies such as Kaposi's sarcoma, non-Hodgkin's lymphoma, primary brain lymphoma, and a number of other clinical findings or diseases indicative of a defect in cell-mediated immunity. In 1987 dementia and a wasting syndrome of inexorable weight loss, persistent, intractable diarrhea, and fever were added to this list. In 1993 invasive cervical cancer became an AIDS-defining condition, and persistent vulvovaginal candidiasis, moderate or severe cervical intraepithelial neoplasia (CIN), and PID were added to the list of symptomatic HIV-related conditions.

Because the HIV epidemic is of relatively early onset, the time course for disease progression is not absolutely known. Large scale epidemiologic studies in adult males suggest that the time from initial infection to diagnosis of AIDS is 8 to 10 years. All infected persons are assumed to eventually acquire AIDS and die from this disease should a permanent cure not be discovered. The interaction between disease progression and factors such as age, lifestyle, and other infections and illnesses is unknown.

HIV is known to be transmitted by the three following major routes: (1) direct blood contact, (2) sexual transmission, and (3) perinatal transmission from an infected woman to her fetus or child either through in utero exposure or at the time of birth. Transmission via infected breast milk also has been documented. Specific activities and lifestyles clearly place one at risk of contracting this disease. Transmission through casual, household contact does not occur.

Injection-drug use using shared needles is the major means by which blood contact leads to HIV infection in the United States. In areas of the country where HIV disease is particularly prevalent among IV drug abusers, most notably New York City and New Jersey, 50% to 60% of IV drug abusers are estimated to be HIV infected. Although medical transfusion of infected blood products accounts for a low level of AIDS cases currently reported, since 1985 screening of blood products has markedly reduced this mode of transmission of HIV.

Semen and cervical and vaginal secretions can contain the virus[283]; transmission of HIV during sexual activity has clearly been documented. Factors influencing rates of sexual transmission are incompletely understood. Heterosexual transmission both from male to female and female to male can occur. Male to female transmission, however, is more efficient. Anal intercourse may be associated with the greatest risk of transmission, although vaginal intercourse can also lead to infection. An exact risk of transmission associated with oral intercourse is unknown.

Increased risk of sexual transmission of HIV has been associated with other STDs, particularly those associated with disruption of mucosal integrity or cervicitis. This list includes syphilis, chancroid, genital herpes, HPV, and to a lesser extent, *T. vaginalis* and *C. trachomatis*.

Other factors influencing the transmission of HIV are poorly understood. Frequency of exposure to the virus, underlying conditions in the exposed individual, and the efficiency of the infecting virus all are factors. Progressive immune suppression likely is associated with greater viral shedding and thus with greater efficiency of transmission. However, all HIV-infected individuals are considered to be potentially infectious.

Diagnosis of HIV infection is typically made by testing for the presence of antibody to HIV. The virus can be inconstantly cultured from blood and from various secretions of an infected individual, but the presence of virus is unpredictable, and cultures are time consuming, expensive, and not generally available.

Antibody testing is conducted first by performing an efficient, inexpensive, very sensitive ELISA test. If the results are positive for HIV, the test is repeated a second time to decrease the likelihood of false-positive reactions, which initially may be as high as 4:1. If the results again are abnormal, a more specific assay that detects exact viral antigen patterns, typically the Western Blot, must be performed. The vast majority of serologic conversions take place within 6 months of initial viral infection.

Certain gynecologic conditions are of concern to HIV-infected women. These are as follows:

1. Squamous cell abnormalities of the lower genital tract are seen more frequently in HIV-infected women than in non-HIV infected women from similar backgrounds.[264] Rates of CIN and vulvar intraepithelial neoplasia are increased. CIN associated with evidence of HPV is particularly prevalent.[106] CIN can be more rapidly progressive, high grade, recurrent, and associated with multifocal lesions in the lower genital tract, particularly in HIV-infected women who are the most immune suppressed.[143] More frequent Papanicolaou smears and more liberal use of colposcopy are proposed. Close follow-up after treatment and innovative therapies are essential to the treatment of recurrent disease. Invasive cervical cancer is documented as a cause of death in some HIV-infected women.
2. PID resulting in hospitalization is associated with HIV-seroprevalence rates of 6% to 16% in studies in the United States.[93, 207] Whether or not PID is more prevalent in HIV-infected women is not clear. However, when PID does occur, indications suggest that it may result in a more aggressive disease, more hospitalizations, prolonged antibiotic therapy, and a greater need for surgical cure.
3. Some HIV-infected women develop severe or multiple recurrent episodes of symptomatic vulvovaginal candidiasis. Occasionally, this condition is the presenting complaint of symptomatic disease.[102] The exact prevalence of this problem and its association with the degree of immune suppression is unclear. There is a concern that some cases of recurrent disease may be caused by nonalbicans species of *Candida*. Women symptomatic from recurrent candidiasis are often treated with intermittent, chronic-suppressive therapy either by vaginal antifungals or by oral fluconazole.
4. Other STDs should be considered in cases of HIV infection. Positive serologic tests for syphilis are a major risk factor for HIV infection in women, and all women with syphilis should be screened for HIV. Initial nonprimary and recurrent episodes of genital herpes can result in atypical, large, very painful lesions that last for prolonged periods of time. Any ulcer of the lower genital tract even in women without a history of prior herpes or current sexual exposure should be cultured for herpes. If positive, treatment with a high dose of acyclovir is indicated.

Currently no effective cure for HIV infection exists. Many antiretroviral agents which delay disease progression and treat associated conditions are in various stages of use and development. Treatment is assumed to be most effective during asymptomatic infection. Medical efforts are now aimed at preventing associated illnesses. Major public health efforts are directed at primary prevention of the disease by educating people about disease transmission and about modification of activities to avoid transmission. Success of such efforts depends on suppressing the fear of the disease, fostering acceptance of such efforts by all segments of society, and committing all possible financial and human resources toward these goals.

REFERENCES

1. Agarwal J, Gupta JK: Female genital tuberculosis: a retrospective clinicopathologic study of 501 cases, *Indian J Pathol Microbiol* 36:389-397, 1993.
2. Anderson J et al: Primary and secondary syphilis: 20 years' experience. 3. Diagnosis, treatment, and follow-up, *Genitourin Med* 65:239-243, 1989.
3. ACOG: Technical Bulletin: Antimicrobial therapy for gynecologic infections, No. 153—March 1991, *Int J Gynaecol Obstet* 38:131-139, 1992.
4. Ashley R et al: Inability of enzyme immunoassays to discriminate between infections with herpes simplex virus types 1 and 2, *Ann Intern Med* 115:520-526, 1991.
5. Bacterial vaginosis: conference proceedings, Seattle, August 8, 1990, *Am J Obstet Gynecol* 169:441-482, 1993.
6. Barbone F et al: A follow-up study of methods of contraception, sexual activity, and rates of trichomoniasis, candidiasis, and bacterial vaginosis, *Am J Obstet Gynecol* 163:510-514, 1990.
7. Bartlett JG et al: Quantitative bacteriology of the vaginal flora, *J Infect Dis* 136:271-277, 1977.
8. Bartlett JG et al: Cervical and vaginal bacterial flora: ecological niches in the female lower genital tract, *Am J Obstet Gynecol* 130:658-661, 1978.
9. Bassa AG et al: Granuloma inguinale (donovanosis) in women: an analysis of 61 cases from Durban, South Africa, *Sex Transm Dis* 20:164-167, 1993.

10. Becker LE: Lymphogranuloma venereum, *Int J Dermatol* 15:26- 33, 1976.
11. Berkley SF et al: The relationship of tampon characteristics to menstrual toxic shock syndrome, *JAMA* 258:917-920, 1987.
12. Beutner KR, Becker TM, Stone KM: Epidemiology of human papillomavirus infections. *Dermatol Clin* 9:211-218, 1991.
13. Billstein SA, Mattaliano VJ Jr: The nuisance sexually transmitted diseases: molluscum contagiosum, scabies, and crab lice. *Med Clin North Am* 74:1487-1505, 1990.
14. Bohach GA et al: Staphylococcal and streptococcal pyrogenic toxins involved in toxic shock syndrome and related illnesses, *Crit Rev Microbiol* 17:251-272, 1990.
15. Bonnez W et al: Efficacy and safety of 0.5% podofilox solution in the treatment and suppression of anogenital warts, *Am J Med* 96:420-425, 1994.
16. Brock BV et al: Frequency of asymptomatic shedding of herpes simplex virus in women with genital herpes, *JAMA* 263:418-420, 1990.
17. Brown ST, Zaidi A, Larsen SA: Serologic response to syphilis treatment: a new analysis of old data, *JAMA* 253:1296-1299, 1985.
18. Brunham RC et al: Etiology and outcome of acute pelvic inflammatory disease, *J Infect Dis* 158:510-517, 1988.
19. Brunham RB et al: Mucopurulent cervicitis: the ignored counterpart of urethritis in the male, *N Engl J Med* 311:1-6, 1984.
20. Bryson Y et al: Risk of acquisition of genital herpes simplex virus type 2 in sex partners of persons with genital herpes: a prospective couple study, *J Infect Dis* 167:942-946, 1993.
21. Buchan H et al: Morbidity following pelvic inflammatory disease, *Br J Obstet Gynaecol* 100:558-562, 1993.
22. Burgoyne RA: Lymphogranuloma venereum, *Prim Care* 17:153-157, 1990.
23. Burkman R et al: The relationship of genital tract actinomycetes and the development of pelvic inflammatory disease, *Am J Obstet Gynecol* 143:585-589, 1982.
24. Burnakis TG, Hildebrandt NB: Pelvic inflammatory disease: a review with emphasis on antimicrobial therapy, *Rev Infect Dis* 8:86-116, 1986.
25. Campion MJ: Clinical manifestations and natural history of genital human papilloma virus infection, *Obstet Gynecol Clin North Am* 14:363-388, 1987.
26. Caplan LR, Kleeman FJ, Berg S: Urinary retention probably secondary to herpes genitalis, *N Engl J Med* 297:920-921, 1977.
27. Carney O et al: A prospective study of the psychological impact on patients with a first episode of genital herpes, *Genitourin Med* 70:40-45, 1994.
28. Carpenter CC et al: Human immunodeficiency virus infection in North American women: experience with 200 cases and review of the literature, *Medicine* 70:307-325, 1991.
29. Cates W Jr, Wasserheit JN: Genital chlamydial infections: epidemiology and reproductive sequelae, *Am J Obstet Gynecol* 164:1771-1781, 1991.
30. Centers for Disease Control: Toxic-shock syndrome: United States, 1970-1980, *MMWR* 30:25-33, 1981.
31. Centers for Disease Control: Antibiotic-resistant strains of *Neisseria gonorrhoeae*: policy guidelines for detection, management, and control, *MMWR* 36(Suppl5):1S-18S, 1987.
32. Centers for Disease Control: Continuing increase in infectious syphilis: United States, *MMWR* 37:35-38, 1988a.
33. Centers for Disease Control: Syphilis and congenital syphilis: United States, 1985-1988, *MMWR* 37:486-489, 1988b.
34. Centers for Disease Control 1993: Sexually transmitted disease guidelines, *MMWR* 42:1-102, 1993.
35. Chirgwin K et al: HIV infection, genital ulcer disease, and crack cocaine use among patients attending a clinic for sexually transmitted diseases, *Am J Public Health* 81:1576-1579, 1991.
36. Classen DC et al: The timing of prophylactic administration of antibiotics and the risk of surgical-wound infection, *N Engl J Med* 326:281-286, 1992.
37. Committee on Public Health: Statement on treatment of gonorrhea-penicillin is passé: the New York Academy of Medicine, *Bull N Y Acad Med* 65:243-246, 1989.
38. Corey L: First-episode, recurrent, and asymptomatic herpes simplex infections, *J Am Acad Dermatol* 18:169-172, 1988.
39. Corey L et al: Genital herpes simplex virus infections: clinical manifestations course and complications, *Ann Intern Med* 98:958-972, 1983.
40. Corey L, Spear PG: Infections with herpes simplex viruses (2), *N Engl J Med* 314:749-757, 1986.
41. Corriere JN Jr: Avoiding overkill in diagnosis and treatment of lower urinary tract infections, *Urology* 32(Suppl2):17-21, 1988.
42. Crombleholme WR et al: Efficacy of single-agent therapy for the treatment of acute pelvic inflammatory disease with ciprofloxacin, *Am J Med* 87(5A):142S-147S, 1989.
43. Criteria for diagnosing and grading of salpingitis, *Obstet Gynecol* 61:113, 1983, (editorial).
44. Dalaker K et al: *Chlamydia trachomatis* as a cause of acute perihepatitis associated with pelvic inflammatory disease, *Br J Vener Dis* 57:41-43, 1981.
45. Daly JW, King R, Monif GRG: Progressive necrotizing wound infection in postirradiated patients, *Obstet Gynecol* 52(Suppl):5-8, 1978.
46. Dangor Y et al: Accuracy of clinical diagnosis of genital ulcer disease, *Sex Transm Dis* 17:184-189, 1990.
47. Davis JP et al: Toxic-shock syndrome: epidemiologic features, recurrences, risk factors, and prevention, *N Engl J Med* 303:1429-1435, 1980.
48. Edelman DA, Berger GS: Contraceptive practice and tuboovarian abscess, *Am J Obstet Gynecol* 138:541-544, 1980.
49. Epstein WL: Molluscum contagiosum, *Semin Dermatol* 11:184-189, 1992.
50. Eschenbach DA: Bacterial vaginosis and anaerobes in obstetric-gynecologic infection, *Clin Infect Dis* 16(Suppl4):S282-287, 1993.
51. Eschenbach DA, Harnisch JP, Holmes KK: Pathogenesis of acute pelvic inflammatory disease: role of contraceptive and other risk factors, *Am J Obstet Gynecol* 128:838-850, 1977.
52. Eschenbach DA, Holmes KK: Acute pelvic inflammatory disease: current concepts of pathogenesis, etiology, and management, *Clin Obstet Gynecol* 18:35-50, 1975.
53. Eschenbach DA et al: Polymicrobial etiology of acute pelvic inflammatory disease, *N Engl J Med* 293:166-171, 1975.
54. Eschenbach DA et al: Diagnosis and clinical manifestations of bacterial vaginosis, *Am J Obstet Gynecol* 158:819-828, 1988.
55. Farley TM et al: Intrauterine devices and pelvic inflammatory disease: an international perespective, *Lancet* 339:785-788, 1992.
56. Faro S: Lymphogranuloma venereum, chancroid, and granuloma inguinale, *Obstet Gynecol Clin North Am* 16:517-530, 1989.
57. Ferenczy A et al: Latent papillomavirus and recurring genital warts, *N Engl J Med* 313:784, 1985.
58. Fidel PL Jr et al: Systemic cell-mediated immune reactivity in women with recurrent vulvovaginal candidiasis, *J Infect Dis* 168:1458-1465, 1993.
59. Fihn SD: Behavioral aspects of urinary tract infection, *Urology* 32(Suppl3):168, 1988.
60. Fihn SD et al: Association between diaphragm use and urinary tract infection, *JAMA* 254:240-245, 1985.
61. Fiumara NJ: Treatment of seropositive primary syphilis: an evaluation of 196 patients, *Sex Transm Dis* 4:92-95, 1977a.
62. Fiumara NJ: Treatment of secondary syphilis: an evaluation of 204 patients, *Sex Transm Dis* 4:96-99, 1977b.
63. Fiumara NJ: Reinfection primary, secondary, and latent syphilis: the serologic response after treatment, *Sex Transm Dis* 7:111-115, 1980.

64. Fong IW, McCleary P, Read S: Cellular immunity of patients with recurrent or refractory vulvovaginal moniliasis, *Am J Obstet Gynecol* 166:887-890, 1992.
65. Fonts AC, Kraus SJ: *Trichomonas vaginalis*: reevaluation of its clinical presentation and laboratory diagnosis, *J Infect Dis* 141:137-143, 1980.
66. Fowler JE Jr: Urinary tract infections in women, *Urol Clin North Am* 13:673-683, 1986.
67. Frenkel LM et al: Clinical reactivation of herpes simplex virus type 2 infection in seropositive pregnant women with no history of genital herpes, *Ann Intern Med* 118:414-418, 1993.
68. Friedland GH, Klein RS: Transmission of the human immunodeficiency virus, *N Engl J Med* 317:1125-1135, 1987.
69. Friedrich EG Jr: Current perspectives in candidal vulvovaginitis, *Am J Obstet Gynecol* 158:985-986, 1988.
70. Galask RP: Vaginal colonization by bacteria and yeast, *Am J Obstet Gynecol* 158:993-995, 1988.
71. Galask RP, Larsen B, Ohm MJ: Vaginal flora and its role in disease entities, *Clin Obstet Gynecol* 19:61-81, 1976.
72. Gardner HL: *Haemophilus vaginalis* vaginitis after 25 years, *Am J Obstet Gynecol* 137:385-391, 1980.
73. Gershman KA, Rolfs RT: Diverging gonorrhea and syphillis trends in the 1980s: are they real? *Am J Public Health* 81:1263-1267, 1991.
74. Gilstrap LC et al: Gonorrhea screening in male consorts of women with pelvic infection, *JAMA* 238:965-966, 1977.
75. Gjonnaess H et al: Pelvic inflammatory disease: etiologic studies with emphasis on chlamydial infection, *Obstet Gynecol* 59:550-555, 1982.
76. Goldberg LH et al: Long-term suppression of recurrent genital herpes with acyclovir: a 5-year benchmark, *Arch Dermatol* 129:582-587, 1993.
77. Golde SH, Israel R, Ledger WJ: Unilateral tuboovarian abscess: a distinct entity, *Am J Obstet Gynecol* 127:807-812, 1977.
78. Granato PA, Franz MR: Use of the gen-probe page system for the detection of *Neisseria gonorrheae* in urogenital samples, *Diagn Microbiol Infect Dis* 13:217-221, 1990.
79. Graves A, Gardner WA Jr: Pathogenicity of *Trichomonas vaginalis*, *Clin Obstet Gynecol* 36:145-152, 1993.
80. Guinan ME et al: The course of untreated recurrent genital herpes simplex infection in 27 women, *N Engl J Med* 304:759-763, 1981.
81. Ha HK et al: Abdominal actinomycosis: CT findings in 10 patients, *AJR Am J Roentgenol* 161:791-794, 1993.
82. Handsfield HH et al: Criteria for selective screening for *Chlamydia trachomatis* infection in women attending family planning clinics, *JAMA* 255:1730-1734, 1986.
83. Haverkos HW, Edelman R: The epidemiology of acquired immunodeficiency syndrome among heterosexuals, *JAMA* 260:1922-1929, 1988.
84. Hemsell DL: Infections after gynecologic surgery, *Obstet Gynecol Clin North Am* 16:381-400, 1989.
85. Henry-Suchet J, Loffredo V: Chlamydial and *Mycoplasma* genital infection in salpingitis and tubal sterility, *Lancet* 1:539-543, 1980.
86. Hibbs JR et al: Emergency department-based surveillance for syphilis during an outbreak in Philadelphia, *Ann Emerg Med* 22:1286-1290, 1993.
87. Hill GB: The microbiology of bacterial vaginosis, *Am J Obstet Gynecol* 169:450-454, 1993.
88. Hilton E et al: Ingestion of yogurt containing *Lactobacillus acidophilus* as prophylaxis for candidal vaginitis, *Ann Intern Med* 116:353-357, 1992.
89. Hillier SL: Diagnostic microbiology of bacterial vaginosis, *Am J Obstet Gynecol* 169:455-459, 1993.
90. Hillier SL et al: The relationship of hydrogen peroxide-producing lactobacilli to bacterial vaginosis and genital microflora in pregnant women, *Obstet Gynecol* 79:369-373, 1992.
91. Hillis SD et al: Delayed care of pelvic inflammatory disease as a risk factor for impaired fertility, *Am J Obstet Gynecol* 168:1503-1509, 1993.
92. Hillis SD et al: Risk factors for recurrent *Chlamydia trachomatis* infection in women, *Am J Obstet Gynecol* 170:801-806, 1994.
93. Hoegsberg B et al: Sexually transmitted diseases and human immunodeficiency virus infection among women with pelvic inflammatory disease, *Am J Obstet Gynecol* 163:1135-1139, 1990.
94. Hoffman MS et al: Advanced actinomycotic pelvic inflammatory disease simulating gynecologic malignancy: a report of two cases, *J Reprod Med* 36:543-545, 1991.
95. Holmes KK, Counts GW, Beaty HN: Disseminated gonococcal infection, *Ann Intern Med* 74:979-993, 1971.
96. Holton PD et al: Prevalence of neurosyphilis in human immunodeficiency virus-infected patients with latent syphilis, *Am J Med* 93:9-12, 1992.
97. Hook EW III, Holmes KK: Gonococcal infections, *Ann Intern Med* 102:229-243, 1985.
98. Hoosen AA, Bassa A, Moodley J: Granuloma inguinale (donovanosis): an analysis of 64 cases from Durban, South Africa, *Int Conf AIDS* 8:91, 1992.
99. Hovelius B, Mårdh PA: *Staphylococcus saprophyticus* as a common cause of urinary tract infections, *Rev Infect Dis* 6:328-337, 1984.
100. Hunter CA, Long KR: Vaginal and cervical pH in normal women and in patients with vaginitis, *Am J Obstet Gynecol* 75:872-874, 1958.
101. Hutchinson CM, Hook EW III: Syphilis in adults, *Med Clin North Am* 74:1389-1416, 1990.
102. Iman N et al: Hierarchical pattern of mucosal candida infections in HIV-seropositive women, *Am J Med* 89:142-146, 1990.
103. Interferon for treatment of genital warts, *Med Lett Drugs Ther* 30:70-72, 1988a.
104. Jacobson L, Westrom L: Objectivized diagnosis of acute pelvic inflammatory disease: diagnostic and prognostic value of routine laparoscopy, *Am J Obstet Gynecol* 105:1088-1098, 1969.
105. Jessamine PG, Ronald AR: Chancroid and the role of genital ulcer disease in the spread of human retroviruses, *Med Clin North Am* 74:1417-1431, 1990.
106. Johnson JC et al: High frequency of latent and clinical human papillomavirus cervical infections in immunocompromised human immunodeficiency virus-infected women, *Obstet Gynecol* 79:321-327, 1992.
107. Johnson RE et al: A seroepidemiologic survey of the prevalence of herpes simplex virus type 2 infection in the United States, *N Engl J Med* 321:7-12, 1989.
108. Jones RB et al: Recovery of *Chlamydia trachomatis* from the endometrium of women at risk for chlamydial infection, *Am J Obstet Gynecol* 155:36, 1986.
109. Joseph AK, Rosen T: Laboratory techniques used in the diagnosis of chancroid, granuloma inguinale, and lymphogranuloma venereum, *Dermatol Clin* 12:1-8, 1994.
110. Jovanovic R, Congema E, Nguyen HT: Antifungal agents versus boric acid for treating chronic mycotic vulvovaginitis, *J Reprod Med* 36:593-597, 1991.
111. Kain KC, Schulzer M, Chow AW: Clinical spectrum of nonmenstrual toxic shock syndrome (TSS): comparison with menstrual TSS by multivariate discriminant analysis, *Clin Infect Dis* 16:100-106, 1993.
112. Kamwendo F et al: Gonorrhea, genital chlamydial infection, and nonspecific urethritis in male partners or women hospitalized and treated for acute pelvic inflammatory disease, *Sex Transm Dis* 20:143-146, 1993.
113. Kandula PV, Wenzel RP: Postoperative wound infection after total abdominal hysterectomy: a controlled study of the increased duration of hospital stay and trends in postoperative wound infection, *Am J Infect Control* 21:201-204, 1993.
114. Kass EH: Chemotherapeutic and antibiotic drugs in the management of infections of the urinary tract, *Am J Med* 18:764-781, 1955.

115. Kass EH, Finland M: Asymptomatic infections of the urinary tract, *Trans Assoc Am Physicians* 69:56-64, 1956.
116. Kelaghan J et al: Barrier-method contraceptives and pelvic inflammatory disease, *JAMA* 248:184-187, 1981.
117. Kent GP et al: Screening for *Chlamydia trachomatis* infection in a sexually transmitted disease clinic: comparison of diagnostic tests with clinical and historical risk factors, *Sex Transm Dis* 15:51-57, 1988.
118. Kinghorn GR: Genital herpes: natural history and treatment of acute episodes, *J Med Virol* 1:33-38, 1993.
119. Klein TA, Richmond JA, Mishcell DR Jr: Pelvis tuberculosis, *Obstet Gynecol* 48:99-105, 1976.
120. Komaroff AL: Acute dysuria in women, *N Engl J Med* 310:368- 375, 1984.
121. Krebs HB, Helmkamp BF: Treatment failure of genital condylomata acuminata in women: role of the male sexual partner, *Am J Obstet Gynecol* 165:337-339, 1991.
122. Krettek JE et al: *Chlamydia trachomatis* in patients who used oral contraceptives and had intermenstrual spotting, *Obstet Gynecol* 81:728-31, 1993.
123. Krieger JN et al: Diagnosis of trichomoniasis: comparison of conventional wet-mount examination with cytologic studies, cultures, and monoclonal antibody staining of direct specimens, *JAMA* 259:1223-1227, 1988.
124. Lafferty WE et al: Recurrences after oral and genital herpes simplex virus infection: influence of site of infection and viral type, *N Engl J Med* 316:1444-1449, 1987.
125. Landers DV, Sweet RL: Current trends in the diagnosis and treatment of tuboovarian abscess, *Am J Obstet Gynecol* 151:1098-1110, 1985.
126. Landesman S et al: Serosurvey of human immunodeficiency virus infection in parturients, *JAMA* 258:2701-2703, 1987.
127. Larsen B, Galask RP: Vaginal microbial flora: practical and theoretic relevance, *Obstet Gynecol* 55(Suppl):1005-1135, 1980.
128. Larsson PG et al: Incidence of pelvic inflammatory disease after first-trimester legal abortion in women with bacterial vaginosis after treatment with metronidazole: a double-blind, randomized study, *Am J Obstet Gynecol* 166:100-103, 1992.
129. Latif AS, Mason PR, Paraiwa E: The treatment of donovanosis (granuloma inguinale), *Sex Transm Dis* 15:27-29, 1988.
130. Lee NC, Rubin GL, Borucki R: The intrauterine device and pelvic inflammatory disease revisited: new results from the Women's Health Study, *Obstet Gynecol* 72:1-6, 1988.
131. Lee NC, Rubin GL, Grimes DA: Measures of sexual behavior and the risk of pelvic inflammatory disease, *Obstet Gynecol* 77:425-430, 1991.
132. Lee TJ, Sparling F: Syphilis: an algorithm, *JAMA* 242:1187-1189, 1979.
133. Lewis JS et al: Direct DNA probe assay for *Neisseria gonorrhoeae* in pharyngeal and rectal specimens, *J Clin Microbiol* 31:2783-2785, 1993.
134. Lightfoot TW, Gotschlich EC: Gonococcal disease, *Am J Med* 56:347-356, 1974.
135. Lin JS et al: Underdiagnosis of *Chlamydia trachomatis* infection: diagnostic limitations in patients with low-level infection, *Sex Transm Dis* 19:259-265, 1992.
136. Linder JGEM, Plantema FHF, Hoogkamp-Korstamje JAA: Quantitative studies of the vaginal flora of healthy women and of obstetric and gynaecological patients, *J Med Microbiol* 11:233-241, 1978.
137. Lossick JG: Treatment of sexually transmitted vaginosis/vagnitis, *Rev Infect Dis* 12(Suppl6):S665-S681, 1990.
138. Lossick JG, Kent HL: Trichomoniasis: trends in diagnosis and management, *Am J Obstet Gynecol* 165:1217-1222, 1991.
139. Lugo-Miro VI, Green M, Mazur L: Comparison of different metronidazole therapeutic regimens for bacterial vaginosis: a meta-analysis, *JAMA* 268:92-95, 1992.
140. Lynch PJ: Sexually transmitted diseases: granuloma inguinale, lymphogranuloma venereum, chancroid, and infectious syphilis, *Clin Obstet Gynecol* 31:1041-1052, 1978.
141. Lynch PJ: Condylomata acuminata, *Clin Obstet Gynecol* 28:142-151, 1985.
142. Magder LS et al: Factors related to genital *Chlamydia trachomatis* and its diagnosis by culture in a sexually transmitted disease clinic, *Am J Epidemiol* 128:298-308, 1988.
143. Maiman M et al: Human immunodeficiency virus infection and invasive cervical carcinoma, *Cancer* 71:402-406, 1993.
144. Marchbanks PA, Lee NC, Peterson HB: Cigarette smoking as a risk factor for pelvic inflammatory disease, *Am J Obstet Gynecol* 162:639-644, 1990.
145. Mårdh P-A: The vaginal ecosystem, *Am J Obstet Gynecol* 165:1163-1168, 1991.
146. Mårdh P-A, Westrom L: Tubal and cervical cultures in acute salpingitis with special reference to *Mycoplasma hominis* and T-strain mycoplasmas, *Br J Vener Dis* 46:179-186, 1970.
147. Mårdh P-A, Westrom L: Adherence of bacteria to vaginal epithelial cells, *Infect Immunol* 13:661-666, 1976.
148. Mårdh P-A et al: *Chlamydia trachomatis* infection in patients with acute salpingitis, *N Engl J Med* 296:1377-1379, 1977.
149. Marshburn PB, Trofatter KF Jr: Recurrent condyloma acuminatum in women over age 40: association with immunosuppression and malignant disease, *Am J Obstet Gynecol* 159:429-433, 1988.
150. McCormack WM: Pelvic inflammatory disease, *N Engl J Med* 330:115-119, 1994.
151. McLellan R et al: The clinical diagnosis of trichomoniasis, *Obstet Gynecol* 60:30-34, 1982.
152. Mead PB: Cervical-vaginal flora of women with invasive cervical cancer, *Obstet Gynecol* 52:601-604, 1978.
153. Mead PB: Epidemiology of bacterial vaginosis, *Am J Obstet Gynecol* 169:446-449, 1993.
154. Meisels A: Dysplasia and carcinoma of the uterine cervix. IV. A correlated cytologic and histologic study with special emphasis on vaginal microbiology, *Acta Cytol* 13:224-234, 1969.
155. Meleney FL: Bacterial synergism in disease processes, *Ann Surg* 94:961-981, 1931.
156. Meltzer RM: Necrotizing gasciitis and progressive bacterial synergistic gangrene of the vulva, *Obstet Gynecol* 61:757-760, 1980.
157. Mertz GJ et al: Prolonged continuous versus intermittent oral acyclovir treatment in normal adults with frequently recurring genital herpes simplex virus infection, *Am J Med* 85:14-19, 1988a.
158. Mertz GJ et al: Transmission of genital herpes in couples with one symptomatic and one asymptomatic partner: a prospective study, *J Infect Dis* 157:1169-1177, 1988.
159. Mertz GJ et al: Risk factors for the sexual transmission of genital herpes, *Ann Intern Med* 166:197-202, 1992.
160. Mindel A et al: Primary and secondary syphilis, 20 years' experience. 2. Clinical features, *Genitourin Med* 65:1-3, 1989.
161. Mittendorf R et al: Avoiding serious infections associated with abdominal hysterectomy: a metaanalysis of antibiotic prophylaxis, *Am J Obstet Gynecol* 169:1119-1124, 1993.
162. Morse SA: Chancroid and *Haemophilus ducreyi*, *Clin Microbiol Rev* 2:137-157, 1989.
163. Muller M, Lossick JG, Gorrell TE: In vitro susceptibility of *Trichomonas vaginalis* to metronidazole and treatment outcome in vaginal trichomoniasis, *Sex Transm Dis* 15:17-24, 1988.
164. Muller-Schoop JW et al: *Chlamydia trachomatis* as possible cause of peritonitis and perihepatitis in young women, *Br Med J (Clin Res)* 1:1022-1024, 1978.
165. Nahmias AJ, Roizman B: Infection with herpes simplex viruses 1 and 2, *N Engl J Med* 289:667-674, 719-725, 781-789, 1973.
166. Nettleman MD, Jones RB: Cost-effectiveness of screening women at moderate risk for genital infections caused by *Chlamydia trachomatis*, *JAMA* 260:207-213, 1988.

167. Nguyen HN, Eisenkop SM, Grimes DA: Ureteral obstruction and hydronephrosis as a complication of tuboovarian abscess: a case report, *J Reprod Med* 33:835-837, 1988.
168. Nolan TE et al: Necrotizing surgical infection and necrotizing fasciitis in obstetric and gynecologic patients, *South Med J* 86:1363-1367, 1993.
169. Nugent RP, Krohn MA, Hillier SL: Reliability of diagnosing bacterial vaginosis is improved by a standardized method of gram stain interpretation, *J Clin Microbiol* 29:297-301, 1991.
170. Oosthuizen AP, Wessels PH, Hefer JN: Tuberculosis of the female genital tract in patients attending an infertility clinic, *S Afri Med J* 77:562-564, 1990.
171. Oriel JD: Genital warts, *Sex Transm Dis* 4:153-159, 1977.
172. Oriel JD et al: Genital yeast infections, *Br Med J (Clin Res)* 4:761-764, 1972.
173. Paavonen J et al: Prevalence and manifestations of endometritis among women with cervicitis, *Am J Obstet Gynecol* 152:280-286, 1985.
174. Pabst KM et al: Disease prevalence among women attending a sexually transmitted disease clinic varies with reason for visit, *Sex Transm Dis* 19:88-91, 1992.
175. Padian N et al: Male-to-female transmission of human immunodeficiency virus, *JAMA* 258:788-790, 1987.
176. Panke ES et al: Comparison of gen-probe DNA probe test and culture for the detection of *Neisseria gonorrhoeae* in endocervical specimens, *J Clin Microbiol* 29:883-888, 1991.
177. Parsons CL: Urinary tract infections, *Clin Obstet Gynecol* 12:487-496, 1985.
178. Parsons CL: Lower urinary tract infections in women, *Urol Clin North Am* 14:240-250, 1987.
179. Patsner B, Giovine AP: Pelvic actinomycosis presenting as a primary retroperitoneal mass: a case report, *J Reprod Med* 38:159-162, 1993.
180. Peacock JE Jr et al: Intravenous acyclovir therapy of first episodes of genital herpes: a multicenter double-blind, placebo-controlled trial, *Am J Med* 85:301-306, 1988.
181. Pearlman MD, McNeeley SG: A review of the microbiology, immunology, and clinical implications of *Chlamydia trachomatis* infection, *Obstet Gynecol Surv* 47:448-461, 1992.
182. Peterson CS, Gerstoft J: Molluscum contagiosum in HIV-infected patients, *Dermatology* 184:19-21, 1992.
183. Peterson HB et al: Pelvic inflammatory disease: key treatment issues and options, *JAMA* 266:2605-2611, 1991.
184. Pheifer TA et al: Nonspecific vaginitis: role of *Haemophilus vaginalis* and treatment with metronidazole, *N Engl J Med* 298:1429-1434, 1978.
185. Phillips RS et al: Should tests for *Chlamydia trachomatis* cervical infection be done during routine gynecologic visits? *Ann Intern Med* 107:188-194, 1987.
186. Phillips RS et al: Gonorrhea in women seen for routine gynecologic care: criteria for testing, *Am J Med* 85:177-82, 1988.
187. Phillips RS et al: *Chlamydia trachomatis* cervical infection in women seeking routine gynecologic care: criteria for selective testing, *Am J Med* 86:515-520, 1989.
188. Phillips RS et al: Should women be tested for gonococcal infection of the cervix during routine gynecologic visits? An economic appraisal, *Am J Med* 86:297-302, 1989.
189. Phillips RS et al: The effect of cigarette smoking, *Chlamydia trachomatis* infection, and vaginal douching on ectopic pregnancy, *Obstet Gynecol* 79:8590, 1992.
190. Plummer FA et al: Cofactors in male-female sexual transmission of human immunodeficiency virus type 1, *J Infect Dis* 163:233-239, 1991.
191. Polk BF: Antimicrobial prophylaxis to prevent mixed bacterial infection, *J Antimicrob Chemother* 8:115-129, 1981.
192. Polk BF et al: Randomised clinical trial of perioperative cefazolin in preventing infection after hysterectomy, *Lancet* 1:438-441, 1980.
193. Quinn TC et al: The association of syphilis with risk of human immunodeficiency virus infection in patients attending sexually transmitted disease clinics, *Arch Intern Med* 150:1297-1302, 1990.
194. Radcliffe KW, Daniels D, Evans BA: Molluscum contagiosum: a neglected sentinel infection, *Int J STD AIDS* 2:416-418, 1991.
195. Reed BD: Risk factors for candida vulvovaginitis, *Obstet Gynecol Surv* 47:551-560, 1992.
196. Reed SD, Landers DV, Sweet RL: Antibiotic treatment of tuboovarian abscess: comparison of broadspectrum β-lactam agents versus clindamycin-containing regimens, *Am J Obstet Gynecol* 164:1556-1561, 1991.
197. Reid G, Sobel JD: Bacterial adherence in the pathogenesis of urinary tract infection: a review, *Rev Infect Dis* 9:470-487, 1987.
198. Reid R et al: Sexually transmitted papillomaviral infections. I. The anatomic distribution and pathologic grade of neoplastic lesions associated with different viral types, *Am J Obstet Gynecol* 156:212 222, 1987.
199. Rice RJ, Thompson SE: Treatment of uncomplicated infections due to *Neisseria gonorrhoeae*, *JAMA* 255:1739, 1986.
200. Richens J: The diagnosis and treatment of donovanosis (granuloma inguinale), *Genitourin Med* 67:441-452, 1991.
201. Rolfs RT, Galaid EI, Zaidi AA: Pelvic inflammatory disease: trends in hospitalizations and office visits, 1979 through 1988, *Am J Obstet Gynecol* 166:983-990, 1992.
202. Romanowski B et al: Serologic response to treatment of infectious syphilis, *Ann Intern Med* 114:1005-1009, 1991.
203. Ronald AR, Corey L, McCutchan JA, Handsfield HH: Evaluation of new antiinfective drugs for the treatment of chancroid, *Clin Infect Dis* 15(Suppl1):S108-S114, 1992.
204. Ronald AR, Plummer FA: Chancroid and *Haemophilus ducreyi*, *Ann Intern Med* 102:705-707, 1985.
205. Rubin GL, Ory HW, Layde PM: Oral contraceptives and pelvic inflammatory disease, *Am J Obstet Gynecol* 114:630-635, 1982.
206. Rudolph AH: Examination of the cerebrospinal fluid in syphilis, *Cutis* 17:749-752, 1976.
207. Safrin S et al: Seroprevalence and epidemiologic correlates of human immunodeficiency virus infection in women with acute pelvic inflammatory disease, *Obstet Gynecol* 75:666-670, 1990.
208. Safrin S et al: Long-term sequelae of acute pelvic inflammatory disease: a retrospective cohort study, *Am J Obstet Gynecol* 166:1300-1305, 1992.
209. St John RK, Brown ST: International symposium on pelvic inflammatory disease, *Am J Obstet Gynecol* 138:845-1112, 1980.
210. Sanders LL Jr, Harrison HR, Washington AE: Treatment of sexually transmitted chlamydial infections, *JAMA* 255:1750-1756, 1986.
211. Saracoglu OF, Mungan T, Tanzer F: Pelvic tuberculosis, *Int J Gynaecol Obstet* 37:115-120, 1992.
212. Schacter J: Chlamydial infections, *N Engl J Med* 298:428-435, 490-495, 540-549, 1978.
213. Schaeffer AJ: Recurrent urinary tract infection in the female patient, *Urology* 32(Suppl3):12-15, 1988.
214. Schiffer MA et al: Actinomycosis infections associated with intrauterine contraceptive devices, *Obstet Gynecol* 45:67-71, 1975.
215. Schmid GP: The treatment of chancroid, *JAMA* 255:1757-1762, 1986.
216. Schmid GP et al: Chancroid in the United States: reestablishment of an old disease, *JAMA* 258:3265-3268, 1987.
217. Scholes D, Dailing JR, Stergachis AS: Current cigarette smoking and risk of acute pelvic inflammatory disease, *Am J Public Health* 82:1352-1355, 1992.
218. Schuchat A, Broome CV: Toxic shock syndrome and tampons, *Epidemiol Rev* 13:99-112, 1991.
219. Schulte JM, Martich FA, Schmid GP: Chancroid in the United States, 1981-1990: evidence for underreporting of cases, *MMWR CDC Surveill Summ* 41:57-61, 1992.

220. Schwartz JJ, Myskowski PL: Molluscum contagiosum in patients with human immunodeficiency virus infection: a review of 27 patients, *J Am Acad Dermatol* 27:583-588, 1992.
221. Scott WC: Pelvic abscess in association with intrauterine contraceptive devices, *Am J Obstet Gynecol* 131:149-156, 1978.
222. Shands KN, Schmid GP, Dan BB: Toxic-shock syndrome in menstruating women: association with tampon use and *Staphylococcus aureus* and clinical features in 52 cases, *N Engl J Med* 303:1436-1442, 1980.
223. Sheffield PA et al: The association between *Chlamydia trachomatis* serology and pelvic damage in women with tubal ectopic gestations, *Fertil Steril* 60:970-975, 1993.
224. Sobel JD: Recurrent vulvovaginal candidiasis: a prospective study of the efficacy of maintenance ketoconazole therapy, *N Engl J Med* 315:1455-1458, 1986.
225. Sobel JD: Pathogenesis and treatment of recurrent vulvovaginal candidiasis, *Clin Infect Dis* 14(Suppl1):S148-S153, 1992.
226. Sobel JD: Candidal vulvovaginitis, *Clin Obstet Gynecol* 36:153-165, 1993.
227. Soper DE: Diagnosis and laparoscopic grading of acute salpingitis, *Am J Obstet Gynecol* 164:1370-1376, 1991.
228. Soper DE et al: Observation concerning the microbial etiology of acute salpingitis, *Am J Obstet Gynecol* 170:1008-1014; discussion 1014-1017, 1994.
229. Soper DE, Bump RC, Hurt WG: Bacterial vaginosis and trichomoniasis vaginitis and risk factor for cuff cellulitis after abdominal hysterectomy, *Am J Obstet Gynecol* 163:1016-1021, 1990.
230. Souney P, Polk BF: Single-dose antimicrobial therapy for urinary tract infections in women, *Rev Infect Dis* 4:29-34, 1982.
231. Spence MR: The treatment of gonorrhea, syphilis, chancroid, lymphogranuloma venereum, and granuloma inguinale, *Clin Obstet Gynecol* 31:453-465, 1988.
232. Spence MR, Adler J, McLellan R: Pelvic inflammatory disease in the adolescent, *J Adolesc Health Care* 11:304-309, 1990.
233. Spiegel CA: Bacterial vaginosis, *Clin Microbiol Rev* 4:485-502, 1991.
234. Spiegel CA et al: Anaerobic bacteria in nonspecific vaginitis, *N Engl J Med* 303:601-607, 1980.
235. Spinillo A et al: Epidemiologic characteristics of women with idiopathic recurrent vulvovaginal candidiasis, *Obstet Gynecol* 81:721-727, 1993.
236. Stamey TA: Recurrent urinary tract infection in female patients: an overview of management and treatment, *Rev Infect Dis* 9(Suppl2):S195-210, 1987.
237. Stamm WE: Diagnosis of *Chlamydia trachomatis* genitourinary infections, *Ann Intern Med* 108:710-717, 1988a.
238. Stamm WE: Protocol for diagnosis of urinary tract infection: reconsidering the criterion for significant bacteriuria, *Urology* 32(Suppl2):6-12, 1988b.
239. Stamm WE et al: Causes of the acute urethral syndrome in women, *N Engl J Med* 303:409-415, 1980.
240. Stamm WE et al: Treatment of the acute urethral syndrome, *N Engl J Med* 304:956-958, 1981.
241. Stamm WE et al: Diagnosis of coliform infection in acutely dysuric women, *N Engl J Med* 307:463-468, 1982.
242. Stamm WE et al: Effect of treatment regimens for *Neisseria gonorrhoeae* on simultaneous infection with *Chlamydia trachomatis*, *N Engl J Med* 310:545-549, 1984.
243. Stergachis A et al: Selective screening for *Chlamydia trachomatis* infection in a primary care population of women, *Am J Epidemiol* 138:143-153, 1993.
244. Stone HH, Martin JD: Synergistic necrotizing cellulitis, *Ann Surg* 175:702-711, 1972.
245. Stone KM et al: Treatment of external genital warts: a randomised clinical trial comparing podophyllin, cryotherapy, and electrodesiccation, *Genitourin Med* 66:16-19, 1990.
246. Stone RL, Schlievert PM: Evidence for the involvement of endotoxin in toxic shock syndrome, *J Infect Dis* 155:682-689, 1987.
247. Strom BL et al: Sexual activity, contraceptive use, and other risk factors for symptomatic and asymptomatic bacteriuria, *Ann Intern Med* 107:816-823, 1987.
248. Sweet RL: New approaches for the treatment of bacterial vaginosis, *Am J Obstet Gynecol* 169:479-482, 1993.
249. Sweet RL et al: Use of laparoscopy to determine the microbiologic etiology of acute salpingitis, *Am J Obstet Gynecol* 134:68-78, 1979.
250. Sweet RL et al: The occurrence of chlamydial and gonococcal salpingitis during the menstrual cycle, *JAMA* 255:2062-2064, 1986.
251. Sweet RL et al: Evaluation of new antiinfective drugs for the treatment of acute pelvic inflammatory disease, *Clin Infect Dis* 15(Suppl1):S53-S61, 1992.
252. Telzak EE et al: HIV-1 seroconversion in patients with and without genital ulcer disease: a prospective study, *Ann Intern Med* 119:1181-1186, 1993.
253. Thomason JL, Gelbart SM, Broekhuizen FF: Advances in the understanding of bacterial vaginosis, *J Reprod Med* 34:581-586, 1989.
254. Thomason JL, Gelbart SM, Scaglione NJ: Bacterial vaginosis: current review with indications for asymptomatic therapy, *Am J Obstet Gynecol* 165:1210-1217, 1991.
255. Thomason JL et al: Statistical evaluation of diagnostic criteria for bacterial vaginosis, *Am J Obstet Gynecol* 162:155-160, 1990.
256. Thompson SE et al: The microbiology and therapy of acute pelvic inflammatory disease in hospitalized patients, *Am J Obstet Gynecol* 36:179-186, 1980.
257. Todd J et al: Toxic-shock syndrome associated with phage-group-1 staphylococci, *Lancet* 2:1116, 1978.
258. Tofte RW, Williams DN: Clinical and laboratory manifestations of toxic shock syndrome, *Ann Intern Med* 96:843-847, 1982.
259. Townsend DE, Smith LH, Kinney WK: Condylomata acuminata: roles of different techniques of laser vaporization, *J Reprod Med* 38:362-364, 1993.
260. Turnbull AE, Cohen ME: Case report: pelvic actinomycosis with the development and resolution of a rectosigmoid stricture, *Clin Radiol* 43:420-422, 1991.
261. U.S. Preventive Services Task Force: screening for sexually transmitted diseases, Washington, DC, *Am Fam Physician* 42:691-702, 1990.
262. Valicenti JE et al: Detection and prevalence of IUD-associated actinomyces colonization and related morbidity, *JAMA* 247:1149-1152, 1982.
263. Van Slyke KK, Michel VP, Rein MF: Treatment of vulvovaginal candidiasis with boric acid power, *Am J Obstet Gynecol* 141:145-148, 1981.
264. Vermund SH et al: High risk of human papillomavirus infection and cervical squamous intraepithelial lesions among women with symptomatic human immunodeficiency virus infection, *Am J Obstet Gynecol* 165:393-400, 1991.
265. Wager GP: Toxic shock syndrome: a review, *Am J Obstet Gynecol* 146:93, 1983.
266. Walker CK et al: Pelvic inflammatory disease: metaanalysis of antimicrobial regimen efficacy, *J Infect Dis* 168:969-978, 1993.
267. Walters MD et al: Antibodies to *Chlamydia trachomatis* and risk for tubal pregnancy, *Am J Obstet Gynecol* 159:942-946, 1988.
268. Washington AE, Arno PS, Brooks MA: The economic cost of pelvic inflammatory disease, *JAMA* 255:1735-1738, 1986.
269. Washington AE, Johnson RE, Sanders LL: *Chlamydia trachomatis* infections in the United States: what are they costing us? *JAMA* 257:2070-2072, 1987.
270. Washington AE, Katz P: Cost of and payment source for pelvic inflammatory disease: trends and projections, 1983 through 2000, *JAMA* 266:2565-2569, 1991.
271. Webster LA, Berman SM, Greenspan JR: Surveillance for gonorrhea and primary and secondary syphilis among adolescents: United States, 1981-1991, *MMWR CDC Surveill Summ* 42:1-11, 1993.
272. Webster LA, Rolfs RT: Surveillance for primary and secondary syphilis: United States, 1991, *MMWR CDC Surveil Summ* 42:13-19, 1993.

273. Weck PK, Buddin DA, Whisnant JK: Interferons in the treatment of genital human papillomavirus infections, *Am J Med* 85:159-164, 1988.
274. Weinberger MN, Harger JH: Accuracy of the Papanicolaou smear in the diagnosis of asymptomatic infection with *Trichomonas vaginalis*, *Obstet Gynecol* 82:425-429, 1993.
275. Weinstock HS et al: *Chlamydia trachomatis* infection in women: a need for universal screening in high prevalence populations? *Am J Epidemiol* 135:41-47, 1992.
276. Westrom L: Effect of acute pelvic inflammatory disease on fertility, *Am J Obstet Gynecol* 121:707-713, 1975.
277. Westrom L et al: Pelvic inflammatory disease and fertility: a cohort study of 1844 women with laparoscopically verified disease and 657 control women with normal laparoscopic results, *Sex Transm Dis* 19:185-192, 1992.
278. Wiesner PJ, Thompson SE: Gonococcal diseases, *Dis Mon* 26:1-44, 1980.
279. Witkin SS: Immunology of recurrent vaginitis, *Am J Reprod Immunol Microbiol* 15:34-37, 1987a.
280. Witkin SS: Transient, local immunosuppression in recurrent vaginitis, *Immunol Today* 8:360, 1987b.
281. Witkin SS: Immunologic factors influencing susceptibility to recurrent candidal vaginitis, *Clin Obstet Gynecol* 34:662-668, 1991.
282. Witkin SS, Jeremias J, Ledger WJ: A localized vaginal allergic response in women with recurrent vaginitis, *J Allergy Clin Immunol* 81:412-416, 1988.
283. Wofsy GB et al: Isolation of AIDS-associated retrovirus from genital secretions of women with antibodies to the virus, *Lancet* 1:527-529, 1986.
284. Wolner-Hanssen P et al: Association between vaginal douching and acute pelvic inflammatory disease, *JAMA* 263:1936-1941, 1990.
285. Wolner-Hanssen P et al: Clinical manifestations of vaginal trichomoniasis, *JAMA* 261:571-176, 1989.
286. Wolner-Hanssen P et al: Decreased risk of symptomatic chlamydial pelvic inflammatory disease associated with oral contraceptive use, *JAMA* 263:54-59, 1990.
287. Wolner-Hanseen P et al: Laparoscopy in women with chlamydial infection and pelvic pain: a comparison of patients with and without salpingitis, *Obstet Gynecol* 61:299-303, 1983.
288. Wysoki RS, Majmudar B, Willis D: Granuloma inguinale (donovanosis) in women, *J Reprod Med* 33:709-713, 1988.
289. Yliskoski M et al: Cryotherapy and CO_2-laser vaporization in the treatment of cervical and vaginal human papillomavirus (HPV) infections, *Acta Obstet Gynecol Scand* 68:619-625, 1989.
290. Zimmerman HL et al: Epidemiologic differences between chlamydia and gonorrhea, *Am J Public Health* 80:1338-1342, 1990.

Chapter 22

CONCEPTION CONTROL

Rapin Osathanondh

The practice of birth control can be traced back to ancient societies of different racial and religious origins.[194] At the present time, voluntary prevention of pregnancy (contraception) and termination of unwanted pregnancy (therapeutic induced abortion) is widely accepted for medical (parental or fetal indications) and socioeconomic reasons. In spite of the rapid advancement in reproductive biology, there still exist four general problems regarding birth control that may or may not be resolved in our time.

1. **There is no ideal contraceptive method**. All contraceptive methods available in the United States are safer than no contraception. However, it is impossible to make a contraceptive that is 100% effective, easy to use, reversible, and has no side effects. For each woman, any method of contraception has advantages and disadvantages as well as relative and absolute contraindications. A suitable method means that its benefits far outweigh the risks. For example, statistical calculations by Tietze and Lewit in the past decade suggested that the safest contraceptive practice for women at any age in the United States is the diaphragm or condom.[290] This practice can be backed by early, legal abortion should the method fail.[197,289,290] Unfortunately, induced abortion may be costly or inaccessible in many localities. To guard against pregnancy and sexually transmitted diseases (STDs), a combination of the low-dose oral contraceptive pill and the use of a latex or polyurethane condom may represent the safest choice for women under 40 years of age who do not smoke cigarettes.
2. **Women who use contraceptives should see a gynecologist at least once a year**. Contraceptive-related problems may occur as a direct or indirect result of contraceptive use. Increased coital activity or an increased number of sexual partners may necessitate switching from one method of contraception to another. For example, studies before and after the use of the oral contraceptive pill showed an increased incidence of bacteriuria in some women, with a tendency for repeated bladder infections.
3. **The efficacy of most contraceptives is dependent on the motivation of the user**. The actual-use effectiveness may not be applicable in many circumstances. For some women, an intrauterine device may be more effective than the pill because of poor dosing compliance. For many women, the *natural family planning method* (abstinence or the rhythm method) is in fact unnatural and often results in high failure rates.
4. **There is an epidemic of unintended pregnancies in teenagers in the United States**. There has been a trend toward earlier and more frequent unprotected intercourse among teenagers. An annual occurrence of over one million unintended pregnancies in teenagers in the population of the United States is considered high when compared with that in other industrialized nations. Epidemiologic data reveal that marriages of teenagers generally lead to eventual separation or divorce, less education, and low-paying jobs or no jobs. Recent national statistics revealed an average of one out-of-wedlock child for every five live births. Moreover, there are approximately three million women 15 to 44 years of age who do not want to conceive yet currently do not practice contraception. This is a serious public health problem and a great concern for society.

ORAL CONTRACEPTIVES

Birth control pills (*the pill*) represent the most studied class of medications since 1960. Oral contraceptives (OCs) are taken daily by over 50 million women, most of whom are not at risk of developing serious side effects. The pill is very effective in preventing unwanted conception, with a crude contraceptive efficacy (Pearl Index) of less than two pregnancies per 100 women-years. Its effects are reversible and there are many noncontraceptive health benefits (Table 22-1), some of which will last for years after use.[9,15,28,29,36,37,42,48,59,80,95,123,124,135,155,192,206,209,224,236,280,293,300,301,314,319] Most OCs contain ethinyl estradiol, a synthetic estrogen, and a progestin (progesterone-like substance). These are called *combined* or *combination OCs*. In the United States, since October 1988 each combined OC tablet contains 20 to 50 μg of ethinyl estradiol or a pharmacologically similar steroid mestranol (Fig. 22-1) plus one of the six progestins: norgestrel, norethindrone, norethindrone acetate, ethynodiol diacetate, desogestrel, or norgestimate. A much less popular type of OC contains a small dose of progestin without estrogen and is known as the ***minipill***. Unless the word minipill is specifically mentioned in this text, OC is generally understood to be the combined pill.

Administration and types of OC

The first tablet is usually taken on day 5 of menses, followed by one tablet per day for 21 days. For simplicity or better protection, some brands are begun either on the first day of bleeding or the first Sunday of the menstrual cycle. Withdrawal (anovulatory) bleeding generally occurs 3 to 5 days after the 21-day regimen, and the routine is begun again on day 5 of the new cycle. Thus there is 1 week off the routine with every 3 weeks on the routine. Most pharmaceutic manufacturers also provide a nonstop 28-day OC package in which the last seven tablets are hormonally inert placebos.

Table 22-1. Patient consent form for obtaining birth control pills

Birth control pills (the pill), or oral contraceptives, are being used every day by more than 50 million women around the world for the prevention of unwanted pregnancy. There are many health benefits of taking birth control pills besides the prevention of pregnancy (noncontraceptive benefits). There are also risks associated with taking the pill. However, these risks (for stroke, blood clots, heart attack) are seen mostly among women older than 35 years and especially among women 35 years or older who smoke. The risk for younger women is very small. According to the U.S. Food and Drug Administration, an increased risk of breast cancer has not been demonstrated among pill users, but there may be a slight increase in the risk for cancer of the cervix. All women must have a Papanicoloau (Pap) test at least once every year. Also, be sure to read the package insert that comes with your birth control pills.

Noncontraceptive benefits

1. The pill usually reduces menstrual cramps.
2. The pill generally protects women against having breast problems that are not cancer, cysts in the ovary, endometriosis (a disease that may cause severe menstrual cramps and infertility), and cancer of the ovary and the womb (uterus).
3. The pill decreases bleeding from the uterus and also reduces the risk of iron deficiency anemia in some women who bleed a lot during their periods and in those who bleed irregularly.
4. The pill may protect against rheumatoid arthritis.

Side effects

Minor side effects

Stay on the pill through the third package cycle. Minor side effects, if they occur will usually go away by then. If not, consult a physician or a nurse. A different brand may agree with you better.

1. Bleeding or spotting between periods
2. Nausea (try taking the pill at bedtime to avoid feeling sick)
3. Weight gain from fluid retention
4. Weight gain or loss due to change in appetite (should not be more than 2.3 kg [5 lb])
5. Breast tenderness, mild headaches, tiredness, or mood changes
6. Increased blood pressure
7. Enlargement of fibroid tumors in some women
8. Scant flow (less and less monthly bleeding) or missed periods
9. Decreased sex drive (however, most pill users report increased sex drive)
10. Acne (pimples) (however, most pill users see a decrease in acne problems) or a redness or darkening of the skin over the cheeks
11. Eye irritation in some pill users who wear contact lenses

More serious side effects

These are rare. Notify a physician immediately if they do occur.

1. Severe abdominal pain or discomfort (as a result of a gallbladder problem, a rare tumor in the liver, or blood clots in the bowel)
2. Severe chest pain or shortness of breath (as a result of blood clots in the heart or lungs)
3. Severe leg pain (as a result of stroke or other problems in the brain)
4. Severe headache (as a result of stroke or other problems in the brain)
5. Eye problems such as blurred vision (as a result of blood clots or an inflamed nerve in the eye)

PATIENT'S STATEMENT

I have read the above and understand that there are benefits and risks associated with the use of birth control pills. I choose to take the pill because I believe that the benefits for me are greater than the risks.

____________________________ __________________

Patient's Signature Date

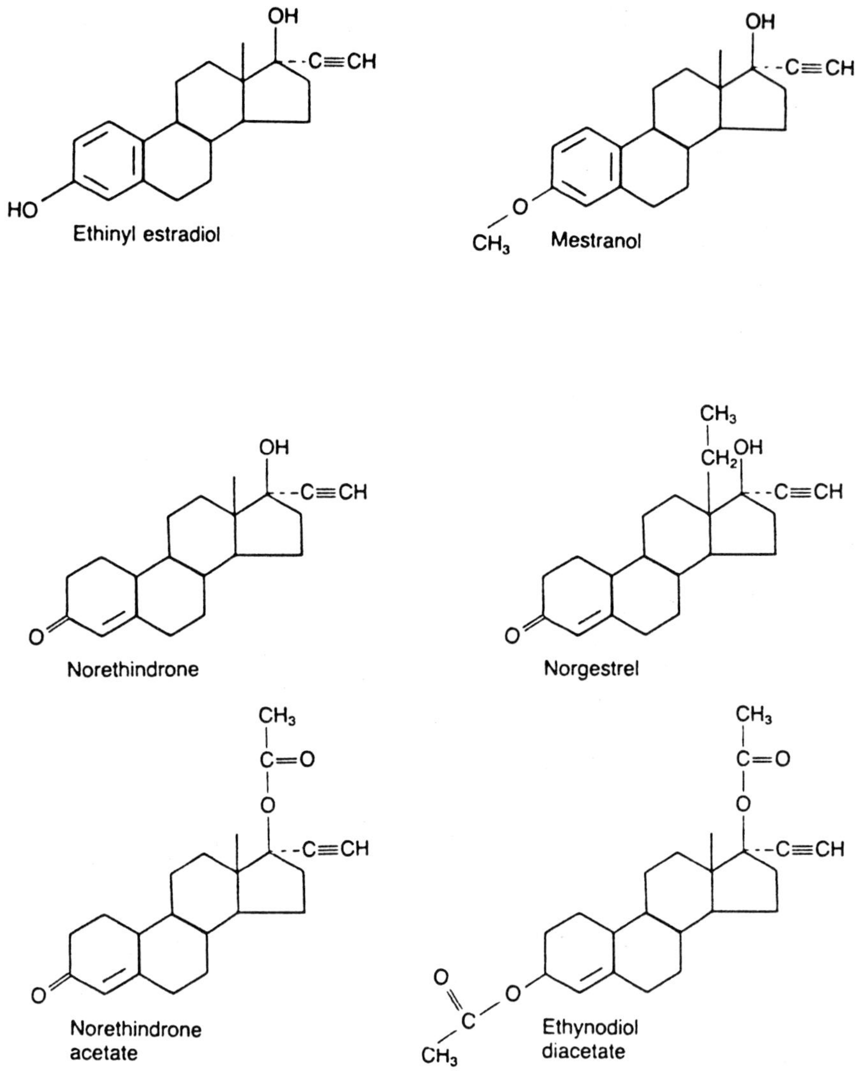

Fig. 22-1. Synthetic steroids used in oral contraceptives sold in the United States today. Estrogens: ethinyl estradiol and mestranol. Progestins: norethindrone, norethindrone acetate, norgestrel, and ethynodiol diacetate. (Courtesy Dr. PG Stubblefield)

The latter packaging system eliminates the need to remember the on or off intervals. Since each of the 21 hormonally active tablets contain the same amount of estrogen and progestin, this conventional OC is known as monophasic.

Because of recent publicity regarding the metabolic side effects of progestins, the biphasic and triphasic pills were produced to lower the total amount of progestin while mimicking the hormonal peak and trough levels within the physiologic menstrual cycle.[73] Of the five types of multiphasic pills (Table 22-2), only one formulation contains slightly varying amounts of estrogen, while three others put 35 μg of estrogen in each hormonally active tablet. To date there are no well-controlled studies with solid evidence for overall superiority of the multiphasic over the common monophasic low-dose pills. Theoretically these multiphasic formulations may represent the safest choice for potential pill users.

Mechanisms of action

The low daily dosage of two synergistic steroids in the pill prevents ovulation by centrally inhibiting the midcycle pituitary gonadotropin surge.[95,195,232,280] The pituitary gland may be unable to respond to the hypothalamic gonadotropin-releasing hormone while the woman is on an OC.[60] This central effect consequently obliterates the endogenous (ovarian) estrogen and progesterone production and commonly leads to a diminished endometrial proliferation. In the OCs with lesser amounts of estrogen, occasional small surges of gonadotropins may appear. However, such levels are usually

Table 22-2 Oral contraceptives available in the United States

Monophasic combination OC	Estrogen (g)	Progestin (mg)	Cost ($)*
Loestrin 1/20	EE20	Norethindrone acetate 1	22
Desogen, Orthocept	EE30	Desogestrel 0.5	18,21
Loestrin 1.5/30	EE30	Norethindrone acetate 1.5	22
Levlen, Nordette	EE30	D-norgestrel 0.15	19,22
Lo/Ovral	EE30	DL-norgestrel 0.3	22
Brevicon, Genora 0.5/35, Modicon, N.E.E. 0.5/35	EE35	Norethindrone 0.5	8-22 Generic 6
Demulen 1/35	EE35	Ethynodiol diacetate 1	21
Genora 1/35, Gynex 1/35, Jenest-28, N.E.E. 1/35, Nelova 1/3, Norcept-E 1/35, Norethin 1/35E, Norinyl 1 + 35, Ortho-Novum 1/35	EE35	Norethindrone 1	6-20 Generic 6-12
Ovcon 35	EE35	Norethindrone 0.4	21
Ortho-Cyclen	EE35	Norgestimate 0.25	21
Ovral	EE50	DL-norgestrel 0.5	34
Norlestrin 1/50	EE50	Norethindrone acetate 1	21
Norlestrin 2.5/50	EE50	Norethindrone acetate 2.5	22
Demulen 1/50	EE50	Ethynodiol diacetate 1	24
Ovcon 50	EE50	Norethindrone 1	23
Genora 1/50, N.E.E. 1/50 M, Norethin 1/50 M, Norinyl 1 + 50, Ortho-Novum 1/50			
Biphasic Combination OC	M50	Norethindrone 1	10-20 Generic 6
N.E.E. 10/11, Nelova 10/11, Ortho-Novum 10/11			
Triphasic Combination OC	EE35	Norethindrone 0.5 (days 1-10), 1 (day 11-21)	10,14,22
Tri-Levlen, Triphasil	EE30-40-30	D-Norgestrel 0.05 (days 1-6), 0.075 (days 7-11), 0.125 (days 12-21)	17,19
Ortho-Novum 7/7/7	EE35	Norethindrone 0.5 (days 1-7), 0.75 (days 8-14), 1 (days 15-21)	20
Tri-Norinyl	EE35	Norethindrone 0.5 (days 1-7), 1 (days 8-16), 0.5 (days 17-21)	20
Ortho Tri-Cyclen	EE35	Norgestimate 0.18 (days 1-7), 0.215 (days 8-14), 0.25 (days 15-21)	21
Progestin only (minipill)			
Micronor, Nor-QD	None	Norethindrone 0.35	25,24
Ovrette	None	DL-norgestrel 0.075	22

*Cost to the pharmacist for 1 month's use, rounded to the dollar, is based on the average wholesale price in the updated Drug Topics Red Book (1993).
EE = ethinyl estradiol; M = mestranol, a methyl ester of EE that is converted by the liver into EE
(Osathanondh R: Combination oral contraceptives. In Bardin CW, editor: *Current therapy in endocrinology and metabolism*, ed 5, Toronto, 1994, BC Decker/Mosby Yearbook.)

insufficient to stimulate ovarian follicles.[101,329] A much debated report of ovarian retention cysts in the users of low-dose pills may challenge this general rule.[24]

Peripherally, OCs also exert antinidation effects involving decreased oviductal function, endometrial glycogen content, and cervical mucus.[95,159,161,232,294] These peripheral effects are probably responsible for the major contraceptive effect of the minipill. The scant, dry, cervical mucus renders the cervix impermeable to penetration by sperm. Furthermore, atrophic, out-of-phase endometrium with resultant amenorrhea is not an uncommon finding. The minipill regimen does not totally abolish surges of luteinizing hormone (LH) or ovarian estrogens. However, it may partially block the central positive-feedback response to endogenous estrogens, resulting in inadequate amplitudes of pituitary LH surges.[95,159,163] Nevertheless, the reported pregnancy rate of two to seven per 100 women-years with this nonstop microdose progestin regimen is considerably higher than that observed with the combination OC. Irregular vaginal bleeding and increased ectopic pregnancy rates among failure cases further reduce the minipill's popularity. At present, the minipill may be appropriate for those few women with cardiovascular disease who cannot tolerate any estrogenic stimulation of their renin-angiotensin-aldosterone axis and those with known hypersensitivity to synthetic estrogens.

Advantages

OCs provide noncontraceptive benefits to the appropriate user and her society. The pill protects the individual user from life-threatening ectopic pregnancy, reduces primary dysmenorrhea, and reduces the risks of benign and malignant gynecologic problems as listed in a simplified patient consent form in Table 22-1. Society also benefits from the annual reduction of over 50,000 hospitalizations and office visits, according to studies in Britain and the United States.[15,42,245] After only 1 year of use, pill users may be protected from developing endometrial and ovarian cancer for 10 years.[15,28,29] The progestin in OCs reduces the number of estrogen and progesterone receptors in the endometrium. Furthermore, since ovulation does not occur, mitotic activity in the ovary, which is repeatedly high at the time of ovulation, is inhibited. There may be a delay in the return of ovulation following the cessation of OC use with an initial prolongation of the follicular phase or a shortened luteal phase.[231] In most cases menses resume within 3 months and fertility returns to the preexisting rate by the end of 2 years. If regular menstruation does not return within 6 months after cessation of OC, a hormonal evaluation is indicated. These particular users may have preexisting, slow-growing, pituitary microadenomas that can be treated successfully. The pill itself does not cause pituitary tumors.[220,265] Weight change, stress, or undiagnosed pregnancy may explain the postpill amenorrhea in other cases.

Disadvantages, side effects and contraindications

The pill must be taken daily and is considered a mild teratogen.[134,144,153] The users must devise their own systems to ensure daily compliance. The pill should be taken at the same time every day. In addition, a backup method such as condoms or contraceptive sponges should be utilized concomitantly in the first cycle of use when low-estrogen OCs may not provide full protection. Lowering the content of ethinyl estradiol in each tablet from 50 to 30 mg significantly increased the pregnancy rate in users.[145] The lower the hormonal content, the less danger from unwanted side effects but the higher the failure rate. Most gynecologists advise the user to take the previous day's pill if she forgets to take one pill and to take two pills each day for 2 days if she forgets to take two pills. If the user forgets 3 days in a row, the pill may not be an appropriate contraceptive method.

Another disturbing side effect that can occur with or without missing the dose is intermittent or irregular breakthrough uterine bleeding (BTB). Most women do not mind having menses or amenorrhea as long as these symptoms are predictable. Therefore, careful precounseling on this possible side effect of OC is essential for successful therapy. BTB during the first few months may resolve without treatment. Nonetheless, irregular bleeding could be a warning symptom that the efficacy of the OC may be compromised in a particular user. A careful history should be obtained to rule out pregnancy, infection, or neoplastic bleeding. In many instances, a watchful expectation may be preferred to the conventional double-dosing or adding more estrogen. Serious estrogen-related thromboembolic disorders appear to be dose dependent. If BTB exists or if it first occurs several months after the initiation of the pill, switching to a more progestogenic pill usually solves the problem. The use of norgestrel-containing OC may lessen the problem with irregular bleeding.[67,229] The alternative of adding a low dose of estrogen or switching to a more estrogenic pill should be tried only after other approaches fail.[315]

Other estrogen-induced side effects that are listed in the patient consent form's section on the minor side effects of OCs (Table 22-1) include nausea, vascular headaches, elevated blood pressure, weight gain as a result of fluid retention, tender breasts (mastalgia), increased mucoid vaginal discharge, cervical erosion (ectropion), or polyposis.[96] A mild increase in blood pressure may occur because of the activation of the renin-angiotensin-aldosterone system, hypervolemia, and decreased prostacyclin.[214] If the diastolic blood pressure is elevated (over 90 mm Hg) in response to OC use, discontinuation should be considered. Synthetic estrogens in the pill induce increased hepatic proteins (renin substrate, binding globulins, and most blood-clotting factors) and decreased antithrombin III and plasminogen activators (Table 22-3).[88,150,168,258,310] Hypercoagulability will occur in pill users with a familial deficiency of antithrombin III. An

Table 22-3. Some laboratory values that are influenced by the use of combination oral contraceptive pills

- Values that may be increased
  - Hematologic
    - Clotting factors (I, II, VII, VIII, IX, X, and XII)
    - Antiplasmins and antiactivators of fibrinolysis
    - Erythrocyte sedimentation rate
    - Red and white blood cells and platelets
    - Iron and iron-binding capacity
  - Hepatic proteins and related tests
    - α_1-globulins, α_2-globulins, and various binding globulins
    - Renin, angiotensin, angiotensinogen, and aldosterone
    - Bromosulfophthalein, bilirubin, and alkaline phosphatase
    - Transaminases and transpeptidase
    - Coproporphyrin and porphobilinogen
  - Hormonal
    - Growth hormone and insulin (and blood glucose)
    - Urinary total estrogens
  - Sterol and lipid
    - Vitamin A
    - Triglycerides and phospholipids
    - Low-density lipoprotein—cholesterol
  - Others
    - α_1-antitrypsin, C-reactive protein, serum copper, and ceruloplasmin
    - Urinary xanthuric acid
    - Positive results for antinuclear antibody and lupus erythematosus preparation
- Values that may be decreased
  - Hematologic
    - Folate and vitamin B_{12}
    - Antithrombin III and fibrinolytic activity
  - Hormonal
    - Lutenizing and follicle-stimulating hormones
    - Urinary preganediol and 17-ketosteroids
    - Triiodothyronine resin uptake
  - Others
    - Glucose tolerance, zinc, magnesium, and ascorbic acid
    - High-density lipoprotein—cholesterol (HDL-C)
    - Hepatoglobulin and cholinesterase

undisputed pill-induced human tumor is hepatic adenoma. This tumor is related to the use of synthetic estrogens (3.4 per 100,000 women/year).[223,255,261] Epidemiologic studies also disclosed twofold to fourfold increases in the diagnoses of cholelithiasis, postoperative deep vein thrombosis, pulmonary embolism (1 in 30,000 women/year), and cerebral thrombosis (1 in 30,000 women/year) among users of OCs with greater than 50 μg of synthetic estrogen, when compared to nonusers.[95,192,215,222,228,242,273,307,308] The overall annual risk of venous thromboembolism may be one to two cases per 1000 current users, depending on the estrogen content in the pill, blood type, and perhaps race and lifestyle. This risk is lower in women with type O blood type.[128] The risk disappears after cessation of the pill and is not related to the length of use of the pill. The effects of estrogen in reducing the activity of antithrombin III and plasminogen activators are dose related.[168,310,315, Lidegaard, 1993]

Untoward events related to progestins are decreased menses, reduced vaginal secretion, weight gain due to increased appetite, acne, leg cramps, fatigue, and sleepiness. BTB, chloasma, depression or mood change, and hypertension may also be related to progestins. Depression in some pill users may be due to pyridoxine deficiency with the resultant increase in xanthurenic acid. Certain medications including long-term antibiotics, anticonvulsants, and some sedatives make OCs less effective.[70,173,192,195,224,284] The most notorious is the antituberculous drug rifampin. Increased hepatic microsomal activity results in increased OC metabolism and decreased contraceptive effectiveness. Additionally, disturbed intestinal function (enterohepatic circulation) or colonic bacterial milieu may lower the pill's efficacy. Commonly prescribed drugs that may decrease the contraceptive effect of the pill include barbiturates, carbamazepine, primidone, phenytoin, long-term tetracycline, and griseofulvin. Backup contraceptive methods and the use of a 50 μg-estrogen pill may be required. Note also that the pill may delay the elimination of theophylline drugs and it may decrease the efficacy of oral anticoagulant preparations.

The long-term metabolic effects of progestins were recently the subjects of arguments with regard to the lowering of serum high-density lipoprotein (HDL) cholesterol and its consequence.[5,13,19,42,74,88,98,137,152,169,177,180,192,214,215,222,228,243,273] One study revealed an increased mortality rate among pill users 25 to 34, 35 to 44, and over 45 years of age because of circulatory diseases. Others showed an increased risk of coronary thrombosis and nonfatal myocardial infarction among pill users who were over 30 years of age. However, close scrutiny later revealed that the risk was limited to those with hypertension, diabetes, and hyperlipidemia. The greatest risk estimated to be 1 in 5000 women/year was actually found among pill users over 35 years of age who were smokers. Interestingly, the risk of coronary heart disease is not increased in former pill users and not correlated with the duration of OC use.[275] The latter finding perhaps suggests that pill-induced coronary vascular changes may be thrombotic and not atherogenic in origin.[15] Progestins in the pill are associated with an increased risk of atherosclerosis, since they tend to lower the levels of serum HDL and HDL_2.[5,13,15,19,74,88,180] In contrast, exogenous estrogens in the pill tend to raise HDL. Thus the effects of a combination OC on the user's lipid profile may depend on the variable interactions between the relative estrogenicity of the estrogen versus the antiestrogenicity and androgenicity of the progestin and the dose of the two hormones. Note, however, that the potency of a progestin in terms of delayed menses, withdrawal bleeding, or endometrial glycogen vacuoles may not be applicable in different women.[42,95,145,195] Furthermore some progestins have inherent estrogenic activity as they are converted in the body to estradiol. Norethynodrel, the first-generation progestin used in OCs was highly estrogenic. All progestins in OC are synthetic derivatives of 19-nortestosterone (meaning no carbon 19). The addition of an ethinyl group to carbon 17 results in an orally active steroid norethindrone as well as other estranes progestins which include norethynodrel, norethindrone acetate, ethynodiol diacetate, lynestrenol, norgestrienone, norgesterone, and quingestanol acetate. More potent progestins (the gonanes) contain an ethyl group at carbon 13 (e.g., norgestrel and desogestrel). The active form of norgestrel is d-norgestrel (levonorgestrel). This 19-norsteroid stays in the body longer than other progestins. Unlike other progestins, levonorgestrel is unique in that its oral administration does not bring about any effects of first-pass hepatic metabolism. The third group of progestins (the pregnanes) are derivatives of 17-OH-progesterone such as chlormadinone acetate, medroxyprogesterone acetate, megestrol acetate, and cyproterone acetate. There are at present 13 progestins utilized in over 300 brand names of steroid contraceptives in various countries. Third-generation progestins such as desogestrel, gestodene, and norgestimate (Figure 22-2) are less androgenic and may be associated with estrogen-induced side effects such as breast tenderness.[230] OCs that contain desogestrel may be the most beneficial for women with idiopathic hirsutism and selected patients with polycystic ovary syndrome.[167,233,247,266] Desogestrel lacks intrinsic androgenicity.[167,247] It does not interfere with the estrogen's capacity to induce an increase in sex hormone-binding globulin.[8] Consequently, combination OCs containing desogestrel increase the binding capacity for androgens. This leads to a substantial decrease in free testosterone and free 5a-dihydrotestosterone.[233] Active metabolites of desogestrel and norgestimate are 11-methylene-levonorgestrel (3-ketodesogestrel) and norgestrel-related compounds, respectively.

While the use of OCs reduces the incidence of benign breast disease, limited epidemiologic and laboratory data emerge almost every year to suggest an increased risk of breast cancer in pill users.[131,164,175,176,178,217,218,256,281,283] Specifically, worrisome findings with regard to breast cancer in pill users came out after the 1984 exoneration of the pill by the United States Food and Drug Administration panel of

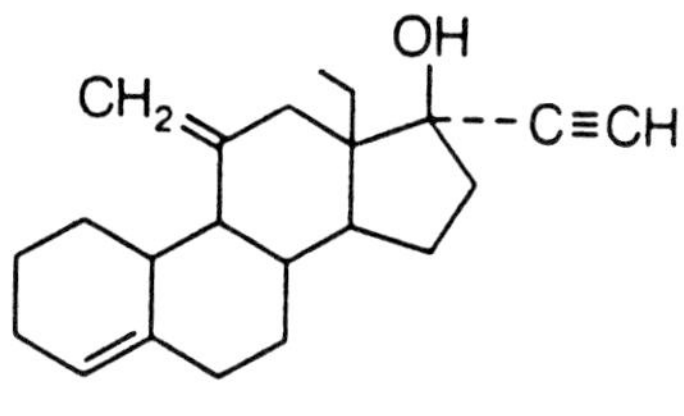

Desogestrel

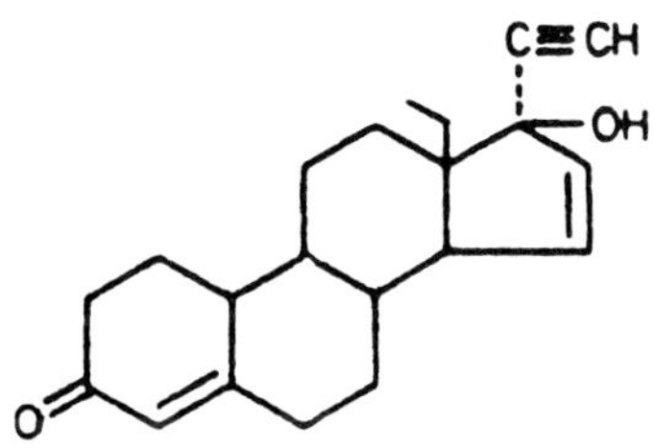

Gestodene

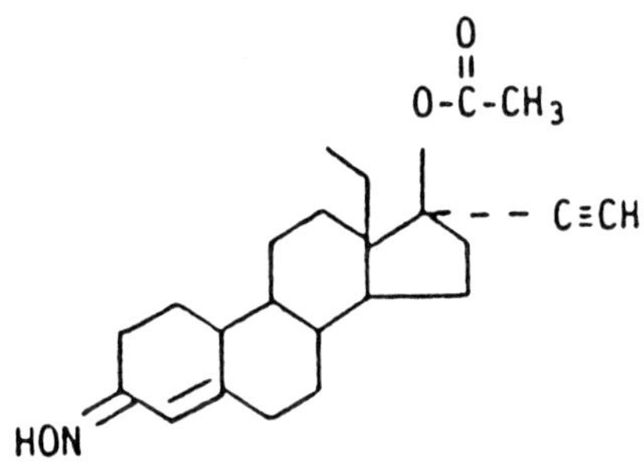

Norgestimate

Fig. 22-2. New progestins not yet available in the United States.

experts.[10,16,27,35,116,127,146,152,156,205,211,235,252,253,274,288,296,304,305] Because OCs have been available since 1960 and because the peak incidence of female breast cancer occurs at 55 to 74 years of age, any long-term latency effects of early pill use may not show up in this decade. Data implicating OC use with increased risks of cervical cancer[42,126,152,241,276,307,309,320] and malignant melanoma have also appeared.[276] Epithelial abnormalities of the uterine cervix in many OC users are a matter of concern among epidemiologists with regard to the transmission of the papilloma and human immunodeficiency viruses and *Chlamydia trachomatis*.[166,219,313,322] Definite conclusions on the risks of breast and cervical cancer and malignant melanoma among pill users cannot be drawn based on presently available data, because study designs have not accounted for the presence and influence of important confounding factors.[282] It is accepted, however, that breast and some other gynecologic tumors as well as certain adenocarcinomas and adenomas may be stimulated by sex steroids. Therefore, women with a present or past history of such tumors should not use the pill.

The American College of Obstetricians and Gynecologists lists the following as absolute contraindications to the pill: thromboembolism or thrombotic disease, active and/or chronic liver disease, undiagnosed uterine bleeding, pregnancy, breast cancer, and estrogen-dependent neoplasia. Other strong contraindications should include a history of coronary heart disease, stroke, hypertension, dyslipidemia (especially type II hyperlipoproteinemia), smokers over 40 years of age, cyanotic heart disease, sickle cell disease, severe headaches, active gall bladder disease, and conditions requiring total immobilization.[5,15,42,74,82,88,98,137,169,177,180,192,214,222,273,307] A rare type of headache which is associated with papilledema (pseudotumor cerebri or idiopathic intracranial hypertension) contraindicates the use of any contraceptive steroid.

Relative contraindications include smokers over 35 years of age, moderate or severe cervical intraepithelial neoplasia, migraines, and certain types of diabetes mellitus. Diabetic women with elevated blood pressure, nephropathy, or retinopathy must be discouraged from using the pill. Many women with well-controlled diabetes or migraines have tolerated OC use and are happy with it. The use of a low-dose OC does not appear to alter the pill user's tolerance to a 75-gram oral glucose load.[133] Impaired carbohydrate metabolism occurs with a high-dose formulation that contains norgestrel.[62] OC-induced insulin resistance is manifested by reduced peripheral tissue insulin sensitivity and may ameliorate with time.[133]

BARRIER METHODS AND SPERMICIDES

Condoms (prophylactics)

The condom is without doubt the most popular but underreported mechanical contraceptive method for various justifiable reasons. It is disposable, convenient to use, inexpensively sold over the counter (OTC), and may help prevent the spread of STDs. It should be used by pregnant women who have or are at risk for STDs.[94] Its use may be indicated even though the couple is sterile. Regarding the feared viral transmission, condoms made of latex appear superior to other materials. However, the perfect barrier material has not yet been invented. An allergic reaction to latex is uncommon but can be life threatening. Furthermore, latex materials can be destroyed by oil-based intravaginal medications. A newly approved condom made of polyurethane appears to be thinner and stronger than the latex rubber and may circumvent the allergy or incompatibility problem. The chance of failure may be further reduced when the condom is prelubricated with a spermicide. The failure rate was estimated to be 3 per 1000, with perfect use. Condoms cover the penis during coitus and serve as a reservoir to prevent the deposition of semen in the vagina. The prototype of a condom made of animal products, prior to the vulcanization of rubber, has been in use for centuries. Failures are related to the material itself or the manufacturing process, and the user's technical or mental difficulties (e.g., wearing the condom after some semen has been released into the vagina, or sperms escaping out as a result of failure to withdraw before detumescence). Besides improper technique, the actual failure rates of barrier contraceptives are often influenced by inconsistent use.

Spermicidal agents

Most vaginal spermicides contain nonoxynol-9, a surface-active, nontoxic detergent that immobilizes sperm. It is available as a cream, jelly, aerosol foam, foaming tablet, and suppository. Another formulation comes in the form of a semitransparent square of contraceptive film which dissolves at body temperature into a gel. Each product comes in 1% or 100 mg but some contain as high as 5% or 28% of nonoxynol-9. It is also convenient and inexpensive, with a theoretical failure rate of 5 pregnancies per 100 women-years. No association has been established between the use of vaginal spermicides and birth defects.[112,165,311] These agents are considered microbicidal and may lower the risk of most STDs. They also disrupt the cell membrane integrity of the mucosa, especially with repeated applications within a short period of time. Vaginal or penile irritation because of local hypersensitivity to nonoxynol-9 may occur in some users but this adverse effect is not common.

Another type of spermicide that shows promising results in clinical trials is propranolol.[333] This drug kills sperms on contact. Its spermicidal property was first discovered in hypertensive men who became azoospermic following propranolol therapy. Among many 3b-sympathomimetic antagonists tested, propranolol showed the strongest spermicidal effect. The mechanism for this effect may be related to the drug's lipophilic activity.[121,213]

Intravaginal devices

The diaphragm is a barrier between the lower vaginal canal and the cervical canal. It is a circular patch made of latex rubber and held by a circular, collapsible, metal frame with a memory like a spring. The user must compress this circular spring rim to flatten and elongate it so that it can slip into the vagina while the user is in a squatting or one-thigh-up position. There are four types of rim: coil, flat, wide-seal, or arcing. The latter may be the easiest to insert correctly for full coverage of the cervical os. It comes in nine sizes based on the diameter of the circular rim (from 50 to 90 mm at 5-mm increments). The three sizes in the middle range (65, 70, and 75) will fit most women. The proper size is determined by a vaginal examination and trial with fitting rings. The correct size should be adequately large but not interfere with urination. The device rests in place under the urethra. Women with frequent cystitis may not be good candidates for using a diaphragm.[79,227] Anatomic changes such as marked weight gain or loss or development of vaginismus may require refitting for a proper size of diaphragm. Proper retention of the device may not be possible in women with pelvic floor relaxation disorders and procidentia. If used correctly and with high motivation and compliance, its failure rate is theoretically less than 3 pregnancies per 100 women-years. Spermicidal jelly should be applied on each side of the diaphragm before its insertion and the device left in for at least 6 hours after intercourse. It is then removed, washed, dried, and put away until the next usage. It must not be dusted with talcum powder, since talc may increase the risk of ovarian cancer. Diaphragm use may lower the risk of pelvic inflammatory disease (PID) and cervical epithelial neoplasia (CIN).[47,138,285] There is controversy regarding any association of toxic shock syndrome (TSS) and diaphragm use.

The cervical cap is much smaller than the diaphragm (Fig. 22-3) and must fit tightly over the cervix. It has a soft, non-metal rim with an external diameter that ranges from 22 to 35 mm. Its cup-like shape fits onto the body of the cervix with the circular rim toward the fornix. The Prentiff cavity rim that is manufactured in England slowly gained acceptance in the United States. Koch in Boston, who has been an active investigator, advises the use of a spermicidal jelly with a high (3% to 5%) concentration of nonoxynol-9 on the cervical side for contraceptive efficacy plus suction-cup effect.[141] Such potent spermicides include Ramses (5%), Koromex (3%), or Shur-Seal (2%). It can be left in place for several days and must be removed if vaginal or menstrual bleeding occurs. Initial users should have a Pap smear taken before the fitting and another taken 3 months thereafter. The increased risk of cervical erosion and CIN among cap users has been a concern. Other problems include the widely different sizes and shapes of the cervix and the difficulty in patient education toward the correct placement of the cap

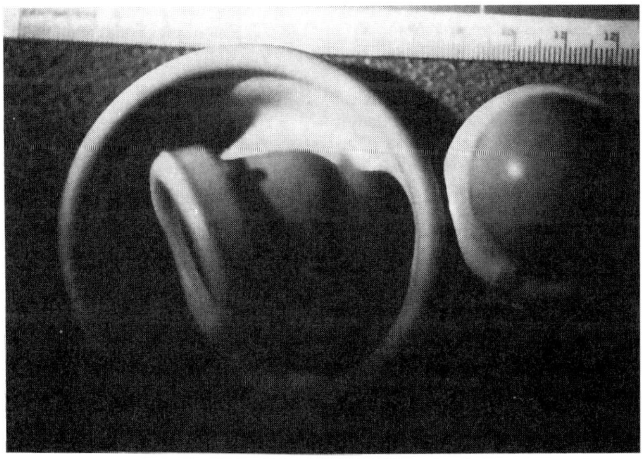

Fig. 22-3. Cervical caps (Prentiff Cavity Rim) compared with a diaphragm.

relative to the diaphragm. Many women have great difficulty in finding their cervix. Others do not like to touch their own genitals especially in certain cultures. On rare occasions when a user cannot remove her cap, a vaginal speculum is required. The cap will drop out of its place once the speculum is open inside the vagina. The cap's failure rate of 8 to 20 pregnancies per 100 women-years is higher than that of the diaphragm. Several designs of custom-fit caps are under clinical trials. Such caps have a one-way valve to permit the outflow of the uterine and cervical secretions while blocking sperm entrance.

The vaginal contraceptive sponge is a one-size-fits-all disposable barrier that is made of polyurethane containing one gram of nonoxynol-9 (enough for multiple acts of coitus). It is a convenient OTC product of modest price and will remain fully effective during 24 hours of use. Its failure rate is comparable to that of the diaphragm. Each sponge has a built-in loop for easy removal. The sponge is placed under tap water and immediately inserted into the vagina. Users are at a reduced risk of STD except for candidiasis.[237] The risk of nonmenstrual TSS of 1 case per 2 million sponges is very low.[76]

The female condom is another type of mechanical barrier which has been utilized off and on since the beginning of this century. The type that has received FDA approval is a disposable seamless polyurethane device that fits loosely inside the vagina and covers the perineum. It has flexible rings at both ends. The inner ring at the closed end can be compressed and pushed into the vagina to cover the cervix. It is soft, prelubricated, and aimed to prevent any contact with body secretions for the man and the woman. However, additional lubricant may be required to prevent dislodging and unpleasant noises during use. Its contraceptive efficacy is probably comparable to that of the diaphragm (based on limited premarketing data). The rebirth of the female condom reflects the need for more protection against viral transmission. In fact, barrier contraceptives have gained immense popularity even though some users consider these barriers messy or inconvenient. Such methods require manipulation of the genitalia at or near the time of coitus and thus require serious motivation for successful use.

Intrauterine devices

The intrauterine contraceptive device (IUD) represents a highly effective means of birth control for a well-selected group of women.[158] It is a small plastic T-shaped rod or tiny circular ring that is made to fit easily inside the uterus. With an IUD in place, the uterus and oviducts become hostile to the sperm, oocyte, and fertilized ovum.[321] Consequently, 96% to 99% of all women wearing an IUD for a year will not conceive. IUD use is not associated with unwanted metabolic effects and one device lasts a long time when compared to other reversible contraceptive methods. It is appropriate for women at low risk of STD, since its use is associated with an increased risk of PID and tubal infertility.[49,54] Since the IUD effectively prevents pregnancy, its use will not increase the overall incidence of tubal pregnancy. In fact, the incidence of ectopic pregnancies among 1000 women

Table 22-4. Patient consent form for intrauterine contraceptive device (IUD) insertion

Intrauterine contraceptive devices are an effective means for birth control, especially for women older than 25 years of age who already have children. However, there are certain problems with IUDs which you must know about if you are considering having one inserted.

1. Sometimes women become pregnant, even with the IUD in place (2 to 4 pregnancies per 100 women per year). Women who become pregnant while using an IUD are more likely to have a miscarriage or premature delivery if the pregnancy continues and occasionally can develop a serious kind of infection in the uterus. Therefore, in the event you become pregnant with an IUD in place, the termination of the pregnancy should be strongly considered.
2. Women who become pregnant while using an IUD have a slightly increased chance that the pregnancy may occur in the tube (ectopic pregnancy). Ectopic pregnancy is a serious condition that requires surgery or a toxic drug for its treatment. Therefore, if you think you are pregnant with an IUD in place, you must report to your doctor without undue delay.
3. Having an IUD slightly increases your risk of developing an infection in the fallopian tubes. Some of the infections can be serious and may result in infertility. Your risk for a tubal infection is greatly increased if you have more than one male partner. This risk for an IUD-related infection is low in women in a mutually monogamous relationship.
4. Many women with an IUD will find that their menstrual pattern is changed and that they have bleeding between periods or that the menstrual period is heavier and more painful. You should consult your doctor if you have lower abdominal pain, abnormal vaginal discharge or bleeding, and if you think you are pregnant or have a sexually transmitted infection.
5. Sometimes the IUD can be expelled (it falls out).
6. Sometimes the IUD perforates the uterus (it makes a hole in your womb) at the time of insertion.

PATIENT'S STATEMENT

I have read the above and understand that there are risks associated with the use of an IUD. I have also read and signed the necessary form provided by the IUD manufacturer. I choose to use this method of contraception because I feel that the benefits for me are greater than the risks.

____________________ __________

Patient's signature Date

who use IUDs is significantly lower than would be the case among 1000 women who do not use contraceptives. However, a high incidence of ectopic pregnancy has been observed among women who conceive while using an IUD, particularly the type that releases progesterone or d-norgestrel.[63] This may be analogous to the increased risk of ectopic pregnancy among minipill failure cases. Women who had an ectopic pregnancy or venereal disease such as gonorrhea or chlamydia should not use an IUD (Table 22-4).

Of all the FDA-approved IUDs, only two kinds are available in the United States: the Copper T-380A (effective up to 10 years) and the Progestasert (effective for 1 year). Both types are T-shaped and radiopaqe but they differ in many aspects. The copper-containing IUD is superior to the noncopper device in contraceptive efficacy and perhaps lower relative risk of PID.[49,269,332] Regarding the influence of the type of device on the risk of PID, the worst record was observed with the Dalkon Shield and was attributed to poor design.[158] A significantly increased risk of PID in IUD wearers was observed during the first few months after insertion.[22] After that period this risk may not be increased in copper IUD wearers, especially those at low risk of contracting STDs. Salpingitis occurring more than a few months after insertion is likely a result of an STD and not the IUD.[148] Women at high risk for developing PID include, in respective order of significance, those with a prior history of PID or STD, with multiple sexual partners, who are nulliparous and under 25 years of age and single.[46,179] They should be discouraged from using the IUD. Those at the lowest risk of developing PID are parous women in a stable and mutually monogamous relationship. Because of its lack of metabolic effects, a copper-containing IUD may be ideal for an older parous woman who smokes cigarettes and does not want permanent sterilization.

Mechanism of action. The IUD prevents fertilization and implantation by several postulated mechanisms, all of which are promptly reversible upon the removal of the device. The IUD alters the intrauterine environment by inducing a local, sterile, inflammatory response (foreign body reaction).[181] It is believed that leukocyte infiltration leads to an environment that is hostile to the oocyte, sperm, and fertilized ovum. Studies of daily serum hCG levels in the luteal phase using highly sensitive assays led to the conclusion that implantation did not occur in IUD wearers.[257,262,318] A controlled study of oocytes that were retrieved via tubal flushing strongly suggests that the IUD also inhibits the fertilization process.[321] Sperm may not reach the oocyte or are unable to penetrate the oocyte coverings. Alternatively, an adverse tubal environment may damage the oocyte. Macrophage destruction of oocytes was shown in copper IUD wearers. Copper may interfere with oocyte release or fimbria function, accelerate transport, or induce premature lysis of the ovum. In contrast to progesterone, copper inhibits the enzyme prostaglandin dehydrogenase in the local tissues.[139] The amount of copper absorbed into the systemic circulation is minute relative to the minimum daily dietary requirement. There have been rare cases of allergic skin lesions with pruritus as a result of intrauterine copper, which can be confirmed by standard skin tests.[234]

Insertion technique. The optimal time to insert an IUD is during menses, when a woman is least likely to be pregnant. The IUD user should have an opportunity to become acquainted with the instructions and the informed consent form, before the day of visit. Some women may require local anesthetic (paracervical block), especially when the insertion is done on a day in the cycle between menses. A bimanual pelvic examination is performed to determine the uterine size and position. The cervix is exposed with a speculum, cleansed with a local antiseptic, and its anterior lip is grasped with a tenaculum. Gentle traction to straighten the angle between the cervical canal and the uterine cavity is followed by a probing of the uterine cavity with a uterine sound to determine the internal direction and depth. The short-bladed Moore-Graves speculum may be required in the case of acute anteflexion. The device is loaded into its inserter and gently slipped through the cervical canal. It is then freed within the uterine cavity by withdrawing the inserter tube over the plunger. This withdrawal technique reduces the risk of a uterine perforation. Women wearing an IUD should report without delay any lower abdominal pain, fever and chill, unusual vaginal bleeding or spotting, pain during intercourse, or unpleasant vaginal discharge. A brief office visit should be offered 3 months after the insertion of the IUD. This should be followed by an annual checkup and a cytologic cervical smear.

Disadvantages, adverse effects, contraindications. Dysmenorrhea and increased menstrual flow are frequent IUD-related problems that may improve with the short-term intermittent use of a nonsteroidal antiinflammatory drug (NSAID) such as ibuprofen or naproxen. This class of drugs (type I inhibitors) inhibits the biosynthesis of cyclic endoperoxides and prostaglandin E and F series. If these problems persist or worsen, the device should be removed and the patient should be offered another choice of contraceptive. A new IUD has been designed so that its side arms will open and close with the uterine relaxation and contraction, with the hope of lowering the IUD-related dysmenorrhea incidence. Progestin-releasing IUDs were originally intended to alleviate both bleeding and dysmenorrhea problems. Unfortunately, such devices have been shown to increase the total number of days of bleeding and the incidence of midcycle spotting, even though the volume of monthly blood loss is actually reduced. A report by the WHO Task Force on Psychological Research in Family Planning indicated that an increase in the number of days of bleeding may be less acceptable to women than an increase in the volume of bleeding.[321] Another WHO study revealed no difference in dysmenorrhea complaints between the Progestasert and the Copper-7 users.[221] Subsequently those findings from WHO were confirmed by various independent investigators[86,193] who reported similar removal rates between progestin-releasing IUDs and copper or nonmedicated devices.[86,193]

Another IUD-related problem that received a careful review by Gupta and Woodruff concerns a unique organism, *Actinomyces*.[107] Reports have emerged since the past decade on the frequent Actinomyces-positive Pap smears among users of nonmedicated IUDs. There was also a high degree of association between true pelvic actinomycosis and the use of multifilamented, tailed IUDs (which were since discontinued). Although not common, true pelvic actinomycosis is a serious disease. A combination of PID and an Actinomyces-positive Pap smear requires aggressive intravenous therapy with broad-spectrum antibiotics.[298] The failure to obtain prompt clinical improvement would be strongly indicative of tuboovarian abscesses that generally require pelviscopic surgical treatment. Actinomyces-positive Pap smears are less frequently found in conjunction with the use of a copper IUD than with noncopper devices.[68] It has been postulated that copper may adversely affect the microbes, the gametes, and the tubal mucosa.

The reported failure rate of the Copper T-380A is only 1 case annually per 100 users over 25 years of age. However, one of every two current IUD users who conceive will miscarry and one of twenty IUD users who conceive will have an extrauterine pregnancy. With an IUD in place, there is a high risk of sepsis among users who miscarry, particularly when the miscarriage occurs during the second trimester. Women who conceive while using an IUD should have the device removed or consider a therapeutic, induced abortion, since the risks and consequences are serious. An important risk is prematurity with or without sepsis.[292] If an accidental pregnancy occurs after IUD use of more than 2 years, the risk of it being ectopic is high. Besides the IUD, contraceptive methods that predispose a user to ectopic pregnancy should the method fail include minipills, subdermal progestin implants, postcoital estrogen therapy, and most types of female sterilization.

Spontaneous expulsion of an IUD may occur in the first few months, especially during menses. The disappearance of the IUD string, which brings the patient back to her physician, may be the first sign of a lost IUD. Pregnancy must be ruled out, and when in doubt a pelvic ultrasound is very helpful. High-resolution transabdominal and transvaginal ultrasound imaging by an experienced sonographer may reveal an abnormal position of the IUD in the uterine wall or posterior wall of the cervix. In nonpregnant users with the possibility of lost IUD strings versus a lost IUD, x-rays of the abdomen and pelvis will ultimately confirm the absence or presence of the IUD, since most plastic devices have been impregnated with barium sulfate. Ultrasound guidance and alligator forceps (Fig. 22-4) can facilitate the nontraumatic removal of an IUD when the string is not visible.[278] The failure of this method of removal usually suggests that a part of the IUD has perforated the uterine wall, in which case a laparoscopy is indicated. The partial expulsion of the stem of the T-shaped device may occur through the cervical canal. This may be associated with cramps, vaginal or cervical erosion with spotting, lacerations of the penis, and reduced contraceptive efficacy. The device must be removed and replaced.

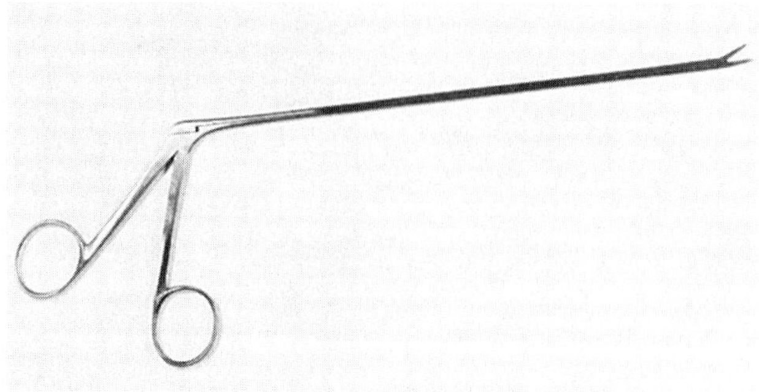

Fig. 22-4. Alligator forceps for IUD removal. (Courtesy Dr. PG Stubblefield.)

In cases of uterine perforation with intraperitoneal protrusion of a copper-containing IUD, the device must be removed without delay because its tissue reactions will rapidly bring about severe adhesions and enclosure by the omentum. The downward displacement of the stem into the endocervix (mostly posteriorly) may require a slight upward dislocation before the whole device can be removed through the cervical canal.

Absolute contraindications to the use of an IUD include a history of PID, STD, ectopic pregnancy, multiple male partners, purulent cervicitis, unresolved cervical neoplasia, undiagnosed genital bleeding, suspected pregnancy, Wilson's disease or known hypersensitivity to copper, valvular heart disease, genital actinomycosis, and any medical disorders predisposing to infection.[46] Relative contraindications include nulliparity, age less than 25 years, unmarried women who are not in a mutually monogamous relationship, recurrent vaginitis, anatomical derangement of the uterus (e.g., congenital anomalies, leiomyoma, cervical stenosis, etc.), painful heavy menses, anemia, rheumatic heart disease, or mitral valve prolapse.[46,321]

POSTCOITAL CONTRACEPTION AND MANAGEMENT OF SEXUAL ASSAULT VICTIMS

The morning-after pill or injection represents the most practical step in terminating the natural development of the fertilized egg(s) after an unprotected sexual intercourse. The original hormonal method of preventing fertilization or implantation of an already fertilized egg was the administration of high doses of a nonsteroidal estrogenic drug, diethylstilbestrol, within 3 days of unprotected coitus (Table 22-5). Morris and van Wagenen were among the first to demonstrate the effectiveness of the morning-after estrogenic pill for intercepting pregnancy in the rape victim.[186] Two decades ago they reported that either diethylstilbestrol or ethinyl estradiol tablets could be administered for this purpose.[187] Other

Table 22-5. Postcoital antifertility treatment from selected clinical trials

Method	Regimen*
DES†	50 mg daily for 5 days
Ethinyl estradiol	5 mg daily for 5 days
Conjugated estrogens	30 mg daily for 5 days or 50 mg daily injection for 2 days
Ovral	Two tablets and two more 12 hr later
Danazol	400 mg and 400 mg 12 hr later
D-norgestrel	0.4 mg within 3 hr of coitus
RU486	Midluteal 50 or 100 mg daily for 4 days regardless of time of coitus
Copper-T IUD	Insertion within 5 days of coitus

*Starting as soon as possible and within 2 or 3 days of coitus unless otherwise stated.
†Not recommended by the manufacturer, according to the package insert.

estrogens that have been effectively utilized are conjugated estrogens, estradiol benzoate, and stilbestrol diphosphate.[43,66,188] Besides exogenous estrogens, a whole host of steroidal and nonsteroidal drugs such as progesterone-receptor blockers, antimetabolites, alkaloids, and prostaglandins can exert antifertility effects when administered postcoitally.[263] These drugs will exert endocrine effects at local and possibly central levels, but the exact single mode of action for each type of morning-after pill has not been conclusively demonstrated.

Postcoital estrogen may prevent pregnancy by several postulated mechanisms, depending on the time of administration in the cycle. A fertilized egg normally reaches the uterine wall in 4 or 5 days, after which implantation of the blastocyst may or may not take place.[52] One out of three midcycle exposures generally results in implantation of the blastocyst, which occurs on or after the sixth day from ovulation. Altered or asynchronic endometrial glandular and stromal development with resultant enzymatic and metabolic derangement such as reduced cellular carbonic anhydrase may render the secretory endometrium nonreceptive to implantation. Disturbances in the endogenous estrogen/progesterone ratio and decreased luteal progesterone may also be responsible for the drug's antifertility effects. A high dose of estrogen given during late follicular phase may suppress ovulation and often prevents the rise in basal body temperature.[99,129] Other hypotheses include interferences with sperm and/or tubal motility, sperm capacitation, fertilization, and viability of the zygote. However, once implantation has taken place, the pregnancy appears to be resistant to most steroids.

The continuation of an unrecognized pregnancy which has been exposed to the morning-after pill may theoretically result in certain birth defects. A controversy exists over whether such birth defects are directly related to the sex steroid exposure during early pregnancy. Nevertheless, the menstrual history should be carefully analyzed prior to any postcoital antifertility treatment. If a question of pregnancy arises, a rapid, specific, and sensitive pregnancy test should be performed and repeated at appropriate intervals. An informed consent form may be obtained before prescribing a specific postcoital antifertility therapy that includes the immediate and late untoward effects of the therapy as well as the recommendation of abortion in the case of treatment failure. The failure rates for most methods are generally less than 2 per 100 isolated courses of treatment. The actual failure rates depend on the time of exposure in the cycle, other factors inherent to each method, and the type of subjects. However, a woman who requests postcoital antifertility therapy may choose to carry her unwanted pregnancy to term, in the event of treatment failure. Interestingly, ectopic pregnancies were diagnosed in 10% of women whose postcoital estrogen therapy had failed.[188,270]

High doses of estrogen often produce an uncomfortable bloated feeling, nausea, vomiting, and swelling of the hands and feet. Estrogen treatment may likely induce spotting or menstrual disturbances for several cycles (i.e., shorter or longer than expected cycles). An antiemetic pill or rectal suppository (e.g., prochlorperazine) should be taken at least one half hour prior to therapy with high doses of estrogen. If vomiting occurs within 1 hour after a dose of estrogen, that dose should be repeated. Morris and van Wagenen reported one serious complication from such high doses of estrogen. A woman with a history of premenstrual fluid retention developed acute pulmonary edema from diethylstilbestrol, which resolved after supportive treatment and the discontinuation of the drug.[188] A history of venous thromboembolism, another possible complication of taking estrogen, certainly contraindicates the use of the estrogenic morning-after pill. Other contraindications to high doses of estrogen include severe hypertension and hepatic impairment.

The routine use of high doses of unopposed estrogen has been discouraged for the past decade not only because of its possible venous thromboembolic complications but also because of the recent awareness of its association with genital cancers. Consequently, the most popular morning-after pill to date is a combination of a potent progestin dl-norgestrel with 50 μg of ethinyl estradiol. Postcoital antifertility treatment with this commonly available contraceptive pill (the Yuzpe regimen) consists of 2 tablets followed by 2 more tablets 12 hours later.[33] Like conventional high-dose estrogens, therapy must be initiated 2 or 3 days after an unprotected coitus and preferably with an antiemetic prophylaxis. Two additional tablets should be provided in case one dose is not retained. About half of the women on this regimen may experience the frequent side effects of nausea and vomiting, unless time-release antiemetic pills have been prescribed. This method is highly effective and has fewer side effects with a shorter duration of therapy than the conventional high-dose estrogen regimens.[239]

A potent progestin alone such as d-norgestrel (levonorgestrel) can also be utilized as a morning-after pill.[140] Other progestin that have been successfully tried for this purpose include clogestone, ethynodiol, norethindrone, norgestrienone, quingestanol acetate, and retroprogestagen. These progestins decidualize the endometrium, thus rendering it nonreceptive to implantation. Additionally, they alter the cervical mucus making it hostile to sperm penetration. Other possible antifertility effects are reduced sperm, tubal motility, and tubal secretions. Delayed ovulation and subsequent menstruation may occur with frequent isolated treatment.[44] Increased intrauterine pH following postcoital administration of d-norgestrel appears to be associated with a decreased number of motile sperm in the intrauterine fluid.[140] It should be mentioned among postcoital steroids that not only progestins but also danazol and RU486 have been utilized for this clinical indication.[142,143,250]

In many areas of the world, other than the United States, the postcoital antifertility treatment of choice is the insertion of a copper IUD (preferably a small T-shaped device).[157] The advantages of a copper IUD over steroidal drugs are in its longer, ongoing protection (up to several years if well tolerated) and the shorter duration of nausea or vagal reflex (usually less than 10 minutes). The latter can be blunted with premedication such as doxylamine, diphenhydramine, or other antihistamines with inherent anticholinergic effects. Local anesthetic (a paracervical block) may also be required for those with a tight internal cervical os. Inert (unmedicated) IUDs are not recommended because they require several days to achieve the intended antifertility effects, whereas the released copper provides faster action after insertion. Women with a history of venous thromboembolism may be candidates for a postcoital IUD. A multiparous woman with a mutually monogamous relationship represents an ideal candidate. Most pelvic infections that can be aggravated by the presence of an IUD will likely be diagnosed within 6 months of the insertion, and a good number of such cases are evident shortly after the insertion.[22] The victim of an unprotected coitus should receive an adequate dose of broad-spectrum parenteral antibiotic before the insertion of an IUD. The antibiotic spectrum should cover both gonorrheal and chlamydial infections. Presently under trial is an IUD impregnated with a chlorhexidine antiseptic that is slowly released and may reduce insertion-related pelvic infections. The precautions, instructions, consent form, and follow-up for a postcoital IUD are similar to those for postcoital steroid therapy. Progestin-releasing IUDs should not be used for postcoital contraception in view of the increased risk of ectopic pregnancy and prolonged spotting that is associated with progestin treatment.[63,193]

Management of female sexual assault victims

Sexual assault (rape) victims are mostly female and range from young children to older adults. Rape is the most underreported violent crime. One third of all victims bear evidence of bodily harm besides genital trauma. A reported lifetime incidence of one victim for every ten females is rising annually at an alarming rate, especially among the victims in the older age groups. Rape is generally defined as any natural or unnatural act of sexual intimacy or intercourse, usually by force, threat of bodily injury, or the inability of the victim to give appropriate consent. This definition varies slightly from state to state.

The management of the victim reflects the interplay between the medical and legal professions and includes (1) the diagnosis and treatment of physical and mental trauma with objective documentation of the assault as well as evidence collection and preservation; (2) the prevention of a pregnancy; and (3) the prevention or treatment of an STD. Beyond the acute management, follow-up and appropriate counseling are also important.[109,118]

The victim should be isolated from the mainstream of medical activity but not be left alone for a long period of time. The victim should receive priority, compassionate care, and respect. Most victims feel helpless and degraded, hence a nonjudgemental approach in obtaining a history and the details of the events is crucial. In Massachusetts, the victim (or guardian) must consent to a full management protocol that includes appropriate diagnostic methods, medical treatment, and the collection and release of evidence (e.g., specimens, clothing, photographs, etc.) before that particular sexual assault will be reported (i.e., the decision is the victim's). If possible, a brief description of the assault in the victim's own words should be recorded by only one clinician. Salient data may include the date of last menstrual period, the number of assailants, any lacerations on the victim or assailant that resulted in bleeding, the orifice of penetration with or without ejaculation, the use of any contraceptives, the victim's sexual activity within the last 5 days before the assault, and the victim's activities since the assault (e.g., wiping, washing, bathing or showering, douching, urinating, defecating, vomiting, teeth brushing, or clothes changing). Besides the physical findings on the victim's skin, hair, face, mouth, throat, breasts, abdomen, back, and extremities, the general physical and emotional status should also be recorded. The complaints and findings, including foreign matter, should be recorded or collected in a standard rape kit with meticulous labeling. Pertinent materials to be collected are fingernail scrapings (each in a separate test-tube), foreign pubic hair (from combing), about ten of the victim's pubic hairs (from cutting), and Polaroid photographs. Data related to the assault are kept in a chain-of-evidence pattern.

The pelvic examination must be performed with a nonlubricated, warm, water-moistened, speculum. The examination of the vagina and cervix should be concentrated toward the signs of pregnancy, parity, menstruation, trauma, infection, foreign material, and the nature of the fluid or discharge. The latter (from the vaginal pool) are smeared and dried on glass slides and preserved for evidence. Motile sperm can be identified within 4 to 6 hours in saline preparation of vaginal fluid. However, acid phosphatase tablets are no longer utilized. Cellular antigen matching and modern DNA fingerprinting techniques are highly reliable and specific, even when applied years later on properly preserved specimens. Microbiologic cultures are obtained from each orifice involved in the alleged assault. The risk of contracting an STD is associated with the degree of sexual contact and the number of assailants. The types of STDs associated with sexual assault (in respective order of frequencies) are gonorrheal (up to 13%), trichomonal/monilial/gardnerella (more than 6%), chlamydial (more than 4%), herpetic (up to 4%), and treponemal (less than 1%).[31] The antibiotics of choice for prophylaxis are single-dose parenteral ceftriaxone and metronidazole (with trichomonads or a frothy and malodorous vaginal discharge) followed by 1 week of oral doxycycline.[58,312] In the case of a suspected pregnancy, a highly sensitive (qualitative), urinary pregnancy test that utilizes a specific antibody against β-hCG can be expediently obtained prior to quantitative serum testing. Pregnancy interception and its small or unknown risk of potential damage, in the event of a retained embryo, should be made clear to the victim. The victim's willingness or unwillingness to abort a pregnancy should be ascertained. Finally, the victim should receive appropriate instructions as to when and whom to contact for test results and whether to implement or cancel the postcoital antifertility hormone and antibiotic treatment.

The long-term consequences or prognosis may depend on the type and degree of the assault (power rape, anger rape, sadistic rape), the immediate and follow-up multilevel care provided, the support from family and friends, and the preexistent adaptive behavior pattern.[3,189]

LONG-ACTING PROGESTINS AND OTHER AGENTS

Progestin in certain forms with or without a synthetic estrogen can be injected intramuscularly or subdermally to provide a prolonged contraceptive effect of several months to 5 years.[159,161] Two long-acting injectables approved by the United States FDA are intramuscular depomedroxyprogesterone acetate (DMPA) in microcrystalline suspension and subdermal levonorgestrel (d-norgestrel). These long-acting contraceptives underwent extensive clinical trials. Under development are single-rod subdermal contraceptives (being tried on breast-feeding women), 3-ketodesogestrel, and biodegradable implants. Other long-acting steroid contraceptives contain norethindrone enanthate with estradiol valerate, dihydroxyprogesterone acetophenide with estradiol enanthate, or DMPA with estradiol cypionate. The latter is entering phase III clinical testing in the United States as a once-a-month-injectable contraceptive.

DMPA was synthesized for contraceptive purposes almost 3 decades ago. It was utilized in the sequential type of combination OC which had been discontinued along with other sequential pills. Nowadays, millions of women use intramuscular DMPA for either contraception or estrogen-induced neoplastic and proliferative disorders.[238] The contraceptive dose is 150 mg of deep intramuscular (IM) injections every 12 weeks. The failure rate during the first year of use is less than 7 pregnancies per 1000 women.[136] Part of the reason that DMPA is so effective is that its effect may last slightly longer than 12 weeks. In fact, following a single 150 mg injection, it takes 8 to 9 months for the body to clear DMPA from the blood as a result of the slow release from the injection site.[183] Thus, users who delay receiving the next scheduled injection for a few weeks are still protected against accidental pregnancy. Its mechanisms of action are theoretically similar to those of the minipill. However, DMPA is much more reliable in consistently inhibiting ovulation through its effect on the hypothalamus.[183] Mean serum estradiol levels during different periods of DMPA treatment are suppressed down to those in the early follicular phase of the normal (untreated) cycle. The median estradiol level is notably slightly lower than the mean.[182] Thus, after 5 years of use, a decreased bone density has been observed when compared against age-matched nonusers.[53] After several years of treatment, the resumption of ovulation and fertility may not occur for a year or even longer. Chronic intermenstrual spotting (from atrophic endometrium) may occur in some patients after prolonged use, and treatment is costly.[291] The prolonged use of DMPA induces unfavorable changes in lipid metabolism, which varies among geographic sites.[325] Additionally, a mild glucocorticoid effect in terms of weight gain is observed in most users. Thus, intramuscular DMPA may only be appropriate for thin, multiparous women. Other unwanted effects may include headaches, decreased libido, tiredness, depression, and hair loss. Because each injection is irreversible for 8 months and in utero exposure may be associated with low birthweight infants, this contraceptive method should be provided only during normal menses (Table 22-6). Undiagnosed genital bleeding and known or suspected breast cancer contraindicate the use of DMPA. Short-term use may slightly increase the risk of breast cancer in young women.[323] On the other hand, the use of DMPA may significantly reduce the risk of endometrial cancer.[324]

Subdermal levonorgestrel implant

A subdermal levonorgestrel implant system was developed by the Population Council in New York for long-term contraception. Originally made and approved for use in Finland, the currently available system is composed of six subdermal capsules, each filled with 36 mg of dry crystals of levonorgestrel. This system will release the steroid at a rate decreasing from 80 μg/day during the first year of use to 30 μg/day after the third year, for an effective period of 5 years. Blood levels of levonorgestrel are comparable to those

Table 22-6. Patient consent form for injectable contraception

The Food and Drug Administration has approved an intramuscular injection of Depo-Provera in the buttock, for birth control. Each injection prevents pregnancy for 3 months. At that time, another injection must be obtained if you wish to continue this method of birth control. The drug in the injection (Depo-Provera) has been used for 3 decades in millions of women for other purposes. Pregnancy can be prevented if the injection is given within 5 days after the beginning of a normal period. If you are already pregnant when you receive the injection and your pregnancy is allowed to continue, your baby may have an increased chance (risk) of being smaller than usual (low birth weight). Babies who are born too small frequently have more health problems than those of normal weight. A possible but unproven risk of birth defects is also mentioned by the drug company. Additionally if you are younger than 35 years of age and have a history of breast cancer in your family, you may not want to use this drug. Short-term use may slightly increase the risk of breast cancer in young women, according to studies by the World Health Organization and in New Zealand. On the other hand, the use of Depo-Provera may protect you from cancer of the endometrium (uterine lining).

Common Side Effects

1. The use of Depo-Provera frequently causes irregular periods (sometimes heavy bleeding, spotting, or no periods at all). Such problems usually stop after the drug leaves the system. The bleeding can be helped with estrogen pills.
2. Sometimes Depo-Provera can cause weight gain, headaches, bloating of the abdomen or breast, nervousness, tiredness, or hair loss. If you suffer from an unwanted effect, you will have to wait it out for several months. There is no way to get rid of this drug quickly from your body.
3. Women who use blood-thinning drugs (coumadin, heparin) and women with a prolonged bleeding time, such as those who take a large amount of aspirin or aspirin-like over-the-counter painkillers, should not use Depo-Provera.
4. Women who regularly take antiseizure drugs (carbamazepine, phenytoin) or certain antibiotics (rifamin, tetracycline) should not use this contraceptive method. Depo-Provera users who take tetracycline should use a barrier method such as a condom or diaphragm while on that antibiotic.
5. Depo-Provera does not protect against sexually transmitted diseases. Therefore, you should always use condoms for this protection.
6. The repeated use of Depo-Provera for years may result in a thinning of the uterine lining that would lead to difficulty in resuming periods or conceiving. It could take 9 months or longer for women to get pregnant after they stop using this injection.
7. The use of this birth control method for longer than 5 years may make your bones slightly thinner. Whether or not the actual risk of fracture (broken bones) is increased is not clear because this effect on the bones seems to disappear after discontinuation of the drug.

PATIENT'S STATEMENT

I have read the above and understand that there are benefits and risks associated with the use of Depo-Provera. Additionally, I have read the manufacturer's package insert for patients. Any questions I had were answered. I choose to use Depo-Provera because I feel that the benefits for me are greater than the risks.

______________________________ ______________

Patient's Signature Date

in minipill users or one third of those using the combination OC. The subdermal levonorgestrel implant system is as effective in the first 2 years as female sterilization.[106] The duration of effectiveness may be inversely related to body weight but not to the body mass index. The adverse influence of body weight on the method's duration of effectiveness appears minimal or nonexistent. There are very few contraindications (Table 22-7). Patients should not undergo insertion while bleeding time is prolonged as a result of acute liver disease, heparin, coumadin, or aspirin. Undiagnosed genital bleeding is another contraindication. As with all progestins, a shift of glucose tolerance curves can be observed after use. Thus, brittle diabetics may not be ideal candidates for this method. Although the lipid profile remains intact with use, women of advanced age who smoke cigarettes may not be ideal candidates for this method. A study also suggests that this method may not be effective in the presence of anticonvulsant therapy.[115] An implant user who conceives because of method failure should be evaluated for a possible ectopic pregnancy. Note, however, that the use of the implants or other contraceptives will actually reduce the risk of an ectopic pregnancy. In fact implant users have only one fifth (0.28/1000 women-years) the risk of ectopic pregnancy when compared against that of noncontraceptive users (1.5/1000). When compared against other reversible contraceptives, implants have the highest efficacy and continuation rates.[264,268] This is because the method is convenient (requires no compliance) and probably because users must return to the clinic in order to discontinue the method. One third to three quarters of the patients continue the method after 5 years of use. Continuation rates after 1 year of use range from 76% to 99%. Proper preinsertion counseling is the key to high continuation rates. The failure rate during the first year of use is 6 pregnancies per 1000 women.

Mechanism of actions. Blood levels of 300 to 400 pg/mL of levonorgestrel may centrally blunt the preovulatory surge of LH. Thus, 70% of the users' cycles are anovulatory. The remaining ovulatory cycles (as judged by vaginal ultrasound) are usually associated with decreased peak serum progesterone levels (7 versus 18 ng/mL) which indicate poor ovum or inadequate luteal support or luteinized/unruptured follicles. Peripherally, sperm penetration may be inhibited by a local effect of progestin, which prevents midcycle thinning of the cervical mucus. This effect is seen with a

Table 22-7. Patient consent form for Norplant contraceptive implants

Norplant (levonorgestrel subdermal implants), a long-acting and reversible birth control method, has been used by over a million women worldwide for the prevention of unwanted pregnancy. Each of the six implants is made from a special Silastic rubber commonly used in the body for other purposes. The drug used in Norplant (levonorgestrel) has been used in birth control pills for the past three decades. These implants are inserted beneath the skin of the upper arm using a minor surgical technique. There have been no serious side effects reported from women who were appropriately selected to receive Norplant.

Advantages of Norplant over other birth control methods

1. Norplant lasts 5 years and is statistically more reliable than the pill. Unlike the pill, Norplant contains no estrogen and therefore has fewer side effects than the pill. The first-year discontinuation rate is lower than the pill or IUD.
2. Norplant reduces the total monthly bleeding from the womb (uterus) and the risk of iron deficiency anemia in some women who bleed a lot with periods. The use of Norplant for longer than 1 year generally leads to higher blood counts (hemoglobin and hematocrit) than before insertion.
3. Norplant may reduce menstrual cramps.
4. Norplant may protect against cancer of the endometrium (the lining inside the womb).
5. There is practically no age limit in using Norplant because the amount of drug that is released into the blood circulation is extremely low, when compared to the pill. Consequently, there is little unwanted metabolic effect in the body, except perhaps in cigarette smokers over 45 years of age.

Disadvantages and common side effects

1. Norplant must be surgically inserted (10 minutes) and removed (20 minutes) after 5 years. Thus the initial cost is higher than the pill or IUD. Although it is 99% effective, it must be removed if pregnancy occurs or if the user develops yellow jaundice.
2. Although Norplant can be removed whenever users want to discontinue contraception, removal usually takes longer than insertion. If Norplant was inserted too deeply under the skin, the user may have to undergo the removal procedure twice or undergo ultrasound-guided removal.
3. Some prospective candidates may require antibiotics prior to insertion and removal if they are at risk for infection of heart valves.
4. Rarely, insertion or removal may be complicated by an infection or a prolonged bruise. Most users have a scar about the size of the tip of a pen, and it is unusual to develop a keloid (excessive scarring) or darkening of the skin. An allergic reaction to the antiseptic cleaning fluid or local numbing medicine may also occur.
5. Women who regularly take the following drugs may not be eligible for Norplant: blood-thinning drugs (heparin or coumadin), antiseizure drugs (phenytoin or carbamazepine), and some antibiotics (tetracycline or rifampipn). Norplant users who will take tetracycline for a long period of time must use a barrier method while on that antibiotic. Women with prolonged bleeding time, such as those who take a large amount of aspirin or aspirin-like over-the-counter painkillers, should not use Norplant until the disorder has been treated.
6. Because Norplant effectively prevents pregnancy, it will automatically reduce the risk of ectopic tubal pregnancy. However, in the event of pregnancy occurring because of this method's failure, one out of five pregnancies may occur in the tube (ectopic).
7. The use of Norplant may cause irregular staining or spotting between periods or the lack of a period. Such problems may or may not go away with time. However, occasional blood pregnancy tests may be required. An additional drug or hormone may be used to reduce these irregular bleeding or menstrual problems.
8. While Norplant theoretically prevents cancer of the endometrium, users who are older may have to undergo endometrial biopsy or other minor testing to detect cervical or endometrial cancer. Women with a history of cancer of the breast should not use Norplant.
9. Norplant is not a barrier contraceptive and so does not protect against sexually transmitted diseases.
10. Some Norplant users may develop pimples (acne), headaches, and weight gain or loss as a result of a change in appetite. Other minor side effects, listed in the manufacturer's package insert, are rare.
11. A Norplant user who develops low abdominal pain, pain during intercourse, fever and chills, unpleasant vaginal discharge, or a visual disturbance should contact her physician without delay.

PATIENT'S STATEMENT

I have read the above and understand that there are benefits and risks associated with the use of Norplant. Additionally, I have read the manufacturer's package insert for patients. Any questions I had were answered. I choose to use Norplant because I feel that the benefits for me are greater than the risks.

Patient's Signature	Date

levonorgestrel level as low as 200 pg/mL. Another progestational effect of levonorgestrel may render the endometrium unreceptive to implantation.

Side effects. Irregular uterine bleeding in the form of frequent, abnormal menses, spotting/staining, or amenorrhea constitutes common initial complaints. In the first year of use there appear to be 129 bleeding days on average (versus 70 bleeding days/year among noncontraceptive users). Short-term oral therapy with daily ethinyl estradiol 50 μg, norgestrel, or ibuprofen will significantly reduce the number of abnormal bleeding days.[64] One quarter of the users bleed every 3 to 5 weeks in the first year. By the fifth year, two thirds of the users have regular cycles. Generally, those who start out with amenorrhea or irregular bleeding patterns are not at risk for method failure. On the other hand, users with regular bleeding patterns who suddenly become amenorrheic should undergo a pregnancy test.

Less frequent side effects include headaches, acne, and weight gain. Headaches associated with papilledema may signal an idiopathic intracranial hypertension (pseudotumor cerebri). This requires cessation of steroid contraception and an appropriate neurologic examination. Intractable weight gain or a classic migraine with an aura may also dictate method discontinuation. Acne may be relieved with proper dermatologic care. Because users' gonadotropin levels are not completely suppressed, follicular development still occurs and the resultant serum estradiol levels are indistinguishable from nonusers. Up to one third of users may have persistent follicles. Thus, simple follicular cysts are common and may reach 5 to 7 cm in some cases, but regression usually occurs spontaneously. Other problems reported are depression, irritation, and in rare cases, hyperpigmentation and keloid at the insertion site.

Insertion and removal techniques. Insertion takes only 5 to 10 minutes but must be done correctly to ensure an easy removal. The capsules must be placed subdermally just below the skin on the inner surface of the upper arm. The use of a special template is strongly advised so that the six capsules are in a typical radial (fan-out) pattern and the local anesthetic infiltration is not done in excess. A videotape is readily available from the manufacturer and will adequately cover the insertion techniques and trouble-shooting. Insert the trocar with the skin tented up to insure the superficial placement of the capsule. The beveled tip should be pointed upward so that its sharp end is pointed down. This keeps the advancing trocar from button-holing the skin. The barrel is then withdrawn while the trocar plunger remains stationary, to facilitate the release of the capsule. The capsule is then digitally secured with pressure on the skin, while both the barrel and plunger set are together slowly retracted to the incision site but not beyond for redirection and placement of the next capsule. This trocar withdrawal action will cause the proximal tip of each capsule to pop down and out of the sharp bevel. The insertion should be performed during the normal menses or OC withdrawal bleeding. Insertion during the luteal phase or in the last half of the low-estrogen OC-induced cycle is not advised.

Removal takes 20 minutes or longer, depending on the skill and correct (or typical) alignment of the capsules that were placed years earlier. The removal techniques described here are based upon 2 decades of experience in other countries. The use of a waterproof surgical marker is strongly advised in order to mark on the skin the distal and proximal tips of each capsule that can be palpated digitally. An ample volume of local anesthetic solution (8 mL of 1% lidocaine hydrochloride) is then infiltrated under the proximal tips of the implants. A 1 -cm-long incision is made transversely over the proximal ends of all of the capsules and slightly above the original insertion site. Pressure is applied at the distal end so that the capsule's proximal tip is pushed into the incision area. That tip is then grasped with a small hemostat or Kelly clamp. The fibrous tissue around the silastic tip is then carefully scratched out with the tip of the knife blade or using dry surgical gauze, until the shiny white implant is cleared of any attachment and can be slid out. Patients must be allowed to see and count all of the removed capsules with a record to that effect. If it takes too long to remove one capsule, the patient should be advised to return in 1 month for another attempt, after the bruising and swelling have disappeared. Ultrasonography can be utilized to locate any loose or broken fragments of the capsule. The insertion and removal of the implants (Fig. 22-5), which should soon become available in the United States are easier than the presently available six-capsule system.[141b]

Other long-acting contraceptives under clinical trials include microcapsules, a progestin or combined progestin-estrogen vaginal ring, a once-a-month pill, and a skin patch.[90] The vaginal silastic ring is somewhat interesting since a user can insert and remove it by herself.[240] One ring lasts 3 months. The contraceptive steroid(s), which is easily absorbed by the vaginal mucosa into the systemic circulation is released at a slow and relatively constant rate. It will not work if it is inserted just before coitus. However, after being in use for one cycle, the occasional removal of the vaginal ring for several hours will not decrease contraceptive protection. In a way, the vaginal ring is the opposite of the barrier method in that users can remove this device in anticipation of sexual intercourse and then insert the vaginal ring after coitus. A 3-weeks-on, 1-week-off schedule with the progestin-estrogen ring will bring about monthly withdrawal bleeding similar to the combination OC.

A safe and practical contraceptive pill for men has not been invented. The suppression of spermatogenesis was demonstrated following treatment with exogenous testosterone or a combination of estrogen and testosterone. Unfortunately, the long-term use of testosterone leads to hepatic dysfunction. Chinese physicians utilized a cotton-plant pigment

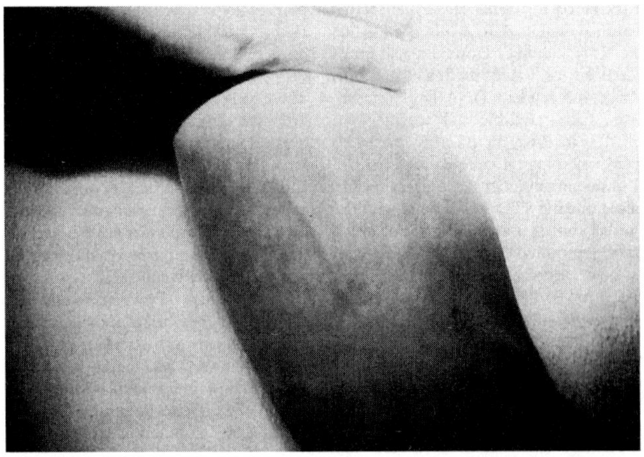

Fig. 22-5. Norplant-2 in situ (inner surface of the patient's upper arm). (Courtesy Dr. PD Darney.)

Gossypol as an injectable or implantable contraceptive for men.[327] Hypokalemia, hepatorenal dysfunction, and irreversible azoospermia were observed in some subjects. Toxicologic data from human trials may prevent the approval for its use in other countries.[71] Another male contraceptive from the Chinese medicinal plant Tripterygium wilfordii was recently analyzed and found to be chlorohydrin. Its effects appear to be reversible.[172]

REVERSIBLE METHODS WITH HIGH FAILURE RATES

Coitus interruptus (withdrawal of the penis before ejaculation) is perhaps the oldest contraceptive practice, according to Catholic theologians and canonists.[194] Besides the demand for extreme self control by the male, the method is not effective in real practice because of the escape of seminal fluid before orgasm, and in many instances, the unavoidable deposition of semen near the vaginal orifice. In other instances, when the woman has not achieved orgasm before penile withdrawal, she may require artificial stimulation for further gratification. Lovemaking modifications for contraceptive purpose include orogenital and anal intercourse. The latter is commonly practiced in certain parts of the world, but most cultures have long condemned anal intercourse as unhealthy.

The postcoital douche, also an ancient contraceptive method, is intended to flush the semen out of the vagina. Water, vinegar solution, and various OTC products were used. Certain douching solutions may possess a spermicidal effect. An example of a folk method is to douche with a diet cola. The carbonated drink actually has an in vitro spermicidal effect.[295] Nevertheless, the effectiveness of a postcoital douche is probably low, since sperm can find their way into the cervical mucus almost instantly following ejaculation, and minutes later they can be found in the oviducts.[259] Thus a postcoital douche is considered an unreliable contraceptive method.

The *rhythm method (periodic abstinence)*, considered unnatural by many couples, is another ineffective way to prevent unwanted conception. A woman's fertile period within each cycle may be crudely estimated from the calendar, basal body temperature, or cervical mucus. Three factors that limit the method's effectiveness appear to be intraindividual variations in cycle length, variations in the length of survival of the sperm, and actual use compliance. There have also been worrisome epidemiologic data implying that an old sperm or an old egg may lead to an imperfect conceptus. However, such fears were not borne out in the Walnut Creek Study.[112]

Prolonged nursing is an unreliable contraceptive method and may turn out to be an unnatural way to nourish a well-grown child.[174] The resumption of ovulation may occur before the first menstrual bleeding, and the antiovulatory effect of lactation varies from woman to woman. Breast feeding mothers should always use a reliable contraceptive such as a condom, diaphragm, sponge, or IUD.

STERILIZATION

Sterilization generally refers to a surgical procedure that is aimed at permanently blocking or removing male or female genital tracts so that fertilization will not occur. The permanency of sterilization should be the main consideration for any user who contemplates undergoing this surgical method of contraception. The reversal of sterilization requires major surgery and is not always successful.[117]

Among the effective methods for birth control, sterilization is the most frequently chosen by fertile men and multiparous women over 30 years of age. In fact, the best contraception for an older multiparous woman in a stable and mutually monogamous relationship is male sterilization (vasectomy).

Vasectomy is an outpatient surgical procedure to occlude a portion of the vas deferens. It requires local anesthetic and usually takes an experienced person 15 minutes in a well-equipped facility. Complications, if they occur, are not serious and include hematoma or sperm leakage, which leads to granulomatous reactions (sperm granulomas). Semen analysis is required 1 and 2 months postoperatively, since two sperm-free ejaculations is considered to be proof of sterility. It may take up to 20 ejaculations. Long-term, deleterious effects of vasectomy have never been proven. The fear of decreased virility or atherosclerosis is unfounded.[26,93,160,171] However, several epidemiologic studies suggest that vasectomy may be associated with an elevated risk of prostatic cancer.[45,91,92]

Like vasectomy, most female sterilization methods are outpatient or day surgery procedures. Nevertheless, female sterilization is not as simple and convenient as a vasectomy, since the female genital tracts are located relatively deep in the pelvis. The risk of death (4 in 100,000) is less than that of one pregnancy and is mostly attributed to anesthetic complications.[162,212] There is also an increased risk of extrauterine pregnancy should the female sterilization fail. Attempts at blocking the oviducts via transcervical (transvaginal) extraperitoneal procedures have been recorded for a century but none is acceptable thus far. Hysteroscopic methods for blocking the oviducts with silicone or caustic chemicals have been offered at some facilities. Such methods never gain popularity because of the high failure rates along with an unacceptable risk of tubal pregnancy.

Female sterilization is commonly achieved by ligation or coagulation, with or without the segmental removal of both oviducts. This tubal sterilization can be performed through two main intraperitoneal routes: the abdominal approach via laparoscopy or minilaparotomy and the vaginal approach via colpotomy or culdoscopy.

Laparoscopic tubal sterilization with bipolar cautery has been the popular choice for interval sterilization in the United States. This method requires elaborate equipment but the procedural time is relatively short. Minilaparotomy has been an excellent choice for sterilization in the postpartum period, when the oviducts are located high in the abdomen. It was also utilized for interval sterilization using local anesthetic with the help of a uterine elevator device.[204] The latter technique is suitable in developing countries where most multiparous women are thin. With a thin abdominal wall, the required amount of local anesthetic will not exceed an allowable limit. The vaginal tubal sterilization is not commonly performed because the method requires considerable technical expertise, since intraperitoneal visualization is limited when compared to other interval sterilization methods. There is also an increased risk of ascending infection from the vagina when compared to abdominal incisions. Thus, broad spectrum intravenous antibiotics should be given for prophylaxis in women who are undergoing vaginal tubal ligation.

The careful selection of the candidates, with a discussion and a simplified consent form for tubal sterilization (Table 22-8) may obviate later regrets for both the patient and physician. Ideal candidates are multiparous women over 25 years of age. Nulliparous women and those younger than 25 years of age may, with a legitimate medical indication, benefit from sterilization provided that they have been counseled by another appropriate authority besides the operating gynecologist.[113]

Laparoscopic Tubal Sterilization (see also Chapter 26 on laparoscopy).

Bipolar electrocoagulation is the method of choice using the two-puncture technique with general endotracheal anesthetic. It is much safer than the unipolar coagulation in avoiding accidental thermal injury to the bowel or neighboring structures, because the electric current will heat and coagulate only the oviductal tissues within the jaws of the electrocoagulation probe. Several contiguous fulgurations are preferred to the transection or segmental removal. The two-puncture technique offers better visualization and ease of manipulation of intraabdominal organs. Immediate complications include anesthetic-related problems, damage to internal organs, and hemorrhage. Other problems that may occur following discharge are infection, hematoma, adhesions, unrecognized bowel injury, luteal phase pregnancy, and recanalization that results in intrauterine or ectopic pregnancy.[190,251] Suboptimal anesthetic technique such as mask inhalation may result in fatal aspiration pneumonitis, since pneumoperineum tends to induce regurgitation and the aspiration of gastric contents. Local bleeding may occur if the

Table 22-8. Patient consent form for tubal sterilization

Tubal sterilization is a surgical procedure to block the fallopian tubes so that fertilization will not occur. This procedure is more effective than any other birth control method but should be chosen only if you are sure that you want no more children, because your tubes will become permanently blocked. Occasionally, women who have had tubal sterilization change their minds and want more children. Major surgery to reconstruct the tubes or in vitro fertilization is then necessary but is not always successful.

Tubal sterilization can be performed by a laparoscopic procedure that requires small punctures of the abdomen or by a minilaparotomy procedure that requires a small surgical opening of the abdomen. The types of tubal sterilization include excision and ligation, surgical relocation of the tubes, and constriction of each tube within a tight band or by the passing of an electric current through the tubes. In general, complications of tubal sterilization may involve infection, bleeding, injuries to internal organs, or anesthetic complications. Damage to the bowel or blood vessels requiring major surgery and blood transfusion could happen, but these life-threatening complications are rare.

Your physician will discuss the choice of procedure most suitable for you based on its avantages and disadvantages, while balancing the possible risk of spontaneous healing that allows the tubes to open again against the complexity and complications of the various procedures. Spontaneous opening of the blocked tubes occurs in about 2 cases per 1000 operations performed and may occur less often after surgical relocation of the tubes when performed following childbirth or at the time of cesarean section. If your tubes heal in a way that leaves an opening, pregnancy may occur months or even years later. Such pregnancies can develop outside the womb (ectopic pregnancies) and cause severe bleeding. It is difficult to predict which women may develop these complications; therefore, you should report any irregularities of your period or pregnancy symptoms to your physician after tubal sterilization.

It is also possible that women may be pregnant at the time of tubal sterilization, especially those whose periods were not normal or those having the operation in the last 2 weeks of their menstrual cycle. Your physician may perform a blood pregnancy test around the time of the operation if needed, but again, you should report any irregular periods or pregnancy symptoms to your physician after the tubal sterilization procedure.

Planned procedure:

Comments:

PATIENT'S STATEMENT
I have read this consent form and understand that there are failure rates and risks associated with tubal sterilization. My physician has discussed the advantages and disadvantages of tubal sterilization. I consent to the planned procedure.

______________________	______________________
Patient's Signature	Witness' signature
Date	

tissue coagulation is inadequate. A major, life-threatening hemorrhage is rare and requires immediate laparotomy to repair the lacerations of the blood vessels. A blood transfusion may also be required. Unrecognized bowel burns may subsequently lead to symptoms analogous to a ruptured appendix.[316] Bowel burns are rare with the use of regularly inspected and well-maintained, bipolar instruments. Luteal-phase pregnancy may be avoided if sterilization is performed during the first half of the cycle. The failure rate of most female sterilization methods is generally quoted as 2/1000 operations performed. Most failures result from recanalization of the oviduct. However, if the procedure is hastily done without identifying the entire length of the oviduct to its fimbriated end, a round ligament could be mistaken for an oviduct. A high incidence of ectopic pregnancy has been reported with failures of electrocoagulation, especially after the obsolete unipolar method (51%).[162] Nevertheless, the general safety of laparoscopic sterilization and the absence of sequela in terms of menstrual or psychosocial problems have been amply documented.[61]

Beside electrocoagulation, mechanical constriction and obliteration of the oviduct can be accomplished with a silastic Yoon band (Falope ring), a spring-loaded Hulka clip, and various other radiopaque, nonelectrical devices. Such devices may not be suitable for use on swollen oviducts (such as in the puerperium) or in the presence of some pelvic adhesions. The Falope ring is suitable for the single-puncture technique that is mostly employed in outpatient laparoscopic sterilization with local anesthetic and for monitored intravenous (conscious) sedation. However, several days of unique postoperative pain (more than that from electrocoagulation) may be expected after the Falope ring application. The Hulka clip is probably the least traumatic to the local tissues but its failure rate is slightly higher than other methods. Major trauma to internal organs can be avoided or substantially reduced with the open laparoscopy technique. This technique is also practical if the procedure has to be performed with local anesthetic. The peritoneum is identified and entered through a small infraumbilical incision using the a blunt, funnel-shaped, Hasson cannula.[114] Blind stabbings of the abdominal wall with a Verres CO_2 needle and a sharp trocar in the conventional laparoscopy are avoided in this open laparoscopy method.

Minilaparotomy

The ligation and transection or resection of a portion of the oviduct may be electively performed during the puerperium and in the nonpregnant interval as well. Electrocoagulation can also be used in the minilaparotomy method of tubal sterilization. The simple tie and cut technique is usually a modification of the Pomeroy method.

There are techniques to relocate and bury the proximal portion of the transected oviduct in order to minimize failure. Uchida of Japan buries the ligated proximal stump of the tube retroperitoneally under the leaves of the broad ligament. The ligated distal stump remains intraperitoneal. The modified Irving method probably has the lowest failure rate, generally quoted as less than 0.1%. It is the sterilization method of choice immediately following a Cesarean delivery. The ligated proximal stump of the tube is buried into the uterine wall near the cornu. The original Irving method of burying the distal stump under the leaves of the broad ligament is not really necessary.

A safe timing for postpartum sterilization should be determined by the obstetrician, the anesthesiologist and the patient. In many circumstances, deferral until the patient is in optimal condition may be the best policy.[2] Parturient and pregnant women in the second or third trimester are at an increased risk of regurgitation and the aspiration of gastric contents. Following natural childbirth, many anesthesiologists prefer a routine waiting period of 6 hours, rather than immediate postpartum sterilization. Any medical, obstetric, neonatal survivability, or infectious problems should override the original plan for immediate or puerperal sterilization.[2] With the advent of 24-hour broad-spectrum intravenous antibiotics for prophylaxis, there is no need for the patient to wait until 6 weeks postpartum before undergoing tubal ligation. In the absence of intrapartum or puerperal infection, minilaparotomy can be performed safely with prophylactic intravenous antibiotics before the complete involution of the uterus. The advantages are the easy access to the oviducts through a small abdominal incision and the patient's convenience in scheduling the surgery during allowable maternity leave.

Minilaparotomy can be performed with local anesthetic for interval sterilization or in conjunction with first-trimester induced abortion. A device such as the Hulka tenaculum or a uterine elevator designed by Osathanondh will allow easy access to the oviduct via a small suprapubic incision.[204] Women who have successfully undergone natural childbirth or surgery with local anesthetic are good candidates. However, the patient should be of average body weight for her height and weigh less than 68 kilograms (< 150 pounds). Hypertension, hyperthyroidism, cardiac arrhythmia, and hypersensitivity to local anesthetics or epinephrine are contraindications. A local anesthetic solution containing a minimal amount of epinephrine is injected into the abdominal wall and the oviducts before ligation or electrocoagulation. A paracervical block anesthetic should be given before applying the uterine elevator or Hulka tenaculum. Intravenous drugs that are helpful include a parasympatholytic agent (such as glycopyrrolate), a sedative (midazolam or droperidol) or an antihistamine (diphenhydramine), and a short-acting opioid (fentanyl citrate). The dosage of these combined medications may be clinically adjusted and should not exceed the maximum allowable limits.

A sterilized woman may undergo a major surgery to unblock her fallopian tubes. The success rate of the tubal reanastomosis depends on the method of sterilization. Those having had the clips, the Silastic bands, or the modified

Pomeroy method, in respective order, are easier to reverse than the Irving, Uchida, or electrocoagulation methods of sterilization. The most difficult to reverse is the blockade after unipolar cautery because of extensive tissue damage and frequent postoperative adhesions. Besides complications inherent to a laparotomy and anesthetics, tubal pregnancy occurs at very high rates, especially after the reversal of unipolar electrocoagulation.[117,316]

Patients with major uterine or pelvic pathology who request sterilization may benefit from a hysterectomy. However, a hysterectomy must not be viewed as a simple method of sterilization, because it carries a higher complication rate than tubal sterilization.

PREGNANCY TERMINATION (THERAPEUTIC INDUCED ABORTION)

Pharmacotherapeutic methods

Agents disrupting chorionic villi. Progesterone receptor blockers represent an important alternative in antifertility therapy. Such antiprogesterones are derivatives of norethindrone and are therefore within the class of 19-norsteroids.

A prototype of antiprogesterone, code-named RU38.486, was synthesized by the Roussel-Uclaf pharmaceutical company in Romainville, France. Specifically, the addition of a functional group dimethylaminophenyl ring into the norethindrone molecule at the 11β-carbon position resulted in this potent compound RU486 that can displace progesterone from its receptors.[6] This receptor blocker appears to have no direct effect on the ovarian production of progesterone. It was approved for use in France, China, and England. In the United States, premarketing trials to evaluate its safety and efficacy are scheduled for 1994 at training sites designated by the Population Council.

RU486 or mifepristone was utilized as an abortifacient in the first quarter of pregnancy, a morning-after pill, and in the treatment of Cushing's syndrome and glaucoma. RU486 can also reduce the size of certain brain tumor cells such as meningioma and meningioblastomas, probably through an obscure fluid-exchange mechanism(s). Additionally, the drug is being tried in the treatment of Alzheimer's disease, endometriosis, and leiomyomata. Its contraceptive efficacy as a once-a-month pill is as yet logistically unreliable.[249]

RU486 effectively antagonizes progesterone actions on the gestational endometrium which leads to the eventual detachment of the chorionic villi and consequent decline in the peripheral blood levels of progesterone and hCG. When administered during midluteal phase, it blocks the effects of progesterone by displacing the natural steroid from its receptors on the secretory endometrium, with the resultant induction of menses. With this method of administration, multiple sites of its action upon the hypothalamic-hypophyseal-ovarian-endometrial axis have been proposed, based on dynamic hormonal studies.[87] In the absence of progesterone, RU486 will exert mild progesterone-like effects (in estrogen-treated postmenopausal women). This leads to a further decrease in the serum gonadotropin levels.[100]

Besides its action within the female reproductive tract, RU486 also binds to the glucocorticoid receptors and thus antagonizes the actions of cortisol. In high doses, this drug may be beneficial in the treatment of Cushing's syndrome. Small and transient compensatory rises in plasma ACTH and cortisol levels were shown following the daily administration of 200 mg of RU486 for 4 days. This course of treatment is required for early pregnancy termination. Alternatively, a single oral dose of 600 mg was employed with slightly less effectiveness.[102] A continued search by German scientists for an ideal antiprogesterone that lacks antiglucocorticoid effects recently produced three other related compounds: ZK112.993, ZK98.734 (Lilopristone), and ZK98.299 (Onapristone) (Fig. 22-6). The latter appears to have much less antiglucocorticoid activity while being a ten times more effective abortifacient than RU486 in preliminary animal studies.[72] Onapristone as well as RU486 are entering clinical trials for cervical ripening and as an adjunct to labor and delivery in Europe.[40]

The oral, or more effectively, parenteral administration of RU486 was shown to induce moderate uterine bleeding with a significant decrease in hematocrit, followed by complete expulsion of early (first quarter) gestational products in 80% of the cases. The remaining 20% of the cases required dilation and curettage (D&C). Bleeding in many cases occurred before the decrease in serum progesterone levels. Successful

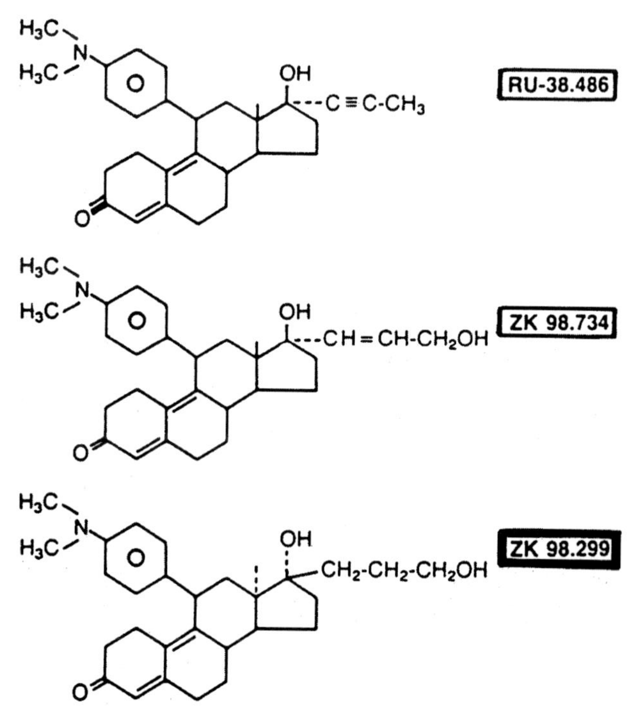

Fig. 22-6. Progesterone receptor blockers.

Table 22-9. Therapeutic abortion at 56 or less days of amenorrhea*

Method	Completion rate
RU486 150 mg/day orally for 4 days	60% (12/20)
PGE_1 analogue 1 mg vaginal pessary every 3 hr up to five doses	97% (29/30)
Vacuum aspiration	96% (27/28)
RU486 as above protocol plus only one dose of PGE_1 on day 3	95% (18/19)

*From Cameron IT, Baird DT: Early pregnancy termination: a comparison between vacuum aspiration and medical abortion using prostaglandin (16, 16 dimethyl-trans-3D_2-PGE_1 methyl ester) or the antiprogestogen RU486, *Br J Obstet Gynaecol* 95:271-276, 1988.)

therapy is associated with an increase in plasma levels of $PGF_{2\alpha}$, myometrial contraction, favorable changes in the uterine cervix, and in some patients, hormonal evidence of luteolysis. However, the most effective pharmacotherapy to terminate an early gestation (and a somewhat later gestation with fetal demise) is the administration of RU486 in combination with an otherwise subtherapeutic dose of a uterotonic prostaglandin (Table 22-9).[23,25] These two different classes of drugs are quite synergistic. A single, low dose of a prostaglandin drug administered toward the end of the course of RU486 treatment will ensure complete abortion without incurring the systemic side effects of prostaglandin. The most common prostaglandin utilized for this purpose is oral or vaginal PGE_1 methyl analog (misoprostol), which induces uterine contraction at all stages of pregnancy.[170] Note that RU486 was not beneficial for terminating ectopic tubal pregnancy in limited, unpublished, clinical trials. Significant concentrations of this drug were experimentally demonstrated in the umbilical plasma during second-trimester therapeutic abortion, which indicates that it is effectively transferred across the placental barrier.[85] It is not known whether this steroid is teratogenic at all. Among the drug-failure cases whose intrauterine pregnancy was not successfully terminated, there has been no fetal abnormality reported to date. The plasma elimination half-life of RU486 is 10 to 25 hours. The data on long-term untoward effects from the repeated administration of RU486 are not available. Its prolonged use could hypothetically lead to unopposed estrogenic stimulation as a result of a blockage of progesterone action. The blood loss and time consumed in medical abortion appear greater than those found in a surgical abortion. Furthermore, RU486 by itself is ineffective for abortion, beyond the first trimester of a normal pregnancy. Another disadvantage of a drug-induced abortion (versus a surgical evacuation) may be the unavailability of pathology specimens, especially in Asian countries where trophoblastic disease is prevalent.

Inhibitors of progesterone biosynthesis such as aminoglutethimide,[246] epostane,[51] or trilostane[302] were tried as moderately effective abortifacients up to 50 days of pregnancy (from the last menstrual period). However, unwanted effects at the therapeutic antifertility dose include adrenocortical suppression, and in many cases, significant uterine bleeding because of incomplete miscarriage.

Aminoglutethimide is a bicyclic chemical compound with two optically active isomers. It inhibits the major steroidogenic enzyme systems (cholesterol side-chain cleavage and aromatase) by blocking the terminal cytochrome P-450s. Besides its adrenal suppressive effects, which can be utilized for medical adrenalectomy, this drug may potentially depress the central nervous system and activate hepatic microsomal enzymes. Trilostane and epostane (Winthrop 24540 and 32729) are 4,5-epoxy steroids structurally related to testosterone and methyltestosterone respectively. Each epoxy steroid blocks the biosynthesis of progesterone by inhibiting the enzyme 3β-hydroxysteroid dehydrogenase, with epostane being less suppressive to the adrenals than trilostane. Nevertheless, a high dose of epostane (800 mg/day for a week) is usually required for an early pregnancy termination. Although therapies with this class of drugs have not led to a subsequent menstrual or ovulational disorder, this group of antifertility agents does not appear as promising as the progesterone receptor blockers.

Inhibitors of folate reductase were utilized as abortifacients. However, these antimetabolites should not be recommended as first-line drugs for terminating a normal intrauterine pregnancy. The required duration of therapy appeared rather lengthy. A prototype oral agent 4-aminopteroylglutamic acid was originally tried for this purpose, over 3 decades ago.[287] All patients in that small series required either a D&C or hysterotomy 5 to 47 days after the initiation of the therapy. Interestingly, one such case of a medically indicated therapeutic abortion with a maternal tuberculosis resulted in a live fetus.

In the past 2 decades, a common parenteral antimetabolite, methotrexate, was successfully employed in the conservative treatment of a placenta accreta. Blood transfusions, uterine packing, and antibiotics were also required in such cases. Stormy, intensive, and protracted hospitalization usually occurred before the patient recuperated with her uterus remaining intact. The availability of sensitive and specific serum hCG measurements together with high-resolution diagnostic ultrasound, led investigators in the Orient, followed by a score of gynecologists in the United States, to use methotrexate in the pharmacotherapy of a small tubal or cervical pregnancy.[77,198,207] It appears that methotrexate works well in destroying abnormal or ectopic trophoblastic cells but is not very effective against a large bulk of normal trophoblastic tissue, unless a prostaglandin drug, misoprostol, is given concomitantly.[50] This is opposite to RU486 that works better on the normal intrauterine trophoblastic cells than on the ectopic ones. The benefit of methotrexate for a tubal pregnancy should be weighed against the as yet unknown long-term sequela of elevated serum hepatic transaminases. Such increased liver enzymes appear reversible upon cessation of the therapy. A fatal idiosyncratic reaction may occur when methotrexate is administered in conjunction with NSAIDs.[277]

Some patients with a small tubal pregnancy do not require any treatment except careful monitoring until the tubal abortion or resorption occurs. Such patients later conceive with normal liveborn offsprings.[30] Therefore, it could be reasoned that some patients reported in those methotrexate-for-ectopic series might have done all right without any treatment at all. Opponents of the methotrexate-for-ectopic treatment modality may label it a radical pharmacotherapy as a result of considering the potential risks from this chemical agent, when compared with their conservative treatment via minilaparotomy (salpingostomy) or pelviscopic surgery. Advocates, on the other hand, believe that any toxic sequela such as liver damage should be negligible based upon the long-term health of the majority of trophoblastic disease patients following oncolytic chemotherapy with methotrexate. The situation is different with a cervical ectopic pregnancy that may present increasing problems for infertility patients.[89] An intrafetal injection of potassium chloride (KCL) is the method of choice for a nonsurgical ablation of the ectopic cervical pregnancy tissue.[81] Unlike methotrexate, which disturbs the implantation site through the abrupt destruction of ectopic trophoblastic tissue, KCL intrafetal injection slowly disturbs the fetal hormonal factors namely hCG, AFP, estriol, and CA-125 as reflected by the changes in maternal serum levels. The end result is a gentle and complete involution of the placental bed within 2 months.[200]

Uterotonic agents. *Prostaglandins* are long-chain 20-carbon derivatives of arachidonic acid that are produced in the human tissues from phospholipids. They bear a common chemical structure of the C20 prostanoic acid that contains a cyclopentane ring between C8 and C12. Biosynthesis of such compounds in the uterine tissues requires a lysosomal enzyme, phospholipase A_2, and a group of microsomal enzymes called prostaglandin synthetase (cyclooxygenase, isomerase, and reductase). Some prostaglandin (PG) drugs that will induce contractions of the gravid uterus include PGE_1 and its methyl analog misoprostol; $PGE_{2\alpha}$ and its synthetic derivatives such as meteneprost potassium and sulprostone; and PGF_2 and its 15-methyl analog. They are extremely thermolabile in soluble form and must be kept below 4° C until use.

PGE_2 (dinoprostone) is available in a suppository (wax) or gel base.[226] The vaginal suppository form of PGE_2 was approved by the United States FDA for labor induction in the case of fetal demise up to 28 weeks of pregnancy. It is readily absorbed through the vaginal mucosa into the systemic circulation with the resultant pharmacologic effects as summarized in Table 22-10. The recommended dosage is 5 to 20 mg clinically adjusted (titrated) at safe intervals (usually every 3 or 4 hours), based upon the optimal uterotonic response versus its undesirable systemic effects. The drug will stimulate the smooth muscles of the gravid uterus and gastrointestinal tract and will disturb the body's thermoregulatory center. Therefore, its common side effects include nausea, vomiting, diarrhea, and fever respectively. Gastrointestinal side effects can be reduced by pretreatment medications with oral diphenoxylate with atropine and an IM antinauseant such as prochlorperazine or phenoxyzine hydrochloride. Fever can be reduced with rectal acetaminophen and a wet body sponge. Unlike $PGF_{2\alpha}$, PGE_2 will dilate the bronchial and most vascular smooth muscles (Table 22-11) resulting in moderate peripheral vasodilation and lowered diastolic blood pressure when large doses are used.[260] Patients with active asthma or compromised cardiopulmonary hemodynamics will tolerate systemic PGE_2 much better than $PGF_{2\alpha}$.

Before labor induction with uterotonic PG, the degree of cervical effacement must be assessed. If the cervix is not well effaced, laminaria pretreatment is indicated regardless of cervical dilation. The induction-to-delivery period is much shorter with adequate laminaria pretreatment of the cervix. After the products of conception are expelled, a routine inspection and gentle exploration of the uterine cavity with a large curette is strongly advised before discharging the patient. This can be accomplished under minimal sedation with or without local anesthetic. Since 1981, multiple laminaria tents plus one dilator were routinely utilized in the overnight preparation of the cervix before the PG induction. With this special pretreatment, there were no cervical lacerations or uterine ruptures in over 7000 consecutive PG-induced midtrimester abortions. The use of a midtrimester dose of PGE_2 on pregnant women in the third trimester could lead to uterine rupture.[210,297] Uterine rupture was also reported after an intraamnionic injection of $PGF_{2\alpha}$ or 15-methyl-$PGF_{2\alpha}$.[34,303] This complication tends to occur when a PG drug is administered in combination with oxytocin treatment. The uterine muscle near term pregnancy may be more sensitive to PG because of an increased number of oxytocin receptors. PG and oxytocin are strongly synergistic and PG itself may induce an increase in oxytocin receptors. Thus, oxytocin should not be administered within 2 hours of the last PG dose.

Following an overnight laminaria preparation of the cervix, PGE_2 suppository can be inserted through the dilated cervical canal as the initial labor-inducing dose. This is done by compressing the PGE_2 wax onto the porous surface of the dilator at its distal pointed end. In order to keep the drug in,

Table 22-10. Systemic effects of prostaglandins

Contraction of pregnant uterus
Fever
Nausea and vomiting
Diarrhea
Increased intraocular pressure
Increased histamine level
Increased platelet aggregation
Decreased noradrenaline level

Table 22-11. Differences between prostaglandin $F_{2\alpha}$ and prostaglandin $E_{2\alpha}$

	$PGF_{2\alpha}$	$PGE_{2\alpha}$
Uterine muscle		
Pregnant	Contract	Contract
Nonpregnant	Contract	Inhibit
Bronchial smooth muscle	Constrict	Dilate
Arterial perfusion		
Coronary	Decreased	Increased
Regional	Decreased	Increased
Arterial pressure		
Systemic	Increased	Decreased
Pulmonary	Increased	Increased
Central venous pressure	Increased	Decreased
Cardiac output and heart rate	Increased	Increased

a large number of laminaria tents must be inserted snugly in the cervical canal immediately following this intrauterine, extraamnionic, lamicel+PGE_2 combination. This initial intrauterine dose may produce less systemic side effects than the vaginal application. The technique can also be used after the rupture of the membranes, provided that all amniotic fluid has been manually expressed out of the uterus with suprapubic pressure.

15(S)-15-methyl-$PGF_{2\alpha}$ (carboprost tromethamine or Hemabate [R]) has been utilized in combination with 64 to 100 mL of hypertonic (23.4% or 4 mEq/mL) saline for intraamnionic abortion in an ambulatory service. This particular prostaglandin analog was approved for IM use in cases of postpartum hemorrhage that are due to atonic uterus.[111] However, parenteral administration may produce severe untoward events including cardiac arrhythmia, bronchoconstriction, pulmonary hypertension, increased intrapulmonary shunting, and arterial oxygen desaturation.[111] Unlike $PGE_{2\alpha}$, PGF_{2a} and its synthetic derivatives will stimulate the uterine contraction even in the nongravid state. Its efficacy following intraamnionic injection for labor induction was described over a decade ago.[65,132] Using a strict protocol of active management, the intraamnionic injection-to-abortion time interval for midtrimester abortion averages 8 hours. Ninety-five percent of prostaglandin abortion cases are safely discharged from the ambulatory unit within 15 hours. The free backflow of clear amniotic fluid must be seen at amniocentesis before the drug is injected into the amnionic sac. This caution is imperative because an accidental leakage of 15-methyl-$PGF_{2\alpha}$ into the systemic circulation may result in cardiopulmonary side effects that will not abate as quickly as those caused by $PGF_{2\alpha}$. A dose-response study revealed that 1.5 mg of 15-methyl-$PGF_{2\alpha}$ and 64 to 100 mL of 23.4% saline are optimal for a midtrimester intraamnionic labor induction protocol. This protocol produces minimal or no systemic side effects when compared to the use of PGE_2 suppositories.

Misoprostol, a methyl analog of PGE_1, was approved by the United States FDA for use in the treatment of peptic ulcer disease. This oral agent has antisecretory activity for up to 5 hours at the usual recommended dose.[184] However, it will exert a significant uterotonic effect at doses above 400 µg.[225] This drug has milder and fewer side effects than other available forms of prostaglandin. It is also the least expensive at the present time. When its use for therapeutic induced abortion during midtrimester is preceded by overnight laminaria preparation of the cervix, this drug has an excellent efficacy and safety profile.[199] Conversely, the use of misoprostol without proper supervision will often lead to tragic sequela.[253b] Misoprostol has been a popular abortifacient in South America and Africa.[18] The protocol requires adequate laminaria preparation of the cervix followed by intraamnionic injection of 64 to 100 mL of 23.4 of saline and oral misoprostol 0.2 to 0.8 mg every 3 hours, based on each individual's uterine activity response. The fetal delivery is accomplished within 12 hours in 95% of the cases.

Oxytocin, a neurohypophyseal hormone, was synthesized for clinical use in the induction of labor beyond the second trimester of pregnancy. Unlike PG, oxytocin is uterotonic only in the presence of an adequate number of oxytocin receptors. It appears more potent than PG in causing the contraction of the myoepithelial cells of the mammary gland. This results in milk ejection. Thus, oxytocin nasal spray is available for stimulating initial milk letdown. Suckling is the only well-defined physiologic stimulus for oxytocin release. Cervical dilation is believed to be another stimulus for its release. Because of its similarity with vasopressin in amino acid sequence, oxytocin has 1/200 the antidiuretic potency of vasopressin. If a concentrated oxytocin solution is to be infused for a prolonged period of time, a limited volume of an electrolyte solution should be used instead of plain dextrose in water. This is to avoid water intoxication with the resultant hyponatremia and its consequences.

In midtrimester abortion, high-dose intravenous oxytocin is effective only when the patient's cervix is near or at full effacement (i.e., 90% to 100%). Oxytocin will exert its uterotonic effect after the uterus has been adequately stimulated by an exogenous PG or other factors. This leads to local endogenous PG production. For midtrimester labor induction with a nonviable fetus, the intravenous oxytocin augmentation protocol requires 60 units in 500 mL of an electrolyte solution at the initial rate of 10 mL/hour (equivalent to 20 milliunits/minute) using an infusion pump. The rate is increased at intervals and in increments of 10 mL/hour up to the limit of 60 mL/hour (120 milliunits/minute).

Two uterotonic agents that have fallen into disuse are buccal oxytocin citrate and an oxytocic alkaloid, sparteine sulfate, for IM injection. The latter is very potent but its uterotonic effect is difficult to titrate. In fact, many ergot alkaloids are potent uterotonic agents. They were used in illegal abortions along with quinine tablets.[224]

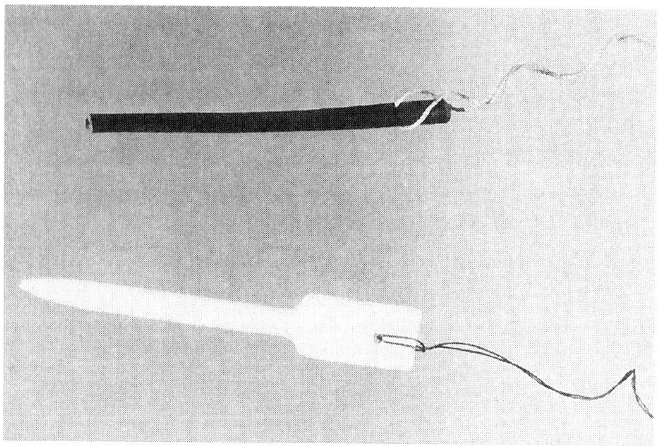

Fig. 22-7. A laminaria tent (dark) shown in comparison with a Lamicel (white).

Hypertonic and locally toxic solutions were utilized for intraamnionic abortions long before the availability of PG drugs. They include 23.4% saline solution, 30% or 40% hyperosmolar urea, and an antiseptic acridine orange (acrinol).[20,130] Originally, hypertonic dextrose solution was also utilized but its use was associated with a high infection rate. An intraamnionic injection of hypertonic or hyperosmolar solutions will induce a cascade of intrauterine events that will lead to prostaglandin release in the local tissues. Effective uterine contractions occur within several hours. Electrolyte and osmolar dynamics in these types of induced abortion have been described by many investigators.[4,20,83,97] Too concentrated or too high a volume of saline solution may result in a life-threatening disseminated intravascular coagulation or hypernatremia if accidentally injected into the uterine circulation.

Agents for softening the cervix. Hygroscopic devices are considered an integral part of a therapeutic abortion beyond the twelfth week of pregnancy. They are placed in the cervical canal in order to achieve gentle and nontraumatic dilation of the cervix. After adequate preparation of the cervix, the uterine evacuation procedure can be expediently accomplished by a trained physician with minimal risk of instrumental trauma and hemorrhage.[11]

A laminaria tent (Fig. 22-7) is a dried stem of seaweed that feels like a wooden stick or a huge toothpick. It is 6 cm long and available in sizes from 2 to 6 mm, based on the cross-section diameter at its tip. The small (2 or 3 mm) diameter laminaria tents are mainly utilized (in large numbers/patient) because of the ease of insertion and greater surface area of exposure than small numbers of large tents. Two small laminarias work better than one large one. They are left in the cervical canal for at least 4 hours but preferably overnight before the uterine evacuation procedure. The insertion technique is described in Table 22-12.

Laminaria was actually utilized in Europe before World War II but quickly abandoned because of sepsis (since it cannot be boiled). Its rebirth in modern-day obstetrics and gynecology came after the availability of gas sterilization

Table 22-12. Laminaria insertion technique

1. Make sure the patient understands that laminaria insertion is the beginning and the most important part of the pregnancy termination procedure. If the patient is 18 weeks or more pregnant, an ultrasound imaging should be done to confirm the gestational age.
2. Do a pelvic examination to record the uterine size and axis, and then change gloves. Put on sterile gloves and insert speculum.
3. Prepare the vagina and cervix with povidone-iodine (Betadine). Use diluted chlorhexidine gluconate (Hibiclens) if the patient is allergic to povidone-iodine.
4. Dip a small, long-stem, cotton swab in povidone-iodine, and gently sound the endocervix with it. Do not go in far beyond the internal os. The brownish staining of the cotton swab stem indicates the length of cervical canal.
5. If necessary, grasp the cervix with a long Allis clamp or straight-ring forceps, taking care to grasp only a small fold of mucosa to minimize the patient's discomfort. A local (paracervical block) anesthetic may be required in the case of cervical stenosis.
6. Grasp the laminaria at the string end with ring forceps and gently insert it until the laminaria tip with the string is flush with the external os. Always use the laminaria with the smallest diameter. For patients who are up to 12 weeks pregnant, insert two laminarias. For patients 13 to 17 weeks pregnant, insert three to five laminarias. For patients 18 weeks or more pregnant, insert three to five laminarias with one Lamicel as tolerated by the patient.
7. Dip a folded 4 by 4 gauze in a small amount of povidone-iodine, lay it over the cervix, and tuck it gently into the fornices. Lay a second (dry) 4 by 4 in. gauze over the first one to pack the laminaria in place. Gently remove the speculum while holding the gauze sponges in place with the ring forceps.
8. Have the patient remain lying in the left lateral position for a few minutes to avoid syncope. Note in the chart the time of insertion and the number of laminarias and sponges inserted.
9. Be certain that the patient understands that she must return for the laminaria removal the next day. Severe infection may result if one set of laminaria is left in situ for more than 48 hours. Inform the patient that the cramping with insertion will subside in a few minutes. Tell her to come back to the hospital at once if the membranes rupture, if bleeding occurs, or if she develops a fever. Forbid coitus. (Some patients have attempted coitus with laminarias in place; hence, give clear instructions against it.) The patient may take one or two acetaminophen tablets as needed for cramping, but aspirin or other prostaglandin synthesis inhibitors should not be used. Give the patient an instruction card that contains the above advice and precautions to read and keep with her in case she forgets the verbal information.

with ethylene oxide and broad-spectrum antibiotics.[69,110,191] The device swells to three to four times its original diameter (Fig. 22-8) and slowly dilates the cervix. Following intracervical placement, the sonographic appearance of the laminaria varies with time because of its hygroscopic nature.[119] While exerting its effect, the laminaria may produce moderate but tolerable crampy pain. Besides its hygroscopic (mechanical) action, the use of the laminaria is associated with significantly increased blood levels of PG metabolites.[328] Following overnight placement, each laminaria tent becomes soft, as large as a cigarette, and easily removable. We prefer laminaria japonica to those from Europe because of its uniform consistency and minimal hour-glass (dumbbelling) effect. Whenever this phenomenon occurs, the removal of such laminarias may be difficult and requires a paracervical block anesthetic. Each laminaria should be grasped with ring forceps, and the forceps rotated 360 degrees before the incarcerated device can be pulled out.

Lamicel is a dried polyvinyl alcohol sponge stick impregnated with magnesium sulfate (Fig. 22-7). This hard, sharp stick will become softened and immediately swells up with a spongy consistency when placed in the cervical canal. Each stick contains 0.2 to 0.5 gm of magnesium sulfate, depending on its diameter. Minimal systemic absorption of magnesium sulfate may occur through the uterine tissue, but blood magnesium levels have not exceeded 4 mg/dL in a testing series. Through some poorly defined histochemical effects, the dilator softens the cervix within 2 hours, making it pliable to gradual dilation with conventional instruments or with multiple laminaria japonica tents. An overnight preparation of the cervix with this dilator plus three to five 4 mm laminarias on the day preceding labor induction significantly shortens the prostaglandin induction-to-delivery interval and has thus far eliminated the risk of cervical rupture or cervicovaginal fistula (Fistula cervicovagnalis laqueatica).[125] Paradoxical to its tocolytic effect, the overnight preparation of the cervix with this magnesium sulfate device may enhance the effectiveness of PG-induced labor. Other investigators have effectively utilized this dilator prior to a suction evacuation of the uterus.

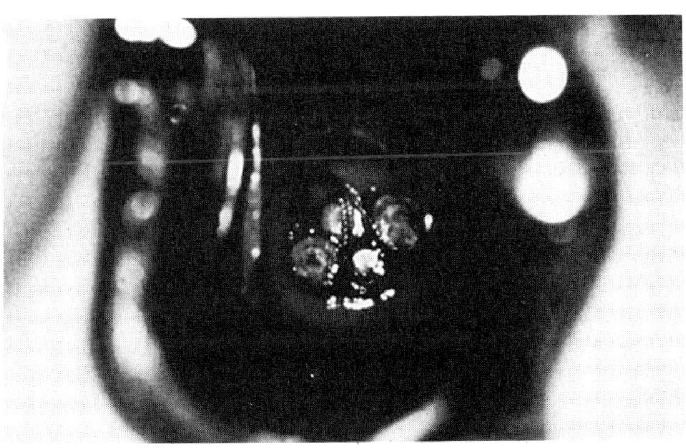

Fig. 22-8. Four laminaria tents that have been in the cervix overnight. (Courtesy Dr. AM Altman.)

Dilapan, another hygroscopic cervical dilator, is a synthetic polymer similar to a soft contact lens. It is recommended by its manufacturer for use within 4 hours of the abortion procedure on patients at or before 16 weeks of pregnancy. When compared to other hygroscopic dilators, this rather gluey and sticky device expands rapidly in and around the cervix. Thus it may be difficult to remove the device within 2 hours of insertion.

Besides hygroscopic devices, intracervical or vaginal PGE_2 and other PG derivatives were successfully utilized for softening the unfavorable (unripe) cervix.[84] Meteneprost potassium, an analog of PGE_2 in suppository form (10 mg) can induce adequate cervical softening within several hours of vaginal administration before a first-trimester induced abortion.[57,202,260] Preparing the cervix with a low dose of PGE_2 or one of its synthetic derivatives will reduce the need for a forceful, instrumental dilation of the cervix prior to uterine evacuation. Minimal but well-tolerated PG-induced side effects should be expected.

Conventional methods of induced abortion

Over one million therapeutic abortions were reported in the United States each year, and there are probably as many unreported menstrual extraction or menstrual regulation procedures routinely performed in physicians' offices. In 1985 approximately one legal abortion was performed for every three live births in the United States.[147] Most therapeutic abortions (95%) employ the vacuum aspiration technique and are safely accomplished in an outpatient facility.[326] It is not a good contraceptive choice but should be used as the last resort. On the other hand, induced abortion is the best therapy to save the mother if she has severe cardiac, renal, metabolic, hepatic, hematologic, or cerebrovascular disease.[12] Appropriate fetal indications range from defects that are incompatible with extrauterine life such as anencephaly, holoprosencephaly, and hypoplasia or agenesis of vital organs, to problems of chromosomal, metabolic, teratogenic, or infectious origin. Unique problems that combine the maternal and fetal indications for terminating the pregnancy are maternal neoplastic diseases requiring radiation or chemotherapy, fetal demise, and chorioamnionitis. With the latter diagnosis, the gravid uterus must be evacuated not only to save the mother, but also to preserve her reproductive capability. The safe termination of a pregnancy beyond 24 weeks from the last menstrual period (LMP) is justified in cases of fetal demise or lethal malformation such an anencephaly.[39,201] Hysterotomy or gravid hysterectomy is rarely indicated when skilled physicians and modern techniques for uterine evacuation are readily available.

In general, complication rates from induced abortion increase with every advancing week of gestation.[103,197,289] Major complications as defined by the Centers for Disease

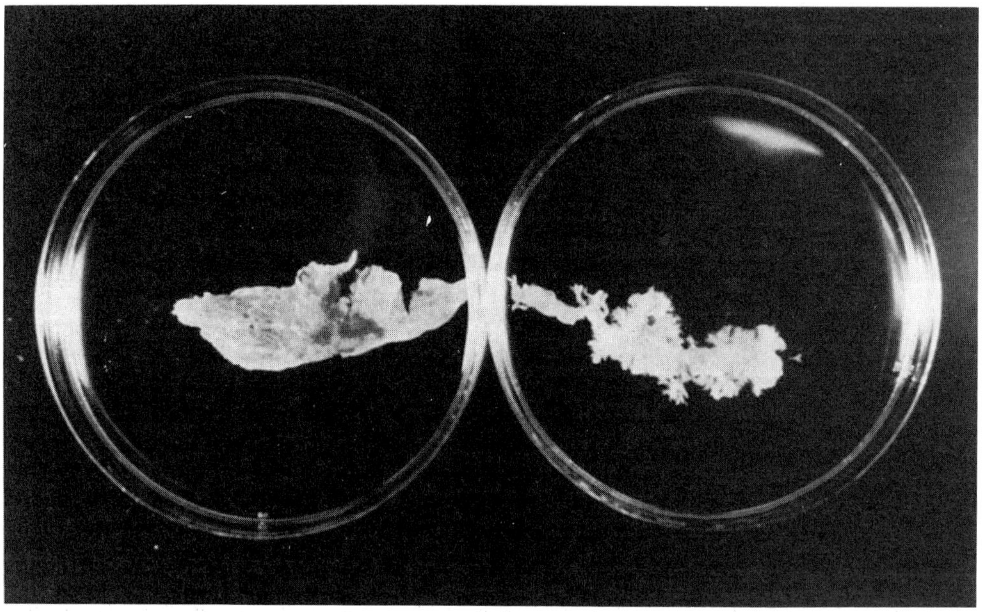

Fig. 22-9. Early pregnancy decidua (*left*) and trophoblastic villi (*right*).

Control Joint Program for the Study of Abortion (JPSA) include cardiac arrest, convulsions, death, endotoxic shock, fever for 3 days or more, hemorrhage necessitating transfusion, hypernatremia, injury to bladder, ureter, or intestine, pelvic infection with 2 or more days of fever and a peak of at least 40°C or with hospitalization for 11 days or more, pulmonary embolism or infarction, thrombophlebitis, major surgical treatment of complications, and wound disruption after hysterotomy or hysterectomy. Other complications not listed by the JPSA include retained pregnancy products or the continuation of pregnancy, hematometra, and coagulopathy.[203,317] Additionally, two or more induced abortions may increase the risk of subsequent first- and second-trimester loss.[120,150,275,149,154,279]

Menstrual extraction (miniabortion, minisuction, or menstrual regulation) is usually performed in a physician's office with a soft, flexible, plastic cannula (sometimes referred to as a Karman cannula). The cannula is attached to a special self-locking syringe or a small suction pump operated electrically or hydrostatically (Vabra aspirator). An experienced operator can perform this miniabortion 6 to 7 weeks after the patient's LMP without anesthetic. Most of the time, a 4-mm cannula or a recently available 3-mm cannula can be inserted into the gravid uterus without instrumental dilation of the cervix. The patient may receive preoperative medications which consist of oral ibuprofen and diazepam (or sublingual lorazepam). An office pregnancy test using a rapid, specific, and sensitive assay is strongly advised before the minisuction in order to avoid unnecessary instrumentation of the uterine cavity. The minisuction evacuation can be accomplished within 5 minutes with an in-and-out movement of the cannula while rotating it 360° around its long axis. After the procedure is complete, the aspirated products of conception (POC) must be carefully inspected for the presence of trophoblastic villous tissue (chorionic villi) (Fig. 22-9). If only the decidual (hypertrophic gestational endometrial) tissue is obtained but the villous structure cannot be identified, an ectopic pregnancy must be ruled out using an appropriate evaluation and treatment protocol. A bleeding (ruptured) tubal pregnancy with signs of peritoneal irritation may be observed shortly after minisuction of the uterine cavity of patients with unrecognized extrauterine gestation.[244] In spite of the obvious presence of villi, all patients should be reexamined several weeks thereafter because of the notoriously high incidence of retained POC or unrecognized continuation of an intrauterine pregnancy. Many authorities advise routine pregnancy testing at the postoperative follow-up visit if the soft plastic catheter was used for miniabortion.

Dilation and suction evacuation (D&E) is the most frequently utilized procedure for terminating a pregnancy 21 to 22 weeks from the LMP.[12,104] D&E beyond 15 weeks of pregnancy should only be done by qualified operators, who possess a high degree of touch-and-feel aptitude. Also an important consideration is the frequency of exposures to late midtrimester D&E which may be unaesthetic and may cause undesirable stress among dedicated staff. The latter problem may be avoided if a labor induction method is routinely available as an alternative.

Almost all of the D&E procedures (99%) are performed using local anesthetic with the use of chloroprocaine hydrochloride instead of lidocaine. Chloroprocaine hydrochloride has a wider safety margin and longer duration of action than lidocaine when injected into highly vascular tissues. Ideally, all D&E should be done with local anesthetic if possible because the procedural blood loss and the incidence of uterine perforation are much less than with general anesthetic. Procedural discomfort is blunted with appropriate intravenous medications and verbal distraction by a special nurse who is trained to coach the patient before and during the procedure. This same nurse simultaneously monitors the patient's vital signs, respiration, and pulse-oxymeter 0_2 saturation. Midazolam not exceeding 2 mg plus fentanyl citrate not exceeding 100 µg is used for the monitored intravenous anesthetic or conscious intravenous sedation. Additionally, 25 mg of diphenhydramine hydrochloride may be required for its mild anticholinergic effects. Vasoactive agents such as atropine, epinephrine, or other pressor drugs such as pitressin are avoided. The cardiogenic risks of such vasoactive substances outweigh the claimed benefits of reducing blood loss or vagal reaction. In fact, many deaths from legal abortion in the United States are reportedly drug related.[32,38] The proper training of the operator under hands-on supervision, and gentle manipulation with adequate dexterity will contribute to the uneventful completion of the procedure with minimal blood loss. The patient must be fasting for at least 6 hours because of delayed gastrointestinal transit especially during late midtrimester. She should not go home by herself after the procedure. An abortion after 12 weeks from the LMP should be preceded by adequate laminaria pretreatment of the cervix.

Blood typing (ABO and Rh), serum antibody screening, and a hematocrit and platelets count are routinely obtained before laminaria insertion. Additionally, cervical cytology and screening for STDs may be indicated in some patients.

At the time of the procedure, an intravenous line is inserted and secured in place for monitored intravenous medications. The no-touch technique is used in which only the portion of the instrument that will be in the uterus is kept sterile throughout the procedure. The operator should wear protective goggles or eyeglasses and a mask. A bimanual palpation of the uterine cervix and fundus should be performed to ascertain the direction of the uterine axis. At this time the sponges and laminaria tents may be digitally removed. The short-blades (Moore-Graves) speculum is required for minimizing the angle between the cervical canal and the uterine axis (Fig. 22-10). The anterior lip of the cervix is cleansed with an antiseptic solution and then injected with 3 mL of 1% chloroprocaine hydrochloride at the 12 o'clock position using a 22-gauge spinal needle. A single-toothed tenaculum is applied vertically with the inner jaw inside the cervical canal, to include the whole thickness of the anterior lip of cervix within the bite. It is important to take a deep enough bite so that the tenaculum will not be inadvertently pulled out and tear through the cervix during the procedure. The rest of the cervix and vaginal fornices are cleansed and the paracervical tissue is injected with 3 mL of the same anesthetic at the 8, 4, 10, and 2 o'clock position. The needle tip should reach the depth of only several millimeters within the submucosal (paracervical) tissue at or near the cervicovaginal junction. Preinjection aspiration is advised in order to avoid inadvertent leakage of the drug into a cervical tributary of the uterine vein. The uterine sound should not be inserted into any gravid uterus before the D&E procedure, since the risk of perforating the thin, soft, uterine wall outweighs any information to be gained. The depth and axis of the uterine cavity change rapidly during the suction evacuation and they should be gently assessed with a large curette but not with the uterine sound. The direction of the already dilated cervical canal can be assessed with a large cotton swab (a scopette). Should there be a need to forcefully dilate the cervix after the removal of the laminarias, dilators with tapered ends such as the Pratt dilator are preferred. The optimal diameter of the cannula for uterine evacuation (Fig. 22-10) generally correlates with the gestational age. For example, a 14-mm cannula is required for a complete evacuation of 13 to 15 weeks of pregnancy from the LMP. Five different sizes of rigid, clear, plastic cannula with internal diameters of 8, 10, 12, 14, and 16 mm are frequently used. The ability to insert a large-bore cannula through the laminaria-pretreated cervix greatly facilitates a safe and expedient D&E beyond the first trimester of pregnancy. However, when the uterine size is greater than 16 weeks, most solid POC must be extracted with the Sopher forceps (Fig. 22-11) because the parts are too large to be aspirated through the cannula. Amnionic membranes can often be easily ruptured with the use of sponge forceps after which amniotic fluid is completely expelled in order to reduce the uterine volume and the depth of uterine cavity. The large-bore cannula is required for the aspiration of the remaining amniotic fluid and for bringing the POC down to the lower uterine segment where the fetal parts can be safely

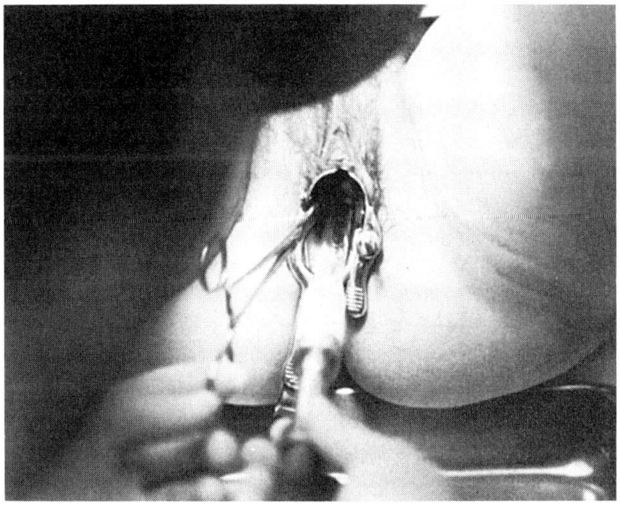

Fig. 22-10. A 16-mm rigid plastic cannula inserted through the cervical canal prior to suction evacuation of midtrimester uterus.

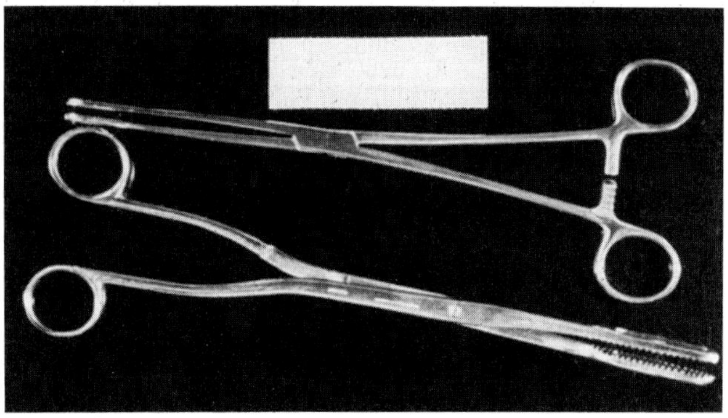

Fig. 22-11. Sopher forceps (*with long jaws*) compared with ordinary ring forceps.

extracted with the Sopher forceps. Ideally, the hinge of the Sopher forceps should be at the level of the cervical canal. Note that the cannula must be connected to the hose and vacuum jar through a specially designed handle. This special handle is the key to the D&E technique since it allows the cannula to be rotated 360° around its long axis while the hose remain immobile. The cannula is initially inserted just beyond the internal cervical os and rotated around the same cervicouterine axis while using a vacuum aspirating pressure of 50 to 60 cm of mercury. Once the intrauterine volume is reduced following the complete drainage of amniotic fluid, this cervico-uterine axis may change (e.g., from midposition to anteflexed or retroflexed). In most instances, the uterine cavity will eventually deviate towards the patient's right side and remain in its resting dextrorotational axis. A gentle exploration of the uterine cavity with a large curette will be required before advancing the cannula slightly deeper (to bring down the parts) and before the use of the Sopher forceps. Only the large curette should be used for this exploration. The operator's left hand may be placed on the abdomen to feel the fundus and to apply a suprapubic pressure. If the fetal calvarium cannot be easily brought down to the safe reach of the Sopher forceps, the patient should be given intravenous oxytocin using the high-dose protocol, and the procedure temporarily halted. The patient can be brought back to the procedure room in 1 or 2 hours when the fetal calvarium is seen or digitally felt at or above the internal cervical os. This second-stage uterine evacuation can be easily and rapidly accomplished without pain or discomfort to the patient. In general, however, uterotonic agent is not administered during the D&E until after the fetal calvarium has been obtained, for fear of trapping it up high or compressing it into the myometrium.[1] The D&E procedure is considered complete after important fetal parts are identified and accounted for. Such fetal parts are the calvarium, spine, and tips of the extremities. Routinely record the fetal foot length to corroborate the gestational age (may use Streeter's data as modified by Moore).[185] The latter correlates well in the patient population. The fetal foot length at 10, 12, 14, 16, 18, 20, and 22 weeks from the LMP are 6, 9, 14, 20, 27, 33, and 39 mm respectively. Induced abortions performed 8 to 10 weeks from the LMP should also yield a recognizable fetal part. Adding 6.5 to the crown-rump length in centimeters will provide an estimation of the gestational age in weeks during the first trimester.

It should be stressed that no descriptive text or manual on the D&E technique can replace proper training with hands-on instruction by a skillful physician. Resident physicians receive a minimum of 6 weeks of daily D&E training by a small number of experienced attending faculty members.[1] This training plus a well-defined protocol and a dedicated nursing staff facilitate the incorporation of the D&E procedure within the emergency-room management of patients with incomplete miscarriage.[14] Such patients safely and expediently undergo D&E with local anesthetic in specially equipped emergency rooms.

Dilation and labor induction is the abortion method of choice when the fetal biparietal diameters (BPD) are measured at 50 to 55 mm. (The fetal BPD increases at an average of 0.43 mm per day or 3 mm per week.) This technique is also indicated whenever a completely well-preserved and intact fetus is to be obtained at the patient's request, usually for personal or genetic counseling reason. On the other hand, several hours of effective labor in a patient whose cervix is not satisfactorily well prepared by laminarias may lead to favorable changes in the cervix and lower uterine segment to allow for a safe and easy D&E procedure. With a strict and active labor induction protocol, the complication rate is much less than that reported by the United States Centers for Disease Control.[103,130] This good record of labor induction protocol is in contradistinction to the national statistics that showed higher serious complication rates with intraamniotic prostaglandin. A complication rate of less than 2% (based on the JPSA criteria) is not higher than that of a late D&E and may be attributed to a protocol which is different from the protocol of others. First, the patient must undergo a laminaria pretreatment of the cervix 20 hours before receiving any prostaglandin drug. Second, ultrasound imaging,[122] and immediate coagulation screening tests, and blood products are available on site.[203] Third, a full-time director of the unit (or a designee) will instantly evaluate and perform the late D&E in case of excessive bleeding or prolonged labor. No patient is allowed to labor longer than 24 hours. Fourth, membranes are artificially ruptured after 3 hours of prostaglandin-induced labor. Oral PGE_1 methyl analog (misoprostol) 200 μg, is used in the morning after at least 20 hours of laminaria preparation of the cervix, along with an intraamniotic injection of 64 to 100 mL of 23.4% hypertonic saline. This procedure is immediately followed by 400 to 800 μg of oral misoprostol every 3 hours based on uterine contraction response. Three hours after the hypertonic with saline injection, the membranes are artificially ruptured. After all of the amniotic fluid is expressed out with suprapubic pressure, the cervical effacement is reassessed. When the cervix is 80% to 90% effaced, a high-dose intravenous oxytocin is administered through an infusion pump using an intermittent regimen (10 minutes on and 10 minutes off). If the cervix is still thick and long, 20 μg of intracervical PGE_2 will be administered with multiple dilators and laminaria tents, to be followed at 3-hour intervals with a PGE_2 vaginal suppository treatment. Finally, the patients undergo a uterine exploration and sharp curettage following the delivery of the placenta. Otherwise, the placenta must be removed using local anesthetic within 2 hours of the fetal delivery.

The second prostaglandin of choice is an intraamnionic instillation of 1.5 mg of 15-methyl-PGF_2 (carboprost tromethamine) followed immediately by 64 to 100 mL of 23.4% saline (4 mEq/mL) using a three-way connecting tube. This procedure is similar to any diagnostic amniocentesis without the use of preoperative medications. However, a local anesthetic is used for infiltrating the abdominal wall because a long (9-cm), large-bore (18-gauge) needle is used to demonstrate a free backflow of clear amniotic fluid before injecting the drugs. Actually, the prostaglandins are inactivated by the normal amniotic fluid. However, the carefully selected pharmacologic dose is in excess and will set off an irreversible chain of intrauterine events leading to myometrial contractions within an hour of administration. The intraamnionic injection produces fewer side effects than the extraamnionic route. Following the artificial rupture of the membranes, pretreatment medications are given at least a half an hour before the first dose of PGE_2 is administered, as described earlier. If the cervical effacement reaches 90%, the high-dose intravenous oxytocin infusion will be initiated as long as it is not within 2 hours of the last dose of PG. Prophylactic antibiotics are not routinely provided. However, broad-spectrum intravenous antibiotics are used liberally in undelivered patients after 10 hours of the artificial or spontaneous rupture of the membranes. Antibiotics are also prescribed following excessive procedural blood loss, if a degree of myometrial injury is strongly suspected, and when a D&E procedure takes longer than 20 minutes to complete. There were some well-controlled trials which favored the routine use of a prophylactic antibiotic but their small study populations limit any conclusive interpretation.[55,208,271,272] High-risk patients are defined as those who may benefit from a course of antibiotic treatment from the time of laminaria insertion on the day before the D&E or labor induction. Such patients are those with fetal demise, placenta previa, habitual abortions, Asherman's syndrome, an intrauterine device, an orthopedic or cardiac prosthesis, trichomonads or koilocytosis on cervical cytology, a history of PID or STD or tubal pregnancy, sickle cell trait or disease, chronic hepatitis, intravenous drug abuse, a tattoo, multiple male partners, and women from a correctional institute. Preoperative prophylaxis is provided against bacterial endocarditis not only for indicated cardiac patients but also for intravenous drug abusers. Additionally, women with a dilated internal os due to an incomplete, inevitable, or missed abortion with vaginal bleeding should receive antibiotics for prophylaxis. The spectrum of prescribed antibiotics should cover *Chlamydia trachomatis*. Twelve percent of women who requested legal abortion at the institution in 1986 had this organism.

The complications of induced abortion are reportedly dependent upon two main factors: the gestational age (too early or too advanced) and the operator's experience (or inexperience). Recent United States national statistics showed that induced abortions performed 7 to 12 weeks from the LMP were associated with fewer complications than those performed before or after this gestational age range, regardless of whether or not the complication rate or severity was a factor.[147,197] Increased risks of uterine trauma and hemorrhage occur in the D&E procedures performed by the resident when compared to those done by the experienced attending physician.[103] Other risk factors include the use of general anesthetic, the failure to adequately prepare the cervix with laminarias, parity, a history of previous abortion, and the woman's age.[105,197,254] With regard to the D&E, the risk of a cervical injury or related trauma is reduced with a history of a prior abortion, the use of laminaria, local anesthetic, and performance by an attending physician.[103,254] This risk is increased with patients who are 17 years of age or less, the use of general anesthetic, and the performance by a physician-in-training. The risk factors for a uterine perforation are similar to those for a cervical injury except that multiparous women have three times the risk of nulliparous women.[33] Fortunately, two thirds of uterine perforations occur in the fundal region and are not associated with acute or uncontrollable hemorrhage. Obese patients and those with repeated cesarean scars may be at an increased risk of uterine perforation. Prompt recognition of this complication is the key to minimizing the damage. Undetected uterine perforation may lead to devastating generalized peritonitis from bowel injury and fatality. Acute problems associated with uterine perforation include lacerations of the uterine vessels, which lead to severe hypovolemia or expanding broad-ligament hematoma, and injuries to intraperitoneal structures. Such problems dictate a prompt laparotomy. A three-way indwelling catheter should be inserted into the urinary bladder before the laparotomy. Thus, methylene blue or indigocarmine can be readily injected intravesically should a bladder injury arise during this life-saving operation. Bleeding vessels can usually be ligated, in which case the uterine trauma is repaired and hysterectomy is not required. If a suction or forceps was applied intraperitoneally, the entire length of bowel should be inspected for any severe contusion or disruption of its blood supply. In the latter situation, an abdominal surgeon may decide to resect and reanastomose the damaged bowel. Most of the time, however, complete bowel rest with the help of intermittent nasogastric suction and broad-spectrum intravenous antibiotics will suffice. If the uterine perforation is promptly diagnosed before any intraperitoneal structure is damaged, the D&E procedure may be continued and readily accomplished under laparoscopic visualization. A delayed diagnosis of slowly expanding broad-ligament hematoma in a hemodynamically stable patient may require only intravenous antibiotics and ultrasound imaging at follow-up intervals. A liquefied infected hematoma can be successfully drained under competent ultrasound guidance to abolish the stormy, febrile course and shorten the patient's incapacitation period. Selective embolization of a damaged uterine vessel was successfully utilized in patients with broad-ligament hematoma and patients with pathology-proven focal placenta accreta after adequate uterine packing and intravenous antibiotic treatment. Such conservative therapies are best preserved for nulliparous patients who fully understand the inherent procedural risks and sign the individualized informed consent form in the chart.

Another type of hemorrhagic complication of induced abortion is coagulopathy. It is not an infrequent problem after a fetal demise of long duration with a large uterine size (beyond 13 weeks) and also after an intraamnionic injection of a high volume of hypertonic saline. Coagulopathy may also occur in rare cases of an otherwise routine D&E beyond 13 weeks for the LMP.[203,317] It is advised that midtrimester abortions be performed near or within a facility where blood products are readily available. Prolonged bleeding from the well-contracting, intact, empty uterus and from the tenaculum site should provoke a high index of suspicion. A tube of blood should be obtained to record the patient's clotting time, which may be prolonged, and abnormal clot retraction or lysis. At the same time, a profile of blood coagulation tests should be immediately obtained. A severe depletion of platelets and fibrinogen that is disproportionate to the minor decrease in hematocrit may promptly confirm this diagnosis. In general, coagulopathy in obstetrical hemorrhage is associated with a severe depletion of circulating fibrinogen before the decline of other clotting factors. A significant leakage of the thromboplastic fetal or trophoblastic tissue into the maternal circulation may be responsible for this postulated consumptive coagulopathy. It is frequently associated with violent uterine contractions or prolonged intrauterine manipulation in the case of D&E for fetal demise. The treatment requires an infusion of cryoprecipitate and fresh plasma.

Another enigmatic complication of D&E which may occur within hours or several days postoperatively is hematometra. Some authorities call this complication the postabortal syndrome or the redo syndrome.[248] It was first reported in 1974 as a unique type of uterine atony with an incidence of one in several hundred D&E cases. This syndrome is characterized by a painful and acutely tender enlargement of the uterus which is full of dark liquid and clotted blood. The patient usually shows facial signs of general distress with sweating and tachycardia but vaginal bleeding is not excessive. A repeat suction evacuation of the uterine cavity will promptly abolish this puzzling phenomenon. Although the cause of this problem is unknown at this time, an ergot and antibiotic drug may be prescribed in such cases for prophylaxis.

An acute drug reaction is a possible complication before or during a D&E procedure. If a toxic dose of the local anesthetic is inadvertently injected into the maternal circulation, convulsions, cardiac arrhythmias, and cardiovascular collapse may follow. The treatment consists of the establishment and maintenance of an airway by endotracheal intubation with adequate ventilation of the patient. Adequate blood pressure is maintained with intravenous fluids and an appropriate sympathomimetic agent, if necessary. However, this particular complication is preventable. Preinjection aspiration as described earlier must be practiced as a routine habit during the induction of a paracervical anesthetic. The D&E should not be commenced within 3 minutes of paracervical anesthetic injections. The use of chloroprocaine hydrochloride and the avoidance of epinephrine (or other pressor substances) in the highly vascular gravid tissues are also observed as part of the protocol. Premedication with 2 mg of intravenous midazolam, a short acting anxiolytic benzodiazepine drug, may prevent a rare syndrome of chest wall stiffness caused by intravenous injection of an opioid such as fentanyl citrate. High doses of the latter drug may lead to a dose-related respiratory depression. Effective intravenous antidotes for fentanyl and midazolam are naloxone hydrochloride 0.4 mg and flumazenil 1 mg respectively.

A rare and unique respiratory embarrassment may occur during a midtrimester D&E, especially with fetal demise of long duration. It is characterized by the signs of respiratory hypersecretion, coughing, and if not promptly corrected, bronchospasm. This syndrome is not related to an amniotic fluid embolism because it is self limited and often occurs in cases of severe oligohydramnios or in dry fetal demise. It is unlike a vasovagal reaction because of the presence of tachycardia and the borderline elevation of the blood pressure. It has been observed in association with violent uterine contractions that produce features analogous to inadvertent intravenous infusion of $PGF_{2\alpha}$. A similar problem was described by Kohorn in collaboration with the New England Trophoblastic Disease Center in 1978 as a trophoblastic embolization syndrome following molar evacuation. The D&E procedure should be temporarily halted and the patient should be turned on her side. Intravenous diphenhydramine 25 mg is slowly administered to reduce the secretion. Epinephrine should not be used for this type of bronchospasm because the patient's blood pressure may become too highly elevated and epinephrine may produce an adverse cardiac effect in this situation.[267] Bronchospasm in such cases is better relieved with an intravenous glucocorticoid such as 4 mg of dexamethasone than with the use of aminophylline, which is slow-acting and produces tachycardia. With assurance and improved ventilation and respiration, the D&E procedure can proceed and be safely accomplished. On the other hand, amniotic fluid embolism can also occur during midtrimester abortion in rare cases, following instrumental disruption of the placenta with a large volume of amniotic fluid in the uterine cavity, or following abruption placentae in cases of labor induction. It is usually associated with the obvious signs of cardiopulmonary collapse and disseminated intravascular coagulation. Prompt arterial blood gas measurement, electrocardiogram, and a ventilation-perfusion radionuclide scan will confirm the diagnosis. Effective resuscitation and successful management will require around-the-clock cardiopulmonary and hematologic care by a team consisting of a competent internist, gynecologist, anesthesiologist, hematologist or blood-bank specialist, nurses, and laboratory personnel in a well-equipped intensive care facility. The uterus must be emptied as soon as the patient's cardiovascular status is reasonably stabilized.

Delayed complications of induced abortion include different degrees of postabortal infection from endoparametritis to pelvic septic thrombophlebitis and thromboembolic events.[21] Infection is usually associated with retained POC. Common symptoms are crampy pain with prolonged vaginal bleeding and low-grade fever. The uterus is tender, slightly enlarged, and boggy. High-resolution ultrasound imaging with a full bladder may confirm or exclude the diagnosis of retained POC. Treatment consists of intravenous antibiotics, an ergot alkaloid, and repeated uterine evacuation if indicated. Patients with a retained pregnancy or retained pregnancy products not infrequently have an unrecognized positional, anatomic, or congenital uterine anomaly. Such patients should undergo a D&E under ultrasound guidance.[122] The latter technique was also useful in a midtrimester D&E with known anatomic derangements and in patients with cervical stenosis.

Controversies exist on the possibility of late sequelae of repetitive induced abortions with regard to premature delivery and low birth weight.[120] Most statistics were derived from patients who have undergone primitive abortion techniques. Increasing experience and opportunities for proper training of physicians in the modern techniques of induced abortion may curtail those problems. Another controversy is related to intrauterine synechiae (Asherman's syndrome) which may involve risk factors that include genetic predisposition and postoperative infection or hematometra. One late sequelae that is theoretically possible is Rh isomune disease.[163] A fail-safe mechanism can be devised in the quality assurance program using the nurse, physician, and patient education to ensure that Rh negative patients will automatically receive adequate doses of Rh immune globulin for prophylaxis within 72 hours of induced abortion or miscarriage.

Selective reduction of multifetal pregnancy

Successful in vitro fertilization, gamete intrafallopian transfer, and aggressive pharmacotherapy of infertility have led to an increase in a gestation with three or more fetuses. With a large number of fetuses in one gestation, each fetus is at a significantly increased risk of premature birth and its serious sequela. The procedures to reduce multiple fetuses to only two (twins) were performed with increasing experience and efficacy using ultrasound guidance. Early methods involved transcervical selective evacuation, transabdominal injection of air or hypertonic saline, needle disruption of a selected conceptus, and selective fetal exsanguination.[78] Currently, the most popular method is an ultrasound-guided transabdominal injection of potassium chloride 4 to 8 mmol (mEq) per embryo at the end of the first trimester. Selective-reduction procedures were also performed in the second trimester for termination of a defective twin. The patient must be informed of the known and unknown risks of losing some or all the fetuses. Such risks were described with and without undergoing the selective-reduction procedure. The risks vary at different gestational ages and increase with an advanced maternal age. These risks include the syndrome of a vanishing twin(s), trapped twin(s), twin-to-twin transfusion, and fetal disseminated intravascular coagulation and porencephaly. Berkowitz described the possible, procedure-related, complications in a two-page informed consent form. Such complications include bleeding, infection, leakage of amniotic fluid, the need for repeating the procedure, the risk of having to undergo a D&E, sterility, and even hysterectomy. Any infertile woman who has taken the risks of infertility treatment may be willing to take any known or unknown risks from the selective reduction of her multifetal pregnancy. With triplets, however, the risk-benefit ratio of undergoing a selective-reduction procedure is unclear, especially at tertiary-care maternity centers where triplets appear to do as well medically (physically) as twins do after birth. In this situation, the individual couple may take into account the quality of the offspring's life and perhaps the cost of upbringing. Thus, complex ethical and legal ramifications of the selective-reduction procedure remain for further debate.

REFERENCES

1. Altman AM et al: Midtrimester abortion by laminaria and vacuum evacuation on a teaching service, *J Reprod Med* 30:601-606, 1985.
2. American College of Obstetricians and Gynecologists Committee on Obstetrics: Postpartum tubal sterilization: appropriate timing of surgery after vaginal delivery, *Committee Opinion* No. 50, 1987.
3. Amir M: *Patterns in forcible rape*, 1971, University of Chicago Press.
4. Anderson ABM, Turnbull AC: Changes in amniotic fluid, serum, and urine following the intraamniotic injection of hypertonic saline, *Acta Obstet Gynec Scand* 47:1-21, 1968.
5. Arntzenius AC et al: Reduced high-density lipoprotein in women aged 40-41 using oral contraceptives, *Lancet* 1:1221-1223, 1978.
6. Baulieu EE, Segal SJ, editors: *The antiprogestin steroid RU486 and human fertility control*, New York, London, Plenum Press (Proceedings of a Conference on the Antiprogestational Compound RU486 held October 23-25, 1984, in Bellagio, Italy.)
7. Beaumont V, Lemort N, Beaumont JL: Evaluation of risk factors associated with vascular thrombosis in women on oral contraceptives: possible role of antisex steroid hormone antibodies, *Artery* 11:331-344, 1983.
8. Bergink EW et al: Binding of a contraceptive progestogen Org 2969 and its metabolites to receptor proteins and human sex hormone-binding globulin, *J Steroid Bioch* 14:175-183, 1981.

9. Berkowitz GS et al: Oral contraceptive use and fibrocystic breast disease among pre- and postmenopausal women, *Am J Epidemiol* 120:87-96, 1984.
10. Black MM et al: Family history, oral contraceptive usage, and breast cancer, *Cancer* 51:2147-2151, 1983.
11. Blumenthal PD: Prospective comparison of dilapan and laminaria for pretreatment of the cervix in second-trimester induction abortion, *Obstet Gynecol* 72:243-246, 1988.
12. Bowers C, Devine PA, Chervenak FA: Dilation and evacuation during the second trimester of pregnancy in a woman with primary pulmonary hypertension, *J Reprod Med* 33:787-788, 1988.
13. Bradley DD et al: Serum high density lipoprotein cholesterol in women using oral contraceptives, estrogens, and progestins, *N Engl J Med* 199:17-20, 1978.
14. Brennan DM, Caldwell M: Dilatation and evacuation performed in the emergency department for miscarriage, *J Emerg Nursing* 13:144-8, 1987.
15. Brenner PF: Oral combination contraceptives. In Bardin CW, editors: *Current Therapy Endocrinology Metabolism-3*, Toronto, 1988, BC Decker.
16. Brooks PG: The relationship of estrogen and progesterone to breast disease, *J Reprod Med* 29:530-538, 1984.
17. Bruce SL, Paul RH, Van Dorsten JP: Control of postpartum uterine atony by intramyometrial prostaglandin, *Obstet Gynecol* 59:47s-50s, 1982.
18. Bughlho, 1993.
19. Burkman RT: Lipid and lipoprotein changes in relation to oral contraception and hormonal replacement therapy, *Fertil Steril* 49 (Suppl):39S-50S, 1988.
20. Burkman RT et al: Intraamniotic urea as a midtrimester abortifacient: clinical results and serum and urinary changes, *Am J Obstet Gynecol* 121:7-16, 1975.
21. Burkman RT, Atienza MF, King TM: Culture and treatment results in endometritis following elective abortion, *Am J Obstet Gynecol* 128:556-559, 1977.
22. Burkman RT and the Women's Health Study: Association between intrauterine device and pelvic inflammatory disease, *Obstet Gynecol* 57:269-276, 1981.
23. Cabrol D et al: Induction of labor with mifespristone after intrauterine fetal death, *Lancet* 2:1019, 1985.
24. Caillouette JC, Koehler AL: Phasic contraceptive pills and functional ovarian cysts, *Am J Obstet Gynecol* 156:1538-1542, 1987.
25. Cameron IT, Baird DT: Early pregnancy termination: a comparison between vacuum aspiration and medical abortion using prostaglandin (16,16 dimethyl-trans-3D_2-PGE_1 methyl ester) or the antiprogestogen RU486, *Br J Obstet Gynaecol* 95:271-276, 1988.
26. Campbell WB: Vasectomy and arterial disease, *J R Soc Med* 81:682-695, 1988.
27. Centers for Disease Control and the National Institute of Child Health and Human Development: Cancer and Steroid Hormone Study: Oral contraceptive use and the risk of breast cancer, *N Engl J Med* 315:405-411, 1986.
28. Centers for Disease Control and the National Institute of Child Health and Human Development: Cancer and Steroid Hormone Study: Combination oral contraceptive use and the risk of endometrial cancer, *JAMA* 257:796-800, 1987.
29. Centers for Disease Control and the National Institute of Child Health and Human Development: Cancer and Steroid Hormone Study: The reduction in risk of ovarian cancer associated with oral contraceptive use, *N Engl J Med* 316:650-655, 1987.
30. Carp HJ et al: Fertility after nonsurgical treatment of ectopic pregnancy, *J Reprod Med* 31:119-122, 1986.
31. Cates W Jr, Blackmore CA: Sexual assault and sexually transmitted diseases. In Holmes KK et al, editors: *Sexually transmitted diseases*, 1984, McGraw-Hill.
32. Cates W Jr, Jordaan HVF: Sudden collapse and death of women obtaining abortions induced with prostaglandin $F_{2\ 3\alpha}$, *Am J Obstet Gynecol* 133:398-400, 1979.
33. Cates W Jr, Schulz KF, Grimes DA: The risks associated with teenage abortion, *N Engl J Med* 309:621-624, 1983.
34. Cederqvist LL, Birnbaum SJ: Rupture of the uterus after midtrimester prostaglandin abortion, *J Reprod Med* 25:136-138, 1980.
35. Centers for Disease Control: Cancer and Steroid Hormone Study: Long term oral contraceptive use and the risk of breast cancer, *JAMA* 249:1591-1595, 1983.
36. Centers for Disease Control: Cancer and Steroid Hormone Study: Oral contraceptive use and the risk of endometrial cancer, *JAMA* 249:1600-1604, 1983.
37. Centers for Disease Control: Cancer and Steroid Hormone Study: Oral contraceptive use and the risk of ovarian cancer, *JAMA* 249:1596-1599, 1983.
38. Centers for Disease Control: Epidemiologic Notes and Reports: Maternal deaths associated with barbiturate anesthetics—New York City, *MMWR* 35:579-587, 1986.
39. Chervenak FA et al: When is termination of pregnancy during the third trimester morally justifiable? *N Engl J Med* 310:501-504, 1984.
40. Chwalisz K: The use of progesterone antagonists for cervical ripening and as a adjunct to labour and delivery, *Human Reproduction* 9(Suppl 1), 1994. (in press)
41. Clarke EA et al: Cervical dysplasia: association with sexual behavior, smoking, and oral contraceptive use? *Am J Obstet Gynecol* 151:612-616, 1985.
42. Connell EB: Oral contraceptives: the current risk-benefit ratio, *J Reprod Med* 29:513-523, 1984.
43. Cook CL, Lance JW, Kraft SL: Pregnancy prophylaxis: parenteral postcoital estrogen, *Obstet Gynecol* 67:331-333, 1986.
44. Craft I et al: Effect of Norgestrel administered intermittently on pituitary ovarian function, *Contraception* 12:589-598, 1975.
45. Cramer DW: Vasectomy and increased risk of prostate cancer, possible hormonal mechanisms, *JAMA* 270:707, 1993.
46. Cramer DW: Infertility in relation to the use of intrauterine devices. In Monif G, editor: *Infectious disease newsletter*, 1989. (in press)
47. Cramer DW et al: The relationship of tubal infertility to barrier method and oral contraceptive use, *JAMA* 257:2446-2450, 1987.
48. Cramer DW et al: Factors affecting the association of oral contraceptives and ovarian cancer, *N Engl J Med* 307:1047-1051, 1982.
49. Cramer DW et al: Tubal infertility and intrauterine device, *N Engl J Med* 312:941-947, 1985.
50. Creinin MD, Darney PD: Methotrexate and misoprostol for early abortion, *Contraception* 48:339-348, 1993.
51. Crooij MJ et al: Termination of early pregnancy by the 3 3b-hydroxysteroid dehydrogenase inhibitor epostane, *N Engl J Med* 319:813-817, 1988.
52. Croxatto HB et al: Studies on the duration of egg transport in the human oviduct. I. The time interval between ovulation and egg recovery from the uterus in normal women, *Fertil Steril* 23:447-458, 1972.
53. Cundy T et al: Bone density in women receiving depot medroxyprogesterone acetate for contraception, *Br Med J* 303:313, 1991.
54. Daling JR et al: Primary tubal infertility in relation to the use of an intrauterine device, *N Engl J Med* 312:937-941, 1985.
55. Darj E, Stralin EB, Nilsson S: The prophylactic effect of doxycycline on postoperative infection rate after first-trimester abortion, *Obstet Gynecol* 70:755-758, 1988.
56. Darney PD: Long-acting hormonal contraception, *Contemp Obstet Gynecol* 32:90-100, 1988.
57. Darney PD, Dorward K: Cervical dilation before first-trimester elective abortion: a controlled comparison of meteneprost, laminaria, and hypan, *Obstet Gynecol* 70:397-400, 1987.
58. Dattel BJ et al: Isolation of *Chlamydia trachomatis* from sexually abused female adolescents, *Obstet Gynecol* 72:240-242, 1988.

59. del Junco DJ, Annegers JF, Luthra HS: Do oral contraceptives prevent rheumatoid arthritis? *JAMA* 254:1938-1941, 1985.
60. Dericks-Tan JSE, Kock P, Taubert HD: Synthesis and release of gonadotropins: effect of an oral contraceptive, *Obstet Gynecol* 62:687-690, 1983.
61. DeStefano F et al: Complications of interval laparoscopic tubal sterilization, *Obstet Gynecol* 61:153-158, 1983.
62. Diamond MP, Wentz AC, Cherrington AD: Alterations in carbohydrate metabolism as they apply to reproductive endocrinology, *Fertil Steril* 50:387-397, 1988.
63. Diaz S et al: Ectopic pregnancies associated with low-dose progestogen-releasing IUDs, *Contraception* 22:259, 1980.
64. Diaz S et al: Clinical assessment of treatments for prolonged bleeding in users of Norplant implants, *Contraception* 42:97, 1990.
65. Dingfelder JR et al: Intraamniotic administration of 15(S)-15-methyl-prostaglandin $F_{2\ 3\alpha}$ for the induction of midtrimester abortion. *Am J Obstet Gynecol* 125:821-826, 1976.
66. Dixon GW et al: Ethinyl estradiol and conjugated estrogens as postcoital contraceptives, *JAMA* 244:1336, 1980.
67. Droegemueller W et al: Triphasic randomized clinical trail: comparative frequency of intermenstrual bleeding, *Am J Obstet Gynecol* 161:1407-1411, 1989.
68. Duguid HLD, Parratt D, Traynor R: Actinomyces-like organisms in cervical smears from women using intrauterine contraceptive devices, *Br Med J* 281:534-537, 1980.
69. Eaton CJ, Cohn F, Bollinger CC: Laminaria tent as a cervical dilator prior to aspiration type therapeutic abortion, *Obstet Gynecol* 39:533-536, 1972.
70. Editorial: Drug interaction with oral contraceptive steroids, *Br Med J* 281:93-94, 1980.
71. Editorial: Gossypol prospects, *Lancet* 1:1108-1109, 1984.
72. Elger W et al: Endometrial and myometrial effect of progesterone antagonists in pregnant guinea pigs, *Am J Obstet Gynecol* 157:1065-1074, 1987.
73. Ellis JW: Multiphasic oral contraceptives—efficacy and metabolic impact, *J Reprod Med* 32:28-36, 1987.
74. Engel HJ, Enge E, Lichtlen PR: Coronary atherosclerosis and myocardial infarction in young women—role of oral contraceptives, *Euro Heart* J 4:1-8, 1983.
75. Eyong E, Buchi K, Elstein M: Effects of 180 25g and 250 25g norgestimate on pituitary—ovarian function and cervical mucus, *Fertil Steril* 50:756-760, 1988.
76. Faich G et al: Toxic shock syndrome and vaginal contraceptive sponge, *JAMA* 255:216-218, 1986.
77. Farabow WS, Fulton JW, Fletcher V Jr: Cervical pregnancy treated with methotrexate, *N C Med J* 44:91, 1983.
78. Farquharson D et al: Management of quintuplet pregnancy by selective embryocide. Program of the 32nd Annual Convention of the American Institute of Ultrasound in Medicine, New Orleans, October 1987.
79. Fihn SD et al: Association between diaphragm use and urinary tract infection, *JAMA* 254:240-245, 1985.
80. Franceschi S et al: Oral contraceptives and benign breast disease: a case-control study, *Am J Obstet Gynecol* 149:602-606, 1984.
81. Frates MC et al: The sonographic diagnosis and conservative treatment of cervical ectopic pregnancies, *Radiology* ,1994. (in press)
82. Freie HMP: Sickle cell diseases and hormonal contraception, *Acta Obstet Gynecol Scand* 62:211-217, 1983.
83. Frigoletto FD, Pokoly TB: Electrolyte dynamics in hypertonic saline-induced abortions, *Obstet Gynecol* 38:647-652,1971.
84. Fruzzetti F et al: Use of sulprostone for induction of preoperative cervical dilation or uterine evacuation: a comparison among the effects of different treatment schedules, *Obstet Gynecol* 72:704-708, 1988.
85. Frydmann R, Taylor S, Ulmann A: Transplacental passage of mifespristone, *Lancet* 2:1252, 1985.
86. Fylling P, Fagerhol M: Experience with two different medicated intrauterine devices: a comparative study of the Progestasert and Nova-T, *Fertil Steril* 31:138-141, 1979.
87. Garzo VG et al: Effects on an antiprogesterone (RU486) on the hypothalamic-hypophyseal-ovarian-endometrial axis during the luteal phase of the menstrual cycle, *J Clin Endocrinol Metab* 66:508-517, 1988.
88. Gaspard UJ: Metabolic effects of oral contraceptives, *Am J Obstet Gynecol* 157:1029-1041, 1987.
89. Ginsburg et al 1994
90. Ginsburg KA, Moghissi KS: Alternate delivery systems for contraceptive progestogens, *Fertil Steril* 49(Suppl):16S-30S, 1988.
91. Giovannucci E et al: A prospective cohort study of vasectomy and prostate cancer in U.S. men, *JAMA* 269:873-877, 1993a.
92. Giovannucci E et al: A retrospective cohort study of vasectomy and prostate cancer in U.S. men, *JAMA* 269:873-877, 1993b.
93. Goldacre MJ, Holford TR, Vessey MP: Cardiovascular disease and vasectomy, *N Engl J Med* 308:805-808, 1983.
94. Goldsmith MF: Pregnancy Dx? Rx may now include condoms, *JAMA* 261:678-679, 1989.
95. Goldzieher JW: Hormonal contraceptives; past, present, future, *Horm Contrac* 75:75-86, 1984.
96. Goldzieher JW et al: A placebo-controlled double-blind crossover investigation of the side effects attributed to oral contraceptives, *Fertil Steril* 22:609-623, 1971.
97. Goodlin RC, Kresch AD: Amniotic fluid osmolality following intra-amniotic injection of saline, *Amer J Obstet Gynecol* 100:839-842, 1968.
98. Gordon T, Castelli WP, Njortland M: HDL as a protective factor against coronary heart disease—the Framingham Study, *Am J Med* 62:707-714, 1977.
99. Gore BZ, Caldwell BV, Speroff L: Estrogen-induced human luteolysis, *J Clin Endocrinol Metab* 36:615, 1973.
100. Gravanis A et al: Endometrial and pituitary responses to the steroidal antiprogestin RU486 in postmenopausal women, *J Clin Endocrinol Metab* 60:156-163, 1985.
101. Grimes DA et al: Ovulation and follicular development associated with three low-dose oral contraceptives: a randomized control trial, *Obstet Gynecol* 83:29, 1994.
102. Grimes DA et al: Early abortion with a single dose of the antiprogestin RU-486, *Am J Obstet Gynecol* 158:1307-1312, 1988.
103. Grimes DA, Schulz KF: Morbidity and mortality from second-trimester abortions, *J Reprod Med* 30:505-514, 1985.
104. Grimes DA et al: Midtrimester abortion by dilatation and evacuation: a safe and practical alternative, *N Engl J Med* 296:1131-1145, 1977.
105. Grimes DA et al: Local vs. general anesthesia: which is safer for performing suction curettage abortions? *Am J Obstet Gynecol* 135:1030-1035, 1979.
106. Gu SJ et al: A 5-year evaluation of Norplant contraceptive implants in China, *Obstet Gynecol* 83:673-678, 1994.
107. Gupta PK, Woodruff JD: Actinomyces in vaginal smears, *JAMA* 247:1175-1176, 1982.
108. Hahn DW, Allen GE, McGuire J: The pharmacological profile of Norgestimate, a new orally active progestin, *Contraception* 16:541-553, 1977.
109. Halbert DR, Darnell-Jones DE: Medical management of the sexually assaulted woman, *J Reprod Med* 20:265-274, 1978.
110. Hale RW, Pion RJ: Laminaria: an underutilized clinical adjunct, *Clin Obstet Gynecol* 15:829-850, 1972.
111. Hankins GD et al: Maternal arterial desaturation with 15-methyl prostaglandin $F_{2\alpha}$ for uterine atony, *Obstet Gynecol* 72:367-370, 1988.
112. Harlap S, Shiono PH, Ramcharan S: Congenital abnormalities in the offspring of women who used oral and other contraceptives around the time of conception, *Int J Fertil* 30:39-47, 1985.

113. Harrison DD, Cooke CW: An elucidation of factors influencing physicians' willingness to perform elective female sterilization, *Obstet Gynecol* 72:570, 1988.
114. Hasson HM: Open laparoscopy: In Zatuchni GI, Daly MJ, Sciarra JJ, editors: *Gynecology and obstetrics*, Philadelphia, 1982, Harper & Row.
115. Haukkamaa, 1986.
116. Hennekens CH et al: A case-control study of oral contraceptive use and breast cancer, *J Nat Cancer Inst* 72:39-42, 1984.
117. Henry A, Rinehart W, Piotrow P: Reversing female sterilization, *Popul Rep* C8:97-123, 1980.
118. Hicks DJ: Rape: sexual assault, *Am J Obstet Gynecol* 137:931-935, 1980.
119. Hirsh MP, Levy HM: The varied ultrasonographic appearance of laminaria, *J Ultrasound Med* 7:45-47, 1988.
120. Hogue CJR, Cates W Jr, Tietze C: The effects of induced abortion on subsequent reproduction, *Epidemiol Rev* 4:66-94, 1982.
121. Hong CY, Turner P: Influence of lipid solubility on the sperm immobilizing effect of 3β-adrenoceptor blocking drugs, *Br J Clin Pharmacol* 14:269-272, 1982.
122. Hornstein MD et al: Ultrasound guidance for selected dilatation and evacuation procedures, *J Reprod Med* 31:947-950, 1986.
123. Hseih CC et al: Oral contraceptive use and fibrocystic breast disease of different histologic classifications, *J Nat Cancer Inst* 72:285-290, 1984.
124. Hulka BS, Chambless LE, Kaufman DG: Protection against endometrial carcinoma by combination-product oral contraceptives, *JAMA* 247:475-477, 1982.
125. Ingvardsen A, Eriksen T: Cervical rupture following prostaglandin-induced midtrimester abortion, *Ugeskr Laeger* 141:3531-3532, 1979.
126. Irwin KL et al: Oral contraceptives and cervical cancer risk in Costa Rica, *JAMA* 259:59-64, 1988.
127. Janerick DT et al: Breast cancer and oral contraceptive use: a case-control study, *J Chron Dis* 36:639-646, 1983.
128. Jick H et al: Venous thromboembolic disease and ABO blood type, *Lancet* 1:539-542, 1969.
129. Johansson EDB: Inhibition of the corpus luteum function in women taking large doses of diethylstilbestrol, *Contraception* 8:27-35, 1973.
130. Kafrissen ME et al: Midtrimester Abortion: intraamniotic instillation of hyperosmolar urea and prostaglandin $F_{2\ 3\alpha}$ vs. dilation and evacuation, *JAMA* 251:916-919, 1984.
131. Kalache A et al: Oral contraceptives and breast cancer, *Br J Hosp Med* 30:278-283, 1983.
132. Karim SMM, Sivasamboo R: Termination of second trimester pregnancy with intraamniotic 15(S)-15-methyl prostaglandin $F_{2\ 3\alpha}$—a 2-dose schedule study, *Prostaglandins* 9:487-494, 1975.
133. Kasdorf G, Kalkhoff RK: Prospective studies of insulin sensitivity in normal women receiving oral contraceptive agents, *J Clin Endocrinol Metab* 66:846-852, 1988.
134. Katz Z et al: Teratogenicity of Progestogens given during the first trimester of pregnancy, *Obstet Gynecol* 65:775-780, 1985.
135. Kaufman DW et al: Decreased risk of endometrial cancer among oral contraceptive users, *Med Intellig* 303:1045-1047, 1980.
136. Kaunitz AM, Rosenfield A: Injectable contraception with depot medroxyprogesterone acetate, *Drugs* 45:857, 1993.
137. Kay CR: Progestogens and arterial disease—evidence from the Royal College of General Practitioner's Study, *Am J Obstet Gynecol* 142:762-766, 1982.
138. Kelaghan J et al: Barrier method contraceptives and pelvic inflammatory disease, *JAMA* 248:184-187, 1982.
139. Kelly RW, Abel MH: Copper and zinc inhibit the metabolism of prostaglandin by the human uterus, *Biol Reprod* 28:883-889, 1983.
140. Kesseru E et al: The hormonal and peripheral effects of d-norgestrel in postcoital contraception, *Contraception* 10:411-424, 1974.
141a. Koch JP: The Prentiff contraceptive cervical cap: a contemporary study of its clinical safety and effectiveness, *Contraception* 25:135-159, 1982.
141b. Koetsawang
142. Kubba AA et al: The biochemistry of human endometrium after two regimens of postcoital contraception: a dl-norgestrel/ethinylestradiol combination or danazol, *Fertil Steril* 45:512-516, 1986.
143. Lahteenmaki P et al: Late postcoital treatment against pregnancy with antiprogesterone RU486, *Fertil Steril* 50:36-38, 1988.
144. Lammer EJ, Cordero JF: Exogenous sex hormone exposure and the risk for major malformations, *JAMA* 255:3128-3132, 1986.
145. Lawson JS et al: Optimum dosage of an oral contraceptive. *Am J Obstet Gynecol* 134:315-320, 1979.
146. Leads from the MMWR (Centers for Disease Control, Atlanta): Oral contraceptive use and the risk of breast cancer in young women, *JAMA* 252:326-327, 1984.
147. Leads from the MMWR (Centers for Disease Control, Atlanta): Abortion surveillance: preliminary analysis—United States, 1984, 1985, *JAMA* 260:3410-3412, 1988.
148. Lee NC, Rubin GL, Borucki R: The intrauterine device and pelvic inflammatory disease revisited: new results from the Women's Health Study, *Obstet Gynecol* 72:1-6, 1988.
149. Levin AA et al: Association of induced abortion with subsequent pregnancy loss, *JAMA* 243:2495-2499, 1980.
150. Lewis JH, Tice HL, Zimmerman HJ: Budd-Chiari syndrome associated with oral contraceptive steroids, *Dig Dis Sci* 28:673-683, 1983.
151. Liddegard, 1993.
152. Lincoln R: The pill, breast, and cervical cancer, and the role of progestogens in arterial disease, *Fam Plann Perspect* 16:55-63, 1984.
153. Linn S et al: Lack of association between contraceptive usage and congenital malformation in offspring, *Am J Obstet Gynecol* 147:923-928, 1983.
154. Linn S et al: The relationship between induced abortion and outcome of subsequent pregnancies, *Am J Obstet Gynecol* 146:135-140, 1983.
155. Linos A et al: Case-control study of rheumatoid arthritis and prior use of oral contraceptives, *Lancet* 1:1299-1300, 1983.
156. Lipnick RJ et al: Oral contraceptives and breast cancer, *JAMA* 255:58-61, 1986.
157. Lippes J, Malik T, Tatum HJ: *The postcoital Copper T.* Paper presented at the Thirteenth Annual Meeting of the Association of Planned Parenthood Physicians, Los Angeles, April 17 1975.
158. Liskin, LS: IUDs: an appropriate contraceptive for many women, *Popul Rep X* (B4):101-135, 1982.
159. Liskin LS: Long-acting progestins—promise and prospects, injectables and implants, *Popul Rep K* 11:17-55, 1983.
160. Liskin LS: Vasectomy—safe and simple, *Popul Rep D* 11:61-100, 1983.
161. Liskin LS, Blackburn R: Hormonal contraception: new long-acting methods, injectables, and implants, *Popul Rep X* V:K57-K87, 1987.
162. Liskin LS, Rinehart W: Minilaparotomy and laparoscopy: safe, effective, and widely used, *Popul Rep C* 8:125-167, 1985.
163. Litvak O et al: Fetal erythrocytes in maternal circulation after spontaneous abortion, *JAMA* 214:531-534, 1970.
164. Longman SM, Buehring GC: Oral contraceptives and breast cancer: in vitro: effect of contraceptive steroids on human mammary cell growth, *Cancer* 59:281-287, 1987.
165. Louik C et al: Maternal exposure to spermicides in relation to certain birth defects, *N Engl J Med* 317:474-478, 1987.
166. Louv WC et al: Oral contraceptive use and the risk of chlamydial and gonococcal infections, *Am J Obstet Gynecol* 160:396-402, 1989.
167. Mall-Haefeli M et al: Klinische und biochemische Resultate bei de Behandlung mit Marvelon-einem neuen steroidalen Ovulationishemmer, *Geburtshilfe Frauenheilkd* 42:215-222, 1982.
168. Mammen EF: Oral contraceptives and blood coagulation: a critical review, *Am J Obstet Gynecol* 142:781-790, 1982.

169. Mann JI, Inman WGW: Oral contraceptives and death from myocardial infarction, *Br Med J* 2:245-248, 1975.
170. Margulies M, Perez GC, Voto LS: Misoprostol to induce labour, *Lancet* 339:64, 1992.
171. Massey FJ et al: Vasectomy and health: results from a large cohort study, *JAMA* 252:1023-1029, 1984.
172. Matlin SA et al: Male antifertility compounds from Tripterygium wilfordii Hook f, *Contraception* 47:387-400, 1993.
173. Mattson RH et al: Use of oral contraceptives by women with epilepsy, *JAMA* 256:238-240, 1986.
174. McCann MR et al: Breast-feeding, fertility, and family planning, *Popul Rep J* 24:525-575, 1981.
175. McPherson K et al: Breast cancer and oestrogen content of oral contraceptives, *Lancet* 1:223, 1984.
176. McPherson K et al: Early oral contraceptive use and breast cancer: results of another case-control study, *Br J Cancer* 56:653-660, 1987.
177. Meade TW, Greenberg G, Thompson SG: Progestogens and cardiovascular reactions associated with oral contraceptives and a comparison of the safety of 50 and 30 mcg oestrogen preparations, *Br Med J* 1:1157-1161, 1980.
178. Meirik O et al: Oral contraceptive use and breast cancer in young women: a joint national case-control study in Sweden and Norway, *Lancet* 2:650-653, 1986.
179. Mishell DR Jr: Contraception by intrauterine device. In Bardin CW, editor: *Current Therapy Endocrinology Metabolism-3*, Toronto, 1988, BC Decker.
180. Mishell DR Jr: Use of oral contraceptives in women of older reproductive age, *Am J Obstet Gynecol* 158:1652-1657, 1988.
181. Mishell DR Jr et al: The intrauterine device: a bacteriologic study of the endometrial cavity, *Am J Obstet Gynecol* 96:119-126, 1966.
182. Mishell DR Jr et al: Estogenic activity in women receiving an injectable progestogen for contraception, *Am J Obstet Gynecol* 113:372, 1972.
183. Mishell DR Jr et al: The effect of contraceptive steroids on hypothalamic pituitary function, *Am J Obstet Gynecol* 128:60, 1977.
184. Monk JP, Clissold SP: Misoprostol, a preliminary review of its pharmacodynamic and pharmacokinetic properties and therapeutic efficacy in the treatment of peptic ulcer disease, *Drugs* 33:1-30, 1987.
185. Moore KL: The developing human: clinically oriented embryology. In *The fetal period: the eighth week to birth*, Philadelphia, 1973, WB Saunders.
186. Morris JM, van Wagenen G: Compounds interfering with ovum implantation and development. III. The role of estrogens, *Am J Obstet Gynecol* 96:804-815 1966.
187. Morris JM, van Wagenen G: Postcoital oral contraception. In Hankinson RKB et al, editors: *Proceedings of the Eighth International Conference,* Santiago, London, 1967, International Planned Parenthood Federation.
188. Morris JM, van Wagenen G: Interception: the use of postovulatory estrogens to prevent implantation, *Am J Obstet Gynecol* 115:101-106, 1973.
189. Nadelson CC et al: A follow-up study of rape victims, *Am J Psychiatry* 139:1266-1270, 1982.
190. Neil JR et al: Late complications of sterilization by laparoscopy and tubal ligation: a controlled study, *Lancet* 2:669-671, 1975.
191. Newton BW: Laminaria tent: relic of the past or modern medical device? *Am J Obstet Gynecol* 113:442-448, 1972.
192. Newton JR, editor: Contraception update, *Clin Obstet Gynecol* 11:551-819, 1984.
193. Nilsson CG et al: Intrauterine contraception with levonorgestrel: a comparative randomized clinical performance study, *Lancet* 1:577-580, 1981.
194. Noonan JT Jr: *Contraception, a history of its treatment by the Catholic theologians and canonists*, 1986, Harvard University Press.
195. Orme ML, Back DS, Breckenridge AM: Clinical pharmacokinetics of oral contraceptive steroids, *Clin Pharm* 8:95-136, 1983.
196. Ortiz A et al: Serum medroxyprogesterone acetate concentrations and ovarian function following intramuscular injection of depot-MPA, *J Clin Endocrinol Metab* 43:32-38, 1977.
197. Ory HW: Mortality associated with fertility and fertility control, *Fam Plann Perspect* 15:57-63, 1983.
198. Ory SJ: Nonsurgical treatment of ectopic pregnancy (Editor's Corner), *Fertil Steril* 46:767-769, 1986.
199. Osathanondh R: Laminaria and misoprostol: safe, simple, and inexpensive method for elective midtrimester pregnancy termination, 1994. (prepublication data)
200. Osathanondh R et al: Elective termination of cervical ectopic pregnancies using ultrasound-guided potassium chloride injection, 1994. (in preparation)
201. Osathanondh R et al: Induction of labor with anencephalic fetus, *Obstet Gynecol* 56:655-657, 1980.
202. Osathanondh R et al: *Prostaglandins for cervical softening and dilatation: recent experience with prostaglandins as dilators*. Program of the Ninth Annual Meeting of National Abortion Federation (Advances in Cervical Dilatation), Boston, June 1985.
203. Osathanondh R et al: Coagulopathy associated with midtrimester D&E, *Adv Plann Parent* 16:30-33, 1981.
204. Osathanondh V: Suprapubic minilaparotomy, uterine elevation technique: simple, inexpensive, and outpatient procedure for interval female sterilization, *Contraception* 10:251-262, 1974.
205. Osborne MP et al.: The relationship between family history, exposure to exogenous hormones, and estrogen receptor protein in breast cancer, *Cancer* 51:2134-2138, 1983.
206. Ostensen M, Husby G: Pregnancy-associated 3α-glycoprotein, oral contraceptives, and rheumatoid arthritis, *Lancet* 1:1391, 1983.
207. Oyer R et al: Treatment of cervical pregnancy with methotrexate, *Obstet Gynecol* 71:469-471, 1988.
208. Park T-K et al: Preventing febrile complications of suction curettage abortion, *Am J Obstet Gynecol* 152:252-255, 1985.
209. Pastides H et al: Oral contraceptive use and fibrocystic breast disease with special reference to its histopathology, *J Nat Cancer Inst* 71:5-9, 1983.
210. Patterson SP, White JH, Reaves EM: A maternal death associated with prostaglandin E_2, *Obstet Gynecol* 54:123-124, 1979.
211. Paul C et al: Oral contraceptives and breast cancer: a national study, *Br Med J* 293:723-726, 1986.
212. Peterson HB et al: Deaths attributable to tubal sterilization in the United States, *Am J Obstet Gynecol* 146:131-136, 1983.
213. Peterson RN, Freund M: Effects of (H^+), (Na^+), (K^+) and certain membrane-active drugs on glycolysis, motility, and ATP synthesis by human spermatozoa, *Biol Reprod* 8:350-357, 1973.
214. Petitti DB, Klatsky AL: Malignant hypertension in women aged 15-44 years and its relation to cigarette smoking and oral contraceptives, *Am J Cardiol* 52:297-298, 1983.
215. Petitti DB et al: Risk of vascular disease in women: smoking, oral contraceptives, noncontraceptive estrogens, and other factors, *JAMA* 242:1150-1154, 1979.
216. Pike MC et al: Breast cancer and oral contraceptives: reply to critics, *Lancet* 2:1414, 1983.
217. Pike MC et al: Breast cancer in young women and use of oral contraceptives: possible modifying effect of formulation and age at use, *Lancet* 2:926-930, 1983.
218. Pike MC et al: Oral contraceptives and breast cancer rates, *Lancet* 1:389, 1984.
219. Piot P et al: AIDS: an international perspective, *Science* 239:573-579, 1988.
220. Pituitary Adenoma Study Group: Pituitary adenomas and oral contraceptives: a multicenter case-control study, *Fertil Steril* 39:753-760, 1983.

221. Pizarro E, Gomez-Rogers C, Rowe PJ: A comparative study of the effect of the Progestasert and Gravigard IUDs on dysmenorrhea, *Contraception* 20:455-466, 1979.
222. Porter JB et al: Oral contraceptives and nonfatal vascular disease, *Obstet Gynecol* 66:1-8, 1985.
223. Porter JB, Jick H: Malignant liver tumor associated with oral contraceptive use, *Pharmacotherapy* 1:160, 1981.
224. Potts M, Diggory P: *Textbook of contraceptive practice*, ed 2, London, 1983, Cambridge University Press.
225. Rabe T et al: Effect of the PGE_1 methyl analog misoprostol on the pregnant uterus in the first trimester, *Geburtshilfe Frauenheilkd* 47:324-331, 1987.
226. Rakhshani R, Grimes DA: Prostaglandin E_2 suppositories as a second-trimester abortifacient, *J Reprod Med* 33:817-820, 1988.
227. Ramahi A, Richardson DA: *Urodynamic changes in women using diaphragms*. Program of the 36th Annual Clinical Meeting of the American College of Obstetricians and Gynecologists, Boston, May 1988.
228. Ramcharan S et al: The Walnut Creek Contraceptive Drug Study: a prospective study of the side effects of oral contraceptives, *J Reprod Med 2* (Suppl 6):345-372, 1980.
229. Ravenholt RT, Kessell E, Speidel JJ: Comparison of the side effects of three oral contraceptives: a double-blind cross-over study of Ovral, Norinyl, and Norlestrin, *Adv Plann Parent* 12:222-239, 1987.
230. Rekers H: Multicenter trial of a monophasic oral contraceptive containing ethinyl estradiol and desogestrel, *Acta Obstet Gynecol Seral* 67:171-174, 1988.
231. Rice-Wray E et al: Return of ovulation after discontinuance of oral contraceptives, *Fertil Steril* 18:212-218, 1967.
232. Rock J, Pincus G, Garcia CR: Effects of certain 19-norsteroids on the normal human menstrual cycle, *Science* 124:891-893, 1956.
233. Rojanasakul A et al: Effects of combined desogestrel-ethinylestradiol treatment on lipid profiles in women with polycystic ovarian disease, *Fertil Steril* 48:581-585, 1987.
234. Romaguero C, Grimalt F: Contact dermatitis from a copper-containing intrauterine contraceptive device, *Contact Dermatitis* 73:163-164, 1981.
235. Rosenberg L et al: Breast cancer and oral contraceptive use, *Am J Epidemiol* 119:167-176, 1984.
236. Rosenberg L et al: Epithelial ovarian cancer and combination oral contraceptives, *JAMA* 247:3210-3212, 1982.
237. Rosenberg MJ et al: Effect of the contraceptive sponge on chlamydial infection, gonorrhea, and candidiasis, *JAMA* 257:2308-2312, 1987.
238. Rosenfield AG: Injectable long-acting progestogen contraception: a neglected modality, *Am J Obstet Gynecol* 120:537-548, 1974.
239. Rowlands S: Morning-after pills, *Br Med J* 285:322-323, 1982.
240. Roy S, Mishell DR: Current status of research and development of vaginal contraceptive rings as a fertility control method in the female, *Res Frontiers Fertil Regulation* 2:1-10, 1983.
241. Royal College of General Practitioners' Oral Contraception Study: Further analysis of mortality in oral contraceptive users, *Lancet* 1:541-546, 1981.
242. Royal College of General Practitioners' Oral Contraception Study: Oral contraceptives and gall bladder disease, *Lancet* 2:957-959, 1982.
243. Royal College of General Practitioners' Oral Contraception Study: Incidence of arterial disease among oral contraceptive users, *Policy Statement R Coll Gen Pract* 33:75-82, 1983.
244. Rubin GL et al: Fatal ectopic pregnancy after attempted legally induced abortion, *JAMA* 244:1705-1708, 1980.
245. Rubin GL, Ory HW, Layde PM: Oral contraceptives and pelvic inflammatory disease, *Am J Obstet Gynecol* 144:630-635, 1982.
246. Salhanick HA: Basic studies on aminoglutethimide, *Cancer Res* 42(Suppl) :3315s-3321s, 1982.
247. Samsioe G: Comparative effects of the oral contraceptive combinations 0.150 mg desogestrel + 0.030 mg ethinylestradiol and 0.150 mg levonorgestrel + 0.030 mg ethinylestradiol on lipid and lipoprotein metabolism in healthy female volunteers, *Contraception* 25:487-504, 1982.
248. Sands RX, Burnhill MS, Hakim-Elahi E: Postabortal uterine atony, *Obstet Gynecol* 43:595-598, 1974.
249. Schaison G: *RU486: antiprogestin and antiglucocorticoid*. Program of the 70th Annual Meeting of the Endocrine Society (New Concept I), New Orleans, June 1988.
250. Schaison G et al: Effects of the antiprogesterone steroid RU486 during midluteal phase in normal women, *J Clin Endocrin Metab* 61:484-489, 1985.
251. Schiff I, Naftolin F: Small bowel incarceration after uncomplicated laparoscopy, *Obstet Gynecol* 43:674-675, 1974.
252. Schlesselman JJ et al: Breast cancer risk in relation to type of estrogen contained in oral contraceptives, *Contraception* 36:595-613, 1987.
253a. Schlesselman JJ et al: Breast cancer in relation to early use of oral contraceptives: no evidence of a latent effect, *JAMA* 259:1828-1833, 1988.
253b. Schonhofer, 1991.
254. Schulz KF, Grimes DA, Cates W Jr: Measures to prevent cervical injury during suction curettage abortion, *Lancet* 1:1182-1184, 1983.
255. Scott LD, Katz AR, Duke JH: Oral contraceptives, pregnancy, and focal nodular hyperplasia of the liver, *JAMA* 251:1461-1463, 1984.
256. Secreto G et al: Increased urinary androgen levels in patients with carcinoma in situ of the breast with onset while taking oral contraceptives, *Cancer Detect Prev* 6:439-442, 1983.
257. Segal SJ et al: Absence of chorionic gonadotropin in sera of women who use intrauterine devices, *Fertil Steril* 44:214-218, 1985.
258. Seligsohn U et al: Factor VII in plasma of women taking oral contraceptives, *Transfusion* 24:171-172, 1984.
259. Settlage DS, Motoshima M, Tredway DR: Sperm transport from the external cervical os to the fallopian tubes in women: a time and quantitation study, *Fertil Steril* 24:655-661, 1973.
260. Shapiro AG et al: Intravaginal administration of 9-deoxo-9-methylene-16,16-dimethyl PGE_2 for cervical dilation prior to suction curettage, *Int J Gynaecol Obstet* 20:137-140, 1982.
261. Shar SR, Kew MC: Oral contraceptives and hepatocellular carcinoma, *Cancer* 49:407-410, 1982.
262. Sharpe RM et al: Absence of hCG-like activity in the blood of women fitted with intrauterine contraceptive devices, *J Clin Endocrinol Metab* 45:496-499, 1977.
263. Shearman RP: Postcoital contraception: a review, *Contraception* 7:459-476, 1973.
264. Shoupe D, Mishell DR: Norplant: subdermal implant system for long-term contraception, *Am J Obstet Gynecol* 160:1286-1292, 1989.
265. Shy KK et al: Oral contraceptive use and occurrence of pituitary prolactinoma, *JAMA* 249:2204-2207, 1983.
266. Siegberg R et al: Sex hormone profiles in oligomenorrheic adolescent girls and the effect of oral contraceptives, *Fertil Steril* 41:888-893, 1984.
267. Silva DA et al: Acute hypertensive response to prostaglandin $F_{2\ 3\alpha}$ during anesthesia administration, *J Reprod Med* 32:700-702, 1987.
268. Sivin I: International experience with Norplant and Norplant-2 contraceptives, *Stud Fam Plann* 19:81, 1988.
269. Sivin I, Tatum HJ: Four years of experience with the TCU 380A intrauterine contraceptive device, *Fertil Steril* 36:159-163, 1981.
270. Smythe AR II, Underwood PB Jr: Ectopic pregnancy after postcoital diethylstilbestrol, *Am J Obstet Gynecol* 121:284, 1975.
271. Sonne-Holmes S et al: Prophylactic antibiotics in first-trimester abortion: a clinical controlled trial, *Am J Obstet Gynecol* 139:693-696, 1981.
272. Spence MR et al: Cephalothin prophylaxis for midtrimester abortion, *Obstet Gynecol* 60:502-505, 1982.

273. Stadel BV: Oral contraceptives and cardiovascular disease, *N Engl J Med* 305:612-618, 672-677, 1981.
274. Stadel BV et al: Oral contraceptives and breast cancer in young women, *Lancet* 2:970-974, 1985.
275. Stampfer MJ et al: A prospective study of past use of oral contraceptive agents and risk of cardiovascular diseases, *N Engl J Med* 319:1313-1317, 1988.
276. Stevens RG, Lee JAH, Moolgavkar SH: No association between oral contraceptives and malignant melanomas, *N Engl J Med* 302:966, 1980.
277. Stockley IH: Methotrexate-NSAID interactions, *Drug Intelligence Clin Pharm* 21:546, 1987.
278. Stubblefield PG, Fuller AF, Foster SC: Ultrasound-guided intrauterine removal of intrauterine contraceptive devices in pregnancy, *Obstet Gynecol* 72:961-964, 1988.
279. Stubblefield PG et al: Fertility after induced abortion: a prospective follow-up study, *Obstet Gynecol* 63:186-193, 1984.
280. Sturgis SH, Albright F: The mechanism of estrin therapy in the relief of dysmenorrhea, *Endocrinology* 26:68-72, 1940.
281. Sturtevant FM: Breast cancer and oral contraceptives, *Lancet* 2:1145, 1983.
282. Swann SH, Petitti DB: A review of problems of bias and confounding in epidemiologic studies of cervical neoplasia and oral contraceptive use, *Am J Epidemiol* 115:10-18, 1982.
283. Swyer GIM: Progestogen "potency" and breast cancer, *Lancet* 2:1416, 1983.
284. Szoka PR, Edgren RA: Drug interactions with oral contraceptives: compilation and analysis of an adverse experience report database, *Fertil Steril* 49(Suppl):31S-38S, 1988.
285. Tatum HJ, Connell-Tatum EB: Barrier contraception: a comprehensive overview, *Fertil Steril* 36:1-12, 1981.
286. Thayssen P, Secher NJ, Arnsbo P: Systolic time intervals and hemodynamic changes during intravenous infusion of prostaglandins $F_{2\,3\alpha}$ and E_2, *Br Heart J* 45:447-456, 1981.
287. Thiersch JB: Therapeutic abortions with a folic acid antagonist 4-aminopteroylglutamic acid administered by the oral route, *Am J Obstet Gynecol* 63:1298-1304, 1952.
288. Thomas DB: Do hormones cause breast cancer? *Cancer* 53:595-604, 1984.
289. Tietze C: New estimates of mortality associated with fertility control, *Fam Plann Perspect* 9:74-76, 1977.
290. Tietze C, Lewit S: Life risks associated with reversible methods of fertility regulation, *Int J Gynaecol Obstet* 16:456-459, 1979.
291. Toppozada M: The clinical use of monthly injectable contraceptive preparations, *Obstet Gynecol Surv* 32:335-347, 1977.
292. Toth M et al: The role of infection in the etiology of preterm birth, *Obstet Gynecol* 71:723-726, 1988.
293. Trapido EJ: A prospective cohort study of oral contraceptives and cancer of the endometrium, *Int J Epidemiol* 12:297-300, 1983.
294. Umapathysivam K, Jones WR: Effects of contraceptive agents on the biochemical and protein composition of human endometrium, *Contraception* 22:425-440, 1980.
295. Umpierre SA, Hill JA, Anderson DJ: Effect of "Coke" on sperm motility, *N Engl J Med* 313:1351, 1985.
296. The U.S. Health and Human Services: Oral contraceptives and cancer, *FDA Drug Bulletin* 14:2-3, 1984.
297. Valenzuela G et al: Uterine rupture at term with vaginal prostaglandin E_2, *Am J Obstet Gynecol* 138:1223-1224, 1980.
298. Valicenti JF et al: Detection and prevalence of IUD-associated actinomyces colonization and related morbidity, *JAMA* 247:1149-1152, 1982.
299. Vandenbroucke JP: Oral contraceptives and rheumatoid arthritis, *Lancet* 2:228-229, 1983.
300. Vandenbroucke JP et al: Oral contraceptives and rheumatoid arthritis: further evidence for a preventive effect, *Lancet* 2:839-842, 1982.
301. Vandenbrouke JP et al: Noncontraceptive hormones and rheumatoid arthritis in perimenopausal and postmenopausal women, *JAMA* 255:1299-1303, 1986.
302. van der Spuy ZM et al: Inhibition of 3β-hydroxysteroid dehydrogenase activity in first trimester human pregnancy with trilostane and WIN 32729, *Clin Endocrinol* 19:521-531, 1983.
303. Vergote I et al: Uterine rupture due to 15-methylprostaglandin $F_{2\,3\alpha}$, *Lancet* 2:1402, 1982.
304. Vessey MP: Exogenous hormones in the aetiology of cancer in women, *J R Soc Med* 77:542-549, 1984.
305. Vessey M et al: Oral contraceptives and breast cancer: final report of an epidemiological study, *Br J Cancer* 47:455-462, 1983.
306. Vessey M, Lawless M, Yeates D: Efficacy of different contraceptive methods, *Lancet* 1:841-843, 1982.
307. Vessey MP, Lawless M: The Oxford Family Planning Association Contraceptive Study, *Clinic Obstet Gynecol* 11:743-757, 1984.
308. Vessey ME, McPherson K, Johnson B: Mortality among women participating in the Oxford Family Planning Association Contraceptive Study, *Lancet* 2:731-733, 1977.
309. Vessey M et al: Neoplasia of the cervix uteri and contraception: a possible adverse effect of the pill, *Lancet* 2:930-934, 1983.
310. von Kaulla E et al: Antithrombin III depression and thrombin generation acceleration in women taking oral contraceptives, *Am J Obstet Gynecol* 109:868-873, 1971.
311. Warburton D et al: Lack of association between spermicide use and trisomy, *N Engl J Med* 317:478-482, 1987.
312. Washington AE, Browner WS, Korenbrof CC: Cost effectiveness of combined treatment for endocervical gonorrhea, *JAMA* 257:2056-2060, 1987.
313. Washington AE et al: Oral contraceptives, *Chlamydia trachomatis* infection, and pelvic inflammatory disease, *JAMA* 253:2246-2250, 1985.
314. Weiss NS, Sayvetz TA: Incidence of endometrial cancer in relation to the use of oral contraceptives, *N Engl J Med* 302:551-554.
315. Wessler S et al: Estrogen-containing oral contraceptive agents: a basis for their thrombogenicity, *JAMA* 236:2179-2182, 1976.
316. Wheeless CR, Katayama KP: Laparoscopy and tubal sterilization. In Mattingly RF, Thompson JD, editors: *Telinde's operative gynecology*, ed 6, 1985, Lippincott.
317. White PF et al: Disseminated intravascular coagulation following midtrimester abortions, *Anesthesiology* 58:99-101, 1983.
318. Wilcox AJ et al: Urinary human chorionic gonadotropin among intrauterine device users: detection with a highly specific and sensitive assay, *Fertil Steril* 47:265-269, 1987.
319. Willett WC et al: Oral contraceptives and risk of ovarian cancer, *Cancer* 48:1684-1687, 1981.
320. World Health Organization: Collaborative study of neoplasia and steroid contraceptives: invasive cervical cancer and combined oral contraceptives, *Br Med J* 290:961-965, 1985.
321. World Health Organization: Mechanism of action, safety, and efficacy of intrauterine devices, *WHO Tech Rep Ser* 753:791, 1987.
322. World Health Organization: Special Programme of Research, Development, and Research Training in Human Reproduction and Special Programme on AIDS: *Report of a meeting on contraceptive methods and HIV infections*, Geneva, 1987.
323. World Health Organization: Collaborative study of neoplasia and steroid contraceptives: breast cancer and depot medroxyprogesterone acetate: a multinational study, *Lancet* 338:833, 1991a.
324. World Health Organization: Collaborative study of neoplasia and steroid contraceptives: depot medroxyprogesterone acetate (DMPA) and risk of endometrial cancer, *Int J Cancer* 49:186, 1991b.
325. World Health Organization: Task Force on Long-Acting Systemic Agents for Fertility Regulation: Special Programme of Research, Development and Research Training in Human Reproduction: a multicentre comparative study of serum lipids and apolipoproteins in long-term users of DMPA and a control group of IUD users, *Contraception* 47:177, 1993.

326. Wu YT: Suction in artificial abortion: 300 cases (Chinese), *Chung-Hua Fa Chan Ko Tsa Chih* 6:447-449, 1958.
327. WU D-F et al: Pharmacokinetics of (±)-, (+)-, and (-)- gossypol in humans and dogs, *Clin Pharmacol Ther* 39:613-618, 1986.
328. Ye BL, Yamamoto K, Tyson JE: Functional and biochemical aspects of laminaria use in first-trimester pregnancy termination, *Am J Obstet Gynecol* 142:36-39, 1982.
329. Young RL et al: A randomized, double-blind, placebo-controlled comparison of the impact of low-dose and triphasic oral contraceptives on follicular development, *Am J Obstet Gynecol* 167:678, 1992.
330. Yuzpe AA, Smith RP, Rademaker AW: A multicenter clinical investigation employing ethinyl estradiol combined with dl-norgestrel as a postcoital contraceptive agent, *Fertil Steril* 37:508-513, 1982.
331. Yuzpe AA et al: Postcoital contraception—a pilot study, *J Reprod Med* 13:53-58, 1974.
332. Zipper JA et al: Metallic copper as an intrauterine contraceptive adjunct to the "T" device, *Am J Obstet Gynecol*, 105:1274-1278, 1969.
333. Zipper J et al: Propranolol as a novel, effective spermicide: preliminary findings, *Br Med J* 287:1245-1246, 1983.

Chapter 23

PEDIATRIC AND ADOLESCENT GYNECOLOGY

Marc R. Laufer
Donald P. Goldstein

Gynecologic treatment of the prepubertal and adolescent patient differs in many respects from the care of the adult woman. Unique problems are encountered in this population, especially in infants and young children, which are usually not seen by the practicing obstetrician-gynecologist. For this reason, it is appropriate that a chapter devoted to the gynecologic problems of this age group be included in a textbook of this scope. Fortunately, the evaluation and treatment of the most common conditions which affect these young patients requires only a minimum of additional knowledge, equipment, and technical skill beyond the capabilities and resources of most gynecologists.

The gynecologic problems encountered in older adolescents are quite similar to those seen in adults. The distinction between these two groups is in the degree of emotional immaturity characteristic of these individuals. The psychologic impact of the first gynecologic examination should not be underestimated. The outcome of this experience may have a profound influence on the care that the patient seeks later.

Providing gynecologic treatment to adolescents undoubtedly is time-consuming and the physician with a busy practice may elect to avoid this population. Adolescents need to be seen by a sensitive person who has time to listen to their needs, give satisfactory explanations, and answer questions in a way that is appropriate to their level of comprehension. These factors are essential to winning their confidence, and more importantly, to improving their compliance.

In this area of gynecologic practice the attitude of the physician is also an important consideration. Children and adolescents are very sensitive to adults' attitudes toward them. The gynecologist must, therefore, feel comfortable in communicating with these patients and their parents and should overcome any reticence about performing an adequate pelvic examination on young children and virginal adolescents. Maintaining a nonjudgmental attitude toward the patient's emerging sexuality is also of utmost importance.

In this chapter, the most commonly encountered gynecologic problems in the pediatric and adolescent age group are discussed. For the most part, those conditions shared with the adult patient are discussed more comprehensively in other chapters. The material is organized according to developmental stages (i.e., prepubertal, pubertal, and post pubertal). The clinical signs and symptoms and management may differ depending on the age group.

OFFICE EVALUATION OF THE CHILD AND ADOLESCENT

Office evaluation of the child

Traditionally, avoidance of the female external genitalia has sometimes prevented parents and physicians from dealing with the total health care of the young girl. Although gynecologic problems are not common among young girls, the physician should always include an inspection of the external genitalia and palpation of the breast as part of the routine physical examination. If the child accepts a brief look at her genitalia as part of the normal physical examination, she is less likely to feel embarrassed or upset by the same examination when she reaches adolescence. In addition, the physician may note smegma or feces in the labial folds, indicating inadequate perineal hygiene. Vaginal discharge or bleeding, pruritis, signs of sexual development, or an allegation of sexual abuse should prompt a more thorough evaluation.

Careful instruction to the parents and child during the examination may prevent the later occurrence of a nonspecific vulvovaginitis. The presence of a cyst, clitoromegaly, early signs of puberty, candida vulvitis, or an abnormality of the hymen may indicate other problems. Errors in diagnosis often result from the lack of a simple inspection.

Healthy dialogue between parents and children on issues of sexuality should begin during the prepubertal years. Parents should be encouraged to answer their young children's questions with simple facts and correct terminology. Physicians should be knowledgeable about the books available at the local library and select appropriate pamphlets for the office.

Obtaining the history. The nature of the history depends on the presenting complaint. If the problem is vaginitis, questions should focus on perineal hygiene, antibiotic therapy, recent infections in the patient or other members of the family, and the possibility of sexual molestation. Behavioral changes and somatic symptoms such as abdominal pain, headaches, and enuresis may suggest abuse. Information on the caretaker should always be elicited. If the problem is vaginal bleeding, the history should include recent growth and development, signs of puberty, use of hormonal creams or tablets (including maternal exposure), trauma, and foreign bodies previously found in the vagina. Although the history is usually obtained chiefly from a parent, the child should be asked questions not only about genital complaints but also about toys or school to put her at ease. Eye contact should be maintained with the child, and it should be stressed that she is an important part of the team. Questions focusing on what has bothered the child (such as itching or discharge) can help the child understand why the examination is important. She should be given the opportunity to ask questions. This time promotes the understanding that the physician is acting in her best interests.

Gynecologic examination. The gynecologic examination should be explained carefully in advance to the parent and the child. It is extremely important to tell the parent that the size of the vaginal opening is quite variable and that the examination will in no way alter the hymen. Often a diagram showing the introitus is helpful because many parents still believe that the virginal introitus is totally covered by the hymen (Fig. 23-1).

Both parent and child should be told that instruments that are specially designed for little girls will be used. The otoscope or hand lens to be used for external examination

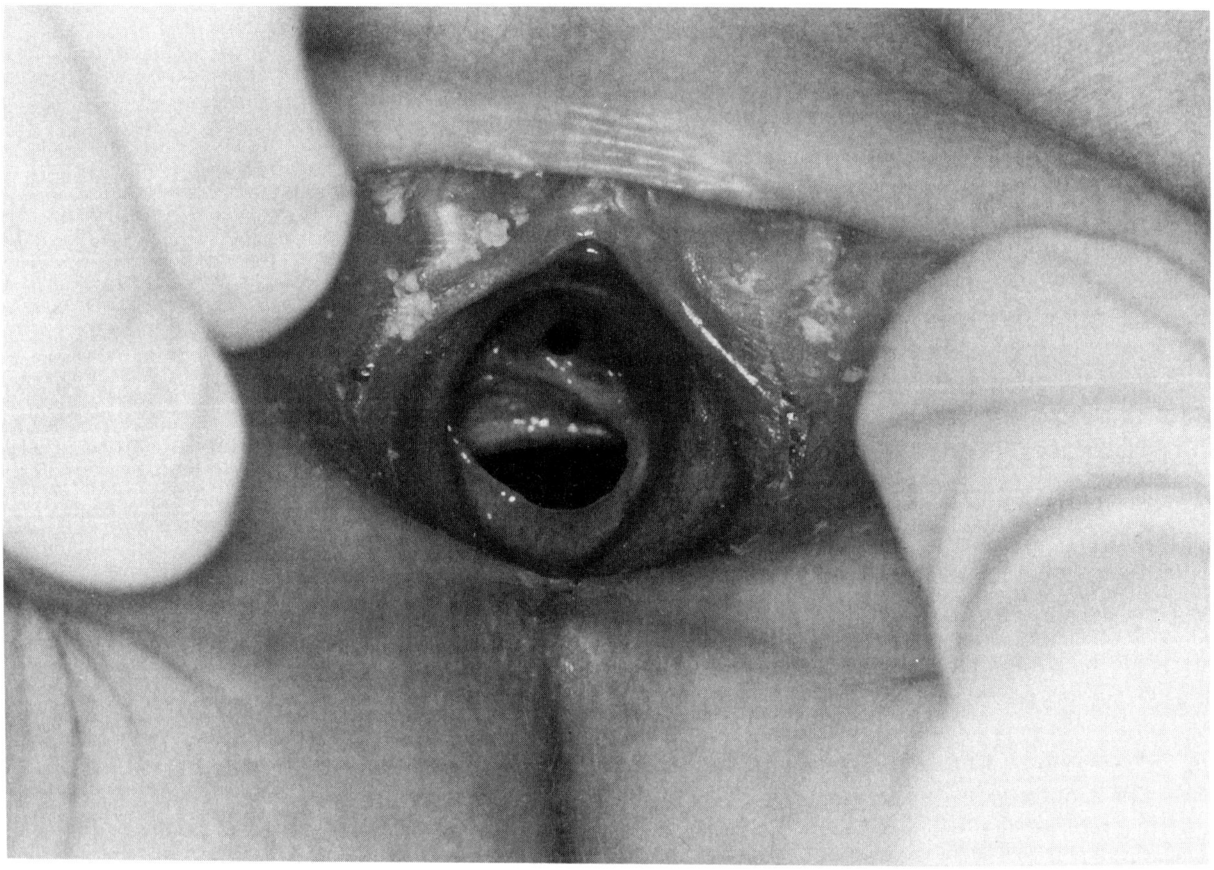

Fig. 23-1. External genitalia of the prepubertal child showing normal anatomy.

should be shown to the child with an emphasis that the physician will use these instruments "to look." If a colposcope will be used for a sexual abuse evaluation, the child should be given a chance to look at the instrument, turn the light on and off, and view fingers or jewelry through the binocular eyepieces to feel comfortable with the examination.

The child can then be offered the choice of whether she wishes to have her parent lift her onto the table or climb "up the big stairs." The parent typically stays in the room to talk with the young child and assist in the examination. Although the father, mother, both parents, or a relative may accompany the child for the assessment, it is the mother who most commonly plays an active role during the examination. The older child should be asked whom she prefers in or out of the room during the examination. Most children and many young adolescents prefer the mother in the room; almost all mid adolescents to late adolescents prefer the mother stay out of the examination room.

The majority of children are comfortable on the examining tables with the mother (or father) sitting close by or holding a hand. Some girls are quite fearful, especially if they have been sexually abused or had a painful genital examination previously. In this case, the mother (or the caretaker bringing the child) can sit on the table in the semireclined position with her feet in stirrups and have the child's legs straddle her thighs. The use of the hand mirror has been found helpful in allowing the child to relax and become an active participant in the examination. If the physician is confident and relaxed, the patient usually cooperates. An abrupt or hurried approach precipitates anxiety and resistance in the child. Sometimes it is necessary to leave the room and return when the patient feels ready.

The examination of a child with gynecologic complaints should include a general pediatric assessment of the child's weight and height, head and neck, heart, lungs, and abdomen. The abdominal examination is often easier if the child places her hand on the examiner's hand; she is less likely to tense her muscles or complain of being "tickled." The inguinal areas should be carefully palpated for a hernia or gonad; occasionally, an inguinal gonad is the testis of an undiagnosed male pseudohermaphrodite. The breasts should be carefully inspected and palpated. The increasing diameter of the areola or a unilateral tender breast bud is often the first sign of puberty.

The gynecologic examination of the child includes inspection of the external genitalia, visualization of the vagina and

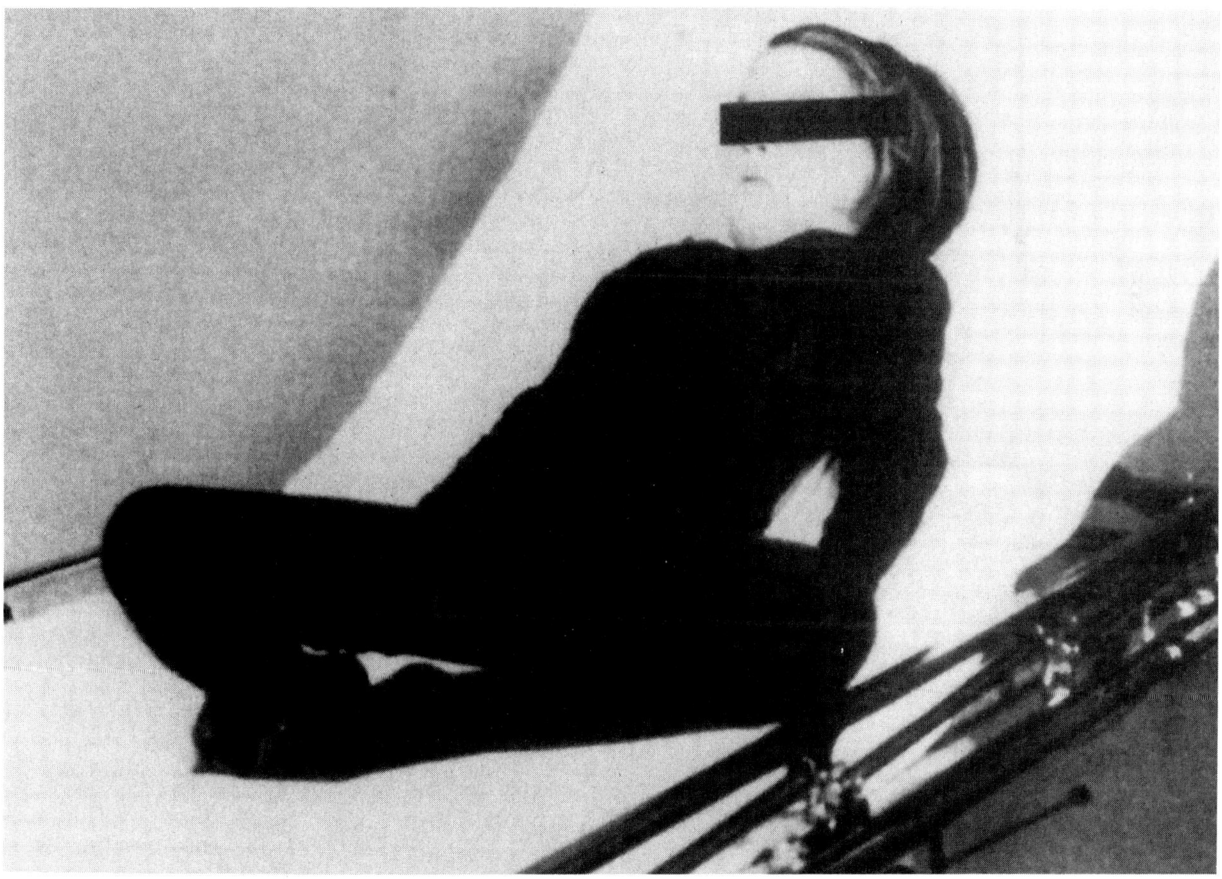

Fig. 23-2. Positioning of the prepubertal child in the frog-leg position (can be flat or with the head of the examining table raised.) (Courtesy Dr. Trina Anglin, Cleveland Ohio).

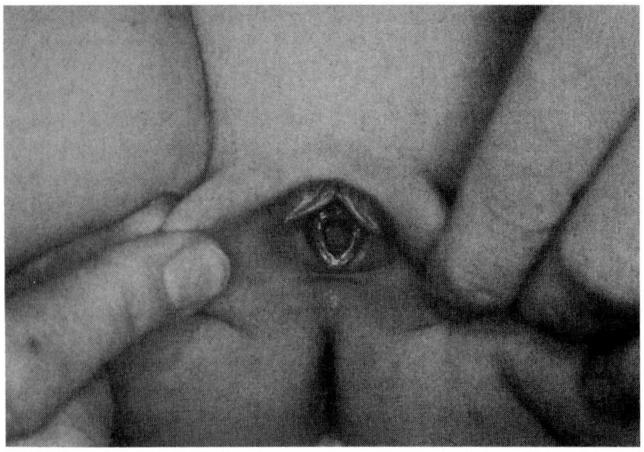

Fig. 23-3. Labial traction maneuver. Ideal for use in newborns and infants to visualize the introitus and lower vagina.

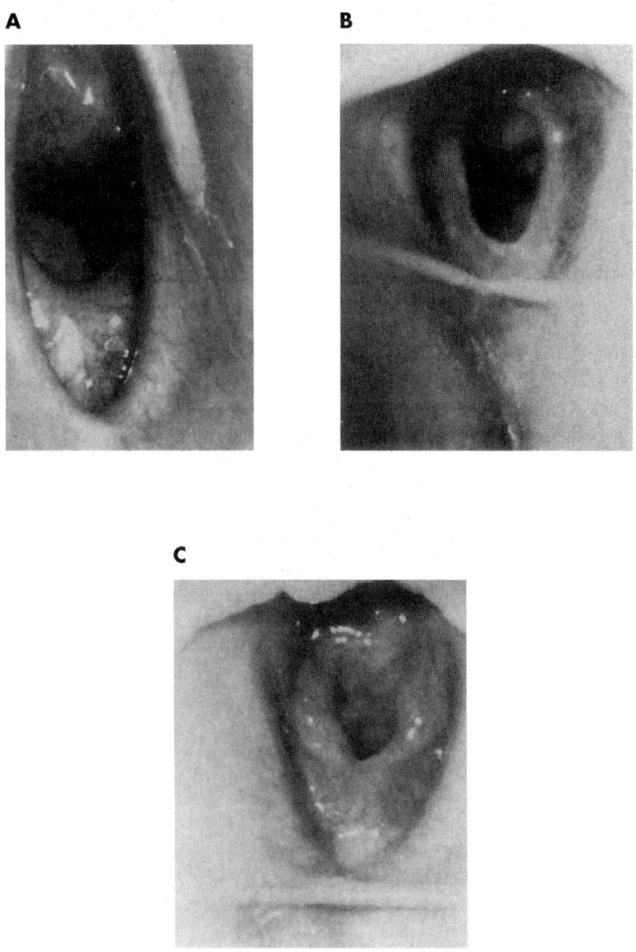

Fig. 23-4. Types of hymens in prepubertal girls. **A**, Posterior rim or crescent hymen. **B**, Circumferential or annular hymen. **C**, Fimbriated or redundant hymen.

cervix, and rectoabdominal palpation.[27] This examination is usually possible without anesthetic if the child has not been traumatized by previous examinations and if the physician proceeds slowly. The child should be told explicitly that "the exam will not hurt." The young child should be examined supine with her knees apart and feet touching in the frog-leg position (Fig. 23-2), or in the lithotomy position with the use of adjustable stirrups. As the external genitalia are inspected, the young child may be less anxious if she assists the physician by holding the labia apart. The physician should note the presence of pubic hair, size of the clitoris, type of hymen, signs of estrogenization of the vaginal introitus, and perineal hygiene. Friability of the posterior fourchette as the labia are separated can occur in children with vulvitis and/or a history of sexual abuse. If the hymenal orifice is still not visible, the labia can be gently gripped and pulled forward (traction maneuver) to view the anterior vagina (Fig. 23-3). A normal clitoral glans in the premenarchal child is on average 3 mm in length and 3 mm in transverse diameter. The vaginal mucosa of the prepubertal child appears thin and red in contrast to the moist, dull pink, estrogenized mucosa of the pubertal child. Frequently the perihymenal tissue is erythematous. The vaginal introitus often gapes open if the child takes a deep breath or coughs; if not, the labia should be pulled gently downward and laterally.[27]

The type of the hymen should be noted using a hand lens or the light and magnification of an otoscope (without a speculum). Hymens can be classified as posterior rim (or crescent), annular, or redundant (Fig. 23-4).[94] The edges of a redundant hymen and the orifice are often difficult to visualize. Congenital abnormalities of the hymen are not uncommon, especially microperforate and septate hymens. The presence of an opening in a microperforate hymen may be difficult to establish without probing with a nasopharyngeal Calgiswab (Spectrum Laboratories, 110 Rankin Rd., Houston, TX 77073) moistened with saline, or a small catheter. Congenital absence of the hymen has not been documented. Acquired abnormalities of the hymen usually result from sexual abuse, and rarely from accidental trauma.

Physicians performing annual physical examinations should visualize the genitalia and the hymen and make a drawing in the office notes of its type. (A change from previously noted anatomy may provide an important clue to ongoing sexual abuse.) The anus and labia should always be examined for cleanliness, excoriations, and erythema. Perianal excoriation often indicates the presence of pinworm infestation.

After the external genitalia have been fully examined, the physician should proceed with visualization of the vagina. In girls more than 2 years old, the knee-chest position provides a particularly good view of the vagina and cervix without instrumentation. The patient is asked to "lie on her tummy with her bottom in the air." She should be reassured that the examiner plans to "take a look at her bottom" but "will not put anything inside her." In the knee-chest position (also used for sigmoidoscopy in older patients), the child rests her head to one side on her folded arms and supports her weight on bent knees (6 to 8 inches apart) (Fig. 23-5). With her buttocks held up in the air she is encouraged to let her spine and stomach sag downward. A pillow can be placed under her abdomen. An assistant or her mother helps to hold the buttocks apart, pressing laterally and slightly upward. As the child takes deep breaths, the vaginal orifice falls open for examination. In 80% to 90% of prepubertal girls, an ordinary otoscope head (without a speculum) provides the magnification and light necessary to visualize the cervix. Small talk about school, toys, and siblings often diverts the child's attention and helps her maintain this position for several minutes without moving or objecting. Because the vagina of the prepubertal child is quite short, the presence of a foreign body or a lesion is often easily ascertained.[29]

An alternative method of visualization is the use of a small vaginoscope, cystoscope, hysteroscope, or flexible fiberopticscope with water insufflation of the vagina. The child is examined supine with her knees held apart. Viscous xylocaine applied to the introitus makes insertion easier. Good visualization of the cervix and vagina is thus possible without general anesthetic. Since it is unlikely that the general physician will have a vaginoscope or cystoscope in the office, examination with a narrow veterinary otoscope speculum with the child in the supine (lithotomy) position can be helpful. A narrow vaginal speculum is rarely useful in examining the older child and only if insertion does not cause pain or trauma. For examinations with anesthetic, a Killian nasal speculum (Codman and Shurtlif, Co., Inc., Randolph, MA) with light source can be used (Fig. 23-6).

If vaginal discharge is present, samples should be obtained for culture, gram stain, saline, and potassium hydroxide (KOH) preparations. Usually, the child prefers to lie on her back with her knees apart and feet together or in stirrups so that she can watch the procedure without becoming excessively anxious.

The child should be allowed to feel a cotton-tipped applicator, Calgiswab, eyedropper, or catheter on her skin before insertion of a sterile device into her vagina. For the prepubertal child, a nasopharyngeal Calgiswab moistened with nonbacteriostatic saline is appropriate. This can be inserted into the vagina painlessly by avoiding the hymenal edges. The child is asked to cough as the examiner inserts the swab. This action distracts the child and makes the hymen gape open. Several samples can be obtained in rapid succession without discomfort. If indicated, a chlamydia culture can be obtained by gently inserting a male urethral swab through the hymen, and scraping the lateral vaginal wall. If multiple samples are needed, as in a rape evaluation, a soft plastic eyedropper or a glass eyedropper with 4 to 5 cm of intravenous plastic tubing attached can be gently inserted through the hymen to aspirate secretions. Alternatively a modified syringe and urethral catheter may be used. The proximal 4-inch end of an intravenous butterfly catheter is inserted into the 4-inch end piece of a number 12 bladder catheter,

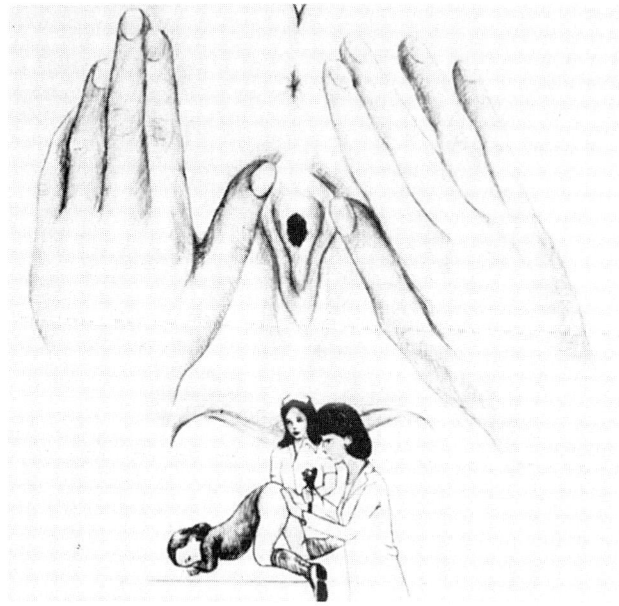

Fig. 23-5. Knee chest position for visualization of vagina with otoscope.

and a syringe is attached. The catheter is slid into the vagina, similar to catheterizing the bladder. One half to 1 mL of sterile saline is injected into the vagina and aspirated.

A culture for *Neisseria gonorrhoeae* should be done on modified Thayer-Martin-Jembec media (Scott Laboratories, Fiskeville, RI 02823) at the time of the examination. Cultures for other organisms are done by placing the moistened Calgiswab into the transport Culturette II with medium (Marion Scientific, Kansas City, MO 64114). The bacteriology laboratory should plate the swab in the standard genitourinary media, which usually includes blood agar, MacConkey, and chocolate media. The laboratory should be notified that the Thayer-Martin-Jembec media being processed is from the vagina of a prepubertal child so that if a *Neisseria* species grows it is properly and unequivocally identified as *N. gonorrhoeae* for medicolegal purposes.[88]

Cultures for *Chlamydia trachomatis* rather than indirect tests and slide immunofluorescent tests are recommended in the prepubertal child because of the possibility of false-positive tests and the association of this organism with sexual abuse. For patients who complain of itching or have suspected yeast infection a Biggy agar (Scott Laboratories, Fiskeville, RI 02823) culture can be incubated and read in the office.

After the samples are obtained, a gentle rectoabdominal examination is done with the patient in stirrups or supine with her legs apart. For bimanual palpation, the examiner places the index or little finger of one hand into the rectum and the other hand on the abdomen. The child can be reassured that this examination will feel similar to having her temperature taken rectally. Except in the newborn period when the uterus is enlarged secondary to maternal estrogen, the rectal

A

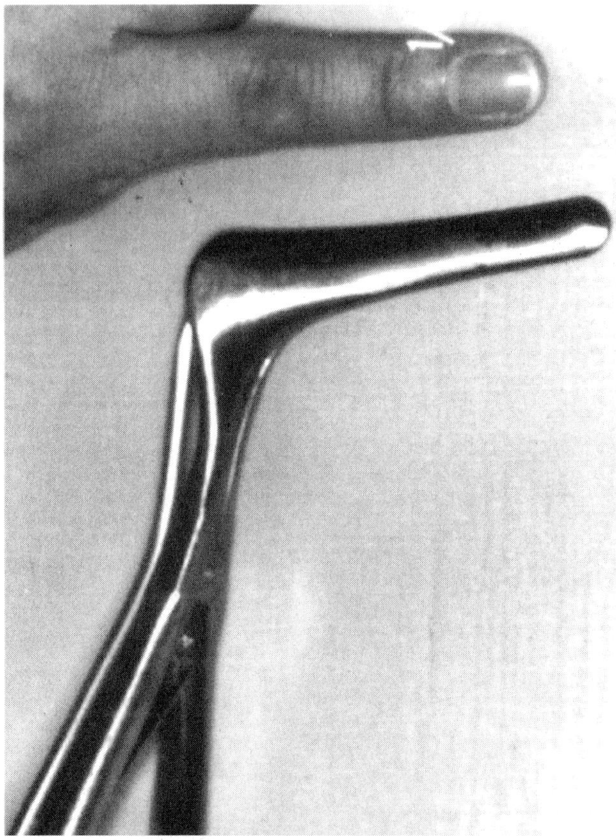

examination in the prepubertal child reveals only the small "button" of the cervix. Because the ovaries are not palpable, adnexal masses should alert the physician to the possibility of a cyst or tumor. As the rectal finger is removed, the vagina should be gently "milked" to promote passage of polypoid tumors or discharge.

After assessing a patient's chief complaint and the results of the examination, the physician should spend time with the parents and child discussing diagnosis, mode of therapy, and necessity of follow-up. Praising the young child for her cooperation and "bravery" helps establish the important doctor-patient relationship for future examinations.

Office evaluation of the adolescent

The evaluation of the adolescent requires additional technical skills, including speculum examination of the vagina and rectal-vaginal-abdominal palpation. More importantly the physician needs the interpersonal skills, sensitivity, and time to establish a primary relationship with the adolescent. The doctor must be willing to see the teenager alone and listen to her concerns.

It is helpful to discuss the special needs of adolescents with the pubescent girl when she reaches her eleventh or twelfth birthday. The parents also need to understand that adolescents require special time to discuss concerns about peer relations, school, family, drugs, alcohol, and sexuality.

B

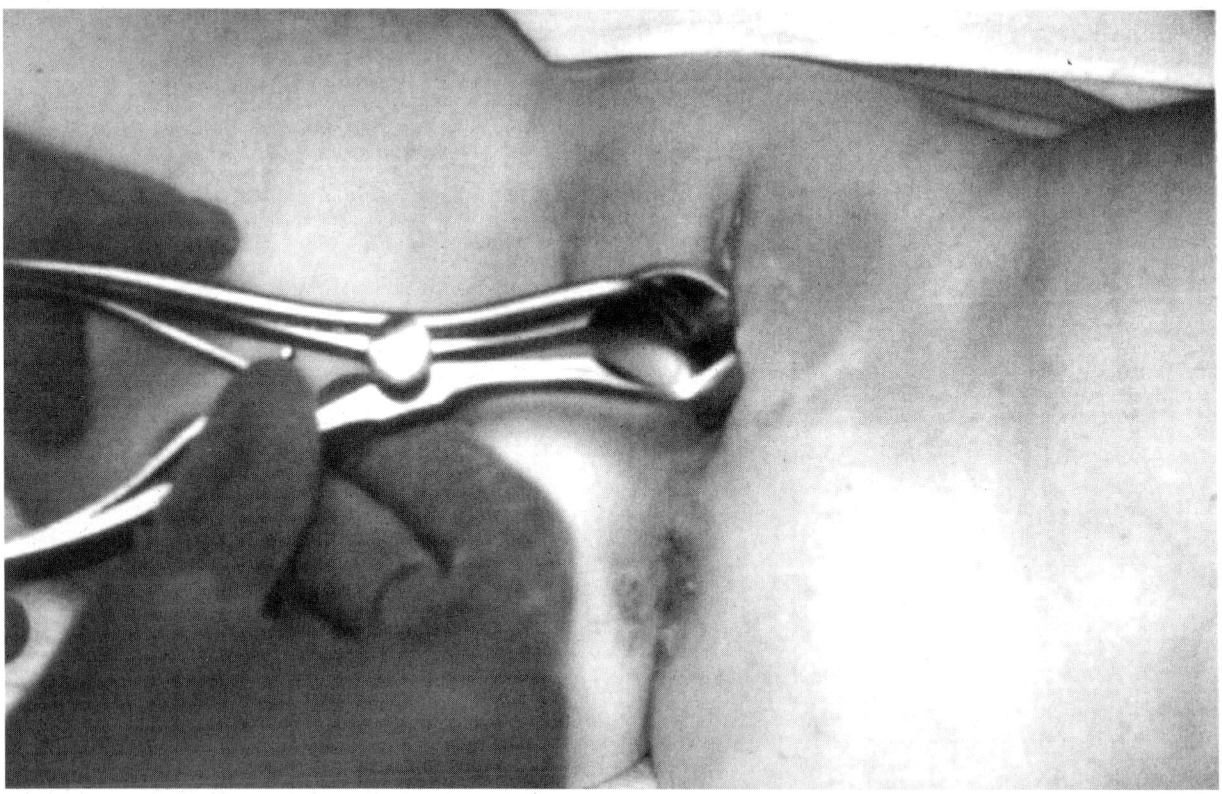

Fig. 23-6. A, Killian nasal speculum with fiberoptic light. **B**, Killian nasal speculum in use during anesthesia examination.

Visits for the well teenager should be on at least an annual basis; a patient with medical or psychologic concerns should obviously be seen more frequently. Parents should be included as much as possible in important medical decisions, but the medical privacy of the adolescent should be respected. Parents should be encouraged to call in advance of an appointment if they have special concerns because an adolescent may be strikingly nonverbal about troubling issues at home or in school. At the same time, parents need help communicating more effectively with the adolescent.

The body changes involved in the development of the prepubertal latency-age girl of 10 years as she changes into the sexually mature woman of 20 years underscore the many issues that arise in the medical care of adolescent girls. The appearance of pubic hair and breast development, over which the girl has no control, can be quite distressing. The fact that these changes occur at the same rate within her peer group may offer some reassurance; however, early or late development can provoke considerable anxiety. A 12-year-old girl who looks 16 may be confronted with heterosexual demands that she is unable to cope with; a 16-year-old girl who looks 10 may be embarrassed to undress in physical education class or to interact with her peer group. Because the young adolescent has many fantasies about her body and its changes, she may ask the same questions at each visit. The older teenager is intellectually more capable of coping with a diagnosis and the physical examination. The physician must therefore be sensitive to the different needs of each patient.

Obtaining the history. The source of the medical history depends on the medical setting and the age of the patient. The older adolescent tends to seek gynecologic care on her own initiative. In a clinic setting, the mother (and father) may be seen by the physician first to ascertain the nature of the chief complaint, as well as the past medical history, school problems, and psychosocial adjustment. More of the visit should be devoted to the teenager alone, since her presenting complaint is quite often different from her mother's concerns.

In the private practice setting, the mother may make the appointment by telephone, and the teenager may arrive alone for the examination. A complete medical history should be obtained on the first visit and should always involve a carefully taken menstrual history and straight-forward questions about sexual relations and birth control.

The physician's approach toward confidentiality should be explicitly stated because few teenagers volunteer a need for birth control.[39] Such discussions should be skillfully handled because repeatedly offering birth control advice may push a young woman into premature sexual relations she may regret. Although the physician may have strong opinions regarding the morality of premarital intercourse, defining the issues under discussion and identifying alternatives may direct the adolescent to an acceptable solution. Concerned medical care sensitive to the patient's needs will hopefully assist her in the development of a healthy body image and responsible sexuality.

Gynecologic examination. Once the history is obtained and the problems identified, the patient should be given a thorough explanation of a pelvic examination. Diagrams or a plastic pelvic model are helpful. During the first examination, the feelings of the adolescent should be acknowledged. Adequate drapes and gowns and allowing the adolescent to control the tempo of the examination will alleviate her concerns. The patient should be given a gown and asked to remove all her clothes, including brassiere and underpants. If she is covered appropriately and approached in a relaxed manner, resistance is unlikely. The presence of a female nurse in the room is often reassuring, especially if the physician is a man. A young adolescent may request that her mother stay with her during a pelvic examination; however, most patients prefer the mother remain in the waiting room. The patients' wishes should be respected.

The general physical examination of a teenage girl should always include a breast examination, inspection of the genitalia, and a careful notation of the Tanner stages of breast and pubic hair development. Demonstrating self-examination of the breast while performing the breast examination often puts the young woman at ease.

A bimanual rectoabdominal examination (in the lithotomy position) should be performed on any teenager with gynecologic complaints or unexplained abdominal pain. A vaginal examination is important to assess irregular bleeding, severe dysmenorrhea, vaginal discharge, in utero exposure to diethylstilbestrol (DES), sexually transmitted diseases, and amenorrhea. Ideally, sexually active patients should have a routine vaginal examination every 6 to 12 months including Pap smears and cultures for gonorrhea and chlamydia. A patient who is not sexually active can begin routine examinations at any age that she feels comfortable initiating gynecologic care, hopefully at least by 17 or 18 years of age. Contrary to popular belief, rarely is a patient unable to fully cooperate during a pelvic examination if she has received a careful explanation about the procedure and its importance in evaluating her individual problem.

The pelvic examination is done with the patient in the lithotomy position with the use of stirrups. A mirror can be offered to the patient. The external genitalia are inspected first; type of hymenal opening, estrogenization of the vaginal mucosa, distribution of pubic hair, and the size of the clitoris are assessed. The pubic hair should be inspected for pediculosis pubis if the patient complains of itching. The inguinal areas should be palpated for evidence of lymphadenopathy. The estrogenized vagina has a moist or thickened, dull pink mucosa in contrast to the thin, red mucosa of the prepubertal child. The normal clitoral glans is 2 to 4 mm in width; a width of 10 mm is considered significant virilization. The hymen in the adolescent girl is estrogenized and thickened. Minor changes resulting from sexual abuse or minor trauma that might have been easily seen in the thin unestrogenized hymen of the prepubertal child may be impossible to visualize in the estrogenized adolescent. Because the hymen is elastic, tampons can be inserted by most adolescents without tearing the hymen. The hymenal opening in the virginal adolescent is large enough usually to allow insertion of a finger for palpation or a small speculum.

An adolescent who has been sexually active may have a hymen without any obvious trauma, may have old or new lacerations of the hymen (down to the base of the hymen), or myrtiform caruncles (small bumps of residual hymen along the lower edge). In the examination of the sexually abused adolescent, the hymenal ring can be examined carefully by running a saline-moistened cotton-tipped applicator around the edges. Any hymenal abnormalities should be discussed with the patient, and the need for, and the timing of, intervention should be decided by the patient after discussion with her physician.

To avoid surprising the patient, a manual or speculum examination should be preceded by a statement such as, "I am now going to touch your bottom" or "I am now going to place this cool metal speculum in your vagina." In the virginal teenager a slow, one-finger examination will determine the size of the introitus and the location of the cervix, and allow subsequent easy insertion of the speculum. It is helpful to warm the speculum and then touch it to the patient's thigh to allow her to feel its "cool metal" quality. The speculum should be inserted posteriorly and downward to avoid the urethra. Applying pressure to the inner thigh while inserting the speculum or finger into the vagina is helpful. If the hymenal opening is small, a Hoffman-Graves adolescent vaginal speculum (11 1/2 x 1 cm) (V. Mueller, 1500 Waullegan Rd, McGaw Park IL 60085) is used to expose the cervix (Fig. 23-7). A latex glove with the tip cut off slipped over the narrow speculum keeps the vaginal walls from collapsing in the virginal girl.

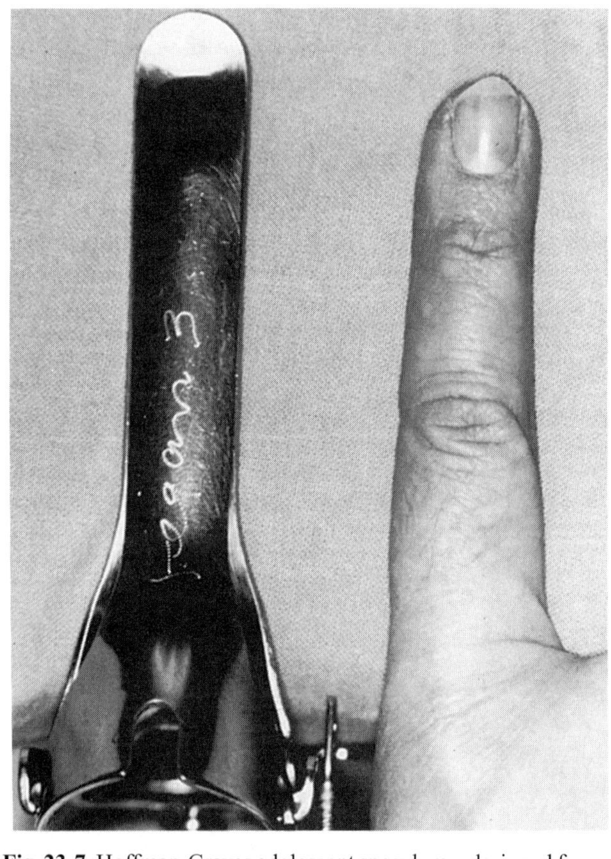

Fig. 23-7. Hoffman-Graves adolescent speculum—designed for use in virginal adolescents because of its narrow gauge and longer blades.

In the sexually active teenager a Pederson vaginal speculum (7/8 x 4 1/2 inches) or occasionally (in the postpartum adolescent) a Graves (1 3/8 x 3 3/4 inches) speculum is appropriate. A child's speculum (5/8 x 3 inches or 7/8 x 3 inches) is rarely ever useful because of its inadequate length and excessive width.

A rectal-vaginal-abdominal examination performed with the index finger in the vagina, the middle finger in the rectum, and the other hand on the abdomen permits palpation of a retroverted uterus and assessment of mobility of the adnexa and uterus.

The uterosacral ligaments should be palpated carefully in patients with pain or dysmenorrhea because tenderness is often found in patients with endometriosis. The patient is usually less anxious if she is told in advance that the rectal examination may produce the sensation that she is "moving her bowels" or "going to the bathroom." Allaying this fear usually elicits better relaxation and cooperation.

In patients with a tight hymen a single bimanual rectoabdominal examination with the index finger pushing the cervix upward allows palpation of the uterus and adnexa. In the relaxed patient a negative examination rules out the possibility of large ovarian masses or uterine enlargement.

After the examination is concluded and the patient has dressed, the physician should sit down and discuss in detail the patient's complaint and what was found on examination. It is essential that the adolescent be treated as an adult capable of understanding the explanation. If a parent has accompanied her, the patient should be asked whether she would like to tell her parent the findings herself or whether she would prefer to have the physician discuss the diagnosis with the parent in her presence. It is extremely important for the patient to know that the doctor and her parent will not have a "secret" about her and that confidential information will not be divulged to her parent.

GYNECOLOGIC PROBLEMS IN THE PEDIATRIC POPULATION

Congenital malformations

Congenital malformations of the female genital tract are usually diagnosed at birth or during adolescence, when reproductive function begins and symptoms develop. Those that are recognized in the infant and young child are external and usually noted either by a parent or the pediatrician. Anomalies diagnosed at menarche are usually those that result in an obstructive condition.

Normal female embryology. By the ninth week of development the embryo has both male (wolffian) and female (müllerian) genital ducts that extend from the mesonephros cranially to the cloaca caudally. A cloaca exists in the human embryo for only a brief period of time; by the seventh gestational week it is divided into rectum and urogenital sinus by descent of the urorectal septum. Normal female internal genitalia develop from the müllerian ductal system as the wolffian ducts regress.

The müllerian ducts develop from an invagination of the coelomic epithelium. These paired ducts are lateral initially but at the future pelvic brim turn in a medial direction to nearly touch in the midline before turning caudally to end on the posterior wall of the urogenital sinus, where the müllerian tubercle forms. Eventually the ducts fuse, forming the primitive uterovaginal canal (Fig. 23-8). The first and second portions of the müllerian ducts eventually form the fimbria and the fallopian tubes, and the distal segment forms the uterus and part of the vagina.

After the müllerian tubercle is formed, two solid evaginations grow from its distal aspect. These are the sinovaginal bulbs and are of urogenital sinus origin. Slightly proximal to the sinovaginal bulbs, growth from the müllerian ducts results in the solid vaginal plate. Growth of the plate and the bulbs changes the urogenital sinus from a long, narrow tube to a broad, flat vestibule, bringing the urethra down to the future perineum.

Canalization of the vaginal plate starts caudally and continues in a cranial direction (Fig. 23-9). It is complete by the fifth month of intrauterine life. The distal portions of the sinovaginal bulbs coalesce to form the hymen. Shortly before birth the central area of the hymen disintegrates, so that it is normally perforate at birth.

The external genitalia form from structures that correlate with development of the male (Fig. 23-10). The external genitalia then differentiate to form normal female external genitalia (Fig. 23-11).

In summary, the uterus is of müllerian origin, as is the proximal four fifths of the vagina. The distal fifth of the vagina and the vaginal epithelium arises from the urogenital sinus.

Ambiguous genitalia in the newborn. Although most clinicians will rarely see an infant with ambiguous genitalia at birth, the need to assess the situation as quickly as possible

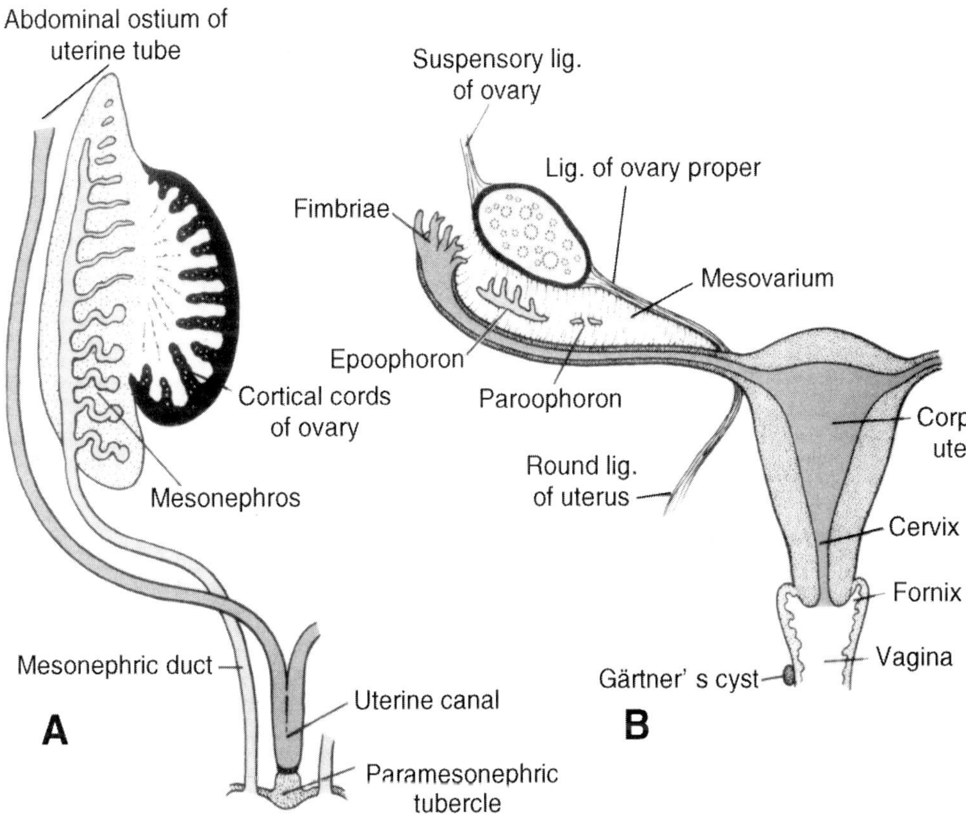

Fig. 23-8. **A**, Schematic drawing of the genital ducts in the female at the end of the 2nd month of development. Note the paramesonephric or müllerian tubercle and the formation of the uterine canal. **B**, The genital ducts after descent of the ovary. The only parts remaining of the mesonephric system are the epoophoron, paroophoron, and Gärtner's cyst. Note the suspensory ligament of the ovary, the ligament of the ovary proper, and the round ligament of the uterus. (From Sadler TW: *Langman's medical embryology*, ed. 6, Baltimore, 1990, Williams & Wilkins.)

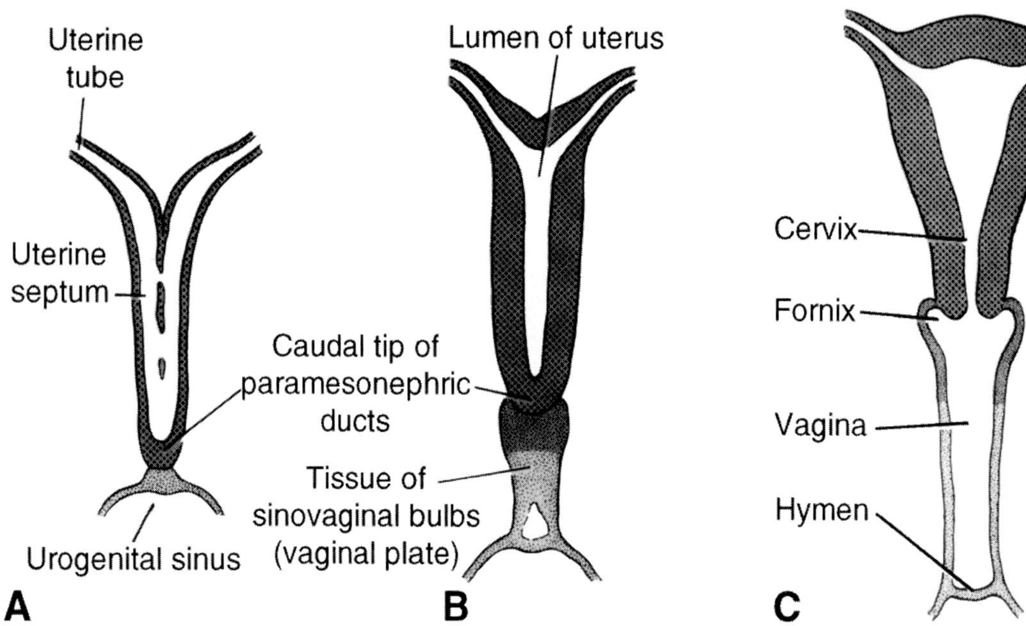

Fig. 23-9. Schematic drawing showing the formation of the uterus and vagina. **A**, At 9 weeks. Note the disappearance of the uterine septum. **B**, At the end of the 3rd month. Note the tissue of the sinovaginal bulbs. **C**, Newborn. The upper portion of the vagina and the fornices are formed by vacuolization of the paramesonephric tissue and the lower portion by vacuolization of the sinovaginal bulbs. (From Sadler TW: *Langman's medical embryology*, ed. 6, Baltimore, 1990, Williams & Wilkins.)

makes this subject essential for inclusion in this chapter. Any deviation from the normal appearance of male or female genitalia should prompt investigation. Incomplete or ambiguous male or female external genitals may be associated with the gonads and genotype of the opposite sex (e.g., the male with androgen insensitivity and the markedly virilized female with congenital adrenal hyperplasia [CAH]). Even a slight doubt that arises in the initial newborn examination should be pursued systematically to prevent a missed diagnosis. Bilateral cryptorchidism, unilateral cryptorchidism with incomplete scrotal fusion or hypospadias, labial fusion, or clitoromegaly require evaluation.

Determining sex assignment. If the physician finds that an infant has ambiguous genitalia, the parents should be reassured that they have a healthy infant, but that because the external genital development is incomplete, tests are necessary to determine the sex. A straightforward explanation of the factors necessary for normal sexual development in utero may be helpful. Most parents will react with dismay and anxiety; they should be reassured that tests will show the cause of the problem and whether their baby is a girl or a boy. The possibility of an intersex disorder (hermaphroditism) should not be raised at this time and speculation about possible sex assignment should be kept to a minimum. Within a few days, or at most 1 to 2 weeks, a definite answer will be possible. The physician should examine the baby in the presence of the parents and explain the common genital anlage for males and females. The concept of an "underdeveloped" boy or "overdeveloped" girl helps parents accept their baby's condition.

Although a diagnosis of the patient's condition requires knowledge of the genotype, assignment of sex is based also on other criteria. The first issue is sexual function and fertility. A girl with CAH may be virilized at birth, yet have normal ovaries and uterus, and is potentially capable of bearing children. Therefore management, including surgery, must aim for female gender identity. When fertility is not possible, as with mixed gonadal dysgenesis (MGD) or male pseudohermaphroditism, decisions are based on surgical requirements for reconstruction of the external genitals. In general, surgical techniques are more suited to clitoral recession, and later the creation of a vagina, than to the construction of a normal male phallus.

Once the decision as to sex of rearing is made, the physician should help the parents accept their infant as a normal boy or girl. If attitudes toward the child's sex remain unequivocal, the child usually assumes his or her gender role without difficulty, regardless of the genotype.

The XX newborn with ambiguous genitalia. The differential diagnosis of XX patients with ambiguous genitalia includes the following: (1) CAH; (2) female pseudohermaphroditism that results from maternal ingesting of drugs, maternal CAH, maternal or fetal virilizing tumor, or idiopathic; and (3) true hermaphroditism.

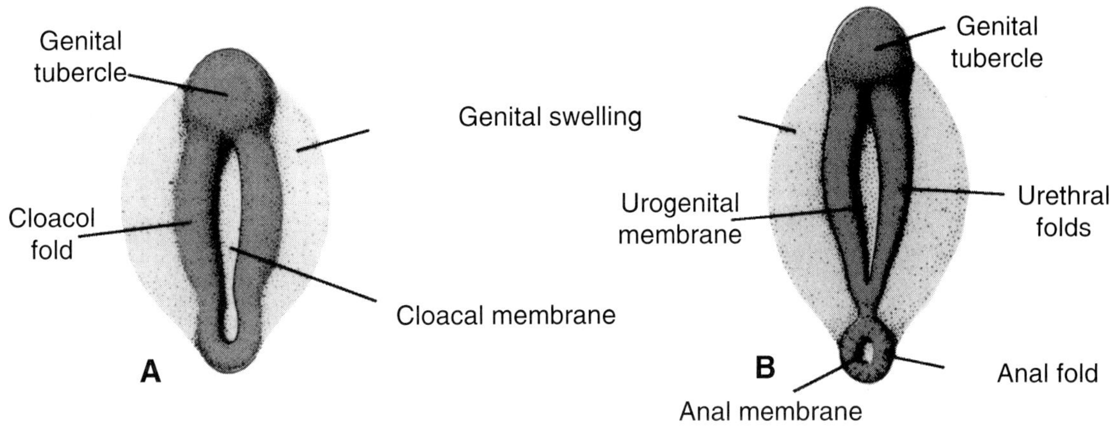

Fig. 23-10. The indifferent stage of the external genitalia. **A**, At approximately 4 weeks. **B**, At approximately 6 weeks. (From Sadler TW: *Langman's medical embryology*, ed. 6, Baltimore, 1990, Williams & Wilkins.)

Congenital adrenal hyperplasia. (CAH) is the most common cause of ambiguous genitalia in the XX newborn. Because of the variability in enzymatic block, ambiguity ranges from labial fusion with or without slight clitoromegaly to a "male phallus" with labial fusion and rugae on the labioscrotal folds.[72,114]

21-hydroxylase deficiency. The enzyme most commonly involved is 21-hydroxylase with a reported incidence of 1 in 5000 to 1 in 15,000.[91,107] The enzyme 21-hydroxylase converts 17-hydroxyprogesterone to 11-deoxycortisol and progesterone to deoxycorticosterone. Because of inadequate cortisol synthesis, ACTH increases, with resultant increased adrenal androgen production. Salt losing is seen in about 50% to 70% of patients with the 21-hydroxylase deficiency because of the severity of the deficiency with decreased aldosterone antagonists.

11β-hydroxylase deficiency. A deficiency of 11β-hydroxylase interrupts the production of cortisol and aldosterone. This results in an increase in the production of ACTH, 11-deoxycortisol, deoxycorticosterone, and adrenal androgens. This syndrome is usually associated with hypertension and moderately increased urinary excretion of pregnanetriol

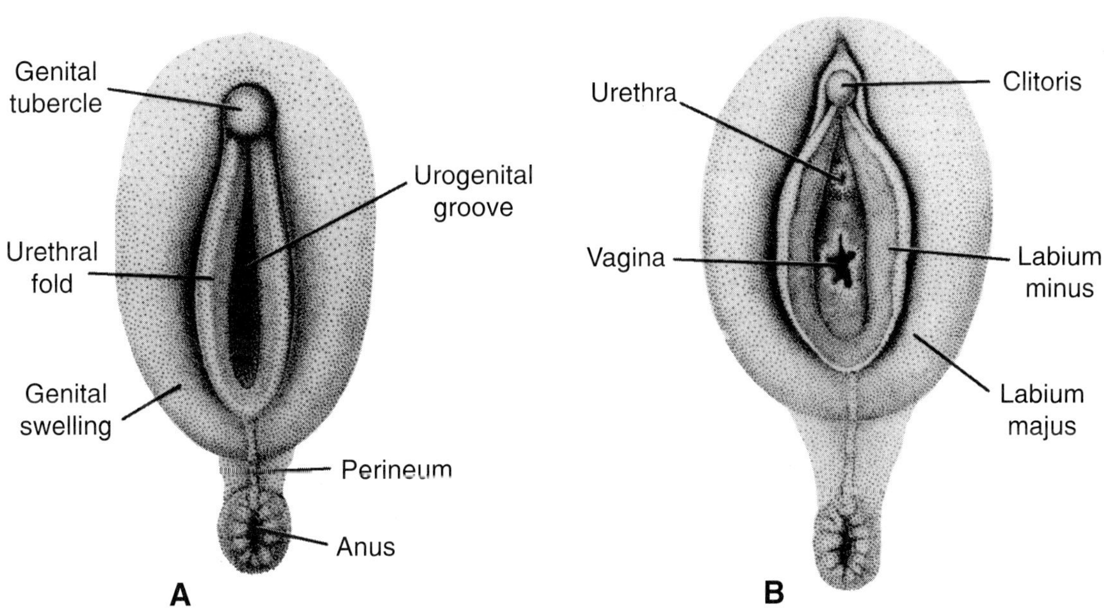

Fig. 23-11. Development of the external genitalia. **A,** In the female at 5 months. **B,** In the newborn. (From Sadler TW: *Langman's medical embryology*, ed. 6, Baltimore, 1990, Williams & Wilkins.)

and the metabolites for 11-deoxycortisol and deoxycorticosterone (tetrahydro-S and tetrahydro-DOC). An affected 46 XX fetus will manifest similar ambiguity of the external genitals.

3β-hydroxysteroid dehydrogenase deficiency. The enzyme 3β-hydroxysteroid dehydrogenase promotes the conversion of pregnenolone to progesterone and 17-hydroxypregnenolone to 17-hydroxyprogesterone. A rare form of CAH, 3β-hydroxysteroid dehydrogenase deficiency, results in severe adrenal insufficiency and increased ACTH levels. This syndrome can result in ambiguous genitalia in both sexes. Virilization of an XX fetus is quite mild because the block is in the initial steps of hormone synthesis so that only the weak androgen dehydroepiandrosterone (DHEA) can be produced in excess, while the more potent androgen testosterone is inadequately produced.

Clinical considerations in CAH. The diagnosis of CAH should be made as soon as possible after birth because of the need to prevent dehydration, hyponatremia, and hyperkalemia with glucocorticoid and mineralocorticoid replacement.

It should be emphasized that XX individuals with CAH are female and are potentially fertile. Thus, regardless of the appearance of the external genitalia, the sex assignment should be female. Surgery may be undertaken for the following: (1) recession of the clitoris, (2) division of the labioscrotal folds, and (3) creation of an adequate vagina. As the buried clitoris can respond with painful erections to high levels of androgens (which may occur with noncompliance of medications during adolescence), recession is usually accompanied by resection of corpora and preservation of the neurovascular bundle with reanastomosis of the glans.[26,50,60,80] This procedure and vaginoplasty in infants whose vagina enters distal to the external urethral sphincter, are usually carried out within the first 6 months of life. In patients with high entry of the vagina into the urethra, vaginoplasty is delayed until 2 years of age. A second vaginoplasty or the use of dilators may be needed during adolescence, the age determined by dialogue with the patient on her readiness to undertake operative and postoperative care. If surgical construction is necessary, postoperative use of dilators is usually necessary to keep the vagina patent until the patient has regular sexual relations.

Other diagnoses of XX neonates. If an infant is XX and has no evidence of CAH, she either has a primary gonadal abnormality, has been exposed to exogenous hormones or a virilizing lesion in the mother. If the mother's history is negative for ingesting of synthetic hormones, then the patient should have a careful physical examination and measurement of urinary and serum androgens.

In the absence of a history of maternal virilization or hormone ingestion, the infant should have an evaluation of internal genital anatomy to determine the gonadal cause of the ambiguous genitalia: true hermaphroditism or idiopathic female pseudohermaphroditism.

The XY newborn with ambiguous genitalia. The differential diagnosis of the infant who is XY includes the following: (1) male pseudohermaphroditism because of defects of testicular differentiation, deficient placental luteinizing hormone (LH) level, Leydig cell agenesis, defects in testosterone synthesis, 5α-reductase deficiency, or receptor defects; and (2) hypogonadotrophic hypogonadism (Kallmann's syndrome).

Increased understanding of the differentiation of the fetal testis and the many steps involved in the development of the normal male has made it possible to diagnose more specifically the kind of syndrome seen in XY girls. The short arm of the Y chromosome is the region responsible for testicular determinants. The exact area of this chromosome responsible for testicular determination is being intensely investigated. The area of the Y chromosome that appears to be the most likely site of sex determination is the "sex-determining region Y" (SRY). This region has been demonstrated in XX males, and is absent in XY females.[7,57,105]

In cases of pure gonadal dysgenesis or Swyer's syndrome (streak gonads, normal stature) the XY female may be diagnosed during adolescence. If during development the human chorionic gonadotropin (hCG) level is deficient (because of a postulated placental insufficiency or inadequate LH level), stimulation of testosterone secretion would be insufficient for complete masculinization. If the testis is unresponsive to hCG or lacks normal Leydig cells (Leydig cell agenesis), the infant will have abdominal testes, an elevated LH level, a female phenotype with short vagina, and an absent uterus. Depending on when during fetal life the testicular regression occurred, patients will have phenotypes ranging from normal females to males with cryptorchidism.

A number of defects in testosterone synthesis have been described. They include deficiencies of 20,22-desmolase; 3β-hydroxy-Δ^5-steroid dehydrogenase; 17α-hydroxylase; 17,20-desmolase, and 17β-hydroxysteroid. The first three defects are also associated with adrenal insufficiency. Patients who have these deficiencies do not have müllerian structures, but the external genitalia are either female or ambiguous.

Failure to produce müllerian-inhibiting factor (MIF) or the lack of MIF receptors will cause persistence of müllerian structures and the presence of a uterus (hernia uteri inguinale) in a male who has unilateral or bilateral cryptorchidism. The development of the wolffian ducts varies among individuals; males are fertile.

The enzyme 5α-reductase is responsible for the conversion of testosterone to dihydrotestosterone, which results in the male differentiation of the external genitalia. Patients with 5α-reductase deficiency (so-called pseudovaginal perineoscrotal hypospadias), an autosomal recessive condition, have a cleft scrotum (hypospadias) and perineal invagination.

Ambiguous genitalia may also be caused by defects in receptor proteins or transcription mechanisms. Complete resistance to the action of testosterone results in the classic picture of androgen insensitivity (sometimes referred to as testicular feminization); the infant appears as a phenotypic female, although occasionally testes are noted early in life. Partial androgen insensitivity results in a spectrum of ambiguous genitalia syndromes at birth and during adolescence; these include the Gilbert-Dreyfus, Reifenstein, Rosewater, and Lubs syndromes. These patients have partial wolffian development, some pubic hair, and partial labioscrotal fusion. Recent research in androgen insensitivity has delineated a number of different syndromes, some with absence of receptors, some with abnormal receptor structure, and some with presumed postreceptor defects. Errors in testosterone biosynthesis may produce a similar phenotype. The pattern of X-linked inheritance coupled with a high LH and testosterone level (especially before and after hCG stimulation) suggests androgen insensitivity.

Cytogenetic studies may help distinguish between patients who have structural defects or dysgenetic testes and those who have structurally normal testes. Many patients in the former group have abnormal sex chromosomes with mosaicism; the patients in the latter group have an XY karyotype. Biochemical studies can pinpoint a diagnosis. Retrograde contrast x-ray studies, ultrasonography, magnetic resonance imaging (MRI), and possibly laparoscopy or laparotomy are necessary to establish the final diagnosis and determine the particular chromatin-negative syndrome present.

Choice of gender identity depends on the external genitalia and the possibility of future coital adequacy. After the sex assignment is definitively made, the gonads that conflict with the assignment should be electively removed. For example, the patient with MGD and 45X/46XY who is given a female sex assignment should have her testis removed to prevent virilization at puberty. Intraabdominal testes should be removed prophylactically in patients with male pseudohermaphroditism and MGD since there is a substantial risk of malignancy, specifically a dysgerminoma or gonadoblastoma in approximately 20% to 30% of cases.[104] In addition, it should be noted that all patients with genital abnormalities should be carefully searched for associated anomalies, especially of the urinary tract.

Introital abnormalities

Masses. The most common abnormality seen in the neonate and young child is a cystic mass at the introitus. It is first observed in the delivery room by the obstetrician, during the neonatal examination by the pediatrician, or by the parent when changing diapers. The mass usually enlarges during crying spells; it is usually cystic, containing a clear or milky mucoid material. The differential diagnosis includes ectopic ureter, hymenal cyst, hymenal skin tag, periurethral cyst, vaginal cyst, or imperforate hymen with mucocolpos/hydrocolpos.

The child should be examined in the frog-leg position, ideally with magnification, using a moistened Q-tip for retraction. The pull-down traction maneuver as shown in Fig. 23-3 opens the introitus so that the origin of the cyst can be ascertained.

Ectopic ureter. If the cyst appears to rise from the periurethral area or anterior vagina, an ectopic ureter should be suspected and pelvic and renal ultrasound scans obtained. If this diagnosis is confirmed, consultation with a pediatric urologist is required. Usually, an intravenous pyelogram (IVP) determines the extent of the anomalous collecting system. High ligation of the ectopic ureter or partial nephrectomy is usually required.

Hymenal, periurethral, and vaginal cysts. Cysts arising from the hymen or periurethral area are usually of the epidermal inclusion variety. Spontaneous resolution is common. If regression does not occur within 3 months, simple marsupialization or electrofulguration is warranted. Before proceeding with surgery, however, urethroscopy should be performed to rule out the presence of a diverticulum of the distal urethra, which would require management by a urologist.

In the newborn period, vaginal cysts can be located posterior to the urethral meatus at the vaginal introitus, arising from the anterior or lateral wall of the vagina, and lined by squamous epithelium. Usually they do not cause pathologic manifestations and can rupture spontaneously, or they disappear after surgical aspiration and removal of a milky white fluid. Occasionally, the cysts grow large enough to obstruct the urethra, causing urinary retention. Operative removal is indicated in such cases. Cysts in the caudal portion of the vagina probably are derived from the epithelium of the urogenital sinus and formed during the last months of gestation. In younger fetuses, multiple cysts can occur in proximal parts of the vagina. They have been considered derivatives of epithelia of the müllerian or wolffian ducts.

Imperforate hymen. When the cystic structure appears to obstruct the vaginal opening and no perforation can be identified, an imperforate hymen with mucocolpos/hydrocolpos is the most likely diagnosis. A mucocolpos/hydrocolpos is due to distention of the vagina with retained secretions which are stimulated by maternal estrogens. The uterus is rarely involved because of the ability of the vagina to distend. The usual presenting symptoms of a massive hydrocolpos in the neonate are a midline lower abdominal mass, urinary retention resulting from bladder angulation, and on occasion respiratory distress. Bilateral hydroureter and hydronephrosis may be detected on an antenatal ultrasound examination. Compression of the ureters at the pelvic brim may also be present.

Respiratory distress may result from pressure on the diaphragm. Lower extremity edema may be caused by compression of the major abdominal veins. One patient has been seen in whom retrograde flow of secretion through the fallopian tubes caused intraperitoneal adhesions and partial bowel obstruction.

The treatment of mucocolpos/hydrocolpos depends on its etiology. If mucocolpos/hydrocolpos is diagnosed, surgery is indicated to avoid late complications of further fluid accumulation and reflux. A simple hymenectomy can be performed in the operating room using a Beaver blade or a needle tip electrocautery. Sutures may be required to maintain patency and avoid a recurrence of the obstruction because of scarring and reclosure of the hymeneal orifice.

Other hymenal abnormalities. Hymenal tags can be present at birth and appear as a fleshy mass protruding from the introitus. They frequently regress when the effects of maternal estrogen have diminished. These lesions may become inflamed and cause vaginal bleeding and discharge. If they are still present at 3 months, they can be removed by electrocautery or cold knife excision.

Inadequate perforation of the hymen, such as septation, microperforation, or cribriform fenestration, is generally asymptomatic in the young child and does not require intervention until puberty when it causes problems with tampon use and/or coitus. Intervention with surgical correction of the hymeneal abnormality is indicated also if it appears to be the cause of recurrent vulvovaginitis and urinary tract infections (UTIs) as a result of stagnation of urine within the partially obstructed vagina. Because most patients with this problem present between the ages of 3 and 6 years, either hymenectomy or hymenotomy and suturing the cut edges with absorbable sutures are satisfactory methods of treatment.

Perineal fissure. Newborns may present with a deep fissure of the median raphe. This area fails to heal spontaneously and remains open and granulating, with purulent drainage because of fecal soiling. The etiology is uncertain, although a perineorectal fistula must be ruled out. Initial treatment is conservative with topical antibiotic ointment such as silver sulfadiazine, protective bland ointments, and silver nitrate applications. If healing does not occur in 2 to 3 months, laser vaporization or excision with primary closure is indicated.

Labia minora hypertrophy or asymmetry. In some instances, one or both labia minora are unusually large, and the patient consults because she notices the anomaly or because of symptoms of irritation associated with exercise. In most of these cases, simple reassurance is necessary. Comparison with asymmetry or hypertrophy of other parts of the body may help the patient to accept this peculiarity. Hygiene counseling and avoidance of tight clothes are usually sufficient to relieve discomfort. If these measures are ineffective, or in the presence of a troublesome cosmetic problem, surgical reduction is in order. This can be accomplished in the ambulatory operating room by simply resecting the redundant labia so that they are symmetrical. Closure of the excised area is best accomplished with a running locking stitch of 3-0 chromic suture (Fig. 23-12). An alternative surgical approach involves identification of labial blood vessels, followed by a wedge resection and reanastomosis as shown in Fig. 23-13.[66]

Clitoromegaly. Clitoral reduction is accomplished surgically in order to gain a functional and cosmetically acceptable clitoris. The procedure for clitoral reduction is described in the section on the management of CAH.

Inguinal ovary syndrome. Inguinal hernias in female infants are generally uncommon, with a male/female ratio of about 6:1. A 1.5-cm firm mass palpated in the groin or vulva usually indicates that the hernia is of the sliding type, where a portion of the wall of the sac is composed of a tube and ovary. It frequently cannot be reduced, but rarely is the blood supply compromised.

Rarely, a girl with a palpable gonad in the labia is actually a male with testicular feminization syndrome. This represents less than 1% of hernias in females. These patients can be identified by the findings of a 46 XY karyotype and the operative findings of testicles. Early identification of these individuals is desirable, although no gender changes should be made because the genitalia are female.

Cloacal anomalies. A cloaca is a common channel into which the products of the gastrointestinal, urinary, and genital tracts empty. The pathogenesis of faulty cloacal division is unknown, but it could result from an arrest in the descent of the urorectal septum, preventing division of the cloaca into the rectum and urogenital sinus. It also stops approximation and fusion of the müllerian ducts, resulting in failure in the formation of the müllerian tubercle and a duplication of the uterus and proximal vagina. The sinovaginal bulbs do not form and the vaginal plate does not enlarge. The urogenital sinus remains in its primitive state as a long, narrow tube, and the urethra empties into the urogenital sinus, high on its anterior wall. The hymen is absent.

A cloacal anomaly involves three major organ systems with complete or partial obstruction of the urinary, genital, or gastrointestinal (GI) tracts. In the absence of other lethal anomalies, urinary tract sepsis resulting from obstruction accounts for the majority of deaths. The five major types of cloacal dysgenesis are as follows:

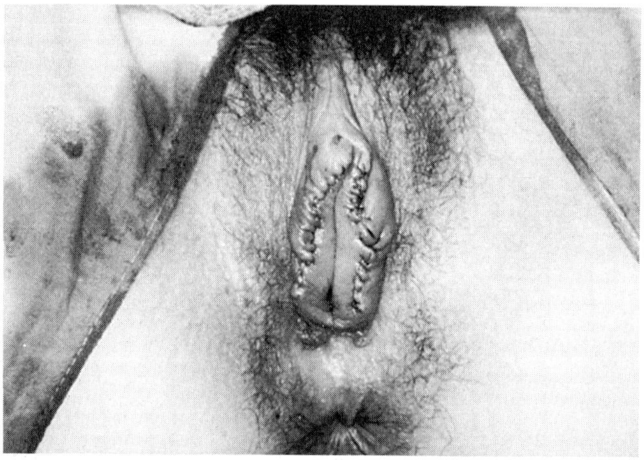

Fig. 23-12. Technique of labial reduction in a patient with symptomatic hypertrophy of labia minora.

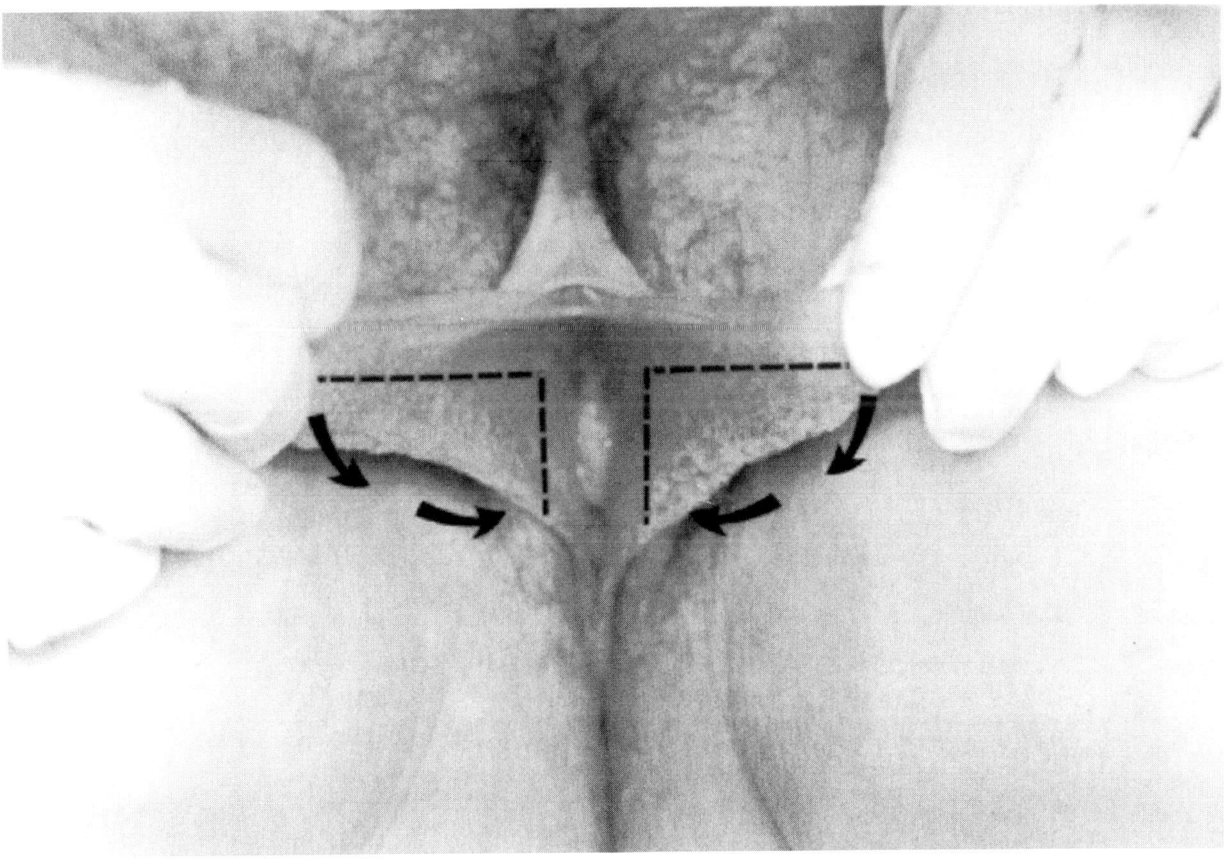

Fig. 23-13. An alternate technique of labial reduction in a patient with symptomatic hypertrophy of labia minora.

1. Type A has a single perineal orifice located between the labia minora. This orifice leads to a long, narrow tube, the cloaca, at the apex of which is an obstructed vagina. The urethral meatus enters the cloaca high on its anterior wall directly across from the posterior rectal fistula.
2. Type B is similar to type A, but the rectal fistula enters the vagina.
3. Type C has a short, broad cloaca.
4. Type D is similar to type A, but a distal vaginal atresia is present.
5. Type E has a high type of imperforate anus, but no rectocloacal fistula.

Other major system anomalies are common, particularly in the cardiovascular, genitourinary, GI, central nervous, and respiratory systems. The most common anomalies are those of müllerian origin; septate vagina, duplication of the uterus, and bicornuate uterus.

The pathognomonic physical finding in cloacal dysgenesis is a single perineal orifice between the labia minora. This opening is the entrance to the cloaca. The urethral meatus and anus are not evident and hydrometrocolpos is often present as an abdominal mass. Reconstruction is complex and best performed by a pediatric surgeon.

Infection

Vulvovaginitis

The normal vaginal environment. The vagina undergoes constant change from birth, through childhood, menarche, reproductive years, menopause, and older ages. Consequently, the types and frequency of inflammatory conditions of the vagina and vulva are different at various ages. At birth the mucous membranes of the vagina and vulva have an adult histologic appearance because of stimulation by circulating maternal estrogens. The cervical, paraurethral, and Bartholin's glands are large and secrete mucus in the immediate neonatal period. The pH is 5 to 7. Within a few weeks, however, the vaginal lining becomes thin and unestrogenized.

Throughout childhood until the immediate premenarchal period, the child is especially vulnerable to vulvovaginitis because of poor estrogenization of the vaginal epithelium. In addition unsupervised and inadequate perineal hygiene contribute to the incidence of vulvovaginitis. It is also well known that compared with older females, these young individuals lack the protection provided by pubic hair and the fat pads of the labia majora. Without these anatomic protections, contaminants and irritants have free access to the sensitive vulvar and vaginal epithelium.

At puberty, estrogen stimulation changes the vaginal epithelium to a thick and stratified squamous epithelium. The subsequent normal flora establishment of the Döderlein's bacillus causes the pH to rise to the 6 to 8 range, which helps to maintain homeostasis and decrease infection.

Presentations of vulvovaginitis. Vulvovaginitis is the most common presenting complaint for a pediatric gynecologist.[44] The symptoms of vulvovaginitis are variable but most often consist of vaginal discharge that varies in quantity, color, and odor. Vulvar pruritus or burning and dysuria are also common complaints.

Whatever the underlying etiology, the examination usually reveals edema, redness, discharge, excoriations, and secondary scratch lesions. The presence of fecal remnants and interlabial debris helps to confirm poor hygiene.

Physiologic leukorrhea. Physiologic leukorrhea occurs at both extremes of childhood. During the neonatal period, maternal estrogens stimulate the newborn's endocervical glands and vaginal epithelium. Characteristically the discharge is grayish, gelatinous, and sticky. In the neonate a small amount of blood may be present because of maternal hormonal withdrawal. This always provides the mother with some anxious moments, but a normal examination and lack of recurrence are reassuring.

During the 6 to 12 months preceding menarche, rising endogenous estrogen secretion is responsible for the appearance of a whitish discharge not associated with irritative symptoms. After appropriate evaluation, it is of great importance to explain to these young women that this is part of the normal process of maturation. Usually breast development and growth acceleration is noted at this time. The unjustified prescription of a vaginal cream or antibiotics serves only to make the patient believe that any vaginal discharge is pathologic and results in multiple unnecessary consultations.

Nonspecific vulvovaginitis. Nonspecific or mixed vulvovaginitis accounts for approximately 70% of vulvovaginal infection in this age group. The etiology can most often be traced to poor local hygiene and fecal contamination. Usually cultures grow predominantly *Escherichia coli* and other anal organisms such as enterococcus.

General hygienic measures are the first step of treatment. Sitz baths in plain warm water should be given two or three times daily followed by thorough drying of the vulvar area with a hair dryer at the lowest speed and heat. A small amount of unscented cornstarch-based powder helps to keep the vulva dry. Only mild, nonperfumed soap should be used and bubble bath should be avoided. Adequate counseling about clothing should also be provided (i.e., only white 100% cotton underpants should be worn; tight-fitting clothes, nonabsorbent fabrics, and wet bathing suits should be avoided). The importance of front-to-back wiping with soft, white, unscented toilet tissue should also be stressed.

Specific vulvovaginitis. A variety of causes of vulvovaginitis are recognized. The differential diagnosis, symptoms, and treatment of the various types are summarized in Table 23-1.

The character of the discharge and other clinical features vary according to the organism responsible; correct diagnosis depends on identification of the offending organism. The most common cause of vulvovaginitis is allergic, but bacterial or viral infections, parasitic infestation, and traumatic vulvovaginitis also occur.

Gonorrhea. Gonococcal infection in the prepubertal child is usually manifested as a purulent vulvovaginitis rather than a cervicitis. The infection may be asymptomatic or be evident as a thin mucoid discharge. Gram stain and culture are important in the evaluation of vaginal discharge in a prepubertal individual. Although the Gram stain is helpful, *Neisseria meningitidis* rarely causes vaginitis; therefore, it is essential that the diagnosis be proved by cultures.

After a diagnosis is made, the child should be interviewed by an experienced social worker, psychologist, or pediatrician to assess the possibility of sexual abuse. Play therapy and repeated interviews may be necessary to establish the history, since in most cases of sexual abuse, the abuser is known to the child and is often a family member. All family members and caretakers of the child may need to be cultured. The source of infection is frequently a male relative, stepparent, or care taker. The mother and sisters frequently are infected. Although it is theoretically possible that *Neisseria gonorrhoeae* can be transmitted by sexual play between siblings and peers, the clinician must strongly suspect sexual abuse in all cases of prepubertal gonorrhea, as almost 100% of cases result from sexual abuse. Because sexual abuse often involves vulvar coitus or oral sex rather than penetration, a physical examination shows a normal hymen in many abused girls. Cultures should be obtained from oral, vaginal, and rectal orifices. Although contacts may be easier to culture and follow-up may be significantly improved if the child is hospitalized, an outpatient approach is taken for most cases. Suspected child sexual abuse must be reported to the mandated state agency.

Before treatment, rectal and pharyngeal cultures for *N. gonorrhoeae* should be obtained from the child with a vaginal gonorrhea, avaginal culture for *Chlamydia trachomatis,* and a serology for syphilis. For children who weigh more than 45 kg, adult schedules for treating cervicitis and urethritis are used. For children who weigh less than 45 kg, recommended regimens are 125 mg of ceftriaxone intramuscularly or spectinomycin 40 mg/kg (maximum 2g) intramuscularly. Coinfection with *C. trachomatis* should be treated with 50 mg of erythromycin/kg/day in four divided doses, or in children older than 9 years adult dosages of doxycycline or tetracycline can be used.

Follow-up cultures of the throat, rectum, and vagina should be taken 7 to 14 days after treatment. Reinfection is likely if the source is not identified and treated. Persistent vaginal discharge in a patient who has been adequately treated and had negative cultures for gonorrhea may indicate a coinfection with *C. trachomatis* that was not adequately treated with single-dose therapy. The family may have been

Table 23-1. Differential diagnosis of specific vulvovaginitis in infancy and childhood

Etiology	Clinical signs	Discharge	Findings	Treatment
Dermatitis/allergy	Red, papular, pruritic vulvar rash	No discharge	Caused by bubble bath or laundry detergent	Discontinue bubble bath; symptomatic care with steroid or antihistaminic creams
Foreign body	Bloody discharge	Purulent, blood tinged, foul smelling	Foreign body identified on pelvic examination	Removal of foreign body
Bacterial				
Gonococcal	Neonate and premenarchal: Bartholin's, Skene's, and cervical glands involved	May have only scant vaginal discharge	Conjunctivitis (neonate), upper genital tract involvement, systemic symptoms, gram-negative, intracellular diplococci in either type	Ceftriaxone, bacterial sensitivities for resistant gonococcus
	Postmenarchal: Severe vulvar edema, purulent discharge	Profuse, yellow-green discharge, intense vulvovaginitis	Upper genital tract not involved	
Staphylococcus aureus	Labial abscesses	Thick, yellow	Abscesses present in other areas	Oxacillin, cephalosporins
Streptococcus pyogenes, ß-hemolytic, group A	Systemic symptoms, vulvar pruritus and redness	Purulent, thin, yellow		Penicillin
Hemophilus influenzae, type B	May be associated with *H. influenzae* infections in more typical areas	Dark yellow, purulent, foul smelling	Rare ininfancy and childhood	Ampicillin
Shigella	Reddened vulva, may be preceded by diarrhea	Severe, purulent vulvovaginitis	*Shigella* from stool and vaginal cultures	Ampicillin
E. Coli [enteropathic]	Preceded by diarrhea	Thin, watery, foul smelling,	Culture *E. coli* from throat, stool, vagina	Local hygiene, amoxicillin,
Fungal *Candida albicans*	Beefy red vulvovaginitis	Profuse, foul smelling, curdy	Budding yeast on wet preparation or Gram stain; search for systemic disease (diabetes) in pre-adolescent; rare in childhood	Topical nystatin
Viral				
Herpes simplex, Type II	Vulvovaginitis and herpetic stomatitis, perineal edema, painful vulvar eruption	Thin, watery	Tender, superficial labial ulcers; enlarged, tender inguinal lymph nodes; diagnosis by rising serum antibody titer or multinucleated giant cells on vaginal cytology; may be primary or recurrent	Symptomatic with local care
Parasitic				
Pinworm	Severe pruritus	Thin, colorless	Usually associated with enteric infestation; diagnosis by seeing worms or ova on fresh smear	Mebendazole
Trichomonas vaginalis	Moderate pruritus	Thin malodorous	Rare before puberty	Metronidazole

noncompliant with the 7-day course of tetracycline or erythromycin.

Only a few cases of salpingitis secondary to *N. gonorrhoeae* have been reported in prepubertal girls; thus no data exist on the best form of treatment. Antibiotics with a similar spectrum as used in adolescent and adult pelvic inflammatory disease (PID) are appropriate; cefoxitin 2 g intravenously every 6 hours, or cefotetan 2 g intravenously every 12 hours plus doxycycline 100 mg intravenously or orally every 12 hours.

Candida albicans. Monilial vulvovaginitis is infrequent in children and is usually associated with recent antibiotic therapy, diabetes mellitus, or HIV disease. The clinical picture is characteristic and consists at the onset of an erythematous vulva with oozing granulomatous lesions that later become crusted. Satellite lesions are present frequently. The cottage cheese appearance of the vaginal discharge is well known. Diagnosis is made by microscopic visualization of mycelia on potassium hydroxide preparation of vulvar exudate or vaginal discharge, or by positive culture on appropriate medium (Biggy Agar). Treatment consists of sitz baths three times daily, followed by vulvar application of an antifungal preparation.

Trichomonas. Although the nonestrogenized vaginal epithelium of the prepubertal child is unfavorable to the growth of *Trichomonas*, this parasite is responsible occasionally for vulvovaginitis. This infection is acquired by direct contact, and the possibility of sexual abuse should be considered, although nonsexual transmission is possible.

The vaginal discharge, characteristically greenish and malodorous, is associated with nonspecific signs of irritation. Treatment consists of oral administration of 10 to 30 mg of metronidazole/kg/day (maximum 125 mg three times daily) for 7 days or 1 gm in a single dose.

Pinworms. *Enterobius vermicularis* (pinworms), a frequent intestinal parasite in children, may occasionally infect the vagina, giving rise to acute inflammatory symptoms and yellow mucopurulent discharge. Diagnosis is suggested by perianal scratching lesions and confirmed by a positive "Scotch Tape Test" result, preferably done in the morning. Because the treatment for pinworms is a single oral dosage and side effects are minimal, some clinicians opt to treat without a definitive diagnosis by a "Scotch Tape Test."

The parasite is usually eradicated by a single dose of 100 mg of mebendazole. All family members should be treated also. Pinworm vulvovaginitis is frequently associated with infection by other anal contaminants, which is approached as discussed above.

Condylomata acuminata. Warty lesions associated with human papillomavirus (HPV) infection are found in infants and young children at concerningly increasing rates. When HPV is present, the possibility of sexual molestation must be ruled out.[22] The incubation period for HPV is believed to be 4 to 12 weeks, but incubation periods of up to 20 months have been reported. In the younger than 20 month age group, one must be suspicious of sexual abuse, but vertical transmission may be the etiology.

DNA probes that identify the viral type may be useful in documentation of the HPV virus in cases that may involve legal matters. HPV types 1, 2, 4, 7, 26, 27, 28, and 29 are associated with the common hand wart. Genital DNA types include 6, 11, 16, 18, 30 to 35, 39, 42 to 44, 48, and 51 to 55. The most common types of 6 and 11 have a high rate of regression and a low rate of persistence. HPV DNA types 16, 18, 31, 33, and 35 are associated with invasive cervical malignancies. Regression of these subtypes is rare; persistence and progression appear to be the rule.

The need to obtain a definitive diagnosis and provide treatment in the least traumatic manner in the child must be considered. For these reasons children may be examined under anesthesia so that a biopsy can be obtained for pathologic documentation and DNA typing. At the same time the condyloma are treated by excision and/or laser vaporization. Visualization of the urinary tract and anal canal is mandatory in cases where recurrence is a problem. A serologic test for syphilis should be done to exclude condylomata lata (secondary syphilis).

Long-term follow-up of children with HPV is important, the long-term implications of this infection at such early ages are not known. It has been well documented that HPV infections are associated with an increased risk of neoplastic changes.[103] Cases of infection with more virulent DNA types present an even more difficult clinical situation because there are no accepted guidelines for the monitoring of these individuals.

Molluscum contagiosum. Molluscum contagiosum usually presents as a small fleshy papule with a central umbilication. The infectious agent is a pox virus that is transmitted by autoinoculation or close contact with an infected individual. Lesions are usually small (2 to 5 mm) and typically appear on the face, trunk, and extremities. The incubation period is 2 to 7 weeks. A definitive diagnosis is made by identification of viral inclusion bodies isolated from the central core of the lesion. The lesion is usually self-limited, but can be treated with destructive procedures such as curettage of the central core, laser therapy, or cryotherapy.

Systemic causes. Vulvovaginitis in children often follows an episode of infection in another part of the body, especially the upper respiratory tract. β-Hemolytic *Streptococcus pyogenes, Streptococcus pneumoniae, Staphylococcus aureus*, and *N. meningitidis* should be treated according to the sensitivity of each organism.

Systemic diseases such as measles, chicken pox, scarlet fever, and HIV disease may have vulvovaginal manifestations. Symptoms usually follow the natural history of the primary disease. Because of scratching and fecal contamination, secondary bacterial infection may occur.

Dermatologic diseases such as *Herpes simplex* and *H. zoster*, eczema, psoriasis, molluscum contagiosum, and poison ivy may also involve the vulvar skin.

Anatomical causes. In some instances, a microperforate hymen, especially when the opening lies high near the urethral meatus, may be responsible for pooling of urine in the vagina. Constant maceration of vulvovaginal tissue causes irritation and often secondary infection. In these cases hymenotomy is curative.

The discharge from ectopic ureters can masquerade as chronic vulvovaginitis. Often these children are erroneously believed to be incontinent or to have enuresis. Workup should consist of pelvic ultrasonography, IVP, and cystoscopy. The treatment is surgical and usually requires either high ligation or excision of the anomalous collecting system or nephrectomy.

Foreign bodies. The presence of an intravaginal foreign body is suggested by a greenish, bloody, and foul-smelling discharge. The most frequent finding is a small piece of toilet paper or stool. Cultures grow mixed flora. Any bloody or malodorous discharge should prompt a thorough vaginal examination, even if anesthesia or analgesia is required. Rarely, the patient complains of abdominal pain because of retrograde flow of infected vaginal secretions into the fallopian tubes, causing peritonitis.

A vaginal foreign body may be a perplexing problem for the clinician, since most are not visible on external examination. Reluctance to perform a pelvic examination in a child makes the diagnosis even more difficult. However, failure to diagnose and remove a foreign body can result in severe PID, peritonitis, and on rare occasions, migration of the foreign body to another area.

Vaginal foreign bodies are most frequently seen between the ages of 3 and 7 years. Usually there is no history of insertion, and virtually any kind of object may be found within the vagina. A forgotten tampon may be the "foreign body" in a menarcheal girl.

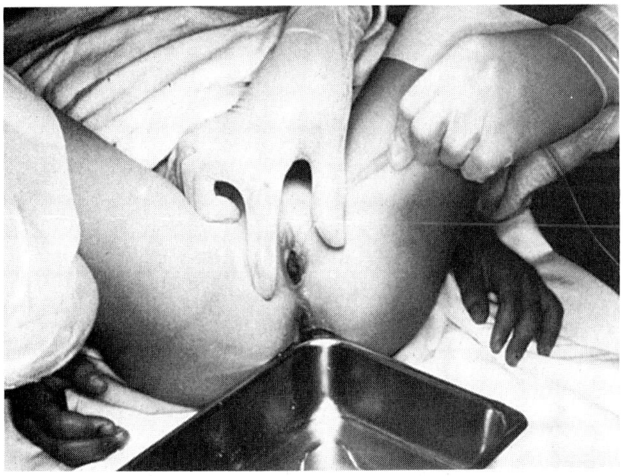

Fig. 23-14. Technique for irrigation of vagina. Used to wash out foreign bodies and debris. Also applicable in examining small children with perineal or labial tears to assess extent of injury.

A foreign body can sometimes be washed out by vaginal irrigation with room temperature saline using IV tubing (Fig. 23-13). Initially, a rectal examination should be done, which frequently reveals the presence of an intravaginal foreign body. If an object is felt, gentle attempts at milking it out may be successful. In girls less than 6 years of age, general anesthesia is most often necessary. Vaginoscopy may be performed with a Killian nasal speculum in the young child. Should vaginoscopy fail to reveal the foreign body, gentle probing of the vagina frequently reveals its presence. Once the object has been removed, the vaginal discharge ceases.

Although most foreign bodies are easily removed, occasionally the object erodes into the vaginal wall. An incision in the mucosa is then necessary to remove it. If a vaginal foreign body has been present for a long period of time, vaginal stenosis may occur.

Labial adhesions. Labial adhesions (synechiae vulvae), a complete or partial fusion of lower labia majora or labia minora in the midline, occur most commonly in girls 6 months to 6 years of age. The cause is unknown but may be related to low circulating estrogen levels and an irritation that erodes the vulvar epithelium, causing the labia to stick together. This concept is supported by the observations that synechiae vulvae is not seen in neonates but is acquired within the first 2 years of life, when the level of circulating estrogen is extremely low, and the use of estrogen creams causes synechiae to disappear.

Occasionally the vaginal orifice is completely covered, causing poor drainage of vaginal secretions and sequestering of urine in the vagina. Parents often become alarmed because the vagina appears "absent."

Diagnosis is made by simple observation. There is fusion of the labia minora and the hymen is not visible. The line of fusion is a thin, transparent membrane which may involve the inner surfaces of the labia. Most frequently, the fusion ends several millimeters behind the clitoris but anterior to the external urethral meatus. There may be several perforations in the membrane, or the adhesions may be partial either anteriorly or posteriorly (Fig. 23-14).

In mild cases no treatment is necessary because the labia usually separate completely at puberty. If symptomatic, they should be treated.

In cases of complete synechia where vaginal or urinary drainage is impaired or the child complains of pain, an estrogen-containing cream should be applied twice daily for 3 weeks followed by once daily for 3 weeks. After 2 weeks of therapy the patient should be seen in follow-up. If the labial adhesion has resolved, then the premarin cream is continued once daily for 1 week. After the discontinuation of the estrogen cream, the use of a bland ointment (e.g., Desitin or White's A and D) is helpful in attempts to keep the labial adhesions from reforming. Occasionally, a repeat course of therapy is necessary. Forceful separation without anesthesia is generally contraindicated because it is traumatic for the child and may cause the adhesions to form again. When

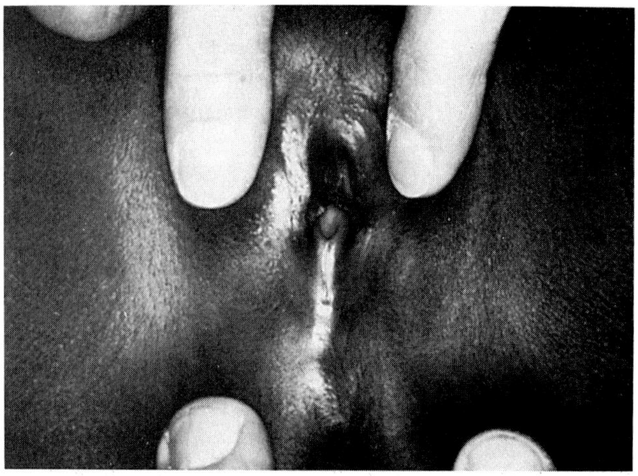

Fig. 23-15. Labial adhesions in a 4-year-old with almost totally fused labia. Note small opening at level of urethra.

Table 23-2. Differential diagnosis of vaginal bleeding in prepubertal children

- Infection
  - Primary
    - Bacterial
    - Fungal
    - Parasitic
    - Viral
  - Secondary
    - Foreign body
    - Reflux of urine
    - Pelvic abscess
    - Fistula
- Trauma
  - Accidental
  - Sexual abuse
- Endocrine abnormalities
  - Newborn bleeding resulting from maternal estrogen withdrawal
  - Isosexual precocity
  - Exogenous hormone ingestion
  - Hypothyroidism
- Anatomical abnormalities
  - Prolapse of urethral mucosa
  - Vaginal and/or uterine prolapse
  - Cervical ectropion
  - Ectopic ureter
- Idiopathic
  - Vulvar dystrophy
  - Vulvitis secondary to irritants
  - Premature endometrial activity
  - Self induced
- Neoplasms
  - Benign
  - Malignant
- Blood dyscrasias
  - Coagulopathy
  - Hematologic neoplasms

estrogen therapy fails, separation is best performed under general anesthetic, followed by application of a bland ointment and gentle separation by the parent at regular intervals. Occasionally separation can be accomplished in the examining room with application of 5% lidocaine gel and manipulation with a cotton swab.

Regardless of the method of treatment, 10% to 15% of synechiae recur. Though spontaneous separation at puberty is the rule, sometimes patients in the midteens are referred because of "hypoplastic labia," but once separation is accomplished under anesthetic, the vulva is found to be quite normal.

Vaginal bleeding

Most girls have their first menstrual period between 9 and 16 years of age. Except for hormone withdrawal bleeding during the first or second week of life, genital bleeding before the age of 9 years is not normal and most likely results from organic causes. Therefore, vaginal bleeding in the prepubertal years should be taken seriously and always carefully assessed.

Classically, vaginal bleeding in childhood is divided as follows: (1) that associated with signs of isosexual precocity, and (2) that not associated with signs of isosexual precocity. However, we find it more useful to classify the problem on the basis of etiologic factors (Table 23-2).

Vulvovaginitis. Vulvovaginitis with or without the presence of a foreign body was the most common cause of vaginal bleeding in 63 patients younger than age 9 years who presented at one gynecology clinic between January 1974 and December 1983 (Table 23-3). When a young child presents with vaginal bleeding, it is mandatory to perform a thorough investigation to rule out the presence of malignancy. It has been the policy to perform an examination under anesthetic as part of the initial workup unless there was complete confidence that full visualization of the cervix and vagina was possible during the outpatient examination.

Coagulation disorder. Hematologic evaluation to rule out coagulation disorders should be performed preoperatively. However, patients with vaginal bleeding resulting from

Table 23-3. Vaginal bleeding in children younger than age 9 years, 1974-1983

Cause	No.	%
Infection	41	65
Trauma	10	16
Endocrine abnormalities	3	5
Anatomical abnormalities	3	5
Blood dyscrasias	3	5
Idiopathic	2	3
Neoplasms	1	2
TOTAL	63	100

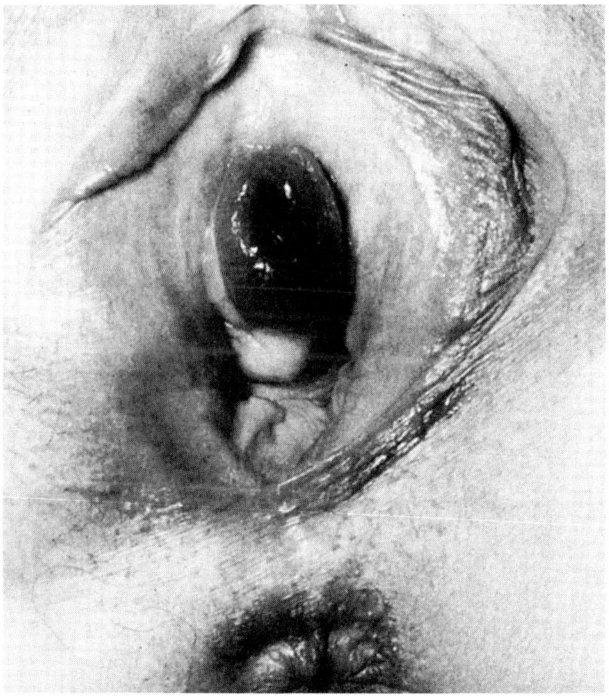

Fig. 23-16. Prolapse of urethral meatus in 9-year-old who presented with bloody discharge and dysuria.

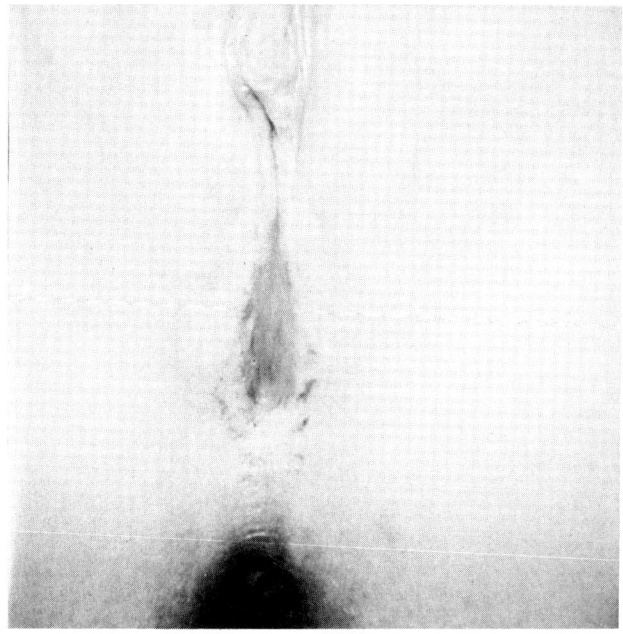

Fig. 23-17. Extensive lichen sclerosus et atrophica in a prepubertal child with characteristic parchment-like skin, chronic ulceration, and secondary inflammation.

blood dyscrasias usually have other signs of bleeding such as epistaxis, petechiae, or hematomas.

Prolapse of the urethra. Occasionally, vaginal bleeding may be a sign of urethral prolapse. Examination reveals the characteristic friable red-blue (doughnut-like) annular mass (Fig. 23-15). The patient may complain of dysuria, bleeding, and pain that developed after coughing, straining, or occasionally trauma. The diagnosis is made by the characteristic shape of the lesion and visualization of the vaginal orifice with the patient in the supine or knee-chest position. Urethral prolapse may resolve spontaneously with sitz baths, but some cases of prolapse require intervention. Because the distal urethra is estrogen dependent, a course of estrogen cream, twice daily for 2 weeks usually results in resolution of the urethral prolapse. If the prolapse does not resolve, surgery may be needed. The CO_2 laser is ideally suited for this condition and appears to be less traumatic than cold knife excision. In cases of prolapse with necrosis of the distal urethra, surgery is the first line of therapy.

Premature menarche. Cyclic vaginal bleeding without signs of pubertal development is rare. Although several girls with this problem have been followed, one of whom has a mother who had the same pattern of bleeding in her prepubertal years, a full examination under anesthesia and an endometrial biopsy is indicated to rule out endometrial pathology. Results of the biopsy usually show only early proliferative endometrium despite the absence of sexual development. Although the etiology of precocious menarche is obscure, it probably results from the prolonged stimulation of unusually sensitive endometrium by weak extragonadal estrogens.

Lichen sclerosus. Lichen sclerosus is an increasingly common disorder in prepubertal children. The reason for this is not certain, although the more prevalent use of synthetic fibers and clinical detergents may be unmasking latent cases in the prepubertal age group. Patients usually complain of itching, irritation, soreness, and dysuria and less commonly of constipation, vaginal discharge, and bleeding. The vulva characteristically has white, atrophic, parchment-like skin, and evidence of chronic ulceration and inflammation from scratching. Often, the involvement of the perianal area along with the labia may give the affected area an hourglass configuration. Secondary infection often occurs. The condition should be distinguished from vitiligo, which causes loss of pigmentation but not inflammation or atrophy.

The diagnosis of lichen sclerosus is made clinically and by examining a biopsy specimen (Fig. 23-16). The treatment aims at elimination of local irritants and any vaginitis present and improved hygiene. Soaps should not be overused; the child should be encouraged to wear cotton underpants and loose-fitting pants or skirts to minimize local maceration and irritation. A short course of topical hydrocortisone ointment for a few weeks is currently used in an attempt to bring the condition under control. Oral medications such as hydroxyzine hydrochloride can be helpful for intense pruritus at bedtime.

The use of 1% hydrocortisone cream applied 1 to 3 times daily meets with excellent results. If needed, testosterone proprianate 2% to 5% in petrolatum gel applied 1 to 3 times daily has been advocated. This medication has been used with an excellent response in some patients. However, the use of topical testosterone is limited by the development of clitoromegaly after 2 to 3 months of treatment.

Severe cases of lichen sclerosus, particularly when associated with extensive excoriation and debris, respond to superficial vaporization with the CO_2 laser (Fig. 23-17). Dramatic results have been seen in a number of patients who failed to respond to more conservative therapy. Laser treatment may interrupt the scratch-itch cycle and allow healing. Most patients, but not all, will note improvement or regression of lesions with puberty.

Clitoral infection. The clitoral hood may occasionally develop an infection with intense edema and erythema. Antibiotics such as dicloxacillin or cephalosporin should be given orally and warm soaks applied. Surgical incision and drainage are necessary if an abscess becomes fluctuant.

Recently a "clitoral tourniquet syndrome" in which a hair had become wrapped around the clitoris, resulting in edema and severe pain, has been described. After removal of the hair, the clitoris returned to normal size. This syndrome is similar to strangulation by hair of other parts of the body, such as fingers, toes, or penis.

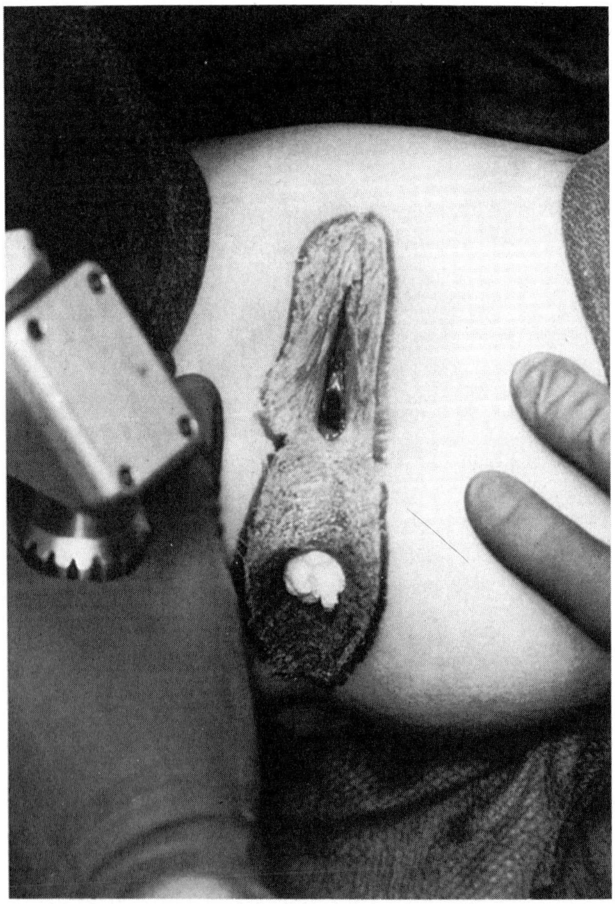

Fig. 23-18. Carbon dioxide laser debridement of adolescent patient with extensive lichen sclerosus at atrophica.

Genital trauma

Trauma to the external genitalia. Female genital trauma is not unusual. The injury may be localized and relatively minor or accompanied by other distant, life-threatening injuries.

The differences between the internal and external genitalia of the child and those of the adult make a perineal injury in a child potentially quite serious. The distance between the perineal skin and the peritoneal cavity is short in the young child. Thus, penetrating injuries can easily damage intraperitoneal organs. The bladder in the infant is an intraperitoneal organ and more easily injured. The urogenital diaphragm, which contains the pudendal nerves and vessels, is very superficial in infants and children. Therefore a relatively superficial laceration can result in massive hemorrhage. Finally, the rectovaginal septum is thin and the perineal body is small; both can be torn easily.

Genital injuries may be accidental, self-induced, or the result of an assault. Straddle injury is responsible for 75% of genital injuries in girls and may be blunt or penetrating. Other common causes are stabbing and automobile accidents. Accidental genital trauma is most common between 4 and 12 years of age.

Because examination of the perineum is often difficult in a bleeding, distraught child, some sedation is advisable. The abdomen must be carefully examined for intraabdominal injury. Abdominal radiographs that include the pelvis may show free air from a perforated viscus, or a pelvic fracture may be evident. A urinalysis should be obtained and checked for blood; if hematuria is present, an IVP and cystogram are indicated. No urine output may indicate an urethral or bladder laceration.

Treatment. Contusions of the perineum and vulva without laceration or bleeding are the most common injury. They may range from a mild ecchymotic area to a large vulvar hematoma that may require surgical intervention. In general, however, a conservative approach in the management of these problems with application of ice packs, analgesic, and bed rest is advocated. An indwelling Foley catheter or suprapubic drainage may be required, depending on the extent of the hematoma. Small lacerations of the labia and hymen usually require suturing; bleeding can be profuse even though the laceration is small.

All lacerations require a thorough examination of the vulva and vagina. This can be accomplished by the use of saline irrigation using IV tubing (Fig. 23-13) directed toward the perineum and into the vagina. Irrigating fluid will wash out the vagina and permit injection of a local anesthetic with epinephrine to decrease bleeding. Absorbable sutures can be inserted immediately. A laceration that does not extend through to the hymen usually does not invade the vagina.

More extensive lacerations always require general anesthesia for both evaluation and treatment. Thus diagnosis and treatment often occur simultaneously. Endoscopic examination of the urethra, bladder, vagina, or rectum is indicated if injuries are adjacent. Most lacerations can be closed primarily, even if extensive, unless fecal contamination is present because of rectal injury. In that event, closure is delayed until appropriate antibiotic treatment and closure of the viscus is accomplished. Using absorbable sutures avoids the need to remove them at a later date.

A particularly difficult injury occurs when the urogenital diaphragm is bluntly compressed against the pubic ramus. A tear in the periurethral structures bleeds profusely and requires a deep mattress suture. Lacerations near or into the urethra require catheterization for 7 to 10 days.

Lacerations into the vaginal fornix may require laparotomy for closure because of the small size of the child's introitus.

A laceration extending in the posterior direction from the introitus should be evaluated for the possibility of sexual abuse, unless there is a history of trauma from an accidental fall on a nail, picket fence, or some other penetrating object. A careful endoscopic search for rectovaginal tears must be carried out prior to closure. Laparotomy is indicated for intra-abdominal injury or for uncontrollable hemorrhage. Tetanus prophylaxis and antibiotic coverage are indicated.

The majority of properly diagnosed and treated genital injuries heal quickly. However, inadequate treatment of lacerations may result in complications from infection. Urethral and vaginal strictures may develop and an unrecognized rectovaginal tear will result in a rectovaginal fistula.

Frequent examinations must be performed until complete healing has occurred. Infection, stricture formation, and delayed hemorrhage occur after adequate treatment in 11% to 25% of cases.

Sexual abuse: the gynecologist's role

Over the past 10 years the number of young girls who are referred for examination because of suspected sexual abuse has markedly increased. The majority of cases of sexual abuse are dealt with most effectively by sexual abuse teams that include a pediatrician, clinical psychologist, social worker, and nurse practitioner. The gynecologist does, however, play a vital role in the assessment, documentation, and treatment of sexually induced infection and trauma.

Great care must be exercised by the physician who is asked to examine a child thought to have been sexually assaulted. Gentle questioning is used to gain enough information necessary to gynecologically evaluate the case. Extensive questioning should be carried out by a qualified clinical psychologist or social worker. The gynecologist's goal is to perform the physical examination and collect the appropriate specimens for the forensic pathologist to evaluate.

The history of the assault is difficult to obtain from the very young child and usually must be obtained from relatives, police, or neighbors. A reliable history can be obtained directly from a child 4 to 5 years of age in most cases. However, the physician must first determine the words used by the child to describe the genitals; this information often is readily obtained from the child's parents.

The sex of the alleged assailant should be determined. Rape refers to the forced act of penetration without consent of the victim. Penetration of the vagina can be caused by a penis or other object such as a finger and thus may involve either a male or female assailant. In addition penetration may involve the mouth or anus.

The examination of the victim requires proper instrumentation; general anesthesia is necessary in infants and children. Table 23-4 outlines the examination of the pediatric patient who has been sexually assaulted.

Colposcopic evaluation of the hymen. The colposcope as a means of documenting sexual trauma is becoming increasingly popular.[75,86,106,109] The advantages to use of the colposcope are as follows: (1) the hymen and vulva can be greatly magnified to detect small changes not visible to the naked eye, and (2) photographs are easily taken at the time of the examination to provide future documentation. The latter prevents the need for repeated examinations when the presence of physical findings is disputed. The problem with the use of colposcopy has been that until recently, normal genital anatomy in prepubertal girls has not been well defined.[5,6,31,38,76] The problem has been compounded by the difficulty in assessing the strength of the association between a history of sexual abuse and variations in the hymenal appearance in individual cases, variations in the 50 states' statutory definition of sexual crimes, and misunderstanding among professionals providing examinations for victims of sexual abuse about the meaning of "penetration."

An atlas of photographs to aid physicians in assessing their own patients is of great benefit. One excellent example of

Table 23-4. Examination of the sexually assaulted patient

1. Obtain consent to examination from parent or guardian, preferably written.
2. Obtain detailed general history: past illnesses, accidents, operations.
3. Obtain detailed specific history: details of alleged incident.
4. Observe: manner, dress.
5. Examine all clothing: remove with physician present; inspect each item separately; retain each item in clean bag; note damage to clothes, staining, soiling, ultraviolet light on underpants, etc.
6. Complete general clinical examination: examine entire body and record all findings; record all injuries, old and new, location, size, description.
7. Examine genitalia; swab vulva and vagina first without lubricant; note injury to labia, hymen, mucosa, thighs, signs of seminal fluid, blood, lubricant.
8. Obtain specimens: buccal swab; blood; saliva; hair; avulsed head hair, loose hairs, pubic hair combings; areas of soiling; fingernail scrapings, clippings; swabs from perineum; vaginal swabs; swabs of anal verge and anal canal.

such an atlas is *Evaluation of the Sexually Abused Child.* The use of the colposcope has greatly increased the physician's knowledge of normal anatomy and fine-tuned visual skills. It is likely that knowledgeable physicians seeing a child for routine annual examination or assessing a genital problem will note changes suggestive of sexual abuse.

The value of the colposcopic examination in the determination of sexual abuse has been a subject of controversy. The percentage of children with a "normal" examination has varied from 16% to 85%, depending on the case mix and age of patients, the definition of normal versus abnormal, and the examiners.[1,11,12,31,83-85,112]

In a clinic survey, children presenting with a history of sexual abuse were compared with children seen for either routine examinations or genital complaints. Girls with a history of sexual abuse were more likely to have scars, friability of the posterior fourchette as the labia were separated, synechiae, and attenuated hymens than girls seen for routine examinations. Hymenal transections or tears, condylomata, and abrasions occurred among only the sexually abused girls. Girls with a history of genital complaints often had findings similar to those of girls with a history of sexual abuse. Vulvar erythema and friability of the posterior fourchette likely occurs secondary to inflammation; scars are probably the result of trauma. Because girls may take months to years to reveal a history of sexual abuse, it is probable that some who were evaluated for vaginitis may have been abused. The finding of a narrow, thin, posterior rim of the hymen in children with vaginitis may mean that these girls had been abused or that this particular anatomical variant may predispose a subset of girls to vaginal contamination and symptoms. In contrast, a narrow rim that has become rounded and scarred with attachment to the vagina likely has resulted from sexual abuse.

The significance of a labial adhesion in a child with a history of sexual abuse is controversial because many normal children have adhesions, and yet it is possible that rubbing and irritation from abuse may also cause agglutination to occur. These adhesions are sometimes mistaken for scars. The difference is usually evident with careful observation; if not, a short trial of estrogen-containing cream which would lyse most labial adhesions but not scars, could be used.

The white midline median raphe evident in some children is frequently confused with a scar in the posterior fourchette. Conditions such as lichen sclerosus, failure of midline fusion from the anus to the posterior fourchette, and ulcerating hemangioma have been confused with trauma from sexual abuse.

Children who have a history of sodomy frequently have no abnormal findings. Minor redness and hyperpigmentation and reflex anal dilation are nonspecific findings that can have other etiologies. More specific findings include scars and distortion of the anus, although the latter can occur with inflammatory bowel disease. Fissures can result from abuse but also from constipation.

The significance of measurements of the diameter of the hymenal orifice is controversial.[31,48,92] The transverse and anteroposterior measurements are influenced by age, relaxation of the child, method of examination and measurement, and type of hymen. The older the child and the more relaxed, the larger the opening. The opening is larger with retraction on the labia and in the knee-chest position than with gentle separation alone in the supine position. The orifice of a posterior rim hymen will appear larger than the opening of a redundant hymen. Because the hymen is distensible, vaginal penetration can have occurred even though the measurement is only 5 mm. In cases of sexual abuse, both anteroposterior and transverse dimensions are measured using a Tine test 5-cm ruler. Some colposcopes have the markings in the eyepiece and direct measurement can be done during the examination. More data on normal children are needed, but a study of 3- to 6-year-old girls found a mean transverse measurement of 2.9 ± 1.3 mm (range 1 to 6 mm) and mean anteroposterior measurement of 3.3 ± 1.5 mm (range 1 to 7 mm). A good rule of thumb is 1 mm for each year of age as the upper limits of normal (e.g., 8 mm for an 8-year-old child), remembering all the caveats of changes with relaxation and position. McCann et al have used a supine traction technique and report a mean horizontal diameter of 5.2 ± 1.4 mm (range 2 to 8 mm) for girls aged 2 years to 4 years 11 months and 5.6 ± 1.8 mm (range 1 to 9 mm) for girls aged 5 years to 7 years 11 months.[76] A large hymenal orifice may be consistent with a history of sexual abuse but should be considered only a part of the evaluation, and not the absolute criterion.

Gynecologic findings during the evaluation. Findings on examination can be classified according to the system described by Muram.[83] These are described as follows: (1) normal; (2) nonspecific (e.g., inflammation, erythema); (3) specific (e.g., acute or healed laceration); and (4) definitive (e.g., presence of sperm).

It has been shown and must be remembered that healing from vaginal and anal trauma is rapid[74,75]; thus the findings on examination may be normal.

Repair of sexual trauma. Another important role for the gynecologist is the evaluation and repair of sexually induced trauma to the perineum in sexually abused children. The extent of the genital injury depends on the nature and size of the penetrating object, the size of the pelvic outlet and vagina, and the force with which penetration is attempted. Thus, injury may range from a simple vulvar or hymeneal tear to a full thickness laceration of the posterior fourchette with intraperitoneal involvement.

It is wise to postpone gynecologic examination until all appropriate cultures and specimens are obtained. Photographic documentation of all traumas is essential. If adequate examination is not possible in the office, clinic, or emergency room, then an examination under anesthesia is mandatory.

In general, the younger and smaller the child, the more widespread the injuries produced by penile penetration because she is less able to resist assault. Thus with the younger child, a lower threshold should be used to initiate an examination under anesthesia.

The only form of resistance to assault may be screaming, which may lead to attempts to silence her. The inner surfaces of the lips should be examined for abrasion or bruising from the lips being forced back against the teeth. Check for loose teeth and damage to the frenulum of the upper lip. Grasping injuries of the arms, thighs, wrists, legs, and ankles are common when the assailant is unknown to the child.

Anorectal injury must be evaluated by examination of the anal canal. Tears in the anorectum are evidence of anal penetration. Bruising and swelling of the anal verge are common findings. Laxity of the anal sphincter is difficult to assess, especially under anesthesia.

After appropriate evaluation, injuries to the female genitalia from assault are treated in the same manner as accidental injuries. The full extent of the injury should be evaluated and then repaired layer by layer with restoration of normal anatomy.

TUMORS

Labial masses

Gynecologic tumors are rare in childhood. They are usually benign and localized to the external genitalia. A few patients with fibromas, lipomas, and myomas have been encountered. They should be surgically excised, generally on an outpatient basis.

Abdominal/pelvic masses

The differential diagnosis of an abdominal/pelvic mass in this age group includes polycystic kidneys, pelvic kidneys, neuroblastomas, intussusception, rhabdomyosarcomas, congenital müllerian abnormalities, and ovarian neoplasms.

Benign ovarian masses

Congenital ovarian cysts. With the more widespread use of sonography in the third trimester, a number of newborn infants are referred for management of cystic masses in the pelvis. These are characteristically single, fluid-filled structures without septation or solid components. Most of these are benign functional cysts that are felt to be the result of maternal estrogen and hCG stimulation of the fetal ovary. They usually resolve spontaneously within 2 to 3 months, but may take up to 1 year to fully resolve. They are generally palpable on rectal examination. If they are large and persistent, they may become palpable abdominally. If the infant appears symptomatic with difficulty feeding or abdominal pain, it may be necessary to intervene. In these cases, aspiration under ultrasound guidance has been successful. Caution should be exercised in transabdominal aspiration because a cystic structure in the pelvis may be due to cysts of other organ systems, such as the urinary tract, mesentery, and paratubal or parovarian structures. Aspirated cyst fluid should be sent for cytologic evaluation. If the cyst is complex, unable to be aspirated, or recurs, then a laparoscopy or laparotomy may be indicated. Care should be taken to perform a procedure that will maintain pelvic anatomy. Thus an ovarian cystectomy should be performed whenever possible with conservation of normal ovarian tissue.

In childhood, multiple small ovarian cysts may be present and are normal. These may be found incidentally on ultrasound evaluation for abdominal pain. These cysts will be simple (without septation, debris, or a thickened capsule) and usually resolve spontaneously.

Other benign masses of the ovary include simple serous or mucinous cysts. Solid tumors of the ovary may be present and are most commonly mature cystic teratomas (dermoids).

Malignant tumors. Ovarian cancer is the most common malignancy (60%) of the female genital tract in the pediatric population. Ovarian cancer accounts for 1% of all pediatric malignancies. The most common malignancy is a germ cell tumor. Germ cell tumors account for 20% of all ovarian malignancies and occur most often in the pediatric age groups.

Germ cell tumors grow rapidly, and commonly present with pain and/or a rapidly enlarging abdominal mass. The most common germ cell tumors are the immature teratoma and the dysgerminoma. Other germ cell tumors include the endodermal sinus tumor, embryonal carcinoma, mixed germ cell tumor, and primary (nongestational) choriocarcinoma.

Other ovarian malignant tumors presenting in childhood include gonadoblastomas and sex cord tumors (granulosa-stromal cell tumors, Sertoli-Leydig cell tumors, gynandroblastoma, and nonspecific stromal tumors).

If a malignant tumor is suspected, tumor markers should be obtained. The common tumor markers and their associated tumors are discussed in detail in Chapter 9.

The management of ovarian malignancies in the pediatric population is directed at conservative therapy with conservation of pelvic anatomy and reproductive function. A staging laparotomy is performed, and staging is according to FIGO staging criteria for adult ovarian malignancies (Chapter 9). A unilateral salpingo-oophorectomy with adjuvant chemotherapy is the treatment of choice.

Vaginal masses in the pediatric population

Benign. Hymeneal tags and other hymeneal abnormalities presenting in children are discussed above, and those presenting in adolescents are discussed below. Benign vaginal polyps may also present in the pediatric population.

Malignant. The malignant tumor involving the vagina, uterus, bladder, and urethra of young children most frequently is rhabdomyosarcoma (sarcoma botryoides). The symptoms include vaginal discharge, bleeding, abdominal pain or mass, or the passage of grapelike lesions. On examination, the tumors appear as prolapse of grapelike masses through the urethra or vagina. A vaginal tag seen on vaginal examination should never be assumed to be benign. Growth of the tumor is rapid and prognosis poor unless the diagnosis is made early and prompt radical surgical excision is performed. Regardless of whether or not there is additional treatment with radiotherapy and/or chemotherapy, prognosis depends on the extent of the disease.

Ovarian transposition for radiation therapy

Radiation-induced gonadal dysfunction is dose dependent.[89] With improvements in longterm survival rates of patients with childhood malignancies it is of increased importance for the pediatric gynecologist to offer options for gonadal protection.

Oophoropexy with the repositioning of the ovaries out of the field of radiation has been well described.[71,97] The oophoropexy can decrease the radiation dose to the ovary and improve gonadal function.[23,69,110,111] Historically this procedure has been performed via laparotomy, but recently a new technique for laparoscopic ovarian transposition for young girls with medulloblastoma was reported.[65] With this procedure it was shown that moving the ovary inferiorly and laterally out of the craniospinal irradiation field decreased the radiation exposure to the pexed ovary to less than 5%. Future studies will need to be performed to document beneficial effects on gonadal protection, although it is hypothesized that the beneficial effects will be similar to that of classic oophoropexy.

GYNECOLOGIC PROBLEMS AT PUBERTY

Normal pubertal development

The prerequisites for the development of normal reproductive function in the female are as follows: (1) normal hypothalamus capable of responding to elevated levels of steroids by appropriate pulsatile secretion of GnRH, (2) a normal pituitary that is sensitive to GnRH and estrogen (or progesterone) and contains a pool of releasable gonadotropins, and (3) normal ovaries capable of secreting steroids (estrogen and progesterone) in response to pituitary gonadotropins (LH and follicle-stimulating hormone [FSH]).

The harmony of the menstrual cycle is a product of an elaborate pubertal process in which the hypothalamic-pituitary-ovarian axis develops concomitant to noted physical changes in the female. It is after the completion of the pubertal process that an individual is fully mature and able to reproduce. The onset of the pubertal event in each individual is variable and influenced profoundly by genetic and environmental factors (e.g., chronic disease and nutrition). The average onset of puberty in the United States is between ages 8 and 13 years which is earlier than the average worldwide; better nutrition is one theory explaining this phenomenon.[35,36] Because the age at the onset of puberty among individuals varies widely (8 to 18 years), bone age correlates best with pubertal age. Therefore, when an individual with delayed or advanced puberty is evaluated, it is important to obtain a bone age study.

To understand the hormone changes during puberty we should review the changes in LH and FSH secretion from the time in utero to puberty. Gonadarche and adrenarche are separate events. Puberty is believed to be controlled by a GnRH sensitivity threshold in the hypothalamus that decreases with increased maturity of the hypothalamic-pituitary axis. Therefore the CNS appears to control the onset of puberty, and thus the secretion of steroid hormones. The first signs of puberty include the commencement of sleep-associated pulsatile GnRH secretion. However, after normal pubertal development has been accomplished, the hypothalamic-pituitary axis becomes subservient to the positive and negative feedback signals from the ovary.

The control of adrenarche is not completely understood, but appears to be under adrenal control. Adrenarche causes pubic and axillary hair growth. The rise in adrenal androgens precedes the growth spurt by 2 years and involves an acceleration in size of the zona reticularis. There is subsequent increased secretion of androgens (DHEA and dehydroepiandrosterone sulphate [DHEAS]).

Pituitary secretion of gonadotropins decreases from about age 4 to 11 years. This is believed to be the result of the development of an intrinsic CNS inhibitory mechanism that suppresses pulsatile GnRH release. Chronologically, the onset of puberty is thus heralded by a decrease in the CNS inhibitory restraint and a decrease in the negative feedback effect. An increase in GnRH secretion and pituitary responsiveness follows.

This responsiveness is demonstrated by the LH response to exogenous GnRH administration (GnRH Stimulation Test). Prepubertal children show a minimal response to GnRH, secreting a small but significant LH peak. Pubertal children and adults have a much greater LH response to GnRH administration. This increase in pituitary reserve and secretion of LH is the hallmark of puberty, and it is elicited before any physical evidence of secondary sexual development. As stated above, the maturational change seen in puberty is sleep-associated pulsatile LH secretion.

The final phase of the maturational changes that take place is the development of cyclic release of LH in response to the positive feedback of estradiol. This elicits the midcycle surge in gonadotropins seen in the normal female menstrual cycle after puberty. A typical cyclic adult pattern is not achieved, however, until these are regular ovulatory events with resulting increased luteal progesterone concentrations (greater than 10 ng/mL).

Concomitant with these changes are differences in adrenocortical functioning, with an increase in adrenal androgen, namely DHEAS (adrenarche). Adrenal maturation, however, is a separate event. In agonadal children, a decrease in basal gonadotropins also occurs at ages 4 to 11 years, attesting to the isolated importance of a maturing CNS inhibitory influence during this period. Adrenarche also occurs in patients with both hypergonadotropic and hypogonadotropic hypogonadism (not hypopituitarism).

"Minimum" weight is another criterion that appears to be associated with normal menstrual function. Losses as little as 10% to 15% of body weight affect the menstrual cycle. A relative degree of body fat is associated with sexual maturation.[34]

Table 23-5. Normal pubertal development milestones

	Age of occurrence	
	Mean	Range
Thelarche	10.9	9.0–13.5
Adrenarche	11.2	9.5–14
Peak height velocity	11.5	9.0–14
Menarche	12.7	11.0–16

A summary of normal pubertal developmental milestones is shown in Table 23-5.

Abnormal pubertal development

A thorough understanding of the normal progression of puberty is essential in the evaluation of patients with precocious puberty. The definition of precocious puberty is the development of secondary sexual characteristics prior to age 8 years. This represents 2.5 standard deviations from the normal.

In normal adolescence, estrogen is responsible for breast development, maturation of the external genitalia, vagina, and uterus, and initiation of menses. An increase in adrenal androgens is associated with the appearance of pubic and axillary hair. Excess androgens of either ovarian or adrenal origin may cause acne, hirsutism, voice changes, increased muscle mass, and clitoromegaly.

Precocious puberty can be divided into three categories as follows: (1) complete or true precocious puberty (GnRH-dependent), (2) incomplete or pseudoprecocious puberty, and (3) extrapituitary gonadotropin production (GnRH-independent).

Premature thelarche. Premature thelarche is most commonly seen among young girls 1 to 4 years of age. Occasionally, neonatal breast hypertrophy fails to regress within 6 months after birth. This persistent breast development is characterized as premature thelarche. The typical child with premature thelarche has bilateral breast buds of 2 to 4 cm with little or no change in the nipple or areola. The breast tissue feels granular and may be slightly tender. In some cases, development is quite asymmetric; one side may develop 6 to 12 months before the other. Growth is not accelerated, and the bone age is normal for height age. No other evidence of puberty appears; the vulva and vagina remain prepubertal without evidence of estrogen effect.

Although it was originally thought that premature thelarche was caused by an increased end-organ sensitivity to low levels of endogenous estrogen, the fact that there are at least transiently elevated serum estrogen levels suggests that small luteinized or cystic graafian follicles may be responsible in some cases. The usual clinical course of regression or lack of progression of breast development correlates with the waning of the estrogen levels as the follicles become atretic.

Treatment consists mainly of reassurance and careful follow-up to confirm that the breast development does not represent the first signs of precocious puberty.

Premature adrenarche. Most patients with premature adrenarche have a slight increase in urinary 17-ketosteroid production and increased plasma DHEA and DHEAS levels, suggesting that hormone biosynthesis in the adrenal gland undergoes maturation prematurely to a pubertal pattern. Although production of these androgens is suppressible by dexamethasone and therefore are dependent on ACTH, the mediator for the change at puberty and in premature adrenarche is unknown.

The assessment of the patient with premature adrenarche is similar to that for heterosexual precocious puberty. The important physical findings are the presence of virilization (pubic hair) and the absence of breast development, or estrogenization of the labia and vagina.

Laboratory tests should include a radiologic examination of the nondominant wrist for bone age, vaginal smear (for maturational index), a 24-hour urine test for free cortisol, and serum DHEAS, testosterone, and 17-hydroxyprogesterone. The clinical studies should be directed at the differential diagnosis which must exclude precocious puberty, congenital adrenal hyperplasia, and an adrenal or ovarian tumor.

Treatment of premature adrenarche is reassurance and follow-up. The child should be examined every 6 months to confirm the original diagnostic impression. In general, pubertal development at adolescence can be expected to be normal but follow-up is necessary to evaluate the progression of a hyperandrogenic state.

Precocious puberty. Puberty is considered precocious if secondary sexual characteristics occur prior to 8 years of age. This occurs in the general population in an incidence of 1 per 5000 to 1 per 10,000. The female/male ratio is between 4:1 and 8:1. This is usually accomplished by accelerated linear growth (advanced bone age). Precocity may be the result of constitutional or organic causes. The majority of cases of isosexual precocious puberty are of a constitutional or idiopathic form (85% of females), and it may be familial. It is, however, vital to distinguish these patients from those who have precocity based on lesions of the brain, ovary, or adrenal glands. Therefore, sexual precocity may be due to central or CNS causes (includes constitutional) or extrapituitary causes (ovarian tumors, adrenal tumors).

Isosexual precocious puberty. In true isosexual precocity, the stimulus for development arises in the hypothalamus and pituitary gland. In response to rising LH and FSH levels, the ovaries produce estrogen. The young girl develops breasts and pubic and axillary hair and begins menstruation, sometimes not in the usual sequence. With the establishment of the cyclic midcycle LH peak, the child becomes potentially fertile.

In isosexual pseudoprecocity, an ovarian tumor or cyst or adrenal adenoma produces estrogen autonomously. The fluctuating estrogen levels result in sexual development and anovulatory menses. In more than 80% of patients with isosexual precocious puberty, the hypothalamic-pituitary axis is activated prematurely for unknown reasons.

Despite the relatively high incidence of constitutional or idiopathic precocious puberty, this diagnosis cannot be made without a thorough evaluation and exclusion of some of the following organic causes:

1. Cerebral disorders (5% to 10% of cases)
2. Ovarian tumors (5% of cases)
3. Adrenal disorders (rare)
4. Gonadotropin-producing tumors (rare)
5. Hypothyroidism (rare)
6. Iatrogenic disorders (rare)

Patient assessment by the gynecologist/reproductive endocrinologist should include a careful history and physical examination and a family history. It is important to perform appropriate studies to rule out cerebral disorders and ovarian tumors, which are the two most common organic causes of this condition.

The first crucial steps in an initial evaluation of precocious puberty are careful history taking (rule out exogenous steroid administration, history of encephalitis, and cerebral trauma) and meticulous physical examination. Blood pressure, accelerated development of thelarche, pubarche, gonadarche, and growth spurt are noted. Skin changes and any café au lait spots are documented. Pelvic and abdominal examination may indicate the presence of an ovarian or adrenal mass, which is further confirmed by ultrasound scanning. Bone radiography documents accelerated linear growth and epiphyseal closure (and also excludes fibrous dysplasia). Skull radiography, computed tomography (CT) scan, or MRI rules out intracranial pathologic lesions. Chemical precocity is indicated by adolescent levels of FSH, LH, and estradiol-17b. These may be found to be elevated only on blood samples obtained at night. Thyroid function tests exclude hypothyroidism. Elevated DHEAS or 17-hydroxyprogesterone points to either possible late-onset CAH or an adrenal neoplasm (especially if documented by scan). In the latter condition, suppression does not occur with a dexamethasone suppression test, whereas suppression does occur in CAH. Increased urinary hCG level may indicate a rare trophoblastic tumor. Exogenous LH and GnRH administration can discriminate between extrapituitary causes of precocity (ovarian tumors) and central causes. The latter will have a pubertal LH response after such stimulation, whereas the former will not. Finally, if the use of exogenous steroids, CNS disease, hypothyroidism, late-onset CAH, McCune-Albright syndrome, and adrenal or ovarian masses are excluded, idiopathic isosexual precocious puberty is the most likely diagnosis.

Treatment and follow-up depend on the diagnosis. Ovarian tumors and CNS tumors require surgical intervention. Idiopathic and CNS-induced precocity can be treated effectively with GnRH agonist therapy. The goals of treatment for precocious puberty are to halt the premature closure of the epiphyses and thus increase final adult height, and to halt the precocious development of secondary sexual development so that the individual is not at increased risk of sexual abuse or other emotionally scarring situations.

Despite the diagnosis of idiopathic precocious puberty, follow-up must continue at least every 6 months to exclude the possibility of organic disease not originally evident. Children with sexual precocity do not automatically manifest intellectual or psychosocial precocity; the degree of psychologic maturity of a young girl is more likely to be related to the life experiences she encounters and transacts.

Heterosexual precocious puberty. Heterosexual precocity arises from excess androgen production from an adrenal or ovarian source, which results in acne, hirsutism, and virilization. The differential diagnosis includes the following: (1) CAH; (2) Cushing's syndrome; (3) adrenal tumors; (4) ovarian tumors, such as Sertoli-Leydig cell tumor, lipoid cell, and Sertoli cell tumors; and (5) rarely, familial precocious puberty with isolated elevation of LH level.

As with isosexual precocity, patients should undergo careful history and physical examination. Laboratory tests should include determination of serum FSH, LH, estradiol, DHEA, DHEAS, testosterone, androstenedione, 17-hydroxyprogesterone, and 17-hydroxypregnenolone values. An ACTH stimulation test should be carried out. Additionally a 24-hour urine should be obtained for cortisol.

The treatment and follow-up of heterosexual precocious puberty is based on the diagnosis. Ovarian and adrenal tumors should be surgically excised, if possible. Patients with CAH should receive glucocorticoid replacement. Follow-up should include careful monitoring of growth every 3 months. If the bone age is not too advanced, breast development may regress with treatment of patients with CAH.

GYNECOLOGIC PROBLEMS IN THE ADOLESCENT POPULATION

Infections

Most gynecologic infections in the adolescent are evaluated and treated in a manner similar to the adult patient (Chapter 21). There are, however, certain aspects of this problem that are unique to the adolescent and deserve special emphasis.

Vulvovaginitis. In the adolescent, vaginitis is a common gynecologic problem despite the fact that the adolescent has developed a more resistent estrogenized vaginal epithelium, pubic hair, and labial fat pads absent in prepubertal patients. The striking difference between prepubertal and adolescent vulvovaginitis is the shift in etiology. Vulvovaginitis in the prepubertal child is often nonspecific and usually results from poor perineal hygiene; vaginitis in the adolescent usually has a specific etiology, often related to sexual contact. A complaint of vaginal discharge may be the presenting symptom of the adolescent with cervicitis secondary to *Neisseria gonorrhoeae*, *Chlamydia trachomatis*, or *Herpes simplex*. In addition to these true infections, physiologic leukorrhea, a normal desquamation of epithelial cells secondary to estrogen effect, is probably the most common cause of discharge in the pubescent girl.

The evaluation of vaginal discharge in the adolescent should include a history of symptoms (pruritus, odor, quantity), other illnesses (e.g., diabetes), recent medications (e.g., broad spectrum antibiotics, birth control pills), and in utero exposure to DES. A history of poorly controlled diabetes mellitus is frequently a clue to the diagnosis of candida vaginitis. The patient should be questioned about recent sexual relations, because treatment failure in an adolescent girl often occurs because of reexposure to an untreated contact. Several infections may coexist; a patient may be adequately treated for one infection and still have a second or third infection. For example, an adolescent may have C. trachomatis cervicitis, Trichomonas vaginitis, and vulvar condylomata. The use of oral broad spectrum antibiotics for the treatment of the vaginitis may be followed by a second infection with *Candida*. In the evaluation of vaginitis, frequently the patient is found to be in need of birth control as well. Although close family contact has been blamed for the spread of some infections, the clinician should assume that most, if not all, cases of trichomonas, condyloma, and genital herpes in adolescents are sexually acquired either through consenting sexual relationships or sexual abuse. The microbiologic flora of the adolescent vagina and cervix is different from those who give a history of sexual activity as opposed to those who deny it.

If a large ectropion is associated with any abnormality of the shape of the cervix or the presence of glandular cells extending into the anterior vaginal wall (adenosis), in utero exposure to DES should be strongly suspected in girls born before 1974.

Although not generally utilized for routine diagnosis of cervical and vaginal infections, the colposcope may be helpful. In patients with sexually transmitted diseases, an endocervical mucopurulent discharge is associated with *N. gonorrhoeae*, *C. trachomatis*, and *Herpes simplex*; ulcers/necrotic areas and increased surface vascularity are associated with *H. simplex*; strawberry cervix (uniformly arranged red spots or stippling of a few millimeters in size, located on the squamous epithelium covering the ectocervix) is associated with *Trichomonas*; hypertrophic cervicitis is associated with *C. trachomatis*; and immature metaplasia is associated with *C. trachomatis* and cytomegalovirus.

Vulvar ulcers and nevi. Determining the etiology of vulvar ulcers is sometimes difficult. The most common causes of ulcers in adolescents are herpes simplex and syphilis. Syphilis is characterized by a painless hard ulcer and a positive rapid plasma reagin (RPR) test by the seventh day of the ulcer. Genital herpes is characterized by painful, usually multiple, shallow ulcers that are positive on Tzanck preparation and viral culture. Inguinal lymph nodes (either unilateral or bilateral) are usually enlarged and tender. Rarely, Epstein-Barr virus infection may cause painful genital ulcers that may occur primarily with mononucleosis.

In the last 5 years, chancroid has reemerged as a potential etiology of genital ulcers. In 1986, 4318 cases were reported, the largest number since 1952.[32] The disease typically presents as multiple purulent ulcers, often with ragged edges, and tender unilateral or bilateral inguinal adenopathy. Diagnosis is made by excluding the diagnosis of genital herpes or syphilis. Culture of *Haemophilus ducreyi* is the only definite means of diagnosis, but special media and conditions are necessary, and thus detection from direct smears of the base of the genital lesion is the method used by most clinicians. The specimen obtained from the ulcer base may involve peeling off the crust or wiping away excess pus (but not extensive cleaning). The cotton swab is used to touch the base first and then the edges of the ulcer. The swab is then rolled onto a slide in a circle about the size of a dime; the slide is air dried and Gram stained. Indirect immunofluorescence of ulcer smears is performed using a monoclonal antibody directed against *H. ducreyi*. A dot-immunobinding serologic test has become available recently. Patients with ulcers and no history of blisters, who do not have herpes or syphilis, and have significant painful inguinal adenopathy, should be suspected of having chancroid and treated with azithromycin 1 g orally in a single dose; ceftriaxone 250 mg IM; or erythromycin base 500 mg orally four times a day for 7 days. A clinical response should be evident within several days. Patients should be seen in 7 days to make sure that ulcer healing is occurring and that adenopathy is less painful. Nodes may become fluctuant in spite of adequate medical therapy and require needle aspiration or drainage. If a response to therapy has not occurred by day 7, the diagnosis may be different (e.g., herpes and chancroid), the patient may be noncompliant with medication, or the organisms resistant to the antibiotic chosen. Sexual contacts should be examined and treated. Genital ulcers are of particular worry in the 1980s and 1990s because of their association with HIV infection.

Lymphogranuloma venereum (LGV) is caused by three serotypes (L-1, L-2, and L-3) of *C. trachomatis*; it is rare and more common in men than women. The ulcer in LGV is the late sequelae (enlarged inguinal nodes and rectal strictures). An LGV titer is used to make the diagnosis.

The diagnosis of carcinoma, pemphigus, or granuloma inguinale generally requires a biopsy. Granuloma inguinale, a rare disease, causes painful ulcerations with red granulation tissue or keloid-like depigmented scars, elephantoid enlargement of the external genitalia, and fistulas.

Ulcers can occur also with chronic fistulas of Crohn's disease; local application of zinc oxide paste may help alleviate symptoms. A course of oral metronidazole has proved beneficial in some patients with chronic fistulas.

The mouth should always be examined in patients with vulvar ulcers. Behcet's disease is a multisystem disease characterized by recurrent oral and genital ulcers, often associated with uveitis, and less commonly, arthritis, phlebitis, and rashes. Although the disease usually does not appear until the third decade of life, rare cases in young children and adolescents have been reported. Therapy is unsatisfactory and includes high estrogen oral contraceptives, corticosteroids, and immunosuppressive agents.

Most darkly pigmented lesions seen on the vulva of adolescent girls represent lentigo, (a benign freckle-like lesion resulting from an increase in the concentration of melanocytes in the basal layer of the epithelium) or a compound, junctional, or intradermal nevus. However, the rare occurrence of melanoma or other form of carcinoma makes it essential to perform an excisional biopsy to establish a benign diagnosis.

Dysuria. Dysuria is a common symptom in adolescent girls and is discussed in this section because vaginitis and vulvar lesions may produce symptoms usually associated with a urinary tract infection (UTI). A careful gynecologic assessment of adolescents who complain of dysuria is necessary. Recent studies in adult women have revealed that only one half of the women with dysuria had bacteriuria with more than 10^5 organisms/mL. Vaginitis, vulvitis, infection with herpes, *N. gonorrhoeae*, *C. trachomatis*, and bacteriuria with fewer than 10^5 organism/mL are responsible for most of the remaining group. The results of a study of 53 adolescent girls (mean age of 17.5 years) presenting with dysuria are shown in Table 23-6. Pyuria on urinalysis was seen most frequently with UTI and trichomonas vaginitis; however, the cases of gonococcal and mixed gonococcal-chlamydial infection (one case of each) also had pyuria. None of the patients who had acute urethral syndrome with unclear cause had pyuria.

Assessment of the adolescent with dysuria should include a history that asks specifically about onset of symptoms, sexual activity (recent and past), symptoms of urethritis in the boyfriend, previous UTIs, and internal dysuria (pain felt inside the body) versus external dysuria (pain felt as urine passes over the inflamed labia). If the patient reports a clear cut external dysuria and discharge, it is highly likely that the symptoms are due to vaginitis or a vulvar cause. Although adult women who have internal dysuria and frequency usually have a UTI, many adolescent girls have vaginitis either alone or in combination with a UTI. In contrast to older women, adolescents are less able to differentiate internal versus external dysuria.

Table 23-6. Etiology of dysuria in adolescent girls

Diagnosis	No. of patients	(%)
Vaginitis from	10	(10)
Candida	8	(15)
Trichomonas	2	(4)
Candida and *Trichomonas*	2	(4)
Bacterial UTI	9	(17)
Bacterial UTI and vaginitis	9	(17)
Other diagnoses		
Herpes progenitals	2	(4)
N. gonorrhoeae	1	(2)
C. trachomatis	1	(2)
N. gonorrhoeae and *C. trachomatis*	1	(2)
Skene's gland abscess	1	(2)
Nonspecific vulvitis	2	(4)
Traumatic urethritis	1	(2)
Urethral syndrome of unclear etiology	4	(8)

The laboratory evaluation of the adolescent with dysuria should include urinalysis, two urine cultures, wet preparations of the vaginal secretions, and cultures for gonorrhea and chlamydia (in sexually active patients). Incubating dip slides in the office is an inexpensive and practical method of screening.

The genitalia should be inspected to exclude urethral or vulvar pathology. Speculum examination should be done for sexually active patients. In virginal patients, samples for wet preparations can be obtained with a saline-moistened, cotton-tipped applicator gently inserted through the hymenal ring. A culture for *Candida* should be done in patients with itching or vulvar erythema in whom the KOH preparation does not reveal *Candida*.

The diagnosis is generally UTI or a specific infection. In patients who have undiagnosed dysuria and persistent pyuria on urinalysis, cultures for *Chlamydia* should be obtained. The patient should ask her partner again about symptoms of urethritis; *C. trachomatis* should be treated in the male at the same time. The patient with pyuria should be treated with a course of antibiotics effective against low count UTIs and *Chlamydia*.

Adolescents with uncomplicated cystitis may be treated with single dose antibiotics or a 3-, 5- or 10-day course. The best studied single doses are amoxicillin 3 gm or trimethoprim/sulfamethizole 320 mg/1600 mg (4 tablets); the cure rate with the latter is slightly higher than the former.

Ultrasonography of the kidneys should be performed in adolescents with complicated UTIs, pyelonephritis, inadequate response to antibiotics, and possibly recurrent cystitis. The lack of response to a single dose of antibiotics can indicate a patient at higher risk of upper tract infection and this may be a good indicator of the need to evaluate the kidneys. In contrast to recommendations in children, vesicocystourethrography is generally reserved for adolescents with an abnormal ultrasonogram (or pyelonephritis).

Patients often have recurrent UTIs in relationship to coitus and especially diaphragm use. Other diaphragms or other methods of contraception may need to be considered. Coitus-related UTI can be treated with frequent voiding (every 2 hours during the day), voiding postintercourse, and suppressive antibiotics. Antibiotic regimens include TMP/SMX 80/160 mg 1/2 tablet daily or 1/2 tablet 3 times per week, postcoital antibiotics, or a single dose therapy with each infection. The use of prophylactic antibiotics is considered cost-effective when women experience more than 2 infections per year. Self-administration of antibiotics at the time of the UTI appears to be most useful in women who are accurate at self-diagnosis and have only 1 to 2 infections per year. A contraindication to self-therapy is the potential failure to reduce the proportion of patients with enterobacterial colonization of the urethra and vagina.

Currently, the patient without pyuria or a diagnosis falls into a small category of those with urethral syndrome of unclear etiology. Antibiotics do not benefit these patients. Studies in the future are likely to shed light on the diagnosis and treatment of this group.

Toxic shock syndrome. Toxic shock syndrome (TSS) received much publicity in the early 1980s as a disease that was occurring in young women primarily in association with one type of tampon. Since then milder cases than the original Centers for Disease Control (CDC) definition have been recognized and newer information on toxin production and risk factors has been forthcoming.

Although the original description of toxic shock suggested a disease of males and females, it is apparent now that this disease predominantly (70% to 80%) affects young menstruating women who use tampons. The disease in menstruating young women is associated with the elaboration of an exotoxin (toxic shock syndrome toxin [TSST-1]) by *Staphylococcus aureus*. *S. aureus* has been cultured from the vagina of 98% of women with TSS versus 7% of controls. TSS has a peak occurrence on the fourth day of the menses and has been associated with continuous tampon use.

Toxic shock syndrome continues to be reported although the associated tampon was removed from the market in 1980. The incidence of TSS since 1980 has been reported to be 2 to 4/100,000 woman-years. Given the current information and the tremendous variability of absorbency of tampons with the current terminology of regular, super, and super plus, mandatory labeling with standardized absorbency would diminish the risk of TSS. Factors which appear to promote the recurrence of TSS are the neutral pH of the vagina during menstruation and the introduction of air into the vagina with the insertion of tampons. However, cases of TSS do occur during menses in women not using tampons.

Contraceptive sponge use and to a lesser extent diaphragm use have been associated with rare cases of TSS. The relative risk of nonmenstrual TSS associated with the sponge has been estimated to be 7.8 to 40. Although in vitro data suggest that *S. aureus* and TSST-1 production are inhibited by the sponge, clinicians should base their counseling on the rare possibility of TSS (the risk of death estimated at 0.1 to 0.6/100,000 woman-years) and discuss the symptoms with each patient using this method of contraception.

The toxin TSST-1 has been isolated in 90% to 100% of menstrual cases of TSS, whereas this toxin has been reported in only 62% of nonmenstrual cases. This suggests that other toxins are involved in the pathogenesis of nonmenstrual TSS. Most individuals develop antibody to TSST-1 by age 20 years. Toxic shock occurs predominantly in the population that lacks antibody, either because of a genetic factor or lack of exposure. Young patients, especially adolescents, would appear to be at increased risk of TSS. This toxin appears to block B lymphocytes from making antibody. Women who have not made antibody to TSST-1 at follow-up are at high risk of recurrence with future menses and tampon usage.

Milder cases of TSS have also been described. To intervene effectively, physicians and patients need to be aware of more minor symptomatology occurring with tampon (or sponge) use. The criteria set up by the CDC to study the epidemiology of TSS is for the more severe manifestations of the syndrome.[77] These criteria are as follows:

1. Fever (temperature > 102° F [38.8° C])
2. Rash (diffuse, macular erythroderma that looks like sunburn)
3. Desquamation 1 to 2 weeks after the onset of the illness, particularly of palms and soles
4. Hypotension (systolic blood pressure < 90 mm Hg for adults, or orthostatic syncope)
5. Involvement of three or more of the following organ systems:
   a. Gastrointestinal (vomiting or diarrhea)
   b. Muscular (severe myalgia or creatinine phosphokinase level greater than twice the upper limits of normal)
   c. Mucous membranes (vaginal, oropharyngeal, or conjunctival hyperemia)
   d. Renal (blood urea nitrogen or creatinine greater than twice the upper limit of normal)
   e. Hepatic (total bilirubin, SGOT, SGPT greater than twice the upper limit of normal)
   f. Hematologic (platelet count < 100,000/mm^3)
   g. Central nervous system (disorientation or alterations in consciousness when fever and hypotension are absent)
6. Negative results on the following tests, if obtained:
   a. Blood, throat, or cerebrospinal fluid cultures
   b. Serologic tests for Rocky Mountain spotted fever, leptospirosis, or measles

Adolescents with any of these symptoms or with vomiting, diarrhea, and rash during menstruation should be instructed to remove the tampon (or diaphragm) and go to the emergency room. Patients with TSS should be managed in the same way as those suffering from other forms of shock, including the administration of fluid. A vaginal examination should be done along with removal of the tampon (if still in place). Gram stain of the vaginal pool should be done. Cultures of blood, rectum, vagina, oropharynx, anterior nares, and urine should be obtained. Penicillinase-resistant antistaphylococcal antibiotics should be administered. Although evidence of benefit is lacking, most clinicians favor irrigating the vagina with saline, povidone-iodine solution, or vancomycin or gentamicin solution.

In patients with deep abscesses in which rapid eradication of toxin-producing staphylococci is unlikely to occur, steroids and immunoglobulin therapy, which has high levels of antibody to TSST-1, are thought to improve outcome.

Because of the approximately 30% risk of recurrence, patients should be warned to avoid tampons for at least 8 months. The presence of high levels of antibody to TSST-1 at follow-up in a patient with no antibody at presentation is reassuring. Serial cultures of the vagina may be difficult to interpret because other strains may be present. Testing for TSST-1-producing strains requires a specialized laboratory.

In the United States the use of all tampons fell initially in response to the publicity about toxic shock in the early 1980s. However, a significant number of young women desire to continue tampon use. There is insufficient knowledge to give absolute guidelines to patients, but the following is suggested: (1) avoiding superabsorbent tampons (this should be easier with mandatory labeling); (2) using tampons intermittently by using pads at night; (3) changing tampons every 4 to 6 hours; and especially (4) removing the tampon and calling a physician if vomiting, diarrhea, rash, or fever occurs. The recommendation about frequency of changing tampons has not been subjected to critical review.

Pelvic inflammatory disease. PID refers to infection in the upper genital tract that involves the fallopian tubes. PID may occur as a sexually-acquired acute salpingitis, a postpartum or postabortal infection, or the chronic sequelae to a previous acute or silent salpingitis.

It has been estimated that 1 million women in the United States are treated for acute salpingitis each year; 16% to 20% of cases occur in adolescents. Adolescents represent an especially high-risk group because they often have multiple sexual partners and have high prevalence of infections with *N. gonorrhoeae* and *C. trachomatis*. Women with multiple partners have a 4.6-fold increased risk of PID. The use of nonbarrier methods of contraception makes adolescents more likely to acquire endocervical infections, and the immaturity of their immune systems appears to increase their susceptibility to ascending infection. It has been estimated that adolescents with a gonococcal or chlamydial endocervical infection have a 30% chance of developing PID, as opposed to a 10% risk in the older woman.

The use of the oral contraceptive pill appears to lessen the risk of gonococcal PID, perhaps because of changes in cervical mucus, lighter menstrual flow, diminished uterine contractions, less retrograde menstruation, and less canal dilation. Because most studies have been limited to hospitalized cases of PID, which represent only 25% of all cases, it is unclear whether the protection of the pill can be generalized to other forms of PID. It has been estimated that the risk of PID in a sexually active 15-year-old is 1 in 8, as contrasted with the risk of a women 24 years and older of 1 in 80. Because a history of previous PID is a risk factor for PID and the sequelae of infertility, ectopic pregnancy, and pelvic pain are related to the number of episodes, it is clear that adolescents deserve prompt attention to complaints that may suggest a diagnosis of PID.

Although in the past, PID has been divided into gonococcal and nongonococcal based on the presence or absence of *N. gonorrhoeae* in the endocervical culture, the most appropriate designations are gonococcal, chlamydial, and nongonococcal, nonchlamydial PID. A positive cervical culture for gonorrhea is found in 20% to 80% of patients with PID.

Chlamydial infection is found in 20% to 45% of patients with PID. Of great concern in the evaluation of adolescents is a recent study that found 40% of patients with asymptomatic endocervical chlamydial infection also have evidence of endometrial infection.[59] The course of chlamydial PID can be subacute and indolent, and adolescents frequently delay seeking medical attention. The sedimentation rate associated with chlamydial PID often is elevated and the tubal damage significant at the time of presentation.

Nongonococcal, nonchlamydial PID involves a number of organisms including coliforms, *Gardnerella vaginalis*, *Hemophilus influenzae*, group B streptococci, Bacteroides species (e.g., *B. fragilis* and *B. bivius*), peptostreptococcus, peptococcus, and *Mycoplasma hominis*. *M. hominis* is frequently cultured from the cervix of women with and without PID; however, it does appear to be responsible for infection in a small number of patients. The flora seen in nongonococcal, nonchlamydial PID is strikingly similar to that occurring in bacterial vaginitis, and thus what has been thought of in the past as a benign condition appears to be a risk factor for PID. It has been suggested that the gonococcus is a precursor for other invaders from the lower genital tract, but anaerobic organisms are frequently found within the first 24 hours of symptoms. Gonococcal and chlamydial PID must be considered to have a polymicrobial etiology and thus antimicrobial therapy must be directed against all the potential organisms.

Diagnosis. The classic picture of acute salpingitis includes lower abdominal pain, vaginal discharge, and fever and chills, usually following the onset of a menses in a sexually active young woman. Symptoms may be less specific and include menstrual irregularities, dyspareunia, vomiting, diarrhea, constipation, dysuria, and urinary frequency. Patients with chlamydial PID are less likely to be febrile and more likely to have long-standing milder symptoms and breakthrough bleeding on oral contraceptives than those with gonococcal or anaerobic PID. The markedly elevated sedimentation rate often contrasts with the mild symptoms of chlamydial PID. The diagnosis of PID is made by finding signs of genital infection, lower abdominal pain, and pelvic tenderness. The abdominal pain and adnexal tenderness are typically bilateral; however unilateral salpingitis has been confirmed by laparoscopy. Pain on cervical motion is usually present but may occur with other pelvic pathology. Rebound tenderness may not be present early in the disease if peritonitis is not present. Liver tenderness caused by perihepatitis may occur in patients even if no pelvic pathology is found. A clinical diagnosis plus a positive culture or rapid diagnostic test for *N. gonorrhoeae* or *C. trachomatis* allows correct diagnosis in 90% of patients. Clearly, a clinician cannot expect all the criteria to be present to initiate therapy; otherwise many adolescents would be undertreated and thus likely to develop sequelae. The most recent criteria for the diagnosis of PID are summarized in Table 23-7.

Laparoscopy has proved invaluable in clarifying the etiologic agents and the clinical accuracy of diagnosis in PID. Laparoscopy is indicated if the diagnosis is in doubt, especially in patients recurrently labelled with PID but never meeting satisfactory criteria. It should be used in research settings also, especially when clinical trials of antibiotics are undertaken. Care should be taken in making sure that cultures taken at laparoscopy are processed so that fastidious organisms will not be missed.

The laboratory tests should include a complete blood count (CBC), sedimentation rate, serologic test for syphilis, Gram stain of the endocervical discharge, cultures or other tests for *N. gonorrhoeae* and *C. trachomatis*, and a sensitive pregnancy test. The CBC may show a normal or elevated white blood cell count. The sedimentation rate is greater than 25 mm/hour in 75% to 80% of patients. The Gram stain of a purulent cervical discharge may reveal gram-negative intracellular diplococci in about one half of patients with gonococcal PID. The finding of 10 or more white cells on a cervical Gram stain (1000 ×) also may be a clue to chlamydial disease. The absence of any white cells in the cervical secretions and vaginal discharge suggests a different diagnosis from PID. A pregnancy test should always be obtained, and the possibility of an ectopic pregnancy considered in the adolescent with acute abdominal pain; it is important to remember that an adolescent may have more than one diagnosis, such as chlamydial PID and ectopic pregnancy. Transabdominal and especially transvaginal ultrasonography can be extremely useful in ruling out other diagnoses and defining masses in the adnexa. Tuboovarian abscesses can be followed in the hospital with sonography.

The diagnosis of PID is sometimes difficult to make. Laparoscopic studies of patients with a presumptive diagnosis of acute salpingitis have concluded that the clinical diagnosis is confirmed by visual inspection in only 60% to 70% of cases.[56] An additional 5% of patients with negative examinations by laparoscopy do have gonococci present in the cervical culture.

Inpatient therapy. Although antibiotic thereby resolves symptoms in most patients, the long-term results of treatment are still far from satisfactory. Given the frequency of noncompliance with medical therapy during adolescence and the risk of future reproductive problems, adolescents should be considered a high priority for inpatient therapy for PID. Some centers admit all adolescents routinely for parenteral therapy. In addition, all patients who have questionable diagnosis, suspected pelvic abscess, upper quadrant pain, peritoneal signs, temperature greater than 38°C or vomiting, are prepubertal or pregnant, and possibly noncompliant to outpatient treatment (including medication and follow-up appointments), or fail to respond to outpatient treatment within 48 hours deserve inpatient therapy.

Table 23-7. Clinical criteria for the diagnosis of acute PID (CDC, 1993)

Minimal Criteria (All 3 must be present)
1. Lower Abdominal Tenderness
2. Adnexal Tenderness
3. Cervical Motion Tenderness

Additional Criteria
1. Oral temperature >38.3°C
2. Abnormal cervical or vaginal discharge
3. Elevated ESR
4. Elevated C-reactive protein
5. Laboratory documentation of cervical infection with N. gonorrhea or C. trachomatis
6. Histopathologic evidence of endometritis on endometrial biopsy
7. Tubo-ovarian abscess on sonography or other radiologic tests, or bimanual examination
8. Laparoscopic abnormalities consistent with PID

In selecting antibiotics for inpatient and outpatient treatment of PID, the clinician must take into account the polymicrobialetiology of the disease, regardless of whether *N. gonorrhoeae* or *C. trachomatis* is cultured. It is especially important to make sure that the antibiotics are known to be effective against chlamydia, since clinical improvement may occur in spite of persistence of positive endometrial cultures for chlamydia. In patients with severe disease or abscess formation, antibiotics effective against anaerobes must be included. The risk of abscess formation and infertility in nongonococcal PID is higher than in gonococcal PID. Antimicrobial regimens that include clindamycin are especially effective in the medical treatment of tuboovarian abscesses.

The CDC Guidelines have recommended one of two regimens:

Regimen A

Cefoxitin 2 g IV every 6 hours or cefotetan 2 g IV every 12 hours,

PLUS

Doxycycline 100 mg IV or orally every 12 hours

NOTE: This regimen should be continued for at least 48 hours after the patient demonstrates substantial clinical improvement, after which doxycycline 100 mg orally 2 times a day should be continued for a total of 14 days. Doxycycline administered orally has bioavailability similar to that of the IV formulation and may be administered if normal gastrointestinal function is present.

Clinical data are limited for other second- or third-generation cephalosporins (e.g., ceftizoxime, cefotaxime, and ceftriaxone), which might replace cefoxitin or cefotetan, although many authorities believe they also are effective therapy for PID. However, they are less active than cefoxitin or cefotetan against anaerobic bacteria.

Regimen B

Clindamycin 900 mg IV every 8 hours,

PLUS,

Gentamicin loading dose IV or IM (2 mg/kg of body weight) followed by a maintenance dose (1.5 mg/kg) every 8 hours

NOTE: This regimen should be continued for at least 48 hours after the patient demonstrates substantial clinical improvement, to be followed with doxycycline 100 mg orally 2 times a day or clindamycin 450 mg orally 4 times a day to complete a total of 14 days of therapy. When tuboovarian abscess is present, many health-care providers use clindamycin for continued therapy rather than doxycycline, because it provides more effective anaerobic coverage. Clindamycin administered intravenously appears to be effective against *C. trachomatis* infection; however, the effectiveness of oral clindamycin against *C. trachomatis* has not been determined.

Alternative inpatient regimens. Limited data support the use of other inpatient regimens, but two regimens have undergone at least one clinical trial and have broad-spectrum coverage. Ampicillin/sulbactam plus doxycycline has good anaerobic coverage and appears to be effective for patients with a tuboovarian abscess. Intravenous ofloxacin has been studied as a single agent. A regimen of ofloxacin plus either clindamycin or metronidazole provides broad-spectrum coverage. Evidence is insufficient to support the use of any single agent regimen for inpatient treatment of PID. Despite concerns about whether the second regimen would cover gonococci and chlamydia, patients treated with these drugs do experience comparable clinical and bacteriologic cure rates of PID.

Most patients with PID respond well clinically to broad-spectrum antibiotics. However, patients with tuboovarian abscesses can be difficult to manage. Such abscesses occur mostly in the third and fourth decades of life but can occur in adolescents as well. Ultrasonography, and in some cases CT and MRI when sonography does not provide adequate information, can be used along with clinical assessment to make the diagnosis and document improvement. Since the diagnosis of abscesses is often difficult in the patient with a tender pelvis, ultrasonography should be used frequently as an aid to the clinician. Anaerobic organisms, particularly *B. fragilis*, are strongly associated with abscess formation.

Laparoscopy is utilized soon after admission in centers obtaining bacteriologic cultures from the fallopian tubes and those centres verifying the diagnosis for inclusion in studies of PID. Laparoscopy is also useful in patients in whom the diagnosis is in doubt at admission or in patients who fail to respond to medical therapy. Surgery is indicated in patients with ruptured abscesses.

With the advent of better anaerobic drug combinations in the last 5 years, probably fewer patients will fail to respond to medical management. Unilateral tuboovian abscesses greater than 8 cm in diameter, and bilateral abscesses, are less likely to respond to medical management alone. Surgical intervention may include percutaneous drainage guided by CT or real-time ultrasound (the majority that have been drained have been unilocular abscesses), transabdominal laparotomy with drainage or extirpation of the abscess with or without unilateral adnexectomy, or total abdominal hysterectomy and bilateral salpingo-oophorectomy. Although long-term data are not available on fertility outcome and are critically needed to evaluate new approaches, some centers have advocated a more aggressive early surgical approach to large tuboovarian abscesses with aspiration of the abscess, gentle washing of the abscess cavity, instillation of antibiotics, and closed drainage to gravity. Other centers have taken a more conservative surgical approach and feel that preservation of fertility is more likely if the patient is treated medically with appropriate antibiotics with performance of surgery later if necessary, when the infection has been thoroughly treated. Fertility after treatment of tuboovarian abscesses with conservative medical and surgical approaches may be 20% to 50%. When surgery is required, all attempts should be made to preserve the uterus and one or both ovaries to maintain options for fertility through in vitro fertilization.

After inpatient parenteral therapy, oral antibiotics, as previously indicated, are continued to complete a 10- to 14-day course. Patients with severe disease including tuboovarian abscesses are usually treated for a longer course with oral clindamycin or a two-drug regimen such as oral doxycycline plus metronidazole. More data are needed on the use of outpatient regimens of ciprofloxacin and amoxicillin-clavulanate.

Following discharge from the hospital, the patient should be seen weekly, and sexual contacts should be identified and treated with regimens effective against both *C. trachomatis* and *N. gonorrhea* to prevent reinfection. Cultures should be repeated 2 to 4 weeks after the completion of therapy. Patients should abstain from sexual relations for 3 to 4 weeks. STD counseling is essential to minimize the chance of reinfection and to protect against other infections such as HPV and human immunodeficiency virus (HIV).

Outpatient therapy. Although most adolescents with PID should be treated as inpatients, the reliable patient with mild signs and symptoms, a temperature less than 38° C, and no vomiting can be treated with either regimen A or B as follows:

Regimen A
Cefoxitin 2 g IM plus probenecid 1 g orally in a single dose concurrently, or ceftriaxone 250 mg IM or other parenteral third-generation cephalosporin (e.g., ceftizoxime or cefotaxime), PLUS, Doxycycline 100 mg orally 2 times a day for 14 days
Regimen B
Ofloxacin 400 mg orally 2 times a day for 14 days, PLUS, Either clindamycin 450 mg orally 4 times a day, or metronidazole 500 mg orally 2 times a day for 14 days

Clinical trials have demonstrated that the cefoxitin regimen is effective in obtaining short-term clinical response. Fewer data support the use of ceftriaxone or other third-generation cephalosporins, but based on their similarities to cefoxitin, they also are considered effective. No data exist regarding the use of oral cephalosporins for the treatment of PID.

Ofloxacin is effective against both *N. gonorrhoeae* and *C. trachomatis*. One clinical trial demonstrated the effectiveness of oral ofloxacin in obtaining short-term clinical response in PID. Despite results of this trial, ofloxacin's lack of anaerobic coverage is of concern; the addition of clindamycin or metronidazole provides this coverage. Clindamycin, but not metronidazole, further enhances the Gram positive coverage of the regimen.

Alternative outpatient regimens. Information regarding other outpatient regimens is limited. The combination of amoxicillin/clavulanic acid plus doxycycline was effective in obtaining short-term clinical response in one clinical trial, but many of the patients had to discontinue the regimen because of gastrointestinal symptoms.

It is essential that the clinician feel comfortable that the patient has the resources to purchase the antibiotics and will return in 48 to 72 hours to assess whether the treatment is effective. A lack of response, vomiting of the antibiotics, or noncompliance should prompt hospitalization. The patient is advised to abstain from intercourse for 3 to 4 weeks and her sexual partner(s) should be seen for appropriate cultures and treatment.

Consequences of acute pelvic inflammatory disease. Infertility, ectopic pregnancies, and chronic abdominal pain are the principal sequelae of acute PID. Thus, the clinician must treat the patient adequately and promptly to prevent recurrences. Women with a first episode of PID have a twofold to threefold increased risk of a second episode of PID compared with women who have never had PID. During the treatment of the infection, it should be explained to the patient how the disease is sexually transmitted and how to prevent recurrences. The importance of monogamous relationships, use of a condom, and treatment of both partners should be stressed. A single episode of gonococcal salpingitis appropriately treated carries a low risk of later infertility, and patients generally can be reassured of this. However, recurrences markedly increase the risk of tubal occlusion.

Tubal occlusion may be more common in nongonococcal infections, although newer data have questioned this. Unfortunately, if the issue of possible infertility is overemphasized to the young adolescent, she may discontinue effective contraception and take risks to prove her own fertility. In general, the more severe the PID, the higher the risk of future infertility.

In addition to infertility, previous salpingitis is a major cause of ectopic pregnancy. Adolescents who have had PID should be counselled about this risk, and ectopic pregnancy should always be considered in the differential diagnosis of the adolescent with acute abdominal pain. The clinician should maintain a high index of suspicion in following the pregnancy of an adolescent with a history of PID.

PID may result in chronic pain. Laparoscopy is necessary to establish the diagnosis and to evaluate the extent of the disease. Adolescents with endometriosis can be incorrectly diagnosed as having PID, and may receive multiple courses of antibiotics before the correct diagnosis is made by laparoscopy.

Therapy must be individualized. Treatment may include the following: (1) an extended course of oral antibiotics such as doxycycline, clindamycin, trimethoprim-sulfamethizole, amoxicillin, or possibly ciprofloxacin; (2) nonsteroidal antiinflammatory drugs for pain; (3) other medicines; (4) oral contraceptives to suppress cyclic ovarian function; and (5) conservative surgery with lysis of adhesions, and if the uterus is retroverted, suspension of the uterus. Cultures should be obtained and the patient treated with appropriate antimicrobial agents for subsequent episodes of PID; the sexual partner must be examined and treated, also.

Sexual assault

In contrast to the pattern of sexual abuse in prepubertal children, sexual abuse during adolescence is more likely to be a one-time assault by a stranger and involve vaginal intercourse. However, even among adolescents the rape may involve an acquaintance or someone the teenager has seen in her neighborhood or school and who was assumed to be a safe individual.[87] In these cases, the adolescent may accept a ride, for example, with that individual and then later be forced into a sexual relationship, often involving intercourse. In other cases, the developmental changes that take place during adolescence may make a long-standing incestuous relationship intolerable; the adolescent then may respond with a sudden disclosure, may seek medical care for somatic symptoms such as abdominal pain or headache, or become involved in impulsive behavior such as running away. A pregnancy may be the first sign of a previous rape or chronic sexual abuse. Therefore it is important to ask adolescents not only whether they have ever had sexual relations but also whether they have ever been forced into a sexual relationship.

In recording the history of the adolescent with alleged sexual assault, it is important to record the date of the visit, sources of the history, who transported the patient to the clinic or hospital, and who knows of the current situation. The date, time, and place of the sexual assault(s) should be recorded. In acute situations, the patient should be asked if she has bathed, douched, or urinated since the assault. Menstrual and contraceptive history should be obtained. The physician should not try to decide whether rape or seduction has occurred on the basis of the patient's emotional response to the trauma, for clearly some patients will be tearful, tense, and hysterical and others will appear controlled or subdued. Questions in terms understood by the patient should focus on what happened and whether vaginal, rectal, or oral penetration occurred. These questions may need to be repeated during the examination when the adolescent is more familiar with the anatomic terms. The patient should be asked if she is aware of any other injuries or symptoms following the attack. A rape protocol should be used to collect evidence. It is extremely helpful if a nurse, preferably an experienced rape victim counselor, can be assigned to the adolescent throughout the 2 to 4 hour stay in the emergency ward and can be present during the history taking and physical examination, and be an ally to the patient. A number of general hospitals now have a rotating system of nurses who have had special training in rape counseling and who are available on an on-call basis to provide such support for the victim. A police officer should not be present during the medical evaluation.

After the history is obtained, the need for a thorough physical examination to assess injury and to collect laboratory specimens should be explained to the patient. The assessment given below applies to the acute sexual assault. When there is a history of an ongoing incestuous relationship in which intercourse has occurred more than 5 days before the physical examination, the search for motile sperm is omitted.

The physical examination should include the following seven steps:

1. A description of the patient's general appearance, emotional state, and especially the condition of the clothing should be recorded. Any clothing that might provide evidence in a legal case should be included in the rape-evidence clothing bag.
2. A general physical examination should note any evidence of bruises, scratches, or lacerations. As noted in the section on Assessment of the Prepubertal Child, debris and dried secretions should be properly collected. The Tanner stage of sexual development should be noted. If the history indicates any attempt of the patient to scratch or fight her ssailant, fingernail scrapings should be obtained with a wooden applicator stick and saved in an envelope.
3. The pelvic examination should include a careful inspection of the perineum, noting any evidence of bleeding or lacerations. A slightly moistened gauze pad should be used to swab any dried secretions, and the location of the dried secretions should be marked on a sketch. A collection paper should be placed under the buttocks of the patient and the pubic hair combed toward the paper to collect any debris. The comb and debris should be placed in the collection envelope. If any foreign hairs are noted, 6 to 12 pubic hairs of the patient should be included and marked. The pubic hair can be cut near the surface to avoid discomfort. The size of the hymenal ring should be noted (e.g., Q-tip size, one finger-breadth, or two finger-breadths). Any evidence of a hymenal tear should be recorded. In most patients, a genital-vaginal examination can be done with a water-moistened adolescent (Huffman) speculum. If the hymen is tight, samples may be obtained from the vagina with a saline-moistened cotton-tipped applicator or long eyedropper. It is extremely important to examine the teenager gently so that the examination does not represent a further trauma. The vagina is inspected for injury and the presence of semen or vaginal discharge. An endocervical culture should be obtained for gonorrhea and chlamydia. If a speculum examination is not done, a vaginal culture for gonorrhea and chlamydia can be obtained by inserting a moistened Q-tip well into the vagina. A Q-tip should be swabbed into the posterior vaginal pool and wet preparations should be done to look for the presence of motile sperm and trichomonads. Another swab from the vaginal pool should be smeared on to two dry slides (frosted at one end so that the patient's name and date can be recorded) and air dried. The swab is placed in a test tube and saved for examination by a police forensic laboratory. If cervical smears also are taken to check for motile sperm, the wet and dry slides should be appropriately marked. A police laboratory can test for acid phosphatase and the blood group antigens of semen and can examine the dry slides for the presence of nonmotile sperm. The anus should be inspected and cultures for gonorrhea and chlamydia obtained. Specimens for sperm and acid-phosphatase determinations should be obtained if there is a history of rectal assault. Anoscopy should be done if rectal bleeding is present or the rectal examination reveals guaiac-positive stool. A bimanual rectal-vaginal-abdominal examination should be done gently to make sure there is no tenderness or enlargement of the uterus to suggest a preexisting pregnancy. Rectal sphincter tone should be assessed, because patients subjected to chronic rectal abuse may have reflex relaxation.
4. If oral-genital contact has occurred, specimens from the girl's mouth should be obtained. A throat swab should be plated in modified Thayer-Martin-Jambec media.
5. Blood should be drawn for a serologic test for syphilis (RPR or VDRL), and a serum specimen frozen to do future testing for HIV and hepatitis B, if indicated.
6. A sensitive urine pregnancy test should be done to detect preexisting pregnancy, especially if the menses are late or irregular or the patient has had previous sexual exposure.

If the patient is unconscious, samples should be obtained from the vagina, rectum, and mouth.

All laboratory specimens for the pathology laboratory or the police should be delivered personally by the doctor or nurse involved in the case, and properly signed receipts should be obtained. Use of a rape evidence kit or rape protocol does not imply that the family or patient must push for prosecution; however, reporting the rape and using a protocol to collect the evidence ensures that the evidence has been appropriately handled and will be admissible in court if prosecution occurs. Under the stress of the crisis, many families may have difficulty deciding whether prosecution will be

Table 23-8. Prophylactic antibiotics in sexual assault (CDC, 1993)

Recommended regimen
Ceftriaxone, 125 mg IM in a single dose
plus
Metronidazole, 2 g orally in a single dose
plus
Doxycycline, 100 mg orally 2 times a day for 7 days

sought; therefore it behooves the physician to obtain evidence that is medically and legally appropriate.

In cases of acute rape, the decision to prescribe antibiotics should be individualized and based on the risks. The benefits of prophylactic treatment for syphilis, gonorrhea, and chlamydia should be discussed with the patient. Current recommendations for prophylactic antibiotics in cases of sexual assault are shown in Table 23-8. In asymptomatic adolescents with long-standing incestuous relationships, the physician should wait for the results of the cultures and blood tests before initiating treatment, unless the perpetrator is known to be infected. Intramuscular ceftriaxone and oral metronidazole is the current treatment regimen of choice. The single dose therapy should be followed by 14 days of tetracycline, doxycycline, or erythromycin. If the initial RPR is negative, a follow-up serologic test for syphilis is necessary if spectinomycin is chosen for gonococcal prophylaxis or no prophylaxis is given. Tetanus toxoid should be given following standard pediatric guidelines for injuries.

"Morning after" therapy should be offered to the postpubertal adolescent who was raped less than 72 hours (preferably less than 48 hours) before being treated. It is important that the patient understand that the medicine should not be used if there is the possibility of a preexisting pregnancy; she should feel ready to have an abortion if she discovers several weeks later that she was in fact pregnant at the time of the combined estrogen-progestin pill administration. A sensitive pregnancy test should be done before medication is given.

A follow-up appointment should be made for 2 weeks later. A repeat pelvic examination is done to assess healing of injuries. The patient should be reassured that her genital anatomy is normal. Patients benefit greatly from drawings that show them the range of hymenal size. The virginal adolescent who has had a forced episode of sexual intercourse may feel considerably relieved to understand that her introitus is not different from some adolescents who have not had intercourse. She needs to be reassured that the assault in no way changes her ability to have normal sexual intercourse in the future or to have normal healthy children. Some older teenagers have had unprotected intercourse because they felt that a rape, which occurred when they were 12 or 13 years old, markedly diminished their reproductive potential.

The extent of the counseling in the aftermath of a sexual assault depends on the initial encounter. For example, in the situation of an isolated episode of exhibitionism or nonforceful genital fondling by a stranger or neighbor, counseling should help integrate the event with a strongly positive view of the future. A case of a long-standing incestuous relationship requires proper reporting and a long-term treatment program. If the young adolescent has been trained to be a sexual object and to give and receive sexual pleasure in order to get approval, the outcome is often poor; such girls are often provocative in foster home settings. Cases of acute sexual assault during adolescence require that the physician discuss the possibility of prosecution and suggest the need for long-term counseling.

The availability of counseling should be stressed to the teenager. Even if she seems nonverbal or appears to be coping well, the counselor often can play an educational and supportive role in the initial interviews. The patient needs reassurance about her intactness and her femininity. She may need the opportunity to tell and retell her story to a caring, sympathetic person. Ideally, an experienced counselor should be available at the time the rape is reported and should be willing to follow up with the patient by telephone or home visits. It is not unusual for a patient to have somatic reactions such as muscle soreness, headache, fatigue, stomach pain, dysuria, sleep disturbances, and nightmares in the first several weeks following a rape. Most rape victims express an extreme fear of physical violence and death. Many older women move and change their telephone numbers.

In the course of counseling, it is important to acknowledge to the patient that she may feel vulnerable and helpless and the rape incident may interfere with her ability to form trusting relationships in the future.

Menstrual disorders

Abnormalities of the pubertal process involve isosexual or heterosexual precocity or delayed puberty. There may be variations on the pubertal process with premature thelarche and premature adrenarche occurring in isolated form. The differential diagnosis of precocious development was discussed previously.

Delayed menarche. The term delayed menarche indicates the absence of menses in females by 18 years of age. This may be classified into three groups: constitutional delay, hypogonadotrophic hypogonadism, and hypergonadotropic hypogonadism.

The majority of patients with delayed adolescent development manifest no demonstrable organic pathologic conditions. The developmental retardation in these individuals represents a normal variation in endocrine function that will usually be rectified by time alone. For this reason, when to commence a diagnostic program is a most perplexing problem. The answer lies in the individualization of each case, taking into account the history, findings of physical examination, and the emotional attitudes of the patient and her family. The practice of initiating therapy to promote sexual development is to be deplored unless adequate diagnostic studies have been undertaken.

The endocrine defect in delayed adolescent development and delayed menarche is the lack of proper estrogenic stimulation necessary for maturation of the accessory sex organs and initiation of uterine bleeding. The secretion of estrogen is dependent on the elaboration of gonadotropin hormones from the adenohypophysis. The secretion of gonadotropins may be diminished or entirely lacking. In these individuals, for reasons unknown, it is assumed that both FSH and LH are held in abeyance.

Malnutrition resulting from starvation or chronic wasting disease may be contributory. Similarly, emotional or psychosomatic factors are known causes of secondary amenorrhea and may act to delay the onset of the puberty. Imbalances of other endocrine organs, such as the thyroid or adrenal glands, also may delay adolescent development and the menarche.

Clinical evaluation of patients manifesting delayed adolescent development should begin with a complete and thorough history and physical examination. Careful scrutiny of the accessory sex organs and the genitalia is mandatory. The internal genitalia may be examined rectally; negligible mental trauma and physical discomfort ensue if the examiner is reassuring and careful. Bone radiographs document bone age. Neurologic and ophthalmologic examinations are indicated if suspicious signs or symptoms such as headaches, scotomata, or diplopia are manifested.

The importance of a thorough rectovaginal examination is emphasized by the fact that delayed menarche may on occasion be due to a congenital mechanical obstruction in the vagina or cervix. Most commonly this is an imperforate hymen, and rectal examination reveals accumulated menstrual discharge in the vagina. Normal menses will immediately follow incision into the hymen and relief of the obstruction.

Assay of gonadotropins will distinguish between pituitary and ovarian failure. An elevated serum gonadotropin level suggests ovarian failure (hypergonadotropic hypogonadism). Diminished levels focus attention on pituitary dysfunction (hypogonadotropic hypogonadism). Plasma FSH levels appear to be the single most reliable assay for the presence or absence of ovarian failure. Estrogens measured in urine or blood are in the range of the prepubertal or postmenopausal female. Yet the function of the endometrium is not altered, since uterine bleeding may be induced by the administration of estrogens alone or estrogens followed by progesterone. As previously stated, the majority of patients with delayed adolescent development manifest no discernible pathologic condition. The prognosis for normal sexual development and reproductive function is excellent. In the absence of proved lesions or hormonal deficiencies, the use of endocrine preparations is deemed advisable. Reassurance, explanation, and passage of time constitute the desired therapeutic regimen. Systemic abnormalities such as obesity, cachexia, infection, and diabetes should be appropriately treated. Adequate psychiatric therapy, if indicated, should be initiated.

Primary amenorrhea. The term primary amenorrhea denotes menarche that has not occurred by 16 years of age. Primary amenorrhea is associated with normal pubertal development in vaginal or müllerian aplasia. Patients who have complete androgen insensitivity may have normal thelarche, but do not have normal hair development and are amenorrheic. In deciphering the cause of primary amenorrhea, it is worthwhile to examine the patient's secondary sex characteristics; if there is good sexual development, then testicular feminization, müllerian agenesis, vaginal atresia, and polycystic ovarian disease are possibilities.

The majority of patients with primary amenorrhea will have hypogonadotrophic hypogonadism or gonadal dysgenesis. Another group will be detected by elevated plasma testosterone levels which indicate some form of polycystic ovary syndrome. The remaining patients with normal breast and uterine development will have prolactin elevation. If the patient is normoprolactinemic, then an intramuscular progesterone or oral medroxyprogesterone challenge test discerns estrogen status. If the patient is estrogenized, withdrawal bleeding occurs. If the progesterone withdrawal test is negative, then further FSH level testing rules out ovarian failure. This final diagnostic category is not primarily associated with primary amenorrhea, but rather with secondary amenorrhea.

Secondary amenorrhea. Secondary amenorrhea denotes loss of menses for more than a 6-month period in a woman who has had previously normal cycles. Oligomenorrhea denotes irregular but consistent periods occurring at intervals of 2 to 5 months. Chronic anovulation usually accompanies secondary amenorrhea or oligomenorrhea. The most common causes for secondary amenorrhea or oligomenorrhea are as follows: (1) hypothalamic dysfunction, (2) hyperprolactinemia, and (3) excess androgen production.

Anorexia nervosa and/or excessive weight loss, malnutrition, stress, sustained systemic illness, and certain levels of exercise activity are all possible causes for hypogonadism. This diagnosis is reached through exclusion, since pituitary, ovarian, and adrenal dysfunction must be eliminated initially. Most patients with hypothalamic amenorrhea have normal puberty. With the onset of amenorrhea, gonadotropins and estrogen levels decrease. Depending on the duration of their disorders and whether or not they have secondary amenorrhea, they may be normoestrogenic or hypoestrogenic. Physical examination serves as a bioassay of estrogen status, because well-cornified, rugated, vaginal epithelium denotes normal estrogen status. Poorly cornified vaginal epithelium with scant cervical mucus denotes a low-estrogen state. The progesterone challenge test produces withdrawal bleeding if the estrogen state is normal.

The three important factors to exclude are pregnancy, a pituitary tumor, and premature menopause. A β-hCG level will preclude pregnancy; LH, FSH, and prolactin level assays and a MRI scan of the pituitary, if necessary, will exclude hyperprolactinemia or hypergonadotropism. Other pathologic processes are, therefore, ruled out and hypothalamic amenorrhea is indicated. Patients should be encouraged to gain weight or decrease exercise activity if these are thought to be causative factors. Hormonal supplementation should be suggested to prevent osteoporosis.

Patients with hypothalamic amenorrhea should be counseled as to the possible causes of their dysfunction. Patients suffering from the effects of excessive dietary restriction, specifically anorectics and bulemics, should receive appropriate psychiatric referral. The care of such individuals is founded on a multidisciplinary approach. There is no long-term effect on the uterus and ovaries in such individuals. This is important, since many worry that they will not be able to maintain a pregnancy if they have had prolonged amenorrhea as a result of exercise or anorexia. However, they should be made aware of the long-term skeletal effects producing osteoporosis resulting from prolonged amenorrhea. Adequate diet, reasonable exercise, and exogenous calcium supplementation help decrease premature onset of osteoporosis.

If amenorrhea or oligomenorrhea are due to hyperprolactinemia, then a careful evaluation of pituitary sellar contents is mandatory. A large pituitary adenoma may be treated medically or removed transphenoidally by an experienced neurosurgeon. The incidence of recurrent hyperprolactinemia is high and patients should be made aware of this. If there is a microadenoma or if no tumor is visible on a sellar CT scan, then medical therapy with bromocriptine is indicated. Therapy should be initiated at the lowest level possible and titrated against serum prolactin levels until the latter are brought into the normal range. A dose of 7.5 mg/day or greater rarely is necessary to bring serum prolactin levels down to the normal range. Yearly CT scans should be performed to rule out suprasellar enlargement of the pituitary.

All hyperprolactinemic patients, even if they are not interested in fertility, should be treated since there is an association between osteoporosis and hypoestrogenemia because of elevated prolactin levels.

Patients with diagnoses of polycystic ovarian syndrome should have intermittent withdrawal of menses with a progestin because of the high incidence of endometrial hyperplasia in this disorder.

Abnormal bleeding

Acute adolescent menorrhagia. Abnormal menstrual bleeding is one of the most common reasons for gynecologic consultation in adolescents. The spectrum of complaints range from minor deviations from the average menstrual pattern to life-threatening hemorrhage. Whatever the seriousness of symptoms, it is usually a subject of great concern for both the patient and her parents and it deserves attentive consideration.

Acute menorrhagia usually occurs quite dramatically and requires prompt management. The clinical picture is that of a pale,anxious teenager who presents at the emergency ward with heavy bleeding of several days' or weeks' duration.

Because dysfunctional uterine bleeding, by definition, occurs on the basis of anovulatory cycles, the teenager in the first years of her menstrual life is the most susceptible candidate.

The differential diagnosis of acute adolescent vaginal hemorrhage is summarized in Table 23-9. Although dysfunctional (anovulatory) uterine bleeding accounts for the largest number of these cases, other etiologies of abnormal genital bleeding should be ruled out systematically.

Pregnancy-related complications are common in adolescents and should be excluded, even in the adolescent who denies sexual activity. These include spontaneous abortions, complications of elective pregnancy termination procedures, ectopic pregnancy, and gestational trophoblastic disease. Occasionally young patients present with third-trimester bleeding in a previously undiagnosed pregnancy.

Though rare, benign and malignant conditions of the genital tract may be responsible for severe hemorrhage. Sarcoma botryoides, which most often occurs in the young child, rarely presents during adolescent years. Bleeding vaginal adenosis, clear-cell adenocarcinoma, extensive ectropion, and cervical or vaginal polyps or hemangiomas may be found on pelvic examination. Uterine neoplasms and endometrial polyps are encountered rarely in this age group. Estrogen-secreting

Table 23-9. Differential diagnosis of adolescent menorrhagia

I. Anovulatory uterine bleeding

II. Pregnancy-related complications
- Spontaneous abortion
- Complications of pregnancy termination procedures
- Ectopic pregnancy
- Gestational trophoblastic diseases
- Bleeding of the third trimester of pregnancy

III. Local genital tract conditions
- Benign and malignant tumors (vagina, cervix, uterus, ovary)
- Infection
- Intrauterine contraceptive devices
- Trauma
- Intravaginal foreign bodies

IV. Systemic causes
- Coagulation disorders
- Thyroid dysfunction
- Diabetes mellitus
- Nutritional disorders, iron deficiency
- Nepatic diseases
- Renal diseases

V. Hormonal
- Oral contraceptives
- Intramuscular
- Subcutaneous

ovarian tumors also can cause endometrial hyperplasia which leads to heavy bleeding, as it can during the perimenopausal age group. PID with associated endometritis and intrauterine contraceptive devices may induce heavy vaginal bleeding. Postcoital or self-imposed traumatic conditions, and intravaginal foreign bodies should be considered also.

Coagulation disorders are probably the most common systemic condition associated with acute menorrhagia. Idiopathic thrombocytopenic purpura, von Willebrand's disease, Glanzmann's disease, thalassemia major, Falconi's anemia, leukemia, side effects of radiation and chemotherapy, and some drugs (anticoagulants, aspirin, hepatotoxic drugs) are possible causes of deficient coagulation mechanisms.[20]

Other systemic conditions possibly associated with menorrhagia include thyroid dysfunction, diabetes mellitus, nutritional disorders, and hepatic and renal diseases.

Patients who present with acute menstrual hemorrhage in their late adolescence should be investigated for other causes of chronic anovulation.

A complete history of recent events as well as premenarchal development should be obtained. In such cases, it is difficult to assess the amount of blood loss because the frightened patient and her over-anxious mother are not objective. Questions about the number of perineal pads or tampons utilized, degree of saturation, the quantity and size of blood clots, and presence of orthostatic symptoms facilitate estimation of blood loss. The normal volume of menstrual bleeding averages 30 to 40 mL and corresponds to 10 to 15 moderately soaked pads or tampons. Information pertinent to all possible causes of vaginal hemorrhage should be obtained.

A complete physical examination should be performed. Special attention must be paid to signs of hypovolemia and anemia, namely pallor, low blood pressure and orthostatic hypotension, tachycardia, and the presence of a functional heart murmur. The abdomen should be carefully palpated for the presence of a mass, localized pain, and/or peritoneal signs. A speculum examination is mandatory to evaluate the amount of bleeding and to rule out any vaginal abnormality and visualize the cervix. In the presence of a tight hymen, blood clots may accumulate and distend the vagina. Finding as much as 500 mL of coagulated blood in the vagina is not unusual. This retrograde accumulation of clots may also account for cervical dilation which can be attributed erroneously to a spontaneous abortion. Internal genital structures are assessed by rectovaginal examination looking for the presence of uterine enlargement and adnexal masses or tenderness.

The laboratory work-up should consist of hemoglobin and hematocrit, platelet count, blood type and cross match, and basic clotting studies including prothrombin time (PT), partial thromboplastin time (PTT) and bleeding time. These specimens should be drawn before the institution of any hormonal therapy or transfusion. A serum β-hCG or other highly sensitive pregnancy test, and cervical cultures for *N. gonorrhea* and *C. trachomatis* should be obtained in every patient. Determination of blood sugar, thyroid function tests and urinalysis are recommended but not essential before treatment is instituted. In certain instances, a pelvic sonogram may be indicated for evaluation of an enlarged uterus or adnexal mass. The need for additional diagnostic studies depends on the clinical assessment of each patient.

Therapy of acute adolescent menorrhagia should aim to control bleeding, restore adequate intravascular volume, correct anemia, treat underlying conditions when present, and prevent recurrence. The method and intensity of therapy obviously depends on the severity of hemorrhage. The adolescent in whom the bleeding is mild to moderate without signs of hypovolemia can be treated on an outpatient basis, provided close follow-up and good compliance are assured. These patients often present with moderate anemia due to prolonged bleeding. In the presence of severe hemorrhage or anemia (hemoglobin less than 8 gm %) or when the patient is hypovolemic, admission is mandatory.

The initial treatment is medical rather than surgical in most patients. Because the primary cause of bleeding is due to unstable endometrium because of fluctuating estrogen levels, the rationale of therapy is to stop the hemorrhage by administering estrogen and stabilize the endometrium with progestogens. Birth control pills may be used effectively in this situation. These are administered at the rate of one pill every 4 hours until the bleeding subsides. If bleeding does not stop within 24 to 36 hours, other causes of bleeding should be considered. In the presence of acute, severe hemorrhage, some centers administer intravenous conjugated estrogens administered at a dose of 25 mg every 4 hours for not more than 3 doses in addition to the oral progestogens. The major side effect of oral progestogen and intravenous estrogen is nausea and vomiting for which anti-nausea medications may be administered prophylactically. Blood is replaced when necessary.

When the bleeding has stopped or decreased appreciably, oral contraceptives are tapered gradually over a period of 7 days and then continued at a rate of one pill per day for 21 days. Withdrawal bleeding will follow the discontinuation of treatment. The patient should be informed that this may be heavy but self-limited.

Dilation and curettage (D&C) is reserved for those cases where medical treatment fails to control the bleeding within 24 to 36 hours. Because the incidence of an intrauterine pathologic abnormality is very small, this intervention is rarely required. In most instances where medical management has failed, endometrial hyperplasia is present. Occasionally, curettings will be scant following a complete endometrial slough.

Two patients have been encountered who did not respond to D&C. In both instances bleeding was controlled by uterine packing. This was carried out using an iodoform gauze which was left in place for 24 hours and then withdrawn slowly. Prophylactic antibiotic coverage should be given in this unusual situation. The only patient who required hysterectomy was a 20 year old woman with artificial heart valves who was anticoagulated.

Close follow-up of these patients is essential to prevent recurrence and provide adequate emotional support. After the initial phase of therapy, the patient may remain anovulatory. Therefore it is advisable to continue these patients on low-dose birth control pills for a period of at least 3 months. The adolescent in need of birth control can be continued on low-dose oral contraceptives. When the risk of unwanted pregnancy is not a concern, the best approach is to start the patient on basal body temperature charts and administer oral progesterones cyclically if the temperature curve is monophasic. A rational regimen is to induce withdrawal bleeding every 6 weeks with a 10-day course of medroxyprogesterone acetate, 10 mg daily. This treatment is usually adequate to prevent endometrial hyperproliferation. Because it does not suppress the hypothalamic-pituitary-ovarian axis it allows the teenager to develop regular, ovulatory cycles on her own. When this occurs the patient may menstruate spontaneously between courses.

Long-term follow up includes correction of anemia with iron supplements and nutritional counselling, and surveillance for spontaneous occurrence of ovulatory cycles. These patients presenting with acute menorrhagia during the perimenarchal period are at greater risk of chronic anovulation, infertility, and endometrial carcinoma.

The emotional aspects of this problem should not be underestimated. For these youngsters, a hemorrhagic event of this type is a very sad way to begin their active reproductive life. Adequate explanation, reassurance, and psychologic support during the acute episode and over the subsequent months will serve to guide these teenagers through their menstrual problems optimistically.

Chronic anovulation

Persistent hypermenorrhea. Cyclic heavy menses is a frequent complaint in adolescents. These patients usually present with more or less regular menstrual cycles, ranging from 4 to 6 weeks, but characterized by excessive bleeding, either in amount or duration.

Although anovulation is the leading etiology of recurrent hypermenorrhea in this population, other causes such as uterine pathologies, coagulation defects, and systemic diseases must be considered.

Besides a thorough history and physical examination, the basic work-up of these teenagers should consist of hemoglobin, hematocrit, and platelet count determination, screening clotting studies, and thyroid function tests.

Therapy depends on the degree of the bleeding abnormality. Patients with mildly increased menstrual flow in whom there is no secondary anemia can be managed expectantly. In these cases, recording of basal body temperature confirms the diagnosis of anovulation. Prostaglandin inhibitors may decrease the amount of bleeding. Adolescents in need of birth control obviously benefit from oral contraception. When treatment is required because of the degree of flow or associated anemia, medroxyprogesterone acetate is prescribed to regulate cycles and induce a progestational effect on the endometrium. In this situation, 10 mg daily is administered from the 6th to the 25th day of each cycle. For most of these young patients, a calendar month schedule (treatment for the first 10 days of each month) is understood more easily. After 3 to 6 months, therapy is discontinued and the patient is observed for spontaneous occurrence of ovulatory cycles. Failure of hormonal therapy is an indication for D&C.

Persistent polymenorrhea. Too frequent periods is a common complaint among this age group. Anovulation is the most frequent cause of polymenorrhea in adolescents. In some patients this menstrual abnormality may also originate from a short follicular phase or corpus luteum dysfunction which usually is self-limiting, until such time as the hypothalamic-pituitary-ovarian axis matures.

The physician should be aware that very often this complaint is unjustified. A thorough history frequently discovers that the patient calculates her intermenstrual interval from the last day of a period to the first day of the next one. The recording of a menstrual calendar and information about normal physiology are usually sufficient to reassure these adolescents.

When cycles are shorter than 21 days, therapy with medroxyprogesterone acetate administered as described above, is indicated. With very short intermenstrual intervals it may be necessary to start the treatment on the 10th day of the cycle for a period of 15 days.

Control of abnormal bleeding in patients on chemotherapy. Abnormal bleeding may occur as a result of chemotherapy in the postmenarchal adolescent with leukemia and low platelet count. The adolescent should be examined gently; ultrasonography may be helpful to exclude pelvic pathology if adequate bimanual examination is difficult in the virginal girl. Hormonal therapy, such as continuous low-dose birth control pills, can be prescribed to induce amenorrhea and endometrial atrophy until the patient has normal platelet function and can cope with normal menses. An option would be the use of GnRH agonists such as those employed for the inductionof amenorrhea.[67]

Premenstrual symptoms. Premenstrual symptoms are commonly reported by adolescents and adult women and include bloating, weight gain, breast soreness, hunger, thirst, fatigue, acne, constipation, hot flushes and chills, difficulty in concentrating, and mood changes in the luteal phase of the cycle. Girls with migraine headaches may suffer an increase in headaches premenstrually and with menses; similarly girls with epilepsy may note an increase in seizure severity and/or frequency premenstrually or with the onset of menses. Retarded girls may have behavior outbursts that are difficult for their caretakers, and psychotic patients may exhibit more uncontrollable actions. Although most adolescents are aware of some premenstrual symptoms, usually reassurance and a few suggestions about diet and exercise are sufficient. Adolescents who experience severe symptoms often are under stress and have other psychosocial issues that need to be addressed. Medical evaluation of the premenstrual symptoms, and psychologic counseling may help. About 20% to 40% of adult women of reproductive age have sufficiently bothersome symptoms to cause a temporary deterioration in interpersonal relationships or job effectiveness; less than 5% of adult women have severe symptoms.

The cause of premenstrual syndrome has been variously attributed to estrogen and progesterone because these symptoms occur in the luteal phase of the cycle and disappear when ovulation is inhibited with the use of GnRH agonists. Because weight may not increase in spite of bloating, changes that the patient notes may occur because of local fluid shifts and bowel wall edema. The release of the opiates may increase appetite and result in unusual food cravings, fatigue, depression, and emotional lability. Later in the cycle the shift toward anxiety and irritability, vague abdominal cramps with loose bowel movements or diarrhea, headaches, and chills and sweats may result from withdrawal of endogenous opiates as hormone levels fall. In sensitive women cyclic exposure to, and subsequent withdrawal from, the central effects of the neuropeptides may result in a cascade of neuroendocrine changes and cause clinical symptomatology.

In the next decade, therapeutic approaches to premenstrual syndrome may be improved by an increased understanding of the pathophysiology. Alteration of the ovulatory menstrual cycle can alleviate symptoms. GnRH agonists can prevent the cyclic progesterone and estrogen production; however, this approach may be more useful as a probe in defining the etiology of the problem than as a long-term treatment because of the potential for osteoporosis in estrogen-deficient patients and menopause symptoms. Preventing ovulation but allowing some estrogen secretion might protect the bones from osteoporosis but would potentially place the endometrium at risk of unopposed estrogen and carcinoma. Danazol may inhibit ovulation but may have undesirable side effects in adolescents. Although oral contraceptives have produced variable results in adult women with premenstrual syndrome, many adolescents, especially those with premenstrual exacerbation of seizures or headaches, show striking improvement on pills low in estrogen and progestin.

For most adolescents premenstrual symptoms are mild and the recognition that they are a real entity can be reassuring. For those troubled by their symptoms, the cyclic occurrence should be established by recording symptoms on a special calendar for 2 to 3 cycles. Otherwise mood alterations and depression occurring through the cycle may be attributed to "premenstrual syndrome" and adequate psychologic intervention not undertaken. A calendar is useful also in deciding which symptoms are most troubling to the patient. Although no controlled studies have demonstrated benefit in diet or exercise, most centers start with this approach because the lifestyle changes are healthy and undoubtedly give the adolescent a sense of control over her life. Patients are instructed to avoid salty foods, alcohol, caffeine, chocolate, and concentrated sweets, and to eat 4 to 6 smaller meals per day during the premenstrual period. A written sheet listing foods to avoid (such as cola, coffee, hot dogs, canned foods, chips) and foods to add to the diet (such as unsalted popcorn, raw vegetables and fruits, skim milk, complex carbohydrates, high fiber foods, low fat meats) is helpful to the young woman. A program of aerobic exercise should be strongly encouraged, and areas of stress should be identified. Many patients experience an increased sense of well-being and control with this type of program.

In adolescents with specific symptoms, drug therapy may be considered after a period of intervention with diet, exercise, and stress reduction. For indications such as edema and weight gain from fluid retention, a mild diuretic such as hydrochlorothiazide 25 to 50 mg once or twice daily during the last week of the cycle (plus supplemental potassium by diet) or spironolactone can be prescribed. Mefenamic acid, 250 mg every eight hours starting on day 18 of the cycle, increased to 500 mg on day 19 of the cycle, lessens fatigue, headache, and general aches and pains; this medication may be especially useful in those patients with severe dysmenorrhea. Other nonsteroidal antiinflammatory drugs (NSAID) used in treating dysmenorrhea may be useful; none of these should be prescribed to the adolescent at risk of pregnancy. Oral contraceptives may be effective in adolescent girls and are especially useful if birth control is also needed.

A variety of other drugs have been used in adult women but none of the studies have focused on adolescents. For example, low-dose danazol (200 mg/day) is beneficial. Alprazolam, 0.25 mg three times daily from day 20 until the second day of menstruation and then tapered by one tablet per day relieves premenstrual symptoms, but concern about patients becoming dependent on this drug and having withdrawal symptoms has made clinicians reluctant to use this group of drugs in adolescents. Bromocriptine has been used in adult women to alleviate breast soreness but this symptoms is rarely a major complaint of adolescents. In adolescents with breast soreness, preference is given to reducing caffeine consumption and a small dose of NSAID's. None of these medications should be prescribed to adolescents at risk of having unprotected intercourse. In addition, adolescents need to be questioned regarding over-the-counter medications. Vitamin B_6 has been popular with some self-help groups. Patients should be cautioned about the toxic potential of this vitamin to cause sensory neuropathy even in low doses.

Dysmenorrhea. Dysmenorrhea is probably the most common gynecologic complaint of adolescents. Dysmenorrhea in adolescents usually is primary (or functional), but can be secondary to endometriosis, obstructing müllerian anomalies, and other pelvic pathology.

In typical histories, the 14- or 15-year-old teenager, 1 to 3 years after menarche, develops crampy lower abdominal pain with each menstrual period. Usually the pains start within 1 to 4 hours of the onset of the menses and last for 24 to 48 hours. In some cases the pain may start 1 to 2 days before the menses and continue for 2 to 4 days into the menses. Nausea or vomiting (or both), diarrhea, lower backache, thigh pain, headache, fatigue, nervousness, dizziness, or rarely syncope may accompany the cramps. Although dysmenorrhea is usually associated with the onset of ovulatory menses, some adolescents may experience cramps from the first few cycles which are often anovulatory, or with episodes of anovulatory dysfunctional bleeding associated with heavy menses and clots.

In the uterus, phospholipids from the dead cell membranes are converted to arachidonic acid which can be metabolized by at least two enzymes; lipoxygenase which begins the production of leukotrienes and cyclooxygenase, which leads to cyclic endoperoxides (PGG and PGH). The cyclic endoperoxides are then converted by specific enzymes to prostacyclin, thromboxanes, and the prostaglandins PGD_2, PGE_2 and PGF_2. Prostaglandin PGF_2 mediates pain sensation and stimulates smooth muscle contraction, whereas PGE_2 potentiates platelet disaggregation and vasodilatation. Exogenously administered PGE_2 and PGF_2 can produce uterine contractions as well as systemic symptoms such as vomiting, diarrhea and dizziness. Although plasma levels of PG are normal in dysmenorrheic women, increased sensitivity or generalized overproduction of prostaglandins may occur.[10]

The PG hypothesis has been further strengthened by the observation that drugs which inhibit prostaglandin synthesis can relieve dysmenorrhea and the associated symptoms. NSAID agents are divided into two classes: carboxylic acids and enolic acids. Enolic-acid agents include phenylbutazone and piroxicam and act by inhibition of the isomerase/reductase step in the production of PGE_2 and PGF_2. Phenylbutazone is not prescribed in dysmenorrhea because of side effects, and piroxicam requires further studies to delineate its role in the therapy of this problem. The carboxylates, most frequently used in the treatment of dysmenorrhea, can be divided into 4 categories: salicyclic acids/esters (aspirin, diflunisal); acetic acids (indomethacin, sulindac, tolmetin); propionic acids (ibuprofen, naproxen, fenoprofen, ketoprofen, flurbiprofen); and fenamates (mefenamic acid, meclofenamate, tolfenamic acid, flufenamic acid). The salicyclic acids and ester appear to inhibit cyclooxygenase but aspirin has little potency compared to some of the other NSAID in reducing prostaglandin synthesis and may increase menstrual flow. Thus aspirin is used less often than previously in the treatment of dysmenorrhea. Indomethacin is the best known drug of the acetic acid group used for treatment of dysmenorrhea, but side effects have prevented its use for most, if not all, patients. Selection is made usually from the two last groups, propionic acids and fenamates, for clinical treatment.

Ibuprofen and naproxen have been most widely studied for the relief of pain in dysmenorrhea. Numerous clinical studies have found these agents to be effective in both adult and adolescent women with pain relief in 67% to 86% of patients. The sodium salt of naproxen has a more rapid absorption than naproxen and can give very rapid relief of symptoms. The newly released prostaglandin inhibitor, flurbiprofen at doses of 50 mg every 6 hours, or 100 mg every 12 hours, also appears to be very effective in the relief of dysmenorrhea.

The fenamates are potent inhibitors of prostaglandin synthesis and can antagonize the action of already formed prostaglandins. This increased activity may give this class of drug a theoretical advantage in treatment although comparative controlled drug trials are not available for a conclusion to be made. A trial of mefenamic acid is useful when propionic acids are ineffective in the individual patient.

Oral contraceptives lessen dysmenorrhea, probably in part related to their antiovulatory actions in addition to their ability to produce endometrial hypoplasia, reduced menstrual flow, and subsequently, less prostaglandins.

In assessing the adolescent with dysmenorrhea, the physician needs to know the patient's menstrual history, timing of the cramps, premenstrual symptoms, and her response to the cramps. Key questions would be: Is she missing school? If so, how many days? Does she miss other activities such as a party? Does she have nausea and vomiting, diarrhea or dizziness? What medications has she used before? What is the nature of the mother-daughter interaction? Did the mother or sister have cramps? Is there a family history of endometriosis? The question about previous medications is particularly crucial because with the availability of ibuprofen over-the-counter, many adolescents have tried this medication, in subtherapeutic doses, and have subsequently discarded the usefulness of ibuprofen.

For the virginal girl of 13 or 14 years of age who has mild cramps the first day of her menses, a normal physical examination, including inspection of the genitalia to exclude an abnormality of the hymen, is reassuring. A speculum examination is not necessary. Treatment includes a careful explanation to the patient of the nature of the problem and a chance for her to ask questions regarding her anatomy. Mild analgesics, such as aspirin, acetaminophen, and especially over-the-counter ibuprofen (200 to 400 mg) usually give symptomatic relief.

Adolescent girls with moderate or severe dysmenorrhea should have a careful pelvic examination. In the majority of adolescents who are carefully prepared, a vaginal examination is atraumatic. In some patients, a rectoabdominal examination in lithotomy position is all that is possible, but even this will exclude adnexal tenderness and masses. The uterosacral ligaments should be palpated carefully for tenderness or the presence of nodules, which would suggest endometriosis. Ultrasonography is useful in defining uterine and vaginal anomalies with obstruction.

If the examination is normal, treatment should be directed at symptomatic relief. The most common approach is to prescribe one of the following NSAID compounds: (1) naproxen sodium 550 mg given immediately, and then 275 mg every 6 hours; (2) naproxen sodium double strength 550 mg twice a day; (3) naproxen 250 to 375 mg twice a day to three times a day; (4) ibuprofen 400 every 4 to 6 hours to 800 mg three times a day with a loading dose of 800-1200 mg; or (5) mefenamic acid 500 mg given immediately, and then 250 mg every 6 hours. As noted above, flurbiprofen 50 mg every 6 hours or 100 mg 2 or 3 times daily and meclofenamate 100 mg initially, followed by 50 to 100 mg every 6 hours are promising.

For most patients effective relief can be obtained by starting the antiprostaglandin medicine at the onset of the menses and continued for the first 1 to 2 days of the cycle (or for the usual duration of cramps). The patient should be told to start as soon as she knows her menses are coming (i.e., the first sign of cramps or bleeding). A loading dose is important in patients with symptoms that are severe and occur rapidly. In this situation, a rapidly absorbed drug such as naproxen sodium would be preferable to naproxen. Generally, giving the medication at the onset of the menses prevents the inadvertent administration of the drug to a pregnant woman. However, a nonsexually active patent with severe cramps may sometimes benefit from starting the drug one or two days before the onset of her menses. A patient may respond to one of these drugs and not another; each should be tried in increasing doses before changing to another drug. Because life stresses may lessen the effectiveness in an individual, patient doses should be based on the response in more than one cycle. Usually medication is prescribed for two to three cycles before changing. Previously the patient may have taken inadequate doses of a medicine, particularly ibuprofen, to obtain relief.

The NSAID compounds should be avoided in patients with known or suspected ulcer disease, gastrointestinal bleeding, clotting disorders (because of effects on platelet aggregation), renal disease, in preoperative patients, and those with allergies to aspirin or NSAIDs or aspirin-induced asthma. All these drugs should be taken with food, even though some patients prefer liquids on the first day of the cycle. The side effects of these drugs appear minimal in short-term use, but the possibility of allergy and gastrointestinal irritation and bleeding should be explained to the patient. Some patients complain of fluid retention or fatigue with these agents.

In some patients, when NSAID drugs are contraindicated or produce undesirable side effects, acetaminophen can be prescribed, often combined with 15 to 30 mg of codeine. Usually only a few pills are needed each month. However, adolescents frequently complain of dizziness and nausea with codeine-containing medications.

The adolescent should be seen initially every 3 or 4 months to evaluate the effectiveness of the medication. Such visits also facilitate the doctor-patient rapport that is essential in the treatment of this problem. Although a few adolescents will use cramps as an excuse to stay out of school or to gain sympathy from the mother, patients should not be made to feel emotionally unstable because they complain of cramps. Some girls can continue to exercise during their menses, others find the discomfort may be too great on the first day. Girls who are involved in competitive sports and have fewer ovulatory menses appear to have less dysmenorrhea.

If dysmenorrhea is relieved by oral contraceptive pills, medication is usually prescribed for 3 to 6 months and then discontinued (frequently during the summer when school attendance will not be disrupted). Often the patient will continue to have relief from cramps for several additional (commonly anovulatory) cycles before the more severe dysmenorrhea recurs. When the cramps recur, a trial of other antiprostaglandin drugs should again be tempted before reinstituting oral contraceptives. The sexually active adolescent with severe dysmenorrhea usually prefers to continue long-term on oral contraceptives. The return of increasingly severe dysmenorrhea in spite of the use of oral contraceptives raises the possibility of organic disease such as endometriosis and calls for a re-evaluation and consideration of laparoscopy for diagnosis.

Pelvic pain

If the patient fails to respond to the antiprostaglandin drugs and continues to have severe pain or vomiting, or at the initial evaluation needs birth control, a course of oral contraceptives should be tried. A pelvic examination is necessary before this medication is prescribed. Cramps are usually substantially, if not completely, relieved with the anovulatory cycles and scantier flow. If severe cramps persist despite three to four cycles of ovulation suppression therapy, or if the examination reveals tenderness or nodularity, laparoscopy is indicated to exclude endometriosis or other organic causes.

Acute pelvic pain. Acute pelvic pain necessitates aggressive management because of the intensity of symptoms and the possibility that a potentially life-threatening condition may exist.

The differential diagnosis of acute pelvic pain in adolescents is summarized in Table 23-10. The gynecologic causes can be divided into three categories: infection, rupture, and torsion. In general, symptoms associated with infection usually develop progressively over a few days. In the cases of rupture or torsion, pain occurs suddenly, and the patient can most often tell precisely at what time symptoms began. Nongynecologic etiologies involve mainly the digestive or the urinary tract.

The history should define the sequence of events, the pain location and its radiation, and associated gastrointestinal, urinary tract, and systemic symptoms. A careful menstrual, contraceptive, and sexual history is also mandatory.

A complete physical examination should be performed. Special attention should be given to the abdomen to localize the pain, define the presence of, and identify peritoneal signs and evidence of bowel obstruction. A pelvic examination must be performed on every patient to determine the uterine size,

Table 23-10. Differential diagnosis of acute pelvic pain in adolescent females

- I. Gynecologic causes
  - A. Infection
    - Pelvic inflammatory disease
  - B. Rupture
    - Follicular cyst
    - Corpus luteum cyst
    - Endometrioma
    - Tumor
  - C. Torsion
    - Ovarian cyst
    - Tube
    - Hydatid of Morgagni
- II. Nongynecologic causes
  - A. Gastro-intestinal
    - Appendicitis
    - Meckel's diverticulitis
    - Gastro-enteritis
    - Mesentery adenitis
    - Intestinal obstruction
  - B. Urinary
    - Cystitis
    - Pyelonephritis
    - Calculi

shape, and symmetry, the presence of adnexal or cervical tenderness, and to identify adnexal masses or thickening.

The basic laboratory workup should include a complete blood count with differential diagnosis, an erythrocyte sedimentation rate (ESR), a complete urinalysis, a urine culture, a pregnancy test, and a cervical culture for *N. gonorrhea* and *C. trachomatis*.

A high white count and/or sedimentation rate suggests the presence of either an infectious or inflammatory process or the presence of ischemia, usually secondary to adnexal torsion or bowel obstruction. Hemoglobin and hematocrit usually are poor indicators of bleeding, since in acute hemorrhage hemodilution may not have occurred. Depending on the type of pregnancy test utilized, it should be remembered that a negative results does not always rule out an early intrauterine or an ectopic pregnancy.

When the pelvic examination is not completely satisfactory, a pelvic ultrasound may be valuable to confirm the presence of a mass, to identify the presence of free fluid in the cul-de-sac, and to localize a suspected pregnancy.

After these first steps have been taken, all patients fall into one of the following situations:

1. There is a definite surgical emergency which necessitates immediate attention. The suspected diagnosis is usually an acute hemoperitoneum, a ruptured appendix, or some other gastrointestinal surgical emergency.
2. The patient is suffering from a medical condition (e.g., urinary tract infection, gastroenteritis, pelvic inflammatory disease, etc.), and adequate treatment is started.
3. The problem needs further investigation (e.g., urinary calculi).
4. The condition remains undiagnosed and whether this patient has PID, an ectopic pregnancy, appendicitis, or a ruptured or torsioned ovarian cyst remains unknown.

At this point, laparoscopy becomes an invaluable diagnostic tool. The potential risk of a surgical diagnostic procedure remains a concern for many physicians. In fact, a laparoscopy provides an immediate diagnosis which allows for appropriate medical or surgical treatment. It is also more cost effective to perform an immediate laparoscopy than to subject the patient to a long period of inpatient observation during which a surgical catastrophe, such as a ruptured appendix or an ectopic pregnancy, remains a possibility. In cases of ruptured ovarian cysts or hemorrhagic corpus luteum, in which there is no more active bleeding, it is possible to aspirate free blood and clots and to ensure hemostasis by fulguration of bleeders. This technique may save the patient several days of agonizing pain and usually allows her to be discharged within 12 hours of the procedure. The advantages of laparoscopy certainly outweigh the minimal surgical risk in these generally healthy teenagers, particularly where appendicitis is a real possibility.[43]

Table 23-11 summarizes the principle laparoscopic diagnosis in 121 patients ages 11 to 17 who presented at Boston Children's Hospital with acute abdominal pain between 1980 and 1986. In general, the most common cause of pain resulted from a complication of an ovarian cyst. It is of interest that the causes of acute abdominal pain in the adolescent do not appear to be age related (Table 23-12).

Chronic pelvic pain. Chronic pelvic pain (CPP) in adolescents is a frequent complaint and a source of frustration for the patient, her parents, and her physician. CPP can be defined as three months or more of constant or intermittent, cyclic or acyclic pelvic pain, which has necessitated at least three separate visits to a physician, and have not resulted in a definite diagnosis. Symptoms are dull or severe pain, dysmenorrhea, dyspareunia, or vaginal pain. Very often these teenagers have been absent from school frequently, have seen a number of physicians, have undergone a number of

Table 23-11. Principal laparoscopic diagnoses in 121 adolescent females 11 to 17 years old with acute pelvic pain. The Children's Hospital, Boston, 1980–1986

	Patients	(%)
Ovarian cyst	47	39
Acute PID	21	17
Adnexal torsion	9	8
Endometriosis	6	5
Ectopic pregnancy	4	3
Appendicitis	13	11
No pathology	21	17

Table 23-12. Age-related prevalence of principal laparoscopic findings in 121 adolescent females 11 to 17 years old with acute pelvic pain. The Children's Hospital, Boston, 1980–1986

	Age 11-13 Pts. (%)	Age 14-15 Pts. (%)	Age 16-17 Pts. (%)
Ovarian cyst	12 (50)	16 (35)	19 (37)
Acute PID	4 (17)	7 (16)	10 (19)
Adnexal torsion	0 (0)	7 (16)	2 (4)
Endometriosis	0 (0)	2 (4)	4 (7)
Ectopic pregnancy	0 (0)	3 (7)	1 (2)
Appendicitis	3 (13)	4 (9)	6 (12)
No pathology	5 (20)	6 (13)	10 (19)
TOTAL	24 (100)	45 (100)	52 (100)

radiologic examinations, and have tried a variety of analgesics without success. Many have already been referred for psychologic or psychiatric evaluation.

The CPP patient, after having been told, often more than once, that nothing is wrong with her, may present with a considerable amount of anger, frustration, or desperation. It is, therefore, important to assure her that all efforts will be made to resolve her problem and that she will not be abandoned or her symptoms dismissed as merely psychosomatic.

Table 23-13 summarizes the differential diagnosis of CPP in adolescent females. It includes many organ systems which can be responsible for pelvic symptoms either directly or by referred pain and those of functional or psychogenic etiology.

An efficient approach to the problem involves taking a thorough history, performing an adequate physical examination, and judiciously using diagnostic studies.

It is essential to review the complete history of the problem, including the description, location, and radiation of the pain, exacerbating and relieving factors, association with the menstrual cycle or with gastrointestinal, urinary and, musculoskeletal symptoms. The medical and surgical history may also provide a clue. All prior diagnostic procedures and trials of treatment should be recorded, and old medical records should be obtained if possible. The familial and social history and the association of the pain episodes with stressful events should be detailed.

A complete physical examination should be performed and the abdomen carefully palpated in search of any masses, tender areas and organomegaly. Special care should be taken to differentiate deep pain from abdominal wall tenderness, especially in patients who have undergone prior surgeries where adhesions to the abdominal wall scar may be present. A skeletal assessment to identify any orthopedic abnormality that may be the cause of referred pelvic pain or associated with a congenital reproductive tract anomaly is also of great importance. A speculum examination should be performed to identify any vaginal or cervical anomaly and to obtain cultures and cytology specimens. The bimanual recto-vaginal-abdominal palpation evaluates the pelvic structures and localizes tender areas. The posterior cul-de-sac should also be assessed for pain and nodularity.

Table 23-13. Differential diagnosis of chronic pelvic pain in adolescent females

I. Gynecologic causes
- Dysmenorrhea (primary, secondary)
- Mittelschmerz
- Endometriosis
- Chronic pelvic inflammatory disease
- Ovarian cyst
- Genital tract malformations
- Pelvic congestion
- Pelvic serositis

II. Gastrointestinal causes
- Constipation, bowel spasms
- Appendiceal fecaliths
- Inflammatory bowel diseases
- Dietary intolerance (lactose)

III. Urinary causes
- Urinary tract infection
- Hydronephrosis
- Urethral stricture
- Urethral caruncle
- Urinary retention

IV. Orthopedic causes
- Lordosis, kyphosis, scoliosis
- Herniation of intervertebral disk

V. Adhesions
- Postoperative
- Post pelvic infection

VI. Psychogenic

The minimal laboratory workup in these patients consists of a complete blood count with differential and ESR, a urinalysis and culture, and cervical cultures for *N. gonorrhea* and *C. trachomatis*. Other hematologic and biochemical studies are ordered depending on clinical indications.

Pelvic ultrasonography may be useful to define a mass, to provide information about a suspected genital tract malformation, and to screen patients in whom a satisfactory pelvic examination is impossible. Routine sonography in every patient is probably not advisable. A pelvic mass detected by ultrasound often is not found during laparoscopy.

No specific rules can be given regarding radiologic examinations. Submitting all these teenagers to pelvic radiation without clinical indications is not advisable. Gastrointestinal, urologic, and orthopedic studies should be ordered on the basis of the diagnostic impression after a thorough history and physical and laboratory workup.

Laparoscopy is invaluable in the diagnosis of CPP. It can diagnose or confirm the presence of organic disease that cannot be demonstrated by physical, radiologic, and sonographic examination. It allows the surgeon to obtain appropriate biopsies and to perform some primary therapy such as fulguration of endometriosis, lysis of adhesions, and aspiration of ovarian cysts. Negative findings at laparoscopy may be equally valuable in that they reassure the patient that no organic disease is present and help her accept the idea that she might have a functional problem that requires medical or psychologic treatment.

Indications for laparoscopy in the evaluation of adolescents with CPP can be summarized as follows:

1. Dysmenorrhea unresponsive to the usual therapy with prostaglandin-inhibitors and/or ovulation suppression.
2. Confirmation or exclusion of clinically suspected endometriosis, chronic pelvic inflammatory disease, pelvic adhesions, appendiceal fecaliths, ovarian cysts, and pelvic serositis.
3. Evaluation of undiagnosed pain after appropriate workup.

At the Children's Hospital, experience with laparoscopy in the diagnosis of CPP in adolescent females revealed that between July 1974 and December 1983, 282 patients ranging in age from 9 to 21 years underwent a diagnostic laparoscopy because of chronic pelvic symptoms.[43] Most of these adolescents had been referred after a negative gastrointestinal and urinary tract workup or because of dysmenorrhea unresponsive to the usual therapy of prostaglandin inhibitors or oral contraceptives. Many of these patients had undergone psychiatric evaluation because of persistent and undiagnosed pain. Cases of chronic pelvic inflammatory disease were not included in the data because this condition is usually suspected on the basis of the past history and the finding of an elevated ESR. In these patients, a laparoscopy is usually performed to confirm the diagnosis and to evaluate its severity rather than to establish the etiology of CPP.

Table 23-14 summarizes the postoperative diagnosis in these patients. Three quarters of the patients had intrapelvic pathology. Endometriosis was the most frequent finding; it was diagnosed in 45% of cases. In most instances, the disease was mild to moderate, with implants located in the posterior cul-de-sac, on the ovaries, and on the lateral pelvic walls. The next most common finding was postoperative adhesions, which was present in 13% of patients and was for the most part secondary to appendectomy or ovarian cystectomy.

One of the most puzzling laparoscopic findings was the presence of pelvic serositis in 5% of the patients. This was characterized by hyperemia and granuloma-like lesions of the pelvic peritoneum and uterine serosa. Peritoneal biopsies revealed the presence of mesothelial hyperplasia with hemosiderin deposits. Peritoneal culture and cytology were normal. The significance of these changes remains unclear. Whether these are signs of very early endometriosis, a reaction to repeated hemoperitoneum secondary to leaking corpus luteum, a hemoperitoneum, a viral infection, or an incidental finding is unknown. These patients are very difficult to treat; because of the small number of cases, no uniform therapy has emerged. Some patients respond to therapy with long-term prostaglandin inhibitors, others to ovulation suppression, and others to steroids. Long-term follow-up hopefully will better define this entity. A few patients with this finding have since developed endometriosis, which was confirmed at subsequent laparoscopy.

Table 23-14. Postoperative diagnosis in 282 adolescent females with chronic pelvic pain. The Children's Hospital, Boston, 1974-1983

	No. of patients	%
Endometriosis	126	(45)
Postoperative adhesions	37	(13)
Serositis	15	(5)
Ovarian cyst	14	(5)
Uterine malformation	15	(5)
Others*	4	(2)
No pathology	71	(25)

*ileitis, infarcted hydatid of Morgagni, pelvic congestion

Other findings included ovarian cysts, uterine malformations of the obstructive type, and cases of ileitis, infarcted hydatid of Morgagni, and pelvic congestion.

No organic disease was documented in 25% of the patients. In this group, pain was attributed to functional bowel disease or to psychogenic factors. Despite apparently normal bowel function, many teenagers with CPP improve when placed on a regimen of stool softeners and increased dietary fiber and fluid intake. The value of a negative laparoscopy should not be underestimated. In many instances the assurance that their pelvic structures are normal is sufficient to improve the symptoms in these adolescents. A significant number of these patients were symptomatically improved after a negative laparoscopy. In a small number of these teenagers, adjunctive psychologic or behavioral modification therapy is necessary.

For the years 1980 to 1983, the results were broken down into age groups (Table 23-15). The incidence of endometriosis among adolescents complaining of CPP increases progressively with age, from 12% in the 11- to 13-year-old group to 54% in patients aged 20 and 21 years. Pelvic serositis was encountered mostly in the 11- to 15-year-old group. Other findings remained fairly constant in all age groups.

Acute and chronic pelvic pain in the adolescent patient must be taken seriously. In the majority of cases an underlying cause can be identified. Under no circumstances should the label of psychogenic pain be proffered without prior negative laparoscopy. Adequate diagnosis and early therapy are essential to improve the quality of life and to preserve the reproductive prognosis in these young patients.

Table 23-15. Age-related incidence of laparoscopic findings in 129 adolescent females with chronic pelvic pain. The Children's Hospital, Boston, 1980–1983

	Age 11-13 No. of pts. (%)	Age 14-15 No. of pts. (%)	Age 16-17 No. of pts. (%)	Age 18-19 No. of pts. (%)	Age 20-21 No. of pts.(%)
Endometriosis	2 (12)	9 (28)	21 (40)	17 (45)	7 (54)
Postoperative adhesions	1 (6)	4 (13)	7 (13)	5 (13)	2 (15)
Serositis	5 (29)	4 (13)	0 (0)	2 (5)	0 (0)
Ovarian cyst	2 (12)	2 (6)	3 (5)	2 (5)	0 (8)
Uterine malformations	1 (6)	0 (0)	1 (2)	0 (0)	1 (0)
Others	0 (0)	1 (3)	2 (4)	1 (3)	0 (0)
No pathology	6 (35)	12 (37)	19 (36)	11 (29)	3 (23)

Treatment of endometriosis in adolescent patients. The importance of finding endometriosis early lies not only in the relief of symptoms but also, hopefully, in the preservation of reproductive potential. The optimal therapy for adolescents and adult women with endometriosis is still debated. The patient needs to understand the pros and cons of each surgical and medical option and that endometriosis commonly recurs. Adolescents need to know that studies in adult women have not shown increased infertility in patients with minimal or mild endometriosis.

The basis of medical therapy for pain is to take advantage of the reliance of endometrial tissue on steroid hormones for growth and function. One strategy is to create an acyclic, low-estrogen environment to prevent bleeding in the implants and to prevent additional seeding of the pelvis during retrograde menstruation. GnRH agonists, similar to those used in treating precocious puberty, can produce a low-estrogen state. The side effects include menopausal symptoms such as hot flushes, vaginal dryness, and decreased libido. The most worrisome side effect of GnRH analogue therapy is decreased bone density, which may be reversible on cessation of therapy. Daily medroxyprogesterone may lessen the menopausal symptoms; research is needed to find potential therapies for maintenance of bone density with an hypoestrogenic environment.

Another strategy is to produce a high-androgen state with androgens or synthetic progestins (with androgenic properties) to produce atrophy of endometriotic implants. This strategy also results in an acyclic low-estrogen state by interrupting ovarian follicular development. This goal can be accomplished by the use of danazol. Although danazol appears to be a very effective drug, many adolescents complain of side effects, which include weight gain, edema, irregular menses, acne, oily skin, hirsutism, and a deep voice change. Other problems with this medication include decreased high-density lipoprotein (HDL) cholesterol, mildly increased insulin resistance, alteration in liver proteins, and androgenic effects on the developing fetus (if the adolescent becomes pregnant while taking the drug). The drug should therefore be avoided in patients with hepatic dysfunction, severe hypertension, congestive heart failure, and borderline renal function. Danazol offers effective contraception at doses of 400 to 800 mg/day; sexually active patients treated with less than 400 mg/day require additional methods of contraception. A six-month course is commonly prescribed, but courses should be individualized. The recurrence rate of symptoms and physical findings in patients treated with danazol is approximately 5% to 20% per year.

Daily oral progestins such as medroxyprogesterone acetate and intramuscular medroxyprogesterone acetate for 6 to 9 months can also be used. The principal complaint in adolescents is weight gain and irregular menses. "Pseudopregnancy" with continuous oral contraceptives for 9 to 12 months may exacerbate symptoms initially because of the swelling of implants secondary to the estrogen in the oral contraceptives. However, with continued use these may give some patients relief of symptoms. A progestin-dominant pill can be initiated; the pill may be doubled or tripled, or estrogen may be added if breakthrough bleeding occurs. Triphasics are not suitable because of the change in progestin dose. The principal problems with the pseudopregnancy are headaches, fluid retention, nausea, weight gain, emotional lability, and hypertension.

A comparison of the different hormonal therapies for endometriosis and their side effects are shown in Table 23-16.

In one clinic, most patients have fulguration of implants using laser (or electrocautery) and lysis of adhesions at the time of laparoscopy. They are then placed on a course of

GnRH agonists for 6 months and switched to cyclic oral contraceptives at the end of the course. Cyclic oral contraceptives are prescribed indefinitely with the hope that scantier menses will lessen the chance of recurrence. Therapy clearly needs to be individualized because adolescents are very conscious of side effects and will become noncompliant. Frequent appointments, support, and careful listening and response to concerns and questions are an important part of medical care. In addition to the endometriosis other diagnoses such as irritable bowel syndrome, lactose intolerance, or psychologic issues must be kept in mind when treating the adolescent with persistent pain. In persistent cases, pelviscopy with fulguration or removal of implants and lysis of adhesions is recommended. The use of a long-term GnRH agonist with hormonal "add-back" therapy[4] may be appropriate for adolescents with persistent chronic endometriosis pain.

Future developments in the treatment of endometriosis may be able to take advantage of the protein growth factors that regulate the epithelial and stromal elements of the endometrium. Modulation of the immune system, which may possibly play a critical role in pain, scarring, and infertility, may offer another method of treating endometriosis.

Obstructing and nonobstructing malformations of the reproductive tract

A large proportion of congenital abnormalities of the female genital tract remain undiscovered until adolescence. These are usually diagnosed when symptoms occur, especially menstrual disorders and coital difficulties, or simply because most patients undergo their first pelvic examination at this time.

Although some congenital malformations become obvious at first glance, the diagnosis of many of these defects requires a high index of suspicion. A thorough understanding of the nature of these anomalies is essential to the gynecologist who deals with the teenage group. Early diagnosis, adequate treatment and appropriate psychologic support and counseling assure the preservation of reproductive function when feasible and allows these adolescents to develop a serene attitude toward their sexuality.

Obstructive defects require immediate attention to remove the obstruction and to stop retrograde menstruation. When there is no obstruction, immediate medical attention is not mandated until reproductive and coital function is desired.

Classification of uterovaginal anomalies. The American Fertility Society has devised a classification scheme of müllerian anomalies based upon the degree of failure of normal development.[2] The system separates the anomalies into groups with similar clinical manifestations and prognoses for fetal salvage upon treatment. This classification system does not include vaginal anomalies but allows the healthcare provider to describe anomalies involving the vagina, tubes, or urinary tract as associated malformations.

Some prefer a simpler scheme based on the presence of an obstructed outflow tract.[93]

Imperforate hymen with hematocolpos (or hydrocolpos). Although the diagnosis of an imperforate hymen

Table 23-16. Comparison of hormonal therapies for endometriosis

Therapy	Resultant hormone state			Side effects
	Acyclic	Hypoestrogenic	Hyperandrogenic	
Progestins	+	+	–	Breakthrough bleeding, depression, bloating, decreased libido
Noncyclic OCP's	+	–	–	Those routinely used for oral contraceptives, nausea, break-through bleeding
Methyltestosterone	+/–	–	++	Virilization, masculinization of a female fetus
Danazol	+	+	++	Weight gain, acne, hirsuitism, voice changes
GnRH agonist	+	++	–	Vasomotor symptoms (hot flushes), bone loss, vaginal dryness
GnRH agonist plus steroid add back	+	?	–	Possible decreased vasomotor symptoms, bone loss, vaginal dryness
Mifepristone	+	+/–	–	Anorexia, nausea, dizziness, somnolence
Oophorectomy	++	++	–	Vasomotor symptoms, bone loss, vaginal dryness

GnRH-gonadotropin-releasing hormone; ++, extremely effective; +, effective; +/–, sporadically effective; –, not effective; ?, questionably effective
From Laufer, MR: Endometriosis in adolescents, *Curr Opin Ped* 4:582-9, 1992.)

should be made long before adolescence, optimally during routine neonatal and pediatric examinations, it is not unusual to see a teenager present with the typical picture of primary amenorrhea, cyclic or acyclic pelvic pain, bulging hymen, and hematocolpos. Hematometra does not usually develop with simple imperforate hymen because the vagina has great distensibility and can accommodate a large amount of blood. It is, however, quite commonly seen with a high transverse septa.

Most cases of imperforate hymen are congenital due to failure of degeneration of central epithelial cells of the hymenal membrane. Rarely, the condition is the result of inflammatory processes before or after birth.

If the vagina and the uterus are not distended by estrogen-induced secretions at the time of birth, the imperforate hymen may remain asymptomatic until after puberty. At that time, the accumulation of menstrual material engorges the vaginal tract, causing pelvic or abdominal pain. It is of historic interest that this condition was known to Aristotle and was mentioned in his treatise on the Generation of Animals:

> We know of instances of women in whom the "os uteri" was grown together and continued so until the time arrived for the menstrual discharge to begin and pain come on; in some, the passage burst open of its own accord, in others, it was separated by physicians; and in some cases, where the opening either was forcibly made or could not be made at all, the patients succumbed.

Most cases of imperforate hymen are diagnosed before the age of 15 years. A cystic mass formed by the enlargement of the vagina and displacement of the uterus can extend above the symphysis and into the abdominal cavity. Abdominal pain is a regular symptom and urinary difficulties, most commonly acute retention, may develop. Many patients who are inadequately examined undergo extensive radiologic evaluation before the correct diagnosis is finally made. Examination of the external genitalia reveals a mass protruding between the labia majora. The bulging mass varies in size, is bluish-red in color, and continuous with the pelvic mass (Fig. 23-19). Constipation results in some cases because of pressure on the rectum from the distended vagina. The surgical therapy consists of hymenotomy, which often reveals a large accumulation of blood (hematocolpos), or secretion (hydrocolpos), depending on the age of the patient. The central part of the hymen should also be excised to for allow for further unobstructed menstrual flow. Needle-tip electrocautery facilitates hemostasis on the hymenal edge. This avoids the need for multiple sutures and minimizes the stricture. The use of a Yankauer suction tip inserted high into the vagina or through the dilated cervix into the uterus facilitates evacuation. At times the wall suction becomes plugged and a high speed suction evacuator is required. Infection is rare once drainage is established, and prophylactic antibody therapy is not required. The distended vagina promptly regresses within days without long-term effects.

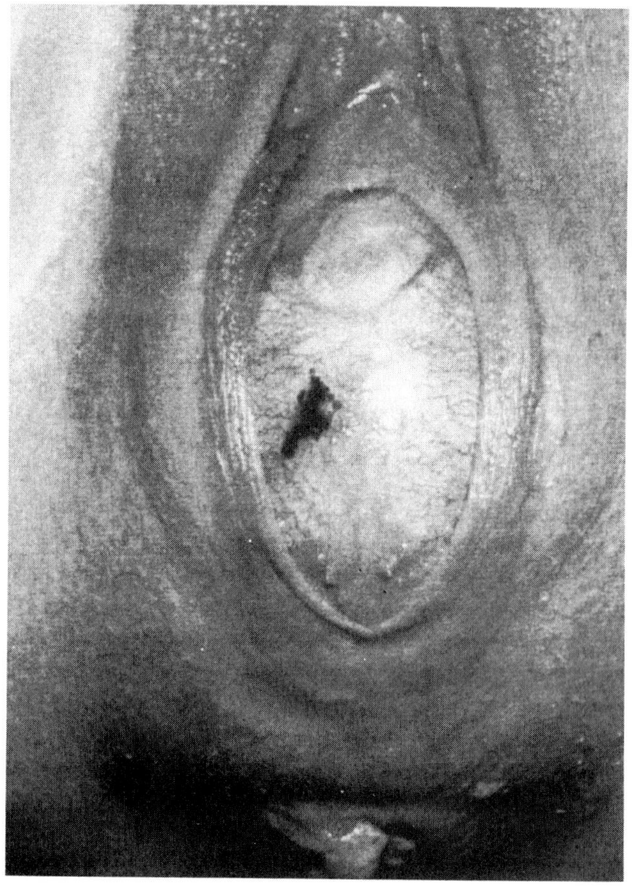

Fig. 23-19. Imperforate hymen in postpubertal patient who presented with abdominal pain, urinary retention, and a large pelvic mass. 850 mL of old blood was evacuated from the vagina after hymenectomy.

Uterine duplication with obstructed hemivagina. Abnormalities of utero-vaginal fusion diagnosed during adolescent years are mostly the obstructing type. These anomalies can be divided into three categories, according to the site of obstruction. At The Children's Hospital, 28 cases of uterine and/or vaginal obstructing duplications revealed that the most commonly encountered anomaly is a didelphic uterus with unilateral vaginal obstruction secondary to a blind vagina.[93] A unicornuate uterus with a contralateral blind horn, either rudimentary or of normal size, is second in frequency. Finally, a small number of patients present with cervical obstruction of one horn of a bicornuate uterus associated with an ipsilateral blind vaginal pouch. Fistulous tracts of various types may connect the blind vagina to a septate cervix and/or to the main vaginal cavity. Intercervical fistulae also have been discovered.

Signs and symptoms depend on the type of the abnormality. Since, in these cases, the obstruction is present only on one side, primary amenorrhea is not a feature.

By far the most common presenting complaint is pelvic pain, either cyclic or acyclic, which is the consequence of unilaterally obstructed menstrual flow and secondary endometriosis. Other frequent symptoms include abnormal vaginal bleeding and purulent discharge usually associated with a fistulous tract connecting the obstructed to the unobstructed side. In the presence of a blind vagina, distention with menstrual blood may give rise to vaginal pain or to the sensation of pressure. During a physical examination, masses corresponding to distended pelvic structures, abnormal uterine shape, and discharge from possible fistulas usually can be visualized or palpated.

The minimal work-up of these patients should include a combined pelvic and renal sonogram and an intravenous pyelogram. In one series, unilateral renal agenesis and other urinary tract abnormalities were found in 75% of the patients. Renal tract abnormalities occur when factors affecting the development of the mesonephric duct or the paramesonephric duct lead to abnormal renal development. Mesonephric duct agenesis would result not only in unilateral agenesis of the wolffian-derived genital structures but also unilateral renal agenesis. Laparoscopy and hysterosalpingography should also be performed to determine the exact nature of the anomaly. MRI appears to accurately assess the anomaly without invasive procedures. Despite its cost, this technique should be seriously considered.

Treatment consists of surgical excision of the vaginal septum. Because the septum may be quite thick, the surgery may be challenging. Generally, abdominal exploration is unnecessary and uterine reconstruction is not indicated. Reproductive performance is related to the type of double uterus unless a delay in diagnosis has resulted in endometriosis or has destroyed tubal function.

Blind uterine horn. Asymmetric obstruction of the uterus such as unicornuate uterus with a noncommunicating uterine anlagen with active endometrium is rare and may present a diagnostic dilemma.

Frequently the patient is considered to have severe dysmenorrhea and treatment with birth control pills or pain medication is instituted before adequate workup is completed. With the advent of ultrasonography and MRI, this omission occurs less frequently and patients are investigated when they respond poorly to medication.

Dysmenorrhea or cyclic abdominal pain from cryptomenorrhea may be the only symptoms. Endometriosis from retrograde menstruation or a tender mass may be present. Removal of the obstructed horn is the procedure of choice and should alleviate symptoms.

Transverse vaginal septum. A vaginal septum is a relatively uncommon anomaly. Septa can be either congenital or acquired, can occur in various positions, and can be multiple. Transverse septa can occur at any level from above the hymenal ring to the junction of the vagina and cervix. Vertical septa can be oriented in an anteroposterior plane (sagittal septum) or in the lateral plane (coronal septum). Finally, septa can be complete or partial, perforate or imperforate.

Transverse vaginal septa occur from lack of complete canalization of the solid primitive vaginal plate or sinovaginal bulbs. Vertical vaginal septa occur in two ways. Failure of the müllerian ducts to fuse results in a duplication of the uterus and vagina. What appears to be a vertical vaginal septum is in fact a duplicated vagina; two vaginal openings are found. In others, incomplete canalization of the vaginal plate in a longitudinal direction results in a septum that may be oriented in either the anteroposterior plane or the lateral plane. The symptoms produced by vaginal septa depend upon the age of the patient, the degree of vaginal obstruction, and the amount of stimulation of the cervical mucous glands by circulating estrogen. The neonate with a completely obstructed vagina resulting from a transverse septum may present with hydrometrocolpos. However, a transverse vaginal septum may not be recognized until the patient reaches menarche when hematocolpos develops. The neonate or older patient with a complete vertical septum may present with a unilateral hydrocolpos or hematocolpos, whereas an older patient with an incomplete vertical septum may seek help for dyspareunia or, if pregnant, for difficulty in delivery.

Symptoms depend on the width and the location of the anomaly. A narrow annular septum usually is a fortuitous finding of no clinical significance and does not require any treatment. On the other hand, primary amenorrhea and early symptoms of obstruction occur in cases of complete septum, and surgical excision is imperative. When the upper and lower vagina communicates only by a small fistulous tract through the septum, the clinical picture is sometimes quite puzzling. These patients may present with dysmenorrhea, irregular vaginal spotting or purulent discharge because of partial obstruction and accumulation of infected blood above the defect. Secondary PID from anaerobic infection may also be the initial mode of presentation. A septum lying low in the vagina is frequently the cause of dyspareunia. Infertility and soft tissue dystocia are unusual presentations of this malformation in the adolescent group.

Surgical correction consists of complete excision of the septum and anastomosis of the upper vagina to the lower vagina. This may prove difficult, depending on the thickness of the septum. MRI may help to define the thickness preoperatively. The utilization of a stent may be necessary when the septum involves a long vaginal segment and primary anastomosis is impossible. Care must be taken not to injure the urethra or rectum. The use of a urinary catheter and a finger in the rectum can guide surgery.

Postoperatively, periodic vaginal examination at six-week intervals should be performed with dilations as necessary. Recurrence is rare if the septum is entirely excised. Postoperatively, stricture may be encountered and subsequent surgery required. A Z-plasty technique helps minimize the problem. In some patients, however, the fallopian tubes will have developed some degree of fibrosis from pyocolpos because of backflow prior to treatment.

Cervicovaginal agenesis. Congenital absence of the cervix can occur in association with vaginal agenesis or with a normal vagina. This rare clinical entity causes early obstructive signs and symptoms characterized by hematometra, tubal regurgitation of menstrual blood with hematosalpingitis, and secondary endometriosis. In many cases, cyclic abdominal pain and amenorrhea are the presenting symptoms. The diagnosis is difficult to make prior to surgery, but ultrasonography and MRI has made this condition more recognizable.

Attempts to preserve fertility by the creation of a fistulous tract between the endometrial cavity and the vagina have been very disappointing.

A conservative surgical approach usually leads to multiple operations, and only two successful pregnancies are reported in the literature. Furthermore, deaths due to sepsis when conservative surgery was attempted, has been reported. The recommended therapy of cervical agenesis, therefore, remains hysterectomy with ovarian conservation, if possible.

Nonobstructing malformations

Longitudinal vaginal septa. Longitudinal vaginal septa most often occur in association with abnormalities of uterine fusion but may sometimes be isolated malformations. Such septa divide the vagina sagittally into equal or unequal parts for its entire or partial length. Surgical excision is indicated when dyspareunia becomes a problem or when childbearing is anticipated.

Uterine agenesis. Absence of the uterus is noted in some apparently female patients who have the syndrome of male pseudohermaphrodism with testicular feminization. These patients are genetic males and have negative sex chromatin and XY karyotype. They do not menstruate and cannot bear children, but their external genitalia are normal female, and they feminize at puberty with good breast development. In rare cases, rudimentary tubes and uteri can be present. Also intraabdominal or inguinal testes with nests of Leydig cells are present.

The uterus is absent also in the majority of male pseudohermaphrodites with ambiguous genitalia. They may have testes situated intraabdominally, in the inguinal canal, or in the scrotum. The vagina can differ in size and length and often communicates with a hypospadiac urethra. A minority of male pseudohermaphrodites with ambiguous external genitalia have a uterus and tubes. This can be of practical importance if, at laparotomy, gonads at the site of ovaries are seen in a child with tubes, uterus, and vagina; such gonads can be testes.

Vaginal agenesis. Failure of development of the müllerian ducts at any time between their origin and their fusion with the urogenital sinus results in failure of development of the uterus and vagina. The Mayer-Rokitansky-Kuster-Hauser syndrome is the most common clinical example of this anomaly. In approximately 90% of patients, the uterus is present in the form of a rudimentary anlagen with congenital absence of the vagina. Some series have included patients with a uterus and an absence of varying lengths of the vagina; however, these patients generally are not considered to have Rokitansky's syndrome. The latter group of patients are more appropriately considered under the group of defects in vertical fusion. The homogeneity and specificity of the Rokitansky syndrome is the absence of a vagina and uterus with a high incidence of urinary tract anomalies. Patients with disorders of vertical fusion have a low incidence of urinary tract anomalies.

Because these patients have a 46XX karyotype and normal ovarian function with normal development of external genitalia and secondary sexual characteristics, they usually present with amenorrhea. Ovulation occurs normally, but because these patients lack a uterus and vagina, menstruation does not occur. An exact genetic etiologic diagnosis has not been elucidated.

A significant number of patients with müllerian agenesis have associated anomalies of the upper müllerian duct system and anomalies of other organ systems. In the classic form of the müllerian agenesis, the uterus is present only in the form of bilateral rudimentary uterine anlagen. These anlagen are located on the lateral pelvic side wall adjacent to the ovaries and are usually connected to the fallopian tubes. However, they are usually not palpable on bimanual examination. The anlagen may or may not have endometrial tissue. Even if the endometrium is functional, the cavity of the anlagen may not communicate directly with the peritoneal cavity as often because of an obstruction located at the junction of the tube and the uterine bulb. Occasionally, anlagen communicate with the peritoneal cavity via the fallopian tubes and active endometrium, if present, may regurgitate into the peritoneal cavity.

Renal anomalies are perhaps the most well-known anomalies associated with Rokitansky syndrome, occurring in about one third of patients. Abnormalities of the skeletal system are reported to occur in 10%.

A serum testosterone level can be obtained to rule out an androgen insensitivity syndrome. A chromosomal analysis can confirm the androgen insensitivity or may be found to be 46XX and thus an aberration of the Rokitansky syndrome. A renal sonogram or IVP is mandatory to define the excretory system and to rule out anomalies. Also, a radiograph can evaluate the lower spine for skeletal anomalies. If symptoms suggest an active uterine anlagen, or if a pelvic mass is present, appropriate studies such as ultrasonography or MRI can differentiate among hematometra, hematocolpos, endometriomas or other cysts.

If functional endometrial tissue is present, symptoms from cryptomenorrhea will begin soon after secondary sexual characteristics start to develop. Surgical removal of the anlagen affords complete relief of symptoms. Occasionally patients will present with dysmenorrhea, but most commonly patients present around the age of 15 or 16 years with primary amenorrhea.

Vaginoplasty is usually performed between the ages of 17 and 20 years when the patient is emotionally mature and intellectually capable of understanding the operative procedure and of partaking in her postoperative care, which is an extremely important variable in terms of outcome.

Psychologic counseling is extremely important in the management of these patients. The single most important factor in determining the success of vaginoplasty is the psychologic adjustment of the patient to her anomaly.

Both surgical and nonsurgical methods for creating a vagina have been described and successfully used.

Nonsurgical methods utilize dilation of the vaginal dimple to create a functional vagina. The first method was described by Robert Frank in 1938 and involves active manipulation by the patient to dilate the neovaginal space. Ingram described a technique of creating a new vagina using dilators specially designed for use with a bicycle seat stool.[55]

In younger, less motivated patients the Frank dilation technique may prove to be very difficult. Several surgical methods of creating a vaginal space have been described. The McIndoe procedure[78] or more appropriately the Abbe-Wharton-McIndoe procedure, is superior to all others. In essence, a skin graft taken from the buttock is placed around a vaginal form of molded plastic, which is then placed into a surgically created space between the vagina and the rectum.[21] It remains for 7 days (Fig. 23-19).[22]

Serious complications associated with the McIndoe procedure have diminished significantly as techniques and experience have improved. Complications, however, still exist. These include morbidity and mortality from anesthesia, infection, and hemorrhage, failure of the graft to take, and formation of postoperative granulation tissue. Fistulas from the lower urinary tract or the rectum into the neovagina have been reported in approximately 4% of patients. Malignancies have also been reported in the neovagina.

Other surgical procedures have been utilized and may be applicable in special cases. Under special circumstances, the vulvovaginal pouch of Williams (Fig. 23-20) or the sigmoid transplant of Pratt may be indicated.

Hymenal anomalies. Incomplete fenestration of the hymenal opening is most often asymptomatic. These patients seek gynecologic treatment because of unsuccessful attempts at inserting tampons or as a result of coital difficulties. With a microperforate hymen, the adolescent may also complain of postmenstrual vaginal spotting or malodorous discharge secondary to incomplete obstruction and poor drainage. Hymenectomy should be performed in all cases.

If the diagnosis is made fortuitously, the patient should be told about this anatomic variant and informed of the

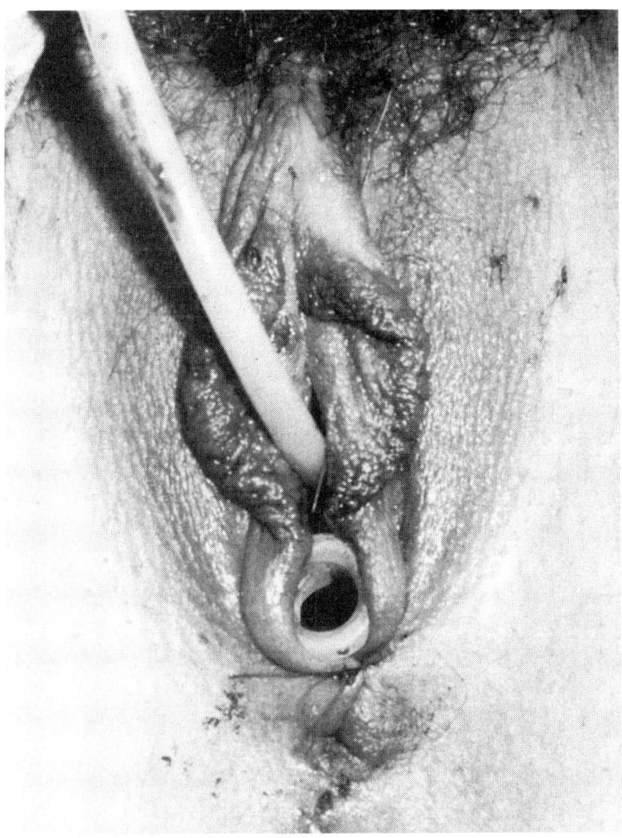

Fig. 23-20. Counsellor stent in place following creation of a neovagina with a split thickness skin graft (McIndoe procedure).

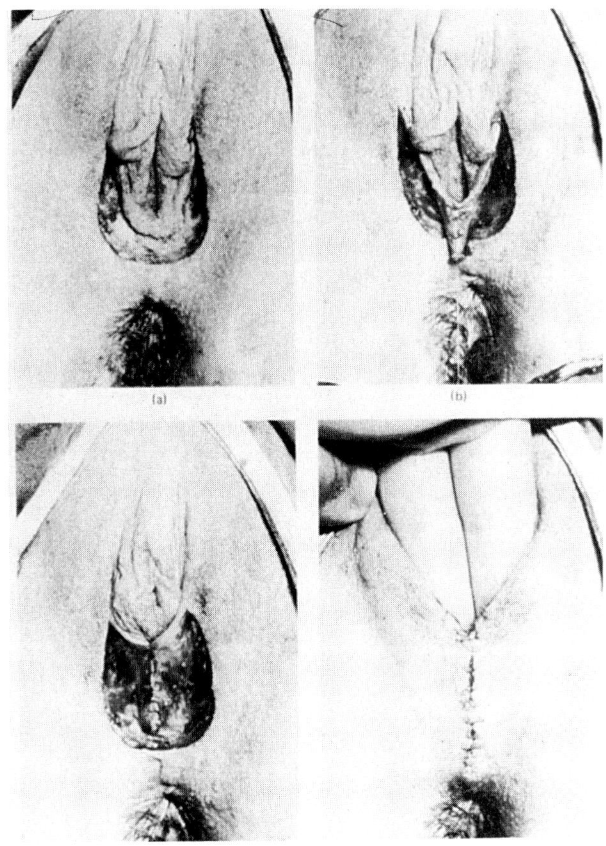

Fig. 23-21. Steps in performing a William's vulvovaginoplasty which creates a functional perinal pouch adequate for intercourse. Used primarily to augment short vaginal or neovagina.

necessity of surgical correction. Performing the procedure during the early teens allows the adolescent to use tampons without problems and may avoid later embarrassment when the patient desires to become sexually active.

Vulvar anomalies. In some instances, one or both labia minora are unusually large and the patient consults because she notices this anomaly or because she experiences symptoms of irritation associated with exercise. In most of these cases simple reassurance is necessary. Comparison with asymmetry or hypertrophy of other parts of the body may help the patient to accept this peculiarity. Hygiene counseling and avoidance of tight clothes are usually sufficient to relieve discomfort. If these measures are ineffective, or in the presence of a troublesome cosmetic problem, surgical reduction is an option. This can be accomplished in the ambulatory operating room by simply resecting the redundant labia so that they are symmetrical. Closure of the excised area is best accomplished with a running locking stitch of 3-0 chromic. The results usually are excellent, and the patients generally are quite pleased (Fig. 23-12). An alternate method is shown in Fig. 23-13.

Gynecologic sequelae of bladder exstrophy

Fortunately, exstrophy of the urinary bladder is an uncommon anomaly. To the parents of such an afflicted newborn infant, the condition is distressing, frightening, and repulsive. The term exstrophy comes from two Greek words; the prefix *exo* means "outside of" and the verb *strophe* means "to twist or turn about." The distraught parents see this condition as a twisted, inside-out urinary bladder accompanied by abnormal genitalia.

Girls with this condition always have a bifid clitoris. Several series report a high incidence of myelomeningocele, which is significant in terms of sphincter incontinence. The distance from the umbilicus to anus is foreshortened. Often the umbilicus is just cephalad to the exotropic bladder, and some are associated with an omphalocele. The anal aperture is often close to the vagina.[18]

Characteristically, the girl with bladder exstrophy presents to the gynecologist following puberty because of abnormalities of the lower abdominal and vulvar area that result from her urologic reconstruction (Fig. 23-22). Examination reveals scarring and deformity of the mons pubis, asymmetry of the labia, a bifid clitoris, and introital stenosis. The upper tract is usually normal. Bladder exstrophy is one of the conditions that leads to congenital prolapse of the uterus; myelodysplasia and spinal bifida are the other two. From the psychologic standpoint, these patients are quite distraught because of their strange appearance and frequently shun their emerging female sexuality. It is quite important, therefore, to reassure them that total reconstruction can be accomplished.

The treatment is surgical and is designed to correct the anomalies. Usually it is necessary to perform a monsplasty, William's vulvovaginoplasty, and Manchester-Fotnerquill procedure in a one-stage operation. The results usually are excellent, and full function is restored. Pregnancy can occur, but delivery should be abdominal because of the abnormal configuration of the bony pelvis and fixation of the uterus.

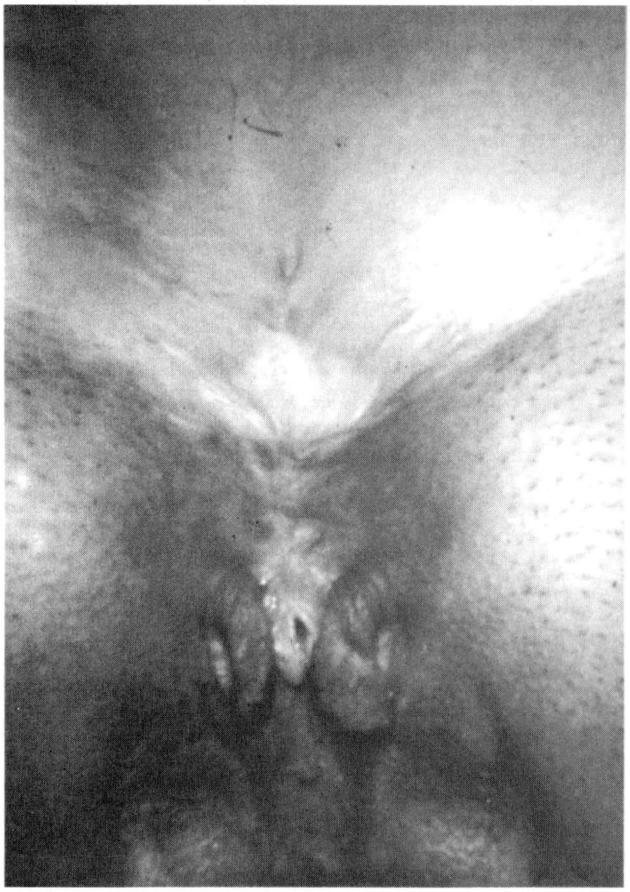

Fig. 23-22. Gynecologic features of bladder exstrophy in adolescent following successful bladder repair.

Cloacal anomalies

The remarkable similarity among otherwise normal individuals with this bizarre type of defect suggests a similar mode of developmental pathology, having its inception as a single localized defect—theoretically in the early development of the mesoderm, which later contributes to the infraumbilical mesenchyme, cloacal septum, and caudal vertebrae. The consequences are as follows: (1) failure of cloacal septation, with the persistence of a common cloaca into which the ureters, ileum, and a rudimentary hindgut open; (2) complete breakdown and exstrophy of the cloacal membrane with exstrophy of the cloaca, failure of fusion of the genital tubercles and pubic rami, and often omphalocele; and (3) incomplete development of the lumbosacral vertebrae with herniation of a grossly dilated central canal of the spinal cord (hydromyelia), yielding a soft, cystic, skin-covered mass over the sacral area, sometimes asymmetric in its positioning (Fig. 23-23). The rudimentary hindgut may contain two appendices, and no anal opening is evident. The small intestine may be relatively short. Cryptorchidism is a usual finding in the male. Affected females have unfused müllerian elements with completely bifid uterine horns and short, duplicated, or atretic vaginas. Most patients have a single umbilical artery, and anomalies of the lower limbs are occasionally present.

Surgical intervention should attempt to reestablish normal function of the urinary, gastrointestinal, and reproductive tracts (Fig. 23-24).

Gynecologic problems in chronic diseases

Adolescents who have chronic diseases and malignancies that were fatal in the past have benefitted from improved medical management and now seek care for a number of gynecologic problems. Even the healthy adolescent girl may have difficulties as she experiences pubertal changes and new sexual feelings; the adolescent with a chronic disease has special needs that must be understood and receive attention. Although only some of the common chronic diseases (cystic fibrosis, end-stage renal disease, diabetes mellitus, Crohn's disease, sickle cell disease, and malignancy) are covered in this chapter, the physician needs to approach every adolescent with a sensitivity to her unique concerns. This sensitivity will enable the physician to treat patients with many other chronic diseases not mentioned. Undoubtedly, an entire text could be devoted to the special gynecologic problems adolescents encounter in coping with a chronic illness.[28]

Cystic fibrosis. Cystic fibrosis is the most common lethal hereditary disease in the Caucasian population. Although previously many children with cystic fibrosis died during infancy and early childhood, many patients with cystic fibrosis now are living through their adolescence and into their reproductive years. Because these adolescents often have low weight for their height and chronic pulmonary infections, they frequently experience a delay in pubertal development and menarchal age.

Adolescents with delayed menarche likely were to be diagnosed with cystic fibrosis earlier in life, have a lower weight for height index, a lower height, and a lower percent of body fat than postmenarchal girls. Because normal levels of sex steroids and gonadotropins usually are reached by most patients in their late teenage years, the adolescent with cystic fibrosis and amenorrhea should receive good medical and gynecologic assessment and supportive counseling. Other causes of amenorrhea, especially pregnancy, should be excluded, and reassurance should be given about the potential for normal menstruation.

The contraceptive choices for the patient with cystic fibrosis are not simple. Although oral contraceptives do not appear to alter pulmonary function, long-term safety data is not available. The risk of fluid retention and other side effects with high-estrogen pills necessitates the prescription of a low-dose pill. Weight, pulmonary and cardiac status, and liver function should be carefully monitored. Patients with preexisting chronic liver disease need careful assessment of the potential risks of pregnancy versus the unknown

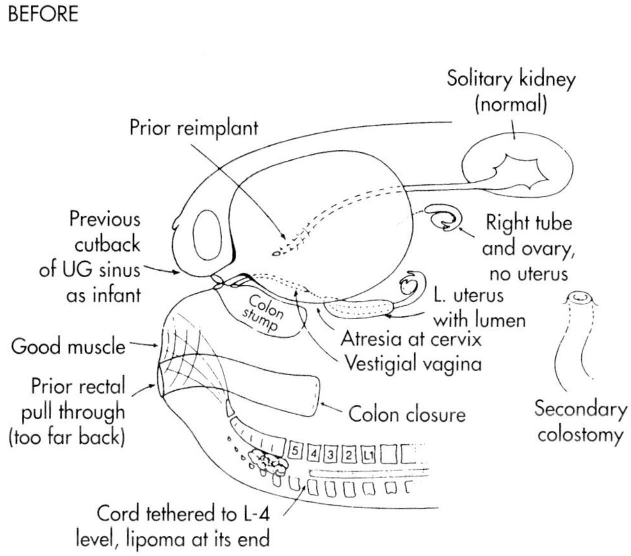

Fig. 23-23. Cloaca anomaly before reconstruction.

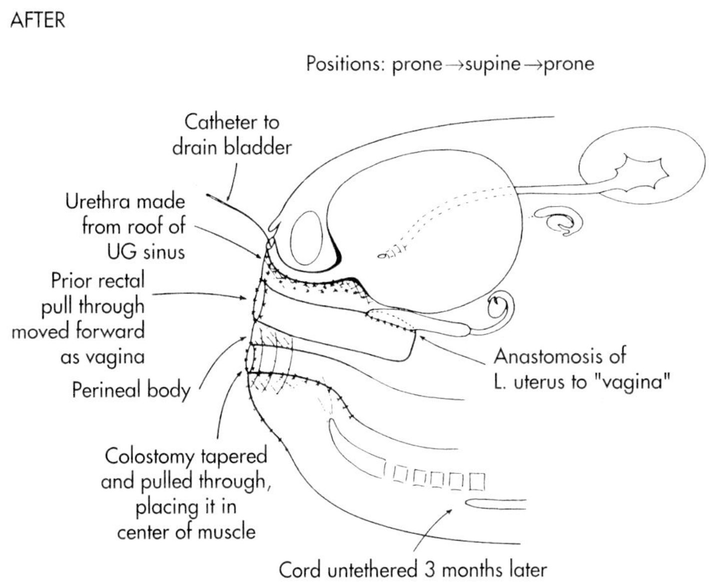

Fig. 23-24. Cloacal anomaly after reconstruction.

risk for potential hepatic effects. For most adolescents with cystic fibrosis, oral contraceptives are well tolerated and offer the many advantages of reliable contraception, diminished menstrual flow, and improved dysmenorrhea. Barrier forms of contraception can be used by the mature adolescent. An intrauterine device (IUD) is not recommended for most nulliparous adolescents and may be especially difficult to monitor in those adolescents with recurrent abdominal pain and severe constipation. Medroxyprogesterone acetate or levonorgestral are also alternatives for these young women. Tubal ligation is an option for the young adult with cystic fibrosis who has made a definitive choice to avoid pregnancy.

Chronic renal disease. Like many patients with other severe chronic diseases, adolescents with end-stage renal disease usually experience a delay in pubertal growth and development and in menarche. Postmenarchal uremic patients on chronic dialysis rarely have regular menses.

Prolactin levels are often elevated in uremic patients on hemodialysis. Hyperprolactinemia appears to be a direct consequence of impaired renal function. Associated with the chronic anovulation of uremia, ovarian cysts occur more commonly in patients on dialysis than in normal women. Ovarian cysts may be asymptomatic or may cause acute symptoms because of torsion or hemorrhage into the cyst (perhaps related to anticoagulant therapy). These ovarian cysts usually respond to hormone suppression therapy or resolve promptly after successful transplantation.

Uremic patients on dialysis usually require no therapy for the amenorrhea other than gynecologic assessment to exclude other etiologies. Although rare, pregnancy can occur in adolescents on dialysis. Adolescents with dysfunctional uterine bleeding require assessment and, depending on the individual, treatment with oral contraceptives or GnRH analogues; if persistent, D&C may be indicated.

It is extraordinarily important for the adolescent who has had a successful renal transplant to understand that ovulation usually returns between 1 and 12 months after renal function approaches normal. Adolescents may not appreciate the increase in fertility and may become pregnant posttransplant because of risk-taking behavior. Contraceptive counseling is paramount. If the adolescent has no contraindications (e.g., hypertension) to the use of oral contraceptive pills, a low-dose formulation can be utilized. In addition medroxyprogesterone acetate or levonorgestral may be an option. The IUD is not a good choice for the immunosuppressed nulliparous adolescent because of the potential for sepsis. Barrier contraception is an acceptable option for the mature adolescent. Patients should have good renal status for a minimum of 2 years after a transplant before undertaking a pregnancy.

Diabetes mellitus. Adolescents with diabetes mellitus are more likely to experience a normal age for menarche than adolescents with other chronic illnesses. Postmenarchal adolescent diabetics may have irregular menses, dysfunctional uterine bleeding, and/or prolonged amenorrhea. Gonadotropin and prolactin levels in amenorrheic diabetics are usually in the lower to normal range despite low estradiol levels, suggesting depression of the hypothalamic-pituitary axis.

Diabetic adolescents are often troubled by recurrent and persistent monilial vulvovaginitis. Improved diabetic control and long-term antifungal vaginal medications can be helpful.

Surprisingly some diabetics who have marked swelling and erythema of the vulva in association with chronic candidiasis complain of few or no symptoms. Condyloma acuminata can be a persistent problem, especially in poorly controlled diabetics. Treatment with 85% trichloroacetic acid may result in suboptimal results. Because some diabetics develop extreme burning and irritation with this medication, the initial application should be limited to only a few warts. Other diabetic patients may have warts that are quite resistant to treatment and may require a combination of improved glucose control, antimonilial vaginal medications, and other forms of treatment such as podofilox, which can be applied by the patient. A carbon dioxide laser can vaporize extensive condyloma acuminata. In addition, the use of electric loop diathermy has been proposed.

Providing contraceptive services to diabetic adolescents involves balancing the risks and benefits of each form of birth control. Oral contraceptives can alter glucose tolerance and lipoprotein levels, and they have been associated with increased vascular complications in diabetics. Although optimally oral contraceptives should be avoided in diabetics, barrier forms of contraception may not be acceptable to the young risk-taking adolescent. Oral contraceptives do not appear to be associated with proliferative retinopathy, but the potential for accelerating the progress of this disorder remains a concern. Thus low-dose oral contraceptives with 20 to 35 μg of ethinyl estradiol and a low-dose progestin with minimal impact on glucose tolerance can be considered for adolescent diabetics, but medical status, blood glucose, and serum lipids should be monitored. Adolescents should be counseled to avoid smoking.

Crohn's disease. Adolescents with Crohn's disease may experience growth failure, pubertal delay, and menarchal delay. In fact, delayed growth may be the first manifestation of Crohn's disease and initially may not be recognized as secondary to a gastrointestinal problem. Gonadotropins and estrogen levels are low and imply a depressed hypothalamic-pituitary axis. Nutritional and medical therapy, and sometimes surgery, to treat active Crohn's disease are important to assure normal pubertal growth and development. Although excess corticosteroids may impair growth, a patient with active Crohn's disease who receives doses that adequately treat the illness often has a growth spurt.

Adolescents with Crohn's disease may experience vulvar and perianal symptoms. Perianal lesions may be the first sign leading to the diagnosis of Crohn's disease. Characteristic vulvar lesions include edema of the labia majora and ulcerations in which skin granulomas are separated from the affected gastrointestinal (GI) tract by normal skin. These ulcerations, which may resemble small herpetic lesions, last for weeks to months. Following proctocolectomy for Crohn's disease, some patients develop vaginal fistulas. A sinus tract may discharge onto the posterior wall of the vagina or directly onto the perineum. These fistulas have responded to long-term metronidazole therapy and to surgery.

Because of the treatment with corticosteroids and immunosuppressive drugs, young women with Crohn's disease may experience recurrent monilial vulvovaginitis and condyloma acuminata. Adolescents can usually take oral contraceptives without difficulty, although an association between the prior use of oral contraceptives and "Crohn's disease" of the colon (but not ulcerative colitis) has been suggested. A small number of cases of colitis associated with rectal sparing and segmental disease but not with granulomas have been attributed to the use of oral contraceptives and have improved after oral contraceptives were stopped. Thus if a patient develops colitis during oral contraceptive use, the pills should be stopped to see if a remission occurs. Patients with true Crohn's disease associated with granulomas on colonic biopsy do not improve with the cessation of oral contraceptives.

Sickle cell disease. Adolescents with sickle cell disease often have a delay in growth and development and in menarche compared with those in their peer group. Adolescents with hemoglobinopathies require contraceptive counseling. Because of the concern for potential thromboembolic phenomenan, including nephropathies and strokes, in patients with vasoocclusive crises combined oral contraceptives should be used with caution. Although the risks of the progesterone-only minipill are unknown, they appear to be well tolerated. Thus levonorgestral and medroxyprogesterone acetate are acceptable options. Other contraceptive choices include barrier contraception and, for some patients, the IUD.

Childhood malignancy. Because many children with malignancies are now surviving into adulthood, it is important for physicians to be aware of the gynecologic problems that occur among these patients. Chemotherapy for leukemia appears to have a minimal impact on later pubertal development and menses in girls diagnosed before puberty. In contrast, girls who are diagnosed with leukemia and treated with chemotherapy after the onset of puberty or menarche may experience a delay in menarche and/or secondary amenorrhea. In almost all cases menses eventually become normal.

Radiation therapy for solid tumors and lymphomas frequently results in permanent ovarian damage and ovarian failure. Data on the long-term survivors of childhood malignancy shows that ovarian failure occurred in 68% of patients who had both ovaries within abdominal radiotherapy fields, in 14% whose ovaries were at the edge of treatment fields, and in none of the patients with one or both ovaries outside an abdominal treatment field.[28] Adolescents with impaired ovarian function may experience either no adolescent sexual development or some estrogen effect at the normal pubertal age accompanied by primary or secondary amenorrhea. Gonadotropin levels are elevated to the menopausal range, and estradiol levels are usually less than 30 pg/mL. Replacement therapy with estrogen and medroxyprogesterone can provide normal sexual development and, in most cases, menses. Some adolescents also develop vaginal adhesions that require dilators and hormonal therapy. Counseling should focus on the potential for normal development and sexual functioning.

Tumors and related disorders

In utero exposure to DES. During the 1950s and early 1960s DES and other nonsteroidal estrogens were given to pregnant women in an attempt to prevent miscarriages. In 1971 Herbst et al reported an association between maternal DES and the later development of clear cell adenocarcinoma of the vagina and cervix in female offspring.[53] Later, adenosis, the presence of glandular (columnar) epithelium of müllerian origin in the vaginal wall (normally stratified squamous epithelium), was described in 36% to 90% of exposed young women.[52] Although adenosis is a benign lesion, the proximity of areas of adenosis to adenocarcinoma in several patients has necessitated the follow-up of all patients with DES exposure.

The number of exposed young women is estimated to range from several hundred thousand to several million. Reliable histories are often difficult to obtain; thus all patients (prepubertal and postpubertal) with abnormal bleeding should have a vaginal examination regardless of history. The gynecologist should:

1. Determine the maternal drug history of all patients.
2. Recommend a gynecologic exam at menarche or age 14 in all patients with a known maternal history of any amount of DES or other nonsteroidal estrogen.
3. Be available for counseling and discussion of the importance of gynecologic follow-up.

This last point is particularly important because mothers often feel extremely guilty about having taken the medication. Some desire to have their daughters checked under some other pretense. The adolescent girl may express great anger toward her mother in making her body imperfect. However, in general, it is much less destructive to a teenager to deal with these issues openly rather than allowing the doctor and mother to have a "secret". Although mothers and daughters are usually seeking reassurance that the vagina is "clean," the high frequency of adenosis indicates that this is not possible. Despite the minimal risk of carcinoma (probably less than 1 in 1000), the long-term risk of the presence of adenosis is unknown.

The following constitutes the gynecologic examination of the teenager exposed in utero to DES:

1. Careful palpation of the vagina.
2. Speculum examination with a Pap smear and Schiller's stain of the vagina.
3. Biopsies as indicated by the Schiller's stain.

If colposcopy is available, follow-up is greatly facilitated. The colposcope allows the whole spectrum of atypia, dysplasia, and carcinoma to be identified. Photos should be taken and then reviewed at subsequent visits. Colposcopy detects more cases of adenosis (80% to 90%) than visual exam (less than 30%) or Schiller's stains (40% to 80%).

Clear cell carcinoma. Although sporadic cases of clear cell adenocarcinoma of the cervix and less commonly of the vagina had been reported prior to the 1960s, the incidence has dramatically risen since 1966 and correlates well with use of DES therapy for problem pregnancies. In all cases nonsteroidal estrogens were started prior to the 18th week of pregnancy.[51] At the time of diagnosis, patients present most commonly with bleeding or discharge but some are asymptomatic. Several of these asymptomatic patients are found to have cancer during routine exam done solely because of a positive maternal history; all these patients are now living.

The average age of diagnosis was the late teenage years. Occasional cases have occurred in prepubertal girls, but all had symptoms of bleeding for weeks to months prior to the diagnosis.

The current recommendation for therapy of stage I and stage II tumors is radical hysterectomy. Metastatic disease is common and implies a poor prognosis.

Benign adenosis. In contrast to the rare occurrence of adenocarcinoma, adenosis is common in young women exposed in utero to DES (36% to 90% of patients). Adenosis is the presence of glandular epithelium of müllerian origin (similar to endocervix and endometrium) in the vaginal wall. Exposure to DES appears to have interfered with the normal differentiation and development of the cervix and vagina.

Several typical gross lesions have been described including (1) a "vaginal hood"—a circular fold that partially covers the cervix, (2) a cock's-comb appearance of the cervix—an irregular peak on the anterior border of the cervix, and (3) erythroplakia—reddish areas that may give the cervix or vagina a "strawberry" appearance.

The observation that adenosis is commonly found adjacent to foci of clear cell adenocarcinoma necessitates careful follow-up of this lesion. Treatment for adenosis is unnecessary because there is good evidence that spontaneous healing occurs. At this time the most prudent course is follow-up exams every 6 to 12 months.

Adnexal masses. Over the past decade, gynecologists have been consulted more frequently about the problem of ovarian masses during childhood and adolescence. The true incidence of this condition has probably not changed, but the increasing use of ultrasonography by pediatricians and family practitioners has led to the detection of many functional cysts that were previously undetected. Even though most of these masses are functional and require only reassurance, true ovarian neoplasms must receive immediate attention and therapy. It is, therefore, important that gynecologists feel comfortable in the evaluation of a child or teenager with an adnexal mass.

The differential diagnosis of adnexal masses includes the enlargement of other reproductive structures and masses of extragenital origin.

All types of ovarian tumors seen in the adult can also be encountered in children and adolescents. The relative incidence of each entity is quite different, however. For example, functional masses are much more frequent in the adolescent because of the high incidence of anovulatory cycles. In this age group, neoplastic tumors are more likely to be of germinal origin rather than of epithelial origin.

Fortunately, only one in ten ovarian tumors is malignant in children and adolescents. It is difficult to obtain accurate statistics regarding the frequency of functional cysts because most studies are based on surgical reviews. Because many patients with functional adnexal enlargement are treated expectantly and never undergo surgery, they are not included in published series.

Studies at the Children's Hospital of 242 children and adolescents operated on for ovarian masses revealed that 31% had a tumor-like condition including follicle, corpus luteum, simple and endometriotic cysts (Table 23-17).[63] Of the 166 cases of primary ovarian tumors, there were 118 (71%) germ cell tumors, of which 78 (66%) consisted of benign mature teratoma. Of 27 epithelial tumors, 85% were benign. Twenty-one (13%) of their patients had a sex cord-stromal tumor which generally are considered to be low-grade malignancies. These results are comparable to other similar reports.

A considerable number of ovarian tumors are asymptomatic and are discovered fortuitously during a routine pelvic examination. Because most young patients do not consult for periodic pelvic examinations, ovarian masses are often detected only when they become large enough to cause symptoms or to be felt by abdominal palpation. Smaller ovarian enlargements are frequently incidental ultrasonographic findings at the time of an examination performed for unrelated symptoms such as pain. This accounts for a large number of consultations for masses which prove to be functional.

Symptoms are usually related to the size of the mass or to mechanical accidents such as rupture, torsion, or hemorrhage. In the young prepubertal girl, pain is abdominal because of

Table 23-17. Pathologic diagnosis of 242 ovarian tumors treated surgically at Children's Hospital Medical Center (Boston) 1928–1982

TUMORLIKE ENLARGEMENTS	76	(31%)
PRIMARY OVARIAN TUMORS	166	(69%)
Germ cell tumors	118	(71%)
mature teratoma	78	
immature teratoma	17	
endodermal sinus tumor	14	
dysgerminoma	8	
choriocarcinoma	1	
Epithelial tumors	27	(16%)
serous	14	
mucinous	12	
mixed	1	
Sex cord stromal tumors	21	(13%)
granulosa	10	
Sertoli-Leydig	7	
thecoma	2	
fibroma	1	
unclassified	1	

From Lack EE, Goldstein DP: Primary ovarian tumors in childhood and adolescence, *Curr Probl Obstet Gynecol* 7(4): , 1984.

the reduced pelvic capacity and the fairly high position of the ovaries. In the older patient, symptoms are more often pelvic. Bladder and ureteral compression may also be encountered with larger masses. Malignant tumors which infiltrate the surrounding tissue may induce bowel obstruction. In cases of mechanical accidents, symptoms develop acutely and usually are characterized by severe pain and peritoneal signs, including nausea and vomiting. In hormone-producing tumors, precocious puberty, menstrual irregularities, or virilization may lead to the diagnosis.

On pelvic examination, the mass usually can be palpated by rectoabdominal examination with the patient in the lithotomy position. As mentioned previously, ovarian tumors in children are often intraabdominal rather than pelvic and should be considered in the differential diagnosis of abdominal masses. Other physical findings depend on the degree of invasion of the tumor and its hormonal activity.

Ultrasonography is invaluable in the diagnosis of ovarian masses. It provides information about the size, location, and consistency of the tumor (i.e., cystic, solid, or complex). Ultrasonography is also useful to determine the presence of free peritoneal fluid or ascites. A radiograph of the abdomen reveals the presence of calcifications, which suggests a diagnosis of dermoid cyst. This information can, however, be obtained by ultrasonography.

The remainder of the workup depends on the clinical picture. In the presence of a solid or hormonally active tumor, blood should be drawn for hCG, α-fetoprotein, CA-125, and estradiol. FSH and LH levels may help to differentiate a true precocious puberty responsible for a functional cyst from an estrogen-secreting tumor inducing a pseudoprecocious puberty. When hirsutism or signs of virilization are present, a testosterone level should be obtained. If malignancy is suspected, a preoperative metastatic workup including chest x-ray, CT scan of the abdomen, and liver function tests should be done.

Ovarian masses in the postmenarchal patient are approached similarly to those in the young adult. An ultrasound examination should be performed on an ovarian mass to confirm the diagnosis and to further define the tumor's characteristics. Because of the high incidence of functional masses, an asymptomatic, purely cystic tumor with a diameter of 6 cm or less is observed for 2 to 3 cycles for spontaneous regression. In these patients the utilization of oral contraceptives or GnRH analog to inhibit ovarian function may accelerate regression and may prevent the appearance of new functional enlargement. Cystic masses that do not decrease in size over a period of three months, that enlarge, or are larger than 6 cm initially, should be operated on. A laparoscopy may be performed prior to laparotomy to confirm the diagnosis. When the cyst appears to be functional and is less than 6 cm in diameter, a puncture-aspiration may be performed. All fluid obtained should be sent for cytologic examination. It is preferable, however, to remove the cyst entirely.

Solid and complex tumors should be removed without delay. A laparoscopy may be performed as the initial procedure to establish the diagnosis, and to help to decide on the optimal incision. In cases of unexpected malignancy laparoscopy allows the surgeon to discuss the extensiveness of the proposed surgery with the patient.

Laparotomy should be performed through an incision large enough to allow excision of the tumor without rupture and according to the principles of ovarian surgery (i.e., peritoneal lavage, complete abdominal exploration, frozen section, and periaortic node dissection when indicated).

Uterine myomas. Uterine myomas occur rarely in teenagers, but have been reported in children as young as 10 years of age. They should be considered in the differential diagnosis of any solid pelvic mass. Ultrasonography is accurate in most cases. Usually treatment with myomectomy is recommended and successful.

A myoma has been encountered in the rudimentary muscular bud in a patient with vaginal agenesis.

Sarcomas of the uterus. Most of the reported malignancies of the uterine fundus in adolescents have been sarcomas; mixed mesodermal tumors are the most common. Mixed mesodermal tumors are neoplasms that arise from malignant epithelial and mesenchymal stromal elements of the uterus. They are classified according to the nature of the sarcomatous component into homologous (tissue normally found in the uterus) or heterologous (tissue not normally found in the uterus, e.g., strained muscle, cartilage, etc.). The tumors are firm and sessile, filling the uterine cavity unlike the grapelike sarcomas of the vagina. These tumors also are usually found in postmenopausal women, but several mixed müllerian tumors have been reported in children and adolescents from 4 to 19 years of age. Patients usually presented with vaginal bleeding and a pelvic mass. The treatment of the tumors requires early diagnosis and radical surgery followed by radiation and chemotherapy tailored to the patient.

Careful staging of the extent of the disease is very important in the treatment and prognosis of children with rhabdomyosarcoma. Pelvic ultrasound and CT can be very useful in evaluating the extent of disease and measuring tumor regression during chemotherapy.

Breast mass

The majority of adolescents who visit the physician's office with a complaint of a breast lump have normal physiologic breast tissue or fibrocystic changes.[47] Adolescents typically have very dense breast tissue. Fibrocystic changes are characterized by diffuse cordlike thickening and by lumps which may become tender and enlarged prior to menses each month. Physical findings tend to change each month; suspected cysts can often be followed clinically.

In contrast to the finding that most breast lumps of adolescents seen in the office settings are normal or simply fibrocystic changes, most breast masses which are excised in this age group are fibroadenomas (Table 23-18).[42] These lesions are typically firm or rubbery, mobile, and have a clearly defined edge. They tend to be eccentric in position and occur more frequently in the lateral breast quadrants than the medial quadrant. The breast mass may remain unchanged or increase in size with subsequent menstrual cycles. Recurrent or multiple fibroadenomas may occur. Giant fibroadenomas may replace most of the breast tissue and, in fact, are often mistaken initially for normal tissue.

Cancer of the breast is extremely rare in children and adolescents. Primary lymphoma may also present as a breast mass in adolescents. Patients with previous radiation therapy to the chest have an increased risk of developing cancer of the breast at a young age and, therefore, require ongoing surveillance. Cystosarcoma phylloides is a rare primary tumor that is sometimes malignant.

A new entity, juvenile papillomatosis, is a rare breast tumor of young women first described by Baey in 1980. The tumor features atypical papillary duct hyperplasia and multiple cysts. The mean age of the patients is 23 years with a range of 12 to 48 years. The localized tumor is often initially mistaken for a fibroadenoma. Twenty-eight percent of the patients have a relative with breast cancer, and 7% have a first degree relative with breast cancer. A small number of patients have breast cancer diagnosed concurrently with the juvenile papillomatosis, and several patients develop cancer at follow-up. Bilateral juvenile papillomatosis may especially increase the risk of developing cancer at a later time. Thus, careful surveillance is indicated in patients with this diagnosis found on excisional biopsy. Papillary hyperplasia without the cystic component of juvenile papillomatosis appears to be a more benign condition in young patients.

Table 23-18. Pathologic diagnosis of 100 breast biopsy specimens

FIBROADENOMA	83	(83%)
adult	58	
juvenile	19	
giant	2	
cellular	2	
papillary	1	
with mixed stroma	1	
FIBROCYSTIC MASTOPATHY	8	(8%)
fibrocystic disease	4	
simple cyst	2	
fibrocystic mastopathy	1	
stromal sclerosis	1	
OTHER	9	(9%)
chronic mastitis	2	
epidermal inclusion cyst	1	
adenomatous hyperplasia	1	
intraductal hyperplasia with focal secretion	1	
capillary hemangioma	1	
fat necrosis	1	
normal fat and breast tissue	1	

If the adolescent presents with the complaint of a breast mass, palpation may make the diagnosis evident in cases such as fibrocystic changes or tenderness with overlying erythema consistent with a breast infection. Trauma may cause a breast mass, but examination immediately following a contusion may locate a preexisting lesion. If the differential diagnosis is a cyst or fibroadenoma, the lesion can be measured and the patient should be instructed to return after her next menstrual period. If the lesion has disappeared, then a cyst was probably present. If the lesion is still present and the patient is cooperative, a needle aspiration of the mass can be performed in the office using a 23 G needle on a 3-cc syringe. A small amount of lidocaine can be used to infiltrate the skin with a 25 G needle. In contrast, a fibroadenoma gives a characteristic "gritty," solid sensation. Any material obtained (even if just on the tip of the needle) should be smeared on a ground glass slide, fixed, and sent for cytologic examination. If the mass collapses after aspiration, it is assumed to be a cyst and the mass is reevaluated in three months. A sonogram of the breast tissue can also help to delineate a fibroadenoma from a cyst and can be used to localize an abscess. Mammography should not be used to evaluate breast masses in the adolescent age group since the breast tissue is very dense, the risk of the patient having carcinoma is negligible, and radiographic features have not influenced clinical management.

When aspiration of a persistent, discrete mass is not feasible or is nonproductive, or when masses are nonmobile and hard, enlarging, tender, or are a source of considerable anxiety, the patient should have an excisional biopsy performed. Unless there are underlying medical conditions, such as cardiac or pulmonary disease, an excisional biopsy can be done in an ambulatory setting under general or local anesthetic, depending on technical considerations and on the patient's preference and ability to cooperate. Because breast scars can be cosmetically deforming, the optimal incision for a lesion near the center of the breast is a radial incision in terms of wound healing and cosmetic results. Periareolar ectopic lobules (Montgomery cysts), which often have clear or dark discharge from the areola (not the nipple), can be excised with a circumareolar incision.

A contusion to the breast may result in a poorly defined, tender mass that resolves over several weeks. A mass from severe trauma may take several months to resolve; occasionally scar tissue remains palpable indefinitely. Fat necrosis may also result from trauma, although the patient may not notice the growing lesion until several months later. A biopsy is indicated in such circumstances. It should be remembered that the examination immediately following a trauma to the breast may locate a preexisting lesion. A sharply delineated, nontender mass is probably unrelated to the recent injury.

REFERENCES

1. Adams J, Ahmad M, Phillips P: Anogenital findings and hymenal diameter in children referred for sexual abuse examination, *Adolesc Pediatr Gynecol* 1:123, 1988.
2. American Fertility Society: Classification of müllerian anomalies, *Fertil Steril*, 49:952, 1988.
3. Baker TG: Radiosensitivity of mammalian oocytes with particular reference to the human female, *Am J Obstet Gynecol* 110:746, 1971.
4. Barbieri RL: Hormone treatment of endometriosis: the estrogen threshold hypothesis, *Am J Obstet Gynecol* 166:740, 1992.
5. Berenson AB, Heger AH, Andrews SE: The appearance of the hymen in newborns, *Pediatrics* 87:458, 1991.
6. Berenson AB, Heger AH, Andrews SE: Morphology of the hymen in twins, *Adolesc Pediatr Gynecol* 4:82, 1991.
7. Berta R et al: Genetic evidence equating SRY and the testis-determining factor, *Nature* 348:448, 1990.
8. Boley SJ: Lesions of the breast. In Holder TW, Ashcroft KW, editors: *Pediatric surgery*, Philadelphia, 1980, WB Saunders.
9. Bongiovanni AM, editor: *Adolescent gynecology: a guide for clinicians*, New York, 1982, Plenum Publishing.
10. Cali RW, Pratt JH: Congenital absence of the vagina, *Am J Obstet Gynecol* 100:752, 1968.
11. Cantwell H: Vaginal inspection as it relates to child sexual abuse in girls under thirteen, *Child Abuse Negl* 7:171, 1983.
12. Cantwell H: Update on vaginal inspection as it relates to child sexual abuse in girls under thirteen, *Child Abuse Negl* 11:545, 1987.
13. Capraro VJ: Gynecologic examination in children and adolescents, *Pediatr Clin North Am* 19:511, 1972.
14. Capraro VJ, Dillon WP, Gallego MB: Microperforate hymen: a distinct clinical entity, *Obstet Gynecol* 44:903, 1974.
15. Carpenter SEK, Rock AJ: *Pediatric and adolescent gynecology*, New York, 1991, Raven Press.
16. Carson SA: Gynecologic problems of adolescence and puberty. In Sciarra JJ, editor: *Gynecology and obstetrics*, Philadelphia, 1984, JB Lippincott.
17. CDC: Sexually transmitted disease: treatment guidelines, *MMWR* 42:7, 1993.
18. Chisholm TC: Exstrophy of the urinary bladder. In Holder TW, Ashcroft KW, editors: *Pediatric surgery*, Philadelphia, 1980, WB Saunders.
19. Christensen EH, Oster J: Adhesions of labia minora (synechia vulvae) in childhood: a review and report of fourteen cases, *Acta Paediatr Scand* 60:709, 1971.
20. Claessons EA, Cowell CA: Acute adolescent menorrhagia, *Am Obstet Gynecol* 193:377, 1981.
21. Counseller VS, Davis CE: Atresia of the vagina, *Obstet Gynecol* 32:528, 1968.
22. Craighill MC: Human papillomavirus infection in children and adolescents, *Seminars in Pediatric Infectious Diseases* 4(2):85, 1993.
23. Damewood MD et al: Induction of ovulation and pregnancy following lateral oophoropexy for Hodgkin's disease, *Int J Gynecol Obstet* 33:369, 1990.
24. Dewhurst CJ: *Practical pediatric and adolescent gynecology*, New York, 1980, Marcel Dekker.
25. Donahue PK, Hendren WH: Intersex abnormalities in the newborn infant. In Holder TM, Ashcroft KW, editors: *Pediatric surgery*, Philadelphia, 1980, WB Saunders.
26. Donahoe PK, Hendren WH III: Perineal reconstruction in ambiguous genitalia infants raised as females, *Ann Surg* 200:363, 1984.
27. Emans SJ: Examination of the pediatric and adolescent female, *Clin Pract Gynecol* 1:1, 1990.
28. Emans SJ: Gynecologic problems in adolescents with chronic diseases, *Clin Pract Gynecol* 1:171, 1990.
29. Emans SJ, Goldstein DP: The gynecologic examination of the prepubertal child with vulvovaginitis: use of the knee-chest postion, *Pediatrics* 65:758, 1980.
30. Emans SJ, Goldstein DP: *Pediatric and adolescent gynecology*, ed 3, Boston, 1989, Little, Brown.
31. Emans SJ et al: Genital findings in sexual abuse: symptomatic and asymptomatic girls, *Pediatrics* 79:778, 1987.
32. Fiumara NJ, Rothman K, Tang S: Reemergence of chancroid as an important STD, *J Amer Acad Dermatol* 15:939, 1986.
33. Frank RT: The formation of an artificial vagina without operation, *Am J Obstet Gynecol* 35:1035, 1938.
34. Fatness and Fertility Sci Am., March 1988; 88.
35. Frisch RE, McArthur JW: Menstrual Cycles: fatness as a determinant of minimum weight for height necessary for their maintenance or onset, *Science* 185:949, 1974.
36. Frisch RE, Revelle R: Height and weight at menarche and a hypothesis of menarche, *Arch Dis Child* 46:695, 1971.
37. Gantt PA, McDonough PG. Dysfunctional bleeding in adolescents. In Barwin BN, Belish S, editors: *Adolescent gynecology and sexuality*, New York, 1982, Masson.
38. Gardner JJ: Descriptive study of genital variation in healthy, nonabused, premenarchal girls, *J Pediatr* 120:251, 1992.
39. Gidwani GP: Establishing a practice in pediatric and adolescent gynecology, *Female Pat* 18:33, 1993.
40. Goldstein DP: Female genital tract. In Welch KJ, editor: *Complications of pediatric surgery*, Philadelphia, 1982, WB Saunders.
41. Goldstein DP, DeCholnoky C, Emans SJ: Adolescent endometriosis, *J Adolesc Health Care* 1:37, 1980.
42. Goldstein DP, Pinsonneault O: Management of breast masses in adolescent females, *Clin Pract Gynecol* 1:131, 1990.
43. Goldstein DP et al: Laparoscopy in the diagnosis and management of pelvic pain in adolescents, *J Reprod Med* 24:251, 1980.
44. Grunberger W, Fisch LF: Pediatric gynecological outpatient department: a report on 600 patients, *Wien Klin Wochenschr* 94:614, 1982.
45. Heald FP, editor: *Adolescent gynecology*, Baltimore, 1966, Williams & Wilkins.
46. Hebeler JR: The abused child. In Holder TW, Ashcroft KW, editors: *Pediatric surgery*, Philadelphia, 1980, WB Saunders.
47. Hein K, Dell R, Caten M: Self-detection of a breast mass in adolescent females, *J Adolesc Health Care* 3:15, 1982.
48. Heger A, Emans SJ: Introital diameter as the criterion for sexual abuse, *Pediatrics* 85:222, 1990.
49. Heger A, Emans SJ: *Evaluation of the sexually abused child*, New York, 1992, Oxford University Press.
50. Hendren WH III, Donahoe PK: Correction of congenital abnormalities of the vagina and perineum, *J Pediatr Surg* 15(6):751, 1980.
51. Herbst A: Clear cell adenocarcinoma of the vagina and cervix: analysis of 170 registry cases, *Am J Obstet Gynecol* 119:713, 1974.
52. Herbst A: A prospective comparison of exposed female offspring with unexposed controls, *N Engl J Med* 292:334, 1975.
53. Herbst A, Ulfelder HJ, Poskanzer CP: Adenocarcinoma of the vagina, *N Engl J Med* 284:878, 1971.
54. Huffman JW, Dewhurst CJ, Capraro VJ: *The gynecology of childhood and adolescence*, ed 2, Philadelphia, 1981, WB Saunders.
55. Ingram JM: The bicycle seat stool in the treatment of vaginal agenesis and stenosis: a preliminary report, *Am J Obstet Gynecol* 140:73, 1981.
56. Jacobson L: Differential diagnosis of acute PID, *Am J Obstet Gynecol*, 138:124, 1980.
57. Jager RJ et al: A human XY female with a frame shift mutation in the candidate testis-determining gene SRY, *Nature* 348:452, 1990.
58. Jirasek JE: Normal sex differentiation. In Sciarra JJ, editor: *Gynecology and obstetrics*, vol 5, Philadelphia, 1991, JB Lippincott.
59. Jones HW Jr, Heller RH: *Pediatric and adolescent gynecology*, Baltimore, 1986, Williams & Wilkins.
60. Jones HW Jr, Verkauf BS: Surgical treatment in congenital adrenal hyperplasia: age at operation and other prognostic factors, *J Obstet Gynecol* 36(1):1, 1970.

61. Koff AK: Development of the vagina in the human fetus, *Contrib Embryol* 24:59, 1933.
62. Kreutner AKK, Hollingsworth DR: *Adolescent obstetrics and gynecology*, Chicago, 1978, Year Book Medical.
63. Lack EE, Goldstein DP: Primary ovarian tumors in childhood and adolescence, *Curr Probl Obstet Gynecol*, 7(4): 1984.
64. Laufer MR: Endometriosis in adolescents, *Curr Opinion in Ped* 4:582, 1992.
65. Laufer MR et al: A new technique for laparoscopic prophylactic oophoropexy prior to cranioplasty irradiation in children with medulloblastoma. *Adolesc Pediatr Gynecol* 1995 (In press).
66. Laufer MR, Galvin WJ: Labial hypertrophy: a new surgical approach. *Adolesc Pediatr Gynecol* 8:39-41, 1994.
67. Laufer MR, Rein MS: Treatment of abnormal uterine bleeding with gonadotropin-releasing hormone analogues, *Clin Obstet Gynecol* 36(3):668, 1993.
68. Lavery JP, Sanfilippo JS, editors: *Pediatric and adolescent obstetrics and gynecology*, New York, 1985, Springer-Verlag.
69. Le Floch O, Donaldson SS, Kaplan HS: Pregnancy following oophoropexy and total nodal irradiation in woman with Hodgkin's disease, *Cancer* 38:2263, 1976.
70. Lewis VG, Ehrhardt AA, Money J: Genital operations in girls with the adrenogenital syndrome, *Obstet Gynecol* 36(1):11, 1970.
71. Mandl AM: A quantitative study of the sensitivity of oocytes to X-irradiation, *Proc R Soc Biol* 150:53, 1958.
72. Marshall WN, Lightner ES: Congenital adrenal hyperplasia presenting with labial fusion without clitoromegaly, *Pediatrics* 66:312, 1980.
73. McCann J: Use of the colposcope in childhood sexual abuse examinations, *Pediatr Clin North Am* 37(4):863, 1990.
74. McCann J, Voris J: Perianal injuries resulting from sexual abuse: a longitudinal study, *Pediatrics* 91:390, 1993.
75. McCann J, Voris J, Simon M: Genital injuries resulting from sexual abuse, *Pediatrics* 89:307, 1992.
76. McCann J et al: Genital findings in prepubertal girls selected for nonabuse: a descriptive study, *Pediatrics* 86:428, 1990.
77. McGregor JA: Toxic shock syndrome. In Sciarra JJ, editor: *Gynecology and obstetrics*, Philadelphia, 1988, JB Lippincott.
78. McIndoe A: Treatment of congenital absences and obliterative conditions of the vagina, *Br J Plast Surg* 2:254, 1950.
79. McIndoe AH, Banister JB: An operation for the cure of congenital absence of the vagina, *J Obstet Gynaecol Br Commonw* 45:490, 1938.
80. Mininberg DT: Phalloplasty in congenital adrenal hyperplasia, *J Urol* 128:355, 1981.
81. Morton KE, Dewhurst CJ: Human amnion in the treatment of vaginal malformations, *Br J Obstet Gynaecol* 93:50, 1986.
82. Muckle CW: Developmental abnormalities of the female reproductive organs. In Sciarra JJ, editor: *Gynecology and obstetrics*, Philadelphia, 1988, JB Lippincott.
83. Muram D: Classification of genital findings in prepubertal girls who are victims of sexual abuse, *Adolesc Pediatr Gynecol* 2:149, 1988.
84. Muram D: Child sexual abuse—genital tract findings in prepubertal girls. I. The unaided medical examination, *Am J Obstet Gynecol* 160(2):328, 1989.
85. Muram D: Child sexual abuse: relationship between sexual acts and genital findings, *Child Abuse Negl* 13(2):211, 1989.
86. Muram D, Elias S: Child sexual abuse—genital tract findings in prepubertal girls. II. Comparison of colposcopic and unaided examinations, *Am J Obstet Gynecol* 160(2):333, 1989.
87. Muram D, Hostetler BR, Jones CE: Adolescent victims of sexual assault, *Female Pat* 18:54, 1993.
88. Murphy M: Sexual abuse in the pediatric and adolescent patient, *Clin Pract Gynecol* 1:31, 1990.
89. Nicholson HS, Byrne J: Fertility and pregnancy after treatment for cancer during childhood or adolescence, *Cancer* 71:3392, 1993.
90. Oberman HA: Breast lesions in the adolescent female, *Pathol Annu* 14:175, 1979.
91. Pang S et al: Worldwide experience in newborn screening for classical congenital adrenal hyperplasia due to 21-hydroxylase deficiency, *Pediatrics* 81:866, 1988.
92. Paradise JE: Predictive accuracy and the diagnosis of sexual abuse: a big issue about a little tissue, *Child Abuse Negl* 13:169, 1989.
93. Pinsonneault O, Goldstein DP: Obstructing malformations of the uterus and vagina, *Fertil Steril*, 44:241, 1985.
94. Pokorny SF: Configuration of the prepubertal hymen, *Am J Obstet Gynecol* 157:157, 1987.
95. Ramenofsky ML: Vaginal lesions. In Holder TM, Ashcroft KW, editors: *Pediatric surgery*, Philadelphia, 1980, WB Saunders.
96. Ravnikar VA: Endocrine disorders. In Kistner RW, editor: *Gynecology—principles and practice*, ed 4, Chicago, 1985, Year Book Medical.
97. Ray GH et al: Oophoropexy: a means of preserving ovarian function following megavoltage radiotherapy for Hodgkin's disease, *Radiology* 96:175, 1970.
98. Reindollar RH, Byrd JR, McDonough PC: Delayed sexual development: a study of 252 patients, *Am J Obstet Gynecol* 140:371, 1981.
99. Rock JA: Surgical correction of uterovaginal anomalies. In Sciarra JJ, editor: *Gynecology and obstetrics*, Philadelphia, 1984, JB Lippincott.
100. Sadler TW: *Langman's medical embryology*, ed 6, Philadelphia, 1990, Williams & Wilkins.
101. Sanfilippo JS: Dysmenorrhea in adolescents, *Female Pat* 18:29, 1993.
102. Sanfilippo JS et al: *Pediatric and adolescent gynecology*, Philadelphia, 1994, WB Saunders.
103. Schiffman MH: Recent progress in defining the epidemiology of human papillomavirus infection and cervical neoplasia, *J Natl Cancer Inst* 84(6):394, 1992.
104. Simpson JL, Photopulos G: The relationship of neoplasia to disorders of abnormal sexual differentiation, *Birth Defects* 12:15, 1976.
105. Sinclair AH et al: A gene from the human sex-determining region encodes a protein with homology to a conserved DNA-binding motif, *Nature* 346:240, 1990.
106. Slaughter L, Brown C: Colposcopy to establish physical findings in rape victims, *Am J Obstet Gynecol* 166:83, 1992.
107. Speiser PW et al: High frequency of nonclassical steroid 21-hydroxylase deficiency, *Am J Hum Genet* 37:650, 1985.
108. Stone SC: Physiology of puberty. In Sciarra JJ, editor: *Gynecology and obstetrics*, vol 5, Philadelphia, 1984, JB Lippincott.
109. Teixeira W: Hymenal colposcopic examination in sexual offenses, *Am J Forensic Med Pathol* 2:209, 1981.
110. Thibaud E et al: Preservation of ovarian function by ovarian transposition performed before pelvic irradiation during childhood, *J Pediatr* 121:880, 1992.
111. Thomas PRM et al: Reproductive and endocrine function in patients with Hodgkin's disease: effects of oophoropexy and irradiation, *Br J Cancer* 33:226, 1976.
112. White S, Ingram D, Lyna PR: Vaginal introital diameter in the evaluation of sexual abuse, *Child Abuse Negl* 13:217, 1989.
113. Williams EA: Congenital absence of the vagina: a simple operation for its relief, *J Obstet Gynecol Br Commonw* 71:511, 1964.
114. Wolff PB et al: Posterior fusion without clitoromegaly in a female with partial 21-hydroxylase deficiency, *J Pediatr* 91:951, 1977.

Chapter 24

PELVIC ULTRASONOGRAPHY

Beryl Benacerraf

During the past several years, pelvic sonography has become an important factor in the armamentarium of gynecologists in evaluating the female pelvis. Sonography is commonly the first test ordered for assessing a wide variety of clinical problems. The most common indications for gynecologic ultrasonography include the following: (1) pelvic pain, (2) abnormal vaginal bleeding, (3) a palpable mass, (4) infertility, (5) a possible ectopic pregnancy, and (6) a follow-up study on known fibroids or adnexal pathology. Recently technologic advances have improved pelvic sonography, and increasing resolution has made the diagnoses more reliable. In addition, the advent of the transvaginal probe has further enhanced the ability to detect pelvic pathology noninvasively. Sonography remains superior to any other radiologic modality for the evaluation of a gynecologic patient.

PREPARATION OF THE PATIENT

Sonography is a tomographic technique which uses thin tomographic slices to visualize anatomy in a given imaging plane, depending upon where the transducer is aimed. Therefore multiple sections of the pelvis are needed, both transversely and longitudinally for a complete examination. A full bladder is necessary so that the gas-filled bowel can be displaced away from the pelvis, since ultrasound cannot penetrate air. Furthermore, the bladder is then juxtaposed against the pelvic organs, creating the best visibility since the fluid-filled bladder enhances sound transmission.

It is possible, however, to overfill the bladder and compress the uterus and ovaries too much.[7] One can therefore manipulate the bladder; if it is too full, it can be partially emptied, if it is not full enough, it can be filled. In some situations the pelvis can be better examined with only a small amount of fluid in the bladder; this is helpful in the examination of fibroids or in the localization of an IUD in an anteverted uterus.[21]

The use of the vaginal probe requires that the bladder be empty so that the pelvic organs can descend in close proximity to the probe. The probe then can be rotated from side to side to evaluate the entire lower pelvis tomographically.

Color Doppler mapping of blood flow can be helpful to evaluate the vascularity of pelvic masses. This is best done transvaginally for the most sensitive Doppler examination.

THE UTERUS

Normal anatomy

The uterus should be the first organ identified in a pelvic sonogram and it is usually centrally located (Fig. 24-1). It appears as a pear-shape structure on a longitudinal scan, just behind the urinary bladder, and contains a midline echogenic stripe depicting the endometrial cavity. In a transverse section, the uterus is round, homogeneous in texture, and contains a central echogenic dot, which is the endometrial cavity in cross-section. The cervix is seen as the lowest extent and narrowest portion of the uterus inferiorly, and the endocervical canal often contains echolucent material that represents mucous. The anteverted uterus is most easily seen transabdominally, even with only a partially full bladder; however, the retroverted uterus can be very difficult to see since it extends away from the ultrasound beam (Fig. 24- 2). The fundus of the uterus may have a hypoechoic texture when the uterus is retroverted as a result of the lack of penetration of sound deep in the pelvis. Transvaginal sonography is necessary for the evaluation of the retroverted uterus, since fibroids can inadvertently be diagnosed when the retroverted uterus is seen transabdominally because of this hypoechoic pattern. The fundus of such a uterus should be examined transvaginally for uterine fibroids and for optimal viewing of the myometrium.

Identifying the central uterine cavity echo is a useful sign for demonstrating that the uterus is empty, therefore

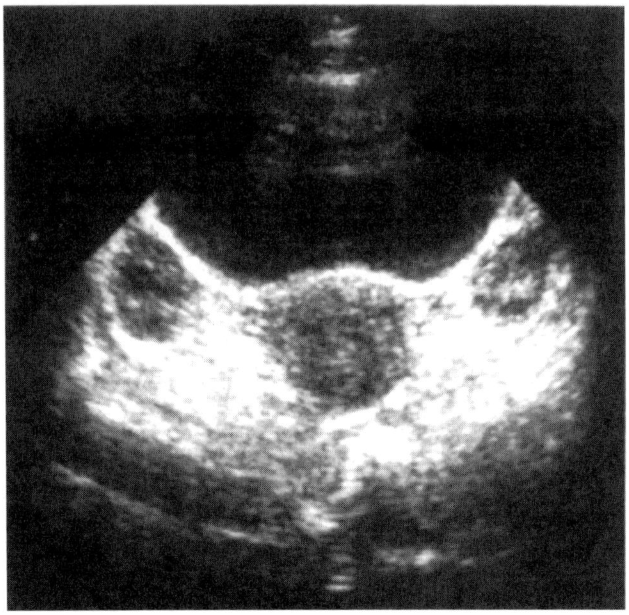

Fig. 24-1. Transverse view through a normal pelvis, showing the uterus centrally located and both ovaries in cross section on either side.

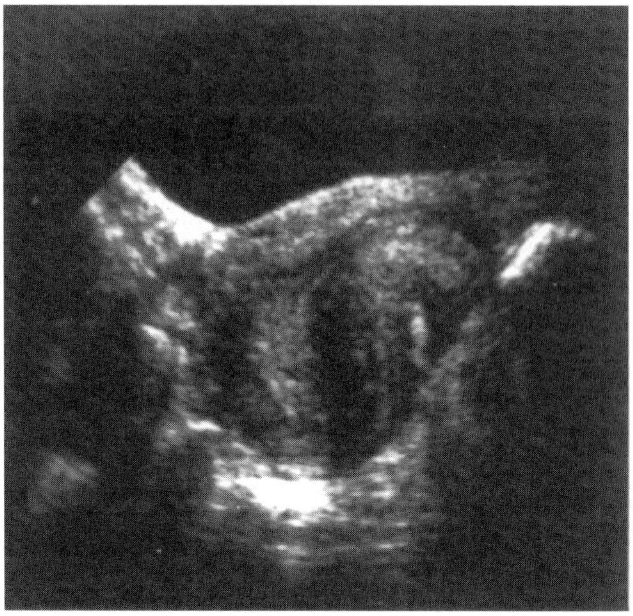

Fig. 24-2. Long axis view of a retroverted uterus. It is possible to follow the increased echogenicity of the endometrium as it extends posteriorly in the retroverted fundus.

excluding intrauterine pregnancy, submucous fibroids, etc. The demonstration of this echo is also helpful in identifying the uterus itself when confusing pelvic pathology is present, such as dense adnexal masses or uterine fibroids.[19] The endometrial echo changes in width during the cycle, from a thin triple-line configuration in the proliferative phase to a marked hyperechoic functional layer in the secretory phase.[41] In the postmenopausal patient who is not receiving hormone replacement, however, an endometrial echo greater than 5 mm in width is considered abnormal, a finding discussed later in this section.[36]

The vaginal probe is very helpful in the evaluation of the uterus and endometrial abnormalities. An early study comparing transvaginal and transabdominal scanning in 29 patients showed that in 23% of the cases, transvaginal scanning provided additional diagnostic information that was not available with the transabdominal technique. In the other 77%, adequate diagnostic information was obtainable by either transabdominal or transvaginal techniques, but in 63% of these cases the quality of the transvaginal image was judged to be superior to that obtained transabdominally.[85]

Congenital abnormalities

Major congenital abnormalities of the uterus are easily detected by transabdominal and transvaginal sonography. More recently, MRI has also proven accurate in the diagnosis of congenital uterine anomalies.[105] The easiest abnormality to identify is the double uterus, or uterus didelphys, where two entirely separate uterine bodies and fundi are seen (Fig. 24-3). It is important not to mistake one of the uterine fundi for an adnexal mass or an ectopic pregnancy when the empty second uterus is visualized.

The bicornuate uterus is identifiable by locating the endometrial echo in a transverse section and by noting that it separates into two discrete portions at the fundus, each surrounded by myometrium (Fig. 24-4). Normally the endometrial echo at the fundus should extend in a line parallel to

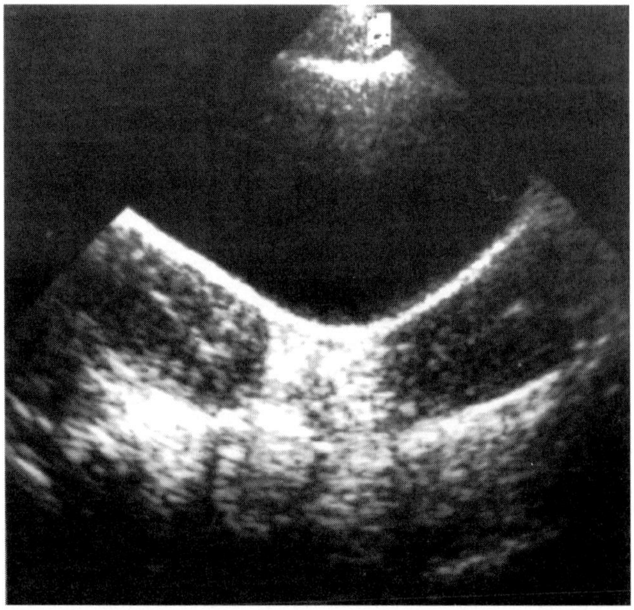

Fig. 24-3. Transverse view through the pelvis of a patient with a double uterus. The two separate uteri are identified on either side of the midline.

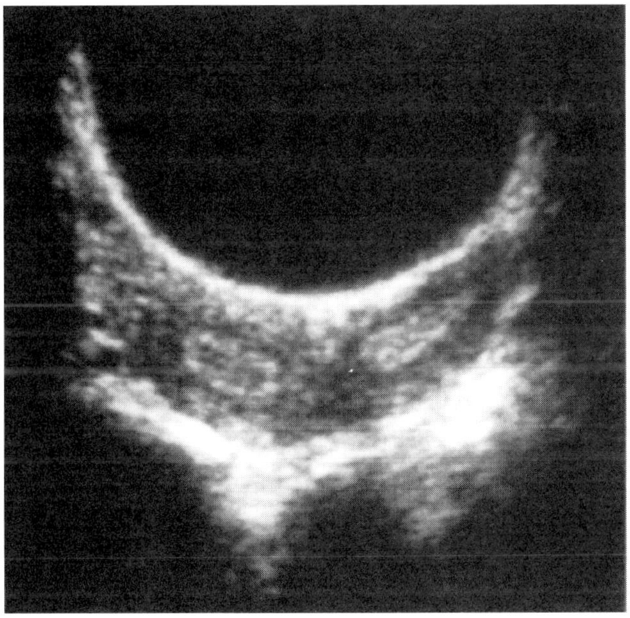

Fig. 24-4. Transverse view through the pelvis of a patient with a bicornuate uterus. Note that the myometrium extends all the way around two separate islands of increased echogenicity, representing the two portions of the endometrial cavity at the fundus.

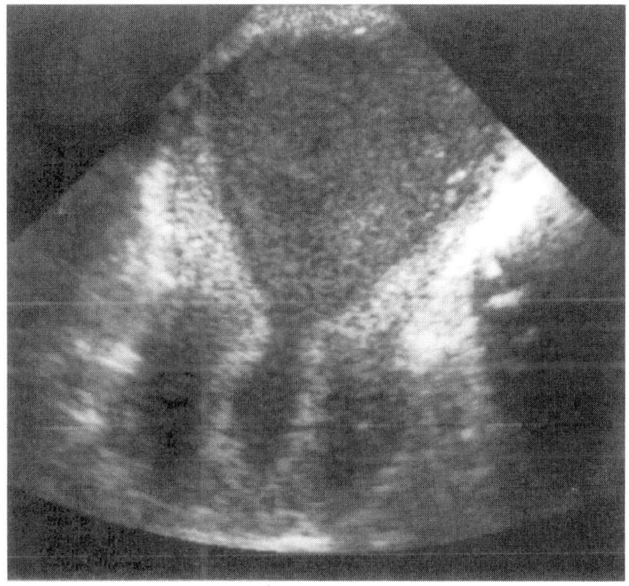

Fig. 24-5. Coronal view of the uterus with a hydrometrocolpos. Note the distended intrauterine cavity at the fundus, extending into a dilated endocervix. The low-level echoes indicate non-clotted blood.

the bladder in transverse section, with no disruption of this line by myometrium in the center. A septated uterus can have an appearance similar to the bicornuate uterus, although a small septum may not be detectable sonographically. The examination of the shape of the intrauterine cavity, however, is better accomplished by hysterosalpingography, particularly for smaller defects. It is important to remember, however, that abnormalities of the müllerian ducts are associated with other genitourinary malformations and that the kidneys should be imaged when a uterine malformation is identified.[77,43,128]

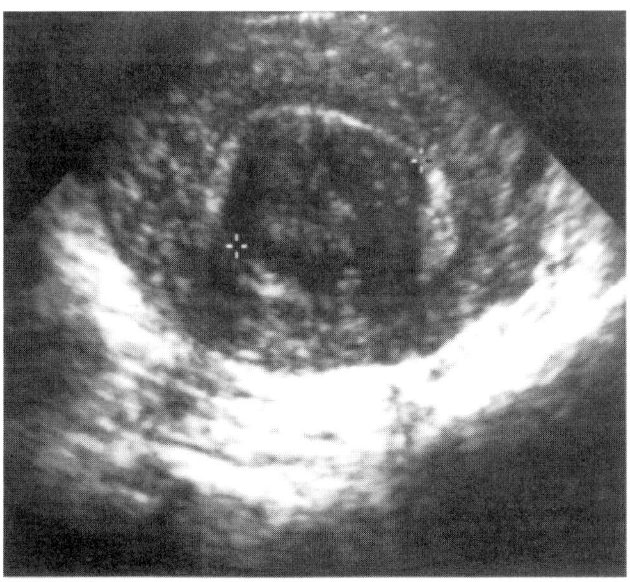

Fig. 24-6. Transverse section through the fundus of the uterus, showing a submucous fibroid (shown by the calipers). The echogenic endometrial stripe is noted, surrounding the fibroid.

Hydrocolpos and hydrometrocolpos result in a large pelvic fluid collection secondary to obstruction of the vagina or uterus. The most common congenital abnormality that causes hydrocolpos or hematocolpos is an imperforate hymen. Sonographically, the fluid collection is usually large and contains low-level echoes, which indicate nonclotted blood or hemosiderin (an appearance similar in texture to an endometrioma) (Fig. 24-5). When a hydrocolpos or hematocolpos is present, the fluid collection will be posterior to the bladder and underneath the uterus in the characteristic location of the vagina. Hydrometrocolpos may be more difficult to diagnose, since it can be confused with an adnexal mass or cyst. The fluid-filled uterus can have a very thin wall and be difficult to recognize as the uterus. In addition, this fluid collection may also contain low-level echoes or material within it which represents blood or blood clots in hematometrocolpos. It is crucial to search for the uterus and to consider this diagnosis if a normal uterus cannot be otherwise located.[149]

Primary amenorrhea is an indication for sonography, and a variety of congenital abnormalities can be diagnosed with this method. Patients with Mayer-Rokitanski-Kruster-Hauser syndrome with vaginal atresia should be evaluated by sonography to determine the extent of the malformations of the internal pelvic organs and kidneys.[115] A spectrum of malformations can be diagnosed definitively by

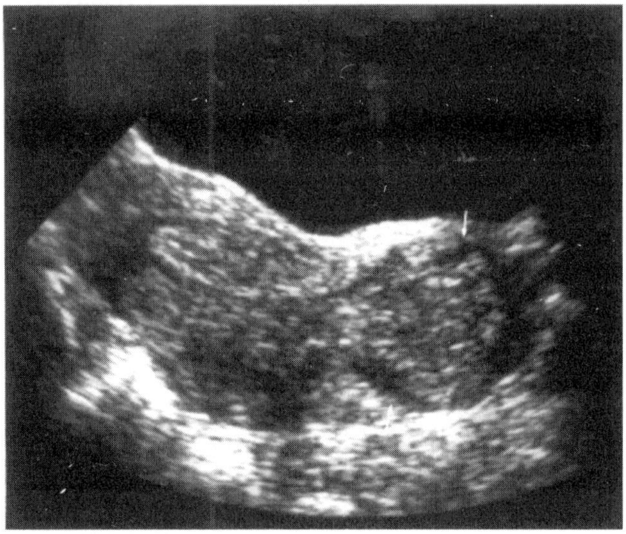

Fig. 24-7. Longitudinal view of the uterus and cervix, showing a prolapsed, submucous, pedunculated fibroid. There is a mass in the upper vagina (arrows), indicating the prolapsed fibroid.

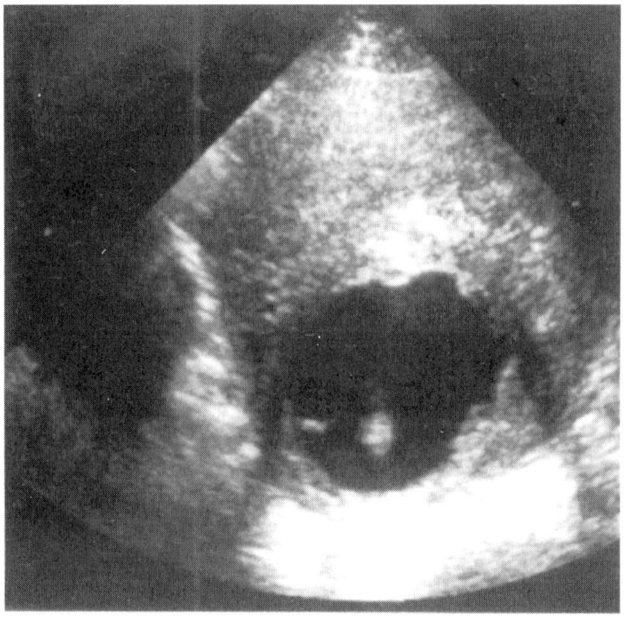

Fig. 24-8. Transverse view through an enlarged uterus, showing an irregular cystic area with some solid material within it. This represents a degenerating fibroid.

ultrasonography including complete absence of the uterus, with pelvic kidneys as the most severe. Patients with Turner's syndrome have a characteristic appearance of the pelvis with a very tiny uterus, both longitudinally and transversely, and unidentifiable ovaries.[127]

Uterine tumors

The most common intrauterine tumor is the fibroid. Leiomyomas can be detected by several sonographic

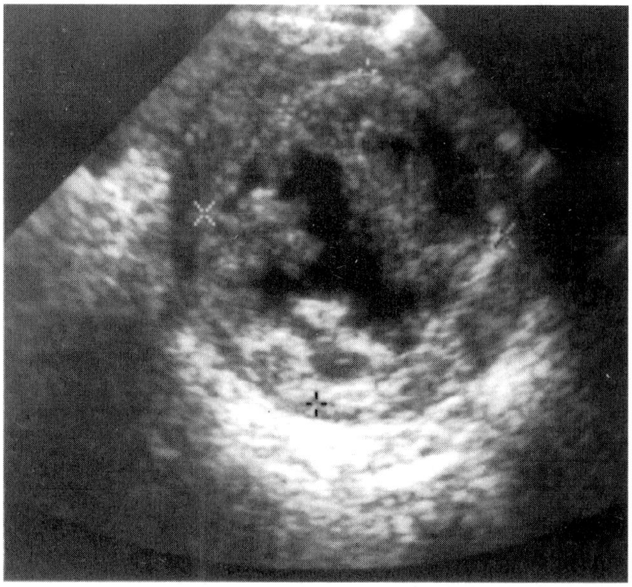

Fig. 24-9. Irregular, complex cystic and solid mass shown by the calipers and located within the uterus. This represents a degenerating fibroid.

features: (1) the uterine contour is often irregular and lobular, (2) the uterus is often enlarged, and (3) the echo pattern of the fibroid itself is most commonly hypoechoic.[48] There are sometimes minimal contour irregularities of the uterus, which may represent a subtle diagnostic sign of a leiomyoma, but with current high-resolution equipment and particularly transvaginal sonography, the contour and exact limits of the fibroids often can be recognized (Fig. 24-6). Transvaginal sonography has helped to determine whether a fibroid is submucous or intramural. Transvaginal sonography has the sensitivity, specificity, and positive predictive value of 100%, 94%, and 81%, respectively, for the prediction of submucous myomas.[32] Hysteroscopy has a similar track record, although it is better at distinguishing myomas from endometrial polyps.[32] Although most fibroids are hypoechoic (but not cystic), some fibroids may be hyperechoic and also may contain calcification. Fibroids can calcify with small specks or clumps of calcium. Alternatively the rim of the fibroid may calcify, similar to the appearance of a fetal head. Pedunculated fibroids may be difficult to diagnose if they occur laterally in the region of the broad ligament. The normal ovary on that side must be identified, to be sure that the solid mass is indeed simply a fibroid.[94] Unless the ovary can be identified with confidence, the possibility of an ovarian mass cannot be excluded. Differentiation between an intramural and a submucosal fibroid depends on the appearance of the endometrial echo (Fig. 24-6). A submucous fibroid will distort this echo and will be located adjacent to it. Rarely, a submucous fibroid will prolapse through the cervix into the vagina and give the appearance of a solid vaginal mass (Fig. 24-7).[144]

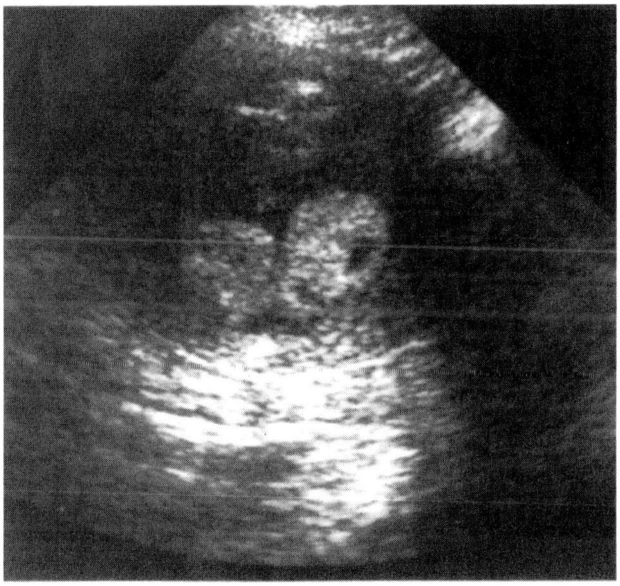

Fig. 24-10. Enlarged uterus containing two irregular, echogenic masses with cystic areas within them. The pathology indicated a leiomyosarcoma.

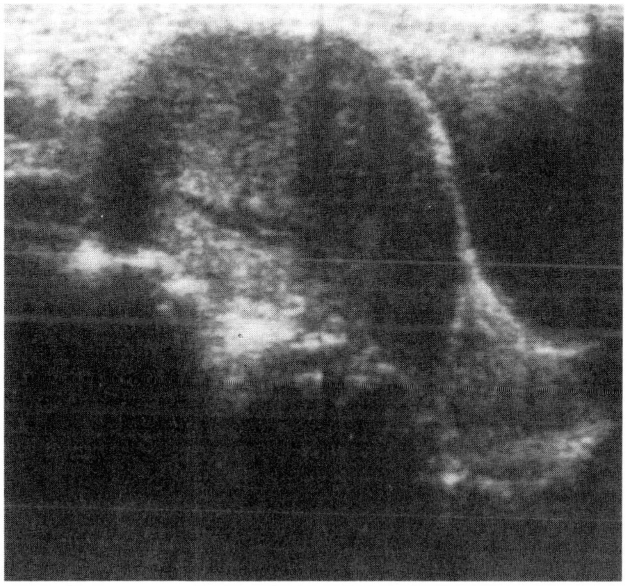

Fig. 24-11. Longitudinal view of an enlarged uterus. There is a symmetry in the position of the endometrial cavity which is more posterior than usually seen. The anterior myometrium is disproportionately wider and heterogeneous, consistent with adenomyosis.

Occasionally, fibroids may degenerate and irregular cystic areas can appear centrally within the fibroid (Figs. 24-8, 24-9). This commonly occurs during pregnancy and may be associated with severe pain. A cystic uterine mass in a nonpregnant patient is a more difficult diagnostic dilemma and should not be assumed to be a degenerating fibroid by sonography alone. Ovarian tumors can invade the myometrium, or rarely fibroids can become sarcomatous and give rise to abnormal uterine fluid collections (Fig. 24-10). Further evaluation is therefore necessary if a cystic fibroid is identified in a nonpregnant patient.

Posterior fibroids are difficult to characterize by transabdominal sonography since there is a decreased penetration of sound in the cul-de-sac, similar to the retroverted uterus. The etiology of a hypoechoic mass in the cul-de-sac may be confusing, particularly if both ovaries cannot be definitively identified. Here again, transvaginal scanning is necessary as a diagnostic modality for the posterior pelvic compartment.

Other rare uterine benign tumors usually have a peculiar sonographic appearance and appear largely cystic rather than solid. An intrauterine mass can be differentiated from an adnexal mass, since a uterine mass will lie within the confines of the uterine wall and be surrounded by serosa rather than being located outside the boundaries of the myometrium.

Adenomyosis is a difficult sonographic diagnosis to make. Adenomyosis can be suspected if the uterus is diffusely enlarged but the myometrial texture and contour appear normal. The myometrial texture can also have a heterogeneous appearance with small echolucent lakes (Fig. 24-11). One study showed that an ultrasonography was able to suggest adenomyosis with a sensitivity of 63%, a specificity of 97%, and a positive predictive value of 71%.[130] Diagnostic errors included three cases of adenomyosis diagnosed as leiomyomas because of the presence of contour and focal uterine abnormalities. Adenomyosis can mimic leiomyomas, particularly when focal, making a definitive sonographic diagnosis very difficult. An occasional patient will have intrauterine fluid collection and a thickened endometrial echo as a manifestation of adenomyosis, although further evaluation of such sonographic findings is necessary to rule out endometrial carcinoma.[76]

Although an occasional intrauterine fluid collection and abnormal endometrial echoes can be secondary to adenomyosis, further evaluation of the patient is necessary, since there is a spectrum of endometrial pathology that can be associated with abnormal endometrial echoes and fluid collection. McCarthy et al studied postmenopausal endometrial fluid collections and found that although malignancy must always be excluded, benign causes of uterine fluid collections were more common than previously reported. Seven-five percent of these postmenopausal patients had benign processes such as endometrial polyps, chronic inflammation of the cervix and endometrium, and inflammatory processes.[83] This is controversial, however, since Breckenridge et al showed widely differing results in a group of 17 postmenopausal patients, 94% of whom had uterine fluid collections associated with active carcinoma of the uterus or cervix (Figs. 24-12, 24-13).[17] Occasionally, the uterus can remain obstructed either by carcinoma of the

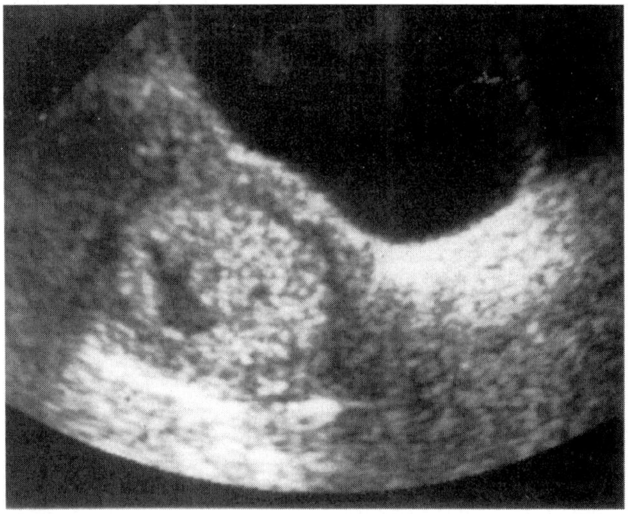

Fig. 24-12. Longitudinal view of the uterus, showing an irregular fluid collection surrounded by marked increased echogenicity with a thickened endometrium. This patient had endometrial carcinoma.

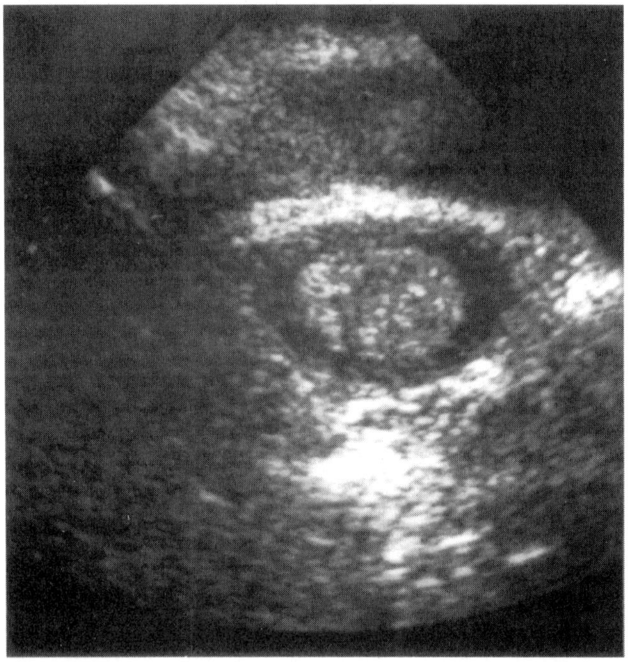

Fig. 24-13. Transverse view of the uterus, showing markedly increased echogenicity centrally in a postmenopausal patient who had endometrial carcinoma.

uterus or cervix or secondary to radiation therapy, which causes a hematometrocolpos. The uterus takes on the appearance of a large thin-walled fluid collection that is easily confused with a mass of ovarian origin. As in hematometrocolpos of the patient with a congenital uterine abnormality, it is important to think of this diagnosis particularly when a normal uterus cannot be otherwise identified.[125] Transvaginal scanning is helpful as an aid in staging carcinoma of the cervix.[22] Transrectal sonography is used in staging for cervical cancer, and in a recent study, the extent of parametrial involvement was diagnosed by transrectal sonography with a sensitivity, specificity, and diagnostic accuracy of 78%, 89%, and 87% respectively.[59]

Abnormal thickening of the endometrial echoes was studied in 12 patients in whom the endometrial cavity echoes were wider than expected. Eighty-three percent of these patients had endometrial pathology, including carcinoma in 33% and normal findings in 17%.[61] As previously stated, the width of the endometrial echo should not exceed 5 mm in the postmenopausal patient and in menstruating patients it should be wide and echogenic only in the secretory portion of the cycle. Although the thickened endometrial echo is a useful sign for the presumptive diagnosis of an endometrial pathology such as carcinoma, many patients with endometrial carcinoma have a normal uterus by ultrasonography. In 10 of 15 cases of proven uterine malignancy, pelvic sonographic studies predicted the diagnosis. This reveals a 67% rate of success for the value of a negative sonogram and an 83% rate of success with a positive sonogram.[24] Chambers et al suggests that although pelvic sonography is not a screening test for uterine malignancy, positive findings should prompt surgical investigation.[24]

More recently, several transvaginal studies of the endometrium in postmenopausal women demonstrated that an endometrial thickness of less than 5mm is not associated with endometrial cancer, particularly in patients who are not on hormonal replacement. The mean endometrial thickness for women with endometrial cancer is greater than 10 mm, mainly 18 mm ± 6 mm.[47,129,138] In women with an endometrial thickness of 5 to 8 mm (intermediate), proliferative endometrium could not be distinguished from hyperplastic endometrium, and in one case there was a low-grade carcinoma.[138] A comparison of transabdominal and transvaginal scanning in the evaluation of the postmenopausal endometrium showed that a 5 mm endometrial thickness was used as a cut-off with both techniques, although the image quality and patient acceptance was much better in the group examined transvaginally. The absence of a full bladder compressing the endometrium and the improved identification of nearby fibroids were additional advantages to the transvaginal approach.[92] Endovaginal ultrasonography also is used to characterize myometrial invasion of endometrial carcinoma. The sensitivity of detecting myometrial invasion of greater than 50% is 79%. The positive predictive value is 100%, however, in all cases where endometrial invasion is suspected to be greater than 50%.[63] Further evaluation of the endometrium, particularly when polyps are suspected, can be done with fluid contrast augmentation where fluid can be injected transcervically into the endometrial cavity during transvaginal sonography. Distention of the cavity is helpful to confirm the presence and location of endometrial polyps and to prepare for hysteroscopic treatment.[132]

Detection of intrauterine contraceptive devices (IUD)

Inability to visualize the string of an IUD is an indication for sonography to determine whether the IUD has perforated, has been expulsed, or has become associated with an intrauterine or ectopic pregnancy. If pregnancy is suspected, a pregnancy test is crucial prior to the sonogram for optimal interpretation. IUDs have a particular type-specific morphology that was recognizable in 94% of patients with Lippe's Loop and in 81% of patients with Copper-7 devices in 1980.[20]

A patient is often sent for localization of the IUD directly after her physician has probed the uterus in an attempt to locate it clinically. In doing so, air can be introduced into the intrauterine cavity, thus simulating a foreign body or IUD. It is contraindicated to probe the intrauterine cavity if the patient is to be sent for a sonogram for localization of an IUD since instrumenting the uterus may confuse the issue.

The IUD is not the only echogenic structure that can be seen within the uterine cavity. Retention of a laminaria or of fetal bones after a therapeutic abortion may have a very similar appearance. This should be kept in mind when an intrauterine echogenic foreign body is seen, so as not to mistake a pathologic foreign body for an IUD.[14,25,58] Uterine perforation by the IUD is readily noticeable when the IUD is traversing the myometrium between the endometrial cavity and the serosa. Occasionally, if it has perforated completely, it can be visualized in the cul-de-sac, although the increased echogenicity of bowel and bowel gas is likely to obscure an IUD located totally outside the uterus. If complete perforation is suspected and if the IUD cannot be visualized sonographically, a pelvic x-ray is helpful to determine whether the IUD has been completely expulsed or whether it is still within the pelvis. Imbedding of the IUD is more difficult to diagnose sonographically since the IUD still would be located in the vicinity of the endometrial echo. Hysterosalpingography is better able to demonstrate imbedding than ultrasonography.[116] Transvaginal sonography may eventually be able to improve the ability of sonography to diagnose imbedding of the IUD.

If the pregnancy test is positive and if the pregnancy is at least 5 weeks in gestation, the gestational sac must be located in the uterus sonographically to confidently exclude an ectopic pregnancy (see the discussion on ectopic pregnancy later in the chapter). If the pregnancy is intrauterine, ultrasonography is helpful in determining the relationship between the position of the gestational sac and the IUD. If the IUD is located in the lower segment it can be easily removed. Removal of IUDs located in very close proximity to the gestational sac or above it is much more hazardous and creates a greater chance of interrupting the pregnancy. Occasionally, IUDs can be removed under sonographic guidance.

Vaginal masses

Cystic vaginal masses are characteristic in their location in that they elevate the floor of the bladder and the uterus still remains intact. Fluid in the vagina can be secondary to hydrocolpos. When seen in the pediatric patient, this may be a result of an imperforate hymen or some other obstructive lesion of the vagina, as discussed earlier in this chapter.[121] It is also possible for a patient to have a double vagina, one of which is obstructed. Sonographic evaluation of the uterus in these patients is crucial since congenital abnormalities of the uterine horns are likely. Gartner's duct cyst is a fairly common vaginal cyst usually diagnosed as an incidental finding during pelvic sonography. The cyst can be single or multiple, lie along the anterolateral aspect of the vaginal wall, and arise in caudal remnants of the mesonephric duct (Fig. 24-14).[84] Solid vaginal lesions are very rare and would be difficult to identify by sonography unless they became large. A prolapsing fibromyoma, however, is easily seen and can be confirmed by a physical examination (Fig. 24-7). The presence of a menstrual tampon is characteristic, since it contains air and creates an acoustic shadow.[84] Small cysts in the region of the cervix usually represent retention cysts or nabothian cysts. These are usually incidental findings during pelvic sonography. Such cysts vary in size from 6 to 20 mm.[40] During a pelvic sonogram, the vagina is normally collapsed and is seen as a linear streak of tissue under the floor of the bladder. Occasionally it can be filled with fluid after douching or secondary to reflux from voiding, mimicking a hematocolpos.

THE ADNEXA

The normal ovaries are usually located between the uterus and lateral side walls (Fig. 24-1). Ovarian volumes can vary

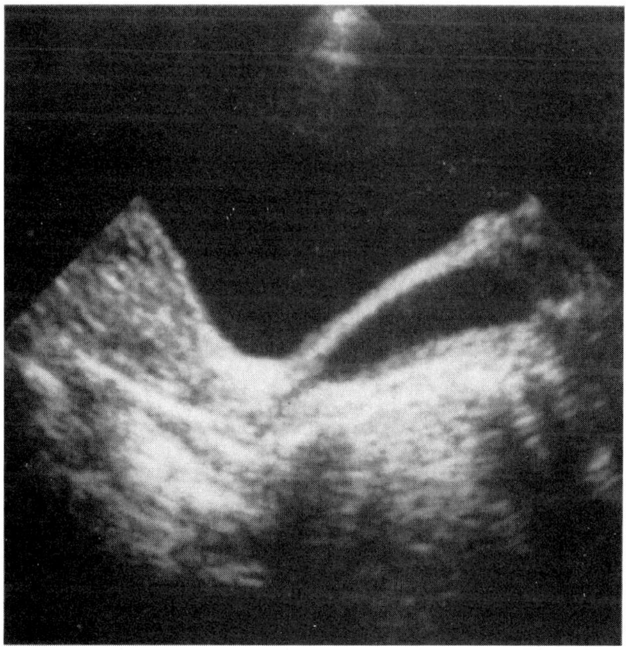

Fig. 24-14. Longitudinal view of the uterus and vagina, showing a tubular fluid collection just underneath the bladder floor in the region of the vagina. This represents a Gartner's duct cyst.

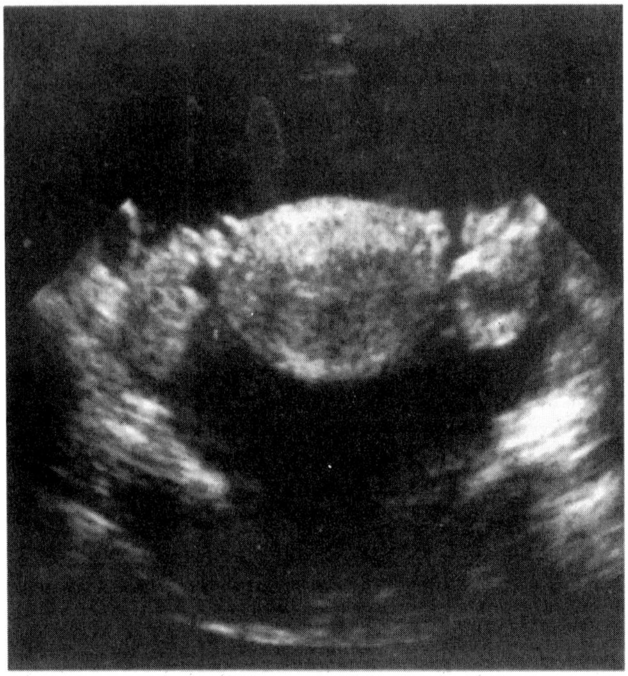

Fig. 24-15. Transverse view of the uterus and adnexa in a patient with a large amount of ascites. Note that the tubes are well seen as a result of surrounding fluid.

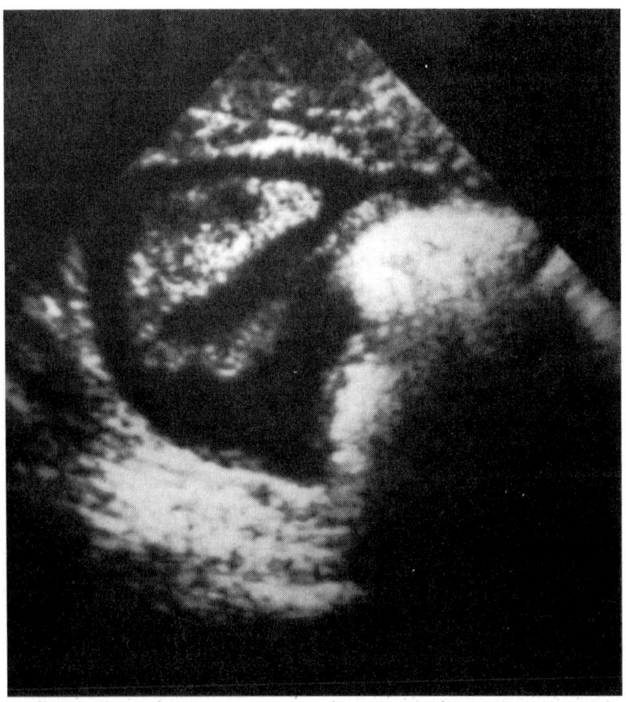

Fig. 24-16. Transvaginal view of the right Fallopian tube, well seen because it is surrounded by fluid in a patient with pelvic ascites.

from 2 to 6 cm^3 in postpubertal patients .[118] Tiny follicles less than 1 cm in size can be identified routinely on the ovaries and are not necessarily considered abnormal. The fallopian tubes are rarely visualized unless they are pathologic or unless there is pelvic ascites (Fig. 24-15). The use of the transvaginal probe has greatly improved the ability to visualize the fallopian tubes and ovaries (Fig. 24-16).[46,139] Early studies showed that transvaginal scanning offered information in 55% of patients additional to that which was obtainable by transabdominal scanning.[139] Lande et al studied 67 patients and concluded that transvaginal sonography added diagnostically useful information in 25 of 28 patients with cystic pathologic changes in the adnexae and that transvaginal sonography was particularly useful in all patients with diseases of the cul-de-sac or fallopian tubes.[69] In further studies done with the transvaginal probe, the image quality was superior to the transabdominal image in 79% to 87% of cases, whereas the transabdominal image was better in 3% to 5% of scans. Both techniques provided equivalent diagnostic information in 60% to 84% of cases; however, individual organs and fine structures were better seen transvaginally.[86] Imaging of the fallopian tubes was particularly helpful using transvaginal scanning and a fluid-filled tube. Tuboovarian inflammatory processes and ectopic pregnancy have been diagnosed with greater accuracy transvaginally.[136]

In addition to imaging the normal adnexae, knowledge of the time of the cycle is helpful. Small amounts of free pelvic fluid can be present during mid-cycle to late-cycle scans. Developing follicles up to 2 cm in size may be seen mid-cycle and should not be confused with ovarian cysts.[30,50] It is sometimes difficult to identify the ovaries sonographically, particularly when they are located in the cul-de-sac, behind a bowel loop, or above the level of the distended bladder. Following the broad ligament from the lateral aspects of the uterus usually leads to the ovaries; this is often very helpful for hard-to-find ovaries.

Ovarian Cysts

A typical ovarian cyst by sonography is completely anechoic with a thin wall and good through transmission, a characteristic of sound as it propagates through water. When such an ovarian cyst is encountered sonographically, it is wise to reexamine the patient one month later since these often represent functional cysts. Hemorrhagic cysts, on the other hand, have a variable appearance. Baltarowich et al described 76 hemorrhagic ovarian cysts, the overwhelming majority of which had good through transmission signifying the basic cystic nature of the lesion. The remainder of the sonographic features are variable and most commonly consist of a heterogeneous mass (83%) that is predominantly anechoic but with hypoechoic material within it. Seventeen percent of hemorrhagic cysts were completely homogeneous, either hypoechoic or hyperechoic (Fig. 24-17).[8] Some hemorrhagic ovarian cysts have thick and irregular walls, 87% have internal echoes, and some even have a few septations.[110] These features are difficult to differentiate from endometriomas, tuboovarian abscesses, and ovarian tumors. Percutaneous ovarian cyst aspiration has been performed using transvaginal sonography, with successful drainage of the cyst.[124] One problem with drainage of ovarian cysts is the difficulty in obtaining adequate cytology on cystic ovarian tumors. Transvaginal ultrasound may actually be more accurate in suggesting malignancy than cytologic evaluation of the cyst's fluid obtained with needle drainage—even after irrigation of the cystic tumor for further cytology.[45]

The simple adnexal cyst in the postmenopausal woman has always been more worrisome because of the usual quiescence of the postmenopausal ovary. Most of the simple clear adnexal cysts in postmenopausal women are benign; in a series of 13 patients, only one had a borderline malignancy.[2,51] In a more recent study of simple adnexal cysts in 184 asymptomatic, postmenopausal women, 53% of the cysts disappeared spontaneously and completely, 28% remained constant in size, 11% enlarged, 3% decreased in size, and 6% both increased and decreased in size over repeated examinations. The largest cyst in the series was 4.7 cm, and it disappeared over time. One patient had an ovarian cancer, but the cyst was an adnexal mass and not a simple cyst.[75] Occasionally, cysts will be identified in the adnexa adjacent to a normal-appearing ovary, representing a paratubal or a paraovarian cyst. Paraovarian cysts are known to arise from the tissues of the broad ligament and may be symptomatic because of their potentially large size.[4]

Not all pelvic cysts are ovarian; inflammatory cysts of the peritoneum can occur in the pelvis, particularly in patients who have had previous surgery (Fig. 24-18). These are usually multiloculated cysts, but their origin is difficult to diagnose sonographically; often the ovaries cannot be visualized, and the patients have had multiple surgical

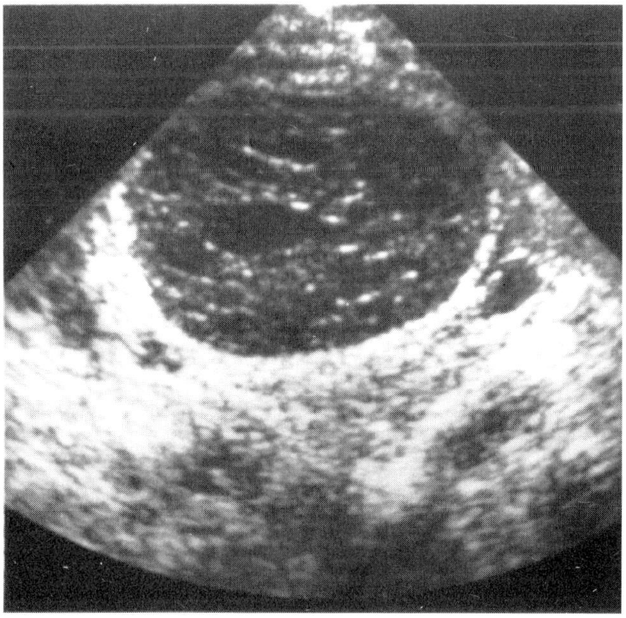

Fig. 24-17. Cystic mass containing stranding and echoes within it in a patient with acute pelvic pain. Presumably this represented a hemorrhagic cyst and was gone within two weeks after the scan.

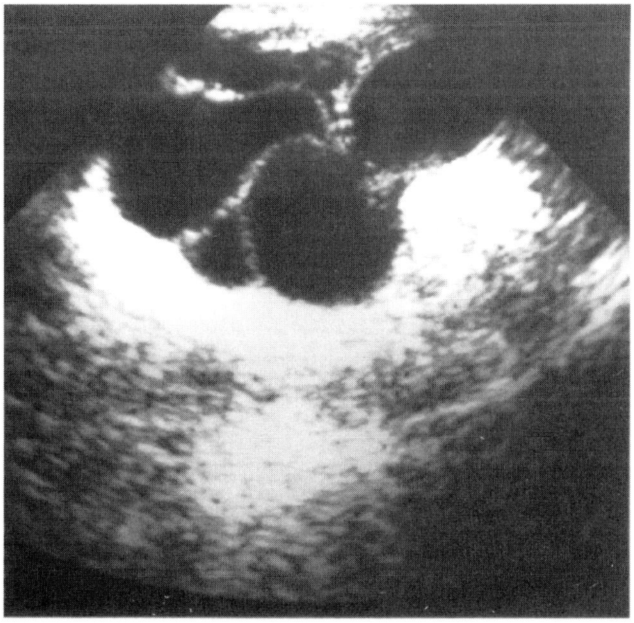

Fig. 24-18. Transvaginal scan of the cul-de-sac in a patient who had undergone multiple pelvic surgeries. At laparotomy, the cystic mass represented multiple adhesions with peritoneal inclusion cysts.

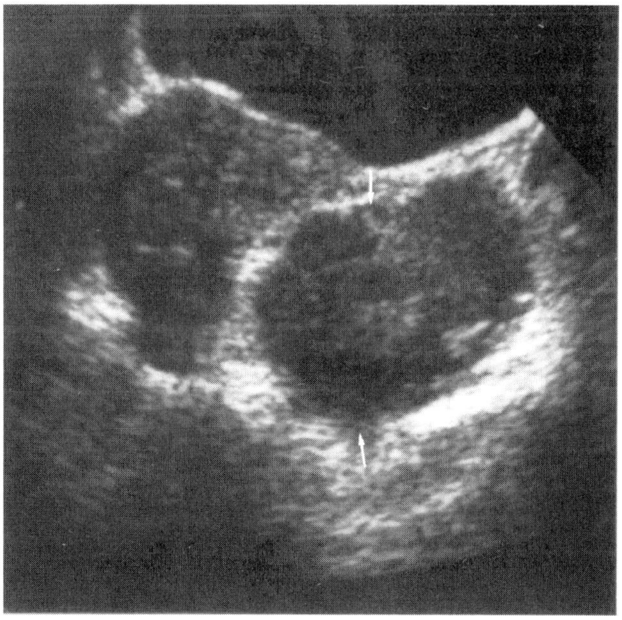

Fig. 24-19. Transverse view of the pelvis, showing a solid mass (arrows) adjacent to the uterus. This mass represented a lymphoma.

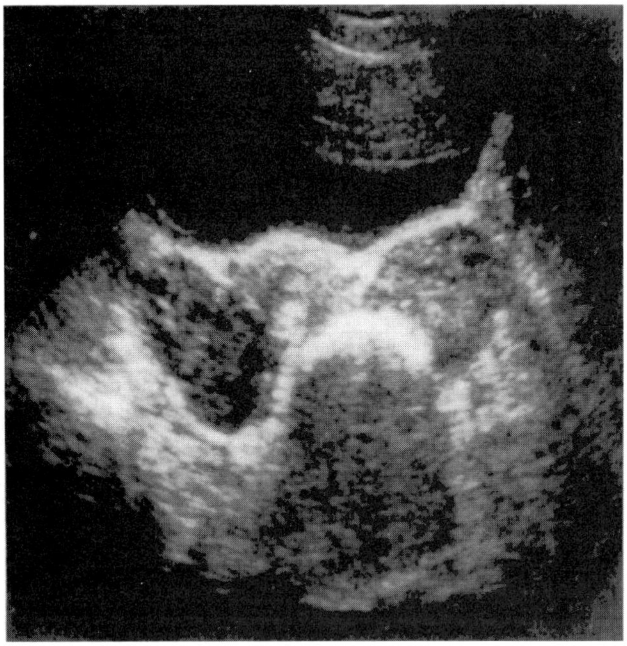

Fig. 24-20. Transverse view of the pelvis in a patient with typical Stein-Leventhal syndrome or polycystic ovaries. The uterus is centrally located and both ovaries are hypoechoic and enlarged.

procedures.[73] Other nongynecologic cystic masses occurring in the pelvis include hydroureters, bladder diverticulae, pelvic kidneys, ectopic ureteroceles, urachal cysts, fixed loops of bowel, iliac artery aneurysms, lymphomas, etc. (Fig. 24-19).[112] Occasionally, the posterior pelvic compartment, or cul-de-sac, is difficult to evaluate; in the past, a water enema was used to delineate the rectum and to attempt to map-out loops of colon which may represent pseudotumors.[68] The use of the transvaginal probe made the water enema obsolete since the probe provides a previously unavailable window to the posterior cul-de-sac.

Polycystic ovarian disease has a wide sonographic spectrum which includes enlargement of the ovaries bilaterally and symmetrically. The cysts can be discretely resolvable and multiple, under 1 cm each in size, or the ovary can have a hypoechoic pattern suggesting that the cysts are too tiny to resolve sonographically (Fig. 14-20). Approximately 30% of cases of polycystic ovarian disease have normal-size ovaries sonographically and, therefore, a normal sonogram cannot exclude this diagnosis.[31,55,152] It is possible to mistake small pelvic varicosities for cystic ovaries. If this is in question, Doppler may be helpful.[148] In general, the mean follicular size is smaller in patients with polycystic ovaries, although the overall ovarian volume is larger; these parameters are the two most helpful discriminators between normal and polycystic ovaries.[103]

Adnexal Masses

In 1977, the accuracy of gray scale sonography in determining the existence, size, and location of a pelvic mass was approximately 91% in 251 cases.[72] Since then, many studies have evaluated the accuracy of sonography for the detection and tissue diagnosis of pelvic masses. Walsh et al in 1979, examined 182 women and found that ultrasonography provided information leading to the correct diagnosis in 56% of cases and contributory data in 23% of patients.[143] This differed from the O'Brien et al study which claimed that the overall performance of sonography was inferior to clinical examination and made the correct diagnosis only 42% of the time.[101] Wade et al studied 900 patients and demonstrated that sonography established the correct diagnosis in 59% of the cases.[140] Today, most investigators agree that there have been major improvements in the sonographic diagnosis of pelvic masses. Requard et al reported that sonography was 97% accurate in the detection of, and 84% correct in the characterization of pelvic masses. In this study, 87% of these tumors were malignant by sonographic criteria.[109] In another study, Herrmann et al reported a positive predictive value of sonography for the detection of malignancy at 73%, whereas benign tumors were predicted correctly in 95% of cases.[56] Ultrasonography was compared with computerized tomography in the evaluation of patients suspected of pelvic masses; both imaging techniques depicted similar pathology and used similar diagnostic criteria.[141] CT did not appear to be superior to ultrasonography in the evaluation of pelvic masses; therefore, sonography is preferred because of the ease and relatively low cost of the technique.

Various criteria have been used in trying to differentiate types of pelvic masses and in making tissue diagnoses, with variable success. In general, anechoic lesions have a high likelihood of being benign tumors, usually cystadenomas; as the percentage of echogenic material increases, the likelihood of malignancy also increases.[26,90] Exceptions include benign teratomas, which are characteristically highly echogenic and reflective.[90,120] Fleischer et al devised criteria for the differential diagnosis of pelvic masses. Ovarian cystadenomas were predominantly cystic and septated (Fig. 24-21). Tuboovarian abscesses were usually complex and predominantly cystic. Dermoid cysts had a characteristic echogenic focus; physiologic ovarian cysts, serous adenomas, and hydrosalpinx were predominantly cystic.[35] Benacerraf et al further refined the criteria for defining benignancy or malignancy of pelvic masses.[9] The most likely lesions to be benign include a clear ovarian cyst with smooth borders, tubular cysts such as a hydrosalpinx, or a solid mass with a separate normal-appearing ovary, such as a fibroid. A clear cyst with slightly irregular borders or a cyst with smooth walls having faint, low-level echoes is more likely to represent an endometrioma. There is a group of cystic masses which are nonspecific in appearance but are usually largely cystic with irregular and thickened walls, although they lack nodularity. These masses may contain solid material within them; an accurate prediction of tissue diagnosis is extremely difficult without a good history. The

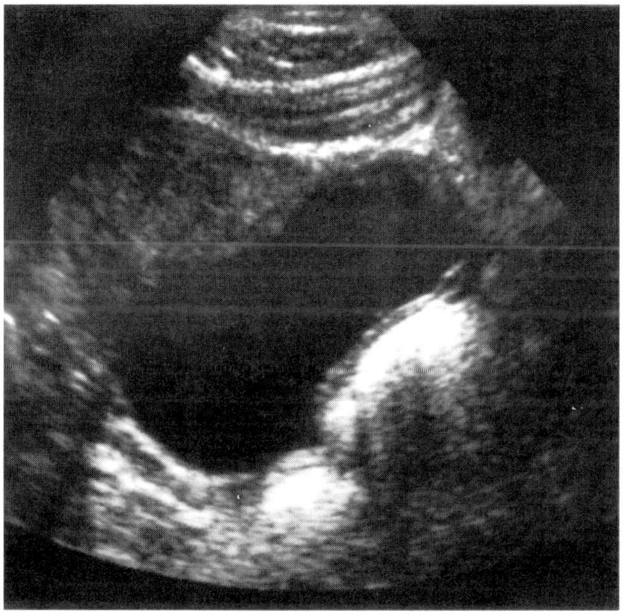

Fig. 24-21A. Transabdominal scan, showing a large left cul-de-sac cyst which appears anechoic.

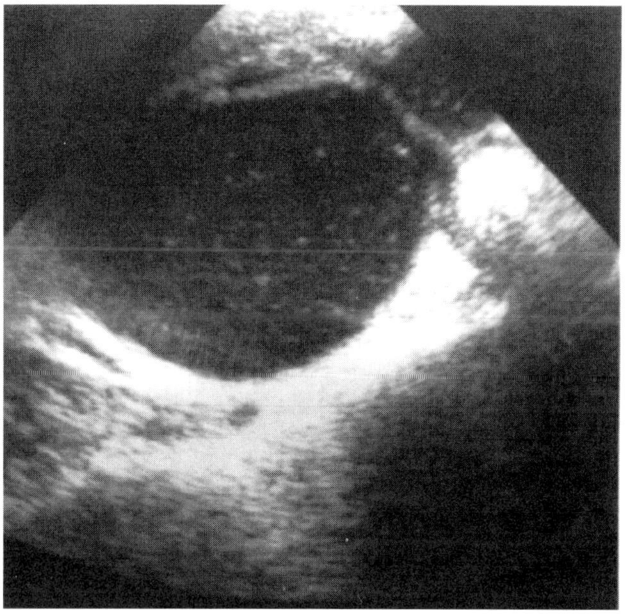

Fig. 24-21B. The transvaginal scan, however, shows that the same cyst contains internal echoes and septations. The pathologic diagnosis was mucinous cystadenoma.

differential diagnoses for such masses would include an endometrioma, a tuboovarian abscess, a benign or malignant tumor of the ovary or fallopian tube, a hemorrhagic cyst, etc. Lesions which are cystic with irregular borders and nodularity are most likely to represent ovarian carcinomas (Fig. 24-22 to 24-24). Solid ovarian enlargement is also suspicious for ovarian tumors, such as dysgerminomas (Fig. 24-25 to 24-27). An irregular cystic mass with ascites is virtually diagnostic of an ovarian malignancy. In a study evaluating pelvic masses in 100 patients undergoing laparotomy, the correct tissue diagnosis was made in 68% of cases, based on the sonographic appearance as described above. The identification of an ovarian malignancy was correct in 24 of 30 patients (80%); the specificity for correctly diagnosing a benign condition was 87%. The positive predictive value of sonography for the diagnosis of an adnexal malignancy was 73%; the negative predictive value for excluding a malignancy by sonography was 91%.[9]

Sonographically the postmenopausal ovaries are usually under 2.5 cubic centimeters in size. In a series of 30 postmenopausal women examined sonographically, both ovaries were visualized in 19 patients.[52] One ovary was seen in three patients and neither ovary could be identified in eight patients. When an ovarian mass is identified in the postmenopausal woman, further workup is indicated; however, the likelihood of malignancy seems to vary with the size of the mass. Only 1 of 32 masses of less than 5 cm was malignant.[117] Of 55 masses, 5 to 10 cm in size, 6 were malignant. Forty of the 63 tumors larger than 10 cm were malignant. The proportion of malignancies also increased with age.[117]

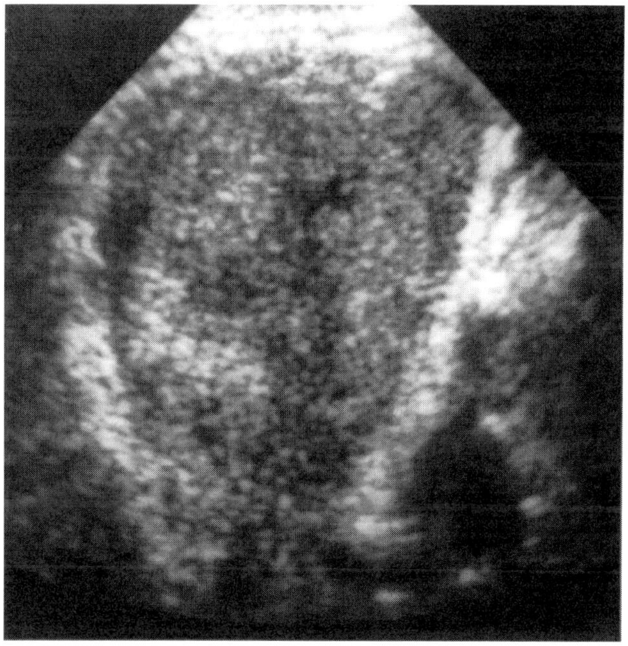

Fig. 24-22. Transvaginal scan of a solid ovarian mass, heterogeneous in texture. This was an ovarian carcinoma at laparotomy.

More recently, investigators have suggested that the neovascularity present in malignant masses can be used to identify malignant characteristics. By color-flow mapping, areas of vascularity can be identified within the mass. Pulsed Doppler then can be applied to the areas of increased vascularity to evaluate the waveform. Investigators suggested

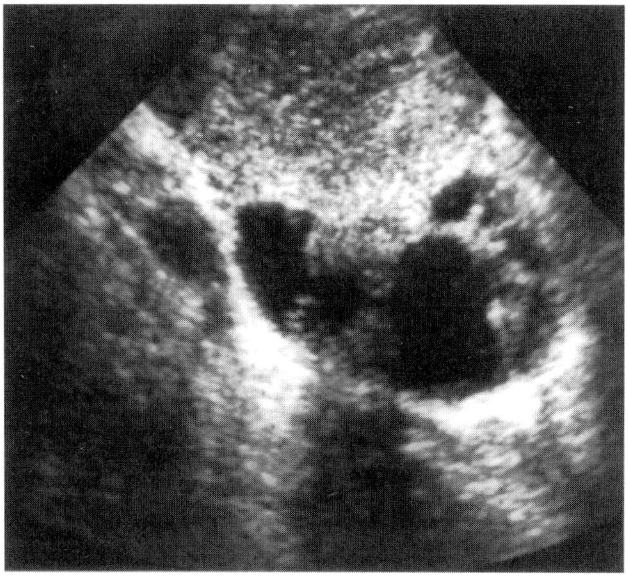

Fig. 24-23. Large, multicystic adnexal mass showing septations and marked solid nodularity with a thickened, irregular border. The patient had cystadenocarcinoma of the ovary.

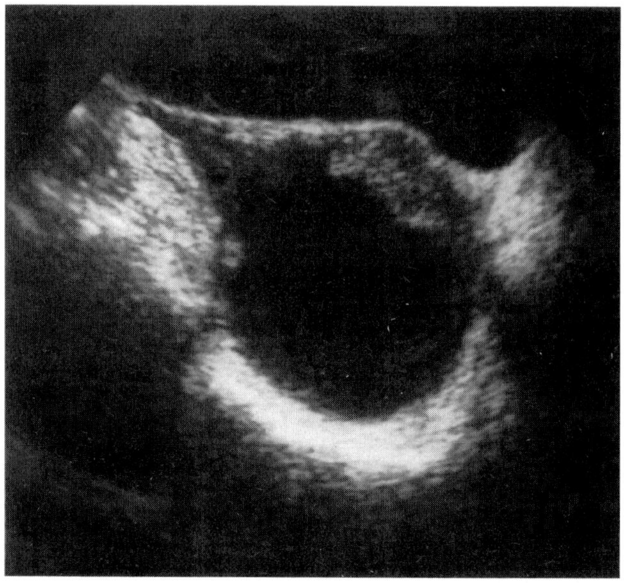

Fig. 24-24. Longitudinal view of an ovarian mass which is largely cystic but which has nodularity of the inner wall with a thickened wall. This was an endometrioma with endometrioid carcinoma.

that a low resistive or pulsatility index with a high level of diastolic flow is characteristic of a malignant lesion and masses with a high resistive with pulsatility index or a low (or sometimes absent) diastolic flow is indicative of a benign process. The decreased vascular resistance in malignant tumors is thought to be secondary to neovascularization and angiogenesis associated with malignant tumors. Recently, there has been much interest concerning the use of color Doppler, in the presence of tumor vascularity, in the differentiation of benign versus malignant ovarian masses. Kurjak et al are strong proponents of transvaginal color Doppler and Doppler waveform, particularly in postmenopausal adnexal masses. In their studies, among 56 malignant adnexal lesions and 624 benign ones proven histologically, 54 of 56 were correctly identified with a Doppler resistance index of less than 0.40 whereas 623 of

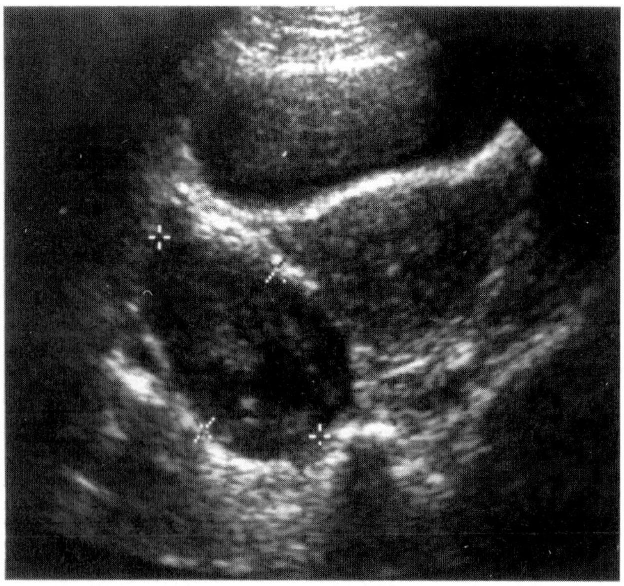

Fig. 24-25. Large, solid mass shown by the calipers in the right adnexa and clearly separate from the uterus. This represents a Brenner's tumor of the ovary.

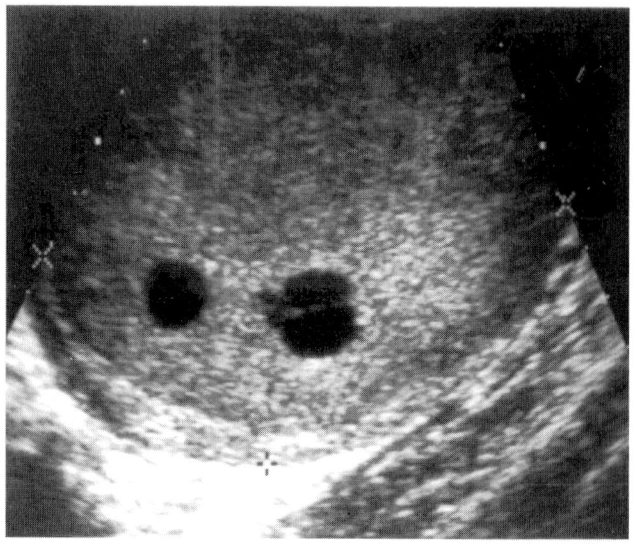

Fig. 24-26. Large, complex ovarian mass shown by the calipers. The mass is largely solid, although it contains two small, rounded, cystic areas. The pathologic diagnosis was Sertoli-Leydig cell tumor of the ovary.

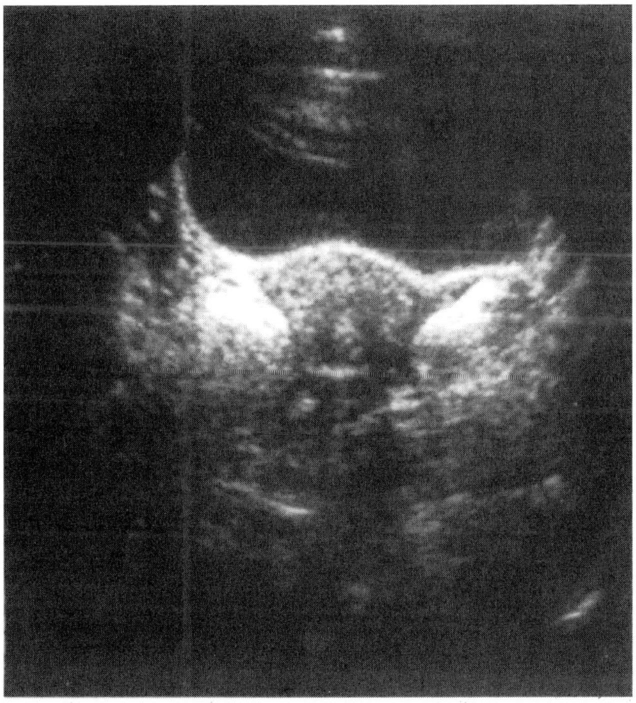

Fig. 24-27. Transverse view of the pelvis, showing a centrally-located uterus. Both adnexa contain markedly echogenic solid masses with well-defined anterior walls and poorly defined posterior walls. These masses represent bilateral dermoid cysts.

624 benign lesions were correctly identified as having a resistance index of greater than 0.40.[66,67] Although Kurjak et al found color Doppler exceedingly useful in differentiating malignant from benign,[65,66] this remains a controversial subject since not all studies reported have been equally successful. There seems to be a variability in the cut-off of the resistance index used for distinguishing benign from malignant lesions. Timor-Tritsch et al used a limit of 0.6 to obtain a sensitivity of 94% for detecting malignancies.[137] Other investigators have used the pulsatility index, at times using a limit of less than 1, and in other studies an index of 1.25.[64,145] It is possible that an accurate cut-off for the waveform does not exist since, according to Tekay and Jouppila, there is enough overlap between the waveform appearances of benign versus malignant lesions such that the cut-offs can vary between 0.4 to 0.8 on the resistance index.[134] Fleischer et al found color Doppler useful in distinguishing benign from malignant lesions in 43 surgically-proven ovarian masses, using a pulsatility index of 1 as a cut-off. They found that although the 32 benign lesions had a higher pulsatility index (1.8 ± 0.8) than malignant masses (0.8 ± 0.6), the benign range and malignant range did overlap—particularly in premenopausal patients.[38,39] Similar results were obtained by Hamper et al showing high pulsatility and resistance indices indicating benign adnexal processes but with considerable overlap between benign and malignant lesions.[53] Schneider et al cautioned the use of Doppler in the detection of ovarian malignancies since 46% of positive Doppler results were false and 37% of benign tumors had low resistance indices suggesting malignancy.[122] It is possible that the location of the vessel being sampled within the ovary may be helpful; the most recent data by Fleischer et al indicate that malignant masses are typically characterized by centrally located vessels with low impedance and without a diagnostic notch in the Doppler waveform. Multiparameter analysis is necessary for the best results in distinguishing benign from malignant ovarian masses. This includes not only Doppler information but also importantly morphologic appearance as well. (Fig. 24-28).[37]

The sonographic appearance of carcinoma of the fallopian tube is entirely nonspecific; and has been described as a complex mass with predominantly cystic components, echoes within it, and wall thickening. These findings could be confused with those of an ovarian tumor, a hydrosalpinx, an inflammatory process, endometriosis of the pelvis, etc.[89,131] Transvaginal ultrasound helps in the detection of fallopian tube carcinoma,[1] and color Doppler reveals areas of neovascularity with a characteristic low impedance in the case of primary adenocarcinoma of the fallopian tube.[126]

Fibromas and thecomas of the ovary also display a broad spectrum of sonographic features, including hypoechoic masses with posterior shadowing, cystic-appearing masses with good through transmission, and echogenic or calcified masses with mixed echogenicity.[5] Krukenberg tumors, which are usually bilateral metastases to the ovaries from a primary neoplasm in the GI tract, can become very large. They usually appear as solid masses containing variable amounts of fluid, mimicking the appearance of a cystadenocarcinoma of the ovary.[3] The bilaterality of these masses should raise the question of metastases rather than ovarian primaries. Abdominal ultrasound is very helpful not only in the examination of the malignant ovarian tumor itself but also in the staging process, since the entire pelvis can be scanned quickly and efficiently, giving valuable results. Sonography can uncover even small amounts of ascites, liver metastases, peritoneal implants, pleural effusions, hydronephrosis, abnormal omentum, etc.[104] The tumor itself, in a series of 57 patients, was usually either solid or mixed solid and cystic, but in no case was the primary malignancy exclusively cystic.[104]

Endometriosis

Endometriosis is a common gynecologic problem of women in their reproductive years. It is defined as the growth of endometrial tissue outside the uterus, and is often responsible for infertility and pelvic pain. Its sonographic manifestations are varied. In a study of 25 patients with 31 lesions characterized at ultrasound, 17 were described as cystic, 4 as polycystic, 5 as mixed, and 4 as solid.[142] Other authors have also experienced difficulty in defining the sonographic characteristics of endometriosis.[24,42,119] More recently, endometriomas have been described as being predominantly cystic but containing homogeneous and faint low-level echoes, which is fairly characteristic of a chocolate cyst (Fig. 24-29).[13] These chocolate cysts can contain echogenic material consistent with clots, a thickened wall, and occasionally some septations, which may make it difficult to differentiate then from an ovarian tumor (Fig. 24-30).

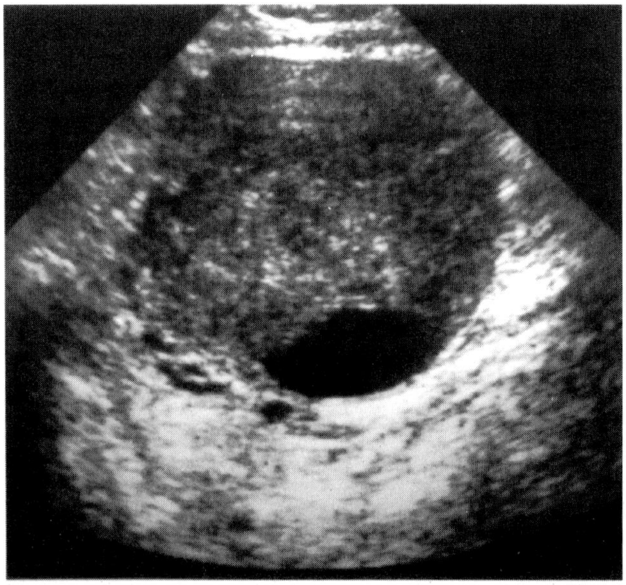

Fig. 24-28A. Solid ovarian mass with a small cystic component in a patient with ovarian cancer.

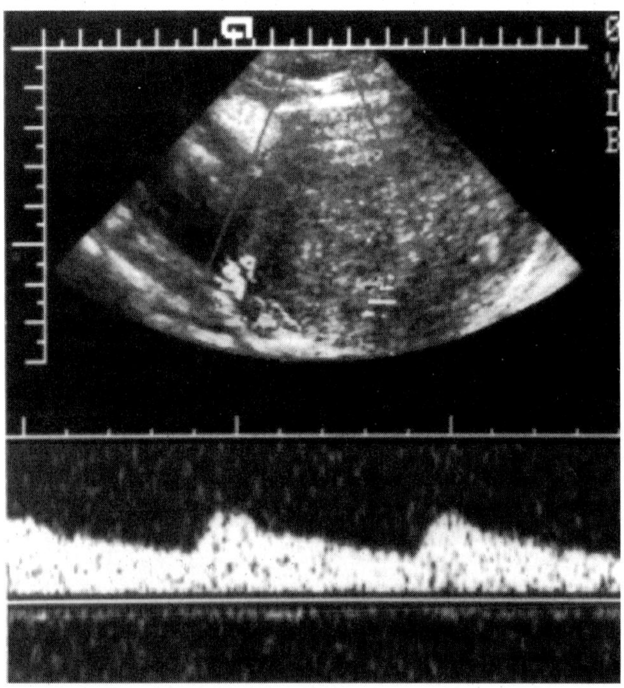

Fig. 24-28B. Within the solid portion of the mass there is evidence of neovascularity with a Doppler waveform showing low impedance flow.

Obtaining a clinical history may be helpful in those cases. Unless the endometriosis is in the form of an endometrioma, sonography may not be reliable in its detection. Tiny endometrial implants or deposits are too small to be visualized by ultrasonography. In some cases small irregular fluid collections in the cul-de-sac can actually represent endometrial implants.

Pelvic Inflammatory Disease

Early signs of pelvic inflammatory disease are difficult if not impossible to identify sonographically. Mild dilation of the fallopian tube is difficult to see; a small amount of free fluid in the cul-de-sac may indicate early pelvic infection. A hydrosalpinx is a tubular fluid-filled structure sonographically, which can have a thick or thin wall. It often has a multicystic appearance because it is folded upon itself and seen in cross section (Fig. 24-31).

A late manifestation of pelvic inflammatory disease is a tuboovarian abscess that is easily imaged by ultrasound as a complex multicystic loculated mass containing both cystic and solid areas and sometimes a small amount of gas with acoustic shadowing behind it (Fig. 24-32 and 24-33). Although the appearance of a tuboovarian abscess may not be specific, a mass, together with lower abdominal pain, leukocytosis, fever, and vaginal discharge, can prompt the correct diagnosis.[70] The accuracy of the diagnosis of a pelvic abscess is excellent, as reported by Taylor et al. They studied 220 patients with a clinical diagnosis of pelvic

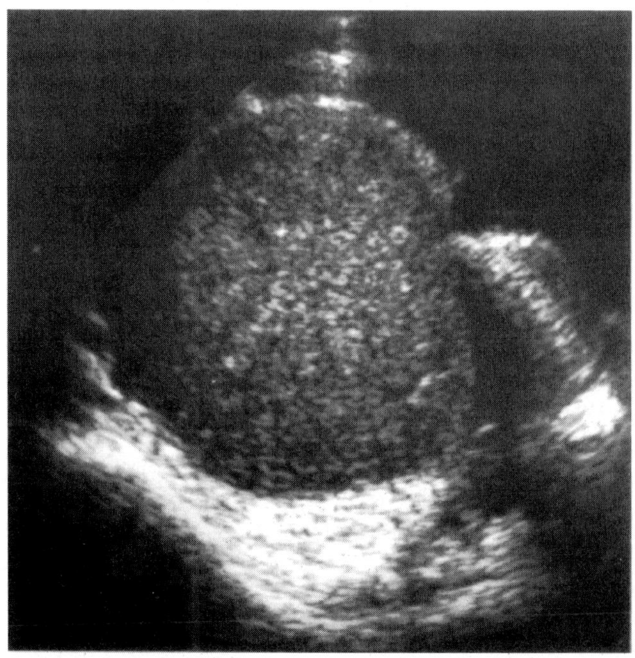

Fig. 24-29. Large, homogeneous mass. Although it appears solid in texture, it is actually cystic as shown by the increased through-transmission of sound beyond it. (Note the increased brightness of the background, beyond the back wall of the mass.) This is a typical appearance of an endometrioma.

abscess and showed that 36 of 40 abdominal and 32 of 33 pelvic abscesses were correctly identified. One hundred and twelve of 113 possible abdominal abcesses and 33 of 34 possible pelvic abscesses were diagnosed correctly.[133]

The typical tuboovarian abscess has shaggy borders and walls that are indistinct, features of inflammatory processes. In addition the pelvis can fill with pus, giving a hypoechoic mass-like effect in the cul-de-sac and adnexa and surrounding the uterus. A similar appearance can result from a blood

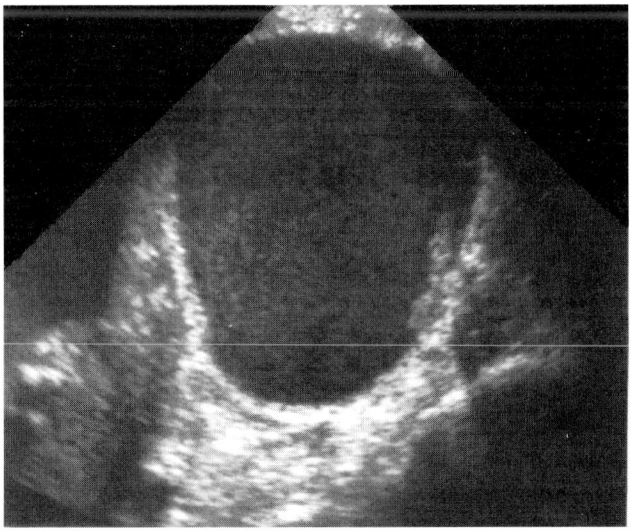

Fig. 24-30. Transvaginal scan of an adnexal cyst which has faint, low-level echoes and a slight irregularity on the inner aspect of one wall. Faint, low-level echoes are characteristic of an endometrioma.

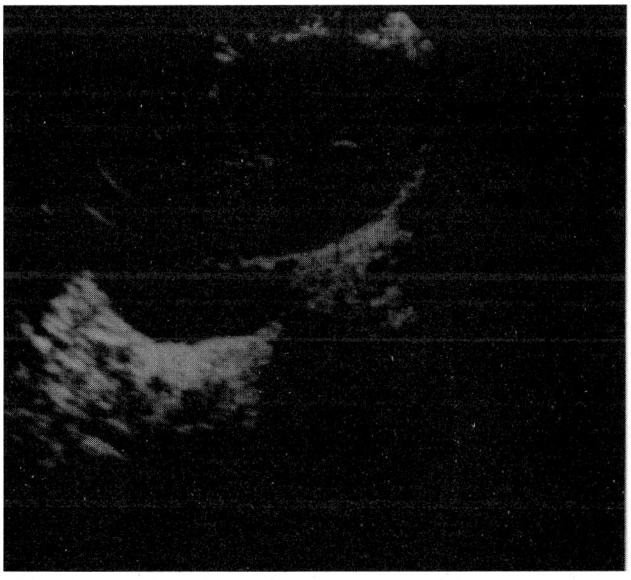

Fig. 24-31. Transvaginal scan of a distended Fallopian tube consistent with a hydrosalpinx.

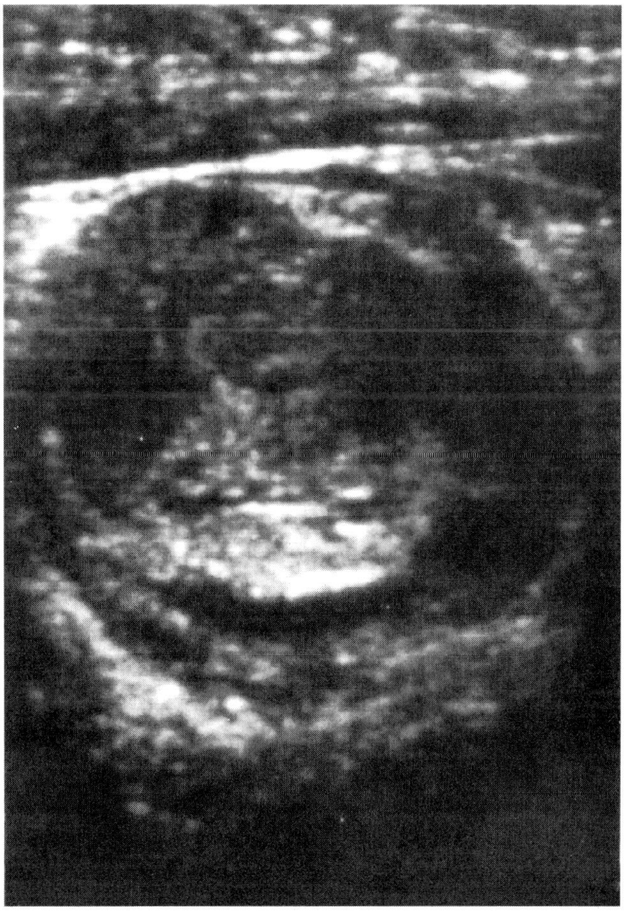

Fig. 24-32. Large, complex mass, mostly solid with a small cystic rim. Although it appears nonspecific, this patient had a tuboovarian abscess.

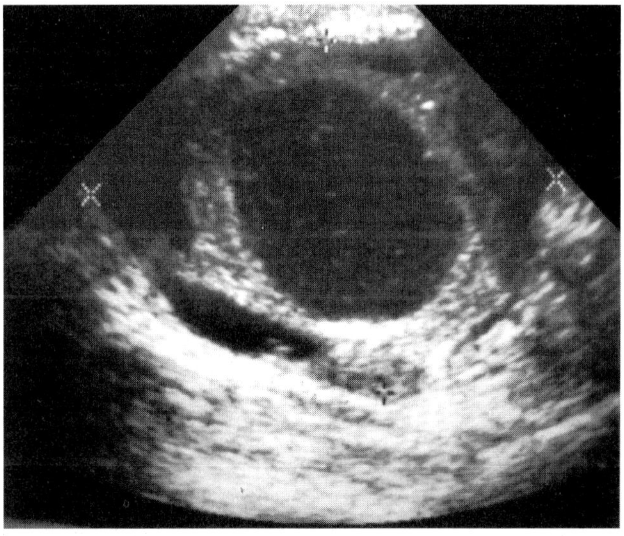

Fig. 24-33. Complex, nonspecific, septated cystic mass in the adnexa of a patient with a tuboovarian abscess.

clot and pelvic hematoperitoneum, which is occasionally seen with a ruptured ectopic pregnancy.[60] An organizing clot, however, is usually more echogenic than the lobulated hypoechoic appearance of pus. Tuboovarian abscesses can successfully be drained, both percutaneously and transvaginally.[95,151]

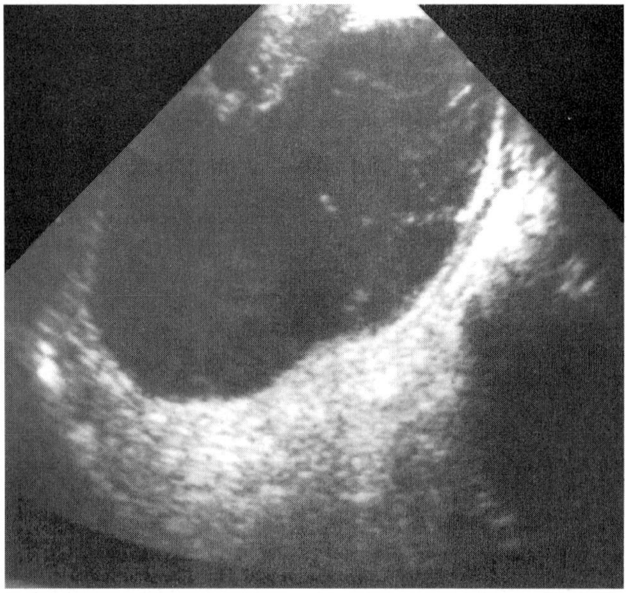

Fig. 24-34. Transvaginal scan of a patient with persistent pain and fever following a hysterrectomy. This large, septated cystic mass represents an organizing hematoma.

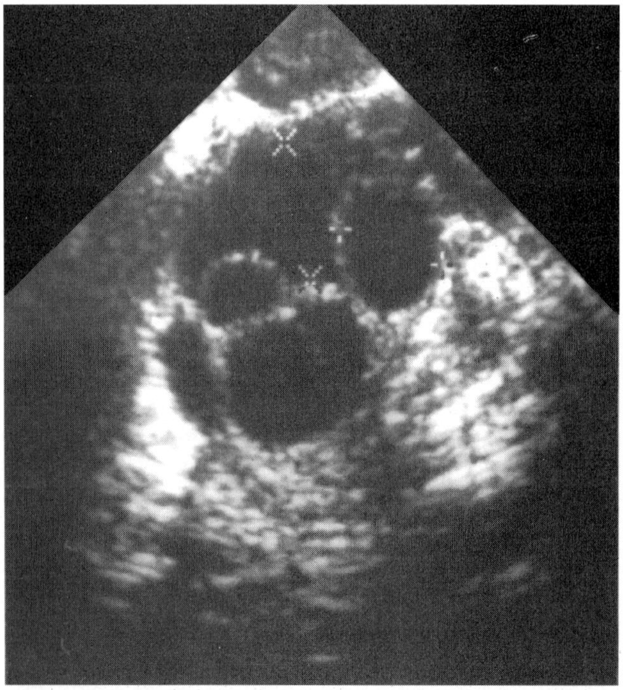

Fig. 24-35. Transvaginal view of an ovary in a patient with ovulation induction. Calipers show the confines of individual follicles.

POSTOPERATIVE COMPLICATIONS

One of the uses of pelvic sonography is to evaluate postoperative patients with surgical complications. Sonography is helpful in evaluating a possible uterine perforation following a D&C. Cunat et al reported a case where ultrasonography demonstrated a loop of small bowel within the intrauterine cavity after a D&C. A loop of ileum had entered the uterine fundus through a laceration; the ultrasonographic appearance prompted immediate operative repair.[29] A pelvic abscess or infected hematoma in posthysterectomy patients can be either solid or cystic, depending on how organized the hematoma has become and whether or not it contains loculations or pockets of pus (Fig. 24-34). Occasionally a hematoma can have a completely solid, echogenic, and lobulated appearance, similar to a fibroid uterus. A posthysterectomy abscess can be drained under direct ultrasound guidance.[82] Ultrasonography enables the surgeon to visualize adequately, drain any loculation, and ensure good positioning of the draining catheter. The ultrasound guidance is done transabdominally to avoid contamination of the surgical field.

Complications after cesarean section include a bladder flap hematoma that is usually hypoechoic with low-level echoes and a thickened wall. It is located between the lower uterine segment and the bladder, at the level of the incision.[6,150] Although it is difficult to differentiate a hematoma from an abscess, the presence of gas within the mass would signify infection. A subfascial hematoma delivery results from extraperitoneal hemorrhage within the prevesicular space, posterior to the rectus muscles but anterior to the peritoneum. Again, the sonographic appearance is predominantly cystic or possibly complex. Subfascial hematomas often occur in association with bladder flap hematomas, although the distinction between these two types of complications must be made if a drainage procedure is contemplated.[147]

ULTRASONOGRAPHY IN INFERTILITY

Sonography has been used extensively in the evaluation of the pelvis for problems of infertility. Some investigators have tried to use the appearance of the endometrial echo in the prediction of fertility. Thickman et al concluded that endometrial thickness was not a useful predictor of patients who would conceive.[135] Brandt et al, on the other hand, believe that endometrial echo abnormalities may be a recognizable cause of infertility.[16] The presence of a homogeneous, hyperechoic endometrium during the luteal phase has been a helpful finding and its absence can be a sign of luteal phase deficiency.[49] Transvaginal evaluation of the endometrium can detect intrauterine adhesions, submucous fibroids, endometrial polyps, and other irregularities in the endometrium. Transvaginal sonography is 98.9% sensitive for detecting endometrial pathology, with a positive predictive value of 94.3%.[91]

Sonography is an ideal method for visualizing developing follicles and for timing ovulation induction with the use of human chorionic gonadotropin (hCG) administration for ovulation. In addition, in a series of 210 patients undergoing sonography for ovulation induction, baseline sonograms demonstrated adnexal abnormalities in 10.7% of cases, a useful adjunct to this technique.[54] Although traditionally the ovaries have been evaluated transabdominally through a full bladder, the transvaginal technique represents a vast improvement in the visualization of the developing follicles (Fig. 24-35). It is also better accepted by patients who are scanned frequently and who want to avoid the repeated discomforts of a full bladder, the inconvenience of drinking fluids, and the delays waiting for the bladder to fill.

Ultrasonography is used (1) to distinguish between the presence of one or more mature follicles; (2) to suggest the possibility of multiple ovulations that risk hyperstimulation and multiple gestations; (3) to indicate the optimal timing for the use of hCG administration, which allows ovulation; (4) to allow detection and confirmation of normal follicular rupture and ovulation; (5) to indicate optimal timing for oocyte retrieval in in vitro fertilization programs; and (6) to assess possible pathologic pelvic conditions such as endometriosis or pelvic inflammatory disease.[87,113]

Patients undergoing treatment with clomiphene citrate or menotropins are scanned every other day or daily, around midcycle, to time the administration of hCG.

Follicles are measured in at least two of their greatest dimensions to obtain an average size. The follicle should be larger than 15 mm, preferably 18 to 20 mm, before hCG is administered to optimize ovulation.[81,102] When hCG was given at a mean follicular diameter of 18 mm, 92% of the cycles were ovulatory and 67% of patients conceived within six ovulatory treatment cycles.[102] Five of the 7 patients who did not conceive were found to have endometriosis at laparoscopy.[102] It is difficult to predict when ovulation will occur; follicles can grow at variable rates, 1 to 3 mm per day. Sonographic signs of imminent ovulation, however, include a line of decreased reflectivity around the follicle in a crenation pattern within the follicle.[107] These findings are helpful when planning artificial insemination or in vitro fertilization.

Clomiphene citrate or menotropins may create ovarian hyperstimulation, which in turn can lead to ovarian torsion, electrolyte imbalance, ascites, and multiple pregnancy. Ovarian enlargement to greater than 5 cm is considered mild hyperstimulation; ultrasonography is used to screen patients who are at risk for this syndrome (Fig. 24-36). When ovaries grow to large sizes with multiple mature follicles, hCG may be withheld to avoid ovulation, thereby minimizing the risk of multiple pregnancy or worsening hyperstimulation syndrome.[79,80,108]

Some patients undergoing ovulation induction remain unsuccessful in becoming pregnant. Ovulation can be confirmed sonographically by acute deflation of the follicle with spillage of the follicular fluid into the cul-de-sac. Free fluid in the cul-de-sac with marked diminution of the follicular size indicates ovulation. When this does not take place, luteinizing of the unruptured follicle occurs. The follicle becomes hazy and filled with echoes; however, it does not decrease in size and no free fluid appears in the cul-de-sac.[28] Investigators have used intraovarian Doppler studies in an attempt to differentiate between ovulatory and anovulatory cycles. After follicular rupture, the intraovarian Doppler flow velocity waveform shows a turbulent flow with a lower resistance index compared with values obtained during the follicular phase of the dominant ovary. In cycles where ovulation did not occur, there was no luteal conversion of the Doppler waveform and the velocity values were similar throughout the cycle.[88] The lack of ovulation can be secondary to the empty follicle syndrome, where no detectable ova is found within the follicle. Transvaginal scanning identified the cumulus oophorus within a dominant ovarian follicle in 152 patients with unmedicated menstrual cycles who were studied because of infertility. Empty follicles were identified in 43% of these patients, which suggests that this is a significant etiologic factor in infertility and can be detected with transvaginal ultrasonography.[57]

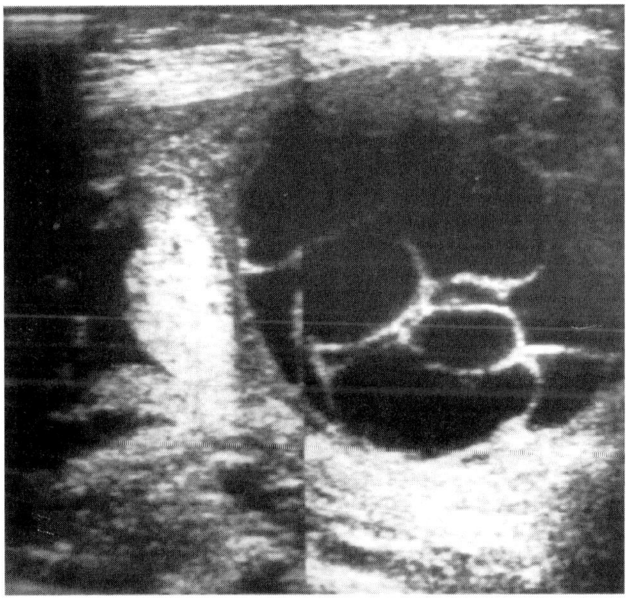

Fig. 24-36. Composite image of an enlarged, hyperstimulated ovary showing multiple, large cysts. The ovary measured 12 cm. Adjacent to this ovary is an early pregnancy (the echogenic placenta is identified next to the ovary) in a patient who underwent ovulation induction for this pregnancy.

Ultrasonography has been used extensively in IVF programs, not only for determining the time when oocyte retrieval should be undertaken, but also as a means of retrieving the oocytes. Outpatient in vitro fertilization using transvaginal ultrasound-guided oocyte retrieval has excellent results. For example, in 61 patients who had oocyte retrievals performed with ultrasound guided transvaginal aspiration of ovarian follicles, 10 patients conceived.[123]

An additional use of sonography to evaluate the infertile patient has been the determination of the fallopian tube patency by injecting fluid into the uterus transcervically and identifying the fluid collecting in the cul-de-sac (Fig. 24-37).[111] Although this technique was useful in the past and avoids x-ray exposure, it is inferior to hysterosalpingography for evaluating the shape of the intrauterine cavity and tubes. Furthermore the patency of both tubes or one tube only will have the same sonographic appearance, since only one tube needs be patent in order for fluid to reach the cul-de-sac.

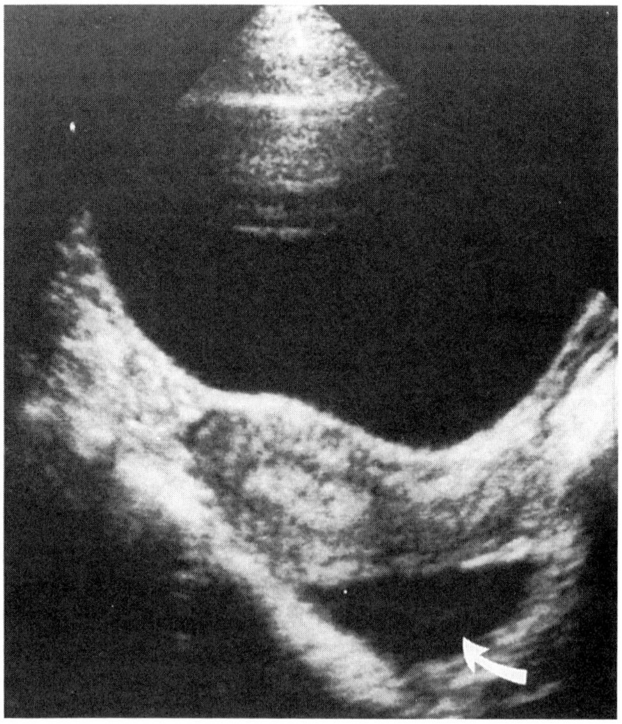

Fig. 24-37. Longitudinal view of the pelvis in a patient with a moderate amount of free fluid in the cul-de-sac (arrow).

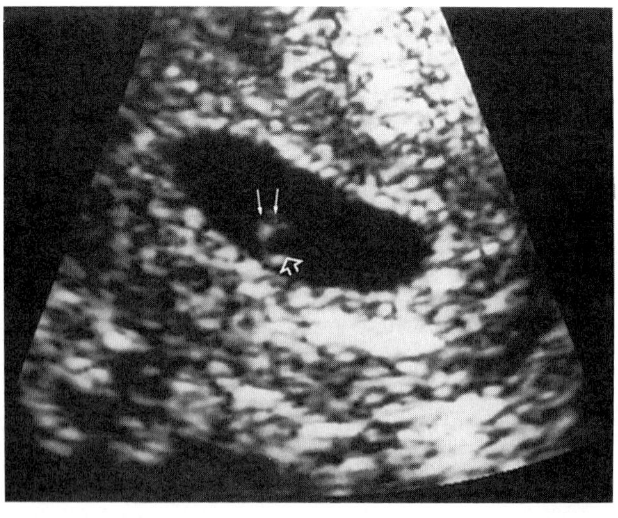

Fig. 24-38. Transvaginal view of a 6-week intrauterine pregnancy. In this magnified image, the yolk sac is indicated by the open arrow and the crown-rump length of the embryo (3mm) is indicated by the two small arrows.

In summary, sonography has permitted dramatic advances in the treatment of infertility. The ability to visualize follicles in different phases of maturation makes it possible to treat problems of ovulation dysfunction and retrieve mature follicles for in vitro procedures without laparoscopy. Sonography also identifies other explanations for the lack of fertility, such as endometriosis, hydrosalpinx, fibroids, etc.

EARLY PREGNANCY

One of the most frequent indications for pelvic sonography is the evaluation of early pregnancy. A gestational sac can be identified by the fifth week of amenorrhea and the embryo by 6 weeks (Fig. 24-38). Cardiac motion should be visible at the time the fetal pole appears. In the past, repeated scanning was necessary to determine a viable from non-viable gestational sac prior to seven weeks since the fetal pole and heartbeat could not normally be visualized. Although a good trophoblastic reaction was encouraging and a sac 2 to 2.5 cm in diameter without a fetal pole was a poor prognostic sign, follow-up scans were often necessary to reliably diagnose a blighted ovum.[12,97] More recently, transvaginal scanning has made the sonographic evaluation of early pregnancy more efficient, by providing better resolution and permitting more reliable and better criteria for the diagnosis of a non-viable pregnancy (Fig. 24-37). Levi et al studied 62 patients and demonstrated that when gestational sacs were 8 mm or larger, the absence of a yoke sac predicted a non-viable pregnancy with a sensitivity of 67% and a specificity of 100%. When gestational sacs were larger than 16 mm, the absence of an embryo predicted a non-viable pregnancy with a sensitivity of 50% and a specificity of 100%. If no cardiac activity could be identified, the sensitivity and specificity for this latter group was 100%.[74] Transvaginal sonography is superior to transabdominal scanning for the evaluation of early pregnancy. The diagnoses (living embryos, missed abortions, blighted ovums, etc.) were correctly predicted in 32 patients who had inconclusive transabdominal sonograms; the transvaginal images were clearer with better resolution, which provided diagnoses with more confidence than their transabdominal counterparts.[106]

Bleeding is the most common indication for pelvic sonography in early pregnancy. Besides determining the viability of the pregnancy, other abnormalities to look for include a blighted twin or a subchorionic collection (Fig. 24-39).[34,44] It is often difficult to tell these two abnormalities apart, since in both cases an echolucent fluid collection will be present adjacent to the gestational sac, which indicates some bleeding. To diagnose a blighted twin the fluid collection adjacent to the viable gestational sac must be sac-like and rounded, since many crescentic fluid collections partly surrounding gestational sacs have been mistaken for blighted twins and actually represent subchorionic bleeding. The diagnosis of a blighted twin carries a good prognosis for carrying the singleton to term. Goldstein et al reported a positive outcome of 80% associated with the presence of subchorionic bleeding.[44] Sonographic follow-up is helpful in these cases. When a viable pregnancy is established by visualizing a fetal pole with a heartbeat, studies have shown that the risk of spontaneous abortion before 20 weeks is 2%.[23]

Sonologists are frequently asked to rule out an ectopic pregnancy. A sonogram, however, cannot be properly interpreted without the results of the β-hCG, since a negative β-hCG essentially rules out any pregnancy. When the pregnancy test is positive, sonography can establish the presence of an intrauterine pregnancy. The mere presence of an intrauterine fluid collection does not necessarily establish the pregnancy, since as many as 20% of ectopic pregnancies can be associated with irregular intrauterine fluid collections such as blood or debris that mimick a gestational sac.[10,78,93] It is often not practical to wait for the appearance of the fetal pole to be sure that the pregnancy is in the uterus. The "double decidual sac sign" is one of the most important criteria for the presence of an intrauterine pregnancy. The double sac consists of two concentric rings partway around the fluid collection; one represents the decidua parietalis or decidua vera, and the other represents the decidua capsularis. This enables the sonologist to discriminate between the actual gestational sac and the uterine cavity itself, which is separate and where a pseudogestational sac would reside.[15,33,98]

When no intrauterine gestational sac can be identified and the pregnancy test is positive, other signs of ectopic pregnancy must be sought. Sometimes the actual ectopic gestation, embryo, and heartbeat will be identified and a definite diagnosis can be made (Fig. 24-40). Nonspecific findings suggesting ectopic pregnancy include an adnexal mass, a fluid collection in the cul-de-sac, or echogenic mass indicating a clot in the cul-de-sac.[18,33] Brown, et al found that 73% of patients with a positive pregnancy test and no intrauterine gestational sac had an ectopic pregnancy. An adnexal ring is also a significant indicator of ectopic pregnancy (Fig. 24-41).[18] It is possible that despite the presence of an ectopic pregnancy, the sonogram can be entirely normal, showing no evidence of adnexal mass. If the patient has a positive pregnancy test but no intrauterine pregnancy and no adnexal masses are identified, an ectopic pregnancy cannot be excluded by imaging alone.[71]

In an attempt to improve our ability to diagnose ectopic pregnancy, the discriminatory β-hCG zone was established at 6000 to 6500 mIU/mL. If the β-hCG is above this level, the absence of an intrauterine gestational sac is virtually

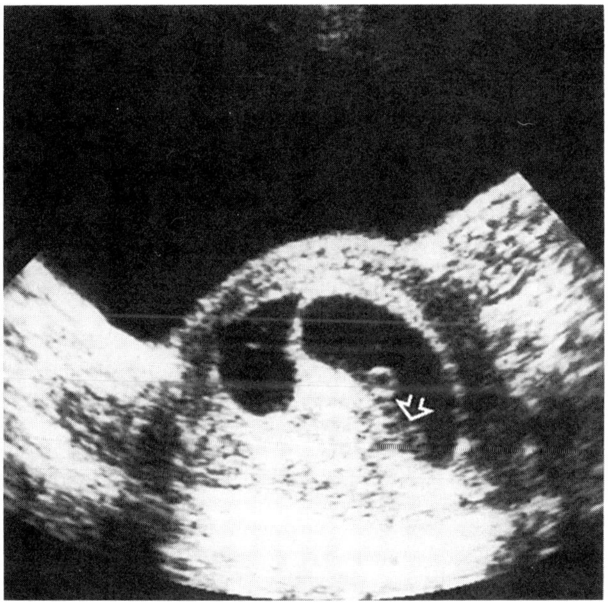

Fig. 24-39. Transverse view of the uterus, showing two different gestational sacs. The arrow indicates the live embryo, just behind the yolk sac. Note that the other gestational sac has a faintly-seen yolk sac but no embryo and represents a blighted twin.

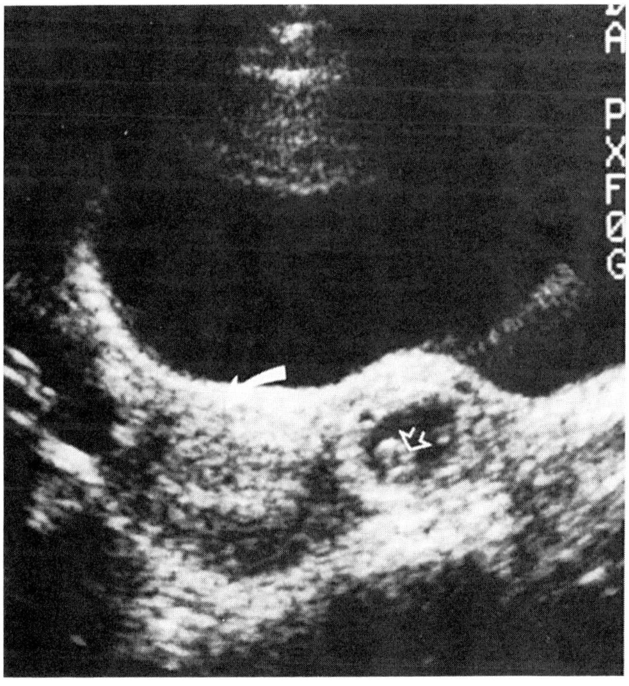

Fig. 24-40. Transverse view of the pelvis, showing an ectopic gestation (open arrow). The curved arrow indicates the empty uterus. This diagnosis was definitive, since extrauterine cardiac motion of the fetus was identified.

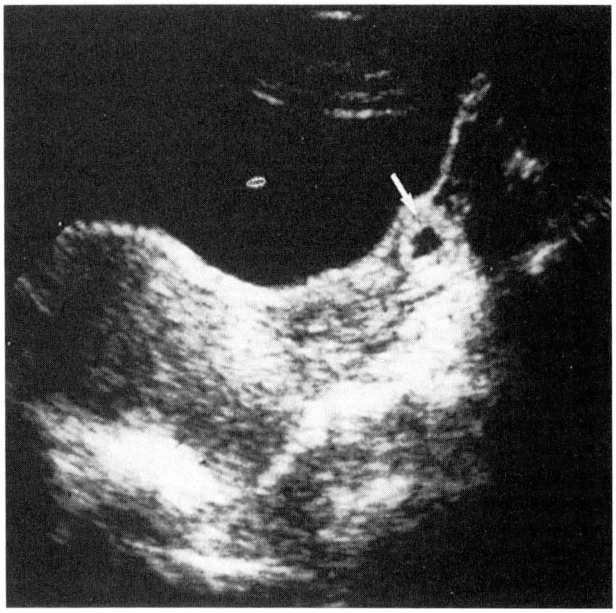

Fig. 24-41. Transverse view of the left adnexa, showing a ring sign (arrow) directly above the left ovary. This represents an ectopic pregnancy.

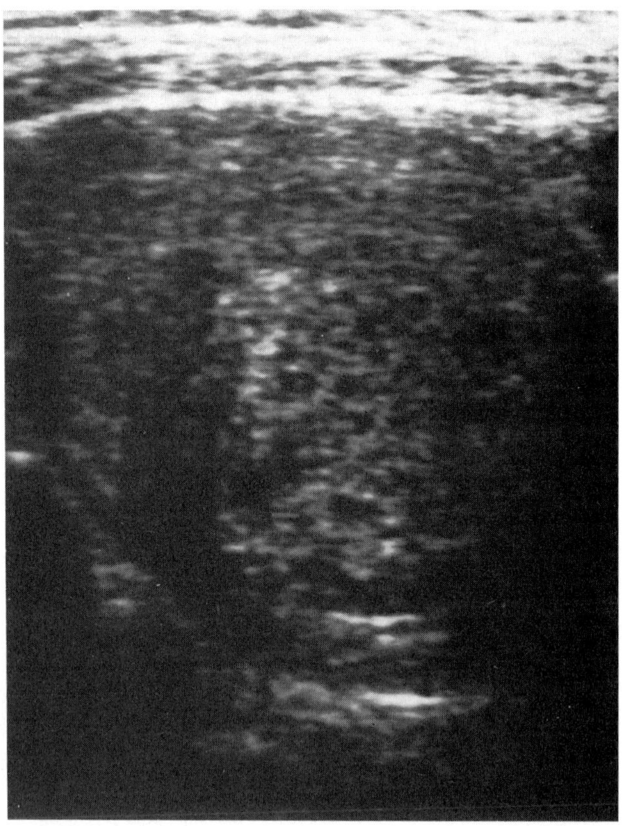

Fig. 24-42. Markedly enlarged uterus, filled with heterogeneous material containing a multitude of very tiny cystic areas. This was a complete mole.

diagnostic of an ectopic pregnancy.[62,114] Since that time, sonographic equipment capable of increased image resolution and greater operator experience have led to using a lower number (1800 mIU/mL) for establishing the presence of an intrauterine pregnancy. Nyberg et al studied 150 women, 76 of whom had intrauterine pregnancy and 55 of whom had a β-hCG exceeding 1800 mIU/mL. In each of these 55 patients, the gestational sac was identified.[96] In comparison, 35 of the 74 patients with ectopic pregnancy had β-hCGs of 1800 mIU/mL or more and had no demonstrable intrauterine gestational sac.[96] This is a more useful number in clinical practice, since ectopic pregnancies tend to have rather low β-hCG levels. With the advent of transvaginal scanning, the level of β-hCG needed to visualize the gestational sac is lower. Nyberg et al again studied 84 women with early pregnancies, comparing the transvaginal sonogram to the β-hCG level. Four of 5 (80%) of these patients with a β-hCG of 500 to 1000, and all of the 17 patients with levels above 1000 mIU/mL had sonograms demonstrating an intrauterine gestational sac. In comparison, none of the patients with ectopic pregnancy had intrauterine gestational sacs, including 17 of 26 women with ectopic pregnancy who had β-hCG levels above 1000 mIU/mL.[100] These data indicate that a gestational sac should be visualized in the uterus using transvaginal scanning when the β-hCG level exceeds 1000 mIU/mL. When the gestational sac is not seen, the patient has a high likelihood of an ectopic pregnancy. Other studies have compared transvaginal with transabdominal sonography in the evaluation of ectopic pregnancy; as expected, transvaginal scanning provided additional information in 60% of cases and less information in 4% of cases compared with transabdominal sonography.[99] It was possible to establish the presence of an extrauterine gestational sac in 10 cases and the extrauterine embryo in 2 cases not observed on transabdominal images.[99] Currently, transvaginal scanning is the standard of care in the evaluation of a possible ectopic pregnancy.

The presence of an intrauterine pregnancy is the most valuable criterion for excluding an ectopic pregnancy sonographically. A simultaneous ectopic and intrauterine pregnancy can occur; although rare (1 in 300,000 pregnancies), this possibility must not be completely forgotten.[11] With the advent of assisted ovulation, the incidence of simultaneous ectopic and intrauterine pregnancy is higher than before and this must be considered when an adnexal mass or free fluid is present in the cul-de-sac, even in the presence of an intrauterine gestational sac. Pregnancies can implant in other ectopic locations such as the cervix, which may lead to large amounts of bleeding, which may be life-threatening.[146] It is important to recognize the cervical gestational sac sonographically, to avoid excess bleeding and maternal morbidity.

Ultrasonography is the most definitive method for the diagnosis of trophoblastic disease. The complete mole has no associated fetus, and the uterus is entirely filled with a heterogeneous mass composed of tiny fluid collections in an echogenic matrix (Fig. 24-42). The uterus is often large for the date, in a patient with a disproportionately elevated β-hCG. Occasionally, fibroid tumors can masquerade as hydatidiform moles, and correlation with the β-hCG is crucial in those cases. Partial moles can have the appearance of a blighted ovum in early pregnancy but with a thickened or hydropic echogenic rim. Later in the first trimester, there may be a viable but usually abnormal fetus. This is most often associated with triploidy. The placenta tends to be large, thickened, and contain many small echolucencies.

Conclusion

Over the past few years, the resolution of sonographic equipment has vastly improved, and sonologists have acquired more experience. In addition the development of the transvaginal probe has enhanced our diagnostic capability, not only because the transducers can come closer to the pelvic organs but also because higher frequency transducers with better resolution can be used. Transvaginal sonography has been crucial in the field of infertility, enabling the IVF patients to undergo easier out-patient egg retrievals. It has also been a major factor in improving diagnostic confidence for the evaluation of early or ectopic pregnancy. Transvaginal scanning has opened a diagnostic window to the posterior cul-de-sac and increased the sensitivity and specificity for the diagnosis of pelvic masses. Furthermore, transvaginal color Doppler has added an additional dimension to the diagnosis of ovarian cancer. Not only are there morphologic criteria for ovarian masses seen sonographically but also there are now Doppler criteria for better sensitivity and specificity in the detection of ovarian malignancy. A complete gynecologic scan still requires a full bladder, however, and the transabdominal component of the scan for visualizing the upper pelvis remains an important part of the pelvic sonogram. Transvaginal sonography is necessary to further evaluate a finding on a transabdominal scan whenever an adnexal mass is encountered or to further define the endometrial stripe. Furthermore, transvaginal sonography can enable us to bypass the full bladder in certain situations, particularly in the evaluation of the emergency patient or in follow-up scans of patients who have already been evaluated transabdominally.

REFERENCES

1. Ajjimakorn S, Bhamarapravati Y: Transvaginal ultrasound and the diagnosis of fallopian tubal carcinoma, *J Clin Ultrasound* 19:116-119, 1991.
2. Andolf E, Jorgensen C: Simple adnexal cysts diagnosed by ultrasound in postmenopausal women, *J Clin Ultrasound* 16:301-303, 1988.
3. Athey PA, Butters HE: Sonographic and CT appearance of Krukenberg tumors, *J Clin Ultrasound* 12:205-210, 1984.
4. Athey PA, Cooper NB: Sonographic features of parovarian cysts, *AJR* 144:83-86, 1985.
5. Athey PA, Malone RS: Sonography of ovarian fibromas/thecomas, *J Ultrasound Med* 6:431-436, 1987.
6. Baker ME, Bowie JD, Killam AP: Sonography of post- cesarean-section bladder-flap hematoma, *AJR Am J Roentgenol* 144:757-759, 1985.
7. Baker ME, Mahony BS, Bowie JD: Adverse effect of an overdistended bladder on first-trimester sonography, *AJR Am J Roentgenol*145:597-599, 1985.
8. Baltarowich OH et al: The spectrum of sonographic findings in hemorrhagic ovarian cysts, *AJR Am J Roentgenol* 148:901-905, 1987.
9. Benacerraf BR et al: Sonographic accuracy in the diagnosis of ovarian masses, *J Reprod Med,* 35:491-495, 1991.
10. Benacerraf B, Parker-Jones K, Schiff I: Decidual cast mimicking an intrauterine gestational sac and fetal pole in a patient with ectopic pregnancy: a case report, *J Repro Med* 29(7):498-500, 1984.
11. Benacerraf BR, Rinehart JS, Schiff I: Sonographic diagnosis of simultaneous intrauterine and ectopic pregnancy, *J Ultrasound Med* 4:321-322, 1985.
12. Bernard KG, Cooperberg PL: Sonographic differentiation between blighted ovum and early viable pregnancy, *AJR Am J Roentgenol* 144:597-602, 1985.
13. Birnholz JC: Endometriosis and inflammatory disease, *Seminars in Ultrasound* 4(3):184-192, 1983.
14. Bourgouin P et al: Sonographic demonstration of post-abortion intrauterine osseous tissue, *J Ultrasound Med* 4:507-509, 1985.
15. Bradley WG, Fiske CE, Filly RA: The double sac sign of early intrauterine pregnancy: use in exclusion of ectopic pregnancy, *Radiology* 143:223-226, 1982.
16. Brandt TD et al: Endometrial echo and its significance in female infertility, *Radiology* 157:225-229, 1985.
17. Breckenridge JW et al: Postmenopausal uterine fluid collection: indicator of carcinoma, *AJR Am J Roentgenol* 139:529-534, 1982.
18. Brown TW et al: Analysis of ultrasonographic criteria in the evaluation for ectopic pregnancy, *AJRAm J Roentgenol* 131:967-971, 1978.
19. Callen PW, DeMartini WJ, Filly RA: The central uterine cavity echo: a useful anatomic sign in the ultrasonographic evaluation of the female pelvis, *Radiology* 131:187-190, 1979.
20. Callen PW, Filly RA, Munyer TP: Intrauterine contraceptive devices: evaluation by sonography, *AJR Am J Roentgenol* 135:797-800, 1980.
21. Carroll R, Gombergh R: Empty-bladder (hysterographic) view on US for evaluation of intrauterine devices, *Radiology* 163:822-823,1987.
22. Carter F et al: Transvaginal sonography as an aid in the clinical staging of carcinoma of the cervix, *J Clin Ultrasound* 20:283-287, 1992.
23. Cashner KA, Christopher CR, Dysert GA: Spontaneous fetal loss after demonstration of a live fetus in the first trimester, *Obstet Gynecol* 70:827-830, 1987.
24. Chambers CB, Unis JS: Ultrasonographic evidence of uterine malignancy in the postmenopausal uterus, *Am J Obstet Gynecol* 154:1194-1199, 1986.
25. Chervenak FA, Amin HK, Neuwirth RS: Symptomatic intrauterine retention of fetal bones, *Obstet Gynecol* 59:58S-61S, 1982.
26. Cohen L, Saggagha R: Echo patterns of benign cystic teratomas by transvaginal ultrasound, *Ultrasound Obstet Gynecol* 3:120-123, 1993.
27. Coleman BG, Arger PH, Mulhern CB, Jr: Endometriosis: clinical and ultrasonic correlation, *AJR Am J Roentgenol* 132:747-749, 1979.
28. Coulam CB, Hill LM, Breckle R: Ultrasonic evidence for luteinization of unruptured preovulatory follicles, *Fertil Steril* 37:524-529, 1982.
29. Cunat JS, Dunne MG, Butler M: Sonographic diagnosis of uterine perforation following suction curettage, *J Clin Ultrasound* 12:108-109, 1984.
30. Davis JA, Gosink BB: Fluid in the female pelvis: cyclic patterns, *J Ultrasound Med* 5:75-79, 1986.
31. el Tabbakh GH et al: Correlation of the ultrasonic appearance of the ovaries in polycystic ovarian disease and the clinical, hormonal, and laparoscopic findings, *Am J Obstet Gynecol* 154:892-895, 1986.

32. Fedele L, Bianchi S, Dorta M: Transvaginal ultrasonography versus hysteroscopy in the diagnosis of uterine submucous myomas, *Obstet Gynecol* 77:745-748, 1991.
33. Filly RA: Ectopic pregnancy: the role of sonography, *Radiology* 162:661-668, 1987.
34. Finberg HJ, Birnholz JC: Ultrasound observations in multiple gestation with first trimester bleeding: the blighted twin, *Radiology* 132:137-142, 1979.
35. Fleischer AC et al: Differential diagnosis of pelvic masses by gray scale sonography, *AJR Am J Roentgenol* 131:469-476, 1978.
36. Fleischer AC et al: Sonographic depiction of normal and abnormal endometrium with histopathologic correlation, *J Ultrasound Med* 5:445-452, 1986.
37. Fleischer AC et al: Assessment of ovarian tumor vascularity with transvaginal color Doppler sonography, *J Ultrasound Med* 10:563-568, 1991.
38. Fleischer AC et al: Transvaginal color Doppler sonography of ovarian masses with pathological correlation, *Ultrasound Obstet Gynecol* 1:275-278, 1991.
39. Fleischer AC et al: Color Doppler sonography of ovarian masses: a multiparameter analysis, *J Ultrasound Med* 12:41-48, 1993.
40. Fogel SR, Slasky BS: Sonography of Nabothian cysts, *AJR Am J Roentgenol* 138:927-930, 1982.
41. Forrest TS et al: Cyclic endometrial changes: US assessment with histologic correlation, *Radiology* 167:233-237, 1988.
42. Friedman H et al: Endometriosis detection by US with laparoscopic correlation, *Radiology* 157:217-220, 1985.
43. Gilsanz V, Cleveland RH, Reid BS: Duplication of the müllerian ducts and genitourinary malformations, *Radiology* 144:797-801, 1982.
44. Goldstein SR et al: Subchorionic bleeding in threatened abortion: sonographic findings and significance, *AJR Am J Roentgenol*141:975-978, 1983.
45. Granberg S, Norstrom A, Wikland M: Comparison of endovaginal ultrasound and cytological evaluation of cystic ovarian tumors, *J Ultrasound Med* 10:9-14, 1991.
46. Granberg S, Wikland M: Comparison between endovaginal and transabdominal transducers for measuring ovarian volume, *J Ultrasound Med* 6:649-653, 1987.
47. Granberg S et al: Endometrial thickness as measured by endovaginal ultrasonography for identifyilng endometrial abnormality, *Am J Obstet Gynecol* 164:47-52, 1991.
48. Gross BH, Silver TM, Jaffe MH: Sonographic features of uterine leiomyomas: analysis of 41 proven cases, *J Ultrasound Med* 2:401-406, 1983.
49. Grunfeld L et al: High-resolution endovaginal ultrasonography of the endometrium: a noninvasive test for endometrial adequacy, *Obstet Gynecol* 2:200-204, 1991.
50. Hall DA et al: Sonographic morphology of the normal menstrual cycle, *Radiology* 133:185-188, 1979.
51. Hall DA, McCarthy KA: The significance of the postmenopausal simple adnexal cyst, *J Ultrasound Med* 5:503-505, 1986.
52. Hall DA, McCarthy KA, Kopans DB: Sonographic visualization of the normal postmenopausal ovary, *J Ultrasound Med* 5:9-11, 1986.
53. Hamper UM et al: Transvaginal color Doppler sonography of adnexal masses: differences in blood flow impedance in benign and malignant lesions, *AJR Am J Roentgenol* 160:1225-1228, 1993.
54. Hann LE et al: In vitro ferilization: Sonographic perspective, *Radiology* 163:665-668, 1987.
55. Hann LE et al: Polycystic ovarian disease: sonographic spectrum, *Radiology* 150:531-534, 1984.
56. Herrmann UJ Jr, Locher GW, Goldhirsch A: Sonographic patterns of ovarian tumors: prediction of malignancy, *Obstet Gynecol* 69:777-781, 1987.
57. Hilgers TW et al: Assessment of the empty folicle syndrome by transvaginal sonography, *J Ultrasound Med* 11:313-316, 1992.
58. Hirsh MP, Levy HM: The varied ultrasonographic appearance of laminaria, *J Ultrasound Med* 1988; 7:45-47.
59. Innocenti P et al: Staging of cervical cancer: reliability of transrectal US, *Radiology* 185:201-205, 1992.
60. Jeffrey R. Brooke, Laing FC: Echogenic clot: a useful sign of pelvic hemoperitoneum, *Radiology* 145:139-141, 1982.
61. Johnson MA, Graham MF, Cooperberg PL: Abnormal endometrial echoes: sonographic spectrum of endometrial pathology, *J Ultrasound Med* 1:161-166, 1982.
62. Kadar N, DeVore G, Romero R: Discriminatory hCG zone: its use in the sonographic evaluation for ectopic pregnancy, *Obstet Gynecol* 58:156-161, 1981.
63. Karlsson B et al: The use of endovaginal ultrasound to diagnose invasion of endometrial carcinoma, *Ultrasound Obstet Gynecol* 2;35-39, 1992.
64. Kawai M et al: Transvaginal Doppler ultrasound with color flow imaging in the diagnosis of ovarian cancer, *Obstet Gynecol* 79:163-167, 1992.
65. Kurjac A, Zalud I, Alfirevic Z: Evaluation of adnexal masses with transvaginal color ultrasound, *J Ultrasound Med* 10:295-297, 1991.
66. Kurjak A et al: Transvaginal color Doppler sonography in the assessment of pelvic tumor vascularity, *Ultrasound Obstet Gynecol* 3:137-154, 1993.
67. Kurjak A et al: Transvaginal ultrasound, color flow, and Doppler waveform of the postmenopausal adnexal mass, *Obstet Gynecol* 80:917-921, 1992.
68. Kurtz AB et al: Ultrasound evaluation of the posterior pelvic compartment, *Radiology* 132:677-682, 1979.
69. Lande IM et al: Adnexal and cul-de-sac abnormalities: transvaginal sonography, *Radiology* 166:325-332, 1988.
70. Landers DV, Sweet RL: Current trends in the diagnosis and treatment of tuboovarian abscess, *Am J Obstet Gynecol* 151:1098-1110, 1985.
71. Lawson TL: Ectopic pregnancy: criteria and accuracy of ultrasonic diagnosis, *AJR Am J Roentgenol* 131:153-156, 1978.
72. Lawson TL, Albarelli JN: Diagnosis of gynecologic pelvic masses by gray scale ultrasonography: analysis of specificity and accuracy, *AJR Am J Roentgenol* 128:1003-1006, 1977.
73. Lees RF et al: Inflammatory cysts of the pelvic peritoneum, *AJR Am J Roentgenol* 131:633-636, 1978.
74. Levi CS, Lyons EA, Lindsay DJ: Early diagnosis of nonviable pregnancy with endovaginal US, *Radiology* 167:383-385, 1988.
75. Devine D et al: Simple adnexal cysts: the natural history in postmenopausal women, *Radiology* 184:653-659, 1992.
76. Lister JE et al: Ultrasound appearance of adenomyosis mimicking adenocarcinoma in a postmenopausal woman, *J Clin Ultrasound,* 16:519-521, 1988.
77. Malini S, Valdes C, Malinak LR: Sonographic diagnosis and classification of anomalies of the female genital tract, *J Ultrasound Med* 3:397-404, 1984.
78. Marks WM et al: The decidual cast of ectopic pregnancy: a confusing ultrasonographic appearance, *Radiology* 133:451-454, 1979.
79. McArdle CR, Sacks BA: Ovarian hyperstimulation syndrome, *AJR Am J Roentgenol* 135:835-836, 1980.
80. McArdle CR et al: Induction of ovulation monitored by ultrasound, *Radiology* 148:809-812, 1983.
81. McArdle C et al: The diagnosis of ovarian hyperstimulation (OHS): the impact of ultrasound, *Fertil Steril* 39:464-467, 1983.
82. McArdle CR, Simon L, Kiejna C: Vaginal drainage of posthysterectomy abscess under direct ultrasonic guidance, *Obstet Gynecol* 63:90S-92S, 1984.
83. McCarthy KA et al: Postmenopausal endometrial fluid collections: always an indicator of malignancy? *J Ultrasound Med* 5:647-649, 1986.
84. McCarthy S, Taylor KJW: Sonography of vaginal masses, *AJR Am J Roentgenol* 140:1005-1008, 1983.

85. Mendelson EB et al: Endometrial abnormalities: evaluation with transvaginal sonography, *AJR Am J Roentgenol* 150:139-142, 1988.
86. Mendelson EB et al: Gynecologic imaging: comparison of transabdominal and transvaginal sonography, *Radiology* 166:321-324, 1988.
87. Mendelson EB et al: The role of imaging in infertility management, *AJR Am J Roentgenol* 144:415-420, 1985.
88. Merce LT et al: Intraovarian Doppler velocimetry in ovulatory, dysovulatory and anovulatory cycles, *Ultrasound Obstet Gynecol* 2:197-202, 1992.
89. Meyer JS et al: Ultrasound presentation of primary carcinoma of the fallopian tube, *J Clin Ultrasound* 15:132-134, 1987.
90. Moyle JW et al: Sonography of ovarian tumors: predictability of tumor type, *AJR Am J Roentgenol* 141:985-991,1983.
91. Narayan R, Goswamy RK: Transvaginal sonography of the uterine cavity with hysteroscopic correlation in the investigation of infertility, *Ultrasound Obstet Gynecol* 3:129-133, 1993.
92. Nasri MN et al: Sonographic depiction of postmenopausal endometrium with transabdominal and transvaginal scanning, *Ultrasound Obstet Gynecol* 1:279-283, 1991.
93. Nelson P, Bowie JD, Rosenberg ER: Early intrauterine pregnancy or decidual cast: an anatomic-sonographic approach, *J Ultrasound Med* 2:543-547, 1983.
94. Nocera RM, Fagan CJ, Hernandez JC: Cystic parametrial fibroids mimicking ovarian cystadenoma, *J Ultrasound Med* 3:183-187, 1984.
95. Nosher JL, Winchman HK, Needell GS: Transvaginal pelvic abscess drainage with US guidance, *Radiology* 165:872-873, 1987.
96. Nyberg DA et al: Ectopic pregnancy: diagnosis by sonography correlated with quantitative hCG levels, *J Ultrasound Med* 6:145-150, 1987.
97. Nyberg DA, Laing FC, Filly RA: Threatened abortion: sonographic distinction of normal and abnormal gestation sacs, *Radiology* 158:397-400, 1986.
98. Nyberg DA et al: Ultrasonographic differentiation of the gestational sac of early intrauterine pregnancy from the pseudogestational sac of ectopic pregnancy, *Radiology* 146:755-759, 1983.
99. Nyberg DA et al: Endovaginal sonographic evaluation of ectopic pregnancy: a prospective study, *AJR Am J Roentgenol* 149:1181-1186, 1987.
100. Nyberg DA et al: Early pregnancy complications: endovaginal sonographic findings correlated with human chorionic gonadotropin levels, *Radiology* 167:619-622,1988.
101. O'Brien WF, Buck DR, Nash JD: Evaluation of sonography in the initial assessment of the gynecologic patient, *Am J Obstet Gynecol* 149:598-602, 1984.
102. O'Herlihy C, Pepperell RJ, Robinson HP: Ultrasound timing of human chorionic gonadotropin administration in clomiphene-stimulated cycles, *Obstet Gynecol* 59:40-45, 1982.
103. Pache TD et al: How to discriminate between normal and polycystic ovaries: transvaginal US study, *Radiology* 183:421-423, 1992.
104. Paling MR, Shawker TH: Abdominal ultrasound in advanced ovarian carcinoma, *J Clin Ultrasound* 9:435-441, 1981.
105. Pellerito JS et al: Diagnosis of uterine anomalies: relative accuracy of MR imaging, endovaginal sonography, and hysterosalpingography, *Radiology* 183:795-800, 1992.
106. Pennell RG et al: Complicated first-trimester pregnancies: evaluation with endovaginal US versus transabdominal technique, *Radiology* 165:79-83, 1987.
107. Picker RH et al: Ultrasonic signs of imminent ovulation, *J Clin Ultrasound* 11:1-2, 1983.
108. Rankin RN, Hutton LC: Ultrasound in the ovarian hyperstimulation syndrome, *J Clin Ultrasound* 9:473-476, 1981.
109. Requard CK, Mettler FA Jr, Wicks JD: Preoperative sonography of malignant ovarian neoplasms, *AJR Am J Roentgenol* 137:79-82, 1981.
110. Reynolds T, Hill MC, Glassman LM: Sonography of hemorrhagic ovarian cysts, *J Clin Ultrasound* 14:449-453, 1986.
111. Richman TS et al: Fallopian tubal patency assessed by ultrasound following fluid injection, *Radiology* 152:507-510, 1984.
112. Rifkin MD et al: Sonography of nongynecologic cystic masses of the pelvis, *AJR Am J Roentgenol* 142:1169-1174, 1984.
113. Ritchie WGM: Sonographic evaluation of normal and induced ovulation, *Radiology* 161:1-10, 1986.
114. Romero R et al: Diagnosis of ectopic pregnancy: value of the discriminatory human chorionic gonadotropin zone, *Obstet Gynecol* 66:357-360, 1985.
115. Rosenberg HK et al: Mayer-Rokitansky-Kuster-Hauser syndrome: US aid to diagnosis, *Radiology* 161:815-819, 1986.
116. Rosenblatt R et al: Uterine perforation and embedding by intrauterine device: evaluation by US and hysterography, *Radiology* 157:765-770, 1985.
117. Rulin MC, Preston AL: Adnexal masses in postmenopausal women, *Obstet Gynecol* 70:578-581, 1987.
118. Sample WF, Lippe BM, Gyepes MT: Gray-scale ultrasonography of the normal female pelvis, *Radiology* 125:477-483, 1977.
119. Sandler MA, Karo JJ: The spectrum of ultrasonic findings in endometriosis, *Radiology* 127:229-231, 1978.
120. Sandler MA, Silver TM, Karo JJ: Gray-scale ultrasonic features of ovarian teratomas, *Radiology* 131:705-709, 1979.
121. Schaffer RM et al: Nonobstructive hydrocolpos: sonographic appearance and differential diagnosis, *Radiology* 149:273-278, 1983.
122. Schneider VL et al: Comparison of Doppler with two-dimensional sonography and CA 125 for prediction of malignancy of pelvic masses, *Obstet Gynecol* 81:983-988, 1993.
123. Schulman JD et al: Outpatient in vitro fertilization using transvaginal ultrasound-guided oocyte retrieval, *Obstet Gynecol* 69:665-668, 1987.
124. Schwimer SR, Marik J, Lebovic J: Percutaneous ovarian cyst aspiration using continuous transvaginal ultrasonographic monitoring, *J Ultrasound Med* 4:259-260, 1985.
125. Scott WW et al: The obstructed uterus, *Radiology* 141:767-770, 1981.
126. Shalan H, Sosic A, Kurjak A: Fallopian tube carcinoma: recent diagnostic approach by color Doppler imaging, *Ultrasound Obstet Gynecol* 2:297-299, 1992.
127. Shawker TH et al: Ultrasonography of Turner's syndrome, *J Ultrasound Med* 5:125-129, 1986.
128. Shenker L, Brickman FE: Bicornuate uterus with incomplete vaginal septum and unilateral renal agenesis, *Radiology* 133:455-457, 1979.
129. Sheth S, Hamper UM, Kurman RJ: Thickened endometrium in the postmenopausal woman: sonographic-pathologic correlation, *Radiology* 187:135-139, 1993.
130. Siedler D et al: Uterine adenomyosis: a difficult sonographic diagnosis, *J Ultrasound Med* 6:345-349, 1987.
131. Subramanyam BR et al: Ultrasonic features of fallopian tube carcinoma, *J Ultrasound Med* 3:391-393, 1984.
132. Syrop CH, Sahakian V: Transvaginal sonographic detection of endometrial polyps with fluid contrast augmentation, *Obstet Gynecol* 79:1041-1043, 1992.
133. Taylor KJW et al: Accuracy of grey-scale ultrasound diagnosis of abdominal and pelvic abscesses in 220 patients, *Lancet* 1:83, 1978.
134. Tekay A, Jouppila P: Validity of pulsatility and resistance indices in classification of adnexal tumors with transvaginal color Doppler ultrasound, *Ultrasound Obstet Gynecol* 2:338-344, 1992.
135. Thickman D et al: Sonographic assessment of the endometrium in patients undergoing in vitro fertilization, *J Ultrasound Med* 5:197-201, 1986.
136. Timor-Tritsch IE, Rottem Shraga: Transvaginal ultrasonographic study of the fallopian tube, *Obstet Gynecol* 70:424-428, 1987.
137. Timor-Tritsch IE et al: Transvaginal ultrasonographic characterization of ovarian masses by means of color flow-directed Doppler measurements and a morphologic scoring system, *Am J Obstet Gynecol* 168:909-913, 1993.
138. Varner RE et al: Transvaginal sonography of the endometrium in postmenopausal women, *Obstet Gynecol* 78:195-199, 1991.

139. Vilaro MM et al: Endovaginal ultrasound: a technique for evaluation of nonfollicular pelvic masses, *J Ultrasound Med* 6:697-701, 1987.
140. Wade RV et al: Reliability of gynecologic sonographic diagnosis, 1978-1984, *Am J Obstet Gynecol* 153:186-190, 1985.
141. Walsh JW et al: Prospective comparison of ultrasound and computed tomography in the evaluation of gynecologic pelvic masses, *AJR Am J Roentgenol* 131:955-960, 1978.
142. Walsh JW, Taylor KJW, Rosenfield AT: Gray scale ultrasonography in the diagnosis of endometriosis and adenomyosis, *AJR Am J Roentgenol* 132:87-90, 1979.
143. Walsh JW et al: Gray-scale ultrasound in 204 proved gynecologic masses: accuracy and specific diagnostic criteria, *Radiology* 130:391-397, 1979.
144. Walzer A, Flynn E, Koenigsberg M: Sonographic appearance of a prolapsing submucous leiomyoma, *J Clin Ultrasound* 11:101-102, 1983.
145. Weiner Z et al: Differentiating malignant from benign ovarian tumors with transvaginal color flow imaging, *Obstet Gynecol* 79:159-162, 1992.
146. Werber J, Prasadarao PR, Harris VJ: Cervical pregnancy diagnosed by ultrasound, *Radiology* 149:279-280, 1983.
147. Wiener MD et al: Sonography of subfascial hematoma after cesarean delivery, *AJR Am J Roentgenol* 148:907-910, 1987.
148. Willard DA: Pelvic varices: sonographic and surgical recognition, *J Clin Ultrasound* 16:265-267, 1988.
149. Wilson DA, Stacy TM, Smith EI: Ultrasound diagnosis of hydrocolpos and hydrometrocolpos, *Radiology* 128:451-454, 1978.
150. Winsett MZ, Fagan CJ, Bedi DG: Sonographic demonstration of bladder-flap hematoma, *J Ultrasound Med* 5:483-487, 1986.
151. Worthen NJ, Gunning JE: Percutaneous drainage of pelvic abscesses: management of the tubo-ovarian abscess, *J Ultrasound Med* 5:551-556, 1986.
152. Yeh HC, Futterweit W, Thornton JC: Polycystic ovarian disease: US features in 104 patients, *Radiology* 163:111-116,1987.

Chapter 25

LAPAROSCOPY, HYSTEROSCOPY, AND LASER SURGERY

Andrew J. Friedman
Marc R. Laufer

LAPAROSCOPY

Laparoscopy (also referred to as peritoneoscopy or pelviscopy) is a procedure that enables the surgeon to visualize or operate on pelvic and abdominal organs endoscopically. This is one of the most frequently performed surgical procedures and has become an essential tool in the diagnosis and treatment of numerous gynecologic conditions. The development of operative laparoscopic equipment and techniques has enabled the pelvic and reproductive surgeon to conduct a wide variety of extensive procedures, previously performed via laparotomy, on an outpatient basis. Laparoscopy results in greater satisfaction among both patients and physicians because of decreased morbidity, mortality, recuperative time, and cost.

History

The first recorded endoscopic procedure was performed in 1805 by Bozzini, who attempted to visualize the urethral mucosa using a simple square-windowed tube and candlelight directed by a concave mirror.[22] Bozzini met with disapproval and was censured by the Medical Faculty of Vienna for "undue curiosity." The first recorded human laparoscopy was undertaken by Jacobaeus of Sweden in 1910.[80] He created a pneumoperitoneum by using a trocar and a cannula and was able to visualize the pelvis with a Nitze cystoscope through the same cannula.

In 1911 Berheim reported on peritoneal cystoscopy performed for the first time in the United States.[173] Ruddock in 1937 reported on 500 laparoscopic cases with a mortality of 0.2% and utilized electrocautery with biopsy forceps.[173] In 1944 Decker introduced a pneumoperitoneum by creating negative intraabdominal pressure with the knee-chest position.[173] "Gaseous distention" of the abdomen was first reported by Palmer in 1946. In 1947 fiberoptics were introduced by Hopkins and Kampany of England.[80] Laparoscopic sterilization by unipolar electrocoagulation was first reported in 1962 by Palmer. Since the early 1970s, numerous advances in equipment and technique have expanded the role of laparoscopy from primarily a diagnostic procedure to one with numerous operative applications.

Equipment

The basic equipment needed for laparoscopy includes a Verres needle (if elected), a primary trocar and cannula, a laparoscope (Fig. 25-1), an insufflator (if elected), a light source, and a camera with a monitor setup. The use of the latter has made it possible to perform more extensive surgeries through the laparoscope. With the use of camera equipment, the surgical assistant can also visualize the procedure and thus can provide the primary surgeon with better support. Some surgeons may choose to use a video cassette recorder for the purpose of documentation or the creation of educational materials.

Laparoscopes range from 1.6 to 13 mm in diameter. The smaller-caliber laparoscopes are adequate for diagnosis and some of the newer small-diameter laparoscopes have optics comparable with that of the larger instruments. Many surgeons prefer larger-diameter (8 to 13 mm) laparoscopes for operative laparoscopy. These larger instruments may have twin-fiber bundles for better illumination, visualization, and

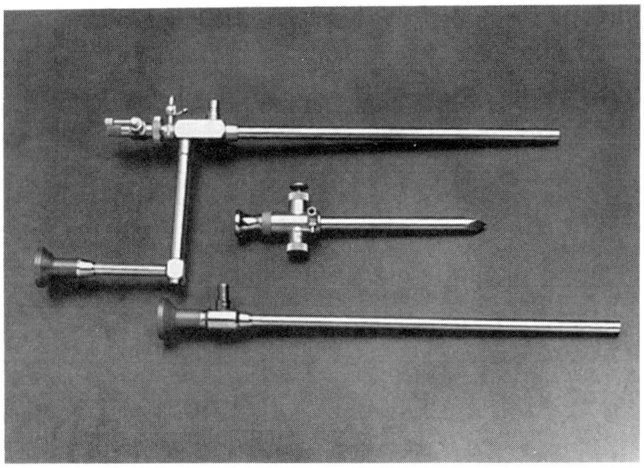

Fig. 25-1. Operative laparoscope, primary trocar, and diagnostic laparoscope. (Courtesy Edward Weck, Princeton, NJ).

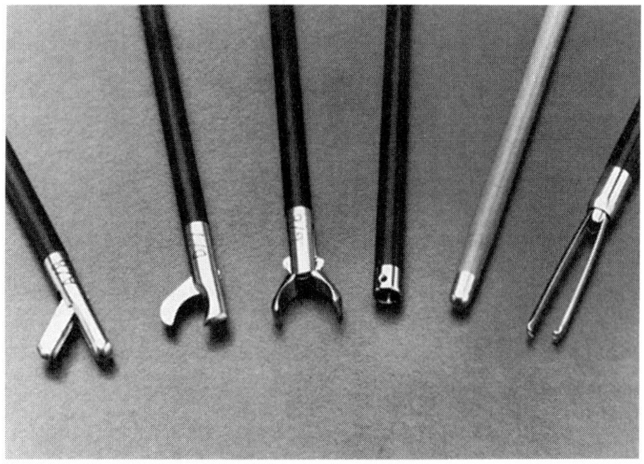

Fig. 25-2. Ancillary laparoscopic instruments including *(from left to right)* punch biopsy forceps, hook scissors, atraumatic grasping forceps, suction-irrigation probe, unipolar cautery probe, traumatic forceps. (Courtesy Edward Weck, Princeton, NJ).

(often) photodocumentation; laparoscopes may also have an operative channel for laser, mechanical, or electrocautery instruments. Larger laparoscopes require primary trocars that have wider tips and need more force than smaller trocars to penetrate the abdomen. Consequently, both the depth of penetration and the risk of visceral injury are increased.[80] To decrease the risk of visceral damage from trocar insertion, disposable trocars with "safety shields" have been designed and marketed. The smaller laparoscopes offer advantages in pediatric and adolescent patients as these instruments weigh less.

Different rates of insufflation of carbon dioxide (CO_2) gas may be used to create the pneumoperitoneum. Most surgeons insufflate CO_2 at 1 L/minute until the pneumoperitoneum is adequate. Laparoscopy units equipped with "high" or "fast-flow" modes are able to insufflate (CO_2) at 3 to 9 L/minute. This rapid insufflation rate is helpful in maintaining an adequate pneumoperitoneum in operative laparoscopic cases where instruments are changed frequently and in cases where the laser plume may be evacuated at intervals. At a given flow rate insufflators may deliver CO_2 by either a pressure-dependent or a pressure-independent mode. The "manual" insufflation mode is pressure independent, maintains a constant flow rate, and is used for establishment of the pneumoperitoneum. The "automatic" mode is pressure dependent, maintains a constant intraperitoneal pressure, and is used once the pneumoperitoneum is established. The higher flow rates of CO_2 are used once the surgeon is sure that the Verres needle is in the peritoneal cavity. The use of an insufflation device (e.g., a Verres needle) has come under scrutiny because complication rates are lower and operative times shorter with direct insertion of the trocar and without the use of a Verres needle for insufflation.[30]

New techniques have been developed for the use of gasless laparoscopy. No insufflation is needed, and the abdominal wall is mechanically elevated (Laparofan, Origin Medsystems, Inc., Menlo Park, CA). This method may be ideal for cases in which increased intraabdominal pressure may compromise the patient (e.g., in the case of severe cardiac or pulmonary disease). In addition to eliminating the need for increased intraabdominal pressure, this method also makes the use of local or regional anesthetic feasible.

The light source in laparoscopy is a fiberoptic cable that transmits intense light from the external source through the laparoscope into the peritoneal cavity. The brightness of the light is a function of both the power of the external source and the diameter of the cable that contains the fiber bundles. Twin fiber bundles produce maximal illumination facilitating photodocumentation and/or video recording. The light source from the cable generates a great deal of heat; if the cable is not attached to the laparoscope, precautions must be taken to prevent the light beam from setting the surgical drapes on fire.

Antifog solutions that increase visibility through the laparoscope are available. Laparoscope warmers are helpful in avoiding fogging of the lens.

Secondary, tertiary, or quaternary puncture sites are often utilized for diagnostic or operative laparoscopy. Each additional site requires a separate trocar and cannula sleeve. Ancillary instruments can then be used at these additional sites for the stabilization and surgical manipulation of pelvic and abdominal structures (Fig. 25-2). These additional parts are available as reusable, disposable, or combination reusable/multiuse equipment.

The most commonly used ancillary instrument is a calibrated probe. The probe may be marked in centimeters and used for the measurement of internal structures that appear magnified through the laparoscopic lens. Probes may be used to stabilize or immobilize pelvic structures or to perform blunt dissection of filmy adhesions. Insulated probes with a metal tip may be used to carry unipolar current for coagulation.

Various forceps may be applied at ancillary puncture sites. Atraumatic forceps allow for delicate handling of tissue, whereas traumatic forceps may be used for stabilization of "hard" tissue that is ultimately destroyed or removed from the peritoneal cavity. Biopsy forceps may be employed to aid in diagnosis. It is important not to use electrocautery for tissue biopsy because it makes an accurate pathologic diagnosis impossible. Bipolar forceps are especially useful for sterilization procedures, coagulation of bleeding sites, and fulguration of endometriotic lesions.

Many types of scissors (i.e., hooked, serrated, "micro") may be used with or without unipolar electrocautery. Cautery should be used to divide vascular structures only when the surgeon has a clear view of the operative field and surrounding tissues so that inadvertent electrical injury to vulnerable viscera is minimized.

Aspirating cannulas come with either blunt ends or pointed "needle" tips. Blunt aspiration cannulas may be used for irrigation or aspiration. A dual-channel, combined irrigation/aspiration instrument is especially useful in the localization of bleeding sites and in "aqua-dissection." Needle-tip aspirators with beveled tips have been used for laparoscopic oocyte harvesting in in vitro fertilization (IVF) procedures; for drainage of ovarian, paraovarian, or paratubal cysts; and for the injection of saline or vasopressin (Pitressin) solutions into pelvic structures (i.e., the mesosalpinx, leiomyomas, and the uterine septa).

Most electrosurgical units contain both unipolar and bipolar modes. In unipolar electrocautery circuitry, the current passes from the generator through the instrument to a ground plate and then back to the generator. Unipolar electrocautery often causes more thermal damage than just the surface area of the distal coagulating tip of the instrument, as the heat from the tip spreads in all directions from the point of contact. In addition, electrical sparks may induce thermal injury in adjacent bowel or other tissues. For these reasons, unipolar cautery must be used with extreme care. In the bipolar system, current is passed from the generator into one insulated jaw of a pair of forceps through the grasped tissue into the second insulated forceps jaw and back to the generator. The passage of current heats and coagulates the grasped tissue in a controlled fashion.

Endocoagulation or thermocoagulation was developed by Semm in 1962.[168] In this technique, hemostasis is achieved by heating the tissue to 100°C to140°C. Endocoagulation may be used to destroy endometriotic implants or to evert serosal edges in a newly created distal salpingostomy.

Endoscopic laser technology is evolving rapidly and is providing new methods of coagulating, cutting, and vaporizing tissue. The four types of lasers used in gynecologic surgery are CO_2, argon, potassium titanyl phosphate (KTP), and neodymium-yttrium aluminum garnet (Nd:YAG or YAG). Lasers may be utilized through an operative channel in the laparoscope or through hollow ancillary instruments.

Endoscopic suturing may be used for certain advanced operative laparoscopic procedures. A Roeder loop (Ethbinder, Ethicon, Somerville, NJ) is a Semm modification of the loop developed by Roeder in the early 1900s for tonsillectomy in children.[166] The Roeder loop may be used for ligation of bleeding sites or for ligation of tissue (e.g., tube, ovary, tube and ovary, pedunculated myoma) before excision. Some new sutures are designed to have the needle placed through the material to be sutured and then through a pretied loop. This method avoids the need for intraabdominal knot tying. Extracorporeal knot tying is a time-consuming but useful method that laparoscopic surgeons can learn with practice. This method is similar to microsurgical tying techniques utilizing two needle graspers.

Stapling devices are available that deliver rows of staples and in some instances cut in between the rows. These instruments are used to ensure hemostasis while removing tissue. The staples are made of titanium and are nonmagnetic; they are considered "safe" for magnetic resonance imaging (MRI) and do not cause significant adhesion formation. Endoscopic absorbable clips of polydioxanone also achieve hemostasis while eliminating the need for time-consuming intraabdominal knotting.

Disposable and reusable instruments are available to place titanium clips. These clips can be used to attain hemostasis or to "tag" structures (e.g., to mark an ovary prior to radiation therapy). Titanium clips offer an advantage over absorbable clips in that the end of the clip does not need to latch in order to work effectively. Thus more difficult placements are possible with these clips. Hernia staples are available to grasp and pull the tissue together (e.g., to repair a fascial hernia).

Tissue may be removed from the abdomen with forceps or a macrospoon. Large or hard pieces of tissue may be morcellated by a 10-mm diameter tissue-punch instrument that stores pieces of tissue in its sheath.[167] Some surgeons make use of a colpotomy incision to remove large pieces of tissue or intact ovarian masses.

Large structures can be removed intact when placed in a plastic specimen pouch. These pouches were developed to avoid spillage of contents from a specimen as it is removed from the peritoneal cavity. Pouches are ideal for ovarian cysts that the surgeon would like to remove without intraperitoneal spillage.

For surgical procedures involving adhesions, peritoneal dissections, or bleeding, a suction/irrigation system is necessary. Suction irrigators (5 mm) with trumpet valves are available in reusable or disposable models. The irrigant should be attached to the upper port and the suction to the lower port. An irrigation pump is useful in maintaining adequate hydraulic pressure for irrigation. Various models of suction irrigators are available with either a single port for suction and irrigation or multiple ports at the end. The single- port model offers the advantage of increased hydraulic force for hydrodissection.

Indications

As experience with operative laparoscopy increases, so does the list of indications for its performance (Table 25-1). The value of laparoscopy for timely, accurate diagnosis and for therapy cannot be overemphasized. Operative laparoscopy can be used for any surgical procedure as long as basic surgical techniques and principles are adhered to and the surgeon has an understanding of the anatomy and a concern for the patient's safety. Surgeons need to be aware of their individual limitations and must know when to ask for assistance and when to convert the laparoscopic procedure into a laparotomy.

The use of operative laparoscopy for procedures that once required a laparotomy can decrease morbidity, length of hospitalization, cost, and recuperative time.

Table 25-1. Indications for laparoscopy

I. Infertility
   A. Diagnostic
      1. Unexplained etiology after thorough evaluation
      2. History of pelvic inflammatory disease (PID), pelvic surgery (including appendectomy), endometriosis
      3. Abnormal hysterosalpingogram
      4. Pelvic mass (or masses) and/or pain on examination
      5. Failure to achieve pregnancy after 6 months of "appropriate" therapy
      6. Second-look laparoscopy after extensive surgery
   B. Operative
      1. Assisted reproductive technology (ART)
      2. Reconstructive tubal surgery
         a. neosalpingostomy
         b. fimbrioplasty
         c. salpingoovariolysis
      3. Uterine suspension

II. Pelvic pain
   A. Acute: Rule out appendicitis, ruptured cyst, ectopic pregnancy, adnexal torsion, PID, etc.
   B. Chronic: Rule out endometriosis, pelvic adhesions, etc.
   C. Uterosacral ligament ablation, presacral neurectomy

III. Tubal sterilization

IV. Pelvic mass
   A. Diagnostic
   B. Operative
      1. Ectopic pregnancy
      2. Ovarian cyst
      3. Endometriosis
      4. Lysis of adhesions
      5. Myomectomy
      6. Oophorectomy, salpingectomy, adnexectomy
      7. Laparoscopic-assisted vaginal hysterectomy
   C. Foreign body retrieval

Contraindications

As experience with laparoscopy has accumulated, the list of contraindications has diminished. However, the gynecologic surgeon must be familiar with these contraindications to maximize safety and minimize procedure-related morbidity. Although all the contraindications for laparoscopy are not uniformly agreed upon, a generally accepted list appears in Table 25-2. Some authorities consider a history of pelvic or abdominal surgery or of any condition that predisposes the patient to extensive adhesions to be a contraindication to laparoscopy. These cases must be judged individually according to the experience of the surgeon and the perceived likelihood of visceral injury. Open laparoscopy may minimize the risk of perforation of a viscus or blood vessel.[84]

Anesthetic

Most authorities consider general endotracheal anesthetic ideal for laparoscopic procedures. It is safe, provides excellent analgesia and muscle relaxation, and is ideally suited for use in cases requiring prolonged surgery or extensive manipulation of pelvic or abdominal structures.

Table 25-2. Contraindications to laparoscopy

I. Contraindications to general anesthetic (e.g., severe cardiopulmonary disease)

II. Hypovolemic shock

III. Contraindications to pneumoperitoneum
   A. Severe cardiopulmonary disease
   B. Large (symptomatic) hiatal hernia

IV. Unacceptably high risk of visceral injury
   A. Severe ileus
   B. Bowel obstruction
   C. Generalized peritonitis with ileus
   D. Advanced pregnancy (>16 wks)
   E. Large (>10 cm) intraabdominal mass
   F. Extreme thinness*

V. Extreme obesity*

VI. Inexperienced surgeon

* Relative contraindications

Local anesthetic has been used successfully for laparoscopic tubal sterilization and may be reserved for the well-prepared patient undergoing a short procedure with minimal intraperitoneal manipulation of tissue.[146] With more extensive surgical procedures requiring increasing amounts of CO_2 for distention, increased intraabdominal and diaphragmatic pressure leads to increased difficulty in spontaneous respiration, making general anesthetic necessary. Local or regional anesthetic can be used more easily in "gasless" laparoscopy.

Postoperative analgesia can be provided with oral narcotics. Peritoneal lidocaine and incisional bupivacaine are safe and effective in reducing postoperative pain.[87]

Technique

After adequate anesthesia is induced, the patient is placed in the dorsal lithotomy position with the buttocks protruding slightly from the table, prepared, and draped, and the bladder is emptied. For procedures that may last longer than 1 hour the insertion of an indwelling Foley catheter is recommended; this device can be removed at the completion of the procedure. A rigid cannula (e.g., Cohen-Eder) placed in the endocervix and affixed to a single-toothed tenaculum that is applied to the anterior cervix will aid in chromopertubation and/or uterine manipulation during the procedure.

For patients in the pediatric age group and for adolescents or adults who are not sexually active, the dorsal supine position can be used, with no instruments placed in the cervix or vagina. The uterus can be manipulated with a blunt probe placed through a suprapubic second puncture site.

A small (2 to 13 mm) vertical or transverse incision is made in the midline in the umbilicus. There are numerous techniques for insertion of the trocar. We prefer to lift the anterior abdominal wall with the assistance of a sponge and with one hand on each side of the umbilicus. Because towel clips create additional punctures that result in additional scars and pain, their use on the sides of the umbilicus should be reserved for morbidly obese patients whose abdominal wall is difficult to lift without assistance. The incision should only be large enough to accommodate the laparoscope and still be occlusive. Alternative incision sites may be chosen if there is a high risk of adhesion formation in the region under the umbilicus (Fig. 25-3). An open laparoscopic technique can be used for patients who have previously undergone surgery involving the upper abdomen. The Verres needle or cannula is inserted through this incision into the abdomen at an angle of approximately 45° pointing toward the most dependent portion of the pelvis (i.e., the hollow of the sacrum) to minimize the risk of injury. The spring-loaded Verres needle ensures penetration of the abdominal wall while decreasing the risk of visceral injury. Proper placement of the needle intraperitoneally is based on the "feel" of the needle going through the peritoneum and a low opening-pressure reading from the insufflator. To ascertain that the Verres needle is in the peritoneal cavity, attach a syringe with 5 mL of saline and observe the free flow of the saline into the abdomen; minimal force should be used.

Insufflation of 2 to 4 L of CO_2 is usually adequate to create a pneumoperitoneum before the trocar insertion. It is important to base adequate insufflation on the amount of abdominal distention rather than on the exact amount of CO_2 insufflated, especially in cases involving children and thin adolescents.

The "opening pressure" at the start of insufflation should be appropriate for the insufflator being used. Higher pressures may indicate extraperitoneal Verres needle placement or partial occlusion of the distal tip of the needle by an intraabdominal structure. During insufflation, intraperitoneal Verres needle placement can be confirmed by documentation of the loss of percussed liver dullness after 1 L has been insufflated. For very thin patients the Verres needle must not be inserted too far, because of potential visceral damage or omental insufflation.

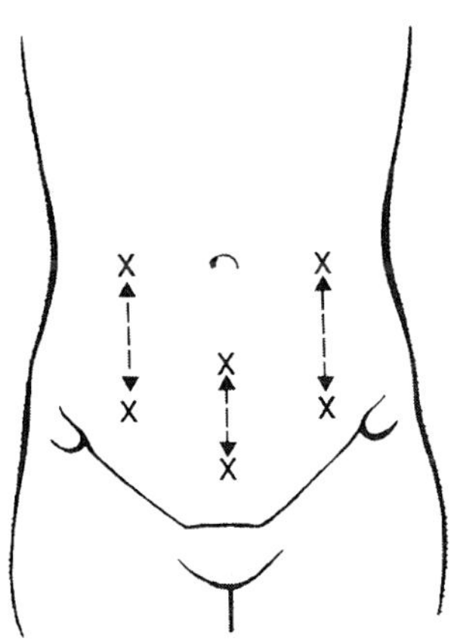

Fig. 25-3. Possible incision sites for the Verres needle.

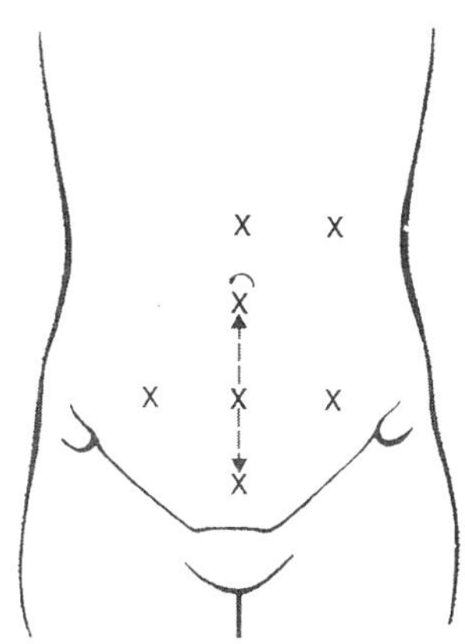

Fig. 25-4. Possible incision sites for ancillary laparoscopic instruments.

Once insufflation is complete, the Verres needle is withdrawn and the laparoscopic trocar and its sheath are introduced into the peritoneal cavity through the same umbilical incision with a twisting motion and with the trocar aimed toward the hollow of the sacrum. The trocar is then removed, the laparoscope is placed into its sheath, and the light cable and insufflation tubing are connected to the laparoscope and its sheath respectively. At this point the surgeon will be able to observe directly whether the laparoscope is in the peritoneal cavity.

The camera equipment is adjusted so that everyone in the operating room can visualize the procedure and give appropriate assistance. It is helpful to dim the overhead lights in the room and to use the surgical lights for the anesthesiologist and the surgical technician.

One or more ancillary punctures may be made if necessary, through separate incisions (Fig. 25-4). Transillumination of the abdominal wall with the distal tip of the laparoscope may localize large vessels before the selection of an ancillary puncture site. When choosing lateral ancillary trocar sites, the surgeon must be familiar with the anatomy of the inferior epigastric vessels to avoid vascular injury. Intraperitoneal visualization can help locate the inferior epigastric vessels that need to be avoided. Hypotensive collapse following trauma to the inferior epigastric artery has been reported.[153] Secondary trocars and cannulas must be inserted under direct laparoscopic visualization to avoid intraperitoneal injury.

If the inferior epigastric vessel is lacerated during the insertion of a secondary port, hemostasis can be attained by multiple means. It is sometimes possible to use bipolar cautery to internally cauterize the bleeding site. A Foley catheter with a 30-cc balloon can be placed through the trocar site and inflated, and the trocar can then be removed. A Kelly clamp can be placed at the level of the skin to hold the Foley balloon tightly against the puncture site. This Foley catheter should be left in place overnight and deflated the next day, with the subsequent discharge of the patient.

Diagnostic laparoscopy

For diagnostic laparoscopic procedures, an orderly and organized survey of the pelvic anatomy will minimize the possibility of missing a subtle but significant finding. Although it is tempting to abandon this organized approach in cases with obvious pelvic pathologic findings, the importance of a disciplined inspection of the pelvis cannot be overstated.

Infertility. A major use of diagnostic laparoscopy is in the evaluation of infertility. Indications for laparoscopy in this setting include (1) abnormal tubal anatomy on a hysterosalpingogram, (2) infertility whose etiology is not apparent after a thorough evaluation (i.e., assessment of ovulation, semen analysis, postcoital testing, and hysterosalpingography), (3) failure to conceive after 6 months of "appropriate" infertility therapy, (4) a history of PID, (5) a history of abdominal or pelvic surgery, and (6) the presence of a pelvic mass. In general, laparoscopy should be the final procedure performed in the basic infertility workup as it is the most invasive.

In several series of cases of diagnostic laparoscopy for primary infertility, no pathology was found in up to 52% of patients, endometriosis was found in 22% to 39%, and tubal or peritoneal factors were found in 9% to 27%.[133] In laparoscopies performed on women with secondary infertility, no pathology was found in 42% to 65%, endometriosis was found in 10% to 25%, and tubal or peritoneal factors were found in 10% to 42%.[133] Several studies of women with infertility and no apparent etiology after a thorough evaluation have documented abnormal pelvic findings in 44% to 75% of those undergoing laparoscopy.[56,58,72,133,144,192] These results underscore the principle that laparoscopy is essential to the complete evaluation of the infertile woman.

It has been suggested that laparoscopy with laser therapy may be superior to laparotomy for the treatment of endometriosis in the infertile patient.[69]

The positive correlation of hysterosalpingographic and laparoscopic findings has ranged from 46% to 84% in various studies.[38,56,68,78,88,133,171] The majority of misdiagnoses were of cornual or proximal tubal occlusion seen on hysterosalpingography, but not found on laparoscopy. Despite the relatively high rate of inaccurate assessment of tubal status by radiographic methods, diagnostic laparoscopy is recommended shortly after hysterosalpingography when findings are abnormal.

Pelvic pain. Laparoscopy is a useful diagnostic tool in the evaluation of pelvic pain. The causes of pelvic pain are numerous, and laparoscopy may clarify the diagnosis. One example is the diagnosis of PID. The presumed clinical diagnosis of PID has been found to be inaccurate with only 65% of the cases confirmed by laparoscopy.[129] In a series of 100 women with chronic pelvic pain who underwent laparoscopy, 83% had associated pelvic pathology; the most frequent findings were pelvic adhesions (38%) and endometriosis (32%).[100] In contrast, only 29% of asymptomatic women undergoing tubal ligation had abnormal findings at laparoscopy.

The laparoscope may be useful in evaluating acute pelvic pain involving ovarian cysts and ruling out ovarian torsion. If ovarian torsion is diagnosed, recent studies have examined the possibility of "untwisting" the torsed ovary and ovarian cystectomy with preservation of the viable adnexa.[197]

For chronic pelvic pain a definitive diagnosis of endometriosis can be made only with a pathologic specimen showing glands and stroma in an ectopic extrauterine location. Visual inspection of lesions or implants may be used to make a diagnosis, but the surgeon must be aware of the appearance of "atypical" endometriotic lesions.[125,127] If a patient is taken to the operating room for a laparoscopic procedure because of chronic pelvic pain and a normal pelvis is visualized, a random peritoneal biopsy from the cul-de-sac should be considered to pathologically identify microscopic endometriosis.[157]

In the adolescent population with chronic pelvic pain, laparoscopic evaluation can result in a definitive diagnosis in 75% of cases.[74] Endometriosis, pelvic adhesions, uterine anomalies, PID, and functional ovarian cysts were the most commonly diagnosed abnormalities in adolescents with chronic pelvic pain.[75]

Operative laparoscopy

The techniques for various operative laparoscopic procedures are beyond the scope of this chapter.[6,80,105,132] Table 25-3 lists surgical procedures performed via laparoscopy. With rapid advances in technology and the development of equipment, this list will continue to expand. In the remainder of this section, clinical experience with some of these procedures will be reviewed.

Tubal sterilization. Laparoscopic tubal sterilization procedures have dramatically increased in popularity over the years. Laparoscopic techniques are associated with lower rates of pelvic and incisional infection and shorter periods of hospitalization and convalescence than are procedures involving laparotomy.[23] Questions have recently been raised as to the possible beneficial effects of laparoscopic tubal ligation and the resulting decrease in the risk of subsequent ovarian cancer.[83,93]

In 1991 a membership survey of the American Association of Gynecologic Laparoscopists revealed recent trends in laparoscopic tubal sterilization procedures.[145] Bipolar coagulation was the most common method of sterilization in 1985, accounting for 56% of laparoscopic procedures; in 1976 this method was used in only 20% of laparoscopic sterilizations. Unipolar coagulation, which accounted for 64% of laparoscopic sterilizations in 1976, was used in only 6% of cases in 1991. Mechanical methods of tubal occlusion such as the ring (27%) and the clip (11%) have increased in popularity in recent years because they are easier to apply, safer, and more readily reversible than when electrocautery methods are used.

Complications requiring laparotomy followed sterilization procedures in 1.6 cases per 1000; the corresponding figure for diagnostic laparoscopic procedures was 3.1 per 1000. The most commonly encountered complication was hemorrhage.[187] In a review of more than 10,000 cases, Bhiwandiwala et al identified very few women who experienced menstrual changes subsequent to sterilization procedures.[21] Among women with changes, equal proportions noted beneficial and adverse effects. The true rate of failure of laparoscopic sterilization is similar to that reported for nonlaparoscopic techniques and ranges from 0.9 to 6.0 per 1000 sterilizations, depending on the technique used.[115] Among pregnancies following laparoscopic sterilization, the

Table 25-3. Operative laparoscopic procedures

I. Tubal sterilization
  A. Electrocautery
    1. Bipolar
    2. Unipolar
  B. Fallope ring
  C. Clip

II. Treatment of ectopic pregnancy
  A. Salpingostomy
  B. Segmental resection
  C. Salpingectomy

III. Treatment of endometriosis
  A. Coagulation and vaporization of implants
  B. Excision of implants
  C. Endometrioma
    1. Drainage
    2. Cystectomy

IV. Lysis of adhesions
  A. Filmy
  B. Vascular

V. Tubal reconstruction
  A. Fimbrioplasty
  B. Terminal salpingostomy

VI. Oocyte harvesting
  A. In vitro fertilization
  B. Gamete intrafallopian transfer
  C. Zygote intrafallopian transfer

VII. Second-look laparoscopy
  A. Ovarian carcinoma
  B. Tubal reconstructive surgery

VIII. Ovarian biopsy
  A. Tissue diagnosis
  B. Karyotype

IX. Ovarian cyst
  A. Drainage
  B. Cystectomy

X. Pelvic inflammatory disease
  A. Diagnosis
  B. Abscess drainage

XI. Myomectomy

XII. Oophorectomy, salpingectomy, adnexectomy

XIII. Laparoscopic-assisted vaginal hysterectomy (LAVH)

XIV. Uterine suspension

XV. Laparoscopic uterosacral ligament ablation (LUNA)

XVI. Removal of foreign body

incidence of ectopic pregnancy is higher after coagulation procedures (29% to 61% of all pregnancies) than after mechanical occlusive techniques (19% to 33%). In addition the risk of ectopic pregnancy is highest the first 2 years after tubal sterilization.[50]

Ectopic Pregnancy. Numerous published reports have described series of cases demonstrating the efficacy of operative laparoscopy in the treatment of ectopic pregnancies. Generally accepted criteria for cases of unruptured ectopic pregnancy amenable to a laparoscopic approach include (1) hemodynamic stability, (2) ectopic gestation 3 cm or less in diameter, (3) adequate pelvic access for laparoscopic visualization and treatment, and (4) agreeability of the patient to close postoperative follow-up including serial beta-human chorionic gonadotropin (ß-hCG) determinations.[46] With extensive surgical experience, more advanced ectopic pregnancies can be managed laparoscopically with salpingostomy or salpingectomy.

Operative laparoscopic procedures can be performed safely in a ruptured ectopic pregnancy, as long as the patient is not hypotensive. If there is a large volume of blood in the pelvis, a wall suction tube can be placed through a 10-mm port to evacuate the blood and the clot. In order not to suction bowel, the omentum, or some other structure, a "safety" hole should be cut in the suction tube approximately 2 feet from its end. The suction will then be active only when a finger is placed over the safety hole. This mechanism is excellent for the evacuation of large clots so that the operative procedure can continue and the source of bleeding can be stopped.

Linear salpingostomy may be performed for unruptured ampullary ectopic pregnancies, whereas linear salpingostomy or segmental tubal resection is reserved for isthmic gestations (Fig. 25-5). Salpingectomy, salpingoophorectomy, or coagulation of the entire gestation may also be performed. Complications following salpingostomy are relatively infrequent and include bleeding requiring laparotomy (2.5%), infection (1.3%), and slowly falling serum ß-hCG levels (12.6%).[46] In a study of a large series of laparoscopically treated ectopic pregnancies, Pouly et al performed 321 conservative laparoscopic procedures on 295 patients.[152] Fifteen patients (4.8%) required either a second laparoscopic procedure or a subsequent laparoscopy for retained trophoblastic tissue. In this series, 76 (64%) of 118 patients desiring a subsequent pregnancy had an intrauterine pregnancy, whereas 26 (22%) had a second ectopic pregnancy.

Numerous prospective randomized studies have documented similar results and complications of laparoscopy and laparotomy in the management of ectopic pregnancies. Patients managed by laparoscopy were shown to have decreased postoperative analgesia requirements, shorter recuperative periods, and shorter durations of hospitalization.[25,119,190]

Methotrexate therapy is an excellent option for the management of persistently elevated ß-hCG levels or of ß-hCG levels that are rising after a laparoscopic procedure.

In most large series, fertility rates following laparoscopic treatment of ectopic pregnancy are approximately 50% to 60%; 10% to 20% of all pregnancies after such treatment are ectopic. These rates are comparable to those reported for procedures utilizing laparotomy.[26,48,174,180]

Endometriosis. Endometriosis is another major indication for operative laparoscopy. Surgical therapeutic procedures should be undertaken during the initial diagnostic laparoscopy to avoid the need for a second operation and anesthetic. Unipolar or bipolar coagulation or laser vaporization may be employed for small implants. For ovarian endometriomas, drainage, puncture, and excision of the cyst wall with drainage and aspiration of its contents, coagulation or vaporization of the cyst base, or oophorectomy or adnexectomy may be performed (Fig. 25-6).[158] Electrocoagulation or laser vaporization of pelvic endometriotic lesions appears to provide relief to the majority of patients with chronic pelvic pain.[85,98]

The results of many studies evaluating the efficacy of laparoscopic treatment of endometriosis in infertile women have been published. Because the majority of these studies suffer from having small populations of patients, short follow-up intervals, inconsistent evaluation of secondary diagnoses, and no randomization, comparisons of laparoscopic treatment, conservative surgery by laparotomy, and medical therapy are difficult to interpret. The study by

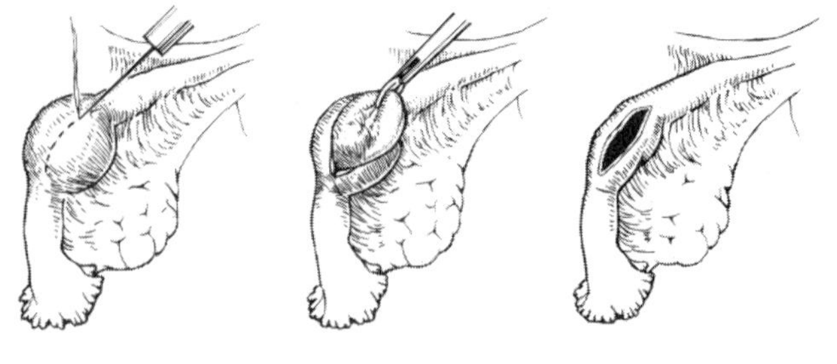

Fig. 25-5. Laparoscopic linear salpingostomy for unruptured ampullary ectopic pregnancy.

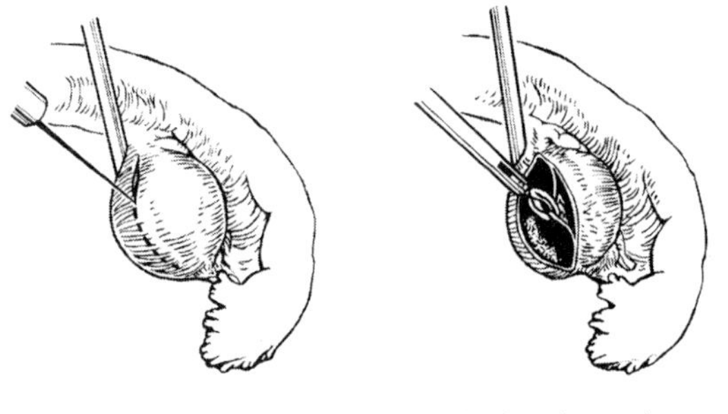

Fig. 25-6. Laparoscopic removal of endometrioma.

Gant comparing the treatment of endometriosis in the infertile population suggested that laparoscopy with laser therapy may be superior to laparotomy.[69] However, additional studies are needed before a definitive statement can be made.

Rates of pregnancy with laparoscopic surgery in stage I and II endometriosis have compared favorably with those with danazol therapy alone[13] and with conservative surgery.[29] In a combined series totaling 348 patients treated with laparoscopic electrocautery and followed for 7 months to 7 years, 162 patients (47%) conceived.[126] Many of these studies failed to control for secondary diagnoses and the stage of endometriosis. In a collected series totaling 374 patients in whom CO_2 laser laparoscopy was evaluated for the treatment of infertility as a result of endometriosis, pregnancy followed therapy in 73% of patients with stage I disease, 66% of patients with stage II disease, and 60% of patients with stage III or IV disease.[126] Laparoscopic treatment of pain, infertility, and pelvic masses resulting from endometriosis may be an acceptable alternative to medical therapy, conservative laparotomy, or both in many cases. The role of preoperative and postoperative medical therapy in combination with laparoscopic surgery needs further study.

Lysis of adhesions. One of the earliest reports of fertility-enhancing laparoscopic surgery was in 1975 by Gomel, who performed salpingolysis and salpingostomy by laparoscopy.[76] Pelvic adhesions may be characterized as thin and filmy or as dense and vascular. The former type of adhesion is easily lysed laparoscopically; the latter type may require cauterization before lysis. It is essential to identify all structures before cutting, coagulating, or vaporizing.[80] There must be sufficient space between structures before lysis of adjoining adhesions especially when coagulation is used, because thermal spread extends beyond visual tissue destruction (Fig. 25-7). The importance of these and other safety measures cannot be overemphasized.

Several published studies have demonstrated comparable efficacy for laparoscopic techniques used for adhesiolysis and conventional laparotomies in infertile women.[61,79,80,95] Gomel reported on laparoscopic lysis of moderate to dense periadnexal adhesions in 92 women of whom 57 (62%) went on to have at least one intrauterine pregnancy, 54 (59%) to have at least one viable birth, and 5 (5%) to have an ectopic pregnancy.[79] Fayez reported pregnancy rates of 72%, 67%, and 50% after laparoscopic ovariolysis, salpingolysis, and salpingoovariolysis respectively.[61] Pregnancy rates after laparoscopic fimbrioplasty have ranged from 31% to 48%.[61,80,130] Laparoscopic terminal salpingostomies may also be performed on hydrosalpinges with laser surgery, electrocautery, or endocoagulation. Tubal patency rates for this procedure have ranged from 31% to 75%, with pregnancy rates of 10% to 44%.[42,77] The low rate of success with this procedure is similar to that reported for conventional laparotomy salpingostomies.[16] Many of these patients may benefit from ART.

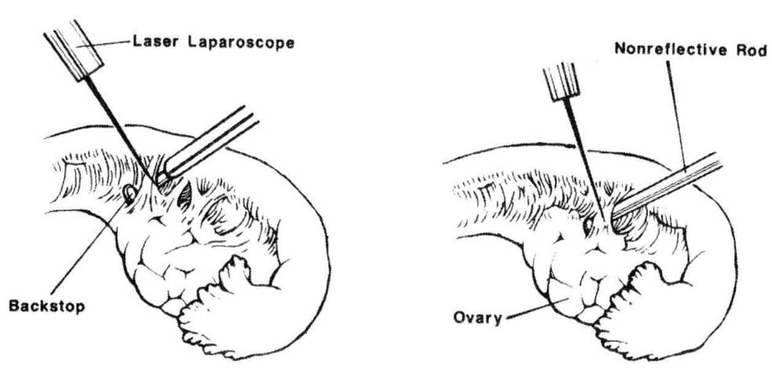

Fig. 25-7. Laparoscopic lysis of tuboovarian adhesions using laser.

Ovarian masses. Ovarian cystectomy can be performed laparoscopically. It is important to assess the likelihood of malignancy before a laparoscopic approach, to decrease the rate of subsequent identification of a malignancy in a laparoscopically excised ovarian neoplasm.[121] Consideration of the patient's age, evaluation of the ultrasound appearance of the mass (e.g., septations, internal echoes, and ascites), and use of serum tumor markers may be helpful.

The use of laparoscopic pouches for excised tissue may eliminate the spillage of potentially malignant cells in the peritoneal cavity.

Adnexectomy. The fallopian tube and/or the ovary can safely be removed by laparoscopy with electrocautery, suture ligatures, or staples. The ureter must be visualized at the time of the procedure to avoid the risk of damage.

Myomectomy. Myomectomy can be performed laparoscopically. Indications for the removal of myomas are still being debated; the need to remove pedunculated myomas is questionable. Myomas can be morcellated or removed through a colpotomy incision. Large myomas or intramural myomas may be difficult to remove laparoscopically because of the risk of bleeding or the inability to adequately reapproximate the myometrium. Myomas whose laparoscopic removal is being planned may be decreased in volume preoperatively with the use of GnRH agonists.

Laparoscopic-assisted vaginal hysterectomy. LAVH has been increasing in popularity for cases in which vaginal hysterectomy would otherwise be difficult (e.g., a history of pelvic adhesions, oophorectomy is desired, and a large fibroid uterus is evident). When a large fibroid uterus is present it is helpful to ligate the infundibulopelvic ligament before uterine morcellation in order to decrease blood loss. These indications can safely convert a proposed abdominal hysterectomy to a vaginal procedure.

Laparoscopic uterosacral nerve ablation. LUNA has been reported in the treatment of chronic pelvic pain.[107,108] In this procedure care must be taken to avoid injury to the ureter, which is found just laterally to the uterosacral ligament. Because of a lack of definitive proof of the benefit of this procedure, patients must be adequately counseled preoperatively as to the risks and proposed benefits.

Laparoscopic presacral neurectomy. Treatment of chronic central pelvic pain with laparoscopic presacral neurectomy (LPSN) has been proposed. The boundaries of the dissection are the bifurcation of the aorta superiorly, the right internal iliac artery and the right ureter on the right, the inferior mesenteric and superior hemorrhoidal arteries on the left, the division of the right and left inferior hypogastric plexus inferiorly, and the periosteum deep. Meticulous dissection is required to maintain hemostasis.

Appendectomy. Appendectomy can safely be performed by a laparoscopic approach with either suture ligatures or stapling devices. Cosmesis is sometimes the goal of such an approach. It is possible to use the umbilical port for the laparoscope and multiple suprapubic ports for the procedure. Thus, the resulting scars are lower on the abdomen than those from the traditional McBurney's incision. Three suprapubic ports with lateral 5-mm ports and a 12-mm port 2 finger breadths above the pubic symphysis are used. The right 5-mm port is used to give counter traction of the cecum superiorly, while the left 5-mm port is used to raise the appendix and move it inferiorly and to the left. The midline 12-mm port is used for the stapling device.

Second-look laparoscopy

Infertility. Following infertility surgery with either electrocautery or laser, a significant percentage of patients will have recurrence of adhesions, which may account for some surgical failures.[52] Some investigators recommend early second-look laparoscopies for lysis of newly formed adhesions 8 days to 12 weeks following the initial operation.[52,156,177,184] Although some investigators have reported significantly fewer ectopic pregnancies following salpingostomy in patients who undergo second-look laparoscopies than in those who do not, there is no difference in viable birth rates.[184] No unanimity exists on the efficacy of second-look laparoscopy for infertility surgery, and some reproductive surgeons have abandoned its practice after discovering that there is no difference in pregnancy rates.[80]

Oncology. Second-look laparoscopy has also been used in patients with ovarian carcinoma to assess their response to chemotherapy.[20,104,151,154,170,196] In each of these studies, the majority of patients with recurrent ovarian carcinoma had positive findings at laparoscopy and thus were spared a more extensive traditional second-look laparotomy. However, a negative laparoscopy is not necessarily predictive of the absence of disease. It should be noted that under these circumstances, laparoscopy carries a high rate of complications, the most common of which is bowel perforation. Berek et al found that 14% of patients had major complications requiring laparotomy.[20]

Gynecologic oncologists have begun to make use of operative laparoscopy for pelvic and periaortic lymph node dissection. This procedure has now been described by numerous authors.[136,155]

Table 25-4. Advantages of operative laparoscopy over laparotomy

1. Higher patient acceptance
2. Decreased operative time
3. Decreased morbidity
4. Decreased length of hospital stay
5. Decreased cost
6. Decreased recovery time

Advantages of laparoscopy

Patient acceptance of operative laparoscopy is high. Some advantages of operative laparoscopy over traditional laparotomies are listed in Table 25-4.

In an analysis of the economic impact of laparoscopic surgery, Levine found a 69% reduction in the length of postoperative stay for operative laparoscopy (0.5 to 2 days) compared with laparotomy (5 to 5.7 days).[106] In addition, women were able to return to full activity 7 to 10 days after laparoscopic surgery, compared with 4 to 6 weeks after traditional laparotomy. A 49% decrease in overall hospital costs was observed in the operative laparoscopy group. Operative time for laparoscopic procedures was also equivalent to or shorter than that for infertility laparotomies. The one important question that remains to be answered is whether the results of surgery are as good with laparoscopy as with conventional laparotomy.

Risks and complications of laparoscopy

Early reports on the safety of laparoscopy estimated the incidence of complications to be 3% to 4%, with the need for laparotomy in 0.73% of cases.[148,149] The most common serious complications in these studies were hemorrhagic episodes (occurring in 0.66% of cases) and penetrating injuries, especially of the gastrointestinal (GI) tract, that resulted from the blind insertion of the Verres needle or trocar (in 0.1% to 0.54% of cases).[34] Another investigator has noted more than 100 cases of major blood vessel injury.[143] In one case report, penetration of the aorta during Verres needle insertion required a transfusion of 22 units of blood and an aortic patch.[37]

Other risks include mechanical trauma, electrical, and heat- or laser-induced injury. Abdominal wall hemorrhage may occur when ancillary puncture sites are placed outside the midline. Occasionally, bleeding from the inferior epigastric vessels leads to hypotensive collapse.[153] Burns from noninsulated portions of unipolar and bipolar cautery may occur in any pelvic structure (e.g., bladder, small and large intestine, ureter, blood vessels). Large bowel perforation or full-thickness burns will require bowel resection and colostomy.

With increasing experience, the incidence of complications has dramatically decreased. Semm reported an overall complication rate of 0.28% in 8943 laparoscopies, 6114 of which were operative cases.[167] Of these, 13 (0.14%) were vascular injuries, 9 (0.1%) were gastric or bowel perforations, 1 (0.01%) was a ureteral injury, and 2 (0.02%) included cardiac arrest. In 10 instances (0.11%), laparotomy was required to treat the complications. No deaths were reported in this series. Daniell estimates the incidence of injury in operative laparoscopy with CO_2 laser to be less than 0.5%.[41] A list of potential complications resulting from laparoscopy is shown in Table 25-5.

Credentialing

With the rapidly changing world of operative laparoscopy or minimally invasive surgery, institutions and organizations such as the American College of Obstetricians and Gynecologists' Committee on Gynecologic Practice are establishing credentialing guidelines.[1] The credentialing process usually involves an extensive didactic course with hands-on experience. Applicants observe a certain number of operative laparoscopies in their institution and are precepted on a certain number of cases. An institutional committee should monitor the credentialing process. These guidelines are intended to decrease surgical complications. A recent study of urologic laparoscopic surgeons found that the rate of complications decreased if surgeons had education beyond an initial course and if they operated with an experienced assistant who was familiar with the technique.[165]

Summary

Both diagnostic and operative laparoscopy are safe procedures when guidelines are observed and the surgeon is aware of the limitations of the techniques. Surgeons must also be aware of their individual limitations and seek additional support when appropriate. With expertise in operative laparoscopy, the gynecologist can offer surgery with decreased morbidity, mortality, recuperative time, and cost.

HYSTEROSCOPY

Hysteroscopy is an endoscopic procedure that enables the surgeon to directly visualize the endocervical canal and uterine cavity. Although not as popular as laparoscopy, it facilitates accurate diagnosis and treatment of numerous gynecologic disorders. This section will introduce the reader to some of the principles and applications of hysteroscopy.

History

Hysteroscopy was first described in 1869 when Pantaleoni, using a 12-mm diameter Desormeaux cystoscope, evaluated a 60-year-old woman who had abnormal uterine bleeding.[141] Using reflected candlelight from a concave mirror, he was able to visualize endometrial polyps and cauterize them with silver nitrate. In 1879 Nitze in collaboration with Leiter, a Viennese instrument maker, added optical lenses to a cystoscope, which increased

Table 25-5. Complications of laparoscopy

I. Induction of pneumoperitoneum
   - A. Extraperitoneal insufflation
   - B. Pneumoomentum
   - C. Penetration of a hollow viscus
   - D. Vascular injury
   - E. Gas embolism
   - F. Subcutaneous emphysema
   - G. Mediastinal emphysema

II. Trocar insertion
   - A. Vascular injury
     1. Abdominal wall (inferior epigastric vessels)
     2. Aorta
     3. Iliac vessels
     4. Mesenteric vessels
     5. Omental vessels
   - B. Injury or penetration of a hollow viscus
   - C. Incisional hernia

III. Operative laparoscopy
   - A. Bleeding
   - B. Mechanical trauma
   - C. Electrosurgical injury
   - D. Laser injury
   - E. Infection

IV. Anesthesia
   - A. Cardiac arrhythmias
   - B. Aspiration

Table 25-6. Indications for hysteroscopy

I. Diagnostic
   - A. Abnormal uterine bleeding
     1. Premenopausal women
     2. Postmenopausal women
   - B. Localization of foreign body (e.g., intrauterine device)
   - C. Infertility
     1. Abnormal hysterosalpingogram
     2. Previous uterine manipulation or surgery
     3. In utero diethylstilbesterol exposure
   - D. Recurrent pregnancy losses
     1. Abnormal hysterosalpingogram
   - E. Secondary amenorrhea with failure of estrogen plus progestin withdrawal bleed
   - F. Evaluation of failed first-trimester elective abortions

II. Operative
   - A. Division of uterine septum (metroplasty)
   - B. Myomectomy
   - C. Removal of endometrial polyp
   - D. Directed biopsy of intrauterine lesion
   - E. Retrieval of foreign body
   - F. Division and excision of intrauterine adhesions (Asherman's syndrome)
   - G. Cauterization of active bleeding site
   - H. Ablation of endometrium for menorrhagia.

illumination and the field of vision.[137] The Nitze principle of endoscopy was not adopted for hysteroscopy until 1908 when David demonstrated the usefulness of hysteroscopy in the diagnosis of uterine disorders.[45] Heineberg first described a water irrigation system in 1908,[86] and Rubin first reported on CO_2 distension of the uterine cavity in 1925.[160] Over the next 60 years, improvements in instruments and the development of fiber optic light sources and ancillary equipment have facilitated the development of hysteroscopy.

Indications

As with laparoscopy, the list of indications for hysteroscopy is increasing. Table 25-6 lists some present-day indications for hysteroscopy. Indications that are still under investigation (i.e., sterilization procedures, salpingoscopy) are not included in this table.

Contraindications

Very few contraindications for hysteroscopy exist. Standard contraindications for this procedure are listed in Table 25-7.

Equipment

The basic equipment needed for hysteroscopy includes a hysteroscope (Fig. 25-8), cervical dilators, a light source, and a distending medium. Operative hysteroscopy requires ancillary instruments that are passed down a channel in the hysteroscope. Different types of hysteroscopes and distending media are discussed below.

Hysteroscopes and light source. There are three basic types of hysteroscopes: rigid panoramic, rigid contact, and "flexible" panoramic. Panoramic hysteroscopy requires a distending medium and a light source, whereas neither of these are required in contact hysteroscopy. The contact hysteroscope collects, traps, and transmits room or directed light through the previously dilated cervical canal.[142] Only surfaces in contact with the tip of the hysteroscope are visible. Vision is not obstructed by blood or other fluids.

The choice of hysteroscope depends upon the goal of the surgeon and the needs of the patient. The telescopes have outer diameters of 2.7 to 4.0 mm with viewing angles of 0°, 12°, 15°, 25°, or 30° off the horizontal. The diameter of the rigid panoramic hysteroscope sheath ranges from 3.3 mm for the smallest diagnostic instruments to 8 mm for some operative hysteroscopes. Hysteroscopes of 5 mm or less in diameter usually require no cervical dilation in premenopausal women. Larger sheaths will allow placement of one or two ancillary instruments. Some sheaths have an Albarron bridge at the distal end allowing ancillary instruments (i.e., a laser fiber, guide wire, or catheter) to be deflected or steered toward a lesion or structure.

The contact hysteroscope is a valuable office instrument that may be used to diagnose endocervical and endometrial pathology.[7] When gentle pressure of the distal end of the hysteroscope is applied to a mucosal surface, even bleeding structures and lesions may be visualized. Contact hysteroscopy is more difficult to master than panoramic hysteroscopy because the surgeon can only view an isolated area and loses spatial orientation and perspective. Complete inspection of the endocervical canal and uterine cavity requires patience and discipline.

"Flexible" hysteroscopes have steerable distal segments which may be deflected over an arc of 130° to 160°. The outer diameter of these hysteroscopes ranges from 3.5 to 4.8 mm. A 1-mm channel allows delivery of CO_2 or 5% dextrose in water (D5W) as a distending medium. The larger flexible hysteroscope has a 2-mm operating channel for biopsy forceps or microscissors. A major advantage of the flexible hysteroscope is the ability to maneuver its distal end around intracavitary structures (e.g., leiomyomata) or

Table 25-7. Contraindications to hysteroscopy

I. Pelvic inflammatory disease
   A. Salpingitis
   B. Endometritis

II. Untreated cervical infection
   A. *Neisseria gonorrhea*
   B. *Chlamydia trachomatis*

III. Contraindications to local or general anesthetic

IV. Pregnancy

V. Invasive carcinoma of the cervix

VI. Inexperienced surgeon

VII. Menstruation*

* Relative contraindication

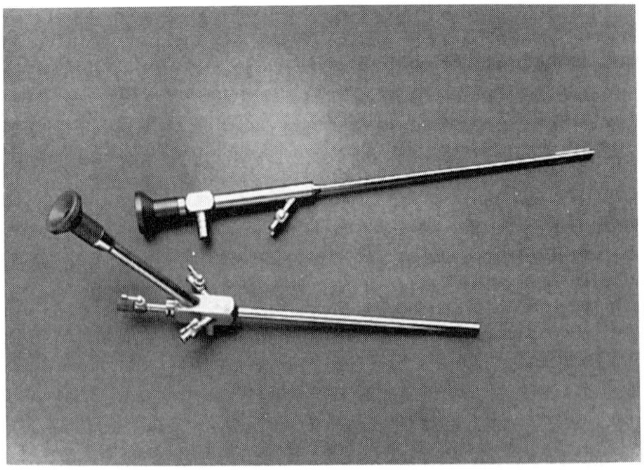

Fig. 25-8. Diagnostic and operative hysteroscopes. (Courtesy Edward Weck, Princeton, NJ).

to visualize eccentrically placed tubal ostia with minimal discomfort to the patient. One disadvantage is that the optics are inferior to that of rigid hysteroscopes and have a "ground glass" quality.

The optics of a hysteroscope consist of a system of lenses transmitting the image and fiberglass that conducts "cold" light. Most sources of cold light are fitted with halogen or xenon lamps with power ranging from 100 to 300 watts. The light is transmitted to the hysteroscope by a fiberglass, loses its heat component entirely, and keeps its intensity. As in the laparoscope, a loss of light occurs at the site of connection of the conduction cord and the hysteroscope.

Distention media. Either gas (i.e., CO_2) or liquid is used to distend the uterine cavity for panoramic hysteroscopy. Liquid distension media may be of low viscosity (e.g., D5W, normal saline, Ringer's lactate, 3.3% sorbitol, or 1.5% glycine) or high viscosity (e.g., dextran 40, dextran 70 [Hyskon Hysteroscopy Fluid]). Each distension medium has different properties which will influence the surgeon's choice.

CO_2 is the only gas used as a distending medium in hysteroscopy. It requires a special insufflator that limits the flow of gas to 100 mL/min for safety reasons. In experiments on German shepherds to evaluate the effect of insufflated CO_2 on acid-base status, Lindemann et al found that there were no changes in pH, pCO_2, or pO_2 after direct insufflation of 200 mL/min into the femoral vein.[111] When CO_2 was insufflated at 400 mL/min, tachypnea and cardiac arrhythmias occurred with no changes in pH, pCO_2, or pO_2. A lethal dosage was established at 1000 mL/min after 60 seconds. The maximal intrauterine pressure must never exceed 200 mm Hg. The insufflator used for laparoscopy should never be used for hysteroscopy. Advantages of CO_2 as a distending medium are its perfect transmission of the image, availability, long history of safety in tubal patency tests, and rapid absorption.[161] Some disadvantages of CO_2 include the need for (1) a complicated, expensive insufflating apparatus, (2) a perfect cervical occlusion with the instrument, (3) extreme care to avoid provoking bleeding or bubbles, and (4) maintaining uterine distention with easy escape of CO_2 through patent tubes. During prolonged procedures, up to 500 mL of the CO_2 may be used.

Low-viscosity liquid can also be used for uterine distention. It is delivered via an intravenous infusion bag by gravity or by either a pressure cuff around the bag of fluid or by using a pump to increase the rate of flow through connecting tubing and into the uterine cavity. The view is initially clear, but the field clouds rapidly, necessitating frequent rinsing. Advantages of low-viscosity media are that they are readily available, inexpensive, and rapidly absorbed through the peritoneal cavity, and the delivery system is simple. Disadvantages include the need for frequent rinsing to maintain a clear image and the use of large amounts of fluids to maintain adequate uterine distention. Electrolyte-containing media cannot be used during electrosurgery. Close monitoring of fluid input and output is necessary to avoid water intoxication, hyponatremia, noncardiogenic pulmonary edema, and seizures when hypoosmotic media is used. The procedure should be terminated when the patient has a positive "water balance" of greater than 1000 mL.

Dextran 70 is a colorless liquid of 70,000 molecular weight with high viscosity and excellent optical qualities.[134] It is the most popular distention medium in the United States and Japan. Dextran 70 is instilled via a 50-mL plastic syringe connected to the hysteroscope with a 25-cm piece of tubing with Luer-Lok connections. Manual pressure is maintained to ensure continuous flow with adequate uterine distention. A dextran pump controlled by a foot-pedal switch operated by the surgeon has been described.[102] Less than 100 mL generally suffice for diagnostic procedures, although more may be necessary for prolonged operative hysteroscopy. The advantages of dextran 70 are that the transmission of light is excellent, only a simple apparatus is required for instillation, and it is immiscible with blood, allowing protracted visibility. Disadvantages of dextran 70 are that it is very viscous, necessitating immediate and thorough washing of instruments to prevent bonding; the rate of absorption in the abdominal cavity is not known; and it may transiently prolong bleeding time, causing plasma volume expansion and resultant high-output left ventricular failure,[139] and occasional allergic reactions, including anaphylaxis. Hysteroscopy with dextran 70 is probably the easiest technique to master and gives the most reproducible results.

Ancillary instruments used in operative hysteroscopy include grasping forceps, biopsy forceps, aspirating cannulas, scissors, coagulating probes and loops, and laser-carrying quartz fibers (Fig. 25-9). Laser fibers may be water or gas-cooled. Several deaths have been reported with gas-cooled Nd:YAG fibers with sapphire tips as a result of gas emboli.[11] With the exception of laser-carrying fibers, most ancillary instruments may be rigid or flexible. For major operative procedures, rigid instruments are preferable. Flexible instruments can be used through a smaller operating shaft even with local anesthetic.

Technique

Before starting hysteroscopy, the patient should be placed in the dorsal lithotomy position, buttocks slightly protruding from the end of the table and elevated about 5°. The speculum should have an opening on one lateral aspect to enable greater manipulation of the hysteroscope. After adequate anesthetic is given, a single-toothed tenaculum is placed on the anterior lip of the cervix and cervical dilation with Hegar's dilators may be performed when using a hysteroscope greater than 5 mm in diameter or when performing hysteroscopy on a postmenopausal woman. It is important not to overdilate the cervix because a good seal between the cervical canal and hysteroscope is essential to maintain adequate uterine distention for panoramic

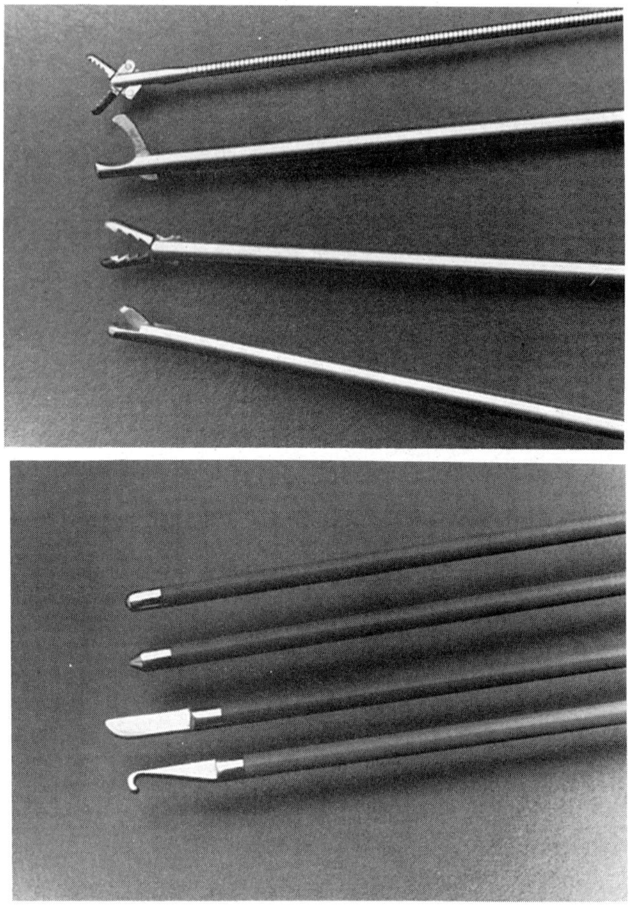

Fig. 25-9. Ancillary hysteroscopic instruments including *(from top to bottom)* grasping forceps, hook scissors, grasping forceps, punch biopsy forceps, unipolar cautery probe, unipolar cautery cone-tipped probe, knife electrode, hook electrode. (Courtesy Edward Weck, Princeton, NJ).

hysteroscopy, especially when CO_2 is used as a distention medium. A cervical adapter is used with CO_2 to prevent CO_2 loss during operative hysteroscopy. The fiber-optic light projector is then adjusted and the tip of the hysteroscope is gently inserted into the cervical canal as the surgeon observes its entrance through the ocular. After exploring the cervical canal, some resistance is encountered just before the uterine cavity is entered.

Just as in laparoscopy, the surgeon must systematically explore the fundus, both horns and ostia, and the lateral, anterior, and posterior walls of the uterine cavity (Fig 25-10). Hysteroscopy is best performed in the postmenstrual or midproliferative phase to avoid encountering heaped up endometrium, which may obscure intracavitary viewing and make operative procedures more difficult. During the proliferative phase, the endometrium appears reddish yellow and assumes a more yellowish hue at ovulation. Throughout the secretory phase the endometrium is reddish purple, swollen, and has wispy projections of tissue going into the cavity.

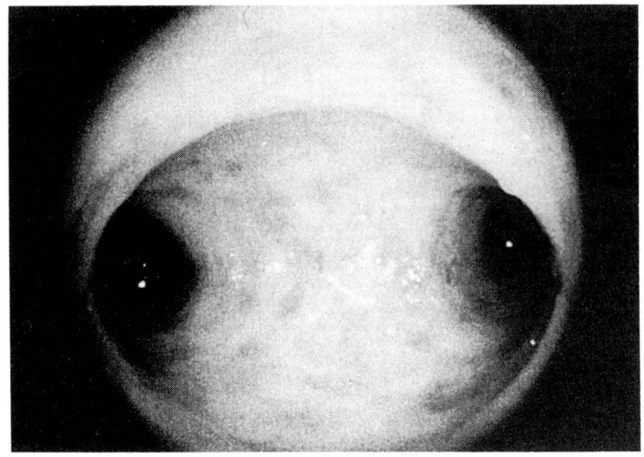

Fig. 25-10. Panoramic hysteroscopic view of normal uterine cavity.

Contact hysteroscopy,[124] and microhysteroscopy with its ability to magnify up to 150 times during contact, may be used to view endocervical and endometrial vascular patterns and histology.[82] These techniques are especially useful in the diagnosis of premalignant or malignant lesions. No distention medium is needed for these techniques.

Anesthetic

Local anesthetic alone or in combination with a systemic analgesic is sufficient and preferable for most hysteroscopic examinations.[2,14] General anesthetic is necessary if concurrent laparoscopy is performed. Some surgeons perform hysteroscopy without any anesthetic,[14] whereas others use analgesic and sedation only. In a series of 1000 patients undergoing microhysteroscopy, 949 (94.9%) required no anesthetic, 12 (1.2%) required local anesthetic, and 41 (4.1%) received general anesthetic (13 of whom had an associated surgical procedure done at the time of hysteroscopy).[175] For conventional hysteroscopy, a paracervical block provides adequate anesthetic in 92% to 96% of patients.[109,122,142,164,169] Gentleness of technique and adequate patient education and preparation will increase the acceptance of local anesthetic, making hysteroscopy an ideal ambulatory procedure. The discomfort experienced by patients is often comparable with that experienced during hysterosalpingography.

Diagnostic and operative hysteroscopy

Over the years the hysteroscope has proven to be an invaluable tool for the gynecologist in diagnosing and treating uterine cavitary disorders. Diagnostic hysteroscopy allows direct visualization of the uterine cavity and enhances the gynecologist's ability to diagnose structural abnormalities over other diagnostic modalities such as hystersalpingography, ultrasonography, and MRI. When operative hysteroscopy is performed, hormonal preparation of the endometrium is often useful to induce atrophy, thereby improving visualization and decreasing vascularity to minimize bleeding. Hormonal medications may be used for 4 to 8 weeks to treat women undergoing operative hysteroscopy and include GnRH agonists, danazol, and synthetic progestins.[24] Treatment with a GnRH agonist has been reported to decrease operating time, intraoperative bleeding, and the amount of distension media required compared with no preoperative medical treatment.[147] Other investigators have advocated "mechanical preparation" of the endometrium (i.e., suction curettage) immediately before performing operative procedures such as endometrial ablation.[71]

Abnormal uterine bleeding. Hysteroscopy is not a substitute for tissue diagnosis. However, hysteroscopic findings will increase the information available to the gynecologist in various clinical situations. Abnormal uterine bleeding in the perimenopausal and postmenopausal woman is a common gynecologic disorder in which hysteroscopy will often provide information that will aid greatly in diagnosis and treatment. Diltation and curettage(D&C) has long been the diagnostic standard for abnormal uterine bleeding. However, even a trained gynecologist curettes at best 70% to 80% of the endometrium.[51] Failure rates in making tissue diagnosis may occur in 36% to 50% of some patient populations.[59,176] Polyps and submucous fibroids are frequently undetected by curettage alone.[28,59,169,194] Hysteroscopic findings correlate highly with histologic results, and hysteroscopy should be considered a basic diagnostic procedure in the diagnosis of abnormal uterine bleeding.

In a series of 853 hysteroscopies performed for abnormal uterine bleeding in perimenopausal (age 45 to 55 years, n = 516) and postmenopausal women (age more than 55 years, n = 337), normal findings were noted in 65% (557 patients).[51] Women in the perimenopausal age group demonstrated normal endometrial architecture in 78% of cases, whereas 45% of postmenopausal women had no pathology. Uterine polyps were noted in 25% of all cases (204 women) or in 10% of perimenopausal and 45% of postmenopausal women. Submucous fibroids were noted in 8% (67) of the patients and comprised 11% of the diagnoses in the perimenopausal and 3% of the postmenopausal age groups. Carcinoma was present in only 0.2% (1) of the perimenopausal women compared with 7% (24) of the postmenopausal women.

In a study comparing hysteroscopy and selected endometrial sampling with D&C, the specificity of both techniques was 100% but the sensitivity of hysteroscopy was greater than that of D&C (98% versus 65%).[114] Endometritis was the only condition missed by hysteroscopic viewing and selected biopsy.

Hysteroscopy combined with D&C can be viewed as a perfected curettage by enabling the surgeon to directly visualize the endometrial cavity.

Infertility. Hysteroscopy may be useful in the diagnosis of uterine causes of infertility and recurrent pregnancy losses. Several studies have demonstrated the increased accuracy of hysteroscopy over hysterosalpingography in this setting.[178,179,188] Coupled with laparoscopy, a thorough anatomic evaluation of the woman of an infertile partnership is possible.[39] In studies comparing hysteroscopy to hysterosalpingography, an accuracy rate of 50% to 62% for the latter has been noted.[188] False-negative diagnoses are uncommon in hysterography, and this method may therefore be used as a screening test for women in the infertility evaluation.

Intrauterine synechiae. Asherman's syndrome, the presence of intrauterine synechiae or scar tissue, is most frequently observed following curettage in a pregnant or recently pregnant uterus (Fig. 25-11).[3] The most common symptoms include amenorrhea, hypomenorrhea, dysmenorrhea, current abortions, and infertility. Although cavitary filling defects noted on hysterography have been used to make the diagnosis, several studies have demonstrated the superiority of hysteroscopy over hysterography in the evaluation of Asherman's syndrome.[122,175] Asherman had the foresight to recognize the potential value of hysteroscopy in the treatment of intrauterine adhesions, as he wrote the following:

> Hysteroscopy, which has so often been mentioned in the literature and just as often discarded, may be of use for this purpose. If it were possible to see the adhesions and to loosen them instrumentally, using the eye as the guide, the ideal method will have been found. We have the intention of trying out the practical application of this theoretical hypothesis.[4]

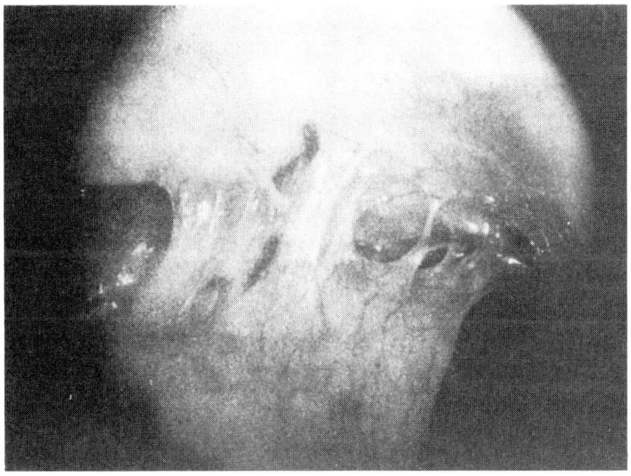

Fig. 25-11. Hysteroscopic view of intrauterine synechiae. (From Salat-Baroux J et al: Postabortal hysteroscopy. In Siegler AM, Lindemann HJ, editors: *Hysteroscopy: principles and practice*, Philadelphia, 1994, JB Lippincott/New York, 1984, Harper & Row.

Today, hysteroscopy is the accepted method for evaluating and treating intrauterine adhesions.[175,188,189] When operative hysteroscopy is used to divide thick intrauterine adhesions, a surgical assistant should perform concurrent laparoscopy to move the bowel away from the uterus and to look for potential uterine perforation. Hysteroscopic scissors, probes, or the unipolar cautery resectoscope can be used to divide adhesions. Postoperative therapy often includes placement of an intrauterine stent (e.g., intrauterine device, Foley catheter) to keep the cavity walls separated, high-dose estrogen treatment for 1 to 2 months, and antibiotics. In a review of the literature, Schenker and Margalioth reported a return of normal menses in 73% to 92% of hysteroscopically treated patients compared with 78% of patients treated by hysterotomy.[162] Conception rates ranged from 47% to 55% in hysteroscopy-treated patients, with 48% to 78% of these patients delivering viable infants. These numbers compared favorably with a 52% conception rate and 76% viable birth rate in those patients treated by hysterotomy.[162] Thus, hysteroscopy is the method of choice in the treatment of the vast majority of cases of intrauterine synechiae.

Myomectomy. Neuwirth reported on hysteroscopic myomectomy in patients with submucous fibroids and menorrhagia (Fig. 25-12).[135] Following resection of fibroids, he inserted and inflated a Silastic balloon into the uterine cavity to tamponade the bleeding raw surface. The balloon was left in place for 24 hours. In his series of 28 patients, 19 (68%) had no recurrence of symptoms following the procedure, and 2 (7%) required a second hysteroscopic myomectomy. Five women (18%) required hysterectomy 2 weeks to 3 years following hysteroscopic fibroid resection for persistent bleeding. Other investigators have since reported a high rate of success in treating menorrhagia by hysteroscopic myomectomy.[90] Preoperative treatment with a GnRH agonist will induce shrinkage of submucous myomas, facilitating hysteroscopic myomectomy.[66] Hysteroscopic myomectomy may be successful in a large proportion of well-chosen patients.

Metroplasty. Hysteroscopic metroplasty may be performed in patients with a uterine septum with a history of recurrent miscarriage or poor obstetrical outcome (Fig. 25-13). In many instances, this approach can replace the more traditional Tompkins or Jones metroplasties. A cystoscopic resectoscope,[49] hysteroscopic scissors,[40,62] or laser may be used to divide the septum.[32,35] Laparoscopy is essential to distinguish between a septate and bicornuate uterus before an operative hysteroscopy. In a comparative study between abdominal and hysteroscopic metroplasty, Fayez performed postoperative hysterosalpingography in 33 patients.[62] Of 14 patients treated by Tompkins metroplasty, 72% had normal uterine cavities, 14% demonstrated incomplete septum excision, and 14% had intrauterine filling defects. The corresponding percentages in the hysteroscopically treated group were 88% normal cavities, 12% incomplete excision, and 0% filling defects. In one study where women undergoing hysteroscopic septal incision were followed postoperatively with serial hysteroscopies and biopsies, complete healing took 2 months' time.[31] In this study, there was only a minimal tendency toward formation of the central fundal adhesions. Most authorites believe that hysteroscopic metroplasty is equal or superior to a transabdominal approach except in cases with thick septa.

Endometrial ablation. Hysteroscopy may also be used for endometrial ablation in cases of menorrhagia or intractable uterine bleeding secondary to coagulopathies. By using this ambulatory surgical procedure in selected patients, a significant decrease could be achieved in the number of hysterectomies performed as a result of abnormal uterine bleeding in the United States each year. Ancillary instruments used to perform endometrial ablation include the Nd:YAG laser,[19,70,73,89,113] the cystoscopic resectoscope,[47] and

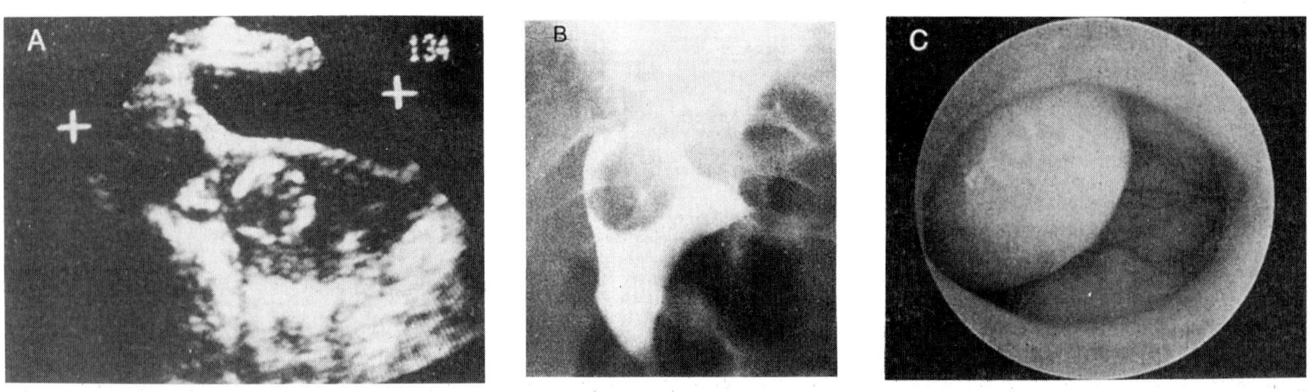

Fig. 25-12. Three views of a submucous leiomyoma. **A,** Ultrasound. **B,** Hysterosalpingogram. **C,** Hysteroscopy. (From Gamerre M, Porto R, Serment H: Hysteroscopy for diagnosis and therapy. In Siegler AM, Lindemann HJ editors: *Hysteroscopy: principles and practice,* Philadelphia, 1984, JB Lippincott/New York, 1984, Harper & Row.

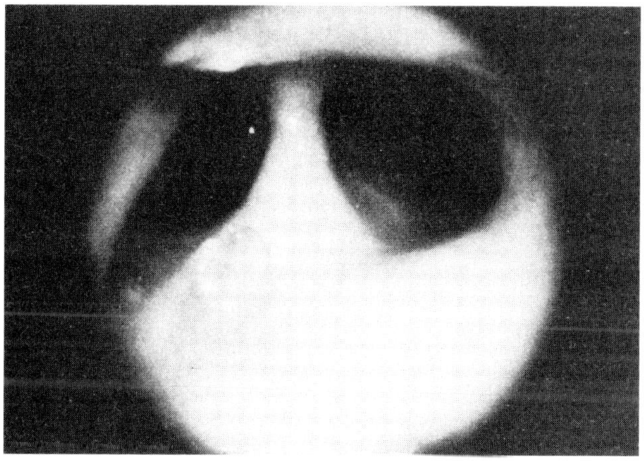

Fig. 25-13. Hysteroscopic view of uterine septum.

the rollerball electrode.[43,183] Reported rates of amenorrhea following endometrial ablation range from 30% to 60% with hypomenorrhea being present in an additional 25% to 35%. In most reports, approximately 8% to 10% of patients are considered treatment failures with no reduction in menstrual flow. Endometrial ablation is less likely to yield satisfactory results if there are multiple submucous leiomyomas or if the uterine cavity is large (i.e., greater than 10 cm). Experienced surgeons do not perform concurrent laparoscopy at the time of endometrial ablation; the risk of uterine perforation is less than 1%,[70] as is the risk of thermal damage to other intraabdominal organs from direct heat transfer through the myometrium.[57,91,92]

Risks and complications of hysteroscopy

Hysteroscopy has a very low rate of complications. In several large series totaling more than 800 patients undergoing hysteroscopy, no complications were reported.[60,123,163] Faulty technique and poor patient selection account for most complications.

Cervical lacerations may result from tenaculum placement, especially with vigorous manipulation. Cervical or endometrial bleeding may result from forceful cervical dilation. Uterine perforation may occur during cervical dilation or intrauterine placement of the hysteroscope. Lindemann reported only 6 fundal perforations in 5220 hysteroscopic examinations.[110]

Intravasation of CO_2 and liquid media may occur. With imperfect gas flow monitors using excessive CO_2 insufflation rates, changes in pH, pCO_2, pO_2 and ECG may occur. In the most extreme cases, a CO_2 embolus may result in the death of the patient. In all cases of CO_2 embolus and death, gas flow rates exceeded 350 mL/min. Following the guidelines listed earlier (i.e., flow rate at 100 mL or less of CO_2/min; peak intrauterine pressure of 200 mm Hg or less), the risk of gas embolism approaches zero.[15] The risks of intravasation of high molecular weight dextran are proportionate to the amount of dextran 70 used. Maddi et al described seven cases of anaphylaxis in patients receiving intravenous high molecular weight dextran.[120] Leake et al reported two cases of noncardiogenic pulmonary edema after operative hysteroscopy with 32% dextran 70.[103] Another reported rare but serious complication is bleeding diathesis.

Infection may result following hysteroscopy. The first reported infection after hysteroscopy was reported by Bumm in 1895.[27] Hysteroscopy may exacerbate latent salpingitis, especially in patients with active cervical infections or a history of salpingitis. Table 25-8 summarizes the complications of hysteroscopy.

Summary

With proper training, good equipment, and rigid adherence to safety standards, hysteroscopy can be an invaluable aid in the diagnosis and treatment of numerous gynecologic disorders. With the development of new equipment and techniques, experimental procedures (i.e., sterilization, embryoscopy, salpingoscopy) will be perfected and added to the growing list of hysteroscopic applications.

LASER SURGERY

Since the invention of the laser almost 30 years ago, laser technology has continued to evolve rapidly, having a significant impact on almost every medical and surgical subspecialty. It is essential for the clinician to have an understanding of the basics of laser-tissue interaction and safety principles to use these tools properly and effectively.

Table 25-8. Complications of hysteroscopy

I. Cervical laceration

II. Cervical or uterine bleeding

III. Uterine perforation
   A. Visceral trauma

IV. Intravasation of distention medium
   A. Carbon dioxide
      1. Acidosis
      2. ECG changes
      3. Cardiac arrest
      4. Death
   B. High molecular weight dextran
      1. Anaphylaxis
      2. Bleeding diathesis
      3. Pulmonary edema
      4. Intravascular volume overload
   C. 5% dextrose
      1. Intravascular volume overload
      2. Pulmonary edema

V. Infection
   A. Salpingitis

Laser physics

Light is energy with a dual nature described both by wave and particle theory. According to wave theory, light may be characterized by wavelength (in Å or nm), frequency (f), and amplitude. The parameters of wavelength and frequency are inversely related, determine the energy level of light, and determine where it falls on the electromagnetic spectrum. Light characterized by long wavelengths (i.e., low frequency) has low energy and falls into the infrared, microwave, or radiowave zone. Conversely, light characterized by short wavelengths (i.e., high frequency) has high energy and includes ultraviolet light, x-rays, and gamma rays.

According to particle theory, light is considered to be a stream of particles of negligible mass called photons, each carrying a quantity (quantum) of energy associated with a specific wavelength of light. When excited by an external energy source, electrons from each element or molecule will jump to a higher energy orbit. Following excitation, electrons fall from high- to low-energy orbits, emitting a photon at a wavelength characteristic for that specific element or molecule. Thus, the wavelength of the light emitted is a function of the type of atom or molecule excited and not a function of the wavelength of light or energy originally used to excite the atom or molecule. If the wavelength of emitted light happens to be within the narrow range of wavelengths of visible light within the electromagnetic spectrum, the emitted light of a specific atom will have a characteristic color.

The word laser is an acronym for light amplification by the stimulated emission of radiation, which is the process by which such a beam is created. Laser light differs from other kinds of light because of three unique properties: (1) it is monochromatic (i.e., the waves are all one wavelength), (2) it is coherent (i.e., all waves are in phase), and (3) it is collimated (i.e., all waves are parallel). Because of these three properties, laser light is able to maintain an intense, focused energy over long distances.

Laser light is created by stimulating a medium of a single pure element or compound and emitting photons simultaneously. This creates a light source that is both monochromatic and coherent. A collimated beam is created by reflecting the light in a resonator tube with reflective mirrors at each end (Fig. 25-14). One mirror is 100% reflective, whereas the other is partially reflective, allowing the laser beam to exit as a series of parallel waves. The waves remain parallel for long distances with only minimal divergence.

Lasing media may be either gas, liquid, or solid. Most lasing media used for gynecologic indications are gas; only the Nd:YAG crystal is solid (Table 25-9).

Laser unit

The laser unit consists of a few essential components. The laser head contains the lasing medium, an excitation source, and an aiming beam. For gas-lasing media, direct electrical current (DC) is often used as the excitation source. For solid-lasing media, incoherent optical flash lamps (i.e., krypton or xenon arc lamps) may be used.

An aiming beam is necessary for lasers with wavelengths outside of the visible spectrum (e.g., CO_2, Nd:YAG). The most commonly used aiming beam is a low-power He-Ne laser that emits light at a wavelength of 632 nm and appears red. The He-Ne beam may be projected coaxially with the surgical laser, giving important information about the integrity of the fiber and delivery system as well as the spot size of the beam at the target tissue. Since the He-Ne wavelength is different from the wavelength of the surgical laser, it will give only an approximation of the characteristics of the surgical beam. When large differences in wavelength exist between the aiming and surgical beams (e.g., CO_2 and He-Ne beams), the aiming beam does a poorer job in approximating the characteristics of the surgical beam.

The bulkiness of most laser units is due to several supporting elements such as a power amplifier, cooling system, and delivery system. Because the process of generating a coherent light beam from an incoherent energy source is inefficient, the electrical current used to excite the lasing medium must be amplified many times. This is accomplished with a high-voltage electrical amplifier.

The inefficiency of creating the laser beam causes tremendous dissipation of heat. Most laser units use a water or air-cooled system to absorb heat and prevent damage of internal components. High-powered and inefficient lasers (e.g., argon) require high volumes of water for cooling, whereas low-powered lasers may be air cooled.

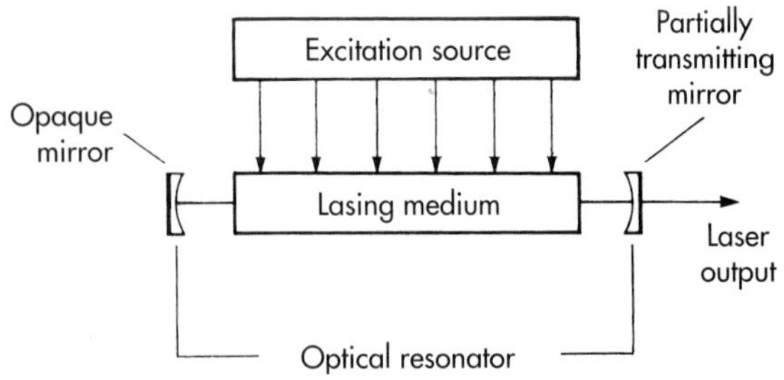

Fig. 25-14. Schematic of the creation of a laser beam.

Table 25-9. Properties of gynecologic lasers

Medium	Phase	Wavelength(s) (nm)	Color
CO_2	Gas	10,600	Infrared
He-Ne	Gas	632	Red
Nd:YAG	Solid	1320	Infrared
		1064	Infrared
Argon	Gas	515	Green
		488	Blue
KTP	Gas	532	Green

A delivery system is needed to transmit the laser beam from the laser head to the target tissue. Some lasers (e.g., argon, KTP, Nd:YAG) may be transmitted by flexible 0.2- to 1-mm diameter flexible quartz optical fibers. The fibers are typically surrounded by tight Teflon sleeves. The main advantage of fiber optic transmission is its flexibility, allowing the surgeon to reach areas of the body otherwise accessible only through open surgery. A disadvantage of fiber optic transmission is that 20% of the generated power is lost through multiple internal reflections along the inner walls of the fiber. In addition, fiber-transmitted laser beams exit the fiber tip with a 10- to 12-degree divergence, decreasing the precision.

A second type of delivery system uses a rigid system of articulated jointed arms with mirrors. This system is used when the laser wavelength (e.g., CO_2) is absorbed by the optical fiber, making fiber-optic transmission impossible. The mirrors in the articulated arms are made of zinc and selenium and have an added reflective coating, because regular glass mirrors would absorb the CO_2 wavelength. Although much bulkier than the fiber-optic delivery system, one advantage of transmission via articulated arms is that the laser still emerges as a collimated beam, thus allowing the beam to be focused with greater precision than an uncollimated beam emerging from an optical fiber. As the precision of focus of the surgical laser increases, the spot size of the laser decreases, increasing the power density of the delivered beam. A smaller spot size increases the predictability, control, and effectiveness of the laser beam.

Laser-tissue interaction of Gynecologic lasers

Carbon dioxide laser. The CO_2 laser is the most frequently used laser in gynecologic surgery and has been used for virtually all indications. It has a wavelength of 10,600 nm, which is almost totally absorbed by water and is not color dependent.[128] In effect, 98% of a CO_2 beam is absorbed within the first 10 μm of tissue (i.e., depth of a few cells), and 99.9% is absorbed within 100 μm.[64] By instantaneously boiling intracellular water, the CO_2 laser "explodes" cells and removes tissue by vaporization (Fig. 25-15). Coagulation resulting from penetration of the CO_2 laser is limited to 100 to 200 μm (Fig. 25-16). Thermal penetration ranges from 200 to 700 μm, depending on the speed at which the operating surgeon guides the laser beam over tissue. Because of its shallow penetration of tissue, the CO_2 laser is characterized by high precision but poor hemostasis. It is able to seal vessels with a diameter of 0.5 mm when focused and 1.0 mm when the spot is defocused.[64] There are other characteristics of the CO_2 laser: (1) there is minimal scattering of energy from the target site, (2) it is absorbed by plastic and glass and reflected by most metals, and (3) the conversion of radiant energy to heat has not been shown to cause genetic mutations of cells.[64] The CO_2 laser requires an He-Ne aiming beam, is delivered by a system of articulated arms and mirrors, and may be used in continuous or pulsed modes. Characteristics of the CO_2, argon, KTP, and Nd:YAG lasers are summarized in Table 25-10.

Argon and KTP lasers. Argon and KTP lasers have wavelengths that are preferentially absorbed by reddish pigments (e.g., heme, melanin) and pass through water. The depth of penetration for both the argon and KTP lasers is 2 mm, and their qualities of precision cutting and coagulation are intermediate between those of the CO_2 and Nd:YAG lasers. Because of their preferential absorption by red pigments, these lasers cause coagulation of blood within the vessel rather than the vessel wall. The specificity of their

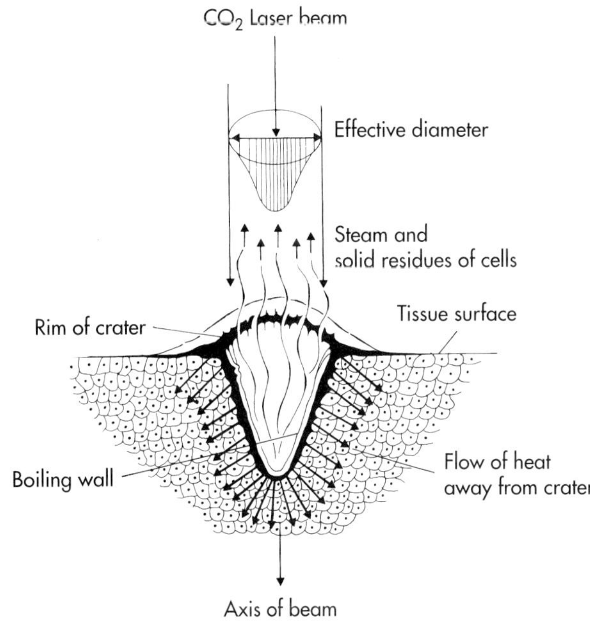

Fig. 25-15. Vaporization of tissue by the CO_2 laser.

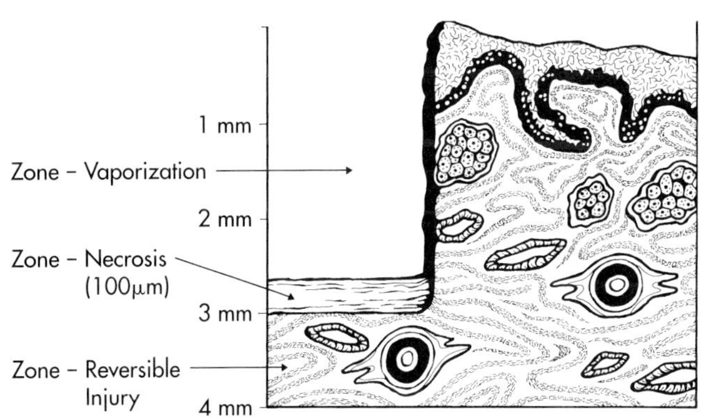

Fig. 25-16. Zones of vaporization, necrosis, and reversible injury by the CO_2 laser.

Table 25-10. Characteristics of gynecologic lasers

	CO_2	Argon/KTP	Nd:YAG
Aiming beam	He-Ne	Argon/KTP	He-Ne
Delivery system	Articulated, rigid mirrors	Fiber	Fiber
Absorption	Water, glass, plastic	Heme, melanin	Proteins
Penetration	0.1 mm	2.0 mm	4-6 mm
Maximum power	100 W	20 W	100 W
Precision cut	+++	+	+
Coagulation	+	++	+++

absorption properties has made these lasers ideally suited for the treatment of endometriosis.[44,98,99] Other investigators have used these lasers for laparoscopic neosalpingostomies, fimbrioplasties, adhesiolysis, and transection of the uterosacral ligaments for pain control.[44,53] These lasers are delivered via fibers and have a green-blue color, thus an aiming beam is unnecessary.

Neodymium: Yttrium-aluminum-garnet laser. The Nd:YAG laser is only minimally absorbed by water, plastic, or glass. It is absorbed by the protein of opaque tissue, with darker tissues showing preferential absorption. The Nd:YAG laser has a deep penetration of 4 to 6 mm of tissue, with significant scatter to adjacent tissues, estimated at up to 25% of the incident energy.[65] The Nd:YAG laser creates a uniform well-defined zone of tissue necrosis with a sharp boundary.[96] It has a more predictable depth of penetration and distribution within the tissue than does electrocoagulation since it does not follow the paths of least electrical resistance within the different tissue types.[96] It will cause thermal necrosis but not vaporization of tissue. Because of its deeper penetrating ability, the Nd:YAG laser is capable of coagulating vessels up to 4 mm in diameter.[64]

The Nd:YAG laser is delivered by a fiber and requires an He-Ne aiming beam. Its main application in gynecology is for hysteroscopic endometrial ablation,[113] although it has been used in the laparoscopic treatment of endometriosis.[116,117]

Laser safety

It is essential that surgeons and assisting personnel working with lasers take formal courses to learn about laser operation, applications, and safety. The major aspects of laser safety will be reviewed in this section.

Lasers with wavelengths greater than 319 nm (i.e., all lasers used in gynecologic practice) emit photoradiation and not ionizing radiation.[64] Gynecologic lasers are therefore not mutagenic, and there have been no reports of carcinoma developing in treated tissue or in health care workers handling the equipment.[64] Some of the materials used to make the laser may themselves be toxic, such as the thallium bromide in experimental CO_2 fibers.[67] However, gynecologic lasers currently marketed do not contain toxic materials.

The laser plume, created from the destruction of tissue, (especially the CO_2 laser) contains chemicals and cell fragments that may be mutagenic or cause irritation of the pulmonary mucosa, which may lead to chronic bronchitis if inhaled.[131] Most investigators believe there is only minimal or no risk from viable cancer cells released into the laser plume by the CO_2 laser.[140] However, more studies need to be performed with the argon, KTP, and Nd:YAG lasers that are less efficient at vaporization. It is advisable to use good ventilation and smoke evacuators with all laser surgery to reduce these potential risks.

Since the collimated laser beam does not lose much power over distance, it is important to fire the laser only when it is aimed at an appropriate target. One must also make certain that there are no shiny surfaces near the operating field that may reflect the beam toward an unplanned target. CO_2 lasers have the highest risk of reflection, and it is recommended to use anodized instruments with a rough matte finish to further decrease this risk.

Eye safety is probably the most important aspect of laser safety. With some lasers, eye injury could result in instantaneous and permanent blindness. The He-Ne aiming beam is the safest of all medical lasers with its low intensity (2 to 5 mW). Protective glasses are recommended but not required for use with this beam; the beam may be hazardous with prolonged direct viewing.

A CO_2 laser is absorbed immediately by the superficial corneal layers and never reaches the retina.[191] If a CO_2 laser beam strikes the retina, it will produce a painful corneal burn that usually heals spontaneously. Glasses (not contact lenses) or goggles with side shields are necessary when this laser is used.

Lasers with wavelengths between 350 and 1400 nm (i.e., argon, KTP, and Nd:YAG lasers) are not stopped by the superficial layers of the cornea and lens and may produce painless but permanent retinal damage.[191] Special goggles marked according to the wavelengths they block must always be used when working with the argon, KTP, or Nd:YAG lasers. The goggles' lens will also be marked with the optical density from a given wavelength (i.e., degree of protection). Goggles are primarily designed to protect the eye from scatter radiation and to afford a short margin of protection from direct-beam exposure.

These protective goggles will reduce the transmission of visible light by 25% to 40%.[159] This property in addition to the color of the goggles (i.e., Nd:YAG goggles are green; argon/KTP goggles are tinted amber) may decrease the visual acuity of the operative field. The surgeon, nurses, anesthesiologists, and patient must wear protective goggles.

The laser unit should be placed in a restricted location, clearly marked, and accessible only by trained personnel. Only trained personnel should manage the laser unit because the high-power voltage amplifier may be a potential electrical hazard. All medical lasers, especially the CO_2 laser, have the potential to ignite flammable objects; all laparotomy pads, towels, and gauze pads must be kept moistened, and flammable gases and prepping materials must not be used. Polyvinyl chloride endotracheal tubes are especially flammable, and several patients have died of severe pulmonary burns when tubes ignited.[112] The importance of proper safety protocols for operative laser cases cannot be overstated.

Laser applications

The actual surgical techniques for the gynecologic indications listed in the following sections will not be covered. For a description of these techniques, the reader is referred to a thorough review of operative techniques.[10]

Vulvar intraepithelial neoplasia (VIN). The stratified squamous epithelium of the vulva is less than 1 mm thick, with the deepest rete peg rarely extending more than 1 mm into the underlying dermis. Vaporization with the CO_2 laser should therefore by performed to a depth of 3 mm only. Because VIN is often a multifocal disease, it may be necessary to treat some patients in stages, waiting 2 weeks between treatments. Several studies have demonstrated remarkable efficacy of CO_2 laser therapy for VIN, with greater than 90% cure rates noted by a 12-year follow-up.[12,182]

Condyloma acuminatum. Condyloma acuminatum is caused by the human papillomavirus, which has been linked to the genesis of lower genital tract neoplasia.[5] The virus proliferates in the prickle and basal cell layers of the epidermis,[101] thus the CO_2 laser may eliminate condylomatous lesions to a depth of 1 mm. Because these lesions may be multifocal and have microwarty epithelial changes, colposcopy may aid in the localization and treatment of condylomata. Warts may be vaporized or excised; this can be accomplished safely in pregnant patients (except for cervical lesions) up to 34 weeks of gestation. In addition, because treatment is limited to the epidermis, there is minimal blood loss and rarely significant scarring. It is important to treat several millimeters of surrounding normal tissue because the papillomavirus often exists in normal tissue around the proliferative lesion. Several series totaling 428 patients have demonstrated greater than 90% cure rates in patients with condylomatous lesions, many of whom had failed multiple courses of medical therapy.[89,33] For vaginal condylomata, a special nonreflective vaginal speculum must be used.

Vaginal intraepithelial neoplasia (VAIN). VAIN is a relatively uncommon preinvasive neoplastic process that is associated with cervical intraepithelial neoplasia (CIN),[81] radiation therapy,[138] chemotherapy, and immunosuppressive therapy. It is usually an asymptomatic lesion that is brought to the attention of the physician by an abnormal Papanicolaou (Pap) smear and investigated with the aid of colposcopy. Lesions may be surgically excised, treated with topical 5-fluorouracil,[193] or in the postmenopausal patient treated with intravaginal estrogens. Stafl et al first reported on the successful treatment of VAIN with CO_2 laser therapy in 1977.[172] Since then, other groups have reported success rates of 84% to 90% with either focal laser therapy or total laser ablation of the vaginal mucosa.[94,181] It is recommended that a 2-mm border of normal tissue be vaporized down to a depth of approximately 2 mm to treat VAIN.

Cervical intraepithelial neoplasia. Laser vaporization of ecto-CIN was one of the first gynecologic applications of the CO_2 laser. In cases of persistently abnormal Pap smears with inconsistent colposcopic findings, endocervical involvement, or when the transformation zone cannot be fully visualized on colposcopic examination, cervical conization may be performed with the CO_2 laser.[54]

In the treatment of ecto-CIN, it is recommended to have a margin extending at least 3 to 4 mm beyond the lesion and transformation zone. Vaporization of the entire transformation zone, including the area of pathology, must be performed with colposcopic guidance to a minimum depth of 6 mm to ensure eradication of CIN lesions extending into cervical crypts. In a series of 514 patients with ecto-CIN (CIN I, II, and III) Wright reported a cure rate of 95.5% after one laser treatment and 99.6% after two vaporization procedures.[195] In a series of 138 laser excisional conizations, Dorsey reported a cure rate of 96%, a mean blood loss of 2 mL, and 6 patients (4.3%) who required emergency visits for delayed heavy vaginal bleeding.[55]

The CO_2 and Nd:YAG lasers are under investigation for the treatment of some invasive gynecologic cancers, thus are not recommended for treatment of these diseases at this time.

Infertility and endometriosis. Laser techniques have been used extensively in female reconstructive pelvic surgery including salpingoovariolysis, fimbrioplasty, terminal salpingostomy, vaporization and excision of endometriosis, myomectomy, metroplasty, and ovarian wedge resection. The CO_2 laser has been used far more frequently than other types of lasers for these indications. Most reports have been anecdotal and uncontrolled with small numbers of subjects, thus making interpretation of true efficacy difficult. This section will provide a brief overview of the use of lasers in female reconstructive pelvic surgery.

Critical aspects in the success of pelvic reconstructive surgery for infertility are the degree of postoperative adhesion formation and the extent of tissue injury. When the CO_2 laser was first used for abdominal reconstructive surgery in 1974,[17] much enthusiasm was generated; laser surgery was touted as potentially superior to conventional surgery (i.e., scalpel, electrocautery) because of its no-touch technique, precision, and minimal tissue injury adjacent to the surgical site. However, in several animal studies comparing the degree of postoperative adhesion formation in laser-treated versus electrocautery-treated animals, no clear advantage has been proved. Some studies have concluded that there is no significant difference in postoperative adhesion formation when CO_2 laser or electrocautery is used.[118,150] Other studies report that the CO_2

laser is superior to electrocautery in reducing postoperative adhesion formation.[18,36,63]

Postoperative adhesion formation after CO_2 laser infertility surgery was evaluated in a prospective multicenter study utilizing early second-look laparoscopy.[52] These investigators found postoperative adhesions in 86% of patients (91 of 106) and concluded that the CO_2 laser was not a panacea for the treatment of tuboperitoneal causes of infertility.

In human studies, both laser and electromicrocautery techniques appear to have comparable efficacy. Tulandi reported pregnancy rates of 53% and 52% in laser (n = 30) and electrocautery (n = 33) salpingoovariolysis procedures respectively, after a 2-year follow-up period.[185] In this study there was a tendency toward a shorter surgery-to-conception interval in laser-treated patients (laser 9.9 months; electrosurgery 13.1 months), although the difference was not statistically significant.

In another comparative study, Tulandi and Vilos reported on the efficacy of laser surgery versus electrosurgery for bilateral hydrosalpinges.[86] Terminal salpingostomies were performed on 67 women, with an intrauterine pregnancy rate of 24% in the laser group (n = 37) and 20% in the electrocautery group (n = 30) after a 2-year follow-up period, demonstrating no statistical difference. As in the salpingoovariolysis study, the surgery-to-conception interval tended to be shorter in the laser group (8.3 months versus 12.1 months), but no statistical difference was reached. Tulandi and Vilos concluded that the CO_2 laser did not offer a distinct advantage over conventional surgery in the treatment of infertility caused by pelvic adhesions or distal tubal occlusion.[186]

Endometriosis is a relatively frequent finding in women with infertility, pelvic pain, or both. Several studies have demonstrated the efficacy of conventional infertility surgery by laparotomy and laparoscopic surgery using electrocautery techniques.[29,126] Although no comparative studies have been performed, CO_2 laser treatment of endometriosis appears to yield results that are similar to or better than these other techniques. In a combined series of 374 infertile patients whose diagnostic evaluations demonstrated only endometriosis, 69% conceived following CO_2 laser laparoscopy.[126] The complication rate for CO_2 laser laparoscopy is less than 0.5%, suggesting that it is quite safe in skilled hands.[41] The KTP, argon, and Nd:YAG lasers have been used in the treatment of endometriosis; preliminary results suggest that these may be safe alternative modes of therapy in selected patients.[44,97,98,116,117] Uterosacral ligament ablation performed by the CO_2 or KTP laser, may be utilized for pain relief in patients with endometriosis.[44]

Summary

The present role of laser surgery remains undefined in gynecologic surgery. Although laser therapy has demonstrated efficacy in lower reproductive tract preinvasive neoplasia, condyloma acuminatum, pelvic reconstructive surgery, and endometriosis, it is unknown whether laser surgery is superior to more traditional surgical modalities. The advantages of less bleeding, decreased tissue handling, and less tissue injury are counterbalanced by the added equipment expense and the need for extra training for surgeons and supporting personnel. Laser surgery does offer an alternative approach in the treatment of many gynecologic disorders, and the evolving laser technology will no doubt add to the present surgical armamentarium.

REFERENCES

1. American College of Obstetricians and Gynecologists: Committee on Gynecologic Practice: *Credentialing guidelines for operative laparoscopy,* No. 106, April 1992.
2. Andersen PK, Stokke DB, Hole P: Carbon dioxide tension in manually ventilated, prone patients, *Anaesthesist* 12:610-613, 1981.
3. Asherman JG: Amenorrhoea traumatica (atretica), *J Obstet Gynaecol Br Emp* 55:23-25, 1948.
4. Asherman JG: Traumatic intrauterine adhesions, *J Obstet Gynaecol Br Emp* 57:892-895, 1950.
5. Aurelian L, Kessler I, Rosenshein NB: Viruses and gynecologic cancers, *Cancer* 48:455-463, 1987.
6. Azziz R, Murphy AA: *Practical manual of operative laparoscopy and hysteroscopy,* New York, 1992, Springer-Verlag.
7. Baggish MS: Contact hysteroscopy: a new technique to explore the uterine cavity, *Obstet Gynecol* 59:350, 1979.
8. Baggish MS: Carbon dioxide laser treatment for condylomata acuminata venereal infections, *Obstet Gynecol* 55:711-715, 1980.
9. Baggish MS: Treating viral venereal infections with the CO_2 laser, *J Reprod Med* 27:737-741, 1982.
10. Baggish MS: *Basic and advanced laser surgery in gynecology,* New York, 1985, Appleton-Century-Crofts.
11. Baggish MS, Daniell JF: Death caused by air embolism associated with neodymium: yttrium-aluminum garnet laser surgery and artificial sapphire tips, *Am J Obstet Gynecol* 161:877, 1989.
12. Baggish MS, Dorsey JH: CO_2 laser for the treatment of vulvar carcinoma in situ, *Obstet Gynecol* 57:371-374, 1981.
13. Barbieri RL, Evans S, Kistner RW: Danazol in the treatment of endometriosis: analysis of 100 cases with a 4-year follow-up, *Fertil Steril* 37: 737-742, 1982.
14. Barbot J, Parent B, Dubuisson JB: Contact hysteroscopy: another method of endoscopic examination, *Am J Obstet Gynecol* 136:721-726, 1980.
15. Bartisch EG, Dillon TF: Carbon dioxide hysteroscopy, *Am J Obstet Gynecol* 124:756-761, 1976.
16. Bateman BG, Nunley WC Jr, Kitchin JD III: Surgical management of distal tubal obstruction. Are we making progress? *Fertil Steril* 48:523-542, 1987.
17. Bellina JH: Gynecology and the laser, *Contemp Obstet Gynecol* 4:24-33, 1974.
18. Bellina JH et al: Carbon dioxide laser and electrosurgical wound study with an animal model: a comparison of tissue damage and healing patterns in peritoneal tissue, *Am J Obstet Gynecol* 148:327-331, 1984.
19. Bent AE, Ostergard DR: Endometrial ablation with the Neodymium: YAG laser, *Obstet Gynecol* 75:923-925,1990.
20. Berek JS, Griffiths CT, Leventhal JM: Laparoscopy for second-look evaluation in ovarian cancer, *Obstet Gynecol* 58:192-198, 1981.
21. Bhiwandiwala PP, Mumford SD, Feldblum PJ: Menstrual pattern changes following laparoscopic sterilization with different occlusion techniques: a review of 10,004 cases, *Am J Obstet Gynecol* 145:684-694, 1983.

22. Bozzini P: *Der Lichtleiter oder Beschreibung einer einfachen Vorrichtung und ihrer Anwendung zur Erleuchtung innerer Hohlen und Zwischenraume des lebenden animalischen Korpers,* Weimar, 1807, Landes-Industrie-Comptoir.
23. Brenner WE: Evaluation of contemporary female sterilization methods, *J Reprod Med* 26:439-453, 1981.
24. Brooks PG, Serden SP, Davos I: Hormonal inhibition of the endometrium for resectoscopic endometrial ablation, *Am J Obstet Gynecol* 164:1601-1608, 1991.
25. Brumsted J et al: A comparison of laparoscopy and laparotomy for the treatment of ectopic pregnancy, *Obstet Gynecol* 71:889-892, 1988.
26. Bukowsky I, Lauger K, Herman A: Conservative surgery for tubal pregnancy, *Obstet Gynecol* 53:709-713, 1979.
27. Bumm E: Diskussion uber die Endometriosis. In Chrobak R, Pfannenstiel J, editors: *Verhandlungen der Deutschen Gesellschaft fur Gynakologie Kongress,* Leipzig, (Wien), 1895, Breitkopf & Hartel.
28. Burnett JE Jr: Hysteroscopy-controlled curettage for endometrial polyps, *Obstet Gynecol* 24:621-623, 1964.
29. Buttram VC Jr: Conservative surgery for endometriosis in the infertile female: a study of 206 patients with implications for both medical and surgical therapy, *Fertil Steril* 31:117-122, 1979.
30. Byron JW, Markenson G, Miyazawa K: A randomized comparison of Verres needle and direct trocar insertion for laparoscopy, *Surg Gynecol Obstet* 177:259-262, 1993.
31. Candiani GB et al: Repair of the uterine cavity after hysteroscopic septal incision, *Fertil Steril* 54:991-994, 1990.
32. Candiani GB et al: Argon laser versus microscissors for hysteroscopic incision of uterine septa, *Am J Obstet Gynecol* 164:87-90, 1991.
33. Caulkins JW et al: Management of condylomata acuminata with the carbon dioxide laser, *Obstet Gynecol* 59:105-109, 1982.
34. Chamberlain G, Beown JC: The report of the working party of the confidential enquiry into gynecological laparoscopy. In *Gynecological laparoscopy,* London, 1978, Royal College of Obstetricians and Gynecologists.
35. Choe JK, Baggish MS: Hysteroscopic treatment of septate uterus with Neodymium:YAG laser, *Fertil Steril* 57:81-84, 1992.
36. Choe JK, Dawood MY, Andrews AH: Conventional versus laser reanastomosis of rabbit ligated uterine horns, *Obstet Gynecol* 61:689-692, 1983.
37. Corson SL: Operating room preparations and basic techniques. In Phillips JM, editor: *Laparoscopy,* Baltimore, 1977, Williams & Wilkins.
38. Cumming DC, Taylor PJ: Historical predictability of abnormal laparoscopic findings in infertile women, *J Reprod Med* 23:295-300, 1979.
39. Cumming DC, Taylor PJ: Combined laparoscopy and hysteroscopy in the investigation of the ovulatory infertile female, *Fertil Steril* 33:475-478, 1980.
40. Daly DC et al: Hysteroscopic metroplasty: surgical technique and obstetric outcome, *Fertil Steril* 39:623-628, 1983.
41. Daniell JF: Operative laparoscopy for endometriosis, *Semin Reprod Endocrinol* 3:353-359, 1985.
42. Daniell JF, Herbert CM: Laparoscopic salpingostomy utilizing the CO_2 laser, *Fertil Steril* 41:558-562, 1984.
43. Daniell JF, Kurtz BR, Ke RW: Hysteroscopic endometrial ablation using the rollerball electrode, *Obstet Gynecol* 80:329-332, 1992.
44. Daniell JF, Miller W, Tosh R: Initial evaluation of the use of the potassium-titanyl-phosphate (KTP/532) laser in gynecologic laparoscopy, *Fertil Steril* 46:373-377, 1986.
45. David C: *L'Endoscopie uterine (hysteroscopie): applications au diagnostic et au traitment des affections intrauterines,* Master's thesis, G Jacques, Paris, 1908, University of Paris.
46. DeCherney AH, Diamond MP: Laparoscopic salpingostomy for ectopic pregnancy, *Obstet Gynecol* 70:948-950, 1987a.
47. DeCherney AH et al: Endometrial ablation for intractable uterine bleeding: hysteroscopic resection, *Obstet Gynecol* 70:668-670, 1987b.
48. DeCherney AH, Romero R, Naftolin F: Surgical management of unruptured ectopic pregnancy, *Fertil Steril* 35:21-24, 1981.
49. DeCherney AH et al: Resectoscopic management of müllerian fusion defects, *Fertil Steril* 45:726-728, 1986.
50. DeStefano F et al: Risk of ectopic pregnancy following tubal sterilization, *Obstet Gynecol* 60:326-330, 1982.
51. Deutschmann C, Lueken RP: Hysteroscopic findings in postmenopausal bleeding. In Siegler AM, Lindemann HJ, editors: *Hysteroscopy: principles and practice,* Philadelphia, 1984, JB Lippincott.
52. Diamond MP, et al: Tubal patency and pelvic adhesions at early second-look laparoscopy following intraabdominal use of the carbon dioxide laser: initial report of the Intraabdominal Laser Study Group, *Fertil Steril* 42:717-723, 1984.
53. Diamond MP, DeCherney AH, Polan ML: Laparoscopic use of the argon laser in nonendometriotic reproductive pelvic surgery, *J Reprod Med* 31:1011-1013, 1986.
54. Dorsey JH: Excisional conization of the cervix. In Andrews AH, Polanyi TG, editors: *Microscopic and endoscopic surgery with the CO_2 Laser,* Boston, 1982, John Wright.
55. Dorsey JH: Excisional conization of the cervix, In Baggish MS, editor: *Basic and advanced laser surgery in gynecology,* Norwalk, CT, 1985, Appleton-Century-Crofts.
56. Drake TS et al: Unexplained infertility—a reappraisal, *Obstet Gynecol* 50:644-649, 1977.
57. Duffy S et al: In vitro studies of uterine electrosurgery, *Obstet Gynecol* 78:213-220, 1991.
58. El-minawi MF et al: Comparative evaluation of laparoscopy and hysterosalpingography in infertile patients, *Obstet Gynecol* 51:29-34, 1978.
59. Englund F, Ingelman-Sundberg A, Westin B: Hysteroscopy in diagnosis and treatment of uterine bleeding, *Gynaecologia* 143:217-220, 1957.
60. Esposito A: Une exploration gynecologique trop negligee: l'hysteroscopie, *Gynecol Pract* 19:165-169, 1968.
61. Fayez JA: An assessment of the role of operative laparoscopy in tuboplasty, *Fertil Steril* 39:476-480, 1983.
62. Fayez JA: Comparison between abdominal and hysteroscopic metroplasty, *Obstet Gynecol* 68:399-403, 1986.
63. Filmar S, Gomel V, McComb P: The effectiveness of CO_2 laser and electromicrosurgery in adhesiolysis: a comparative study, *Fertil Steril* 45:407-410, 1986.
64. Fischer JC: Principles of safety in laser surgery and therapy. In Baggish MS, editor: *Basic and advanced laser surgery in gynecology,* New York, 1985, Appleton-Century-Crofts.
65. Frank F, Hofstetter A, Keiditsch E: Experimental investigations and new instrumentation for Nd:YAG laser treatment in urology. In Bellina JH, editor: *Gynecologic laser surgery,* New York, 1981, Plenum.
66. Friedman AJ et al: A randomized, placebo-controlled, double-blind study evaluating the efficacy of leuprolide acetate depot in the treatment of uterine leiomyomata, *Fertil Steril* 51:251, 1989.
67. Fuller TA: From source to patient: the surgical laser delivery system, *Lasers Surg Med* 3:349-355, 1984.
68. Gabos P: A comparison of hysterosalpingography and endoscopy in examination of tubal function in infertile women, *Fertil Steril* 27:238-241, 1976.
69. Gant NF: Infertility and endometriosis: comparison of pregnancy outcomes with laparotomy versus laparoscopic techniques, *Am J Obstet Gynecol* 166: 1072-1081, 1992.
70. Garry R, Erian J, Grochmal SA: A multicentre collaborative study into the treatment of menorrhagia by Nd:YAG laser ablation of the endometrium, *Br J Obstet Gynaecol* 98:357-362, 1991.
71. Gimpelson RJ, Kaigh J: Mechanical preparation of the endometrium prior to endometrial ablation, *J Reprod Med* 37:691-694, 1992.
72. Goldenberg RL, Magendantz HG: Laparoscopy and the infertility evaluation, *Obstet Gynecol* 47:410-416, 1976.

73. Goldfarb HA: A review of 35 endometrial ablations using the Nd:YAG laser for recurrent menometrorrhagia, *Obstet Gynecol* 76:833-835, 1990.
74. Goldstein DP, deCholnoky C, Emans SJ: Adolescent endometriosis, *J Adolesc Health Care* 1:37-41, 1980.
75. Goldstein DP et al: Laparoscopy in the diagnosis and management of pelvic pain in adolescents, *J Reprod Med* 24:251-256, 1980.
76. Gomel V: Laparoscopic tubal surgery in infertility, *Obstet Gynecol* 46:47-55, 1975.
77. Gomel V: Salpingostomy by laparoscopy, *J Reprod Med* 18:265-269, 1977.
78. Gomel V: Salpingostomy by microsurgery, *Fertil Steril* 29:380-384, 1978.
79. Gomel V: *Microsurgery in female infertility*, 1983, Boston, Little, Brown.
80. Gomel V et al, editors: Laparoscopy and hysteroscopy. In *Gynecologic practice*, Chicago, 1986, Year Book Medical.
81. Graham JF, Meigs JV: Recurrence of tumor after total hysterectomy for carcinoma in situ, *Am J Obstet Gynecol* 64:1159-1164, 1962.
82. Hamou J: Hysteroscopy and microhysteroscopy with a new instrument: the microhysteroscope, *Acta Eur Fertil* 12:29-35, 1981.
83. Hankinson SE et al: Tubal ligation, hysterectomy, and risk of ovarian cancer—a prospective study, *JAMA* 270:28138, 1993.
84. Hasson HM: A modified instrument and method for laparoscopy, *Am J Obstet Gynecol* 110:886-889, 1971.
85. Hasson HM: Electrocoagulation of pelvic endometriotic lesions with laparoscopic control, *Am J Obstet Gynecol* 135:115-121, 1979.
86. Heineberg A: Uterine endoscopy, an aid to precision in the diagnosis of intrauterine disease, *Surg Gynecol Obstet* 18:513-520, 1914.
87. Helvacioglu A, Weis R: Operative laparoscopy and postoperative pain relief, *Fertil Steril* 57:548-552, 1992.
88. Hutchins CJ: Laparoscopy and hysterosalpingography in the assessment of tubal patency, *Obstet Gynecol* 49:325-328, 1977.
89. Indman PD: High-power Nd:YAG laser ablation of the endometrium, *J Reprod Med* 36:501-504, 1991.
90. Indman PD: Hysteroscopic treatment of menorrhagia associated with uterine leiomyomas, *Obstet Gynecol* 81:716-720, 1993.
91. Indman PD, Brown WW III: Uterine surface temperature changes caused by electrosurgical endometrial coagulation, *J Reprod Med* 37:667-669, 1992.
92. Indman PD et al: Uterine surface temperature changes caused by endometrial treatment with the Nd:YAG laser, *J Reprod Med* 36:505-512, 1991.
93. Irwin KL et al: Tubal sterilization, hysterectomy, and the subsequent occurrence of epithelial ovarian cancer, *Am J Epidemiol* 134:362-369, 1991.
94. Jobson VW, Homesley HD: Treatment of vaginal intraepithelial neoplasia with carbon dioxide laser, *Obstet Gynecol* 62:90-94, 1983.
95. Jones HW Jr, Rock JA: *Reparative and constructive surgery of the female genital tract*, Baltimore, 1983, Williams & Wilkins.
96. Keiditsch E, Hofstetter A, Rothenberger K: Comparative morphological investigations of the effects of the Nd:YAG laser and electrocoagulation in experimental animal research. In Bellina JH, editor: *Gynecologic laser surgery*, New York, 1981, Plenum.
97. Keye WR, Dixon J: Photocoagulation of endometriosis with the argon laser through the laparoscope, *Obstet Gynecol* 62:383-387, 1983.
98. Keye WR et al: Argon laser therapy of endometriosis: a review of 92 consecutive patients, *Fertil Steril* 47:208-212, 1987.
99. Keye WR Jr, Matson GA, Dixon J: The use of the argon laser in the treatment of experimental endometriosis, *Fertil Steril* 39:26-30, 1983.
100. Kresch AJ et al: Laparoscopy in 100 women with chronic pelvic pain, *Obstet Gynecol* 64:672-674, 1984.
101. Laverty C: Noncondylomatous wart virus infection of the cervix: cytologic, histologic, and electron microscopic features, *Obstet Gynecol Surv* 34:820-829, 1979.
102. Lavy G et al: A new devide to facilitate intrauterine instillation of dextran 70 for hysteroscopy, *Obstet Gynecol* 70:955-957, 1987.
103. Leake JF, Murphy AA, Zacur HA: Noncardiogenic pulmonary edema: a complication of operative hysteroscopy, *Fertil Steril* 48:497-499, 1987.
104. Lele SB, Piver MS: Interval laparoscopy as predictor of response to chemotherapy in ovarian carcinoma, *Obstet Gynecol* 68:345-347, 1986.
105. Leventhal JM: Laparoscopy in female infertility, *Curr Probl Obstet Gynecol Fertil* 9:174-224, 1986.
106. Levine RL: Economic impact of pelviscopic surgery, *J Reprod Med* 30:655-661, 1985.
107. Lichten EM: Three years' experience with LUNA: out-patient laser laparoscopic treatment of dysmenorrhea, *Am J Gynecol Health* 3:144-147, 1989.
108. Lichten EM, Bombard J: Surgical treatment of primary dysmenorrhea with laparoscopic uterine nerve ablation, *J Reprod Med* 32:37-41, 1987.
109. Lindemann HJ: NO_2 hysteroscopy today, *Endoscopy* 11:94-102, 1979.
110. Lindemann HJ: *Atlas der Hysteroskopie*, Stuttgart, FRG, 1980, Gustav Fischer.
111. Lindemann HJ, Mohr J, Gallinat A: Der Einfluss von CO_2-Gas wahrend der hysteroskopie, *Geburtshsilfe Frauenheilkd* 36:153-157, 1976.
112. Lipow M: Laser physics made simple, *Curr Probl Obstet Gynecol Fertil* 9:442-493, 1986.
113. Loffer FD: Hysteroscopic endometrial ablation with the Nd:YAG laser using a nontouch technique, *Obstet Gynecol* 69:679-682, 1987.
114. Loffer FD: Hysteroscopy with selective endometrial sampling compared with D&C for abnormal uterine bleeding: the value of a negative hysteroscopic view, *Obstet Gynecol* 73:16-20,1989.
115. Loffer FD, Pent D: Pregnancy after laparoscopic sterilization, *Obstet Gynecol* 55:643-648, 1980.
116. Lomano JM: Laparoscopic ablation of endometriosis with the YAG laser, *Lasers Surg Med* 3:179-183, 1983.
117. Lomano JM: Photocoagulation of early pelvic endometriosis with Nd:YAG laser through the laparoscope, *J Reprod Med* 30:77-81, 1985.
118. Luciano AA et al: A comparison of thermal injury, healing patterns, and postoperative adhesion formation following CO_2 laser and electromicrosurgery, *Fertil Steril* 48:1025-1029, 1987.
119. Lundorff P et al: Adhesion formation after laparoscopic surgery in tubal pregnancy: a randomized trial versus laparotomy, *Fertil Steril* 55:911-915, 1991.
120. Maddi VI et al: Dextran anaphylaxis, *Angiology* 20:243-246, 1969.
121. Maiman M, Seltzer V, Boyce J: Laparoscopic excision of ovarian neoplasms subsequently found to be malignant, *Obstet Gynecol* 77:563-565, 1991.
122. March CM, Israel R, March AD: Hysteroscopic management of intrauterine adhesions, *Am J Obstet Gynecol* 130:633-637, 1978.
123. Marleschki V: Hysteroskopische Feststellung der spontanen perfusionsschwankungen am menschlichen Endometrium, *Zentralbl Gynakol* 90:1094-1098, 1968.
124. Marleschki V: Geburtserleichterung unter Kontrolle, *Urania* 11:34-38, 1971.
125. Martin DC, editor: *Laparoscopic appearance of endometriosis*, ed 2, vol 1, Memphis, 1990, Resurge Press.
126. Martin DC, Diamond MP: Operative laparoscopy: comparisons of lasers with other techniques, *Curr Probl Obstet Gynecol Fertil* 9:564-617, 1986.
127. Martin DC et al: Laparoscopic appearance of peritoneal endometriosis, *Fertil Steril* 51:63-67, 1989.
128. McKenzie AL: Lasers in surgery and medicine, *Phys Med Biol* 29:619-641, 1984.
129. Method MW et al: Economic considerations in the use of laparoscopy for diagnosing pelvic inflammatory disease, *J Reprod Med* 32:759-764, 1987.

130. Mettler L, Giesel H, Semm K: Treatment of female infertility due to tubal obstruction by operative laparoscopy, *Fertil Steril* 32:384-389, 1979.
131. Mihashi S, Veda S, Hirano M: Some problems about condensates induced by CO_2 laser irradiation. In Atsumi K, editor: *Transactions, 4th Congress of the International Society for Laser Surgery,* Tokyo, 1981, Intergroup.
132. Murphy AA: Operative laparoscopy, *Fertil Steril* 47:1-18, 1987.
133. Musich JR, Behrman SJ: Infertility laparoscopy in perspective: review of 500 cases, *Am J Obstet Gynecol* 143:293-303, 1982.
134. Neuwirth RS: Hysteroscopy. In Friedman EA, editor: *Major problems in obstetrics and gynecology,* vol 8, Philadelphia, 1975, WB Saunders.
135. Neuwirth RS: Hysteroscopic management of symptomatic submucous fibroids, *Obstet Gynecol* 62:509-511, 1983.
136. Nezhat CR et al: Laparoscopic radical hysterectomy with paraaortic and pelvic node dissection, *Am J Obstet Gynecol* 166:864-865, 1992.
137. Nitze M: Uber eine neue Beleuchtungsmethode der Hohlen des menschlichen Korpers, *Wien Med Presse* 20:851-857, 1879.
138. Novak ER, Woodruff JD: Postirradiation malignancies of the pelvic organs, *Am J Obstet Gynecol* 77:667-672, 1959.
139. Oslan A et al: High-output left ventricular failure after dextran use in an operative hysteroscopy, *Fertil Steril* 54:939-941, 1990.
140. Osterhuis JW: *Tumor surgery with the CO_2 laser: studies with the Cloudman S-91 mouse melanoma,* Groningen, Netherlands, 1977, Veenstra-Visser.
141. Pantaleoni D: On endoscopic examination of the cavity of the womb, *Med Press Circ* 8:26-32, 1869.
142. Parent B, Barbot B, Doeufleu B: *Hysteroscopie de contact: documentation scientifique,* Paris, 1976, Laboratories Roland Marie SA.
143. Penfield AJ: Vascular injuries and their management. In Phillips JM, editor: *Endoscopy in gynecology,* Downey, CA, 1978, American Association of Gynecologic Laparoscopists.
144. Peterson EP, Behrman SJ: Laparoscopy of the infertile patient, *Am J Obstet Gynecol* 36:363-368, 1970.
145. Peterson EP et al: Laparoscopic sterilization: American Association of Gynecologic Laparoscopists' 1991 membership survey, *J Reprod Med* 38:574-576, 1993.
146. Peterson HB et al: Local versus general anesthesia for laparoscopic sterilization: a randomized study, *Obstet Gynecol* 70: 903-908, 1987.
147. Perino A et al: Role of leuprolide acetate depot in hysteroscopic surgery: a controlled study, *Fertil Steril,* 59:507-510,1993.
148. Phillips J, Keith D, Hulka B: Gynecologic laparoscopy in 1975, *J Reprod Med* 16:104-111, 1976.
149. Phillips J, Keith D, Keith L: Survey of gynecologic laparoscopy for 1974, *J Reprod Med* 15:45-51, 1975.
150. Pittaway DE, Maxon WS, Daniell JF: A comparison of the CO_2 laser and electrocautery on postoperative intraperitoneal adhesion formation in rabbits, *Fertil Steril* 40:366-370, 1983.
151. Piver MS et al: Second-look laparoscopy prior to proposed second-look laparotomy, *Obstet Gynecol* 55:571-573,1980.
152. Pouly JL et al: Conservative laparoscopic treatment of 321 ectopic pregnancies, *Fertil Steril* 46:1093-1097, 1986.
153. Pring DW: Inferior epigastric haemorrhage, an avoidable complication of laparoscopic clip sterilization, *Br J Obstet Gynaecol* 90:480-482, 1983.
154. Qu JY, Sun AD, Lien LC: Laparoscopy in the diagnosis and management of ovarian cancer, *J Reprod Med* 29:483-488, 1984.
155. Querleu D, Leblanc E, Castelain B: Laparoscopic pelvic lymphadenectomy in the staging of early carcinoma of the cervix, *Am J Obstet Gynecol* 164: 579-581,1991.
156. Raj SG, Hulka JF: Second-look laparoscopy in infertility surgery: therapeutic and prognostic value, *Fertil Steril* 38:325-328, 1982.
157. Redwine DB, Yocom LB: A serial section study of visually normal peritoneum in patients with endometriosis, *Fertil Steril* 52:149-151, 1989.
158. Reich H, McGlynn F: Treatment of ovarian endometriomas using laparoscopic surgical techniques, *J Reprod Med* 31:577-583, 1986.
159. Rockwell RJ: Laser safety and training: reviewing risks and safety protocols. In Breedlove B, editor: *Clinical lasers: expert strategies for practical and profitable management,* Atlanta, 1985, American Health Consultants.
160. Rubin IC: Uterine endoscopy, endometroscopy with the aid of uterine insufflation, *Am J Obstet Gynecol* 10:313-318, 1925.
161. Rubin IC: *Uterotubal insufflation,* St. Louis, 1947, CV Mosby.
162. Schenker JG, Margalioth EJ: Intrauterine adhesions: an updated appraisal, *Fertil Steril* 37:593-610, 1982.
163. Schroeder C: Uber den Ausbau und die Leistungen der Hysteroskopie, *Arch Gynaekol* 156:407-413, 1934.
164. Sciarra JJ, Valle RF: Hysteroscopy: a clinical experience with 320 patients, *Am J Obstet Gynecol* 127:340-345, 1977.
165. See WA, Cooper CS, Fisher RJ: Predictors of laparoscopic complications after formal training in laparoscopic surgery, *JAMA* 270:2689-2692, 1993.
166. Semm K: Tissue-puncher and loop ligation: new aids for surgical-therapeutic pelviscopy, *Endoscopy* 10:119-125, 1978.
167. Semm K: *Endoscopic intraabdominal surgery,* Kiel, 1984, Christina-Albrechts-Universität.
168. Semm K, Mettler L: Technical progress in pelvic surgery via operative laparoscopy, *Am J Obstet Gynecol* 138:121-126, 1980.
169. Siegler AM, Kemmann EK, Gentile GP: Hysteroscopic procedures in 257 patients, *Fertil Steril* 25:1267-1271, 1976.
170. Smith WG, Day TG Jr, Smith JP: The use of laparoscopy to determine the results of chemotherapy for ovarian cancer, *J Reprod Med* 18:257-260, 1977.
171. Snowden EU, Jarret JC II, Dawood MY: Comparison of diagnostic accuracy of laparoscopy, hysteroscopy, and hysterosalpingography in evaluation of female infertility, *Fertil Steril* 41:709-713, 1984.
172. Stafl A, Wilkinson EJ, Mattingly RF: Laser treatment of cervical and vaginal neoplasia, *Am J Obstet Gynecol* 128:128-132, 1977.
173. Steptoe PC: *Laparoscopy in gynecology,* Edinburgh, 1967, E & S Livingstone,
174. Stromme WB: Conservative surgery for ectopic pregnancy, *Obstet Gynecol* 41:215-220, 1973.
175. Sugimoto O: Diagnostic and therapeutic hysteroscopy for traumatic intrauterine adhesions, *Am J Obstet Gynecol* 131:539-544, 1978.
176. Surrey MW, Aronberg S: Hysteroscopic diagnosis of abnormal uterine bleeding: a clinical study. In Siegler AM, Lindemann HJ, editors: *Hysteroscopy: principles and practice,* Philadelphia, 1984, JB Lippincott.
177. Surrey MW, Friedman S: Second-look laparoscopy after reconstructive pelvic surgery for infertility, *J Reprod Med* 27:658-663, 1982.
178. Taylor PJ: Correlations in infertility: symptomatology, hysterosalpingography, laparoscopy, and hysteroscopy, *J Reprod Med* 8:339-344, 1977.
179. Taylor PJ, Cumming DC: Laparoscopy in the infertile female, *Curr Probl Obstet Gynecol* 2:3-32, 1979.
180. Timonen S, Nieminen V: Tubal pregnancy: choice of operative method of treatment, *Acta Obstet Gynecol Scand* 46:327-331, 1967.
181. Townsend DE et al: Treatment of vaginal carcinoma in situ with the carbon dioxide laser, *Am J Obstet Gynecol* 143:101-104, 1982a.
182. Townsend DE, Levine RU, Richart RM: Management of vulvar intraepithelial neoplasia by carbon dioxide laser, *Obstet Gynecol* 60:97-102, 1982b.
183. Townsend DE et al: "Rollerball" coagulation of the endometrium, *Obstet Gynecol* 76:310-313, 1990.
184. Trimbos-Kemper TCM, Trimbos JB, van Hall EV: Adhesion formation after tubal surgery: results of eighth-day laparoscopy in 188 patients, *Fertil Steril* 43:395-399, 1985.
185. Tulandi T: Salpingoovariolysis: a comparison between laser surgery and electrosurgery, *Fertil Steril* 45:489-491, 1986.

186. Tulandi T, Vilos GA: A comparison between laser surgery and electrosurgery for bilateral hydrosalpinx: a 2-year follow up, *Fertil Steril* 44:846-847, 1985.
187. Uribe-Ramirez LC et al: Outpatient laparoscopic sterilization: a review of complications in 2000 cases, *J Reprod Med* 18:103-108, 1977.
188. Valle RF: Hysteroscopy in the evaluation of female infertility, *Am J Obstet Gynecol* 137:425-431, 1980.
189. Valle RF, Sciarra JJ: Current status of hysteroscopy in gynecologic practice, *Fertil Steril* 32:619-623, 1979.
190. Vermesh M et al: Management of unruptured ectopic gestation by linear salpingostomy: a prospective randomized clinical trial of laparoscopy versus laparotomy, *Obstet Gynecol* 73:400-408, 1989.
191. Winburn DC: *Practical laser safety,* New York, 1985, Marcel Dekker.
192. Wood GP: Laparoscopic examination of the normal infertile woman, *Obstet Gynecol* 62:642-643, 1983.
193. Woodruff JD, Parmley TH, Julian CG: Topical 5-fluorouracil in the treatment of vaginal carcinoma in situ, *Gynecol Oncol* 3:124-128, 1975.
194. Word B, Gravlee LC, Wideman GL: The fallacy of simple uterine curettage, *Obstet Gynecol* 12:642-645, 1958.
195. Wright VC: Laser vaporization of the cervix for the management of cervical intraepithelial neoplasia. In Baggish MS, editor: *Basic and advanced laser surgery in gynecology,* New York, 1985, Appleton-Century-Crofts.
196. Xygakis AM et al: Second-look laparoscopy in ovarian cancer, *J Reprod Med* 29:583-585, 1984.
197. Zweizig S et al: Conservative management of adnexal torsion, *Am J Obstet Gynecol* 168:791-795, 1993.

D

H

I

J

K

L

O

P